MOSBY'S CANADIAN TEXTBOOK FOR THE SUPPORT WORKER

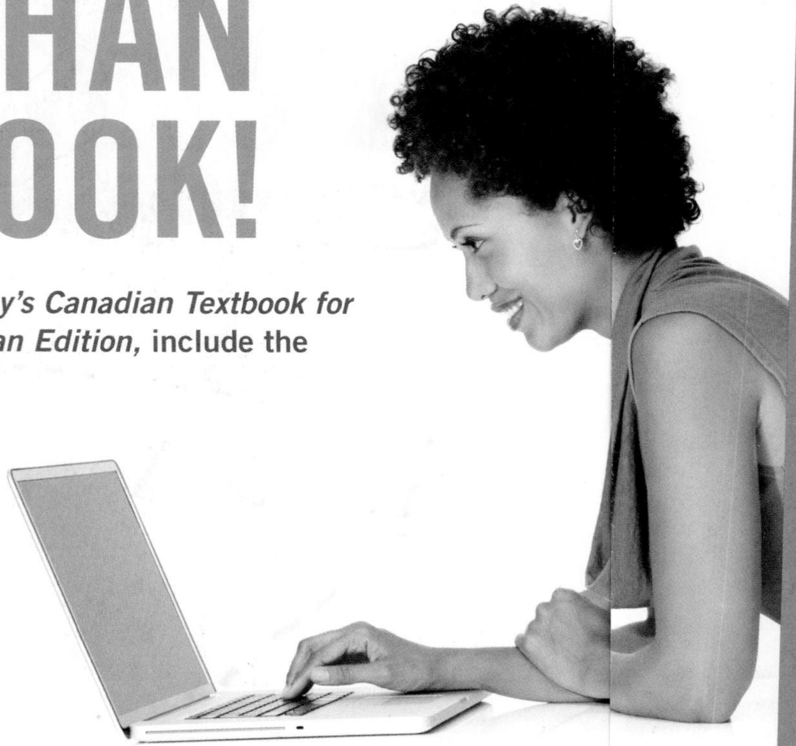

FOURTH CANADIAN EDITION

MOSBY'S CANADIAN TEXTBOOK FOR THE SUPPORT WORKER

Sheila A. Sorrentino **RN, PhD**
Delegation Consultant
Anthem, Arizona

Leighann N. Remmert **RN, MS**
Certified Nursing Assistant Instructor
Williamsville, Illinois

Mary J. Wilk **RN, GNC(C), BA, BScN, MN**
Professor and PSW Program Coordinator
Fanshawe College, London, Ontario

ELSEVIER

ELSEVIER

This adaptation of *Mosby's Textbook for Nursing Assistants*, Ninth Edition, by Sheila A. Sorrentino and Leighann N. Remmert is published by arrangement with Elsevier Inc.

ISBN: 978-0-323-31974-4 (softcover)
ISBN: 978-0-323-31975-1 (hardcover)

Notices

The content and procedures in this book are based on information currently available. They were reviewed by instructors and practising professionals in various regions of Canada. However, agency policies and procedures may vary from the information and procedures in this book. In addition, standards and guidelines may change as new information becomes available. Other federal, provincial, and territorial agencies also may issue new standards and guidelines, as may accrediting agencies and national organizations.

You are responsible for following the policies and procedures of your employer and the most current standards, practices, and guidelines as they relate to the safety of your work.

To the fullest extent of the law, neither the Publisher nor the authors or editors assume any liability for any injury and/or damage to persons or property as a matter of products liability, negligence, or otherwise or from any use or operation of any methods, products, instructions, or ideas contained in the material herein.

The Publisher

Library and Archives Canada Cataloguing in Publication

Sorrentino, Sheila A., author
Mosby's Canadian textbook for the support worker / Sheila A. Sorrentino RN, PhD (Delegation Consultant, Anthem, Arizona), Leighann N. Remmert, RN, MS (Certified Nursing Assistant Instructor, Williamsville, Illinois), Mary J. Wilk RN, GNC(C), BA, BScN, MN (Professor and PSW Program Coordinator, Fanshawe College, London, Ontario). – Fourth Canadian edition.
Includes bibliographical references and index.
ISBN 978-1-77172-043-4 (paperback)
1. Nurses' aides–Textbooks. 2. Nurses' aides–Handbooks, manuals, etc. 3. Care of the sick–Textbooks. I. Wilk, Mary J., author II. Remmert, Leighann N., author III. Title. IV. Title: Canadian textbook for the support worker. V. Title: Textbook for the support worker.

RT84.S67 2017 610.7306'98 C2016-905586-8

Vice President, Publishing: Ann Millar
Content Strategist (Acquisitions): Roberta A. Spinosa-Millman
Developmental Editor: Joanne Sutherland
Publishing Services Manager: Jeff Patterson
Book Production Specialist: Bill Drone
Copy Editor: Cathy Witlox
Cover Design: Brett J. Miller, BJM Graphic Design and Communications
Cover Image: Praisaeng/Shutterstock, Inc.
Interior Design: Maggie Reid
Typesetting and Assembly: Toppan Best-set Premedia Limited

Elsevier Canada
420 Main Street East, Suite 636, Milton, ON Canada L9T 5G3
416-644-7053

Printed in Canada

3 4 5 6 21 20 19

Ebook ISBN: 978-1-77172-107-3

In memory of my mom
December 21, 1918–October 14, 2015
A beautiful woman with amazing inner strength
She is with my dad and their babies now
Love you, Mom

Sheila

To my baby girl
Ava Leigh Remmert
Born February 18, 2015
You remind me daily how precious life is
With all my love,

Leighann (Mom)

I wish to dedicate this book to my writing partner, Rosemary Newmaster, who sadly passed away and was unable to join me on this latest journey; my loving parents, Michael and Natalia Wilk; my husband, Gord, and children, Andrew, Julie, and Brett; and my siblings, Carol and Mike. You are my supports, my inspirations, and my best friends. Thank you for your patience, your love, and your laughter. I also wish to acknowledge my father-in-law, J. Harvey Peterson, for his inspiring courage; my Fanshawe College colleagues; and my students, past and present. Thank you—all of you—for helping me become the person I am today.

Mary Wilk

The content and procedures in this book are based on information, standards, and guidelines currently available. They were reviewed by instructors and practising professionals in various regions of Canada. However, agency policies and procedures may vary from the information and procedures in this book. In addition, research and new information may require changes in standards and practices.

You are responsible for following the policies and procedures of your employer and the most current standards, practices, and guidelines as they relate to the safety of your work.

Contents

About the Authors

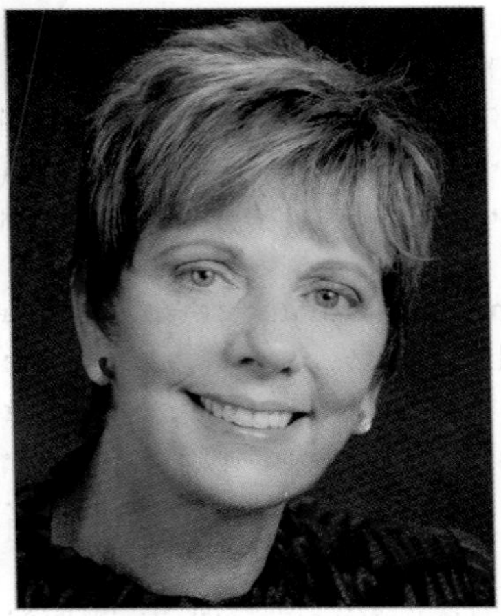

SHEILA A. SORRENTINO, RN, PHD

Sheila A. Sorrentino was instrumental in the development and approval of CNA-PN-ADN programs in the Illinois community college system and has taught at various levels of nursing education—nursing assistant, practical nursing, and baccalaureate and higher degree programs. Her career includes experiences in nursing practice and higher education—nursing assistant, staff nurse, charge and head nurse, nursing faculty, program director, assistant dean, and dean.

A Mosby author and co-author of several assistant titles since 1982, Dr. Sorrentino's titles include:

- *Mosby's Textbook for Nursing Assistants* (eds. 1–9)
- *Mosby's Essentials for Nursing Assistants* (eds. 1–5)
- *Mosby's Textbook for Long-Term Care Nursing Assistants* (eds. 1–6)
- *Mosby's Textbook for Nursing Assistive Personnel* (eds. 1–2)
- *Mosby's Basic Skills for Nursing Assistants*
- *Mosby's Textbook for Medication Assistants*

She was also involved in the development of and early version of *Mosby's Nursing Assistant Video Skills* and *Mosby's Nursing Video Skills*, winner of the 2003 *American Journal of Nursing* Book of the Year Award (electronic media). An earlier version of the nursing assistant skills videos won an International Films Award on caregiving.

Dr. Sorrentino has a Bachelor of Science degree in nursing, a Master of Arts degree in education, a Master of Science degree in nursing, and a PhD in higher education administration. She is a member of Sigma Theta Tau International, the Honor Society of Nursing. Her past community activities include the Rotary Club of Anthem (Anthem, Arizona), the Provena Senior Services Board of Directors (Mokena, Illinois), the Central Illinois Higher Education Health Care Task Force, the Iowa–Illinois Safety Council Board of Directors, and the Board of Directors of Our Lady of Victory Nursing Center (Bourbonnais, Illinois).

She received an alumni achievement award from Lewis University for outstanding leadership and dedication in nursing education. She is also a member of the Illinois State University College of Education Hall of Fame.

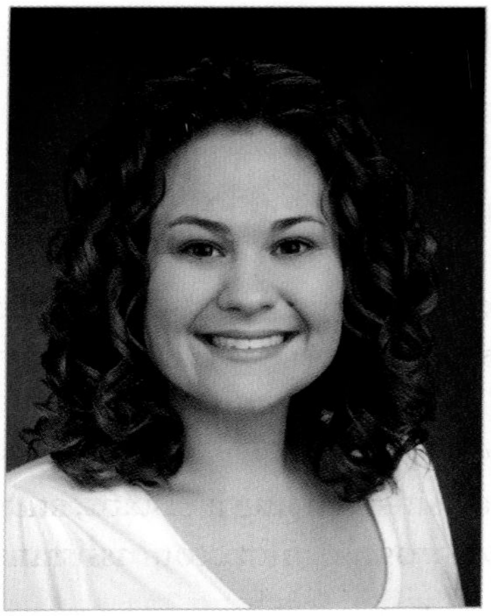

LEIGHANN N. REMMERT, RN, MS

Leighann N. Remmert is a nursing assistant instructor in central Illinois. She has taught adult learners and high school nursing assistant students in the classroom and clinical settings.

Leighann has a Bachelor of Science degree in nursing from Bradley University (Peoria, Illinois) and a Master of Science degree in nursing education from Southern Illinois University Edwardsville (Edwardsville, Illinois). Leighann's clinical background includes the roles of nursing assistant/tech, nurse extern, staff nurse, charge nurse, nurse preceptor, and trauma nurse specialist. She acquired diverse clinical experience as a nursing assistant/tech and extern at St. John's Hospital (Springfield, Illinois). As an RN, Leighann concentrated in the area of emergency nursing at Memorial Medical Center (Springfield, Illinois). She is a member of Sigma Theta Tau International, the Honor Society of Nursing, and the Certified Nursing Assistant Educator Association (Illinois, Central Region).

Leighann supervised, instructed, and evaluated student learning in various long-term care and acute-care settings as a clinical nursing instructor at the Capital Area School of Practical Nursing (Springfield, Illinois). As a nursing assistant instructor, Leighann guides students in acquiring the skills and knowledge needed to succeed as nursing assistants. Through her teaching, she emphasizes the importance of professionalism and work ethics, safety, teamwork, communication, and accountability. Valuing the role of the nursing assistant and treating the client with dignity, care, and respect are integral to her instruction in the classroom and clinical settings.

Leighann is co-author of *Mosby's Textbook for Nursing Assistants* (eds. 8–9), *Mosby's Essentials for Nursing Assistants* (eds. 4–5), and *Mosby's Textbook for Medication Assistants*. She was a consultant on *Mosby's Textbook for Long-Term Care Nursing Assistants* (ed. 6) and served as a content advisor for *Mosby's Nursing Assistant Video Skills* (version 4.0).

Leighann and her husband, Shane, have two daughters, Olivia and Ava. Leighann and Shane are active in various ministry areas at Elkhart Christian Church (Elkhart, Illinois). Leighann is certified as a Basic Life Support instructor and teaches CPR courses for the church and community.

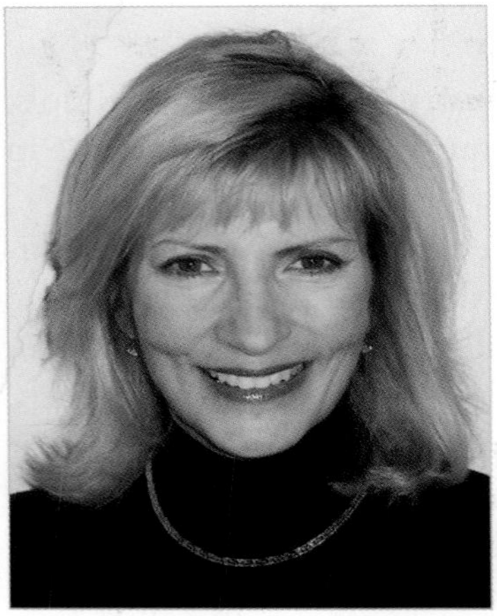

MARY J. WILK, RN, GNC(C), BA, BScN, MN

Mary J. Wilk is currently a professor and coordinator of the Personal Support Worker (PSW) program within the School of Nursing at Fanshawe College. She has been instrumental in the design and implementation of Fanshawe's PSW program curriculum, which is taught throughout the college's seven campuses. In addition, she is actively involved in the Ontario PSW Subcommittee for the Heads of Health Sciences and is chair of the Canadian Association of Continuing Care Educators (CACCE).

Mary has taught at Fanshawe College for over 25 years in the School of Nursing, teaching pharmacology, anatomy and physiology, health promotion, psychiatric nursing, communication, nursing theory, nursing accountability, and clinical nursing in a variety of settings. During her teaching career, she has taught in the PSW, Practical Nurse, Diploma Nurse, Developmental Service Worker, Paramedic, and Recreation and Leadership programs. She was also involved in curriculum development for the Collaborative Nursing program, in affiliation with the University of Western Ontario. Her nursing career includes work experience in emergency, coronary care, intensive care, orthopedic, gynecological, medical–surgical, psychiatric, and gerontological nursing.

Mary has earned a Bachelor of Arts degree, a Bachelor of Science in Nursing degree, and a Master of Nursing degree from the University of Windsor, where she graduated from each program with honours. She also holds a Gerontology Nurse Certificate through the Canadian Nurses Association. She has been a guest speaker numerous times on a variety of nursing and related topics at conferences and workshops at the local, provincial, and national levels.

Canadian Editorial Advisory Board and Reviewers

Elsevier Canada and the author are grateful to our Editorial Advisory Board and reviewers for sharing their knowledge and expertise; for providing their insights about support work and making many valuable content suggestions; and for their diligence in meeting very tight deadlines. Without their efforts, this textbook would not be the true representation of support work across Canada that it is. Their valuable feedback has improved the text immeasurably, and we wish to acknowledge their efforts.

EDITORIAL ADVISORY BOARD

Laura Bulmer, *RN, BScN, MEd*
Professor, Clinical Instructor
Sally Horsfall Eaton School of Nursing
George Brown College
Toronto, Ontario

Judith DeGroot, *MScN, RN*
Program Coordinator and Instructor
Health Care Assistant Program
Kwantlen Polytechnic University
Surrey, British Columbia

Jo Anne MacDonald, *RN, BScN*
Faculty, Continuing Care
Nova Scotia Community College
Port Hawkesbury, Nova Scotia

Ursula Osteneck, *RN, BN, BV/T Ed, MEd, PhD(c)*
Program Head, Continuing Care Assistant
School of Health Sciences
Saskatchewan Polytechnic
Prince Albert, Saskatchewan

Ann Robinson
President of ARC Advantage
Career College Consultancy

Deborah Schuh, *RN, BN, PNC(c)*
Co-Coordinator, PSW Program
Faculty, School of Health and Community Services
Durham College
Oshawa, Ontario

REVIEWERS

Siobhan Bell, *RN, BScN, MN*
Coordinator, Practical Nursing and Personal Support Worker
School of Health and Wellness
Georgian College
Orangeville, Ontario

Mary Cammaert, *RN*
Coordinator, Personal Support Worker Program
Fanshawe College
St. Thomas, Ontario

Linda Clark, *LPN*
Instructor, Health Care Assistant Program
Health and Human Services
Selkirk College
Trail, British Columbia

Natalie Clark, *RN, BScN*
Coordinator, PSW Program
St. Lawrence College
Cornwall, Ontario

Acknowledgements

Textbooks are written and published through the combined efforts of many people. The planning, manuscript development, review, design, and production processes involve the ideas, talents, and contributions of many individuals. I would like to thank Ann Millar, publisher at Elsevier, as well as Joanne Sutherland, freelance editor, for helping me stay sane and focused throughout this entire journey, and Cathy Witlox, copy editor, who has assisted me immensely.

The publisher and I would like also to acknowledge Fanshawe College, as several of the photos in this book were taken at its lab facilities.

Mary J. Wilk

Instructor Preface

In keeping with the approach of the previous edition, the fourth edition of *Mosby's Canadian Textbook for the Support Worker* serves the needs of students and instructors in educational programs taught in community colleges, secondary schools, and private colleges. This textbook has been written to prepare students to function in the role of support worker in communities and facility settings across Canada. It has been prepared entirely *by* Canadians *for* Canadians. Similar to the last edition, this textbook has been written in language that is interesting, easy to read, and easy to understand for most students, regardless of their previous educational background. Because this book is used throughout the country, great care has been taken to use terminology and content that is common and *not* specific to any one area or province or territory.

This textbook is also designed to be an excellent resource for support workers already working in the field—whether in facilities or in community settings—who may have questions about issues they have encountered in their clinical practice. Support workers will learn many new things, experience new situations and new challenges, and even acquire new skills in the course of their work. Whatever the setting, they will find that learning is an ongoing process, and this textbook and its available learning tools will be a valuable resource that will aid them in that process.

While writing this textbook, we consulted a number of legal and health care experts because we recognize the importance of using terminology and concepts that are both accurate and appropriate to Canada. For example, lawyers were consulted to ensure the accuracy of the legal concepts relating to wills, powers of attorney, and end-of-life care. In regard to the content on medication delivery techniques, pharmacists and medical doctors were consulted. In yet another example, in the section on dementia care, mental health specialists and the Alzheimer Society of Canada were consulted and asked for input. Such consultation has resulted in a correct, current, and accurate reflection of today's educational trends and content for support workers.

NEW TO THE FOURTH CANADIAN EDITION

Since the last edition was published, educational and vocational standards for support workers have been released both nationally and within many provinces. To reflect these new standards, as well as anticipated practice trends across Canada, *Mosby's Canadian Textbook for the Support Worker*, Fourth Edition, has been revised, updated, and reorganized while keeping the features that students and instructors have benefited from and depended on. Based on feedback from instructors, the order of the chapters has been revised to make them easier and more intuitive for both instructors and students to follow.

Pedagogical Features

The pedagogy of *Mosby's Canadian Textbook for the Support Worker*, Fourth Edition, has been brought up-to-date and enriched with the addition of new photos and figures reflecting current practice. Another addition has been the ***Critical Thinking in Practice*** questions at the end of each chapter. Each question presents students with a realistic, practice-based challenge and encourages them to find a reasonable solution to the scenario, incorporating their learned knowledge.

The very popular ***Supporting*** boxes that present real-life scenarios embodying the concepts covered in the chapters have been retained. These ***Supporting*** boxes have been valuable tools for students trying to understand the impact that a particular client's health challenge or issue may have on that client, on his or her family or significant others, and on the health care that is required. The scenarios and clients discussed in each of these boxes are adapted from real-life situations, describing clients from different ethnic and cultural backgrounds. Instructors will find these boxes very useful to elicit discussion and dialogue from the class on various issues that students are likely to encounter in the field. The portrayal of these realistic situations allows students to empathize more easily with the clients and, in doing so, adapt these lessons to their own practice. Instructors who would like more information on the issues that are presented in the ***Supporting*** boxes are encouraged to refer to the instructor resources that accompany the textbook.

Indigenous Issues

Indigenous peoples represent a significant and expanding group within Canada and include three groups: First Nations, Métis, and Inuit. **First Nations** refers to Status, Non-Status, and Treaty Indian peoples of Canada. These include the nations, bands, or groups of people who were originally living in Canada before the European explorers began to arrive in the 1600s.

Indigenous issues have been at the forefront of Canadian politics and policy over the past few years. In 2016, Canada adopted the United Nations Declaration on the Rights of Indigenous Peoples (UNDRIP) and also continued to implement the recommendations of the Truth and Reconciliation Commission (TRC) in an effort to address many years of legislated wrongs and inequities against Indigenous people.

While it is too early to report how the TRC recommendations and UNDRIP will influence health policy and practice, they have already influenced the terms that are used to refer to the diverse Indigenous populations in Canada. In support of UNDRIP and the process of healing and reconciliation, the terms *Indigenous people(s)* and *Indigenous health* are used throughout this text to acknowledge the inherent rights and political views of the diverse groups of original peoples with historical and cultural ties to Canada. The term *Aboriginal* does not fully recognize the diversity of Indigenous Peoples but remains in common use. The term *Aboriginal* can be found in this textbook when referring to specific current titles or groups such as *Aboriginal Support Workers* or the *Aboriginal Nurses Association of Canada* (ANAC).

Trends in Support Work

Health care is constantly changing, and this textbook has been revised to reflect new trends and policies that affect support workers throughout Canada. The chapters on body structure and function, and diseases and conditions, have been significantly enhanced to ensure that students have the suitable background of anatomy, physiology, physical changes related to aging, and disease processes. The scope of the chapters on mental health disorders and disorientation, delirium, and dementia have been almost completely rewritten to reflect the changes in the ***Diagnostic and Statistical Manual of Mental Disorders,* Fifth Edition** (*DSM-5*). For example, names of the various disorders have been updated, and the chapters have been expanded to include important discussions on suicide among older adults, post-traumatic stress disorder, and the types of primary and secondary dementias.

An emerging trend in Canada is the expanding role of the support worker, in regard to performing delegated acts and working in acute-care settings, where support workers may have the opportunity to perform increasingly advanced tasks and to problem-solve more than in the past. *Mosby's Canadian Textbook for the Support Worker*, Fourth Edition, has added a new chapter, *Working in Acute Care*, which focuses on practice specific to acute care. Students who read this textbook are frequently reminded about when they should be consulting the client's care plan or their supervisor for instructions.

Perhaps most importantly, this new edition places a stronger emphasis on understanding the role of support workers and their scope of practice. ***Throughout this textbook, students are reminded to check their scope of practice and to be aware of provincial or territorial legislation related to their profession.*** The Appendix at the end of the book outlines the provincial and territorial differences in support worker titles.

GUIDING PRINCIPLES

This textbook is structured around several key ideas and principles:

- ***Support workers provide services in a variety of community and facility settings.*** Because training programs prepare students for a variety of workplaces, multiple workplace settings—long-term care, home care, and hospital settings—are discussed throughout the text, especially in the ***Focus on Home Care*** and ***Focus on Long-Term Care*** boxes and the ***Procedures*** boxes, which highlight information and insights in regard to these settings.

- *Each client is an individual with dignity and value.* Throughout this textbook, students are reminded that each client is a whole person, with physical, emotional, social, intellectual, and spiritual dimensions. Students are encouraged to appreciate the client as a unique individual with a past, a present, and a future. Students are also taught to recognize a client's basic needs and protected rights.

- *An essential part of a support worker's job is to provide compassionate care.* The acronym *DIPPS* helps identify, recognize, and promote the five principles of support work—dignity, independence, preferences, privacy, and safety—which are highlighted in ***Providing Compassionate Care*** boxes, which discuss ways to promote the principles of support work when giving the care described in the chapter.

- *Effective communication skills are necessary to develop good working relationships.* Chapter 5 is devoted to communication skills, and Chapter 39 discusses communication with clients who have speech and language disorders. Case studies and other boxes throughout the text also highlight the importance of clear communication.

- *Support workers must respect the cultural diversity among their clients.* Culture influences people's attitudes and beliefs. Chapter 10 discusses the role of cultural heritage in health and illness practices as well as in other aspects of life, such as communication. ***Respecting Diversity*** boxes throughout the text provide examples of the influence of culture on support care.

- *Students learn best by reading about real-life examples.* Case studies and examples that apply concepts to the real world of support work appear throughout the text. ***Supporting*** boxes discuss ways to solve the problems that may occur in support work in different settings and help students to understand a particular client's health challenge or issue and to empathize with the client.

- *Support workers need to understand their scope of practice and the delegation process.* Because agencies and facilities across Canada vary in the way they utilize support workers, the responsibilities and limitations of support workers are emphasized throughout the text. The text presents many procedures that support workers across the country need to know and points out procedures that require extra training and supervision. Students are advised that they must understand and respect their employer's policies as well as provincial or territorial laws governing scope of practice. Chapter 6 addresses scope of practice and delegation issues; Chapter 8 focuses on ethical principles; and Chapter 9 addresses specific legislation that affects support workers in Canada.

- *Providing safe care is at the core of support work.* Ensuring the client's safety is one of the top priorities in support work and is therefore emphasized throughout the text. The numerous ***Think About Safety*** boxes throughout the textbook list straightforward, easy-to-understand ways to ensure client safety. An entire chapter (Chapter 22) devoted to safety discusses the major types of accidental injuries among clients and measures to prevent them. It also discusses how support workers can take steps to ensure their own safety on the job. Other safety concepts are detailed throughout the book, such as how to prevent the spread of infection (Chapter 23), how to recognize and report abuse (Chapter 16), and the basic principles of body mechanics and safety while moving and transferring clients (Chapter 25).

- *Following the client's care plan is critical to providing good care.* Chapter 14 describes the care-planning process in both facilities and communities. Students are reminded throughout the text that support workers must follow the care plan and their supervisor's directions.

- ***Support workers need to be effective problem solvers.*** Support workers must make decisions throughout their day, such as what to report to their supervisor; how to safely feed a client who may have choking difficulties (Chapter 28); how to safely move and reposition a client (Chapter 25); how to dress and assist a client with activities of daily living (Chapters 30, 31, 32, 33, and 43); and even how to respectfully communicate with clients, taking into account their culture (Chapters 5 and 10), their age (Chapters 19, 20, and 21), or existing physical or mental health challenges (Chapters 16, 35, 36, 37, 38, 39, and 40).

PEDAGOGICAL FEATURES AND DESIGN

Mosby's Canadian Textbook for the Support Worker, Fourth Edition, is presented in an attractive, four-colour, user-friendly design that makes the text easily navigable and the concepts and regulations easy to understand.

- ***Objectives***—explain what is presented in the chapter and what students will learn.
- ***Key Terms***—appear at the beginning of each chapter along with definitions and again in bold print within the body of the chapter, where they are defined in the context of the subject discussed. An alphabetized list of the key terms, together with their definitions, is presented in the Glossary at the end of the book for easy reference. Key terms are set out in bold blue type in the chapters, and other important terms appear in italics for emphasis.
- ***Illustrations and photographs***—are numerous and presented in full colour.
- ***Boxes and tables***—list principles, guidelines, ;igns and symptoms, care measures, and other nformation.
- ***'upporting boxes***—present scenarios about ırticular clients and discuss how support ›rkers make decisions and solve problems.
- ***'se Study boxes***—apply some of the concepts cussed in the text to real-life examples of port workers and clients. They complement ***Supporting*** boxes.
- ***Think About Safety boxes***—provide clear, concise, easy-to-follow advice on how to provide safe care to clients of all ages.
- ***Focus on Children boxes***—provide age-specific information about the needs, considerations, and special circumstances of children.
- ***Focus on Older Adults boxes***—provide age-specific information about the needs, considerations, and special circumstances of older adults.
- ***Focus on Home Care boxes***—highlight information necessary for safe functioning in the home setting.
- ***Focus on Long-Term Care boxes***—highlight information unique to the long-term care setting.
- ***Providing Compassionate Care boxes***—remind students of the principles of support work: respecting and promoting their client's dignity, independence, preferences, privacy, and safety. The acronym *DIPPS* is used to summarize these five principles.
- ***Respecting Diversity boxes***—help students learn to appreciate the influence of culture on health and illness practices and the importance of sensitivity to cultural diversity in support work.
- ***Procedure boxes***—are usually divided into Pre-Procedure, Procedure, and Post-Procedure sections. The format includes steps and rationales to help students learn how and why a procedure is performed. The *Compassionate Care* section at the beginning of most of the Procedure boxes is a reminder of the principles of support work. Asterisks are used to identify steps that are usually not applicable in community settings.
- ***Key Points***—are found at the end of each chapter. This section summarizes the important points from each chapter, providing a good framework for students to study from.
- ***Critical Thinking in Practice boxes***—are found at the end of each chapter. Each question presents a realistic, practice-based challenge to students and encourages them to find a reasonable solution to the scenario.
- ***Review questions***—are found at the end of each chapter after the Key Points section. Answers to the questions are presented (upside down) at the end of the section.

The authors and the publishing team at Elsevier Canada are confident that this text will serve you and your students well by providing the information needed to teach and learn safe and effective care during this dynamic time in Canadian health care.

AN IMPORTANT NOTE ON TERMINOLOGY AND EQUIPMENT

Throughout the book, the generic term ***support worker*** has been chosen to describe a worker who provides personal care and support to clients in a variety of settings. We recognize that, throughout Canada, support workers are designated a variety of titles; these titles may vary provincially, territorially or even locally, and it is expected that instructors will explain this terminology difference to students.

The client and his or her family who receive the services of support workers may also be referred to by different terms, depending on the location and the context of where these services are provided. For example, Mrs. Jones, who is receiving care in her own home (or in an assisted-living facility), would be referred to as a *client* by her caregivers. If she were to be admitted to an acute- or complex-care, continuing care, or subacute care facility—such as a hospital—she would then be called a *patient*. If she needed to live in a continuing care (or long-term care) facility, she would then be called a *resident*.

While the practice in an area or agency might be to refer to the recipient of support services as a ***patient***, ***resident***, ***consumer***, or ***customer***, for the purposes of this textbook, we have chosen to use the term ***client*** for the sake of simplicity and to make it easy for students, who are in the process of learning a large number of terms related to health care that constitute a whole new language. We discuss the issue of differences in terminology in Chapter 3: Workplace Settings. The chapter on medical terminology (Chapter 13) has also been revised to reflect current vocabulary and abbreviation practices used in health care facilities across Canada.

In this text, we have also chosen to use the more generic and widely used term ***long-term care*** (referred to as **LTC** in the field) in the context of care that is ongoing and provides relatively stable assistance to people with their activities of daily living (ADLs). It also relates to any type of home or facility where clients are cared for and supported—long-term care facilities (nursing homes) or even group homes for the developmentally delayed who are not physically or intellectually ill but are unable to care for themselves. While this term is *not* the preferred term in every province or regional area, we use *long-term care* throughout the text because it does not have different (and therefore misleading) meanings from one region to another within Canada. In contrast, the term *complex care* refers to the old terms "intermediate" and "extended" care in British Columbia, while it can mean "acute or subacute care for people with multisystem failure," a completely different meaning, in Ontario. Some provinces use the term *continuing complex care* to mean "ongoing care," while other provinces do not use the term at all. The term *continuing care* is being widely used throughout Canada in this context, but it is a relatively newer term than *long-term care* and therefore not widely recognized in some areas of Canada.

In summary, being aware of the terminology differences existing within this diverse country of ours, instructors (and students) should use whatever term is the choice in their particular region.

It should also be noted that we recognize that a wide range of equipment brands are used across the country, so it is possible that some instructors will find within this textbook photographs that depict a piece of equipment that has never been used in their area. We suggest that clinical instructors provide an opportunity for students to observe the equipment that is more familiar to their own area.

Student Preface

As a support worker, you are a very important member of the health care team because you probably spend more time with your clients than any other member of the team does. Team members rely on your observations, reports, and recordings, especially of any changes in your client. Your clients and their families rely on you to provide professional and safe care. You and the care you give may be the bright spots in a client's day.

This book was designed to help you learn by using its special features, which are described on the following pages. Since the last edition was published, educational and vocational standards for support workers have been released both nationally and within many provinces. To reflect these new standards, as well as anticipated practice trends across Canada, *Mosby's Canadian Textbook for the Support Worker*, Fourth Edition, has been revised, updated, ınd reorganized to assist you, the student. Even after ɔu graduate, the book will continue to be a useful source to you in the field as you gain experience d expand your knowledge.

This preface presents some study guidelines and for using this book effectively. Your instructor probably assign chapters or partial chapters from extbook to read before or after class. When given ding assignment, do you read from the first page e last page without stopping? How much of you read do you remember? Using an efficient system will help you understand and retain all formation that you read. A useful study system ese steps:

view or survey
estion
d and record
te and review

VIEW

ɔu start a reading assignment, preview or assignment to get an idea of what it covers ecall what you already know about the eview the chapter title, headings, subheadings, and terms or ideas in bold print or italics. Also, survey the objectives, key terms, introductory paragraph, boxes, key points, and the review questions at the end of the chapter. Previewing takes only a few minutes. Remember, previewing helps you become familiar with the material.

2 QUESTION

After previewing, you need to form a list of questions to be answered as you read the material. Questions should relate to what might be asked on a test or how the information applies to giving care. Use the title, headings, and subheadings to form questions. Avoid questions that have one-word answers. Questions that begin with *what*, *how*, or *why* are most helpful. While reading, if you find that a particular question does not help you understand and retain the assignment material, change the question to make this step more useful.

3 READ AND RECORD

Reading, which is the next step, is more productive after you have determined what you know already and what you need to learn. The purpose of reading is to:

- Gain new information
- Connect the new information to what you know already

Break the assignment into smaller parts, and as you read each part, try to find answers for the questions you had formulated earlier. Also, mark important information in the text by underlining, highlighting, or making notes, which will remind you later what you need to go back to in order to review and learn. Making notes helps you remember what you have learned. When making notes, write down important information in the text margins or in a notebook. Use words and summary statements that will jog your memory about the material.

After reading the assignment, in order to retain the information, you must organize it into a study guide—in the form of diagrams or charts that show relationships or steps in a process. Much of the information in this text is organized in this manner to help you learn. Note-taking in outline format is also very useful.

The following is a sample outline:

I. Main heading
  1. Second level
  2. Second level
    a. Third level
    b. Third level
II. Main heading

4 RECITE AND REVIEW

Finally, recite and review, using your notes and the study guide, by finding the answers for the questions you formed earlier and any others that may have come up during the reading and as you answered the review questions at the end of the chapter. Answer all questions out loud (recite). If you are unsure about the answers to any of the questions, consult your instructor.

Reviewing is more about *when* to study than *what* to study. You already decided what to study during the preview, question, and reading steps. Your instructor may have emphasized key points from the reading assignment in class. The best times to review both the information in your text and your notes from class are (1) the same day or evening of the class, (2) right after your first study session, (3) 1 week later, and (4) regularly before a quiz or test, midterm, or final exam. Studying the information many times will help you remember it.

Chapter titles and subtitles tell you the subject of the chapter.

CHAPTER 10

Caring About Culture and Diversity

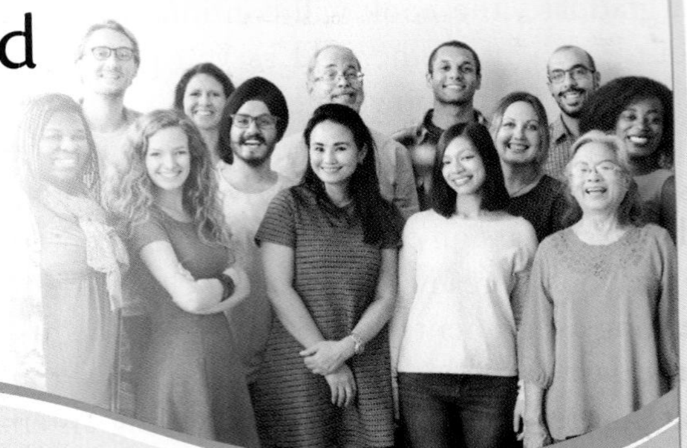

OBJECTIVES

After reading this chapter, the learner should be able to do the following:

- Distinguish among *race* (or *ethnicity*) and *culture*.
- Describe the factors that influence a person's culture.
- Summarize how culture influences a person's attitudes and behaviours.
- Describe how culture may affect communication, family organization, religious convictions, and perceptions about illness and health care.
- Analyze how your own cultural biases may affect your relationships with your clients.
- Apply the information in this chapter in your work by providing culturally sensitive care.

http://evolve.elsevier.com/Canada/Sorrentino/SupportWorker 147

Objectives tell you what is presented in the chapter and what you will learn. As a final review of the chapter, see if you have learned all the information listed in the Objectives.

KEY TERMS

ageism Feelings of impatience, intolerance, or prejudice based on negative attitudes and stereotypes toward a person or group of people because of their age. *p. 151*
assimilate Adopt the traditions of the larger society. *p. 150*
bias A point of view that prevents a person from being impartial. *p. 150*
blended family A couple with two or more children, one or more of whom is the natural child of both members of the couple and one or more of whom is the stepchild of one member of the couple. *p. 154*
cultural competence The ability to interact effectively with people from different cultures or socioeconomic backgrounds. *p. 153*
cultural conflict Negative feelings and conduct that can result when people from one culture try to impose their own set of values and behaviours on people from another culture. *p. 152*
culture The characteristics of a group of people, including the language, values, beliefs, customs, habits, ways of life, rules for behaviour, music, and traditions. *p. 149*
diversity The state of different individuals and cultures coexisting. *p. 148*
ethnic identity The ethnic background a person feels a part of, based usually on similar language and customs. *p. 149*
ethnicity The sharing of a common history, language, geography, national origin, religion, or identity. *p. 149*
ethnocentrism The belief that one's own culture or ethnic group is better or more important than others'. *p. 149*
homophobia Negative attitudes toward or intolerance of homosexuality or people who are identified or perceived as being lesbian, gay, bisexual, transgender, or questioning their sexuality (**LGBTQ**). *p. 152*
LGBTQ An abbreviation that stands for the group of people who identify themselves as lesbian, gay, bisexual, transgender, or questioning their sexuality. *p. 152*
nuclear family A family consisting of a father, a mother, and children. *p. 154*
personal space The area immediately around one's body. *p. 156*
prejudice An attitude that forms an opinion about a person based on his or her membership in a group. *p. 150*
racism Feelings of superiority over, and intolerance or prejudice toward, a person or group of people who may have different physical appearances or cultural practices. *p. 149*
same-sex family A family in which both adults who live together in a loving, intimate relationship are of the same gender. *p. 154*
sexism Feelings of intolerance or prejudice toward a person or group of people because of their gender. *p. 152*
single-parent families Families in which the adult head of the household does not have a partner who shares the home. *p. 154*

This chapter addresses one of the most important values that all support workers—and all caregivers, for that matter—must possess: respect for diversity. Diversity is the state of different individuals and cultures coexisting. During your career as a support worker, you will care for and work with people whose lifestyles, beliefs, customs, and rituals are different from your own. It is necessary that you are always respectful of a person's age, race, gender, occupation, sexual orientation, and lifestyle. ***Respect for diversity is a theme that will be repeated throughout this***

148

Key Terms are important words and phrases in the chapter. The list at the beginning of the chapter includes the definitions for all the terms. Not only do the key terms introduce you to the important terms in the chapter; they are also useful study guides.

Terms in blue bold present the key terms and definitions again within the body of the chapter, which helps reinforce learning. The key terms and their definitions are listed alphabetically in the Glossary at the end of the book (see p. 1101). Whenever you come across a key term again in a later chapter, you can turn to the Glossary for the definition of the term.

Terms in italics present other important terms and information in the text that require special attention.

Focus on Home Care boxes highlight information necessary for providing safe care in the home setting.

CHAPTER 1

FOCUS ON HOME CARE

Assisting the Primary Caregiver

Sometimes you will work closely with the client's primary caregiver. For example, you assist Mrs. Kalopsis with housekeeping and meal preparation so that she can spend more time caring for her husband, who is ill.

Primary caregivers are often relieved to have assistance from the health care team. However, some may have mixed feelings about your presence in their homes. Some people may resent the interruption to their routines or may feel that you are invading their privacy. Some caregivers may also feel that they are failures for needing help or may regret that someone else is accomplishing tasks that they wish they had accomplished themselves.

Try to put the family caregivers at ease by showing that you are there to help, not to take over or judge their housekeeping or caregiving skills. Do not take on tasks that have not been assigned to you. As well, adapt your support work to suit the family's standards and preferences, not your own. Respect the family's routines, schedules, and ways of doing things. Consult with your supervisor if you think the family's wishes may affect safety.

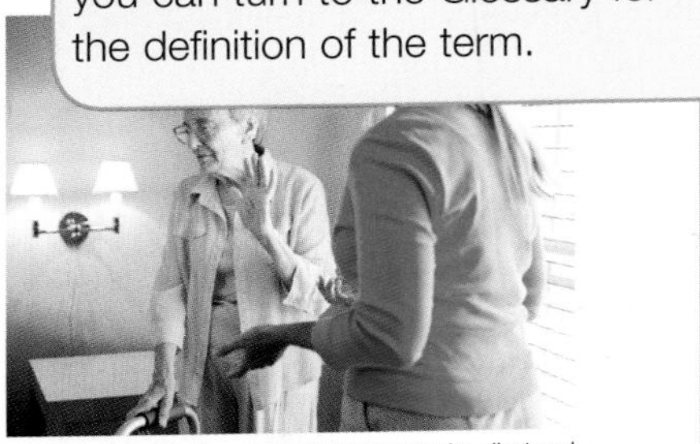

FIGURE 11–2 Tensions may erupt between the client and family members when forced to deal with the challenges of illness and disability. (**Source:** © Golden Pixels LLC/Alamy.)

relationships within the family, including any conflict and potential for conflict. They may help the family deal with stress by working on improving the communication skills and problem-solving abilities of family members. Sometimes bringing them together in a family conference is needed to discuss how the caregiving can impact the entire family. As a support worker, you will be asked to attend such family conferences.

Families in Conflict

When illness or disability occurs, the stress on all family members may be great, and members may have to cope with conflict. Conflicts may take the form of expressions of irritation, anger, bickering, or arguments. Conflict may sometimes be hidden. Adult children may care for aging parents with whom they have unresolved conflicts. Siblings who have not spoken in years may be forced to see one another during a parent's illness. Sometimes, the health care team can help families resolve their difficulties in such situations. Members of palliative care teams are specially trained to help people resolve emotional problems that are causing them distress (see Chapter 7 for managing conflict).

When working with a family, try to be aware of family relationships and any conflicts, communication difficulties, and stressful situations (FIGURE 11–2). It is not part of your role to help families deal with their interpersonal problems, but there are some things you can do in a stressful situation. You could encourage communication without taking sides, or you could defuse (calm) a tense situation—for example, when angry words have been exchanged between the client and a family member, you may suggest to the family member to go out for a cup of coffee (see Chapter 7). Agencies and facilities have policies to guide you in dealing with conflicts you might encounter. You must observe and report on family interactions (see the *Case Study: Family Conflict* box) and also be alert for signs of abuse (see Chapter 16).

Focus on Long-Term Care boxes highlight information unique to the long-term care setting.

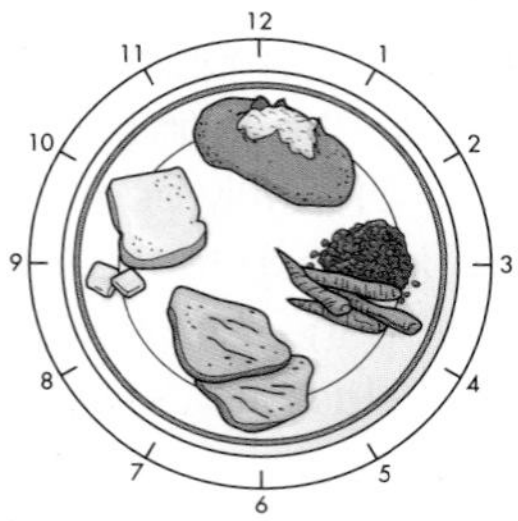

FIGURE 28–5 The numbers on a clock are used to help a client with vision loss locate food on a plate.

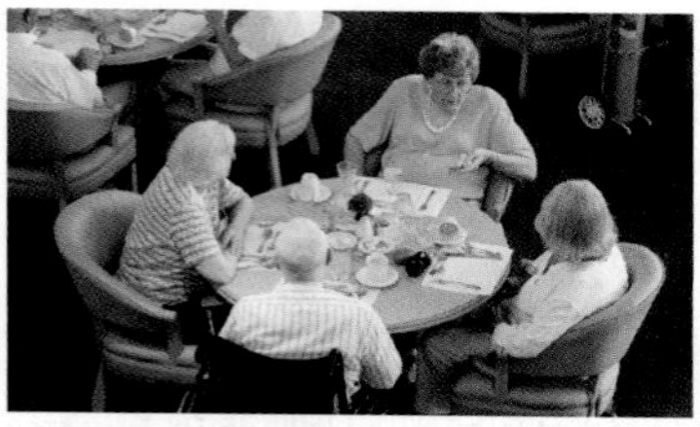

FIGURE 28–6 Clients enjoy a pleasant meal in the dining room. Source: © Dennis MacDonald/maXximages.com.

Serving Meal Trays

Most clients in hospitals eat their meals in their rooms. However, long-term care clients are encouraged to eat in the dining room (see the *Focus on Long-Term Care: Dining Programs* box), but those who are too ill to move about eat in their rooms.

In most provinces and territories in Canada, clients in long-term care facilities must eat in the dining room unless they are ill. If a client wishes to eat in his room, a team conference to discuss the safety issues and risks of eating alone, especially if the client has dysphagia, must be scheduled and must involve the family, client, and staff. A staff member has to be

FOCUS ON LONG-TERM CARE

Dining Programs

Many long-term care facilities have special dining programs:

- ***Social dining***—clients eat in the dining room. Each table has four to six residents (FIGURE 28–6). Food is served as in a restaurant. Depending on the policy of the facility, agency, province, or territory, clients usually sit in the same place for each meal and are not moved except under special circumstances. They establish a relationship with the other clients at their table, and because this relationship is respected, their place is maintained. Follow the dining room seating plan posted in your facility dining room.
- ***Family dining***—food is placed in bowls and on platters, and clients serve themselves as they would at home.
- ***Assistive dining***—some facilities have circular or horseshoe-shaped tables. Clients who need assistance with eating are seated around the tables. In this arrangement, the support worker sits at the centre of the table and is able to feed

Bulleted lists present information in a way that is easy to study and remember.

The client is treated in a hospital coronary care unit (CCU), which has emergency equipment and medications needed to prevent life-threatening complications. The client is kept in the CCU for 2 to 3 days (depending on your area) and then transferred to another nursing unit once stable.

The client who has suffered an MI is allowed to increase his level of activity gradually. Medications and measures to prevent complications are continued. Rehabilitation, with the goal of preventing another heart attack, is begun in a hospital and continued when the client returns home. The rehabilitation includes an exercise program and teaching about medications, dietary changes, activity, and lifestyle modifications. Activities, including sexual activity, return to normal levels slowly, and the client can return to work when advised by the physician.

Congestive Heart Failure

Congestive heart failure (CHF), or simply *heart failure*, is an abnormal condition that occurs when the heart cannot pump blood normally. Blood backs up and causes an abnormal amount (congestion) of fluid in the tissues. CHF may affect the right side, left side, or both sides of the heart.

The right side of the heart receives blood from body tissues and pumps it into the lungs to get oxygen. With right-sided heart failure, blood backs up into the veins. Fluid collection in the body produces weight gain. *Pitting edema* (swelling due to excess fluid in the tissues—see Chapter 28) becomes evident in the feet and ankles, and the neck veins become enlarged. The liver becomes engorged, which impairs its function. Congestion in the abdomen may cause digestive problems, including loss of appetite, abdominal pain, and (eventually) weight loss.

The left side of the heart receives blood from the lungs and pumps it into the rest of the body. With left-sided heart failure, blood collects in lung tissue, resulting in difficulty breathing (*dyspnea*), increased sputum (mucus in the lungs), cough, and gurgling sounds in the lungs. Dyspnea is worse when the client is active or is lying down, so it disrupts sleep. The client may wake up with a feeling of suffocation. Fatigue and weakness in the limbs are common.

In advanced CHF, the brain may not get enough oxygen, causing confusion and behaviour changes. Poor blood flow to the kidneys results in impaired kidney function and low urine output.

CHF can be treated and controlled by medications that can strengthen the heart and reduce the amount of fluid in the body. Treatment also includes a sodium-restricted diet and administration of oxygen. Weight is measured daily to check for weight gain, an early sign of fluid buildup. Most clients with CHF prefer the semi-Fowler's or Fowler's position for ease of breathing. As a support worker, you may be involved in the following:

- Maintaining bed rest
- Measuring intake and output
- Measuring daily weight, ideally before eating and after voiding
- Restricting fluids, as ordered by the physician
- Assisting with transfers or ambulation
- Assisting with self-care activities
- Maintaining good positioning and body alignment according to the care plan
- Applying elastic stockings to reduce leg swelling

See the *Focus on Children: Congestive Heart Failure* and *Focus on Older Adults: Congestive Heart Failure* boxes.

FOCUS ON CHILDREN

Congestive Heart Failure

Congenital heart defects can cause CHF in children. (*Congenital* comes from the Latin word *congenitus*, meaning "to be born with.")

FOCUS ON OLDER ADULTS

Congestive Heart Failure

Because the heart is a muscle and muscles weaken with age, many older people develop CHF. Some may need home care or long-term care.

Older adults with CHF are at risk for skin breakdown. Tissue swelling, poor circulation, and fragile skin combine to increase the risk for pressure ulcers. Effective skin care and regular position changes are essential.

Focus on Children boxes provide information about the needs, considerations, and general circumstances of children.

Focus on Older Adults boxes provide information about the needs, considerations, and special circumstances of older adults.

CHAPTER 10 Caring About Culture and Diversity **153**

CASE STUDY **Cultural Conflict**

Salvinia Di Silva is a 75-year-old widow receiving home care. She and her husband moved from Portugal to Canada in the 1960s with their three young children. For the next 30 years, Mr. Di Silva worked on the assembly line of an automobile factory, while Mrs. Di Silva worked as a dressmaker. They worked long hours to pay for their children's education. All three children now have successful careers and their own families.

Mrs. Di Silva's health began to decline after her husband died. Severe arthritis in her leg and hip progressed to the point that she could no longer walk. A family conference was held, and the children agreed that their mother no longer could care for herself, even with the aid of a support worker. They thought it was unsafe for her to live alone. None of the children felt that they could manage their mother's care and the demands of their own families and careers, so they told their mother that she should consider moving into a long-term care facility.

Her children's suggestion came as a great shock to Mrs. Di Silva. She and her husband had taken care of her mother years before, until her mother's death. Mrs. Di Silva had assumed that one of her children would do the same for her. In Portugal, it was common for children to take care of their older parents. Mrs. Di Silva felt as if she was being cast aside. The idea of leaving her home and moving into a facility with strangers depressed her greatly. Her depression, in turn, caused feelings of guilt and remorse among the Di Silva children, who deeply loved their mother. This situation is an example of conflict between two cultures. Mr. and Mrs. Di Silva had given their children opportunities to enter and succeed in a new culture. But because the children are now a part of the new culture, they, like others in their environment, are less willing to give up their lifestyles to care for their mother in their own homes. They see their friends' parents enjoying living in a retirement facility with other people their own age and hope their mother will also eventually settle in and feel at home there.

that reveals religious affiliation in certain environments. Or a caregiver might serve unfamiliar foods to a client because those foods are common in the caregiver's ethnic background, not the client's.

An individual living within different cultures at the same time can also have feelings of cultural conflict. A child raised in a very modest, religious family may experience cultural conflict when he grows up and moves out of the house to go to school. This person may struggle with trying to live by the family's rules, as expected by his parents, while trying to enjoy some newly found freedoms within his peer group. Refer to the *Case Study: Cultural Conflict* box for an example of cultural conflict experienced by an individual.

Cultural Competence

Cultural competence is the ability of a person to interact effectively with people from different

Case Study boxes apply some of the concepts in the text to real-world examples of support workers and the clients they care for.

Supporting boxes present scenarios depicting situations and problems that support workers may face on a typical day. The boxes discuss how support workers in these cases make decisions and solve problems. Put yourself in the same situation. What would you do?

CHAPTER 20 Caring for the Young **361**

Supporting Jamie: Offering Respite to Family

Jamie is a happy, fun-loving boy who has just celebrated his twelfth birthday. Like many preteens his age, he likes to watch television and listen to music. Jamie is in Grade 8 and is looking forward to attending high school next year. He does well in school, but he is not sure yet about the career he wants to pursue. Jamie is just beginning his growth spurt. His family has noticed that he has grown taller and his voice is getting deeper. He has three younger brothers, and his mother and stepfather care for Jamie when he is home from school.

Jamie has cerebral palsy and is wheelchair dependent. He is often incontinent of urine, so he must wear incontinence products. Because of his ever-increasing size, his mother (who has always been his primary caregiver) has rented a mechanical lift and is able to use it to toilet, bathe, and move Jamie from the bed to his chair. Jamie also requires assistance with eating. He communicates by way of a computer, which sounds out the words that he types using the keyboard.

After putting off surgery on her knee for several years, Jamie's mother is now going to have a total knee replacement and will therefore not be able to care for Jamie for several weeks. You are one of the support workers who will be caring for Jamie in his home during this time. Your duties are to assist with his activities of daily living (ADLs) and occasionally arrange for his wheelchair taxi to drive him to school. You will get to know all of Jamie's family, as they will be home during the afternoon and evening hours when you are there.

Think About Safety boxes provide clear, concise, easy-to-follow advice on how to provide safe care to clients of all ages and keep yourself safe.

Think About Safety

Family Situations That Must Be Reported

- Violent behaviour of a family member (see Chapter 16)
- Frequent visits by "strangers," who seem to make the members of the household fearful or uneasy
- Suspected drug abuse—for example, the presence of instruments or equipment for drug use
- Excessive drinking, as evidenced by the presence of liquor bottles hidden throughout the house or the child's parent or caregiver being inebriated
- Electricity, heat, or water turned off
- Severe shortage of food or clothing—for example, no food in the cupboards or refrigerator, or the child being dressed inappropriately for the weather (such as no coat in winter)
- Illness of a child that has been unreported to you
- Sudden departure of caregiver
- Unexpected return of a family member

Your role in disciplining the child is to:

- Know the rules of acceptable behaviour in each family situation
- Ask an appropriate family member to clarify the rules if you are unsure
- Reinforce existing rules
- Be consistent when using discipline
- Praise the child's efforts at following the rules

Some parents may have very few rules of discipline, or the existing rules may seem too harsh or too loose. In such a case, you should contact your supervisor. New rules may need to be set, but you should not set discipline rules without the guidance of your supervisor.

Punishment

Punishment is a harsh response that occurs when a discipline rule is broken. ***Punishing a child for failing to follow the rules of the household is not your responsibility.*** If a family member asks you to do so, explain that it is against your agency's policy to carry out punishment. Ask the family member to membership. An example of discrimination is using the assumption that "All people who are ______ are lazy" to justify why a certain person is not hired.

Types of Prejudice

In an ethnically and culturally diverse society such as Canada's, prejudices and discrimination should not be tolerated. As a support worker, you will be caring for and supporting all types of people and must be prepared to give all your clients the same high quality of care, regardless of their differences.

Some people stereotype ethnic or cultural groups by assuming they are "all alike" or by believing that everyone in that group acts or behaves in a certain way. A stereotype is an overly simple or exaggerated view of a group of people. An example of a stereotype is "Women are shorter than men." While many women may be shorter than some men, this general statement is certainly not true.

Ageism refers to feelings of intolerance or prejudice toward others because of their age, based on negative attitudes, stereotypes, or impatience (see BOX 10–1). North American society has long fostered

Boxes and Tables present principles, guidelines, signs and symptoms, care measures, and other information, often in a list format, and are useful study guides for reviewing.

BOX 10–1 Ageism and Age Discrimination (Fact Sheet)

The term *ageism* refers to two concepts: a socially constructed way of thinking about older persons based on negative attitudes and stereotypes about aging and a tendency to structure society based on an assumption that everyone is young, thereby failing to respond appropriately to the real needs of older persons.

Ageism is often a cause for individual acts of age discrimination and also discrimination that is more systemic in nature, such as in the design and implementation of services, programs and facilities. Age discrimination involves treating persons in an unequal fashion due to age in a way that is contrary to human rights law. The Ontario Human Rights Code prohibits age discrimination in employment, housing accommodation, goods, services and facilities, contracts, and membership in trade and vocational associations.

Age discrimination is often not taken as seriously as other forms of discrimination. However, it can have the same economic, social, and psychological impact as any other form of discrimination.

To combat ageism it is necessary to raise public awareness about its existence and to dispel common stereotypes and misperceptions about aging. Aging is a highly individual experience and it is not possible to generalize about the skills and abilities of an older person based on age, any more than it is possible to make assumptions about someone based on any other aspect of their identity. Human rights principles require people to be treated as individuals and assessed on their own merits, instead of on the basis of assumptions, and to be given the same opportunities and benefits as everyone else, regardless of age. It is important to recognize that older persons make significant contributions to our society and that we must not limit their potential.

At the same time, ageism can be combated through inclusive planning and design which reflects the circumstances of persons of all ages to

Source: Ontario Human Rights Commission. *Ageism and age* en/ageism-and-age-discrimination-fact-sheet.

insurance plan. The provincial or territorial government finances and plans its health care services, following the five basic principles outlined in the *Canada Health Act*. For example, provincial and territorial governments decide where hospitals or long-term care facilities will be located and organized; how many physicians, nurses, and other service providers will be needed; and how much money to spend on health care services. Provincial and territorial health insurance plans (TABLE 2–1) pay for hospital and physician costs.

HEALTH CARE CHALLENGES, SUPPLEMENTARY SERVICES, AND TRENDS

Challenges

The Canadian health care system has come under stress in recent years. Many factors challenge the country's ability to provide quality, universal health care, and these factors are expected to continue into the future.[4] They include:

- ***Worker shortages.*** Many rural and remote areas face severe shortages of physicians, nurses, and other health care workers. The growing trend of people moving to bigger cities leaves smaller communities in need of educated workers.
- ***Aging of the baby boomer generation (those born between 1945 and 1964).*** The Canadian society is aging. For the older-adult population to live safely and with dignity and independence, the costs of our health care system will rise.
- ***Aging of health care workers.*** Health care workers are also aging. Many studies are investigating the effects of different types of work on older bodies. One finding is that older workers have fewer injuries, but the injuries they have tend to be more severe.[7]
- ***Long waiting lists for surgeries, diagnostics, and medical procedures.*** Long wait times cause stress and a possible worsening of their condition for many clients in need of treatment.
- ***Long waiting times for admission to long-term care facilities.*** Clients who are ill and waiting for long-term care placement must often stay in an acute-care hospital because it is unsafe for them to live at home. Overcrowded hospital units and emergency departments have resulted. To remedy the situation, many hospitals have restructured their care delivery to include continuing care units, where these clients can await long-term care admission.
- ***The steadily rising cost of care.*** Of all the challenges facing the health care system, its rising cost is the greatest. Drugs and technology that help treat diseases and disabilities are better than ever before. However, these advances come at a high price due to the cost of developing them. Building

TABLE 2–1 Provincial and Territorial Health Insurance Programs

Province/Territory	Name of Plan
Alberta	Alberta Health Care Insurance Plan
British Columbia	Medical Services Plan
Manitoba	Manitoba Health
New Brunswick	Medicare
Newfoundland and Labrador	Newfoundland and Labrador Medical Care Plan
Northwest Territories	NWT Health Care Insurance Plan
Nova Scotia	Medical Service Insurance
Nunavut	Nunavut Health Care Plan
Ontario	Ontario Health Insurance Plan
Prince Edward Island	Medicare
Quebec	Assurance maladie (Medicare)
Saskatchewan	Saskatchewan Medical Care Insurance Plan
Yukon	Yukon Health Care Insurance Plan

Source: Health Canada. (2015). *Provincial/territorial role in health.* Retrieved from http://healthycanadians.gc.ca/health-system-systeme-sante/cards-cartes/health-role-sante-eng.php.

CHAPTER 21 Caring for Older Adults 371

Providing Compassionate Care
Supporting Older Clients

- ***Dignity.*** Show respect for your older clients. Avoid using terms, gestures, or a tone of voice that could be considered patronizing (see Chapters 5 and 10). For example, never use the term "girl" when addressing an older female client. Some older clients find it disrespectful to be addressed by their first names, especially by younger people. Ask your clients how they would like to be addressed. Never assume you can use a client's first name, even if you have heard your co-workers use it. Do not talk about the client with others. Do not exchange glances with co-workers when reacting to something an older client has said or done.
- ***Independence.*** Help clients only when necessary. Respect their routines. Do things the way clients are used to doing them. Allow time for rest, and avoid rushing them.
- ***Preferences.*** Older clients have the right to make choices, so you must have their consent for all procedures. They can make decisions regarding their care and also choose when to get up and when to go to bed, what to wear, what activities to participate in, and what to eat. Always ask about and accommodate a client's preferences.
- ***Privacy.*** Provide for privacy, and keep information about the client confidential. All clients should be given privacy when they are visiting with others or using the telephone. Use draping and screening to avoid exposing the client's body during procedures. Provide for privacy during elimination.
- ***Safety.*** Be alert to safety hazards in the client's environment. Practise the safety measures discussed in Chapter 22 to prevent falls, burns, poisoning, and suffocation. Apply restraints only if ordered by a physician and only once the task has been properly delegated to you.

Note that older clients may not show the usual signs of infection such as fever, pain, inflammation, and swelling (see Chapter 23). The only signs may be changes in behaviour, so observe for any such changes, including sudden confusion; urinary incontinence; a fall; or a change in mood, energy levels, or eating habits. Immediately report all changes in your client's behaviour and health to

Providing Compassionate Care boxes highlight how to provide the care discussed in the chapter in a compassionate manner. The first words in the list are bolded and italicized to help you remember DIPPS, the acronym that summarizes the five principles of support work—providing for the client's dignity, independence, preferences, privacy, and safety.

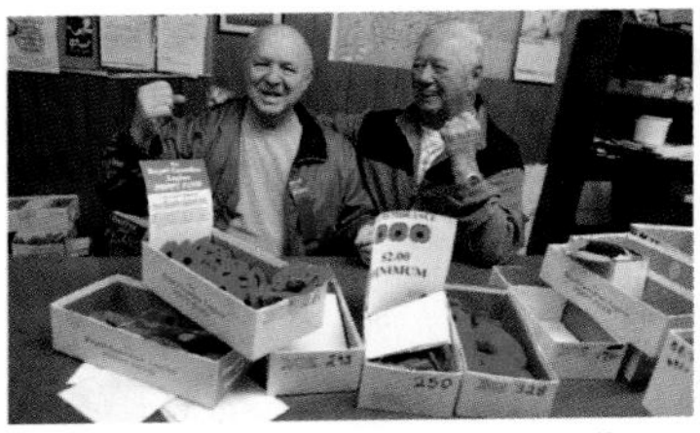

FIGURE 21–2 These retired people volunteer. (**Source:** Michael Stuparyk/GetStock.com.)

enjoyed or the time to take up new ones. However, for people who have never cultivated interests or hobbies outside of their job, retirement can cause a very abrupt and upsetting change of lifestyle that they have difficulties adjusting to.

CHAPTER 12 Promoting Client Well-Being, Comfort, and Sleep 181

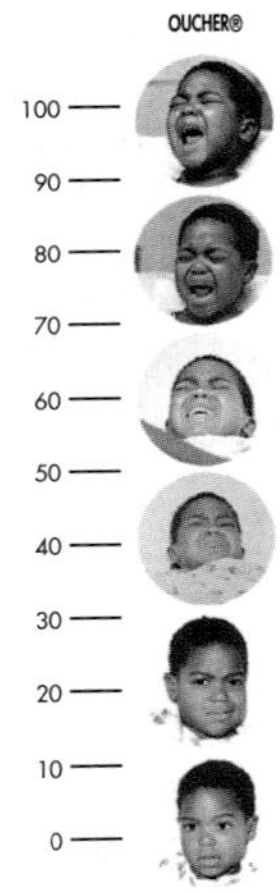

FIGURE 12–11 The Oucher pain scale. (**Source:** Potter, P.A., Perry, A.G., Ross-Kerr, J.C., et al. (2010). *Canadian fundamentals of nursing* (Revised 4th ed., p. 1024). Toronto, ON: Elsevier Canada.)

BOX 12–2 Signs and Symptoms of Pain

Body Responses
- Increased pulse, respirations, and blood pressure
- Nausea
- Pale skin (pallor)
- Sweating (diaphoresis)
- Vomiting

Behaviours
- Changes in speech: slow or rapid, loud or quiet
- Crying
- Gasping
- Grimacing
- Groaning
- Grunting
- Holding the affected body part (splinting)
- Being irritable
- Maintaining one position; refusing to move
- Moaning
- Being quiet
- Being restless
- Rubbing
- Screaming
- Rocking back and forth

Respecting Diversity boxes contain information to help you learn about the various practices of different cultures.

Respecting Diversity

Cultural Aspects of Pain

Culturally acquired patterns of pain responses may also influence the neurophysiological and verbal responses to pain. A client's expectations concerning pain may influence how much pain can be tolerated. Response to pain may be limited by language used to describe or report pain. The degree of pain expression does not necessarily correlate with pain intensity. Preferences for pain-coping strategies are usually determined by culture; thus, nontraditional interventions to manage pain need to be explored with the client. How people view and respond to pain may influence your choice of interventions.

Implications for Support Workers
- Be aware of perceived causal factors of pain (fate, lifestyle, punishment, witchcraft).
- Emotional responses to pain (overt [obvious], stoic [bearing quietly]) vary among and within cultures.
- Words used to express pain vary among cultures (*hurt, ache, discomfort*).
- Personal and social meanings of pain and past pain experiences affect pain perception.
- Definitions of pain change the perception of pain intensity.
- Feelings about pain direct treatment.
- The health care professional's beliefs and expectations regarding pain expression sway pain-management strategies.
- Therapeutic goals of pain management are influenced by cultural beliefs.

Source: Potter, P.A., Perry A.G., Ross-Kerr, J.C., et al. (2014). *Canadian fundamentals of nursing* (5th ed., p. 1026). Toronto, ON: Elsevier Canada.

Making a Closed Bed—cont'd

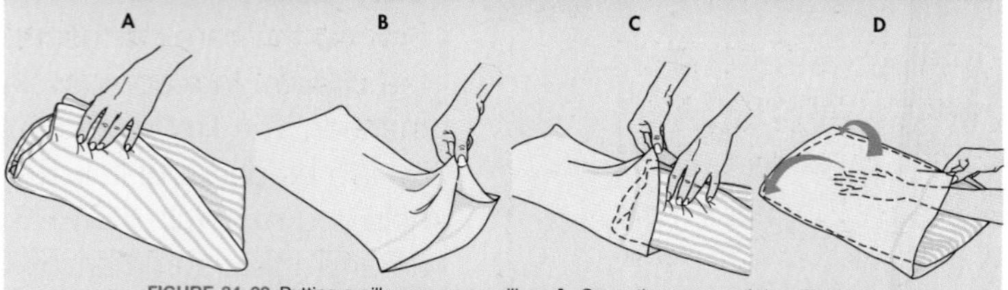

FIGURE 34–22 Putting a pillowcase on a pillow. **A,** Grasp the corners of the pillow to form a "V." **B,** The pillowcase is flat on the bed; the pillowcase is opened with the free hand. **C,** The "V" end of the pillow is guided into the pillowcase. **D,** The "V" end of the pillow falls into the corners of the pillowcase.

29 Put the pillow in the pillowcase (FIGURE 34–22). Fold the pillowcase edges under together, and tuck them in next to the pillow.
This prevents the pillow from slipping out.

30 Place the pillow on the bed. The open, tucked end should be away from the door and the seam of the pillowcase toward the head of the bed.

POST-PROCEDURE

31 Attach the call bell to the bed.*
This provides an easy, safe way for the client to contact staff, if necessary.

32 Lower the bed to its lowest position. Lock the bed wheels.*

33 Follow your employer's policies as to where you put clean leftover linens in your client's room.

34 Remove the laundry bag from the room (if your facility has laundry bags in clients' rooms). Follow employer policy for care of dirty linen.

*Steps marked with an asterisk may not apply in community s

The Open Bed

An *open* bed is made shortly before the bed is to be occupied. Top linens are folded back so that the client can get into bed easily (FIGURE 34–23). An open bed is made when the client is out of bed only for a short time, or it is made just before the client goes to bed.

The Occupied Bed

An *occupied* bed is made while the client is still in the bed (FIGURE 34–24) because the client cannot get

Colour illustrations and photographs visually present key ideas, concepts, and procedure steps and help you apply and remember the written material.

The **Report and Record** step is highlighted in procedures to remind you of the importance of communicating with the rest of the health care team about your actions and observations.

Assisting a Client to Eat Meals From a Food Tray 123

Advocate on behalf of the client's quality of life by promoting:
Dignity • Independence • Preferences • Privacy • Safety *(see BOX 1-4, on p. 17)*

PRE-PROCEDURE

1 Identify the client, according to employer policy
This eliminates the possibility of mistaking one client for another.

2 Perform hand hygiene.

3 Prepare the client for the meal. Assist with handwashing.

4 If indicated in the client's care plan or if requested by your client, provide for privacy.
This ensures dignity for the client. However, most clients benefit from the social interaction that takes place at mealtime.

5 Make sure the tray contains everything needed. Make sure special utensils are included if needed.

PROCEDURE

6 Help the client to a sitting position.
This helps reduce the risk of choking.

7 Place the tray on the overbed table or other table.

8 Remove lids from dishes. Open milk cartons and cereal boxes, cut the meat, and butter the bread if indicated in the care plan (FIGURE 28–7).

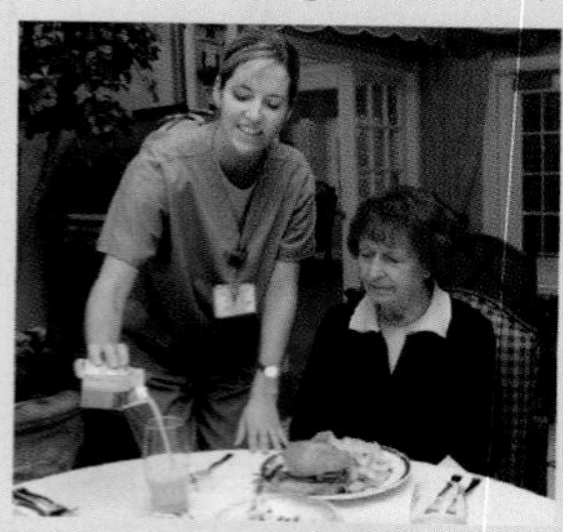

FIGURE 28–7 Open cartons and other containers for the client.

9 Place the napkin, clothes protector (if needed), and utensils within the client's reach.

10 Measure and record intake if ordered (see pp. 595–596). Note the amount and types of foods eaten.

11 Check for and remove any food in the client's mouth (pocketing). Wear gloves.
Pocketing food can lead to choking if kept in the mouth. Pocketing food indicates that the client has difficulty swallowing the food, which must be recorded and reported.

12 Remove the tray.

13 Assist with handwashing. Offer oral hygiene. Wear gloves for this step.
Handwashing decreases the risk for pathogen spread. Oral hygiene can stimulate saliva production, which can assist in chewing food and in digestion.

14 Clean any spills, and change soiled linen.

15 Help the client to return to bed if indicated.

POST-PROCEDURE

16 Provide for safety and comfort.

17 Place the call bell within reach.*
This provides an easy, safe way for the client to contact staff if necessary.

18 Follow the care plan for bed rail use.*
This helps ensure client safety.

19 Perform hand hygiene.

Report and Record your actions and observations, according to employer policy. Include the amount and kind of food eaten.
It is important to monitor the food intake of clients. Documentation is also done for legal reasons and to keep the rest of the health care team informed.

*Steps marked with an asterisk may not apply in community settings.

In the **Procedure boxes**, procedures are presented in a step-by-step format and are divided into Pre-Procedure, Procedure, and Post-Procedure sections for easy studying. The two-column format includes steps and rationales to help you learn both how and why a procedure is performed. Steps that may not apply in community settings are identified with an asterisk. The Compassionate Care sections in the Procedure boxes remind you of the DIPPS principles.

CHAPTER REVIEW

KEY POINTS

- Canada's publicly funded health care system is best described as an interlocking set of 10 provincial and 3 territorial health insurance plans.
- Medicare provides access to universal, comprehensive coverage for medically necessary hospital and physician services. These services are administered and delivered by the provincial and territorial governments and are provided at no additional cost to the client.
- To receive their full share of federal funding for health care, the provincial and territorial health insurance plans must meet the five criteria of the *Canada Health Act*—comprehensiveness, universality, portability, accessibility, and public administration.
- Health care delivery is divided into primary, secondary, and tertiary delivery categories. Primary care is aimed at preventing illness whenever possible. Tertiary health care delivery is the most expensive to deliver.
- Many factors challenge and stress the Canadian health care system. These factors include (1) severe shortages of physicians, nurses, and other health care workers in rural areas; (2) the aging of the baby boomer generation; (3) long waiting lists; and (4) the steadily rising cost of care and new technology, which is the greatest challenge.
- Supplementary health benefits often include prescription drugs, dental care, vision care, medical equipment and appliances, independent-living assistance, and the services of other health care providers, such as chiropractors. The level of coverage varies across the country.
- Residents may have private insurance plans that pay for these supplementary services.
- New trends in health care include (1) alternative care in clinics, (2) health care centres, and (3) home care programs.
- To control costs, provincial and territorial governments are focusing on (1) health promotion and disease prevention and (2) home care.
- Support workers provide most home care support services.
- In most provinces and territories, support services are provided by for-profit and not-for-profit public and private agencies. Every province and territory has a publicly funded home care program, but the funding per client will vary depending on the province's funding policies.
- Home care services are classified by (1) personal care services, (2) home support services, (3) nursing and professional services, and (4) support for IADLs.

CRITICAL THINKING IN PRACTICE

How do the following issues impact our Canadian health care system: (a) escalating costs of care, (b) privatization of services, (c) continuity of care, and (d) electronic health records?[10]

REVIEW QUESTIONS

Answers to these questions are at the bottom of p. 32.

Circle the BEST answer.

1. Canada's health care system is:

Key Points are found at the end of each chapter. This section summarizes the important points from the chapter, providing a good framework for you to study from.

Critical Thinking in Practice exercises present a scenario with questions that require you to think critically and apply what you have learned in the chapter.

32 CHAPTER 2 The Canadian Health Care System

3. Which law ensures that every citizen has access to health care?
   A. The *Medical Care Act*
   B. The *Canada Health Act*
   C. The *Long-Term Care Facilities Act*
   D. The *Hospital Insurance and Diagnostic Services Act*
4. Canadians who travel to other parts of the country still maintain their provincial or territorial health care coverage. Which principle of medicare does this exemplify?
   A. Portability
   B. Universality
   C. Comprehensiveness
   D. Public administration
5. The most pressing cause of health care reform has been:
   A. The Great Depression
   B. Lack of accessibility
   C. Lack of available technology
   D. Rising costs of providing technology, drugs, and services
6. A recent trend in health care is to focus on:
   A. Cutting back on home care services
   B. Opening more hospitals in rural areas
   C. Cutting back on public health policies
   D. Public policy that promotes health and prevents disease
7. Immunization programs are an example of a:
   A. Medicare system
   B. Disease prevention program
   C. Home care service
   D. Facility-based treatment
8. One major focus of home care is to:
   A. Diagnose and treat disease
   B. Enable clients to remain in their own homes
   C. Provide accommodation for people with disabilities
   D. Provide accommodation for acutely ill people who do not want to go into the hospital
9. Home care services provided by support workers might include:
   A. Vacuuming and dusting
   B. Respiratory therapy
   C. Assisting the client with physiotherapy
   D. Assisting the client with banking
10. Which statement about Canadian home care programs is correct?
    A. All home care is free to Canadians.
    B. Provincial government funding is shifting to home care.
    C. Hospital care is a cheaper and better alternative for most people.
    D. All provinces and territories govern their programs in a similar manner.
11. In Canada's provinces and territories, support services are governed by:
    A. Regional health boards
    B. The federal government
    C. Private or not-for-profit agencies
    D. The provincial or territorial government

Answers: 1.D, 2.B, 3.B, 4.A, 5.D, 6.D, 7.B, 8.B, 9.A, 10.B, 11.D

Review Questions are a useful study guide as they provide a means to review the main ideas presented in the chapter. Use them to study for a test or examination. Answers are placed upside down below the questions.

The Role of the Support Worker

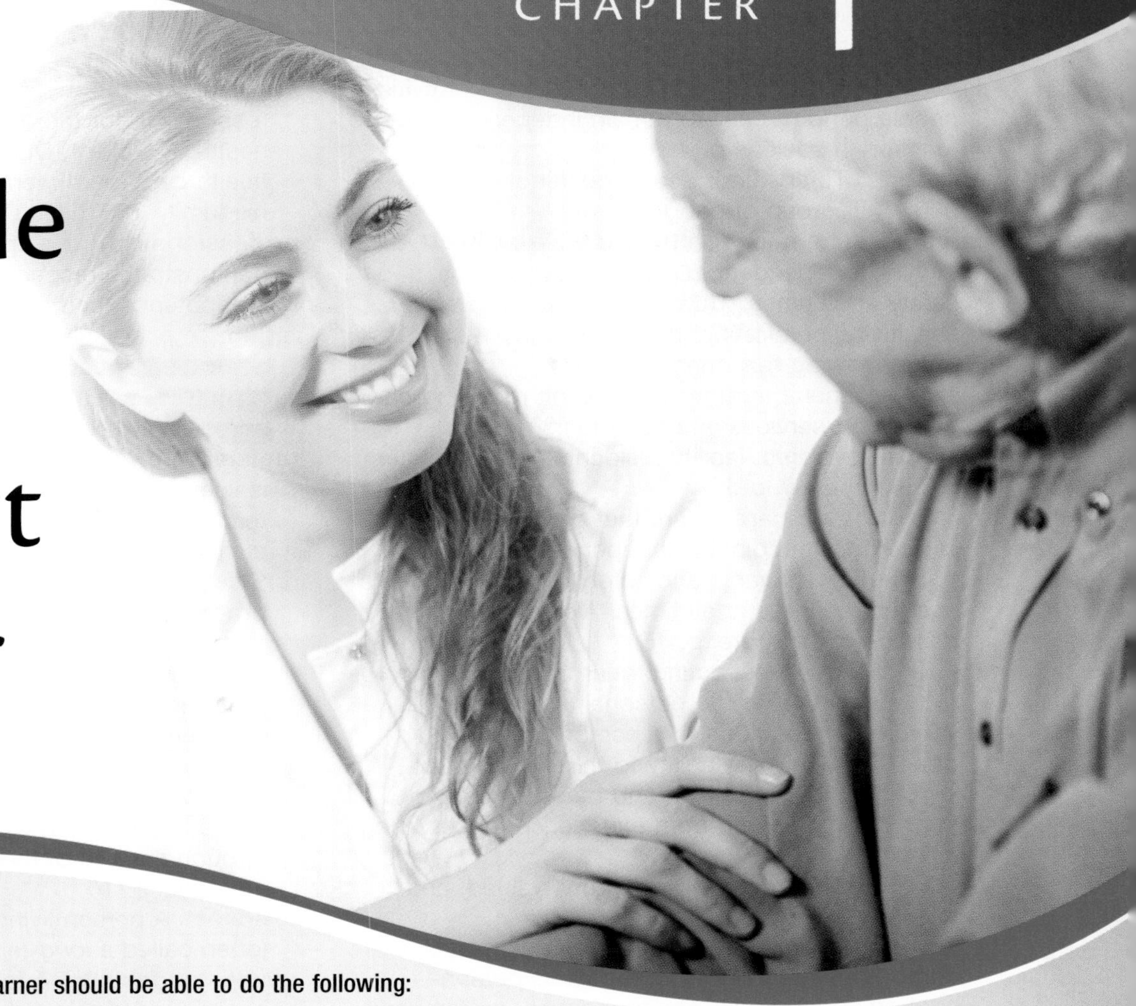

OBJECTIVES

After reading this chapter, the learner should be able to do the following:

- Describe the goal of support work.
- List the principles of compassionate care.
- Describe the main responsibilities of the support worker.
- Identify the role support workers play within the health care team.
- Distinguish between regulated and unregulated health care providers.
- Describe the importance of scope of practice in support work.
- Differentiate between activities of daily living (ADLs) and instrumental activities of daily living (IADLs).
- Describe the significance of having a professional approach to support work.
- Identify the things to consider when thinking critically and solving problems.

KEY TERMS

activities of daily living (ADLs) Self-care activities people perform daily to remain independent and to function in society. *p. 4*

advocate To speak or act on behalf of another person or group of people. *p. 3*

caring Concern for clients' and their families' dignity, independence, preferences, privacy, and safety at all times. True *caring* requires honesty, sensitivity, comforting, discretion, and respect while showing this concern. *p. 16*

client A general term for any person receiving care or support services in a community setting: hospital patients, facility residents, and clients in the community. *p. 9*

compassionate care Care that demonstrates concern for the dignity, independence, preferences, privacy, and safety (DIPPS) of clients and their families at all times. Also known as *person-centred care*. *p. 16*

confidentiality Respecting, guarding, and using discretion in regard to personal and private information about another person. *p. 14*

critical thinking The ability to think clearly and logically, using reflection and reason, based on knowledge obtained from experience, observation, or education. *p. 11*

dignity The state of feeling worthy, valued, and respected. *p. 16*

DIPPS An acronym for the five principles of compassionate care (also known as *person-centred care*): *dignity*, *independence*, *preferences*, *privacy*, and *safety*. *p. 16*

discretion The use of responsible judgement to avoid causing distress or embarrassment to a person. *p. 14*

empathy The ability to recognize, perceive, and have an understanding of another person's emotions by seeing things from his or her viewpoint. *p. 3*

instrumental activities of daily living (IADLs) The complex skills needed to successfully live independently. *p. 4*

licensed practical nurse (LPN) A health care provider licensed and regulated by the province or territory to carry out nursing techniques and provide client care. Known as a **registered practical nurse (RPN)** in Ontario. *p. 13*

patient A person receiving care in a hospital setting. Also known as a *client*. *p. 9*

primary care nurse A primary care nurse is responsible for the ongoing management of the health of a client. Duties include liaising with other health care team members, the client, and her or his family. *p. 13*

professionalism An approach to work that demonstrates respect for others, commitment, competence, and appropriate behaviour. *p. 14*

reflective practice review A review and self-evaluation of care provided with the goal of identifying ways to improve clinical performance and caregiving. *p. 11* Feelings, strengths, and weaknesses

registered nurse (RN) A health care provider who is licensed and regulated by the province or territory to maintain overall responsibility for the planning and provision of client care. *p. 11*

registered practical nurse (RPN) See **licensed practical nurse**. *p. 13*

registered psychiatric nurse (RPN) A nurse who is educated and registered in his or her own province to provide care specifically to individuals whose primary needs relate to mental, emotional, and developmental health. *p. 13*

rehabilitation The process of restoring a person to the highest possible level of functioning through the use of therapy, exercise, or other methods. *p. 10*

resident A person living in a **residential facility** (often called a *long-term care facility*). *p. 9*

residential facility A facility that provides living accommodations and services; includes assisted-living facilities, long-term care facilities, group homes, and retirement residences. *p. 9*

scope of practice The legal limits and extent of a health care worker's role. Scope of practice in a health care field varies from province to province and employer to employer. *p. 11*

social reintegration See **social support**. *p. 4*

social support Equipping a person with the skills and knowledge necessary to successfully live independently outside an institution. Also known as **social reintegration**. *p. 4*

support worker A health care worker who provides services to people, both in facilities and in the community, who need help with their daily activities. *p. 3*

unregulated care providers (UCPs) A broad term applied to staff members who assist nurses and other health care providers in giving care. *p. 11*

Support workers provide care and assistance to clients of any age who have defined health care needs and who require help with their daily activities whether they live in a facility or in the community.[1] The ultimate goal of support work is to improve the quality of life of the client and family by offering support in a safe, kind, sensitive, caring, and understanding manner. Support workers can make a difference in people's lives by alleviating loneliness, providing **empathy**, ensuring comfort, encouraging independence, and promoting the client's self-respect (**FIGURE 1–1**). They support the client and family in a holistic manner by addressing the client's physical, psychological, social, cognitive, cultural, and spiritual needs and **advocate** for the client by speaking or acting on her behalf.

Support workers may work as part of a health care team or work individually with a client. Legislation, employer policies, and a client's condition all influence how support workers function and how much supervision they need. They may collaborate with health care providers or with professionals outside of the health care sector, depending on the needs of their clients. Support workers must use discretion at all times and honour the client's right to confidentiality whenever discussing the client's case with co-workers. Support workers are expected to adapt their work style to the setting and to the needs and wishes of the client receiving care.

UPPORT WORK ACROSS CANADA

he nature of support work varies across the country. ıere are differences in educational programs, work tings, job responsibilities, and terms used to scribe support workers. Some sections of this text y not apply to support work in your particular , province, or territory. If you are unsure about ch parts apply to your area, ask your instructor mployer.

he term **support worker** refers to the worker provides personal care and support services. ever, *assisted-living worker, personal support r, personal attendant, patient care assistant, resi- are aide, resident care attendant, health care aide, care attendant, home support worker, nursing ursing attendant, community health worker, or uing care assistant*—among other titles—may be used in your province or territory to describe similar (but not always equivalent) jobs. The Appendix at the end of this book lists the support worker's titles in each province and territory. Because of the wide variety of titles, the general public may not be aware of what support workers are called in their own province or territory or even within a facility they use. It is the role of support workers, their employing agencies, other health care providers, and their province's or territory's Ministry of Health to inform others of their role and how it fits in their current health care structure.

This list may also include several titles that are not equivalent to one another. For example, in Ontario, developmental service workers (DSWs) play a different role and follow different educational standards than personal support workers (PSWs), and yet both are considered to be *support workers* within the health care team. In some parts of Canada, the term *personal attendant* refers to a worker who is supervised directly by the person for whom he or she provides support services; personal attendants support people with physical disabilities. Educational programs to become a personal attendant are generally shorter than ones for support workers.

Support workers work in a variety of settings (see Chapter 3 for definitions and details of workplace settings). In all settings, support workers ensure the safety of their clients, including those who have cognitive or mental health challenges. Services provided

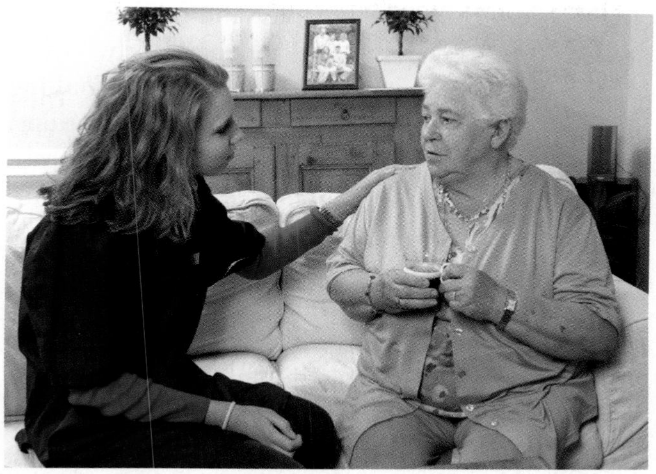

FIGURE 1–1 A support worker comforts a client. (**Source:** Catchlight Visual Services / Alamy Stock Photo)

by support workers to clients in their homes can enable some clients to live independently or with their families. Support workers may also assist clients with **social support**, or **social reintegration**, as they prepare to move into an assisted-living facility or group home. In long-term care facilities, support workers assist clients with complex health challenges. Support workers also provide comfort and end-of-life care to dying clients so that they can die with dignity.

Support Worker Responsibilities

A support worker's general responsibilities, depending on the jurisdiction he or she works in, can be grouped into five categories: (1) personal care, (2) support for nurses and other health care providers, (3) family support, (4) social support, and (5) housekeeping or home management.

Personal Care

Personal care responsibilities include assisting with **activities of daily living (ADLs)**. These are the self-care actions that people perform every day to remain independent and to function effectively in society. Support workers help with daily activities such as eating, bathing, grooming, dressing, and toileting ("elimination"). They assist clients with limited mobility to change positions or move from one place to another and also help promote the client's safety and physical comfort.

In community settings, support workers also assist clients with **instrumental activities of daily living (IADLs)**, which are the complex and necessary skills needed to successfully live independently. These IADLs may include assisting the client with handling finances, assisting with management of medications, arranging transportation, shopping, preparing meals, assisting with using a telephone or other communication devices, and doing housework and basic home maintenance.[2]

The support worker is not responsible for deciding what should or should not be done for the client. However, while providing personal care, the support worker observes for and reports any changes in the client's behaviour or health. Such information is important to share with the health care team.

Support for Nurses and Other Health Care Providers

Support workers assist nurses or other health care team members by following the established care plan for each client; for instance, they may be required to clean equipment, measure and report vital signs, or assist with simple wound care. Support workers might also assist with oxygen therapy, heat or cold applications, and range-of-motion (ROM) exercises. They are often the supervisor's "eyes and ears," meaning that because they are the person who spends the most time with the client, they are most likely to observe or hear things that should be reported to the supervisor, who may be a nurse or another type of health care worker. Observing and reporting are very important parts of the support worker's role and can have a great impact on a client's care.

Support workers may have to consult with other health care providers, such as social workers or physiotherapists, and may also have to consult with other professionals, such as the client's employers, clergy, or teachers, depending on the client's individual care plan.

Family Support

In many facilities, support workers assist with admissions and discharges by introducing the client and family to the facility and helping the client unpack and settle in. In private homes, support workers help families care for loved ones who have health issues or need assistance with ADLs. Some families may need help with preparing meals and doing household chores; other families may need help with child care. Support worker services often give family caregivers a break from their duties.

Social Support

Support workers may help clients participate in social activities. These activities provide the client with enjoyment, recreation, and a chance to meet with friends. They may organize games and outings or may be hired privately to be a client's companion. Support workers may also be responsible for teaching clients to learn to live independently and to cook, clean, or shop by themselves.

Housekeeping or Home Management

Support workers often do a variety of housekeeping tasks in a facility setting, including making beds, delivering meals, tidying up living areas, and maintaining supplies. In a private home, housekeeping is called *home management.* Services depend on the needs of the person and the resources available to provide these services. Duties may include assisting clients with their IADLs, doing light housekeeping, doing laundry, and preparing and serving nutritious meals.

The *A Day in the Life* boxes on pages 5–9 describe three support workers' typical workdays—in the community, in a long-term care facility, and in a hospital setting. In each box, the word *nurse* may mean registered nurse (RN), registered practical nurse (RPN), or licensed practical nurse (LPN), depending on the staffing policies of that particular agency.

A Day in the Life of a Support Worker

In the Community (Home Care)

Each evening, Stephen receives his assignment for the next day from his supervisor. He uses the details in the assignment to plan his day. He consults a city map and plans his route. The people he is assigned to visit have a range of physical, emotional, and social issues and disabilities. Their major issues are briefly described below.

Ms. Lau, 32, has cerebral palsy. She uses a wheelchair. She lives alone. Two days per week, she works outside the home. She receives home care to help her prepare for work.

Mr. O'Connor, 59, is recovering at home from a stroke. He is paralyzed on one side of his body and has a speech–language disorder. His wife is his rimary caregiver. Mr. O'Connor receives home are three mornings a week. Mrs. O'Connor, 51, is work during Stephen's visit.

Mr. Horowitz, 71, has dementia. His wife, 67, is ing for him at home. The couple gets emotional l social support from family and friends. Mrs. rowitz looks after her husband's personal care ls. They receive 2 hours of home care per week ve Mrs. Horowitz a break.

s. Adams, 25, is a single mother on social ance. She is recovering from a Caesarean n. She gets very little social and emotional rt. She has newborn twins and three young n aged 1, 3, and 4 years.

w are the tasks and activities that Stephen ns on a typical day at work.

0830 hours (7:15 a.m. to 8:30 a.m.)

ls to first appointment; arrives at 0730

- Assists Ms. Lau with showering, grooming, and dressing
- Helps Ms. Lau to prepare breakfast, clean up kitchen, and make bed
- Records care provided, including any relevant observations

0830 to 1000 hours (8:30 a.m. to 10:00 a.m.)

- Travels to next appointment; arrives at 0900 hours
- Assists Mr. O'Connor with elimination, bathing, shaving, hair care, and mouth care
- Prepares breakfast for Mr. O'Connor and assists him with eating
- Cleans up kitchen and makes bed
- Takes Mr. O'Connor for a brief walk; he is learning to walk with a cane
- Assists Mr. O'Connor with elimination again
- Records care provided, including any relevant observations

1000 to 1215 hours (10:00 a.m. to 12:15 p.m.)

- Travels to next appointment; arrives at 1015 hours
- Listens to Mrs. Horowitz, who is crying and says she is "worn out"; telephones supervisor, who, in turn, calls the Horowitzes' case manager; case manager schedules a visit
- Assists Mr. Horowitz with elimination, bathing, shaving, hair care, and mouth care
- Cleans kitchen and does light housework in main living areas
- Prepares lunch for Mr. Horowitz and assists him with eating
- Records care provided, including any relevant observations

Continued

A Day in the Life of a Support Worker—cont'd

1215 to 1530 hours (12:15 p.m. to 3:30 p.m.)

- Takes break for lunch
- Travels to next appointment; arrives at 1330 hours, the same time as the public health nurse
- Helps children wash faces and hands
- Prepares lunch for Ms. Adams and the three older children, while the nurse assists Ms. Adams with breastfeeding the infants; feeds 1-year-old
- Helps children with oral hygiene after lunch
- Prepares three dinners; leaves one in the refrigerator and the others in the freezer
- Records care provided, including any relevant observations
- Reports observations from the day to nurse supervisor (would report unusual findings immediately throughout the day to supervisor)
- Drives home

A Day in the Life of a Support Worker

In a Long-Term Care Facility

Claire works on a unit in which the residents, mostly older adults, require help with ADLs. The eight residents assigned to her have a range of physical, emotional, and social issues and disabilities.

Miss McDonald, 94, is partially disabled due to rheumatoid arthritis.

Mr. Schmidt, 82, is recovering from surgery. He has urinary incontinence, which causes him anxiety.

Mrs. Lawson, 88, has a heart condition and osteoarthritis.

Mr. Delgado, 63, is paralyzed on one side due to a stroke. He is unable to speak but is able to understand both written and spoken language.

Mr. Taylor, 71, is in the early stages of Parkinson's disease. He has diabetes and poor vision as well.

Mrs. Sanchez, 81, is partially disabled due to multiple leg and hip fractures. She has osteoporosis. She is also depressed.

Mr. Bouchard, 89, is recovering from pneumonia. He has age-related hearing loss.

Mrs. Khan, 44, is severely disabled due to multiple sclerosis. She has urinary and fecal incontinence.

Below are the tasks and activities that Claire performs on a typical day at work.

0700 to 0715 hours (7:00 a.m. to 7:15 a.m.)

- Receives report from nurse on the conditions of all residents on the unit
- Receives assignment of care requirements, appointments, and activities scheduled for residents
- Plans morning's tasks and activities

0715 to 0845 hours (7:15 a.m. to 8:45 a.m.)

- Helps seven of the residents get out of bed
- Provides partial hygiene care to six residents, a shower for one resident, and a tub bath for another
- Assists with elimination and changes their incontinence briefs
- Assists residents with dressing and accompanies them to the dining room
- Returns to the unit; provides partial hygiene to Mrs. Khan
- Observes that the cut on Mrs. Khan's arm looks red and swollen and feels warm to the touch; makes a written record of it and gives a verbal report to the nurse
- With help from another support worker, moves Mrs. Khan from her bed to a wheelchair
- Transports Mrs. Khan to the dining room for breakfast

Continu

A Day in the Life of a Support Worker—cont'd

- Records care provided, including any relevant observations

0845 to 0930 hours (8:45 a.m. to 9:30 a.m.)

- Assists residents with breakfast, ensuring that all have a nutritious breakfast and that special diets are followed
- Encourages Mr. Taylor, Mrs. Lawson, and Miss McDonald to eat
- Assists Mrs. Khan with eating; transports Mrs. Khan back to her unit
- Returns to dining room and accompanies other residents back to their units
- Records each resident's dietary intake in dietary intake record

0930 to 1130 hours (9:30 a.m. to 11:30 a.m.)

- Reports to nurse that Mr. Taylor (who has diabetes) did not eat
- With assistance, lifts Mrs. Khan and settles her in bed
- Assists residents with mouth care and elimination; changes their incontinence briefs
- Reports on the conditions of residents to replacement support worker; takes a 15-minute break
- Completes hygiene and grooming care for residents who received only partial care before breakfast
- At 1030 hours, accompanies residents to games room
- Makes beds and changes linens
- Repositions Mrs. Khan in bed to prevent pressure ulcers
- Tidies rooms and living areas
- At 1130 hours, accompanies residents back to their units from games room
- Records care provided, including any relevant observations

1130 to 1300 hours (11:30 a.m. to 1:00 p.m.)

- Reports on the conditions of residents to replacement support worker; takes a 30-minute break for lunch
- Checks care requirements for each resident and plans the afternoon's tasks and activities
- Accompanies residents to the dining room
- Supervises residents and assists with feeding, as required
- Accompanies residents back to their units
- Assists residents with elimination and changes their incontinence briefs
- Assists with mouth care
- Makes sure that residents rest after lunch, as directed
- Records care provided, including any relevant observations
- Records each resident's dietary intake in dietary intake record

1300 to 1500 hours (1:00 p.m. to 3:00 p.m.)

- Assists residents with elimination and changes their incontinence briefs
- Greets new resident, Mrs. Griffiths, and her family; introduces them to the facility; assists Mrs. Griffiths with unpacking
- Introduces Mrs. Griffiths to other residents
- Repositions Mrs. Khan
- Comforts Mrs. Griffiths, who is feeling upset and lonely
- Takes Mrs. Sanchez and Mrs. Griffiths for a walk
- Assists residents with elimination and changes their incontinence briefs
- Records care provided, including any relevant observations
- Provides a verbal report to the nurse concerning each client's care

A Day in the Life of a Support Worker

In a Hospital

Gina works on a surgical unit, which is one type of acute care. Most clients on this unit have had surgery for fractures (broken bones). Others have had hip- or knee-replacement surgery. A few are waiting for their surgery. Many of these clients have additional health issues. Gina assists with the care of 10 clients.

Miss Kwan, 66, has a thigh bone (*femur*) fracture.

Mr. McDuff, 76, has a spine fracture and osteoporosis.

Mrs. Sadiq, 46, has shoulder and rib fractures, as well as osteoporosis and quadriplegia.

Mrs. Clark, 85, has a hip fracture. She has osteoporosis and Alzheimer's disease.

Mr. Keene, 44, has thigh bone and knee fractures.

Mr. Cross, 55, had a knee replacement. He has arthritis.

Mrs. Pocza, 82, has a hip fracture and osteoporosis.

Ms. Hill, 35, has multiple fractures; affected are her spine, thigh bone, and ankle.

Mrs. Leblanc, 74, had a hip replacement. She also has diabetes.

Mr. Paes, 82, has a hip fracture. He also has hearing loss.

Below are the tasks and activities that Gina performs on a typical day at work.

0700 to 0710 hours (7:00 a.m. to 7:10 a.m.)
- Receives assignment on care requirements
- Plans morning's tasks and activities

0710 to 0800 hours (7:10 a.m. to 8:00 a.m.)
- Provides hygiene care to four clients, including assisting with oral hygiene and hair care and providing partial bed baths
- Assists with elimination
- Records care provided, including any relevant observations

0800 to 0845 hours (8:00 a.m. to 8:45 a.m.)
- Accompanies dietary staff as they deliver breakfast trays
- Positions and arranges trays for clients; assists clients with eating
- Listens to Mrs. Pocza's concerns about her surgery; calls for the nurse, who answers Mrs. Pocza's questions
- Records clients' food and fluid intakes
- Assists clients with elimination
- Records care provided, including any relevant observations

0845 to 1130 hours (8:45 a.m. to 11:30 a.m.)
- Assists clients with hygiene, elimination, showers, and baths, as required
- Reports on the conditions of clients and care requirements to replacement support worker; takes a 15-minute break
- Makes and changes beds
- Assists with two discharges; helps clients pack
- Helps nurse to reposition clients, as required
- Assists clients with leg exercises and coughing and deep-breathing exercises
- Records care provided, including any relevant observations

1130 to 1300 hours (11:30 a.m. to 1:00 p.m.)
- Reports on the conditions of clients and care requirements to replacement support worker; takes a 30-minute break for lunch
- Checks the condition and care requirements of each client and plans afternoon tasks
- Accompanies dietary staff as they deliver lunch trays
- Positions and arranges trays for clients; assists clients with eating
- Observes that Mr. McDuff's intravenous (IV) fluid is running low; notifies nurse immediately
- Records food and fluid intakes
- Assists clients with elimination and mouth care
- Records care provided, including any relevant observations

Continued

A Day in the Life of a Support Worker—cont'd

1300 to 1500 hours (1:00 p.m. to 3:00 p.m.)

- Removes Mr. Paes's dentures before his medications are given
- Assists clients with elimination
- Observes drainage under Miss Kwan's cast; notifies nurse immediately
- Answers call from nurse; provides comfort to Mrs. Clark, who is upset
- Assists clients with leg exercises and coughing and deep-breathing exercises
- Assists with admitting two clients
- Helps nurse reposition clients, as required
- Records care provided, including any relevant observations
- Provides a verbal report to the nurse who is responsible for each of these clients

(*Note:* In many hospitals, a client is assigned to a primary care nurse. A support worker might be assigned to help care for the clients of several nurses so would have to report observations about the clients he or she works with to each client's primary care nurse.)

People Who Receive Support Services

People receiving health care and support services are known by different terms, depending on the setting. A person receiving care in a hospital is usually called a **patient**. A person living in a **residential facility** is called a **resident**. A person receiving care or support services in the community is called a **client**. *Client* is also an all-encompassing term for people receiving health care or support services: hospital patients, facility residents, and clients in the community.

Whether the individual receiving care is known as a *client*, *patient*, or *resident*, always remember that he or she is a *person*. Every person is unique, with unique fe experiences and situations, desires and opinions. ach will have different needs and different abilities. pport workers work with people from a variety of tures or backgrounds (see Chapter 10). Part of the port worker's job is to accept this diversity among ple. The *Respecting Diversity* boxes that appear ughout this text outline the importance of divers- nd how people's backgrounds influence who they nd what they do.

ents can be grouped according to their issues, and ages:

- ***r adults.*** Aging is a normal process and is not ness or disease. Many older adults enjoy good . However, body changes normally occur the aging process. Social and emotional es may also occur (see Chapter 21). The risks for contracting serious illnesses and becoming disabled increase with age. Most older adults remain at home as long as possible. Others are unable to manage even with assistance and move into a residential facility. Throughout the text, issues relevant to older adults are discussed.
- ***People with disabilities.*** Some people have disabilities due to illness, injury, or conditions present at birth. Disabilities may affect physical functioning, mental functioning, or both. Many adults with disabilities live in their own homes. Many work outside their homes. Support workers might help clients who have disabilities with their ADLs or might be responsible for teaching them how to perform the ADLs independently.
- ***People with medical issues.*** Medical issues include illnesses, diseases, and injuries. These may include short-term (such as a broken bone), long-term (such as diabetes or multiple sclerosis), or progressive and life-threatening (such as some types of cancer) issues.
- ***People having surgery.*** Surgical clients are those being prepared for surgery or who have recently had surgery. Preoperative care includes preparing the client for what to expect after surgery and addressing the client's fears and anxieties. Needs after surgery relate to relieving pain and discomfort, preventing complications, and helping the client adjust to body changes. People recover from surgeries in hospitals or in their homes.

- ***People with mental health issues.*** Mental health issues range from mild to severe. Some people function normally but need help making decisions or coping with life stresses. Others are severely affected and need assistance with ADLs.
- ***People needing rehabilitation.*** **Rehabilitation** is the process of restoring a person to the highest possible level of functioning through the use of therapy, exercise, or other methods. The person may need to regain functions lost due to surgery, illness, or accident. Some hospitals have special rehabilitation units. Many people receiving support at home and in long-term care settings require rehabilitation.
- ***Children.*** When hospital care is needed, children are admitted to the pediatric unit. In some areas of Canada, support workers are hired to work in pediatric units (**FIGURE 1–2**). However, most support work for children occurs in community settings and long-term care facilities. Some children who receive care have physical or intellectual disabilities. Others need care because a parent has a medical challenge or has just had a new baby. The *Focus on Children* boxes and Chapter 20 discuss issues related to caring for children.
- ***Mothers and newborns.*** Complications and difficulties can occur at any time during pregnancy and even up to 6 to 8 weeks following childbirth. Some new mothers need assistance with their own care or with their newborn's care. Most support work with mothers and newborns takes place in the home (see Chapter 19).
- ***People requiring special care.*** Some people who have serious and complex medical conditions need special care and equipment. Hospitals have special care units, including intensive care units, coronary care units, kidney dialysis units, burn units, and emergency departments. In some areas of Canada, support workers are hired to work in these units. Support workers might transport people from one unit to another; take specimens to the lab; assist clients with bathing, feeding, mobility, or toileting; and assist other health care providers with special procedures. In some parts of Canada, support workers are not allowed to provide personal care to clients in unstable or critical conditions.

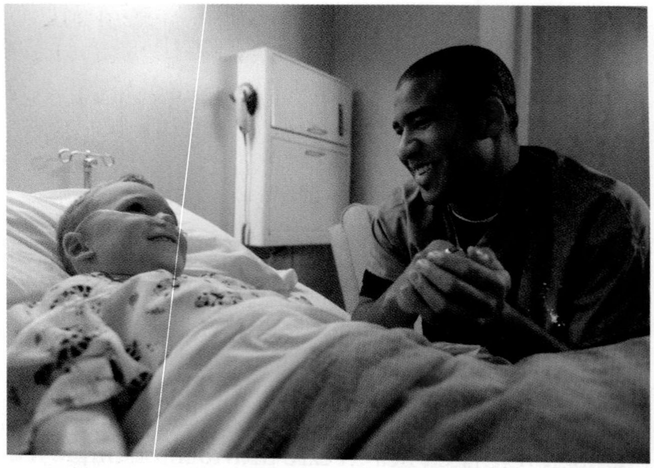

FIGURE 1–2 A support worker provides care to a sick child. (**Source:** RubberBall / Alamy Stock Photo)

THE HEALTH CARE TEAM

A *team* is a group of people working together toward a common goal. Health care teams include professionals with a variety of skills and knowledge who work together to meet the client's needs. Their goal is to provide quality care. Many professionals, including support workers, are involved in the care of one client. Which professionals are involved depends on the needs of the client (**FIGURE 1–3**).

Regulated and Unregulated Workers

Health care professions are either regulated or unregulated. A regulated profession is self-governing. It has a professional organization called a *college*,

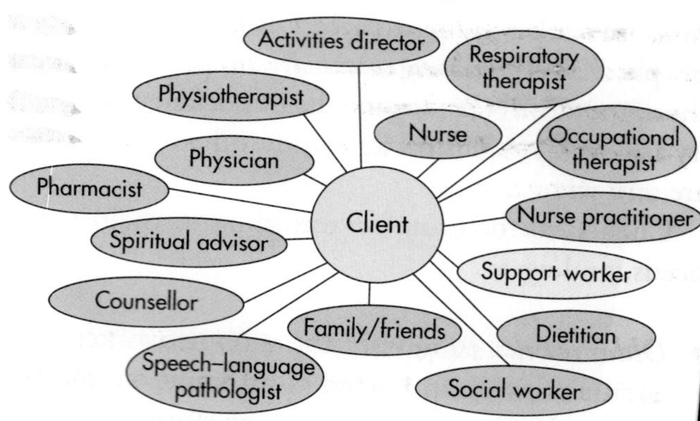

FIGURE 1–3 The support worker is an important member o the health care team. The client is always the focus of th health care team's efforts.

which sets education and licence requirements. It also establishes the scope of practice, code of ethics, and standards of conduct for its members. In the case of a complaint about a member's conduct, the college investigates and, if necessary, disciplines members guilty of misconduct. Each regulated health care profession has legislation that details the roles and responsibilities of its members. Nursing is one of many regulated health care professions.

Unregulated care providers (UCPs) are health care providers who perform clearly identified services under the direction and supervision of a client, family member, regulated health care provider, or employer. However, UCPs are not regulated through legislation and are not members of an organization or professional college that governs their role. While UCPs do not currently follow any official code of ethics, they must adhere to the codes of behaviour dictated by their employers (see Chapter 8, Box 8-1, for *A Sample Code of Ethics for Support Workers*, on pages 119–120). At this point, support workers in most provinces and territories are considered to be UCPs.

TABLE 1–1 describes the titles and positions of the common health care team members. It also specifies whether they are regulated or unregulated workers.

Scope of Practice

Support workers must understand what to do, what not to do, and the legal limits of the support worker role in order to protect clients from harm—in other words, they must understand their **scope of practice**.

Never act beyond the legal limits of your role. Also, never perform a function or task that you have not been trained to do. If you perform a task that is outside these limits, you could harm a client and create serious legal problems for yourself and your employer.

Three sources of information about scope of practice are as follows:

1. ***Educational program***. The support worker educational program includes information on the scope of practice for support work in that province or territory. Many provinces now follow either the national or provincial program standards, which dictate what support workers should be taught in their educational programs. Students will learn about the laws and the support worker's professional responsibilities in their part of the country and, if necessary, should ask their instructors if they require any clarification.
2. ***Employer's policies***. Every employer has written policies that establish what can and cannot be done. These policies should be read carefully before starting work.
3. ***Supervisor.*** On the job, the supervisor is the best source of information. It is far better to ask for direction than risk harming a client, so never hesitate to ask questions or request clarification about any procedure.

Professional Development and Lifelong Learning

Being a professional requires critical thinking and reflective practice review. **Critical thinking** is the ability to think clearly and logically, using reflection and reason, based on knowledge obtained from experience, observation, or education. A **reflective practice review** is a self-evaluation of care provided with the goal of identifying ways to improve clinical performance and caregiving.

Health care is an ever-changing field. It is the responsibility of every professional in the field to ensure that all clinical skills and knowledge are up to date since their own health and safety and the health and safety of co-workers and clients are at stake. Depending on the region, many postgraduate certificate courses and workshops may be available to support workers, such as dealing with conflict, providing palliative care, or assisting with medications. Support workers also need to be aware of the scope of practice in their province or territory since some, in particular situations, have been asked to perform tasks that are not within the support worker's scope.

The Supervision of Support Workers

In facilities, in the community, or in private homes, support workers may be supervised by a nurse or other health care provider. A **registered nurse (RN)** is licensed and regulated by the province or territory to maintain overall responsibility for the planning and provision of client care. Some RNs have

TABLE 1–1 Support and Health Care Team Members

Title	Description	Regulated/Unregulated
Aboriginal support worker	Assists First Nations, Métis, and Inuit clients; provides education on diabetes prevention and management; provides guidance on self-care management; facilitates discharges from and admissions to health care facilities; organizes services	Unregulated
Activities director	Assesses, plans, and implements recreational activities based on clients' needs	Unregulated; provincial or territorial educational requirements vary
Dietitian	Assesses and plans for nutritional needs; teaches clients about nutrition, food selection, and preparation	Regulated
Nurse practitioner	Diagnoses; treats clients with simple injuries and illnesses; is a registered nurse with advanced education and additional responsibilities for management of client care	Regulated
Occupational therapist	Focuses on rehabilitation; teaches clients skills needed to perform ADLs; designs adaptive equipment for ADLs	Regulated
Pharmacist	Fills medication orders written by physicians; monitors and evaluates drug interactions; consults with physicians and nurses about drug actions and interactions	Regulated
Physician	Diagnoses and treats clients with illnesses and injuries	Regulated
Physiotherapist (Physical therapist)	Focuses on rehabilitation; assists clients with musculo-skeletal impairments; focuses on restoring function and preventing disability from illness or injury	Regulated
Recreational therapist	Focuses on improving the quality of the client's life through leisure and recreation-related activities such as arts and crafts, drama, music, dance, sports, games, and field trips	Unregulated
Registered nurse (RN)	Assesses; makes nursing diagnoses; plans, implements, and evaluates nursing care; tends to clients who have unstable health conditions; provides direct client care; administers medications; supervises support workers	Regulated

Continued

TABLE 1–1 Support and Health Care Team Members—cont'd

Title	Description	Regulated/Unregulated
Registered practical nurse/Licensed practical nurse (RPN/LPN)	Assesses; makes nursing diagnoses; plans, implements, and evaluates nursing care; tends to clients who have stable health conditions; provides direct client care; administers medications; supervises support workers	Regulated
Registered psychiatric nurse (RPN)	Provides care to individuals whose primary needs relate to mental, emotional, and developmental health; works independently or in cooperation with other health care providers (e.g., psychiatrists, physicians, psychologists, social workers, recreational therapists, and occupational therapists) to develop or implement therapeutic programs	Regulated
Respiratory therapist	Focuses on rehabilitation; assists in treatment of lung and heart disorders; gives respiratory treatments and therapies	Regulated
Social worker	Helps clients and families deal with social and emotional issues related to illness and recovery	Varies according to province or territory
Speech–language pathologist (therapist)	Focuses on rehabilitation; evaluates speech and language; and treats people with speech, voice, hearing, communication, and swallowing disorders	Regulated
Spiritual advisor	Assists clients and families with spiritual needs	Determined by religious order
Support worker	Assists clients with personal care, family responsibilities, social and recreational activities, and housekeeping or home management; provides personal care and assistance with ADLs	Unregulated

university degrees and even postgraduate education. Others have community college diplomas. RNs assess clients, make nursing diagnoses, develop care plans, and implement and evaluate nursing care. They also carry out physicians' orders. An RN is usually a team leader of the health care team, which includes RPNs or LPNs (see below), support workers, and other allied health care providers.

A **licensed practical nurse (LPN)**, also known as a **registered practical nurse (RPN)**, is licensed and regulated by the province or territory to carry out basic nursing procedures and provide client care. RPNs and LPNs have a community college diploma, and, like RNs, they must hold a current nursing registration in the province that they practise in. RPNs or LPNs function in a decision-making position when caring for stable clients with uncomplicated health issues, but when providing care to clients with serious and unstable health issues, they assist RNs and help with complex procedures. RPNs and LPNs often supervise support workers.

Some clients, particularly in a residential environment, may be assigned to a **primary care nurse**, who is responsible for the ongoing management of the health of a client. Duties of this nurse include liaising with other health care team members, the client, and her or his family. In an acute-care environment, the primary care nurse may or may not be directly involved in providing the client care on a daily basis but will oversee the work of those who do, including the support worker.

In some situations, a support worker may be supervised by a professional other than an RN, RPN, or LPN. For example, in the recreation department of a long-term care facility, support workers may report to a recreational therapist. In the community, a supervisor may be a social worker, a physiotherapist, or another health care provider.

Some support workers are hired and supervised directly by clients. These support workers must be particularly aware of provincial or territorial legislation that limits the tasks and procedures they can perform.

BEING A PROFESSIONAL

Professionalism is an approach to work that demonstrates respect for others, commitment, competence, and appropriate behaviour. Being cheerful and friendly, keeping work schedules, performing tasks competently, and being helpful are all part of a professional approach. To be a true professional, you must demonstrate the following:

- ***Positive attitude.*** You need to show a good attitude about your job. The work you do is very important. People rely on you to give efficient care and support. You need to believe that you and your work are valuable and show that you enjoy your work. Be enthusiastic, considerate, courteous, honest, and cooperative. Speak in a professional manner, and avoid the use of slang terms or profane language. Always think before you speak, do not gossip, and do not complain. Your words reveal your attitude. BOX 1–1 lists some statements to avoid so as not to show a negative attitude.
- ***Sense of responsibility.*** Never blame others for your problems or mistakes at work. Admit your errors, accept constructive criticism, and learn from others. Always report to work when scheduled and on time. Everyone on the team, including the client, is affected when even one person is late. Have a plan ready for times when you are urgently needed at home or your transportation is unavailable. Inform your supervisor immediately if you will be late or unable to work. Also, be sure to finish assigned tasks before you leave for the day. The client's care cannot be neglected for any reason. In the case that you cannot finish your assignment, promptly explain why to your supervisor.
- ***Professional appearance.*** A professional, appropriate appearance shows respect for the people in your care, your co-workers, and yourself. It indicates that you take your job seriously. Your appearance includes your clothes, grooming, and hygiene (BOX 1–2 and FIGURE 1–4).
- ***Discretion about client information.*** **Discretion** means showing good judgement about what you say, how you say it, when you say it, and where you say it. You need to judge when information should be kept private and when it should be shared. Information about a client is confidential. **Confidentiality** means respecting and guarding personal and private information about another person. Information should be shared only among the health care team members involved in the client's care. Information about your employer, your co-workers, and other clients is also private. For example, you must never talk with a client about another client, even if you avoid using names. Also, avoid talking about clients, co-workers, and your employer where you can be overheard; if you need to discuss a client's care with team members, make sure that other clients, families, and visitors cannot hear you. People overhearing may think you are talking about them or

BOX 1–1 Statements That Show a Negative Attitude

- "I can't. I'm too busy. Can't somebody else help?"
- "I didn't do it."
- "It's not my fault."
- "Don't blame me."
- "It's not my turn. I did it yesterday."
- "Nobody told me."
- "I work harder than anyone else."
- "No one appreciates what I do."

BOX 1–2 Practices for a Professional Appearance

- Follow your employer's dress code policies.
- Wear a clean, well-fitting, modest, and wrinkle-free uniform.
- Wear a name badge or photo ID, per your employer's policy.
- Wear clean stockings or socks that are in good repair.
- Wear comfortable and clean shoes that give you good support. Shoes should provide a safe barrier for your feet from spills and body fluids.
- Ensure that your underclothing cannot be seen through your uniform.
- Keep your hair away from your face and up off your collar.
- Use makeup sparingly. Avoid chewing gum.
- Be aware that cigarette smoke and cooking odours can be absorbed into your uniform. These odours can be unpleasant to many clients.
- Do not wear perfume, cologne, or aftershave. Strong scents may cause nausea or breathing problems in some clients.
- Keep fingernails clean, short, and neatly shaped. Long nails can scratch the client. Artificial nails present an infection risk to clients, so they are ot appropriate for support workers in any tting.
- o not wear jewellery (even if parts of your dy are pierced). Jewellery may scratch or ise injury to your client and yourself and may e infection-control risks. It may offend some nts as well.
- ending on your agency's policies, you may ked to cover tattoos that may offend some ts.

mily members. This assumption can lead iformation and confusion, which can be ıg to those affected.

learning. Equipment and techniques for clients can become outdated, and it is ısibility of *all* caregivers to keep current information that affects the care they eep your knowledge up to date, attend workshops and in-services that are offered by your employer, get clarifications from your supervisor, and read up about new equipment or practices that you are uncertain about.

- ***Advocating for the client.*** Support workers will often make important observations about the client or family, and these observations must be communicated to the health care team. Sharing this information is especially important if a client is unable to speak for him- or herself. It is also the responsibility of professionals to avoid taking shortcuts in their care, as doing so may seriously harm the client. Shortcuts include taking longer breaks, skipping tasks listed on the client's care plan, or failing to apply theory on hygiene learned in school to client practice.
- ***Discretion about personal matters.*** Discretion in support work includes keeping personal matters out of the workplace. Your role is to focus on your clients and the task at hand. Do not discuss with clients your family matters and personal problems or the problems of others (BOX 1–3). ***No matter***

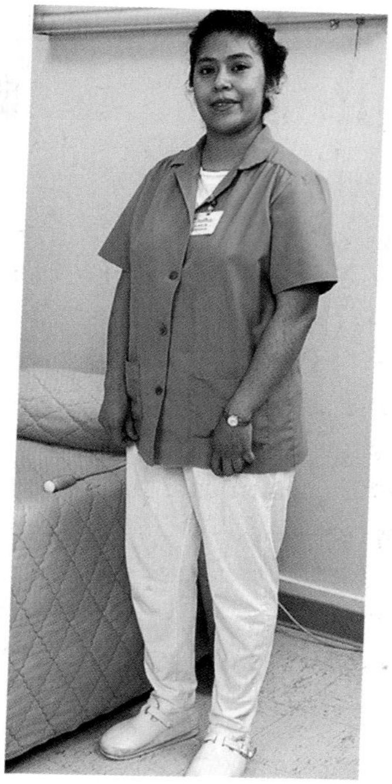

FIGURE 1–4 This support worker is well groomed. Her uniform and shoes are clean. Her hair is worn in a simple style and is kept out of her face and off her collar. She is not wearing any jewellery, except a watch. Her name tag is easily visible and approved by her employer. (**Source:** Sorrentino, S.A. (2000). *Mosby's textbook for nursing assistants* (5th ed., p. 37). St. Louis, MO: Mosby.)

BOX 1–3 Keeping Personal Matters out of the Workplace

- Make personal calls only during scheduled breaks. Use a client's phone *only* for urgent matters. Always ask for permission before using a client's phone.
- Do not discuss your personal problems at work.
- Do not let your family and friends visit you at work.
- Arrange your personal appointments outside of your scheduled work hours.
- Do not use your employer's supplies or equipment for personal matters.
- Do not try to raise funds at work, even if the funds are for a good cause.

how well you think you know a client, remember that your relationship must remain professional. It would be inappropriate to discuss your personal problems with your client.

- ***Using acceptable speech and language.*** The way you speak at home and in casual social settings may not be appropriate for a work setting. Even if you are speaking with a co-worker, others could hear you and be offended by what you say or how you say it. Your speech and language must remain professional while you are on the job. To avoid offending clients or co-workers, never use foul, vulgar, or abusive language. Also, avoid using slang. Speak gently and clearly; never yell or shout. And never fight or argue with clients, their family members, or your co-workers.

THE GOAL OF SUPPORT WORK: COMPASSIONATE CARE

Compassionate care (also known as *person-centred care*) or **caring** means having concern for the dignity, independence, preferences, privacy, and safety of clients and their families at all times. The goal of support work is to demonstrate true compassionate care by following this principle and treating clients with kindness, honesty, sensitivity, comfort, discretion, respect, and understanding. Many people who require support are coping with serious illness, disability, personal issues, or challenges, and they depend on the care given to them for survival and improved quality of life. The acronym **DIPPS** is a reminder of the five principles of compassionate care—**D**ignity, **I**ndependence, **P**references, **P**rivacy, and **S**afety—which is the goal of support work:

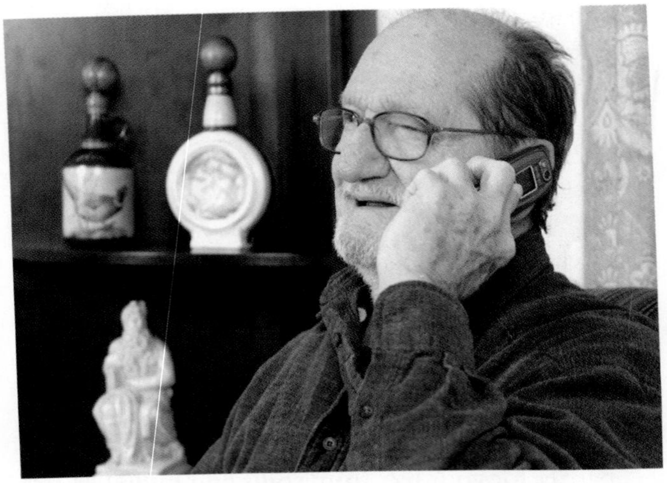

FIGURE 1–5 A client talks privately on a telephone. (**Source:** Sorrentino, S.A. (2008). *Mosby's textbook for nursing assistants* (7th ed., p. 137). St. Louis, MO: Mosby.)

- ***To preserve their dignity.*** **Dignity** is the state of feeling worthy, valued, and respected. People need to feel dignified.
- ***To live independently.*** Clients need to do what they can for themselves.
- ***To express their preferences.*** Clients need to make choices and explain how they want to have things done.
- ***To preserve their privacy.*** Clients need to know that their bodies and their affairs are treatec respectfully and protected from public viev (**FIGURE 1–5**).
- ***To be safe from harm.*** Clients need to live in a environment that is as hazard free as possible. The also need to feel secure about the care provided.

When well and able-bodied, most people take t fulfillment of the five needs listed above for grante When they have disabilities or suffer serious illness however, these needs may be more difficult to fulf Those who rely on others for personal care may wo about losing their dignity, and they may not feel f to express their wishes. For example, clients living long-term care facilities may have to eat wha provided and socialize only at prearranged times. They may share a room with another client and find that private moments are rare. Safety concerns are serious issues for clients with illnesses or disabilities. For example, they may worry about reaching the bathroom without falling.

Clients with illnesses or disabilities do not all have the same needs. However, most have at least some of the needs just discussed. To help you recognize clients' needs, *Providing Compassionate Care* boxes throughout the text discuss the goal of support work, which is to follow the principles of compassionate care when performing procedures with clients (**BOX 1–4**).

BOX 1–4 DIPPS—Principles of Compassionate Care, the Goal of Support Work

When performing every procedure listed in this textbook, it is important to advocate on behalf of the client's quality of life by promoting:

Dignity • **I**ndependence • **P**references • **P**rivacy • **S**afety

To do so, take the following steps:

- Check the client's care plan before starting any procedure to familiarize yourself with the client's preferences and safety considerations.
- Knock before entering the client's room.
- Address the person by name, and introduce yourself using your name and title.
- Explain the procedure before starting and explain each step throughout the procedure. Informed clients are usually more willing to assist and less likely to react out of fear. Accordingly, they are less likely to injure themselves or their caregivers during the procedure.
- Obtain the client's consent for any procedure before starting.
- Protect the person's rights throughout the procedure, including the person's right to privacy.
- Identify the client's ability to perform the procedure and guide the client to self-assist so as to remain as independent as possible.
- Handle the person gently during the procedure and observe safety guidelines at all times to minimize the risk for injury to the client or to yourself.
- Follow standard practice to decrease the risk for pathogen spread.

CRITICAL THINKING, DECISION MAKING, AND PROBLEM SOLVING

Support workers think critically and make many decisions in the course of a workday. For example, they estimate the time each task will take and plan the best way to complete their work on time, taking into account the various needs of the client. Many decisions involve critical thinking in order to solve problems.

When solving problems, consider the following:

- ***The goal of support work.*** Solutions to problems should not compromise the five principles of compassionate care: dignity, independence, preferences, privacy, and safety, or DIPPS.
- ***'he client's viewpoint.*** Involve clients in solving roblems that concern them. Examine the problem om the client's point of view.
- ***ope of practice.*** Learn and observe the rules of ur workplace. Know the limits of your role.
- ***pervisor's viewpoint.*** Decide if the problem is that you can handle on your own or one that r supervisor should handle. Your supervisor ıld provide guidance about which problems can deal with on your own.

cal thinking, decision making, and problem are crucial to the support worker's role but are often difficult when a person is new to the job. To help you with the problem-solving process, this text includes *Supporting* boxes that present examples of problems faced by support workers and how the problems were solved.

CHAPTER REVIEW

KEY POINTS

- The ultimate goal of support work is to improve the client's quality of life by following the principles of compassionate care (DIPPS). The support worker tends to the person's needs, which include physical needs as well as helping to relieve loneliness, providing comfort, encouraging independence, and promoting the person's self-respect. A support worker's services to people in their homes help them remain independent and continue to live with their families. Support workers make a difference in people's lives.
- Support workers can work in community-based or facility-based settings. Duties will vary according to the setting.
- Most of a support worker's responsibilities can be grouped into five categories: (1) personal care, (2) support for nurses and other health care providers, (3) family support, (4) social support, and (5) housekeeping or home management.
- Depending on their setting, people receiving health care and support services are known by different terms, such as patient (in a hospital), resident (in a residential facility), or client (in the community).
- The people supported can be grouped according to their problems, needs, and ages.
- At this point, support workers in most provinces and territories are still considered health care providers not regulated through legislation, or unregulated care providers (UCPs). Support workers are accountable to their supervisors, employers, and clients; they do not presently have an organization or college that governs their role. Regulated care providers are health care providers licensed and regulated by the province or territory to carry out care that is within their scope of practice.
- There are many members of the health care team, with the client always at the centre of care.
- It is important that support workers understand their scope of practice and never act beyond their role.
- In many settings, support workers are supervised by nurses or other professionals.
- Professionalism includes having a positive attitude, a sense of responsibility, a professional appearance, being discreet about client information, being a lifelong learner, advocating for the client, being discreet about personal matters, and using acceptable speech and language.
- While discussing the client with co-workers, support workers must use discretion at all times and honour the client's right to confidentiality. Confidentiality means respecting and guarding personal and private information about another person.
- Part of being a professional, reflective practice reviews consist of a review and self-evaluation of any care provided and identification of ways to improve clinical performance.
- When thinking critically, making decisions, and solving problems, support workers must consider the principles of compassionate care (DIPPS), the client's viewpoint, their scope of practice, and their supervisor's viewpoint.

CRITICAL THINKING IN PRACTICE

In the clinical setting, a resident asks you to help her move from her wheelchair to bed. You have not learned how to perform transfers yet. How will you respond? What will you do? As a student, what rules must you follow to protect patients and residents?

REVIEW QUESTIONS

Answers to these questions are at the bottom of p. 19.

Circle the BEST answer.

1. Activities of daily living (ADLs) are:
   A. Social and recreational activities
   B. Activities that support workers perform to prevent injuries
   C. Physical exercises that people perform daily to keep themselves fit
   D. Self-care activities that people perform daily to remain independent and to function in society

2. Which of the following is a way in which support workers assist nurses or other health care team members?
A. Assess the client's needs
B. Order range-of-motion exercises
C. Witness legal signatures on permission forms
D. Report changes in the client's behaviour or health

3. *Resident* is a term used to describe a person who is receiving care at:
A. Home
B. A long-term care facility
C. An outpatient clinic
D. A hospital

4. The main focus of the health care team is to:
A. See as many clients as possible
B. Provide quality care for the client
C. Complete assigned tasks as quickly as possible
D. Find a cure for the client's illness or condition

5. Support workers are:
A. Unregulated care providers
B. Licensed health care workers
C. Members of a professional college
D. Members of a regulatory body

. *Scope of practice* means:
A. The tasks that are assigned by your supervisor
B. The tasks that a client asks you to perform
C. The effort you put into performing a task or procedure
. The legal limits of your role

ofessionalism is:
A term used to describe workplace settings
An approach to work that demonstrates respect for others, commitment, competence, and appropriate behaviour
A commitment made by regulated rofessionals
nother term for confidentiality

8. Which of the following is true?
A. You can use a client's phone to make personal calls.
B. Friends can visit you at work.
C. You must follow your employer's dress code policies.
D. Sharing your personal problems with a client shows compassion.

9. In a long-term care facility, the client's information should be shared among:
A. Health care team members involved in the client's care
B. Health care team members and friends who visit the client
C. Family and friends of the client
D. All staff members at the facility

10. *Compassion* means:
A. Keeping one's feelings to oneself
B. Approaching your work with enthusiasm
C. Taking pity on those who are less fortunate
D. Caring about another's misfortune and suffering

11. The acronym DIPPS stands for:
A. Disability, independence, preferences, policies, sympathy
B. Dignity, independence, preferences, privacy, safety
C. Discretion, individuality, pity, privacy, support
D. Disability, individuality, pity, privacy, scope of practice

12. Which is false? When solving problems, you should:
A. Consider your scope of practice
B. Consider the principles of compassionate care
C. Discuss the problem with the client
D. Not involve the client to prevent causing more problems

Answers: 1.D, 2.D, 3.B, 4.B, 5.A, 6.D, 7.B, 8.C, 9.A, 10.D, 11.B, 12.D

ner image: Photographee.eu/Shutterstock.com

CHAPTER 2

The Canadian Health Care System

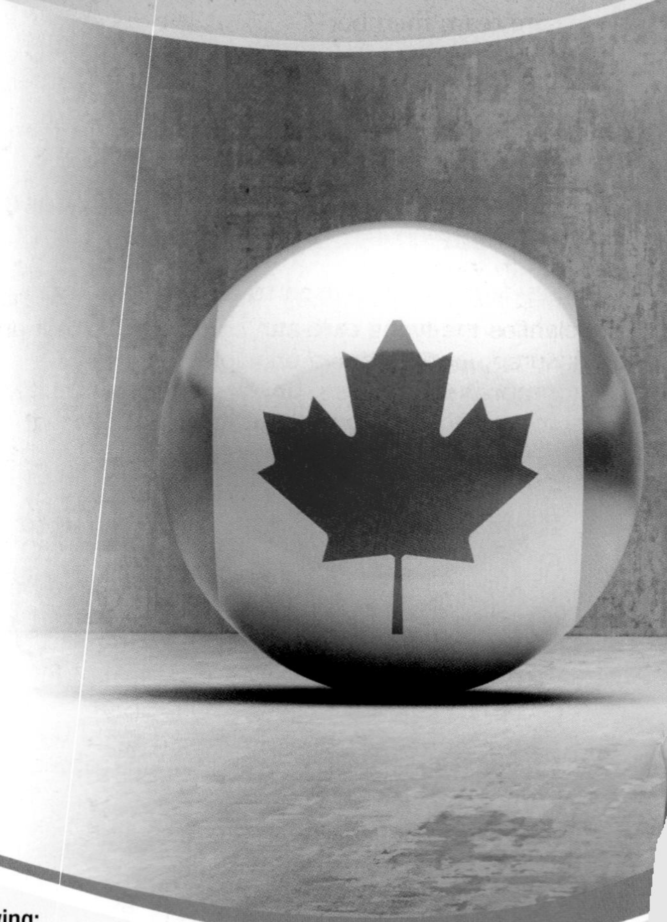

OBJECTIVES

After reading this chapter, the learner should be able to do the following:

- Describe medicare and how it has evolved.
- Identify the federal, provincial, and territorial roles in the Canadian health care system.
- Summarize the principles of medicare described in the *Canada Health Act*.
- Differentiate among primary, secondary, and tertiary health care deliveries.
- Identify how the focus of the Canadian health care system is shifting to home care.
- Explain why health promotion and disease prevention are important functions of the Canadian health care system.
- Recognize the emerging importance of home care and the support worker's role in providing some of these services.

KEY TERMS

accessibility A principle of the *Canada Health Act* that states that people must have reasonable access to insured health care services. *p. 24*

benefits Types of assistance that are provided through available insurance premiums. An example of a benefit is a dental procedure without any additional cost to the consumer. *p. 27*

Canada Health Act (1984) Federal legislation that clarifies the types of health care services that are insured; it outlines five principles (**comprehensiveness**, **universality**, **portability**, **accessibility**, and **public administration**) that must be met by provinces and territories to qualify for federal health funding. *p. 22*

comprehensiveness A principle of the *Canada Health Act* that states that all necessary health services, including hospitalization and access to physicians and surgical dentists, must be insured. *p. 24*

disease prevention Strategies that prevent the occurrence of disease or injury. *p. 28*

health promotion A strategy for improving the population's health by providing the necessary information and tools for individuals, groups, and communities to make informed decisions that promote health and wellness. *p. 28*

home care Health care and support services provided to people in their places of residence. *p. 28*

medicare Canada's national health care insurance system, which publicly funds the whole cost of medically necessary health services for permanent residents. *p. 21*

portability A principle of the *Canada Health Act* that states that residents continue to be entitled to coverage from their home province even when they live in a different province or territory or outside the country. *p. 24*

primary health care delivery The first point of contact people have with the health care system. It could be through a doctor, a nurse, or another health care provider or perhaps through phone- or computer-based services. *p. 25*

public administration A principle of the *Canada Health Act* that states that provincial health insurance must be administered by a public authority on a nonprofit basis. *p. 24*

secondary health care delivery An intermediate level of health care that includes diagnosis and treatment. It is performed in a hospital that has specialized equipment and laboratory facilities. *p. 25*

Telehealth Medical telephone call centres through which nurses give advice to callers about health concerns. *p. 25*

tertiary health care delivery The specialized, highly technical level of health care that takes place in large research and teaching hospitals. *p. 25*

universality A principle of the *Canada Health Act* that states that all residents are entitled to the same basic level of health care services across the country. *p. 24*

lth care is of great importance to Canadians. Canadians believe that quality health care d be available to all citizens, regardless of their to pay. Canada's national health insurance , known as **medicare**, was developed to this goal. Medicare uses provincial or territ- xes and federal taxes to pay for all medically y health services for all permanent residents. workers have an increasingly important role anada's changing health care system.[1]

THE EVOLUTION OF CANADA'S HEALTH CARE SYSTEM

In the first part of the twentieth century, individuals in Canada were expected to pay the entire amount of their doctors' bills and hospital fees. Often, there were no "set fees"; that is, for the same treatment, a physician could charge one patient a certain amount and another an entirely different fee, depending on what the physician thought the patient could afford

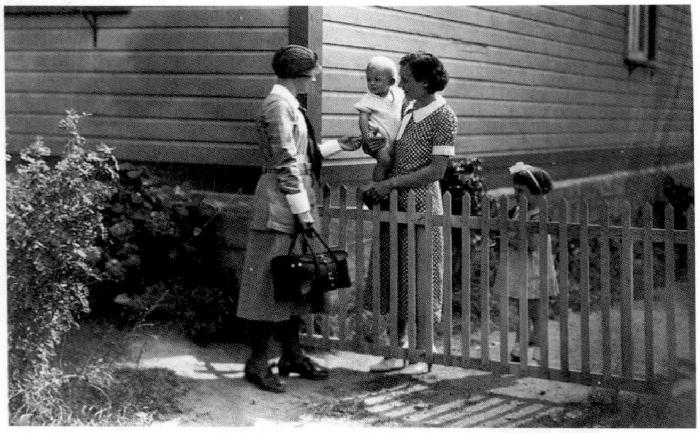

FIGURE 2–1 In the first part of the twentieth century, charitable services were provided by community agencies such as the Victorian Order of Nurses for Canada. (Courtesy VON Canada (Victorian Order of Nurses)).

to pay. Those who could not afford to pay had to access charity services through community agencies such as the Victorian Order of Nurses, the Red Cross, and local churches (**FIGURE 2–1**), and some just went without health care.

The Great Depression of the 1930s had a dramatic effect on Canada's health care system. Families struggled to feed, clothe, and house their members and could not possibly pay their medical bills. A serious illness or stay in a hospital caused financial disaster for many. The cost of care prevented others from even seeking medical treatment, so those with illnesses and disabilities would instead depend on family members and neighbours to provide care.

These hardships inspired Canadians to create a prepaid medical and hospitalization insurance plan. In 1947, under Premier Tommy Douglas, Saskatchewan became the first province to introduce a public insurance plan that covered the costs of hospital services (**BOX 2–1**). By 1961, all 10 provinces and 2 territories agreed to provide coverage for inpatient hospital care. The federal government paid about half the cost of hospital and diagnostic services for each province and territory while provincial and territorial governments paid the other half. By 1972, all provinces and territories extended their insurance plans to also cover medical services provided outside hospitals. Again, provincial and territorial governments and the federal government shared the health care expenses roughly equally. Modern medicare began that year, giving all permanent residents free access to the same quality of hospital and medical care, regardless of their personal financial status.

For Indigenous people in Canada, universal health care access has been an evolving objective (see **BOX 2–2** on page 24). Challenges to delivering health care, such as geography, lack of organization, language or cultural barriers, and socioeconomic status, have been recognized. However, access that is culturally sensitive and inclusive is improving through new strategies.[2]

CANADA'S CURRENT HEALTH CARE SYSTEM

Canada's publicly funded health care system is best described as an interlocking set of health insurance plans, with the federal government and the 10 provincial and 3 territorial governments sharing responsibilities within Canada's health care system. The provincial and territorial governments fund health care services with assistance from the federal government. To receive their full share of federal funding for health care, provincial and territorial medicare plans must meet five criteria—comprehensiveness, universality, portability, accessibility, and public administration (see **BOX 2–3** on page 24)—that are provided in the federal government's **Canada Health Act**.

Medicare provides access to universal, comprehensive coverage for medically necessary hospital and physician services. These services are administered and delivered by the provincial and territorial governments to Canadian residents with no payment necessary upon delivery of the service.

The responsibility for First Nations, Métis, and Inuit peoples' health services is shared by federal, provincial, and territorial governments and Indigenous organizations. Together with these organizations and communities, Health Canada carries out many activities to help people of all ages stay healthy and to prevent persistent and contagious diseases. Improvements have occurred as a result of efforts to extend lifespan and prevent infant deaths. However, gaps still remain in the overall health status of indigenous peoples compared with that of other Canadians. For example, the occurrence of suicide, injury, and diabetes are higher among First Nations, Métis, and Inuit people than the Canadian average.

Many other organizations and groups, includin health care providers' professional associations as we

BOX 2–1 Tommy Douglas, the "Greatest Canadian"

In the spring of 2004, the Canadian Broadcasting Corporation (CBC) invited Canadians to submit their nominations for the "Greatest Canadian" of all time. Canadians responded with thousands of worthy suggestions, including Terry Fox, a courageous young man who ran across Canada to champion cancer research; scientists; athletes; and prime ministers who have contributed to Canada's history. After 6 weeks of voting, Canadians chose Tommy Douglas. You might be wondering who he was and why Canadians are grateful for his contributions to this country.

Thomas Clement Douglas (1904–1986) was elected to office in June 1944 and, with his party, the Co-operative Commonwealth Federation (CCF), was given the difficult task of reorganizing Saskatchewan's post-war employment, social, and public health policies. Douglas's reforms became his legacy, as they formed the basis for Canada's social and health care policies, which continue to exist today.

He made many contributions to the province of Saskatchewan and to the whole country. For example, as health minister (1944–1948), he took the first steps toward what we now call medicare by:

- Creating a universal and compulsory hospital insurance program for Saskatchewan, the first in Canada, beginning what Canadians now know as *health insurance programs*
- Establishing a minimum wage and ensuring a maximum 44-hour workweek and paid 2-week vacation leave, rights some workers take for granted today
- Overseeing increases in old-age pensions and mother's allowance
- Legislating that medical and hospital benefits be given to welfare recipients at no out-of-pocket cost to them at the time of care

These are just a few of the many contributions that Tommy Douglas made. Without him, Canada would be a very different country today. We can all be grateful for the role he played in making Canada the country that it is.

Source: Tommy Douglas Research Institute. (2007). *The greatest Canadian*. Retrieved from http://www.tommydouglas.ca/tommy/greatest_canadian.

as organizations involved with accreditation, education, research, and voluntary assistance, contribute to health care delivery in Canada. Public health, too, is a shared responsibility. While public health services ıre generally delivered at the provincial, territorial, ıd municipal levels, the federal Public Health ɟency of Canada acts as a focal point for disease ·vention and control and for emergency response ıutbreaks of infectious diseases.

Federal Role

ːderal government is responsible for:

- ıinistering the *Canada Health Act* and provid- ›rovincial funding
- ding direct delivery of health care services to ic groups, such as First Nations people living on reserves; Inuit peoples; serving members of the Canadian Forces and the Royal Canadian Mounted Police (RCMP); eligible veterans; and inmates of federal penitentiaries[4]
- Developing and carrying out government policy and programs that promote health and prevent disease; for example, the federal government approves drugs, assesses health risks posed by environmental hazards, and provides funds to support public health programs such as prenatal health education[5]
- Transferring tax money to the provinces and territories to share the cost of medically necessary health care services
- Prohibiting service providers (such as physicians) from billing clients extra charges and user fees and ensuring that all the provinces and territories provide the same quality and type of care

BOX 2–2 Health Canada's Role in Indigenous Health Care

1945	Health services for this population were transferred from the Department of Indian Affairs to Health Canada.
1962	Through the new Medical Services Branch, Health Canada started to provide direct health services to First Nations people on reserves and to the Inuit in the North.
1974	A governmental policy acknowledged that although no treaty required the government to provide health care to Aboriginal people, Health Canada would ensure the availability of services.
1979	A new Indian Health Policy stated that uninsured benefits would rely upon "professional medical and dental judgment" and recognized "the need for community development, a strong relationship between First Nations people, the federal government, and the Canadian health system."
Mid-1980s	Work began to have First Nations, Métis, and Inuit communities control more of their own health services.
1998	"Gathering Strength—Canada's Aboriginal Action Plan" emphasized Health Canada's commitment to diabetes and tuberculosis initiatives, the development of the Aboriginal Healing Foundation, and a healing strategy related to Indian residential schools, in partnership with the Department of Indian Affairs.
2000	The Medical Services Branch was renamed the First Nations and Inuit Health Branch.

BOX 2–3 The Principles of Medicare, as Listed in the *Canada Health Act* (1984)

1. **Comprehensiveness.** The insurance plan must pay for all medically necessary services. In a hospital, all necessary drugs, supplies, and diagnostic tests are covered. A range of necessary services provided outside a hospital are also covered.
2. **Universality.** Every permanent resident of a province or territory is entitled to receive the insured health care services provided by the plan on similar terms and conditions.
3. **Portability.** People can keep their health care coverage even if they are unemployed, change jobs, relocate between provinces and territories, or travel within Canada or abroad. However, if they are moving, it is their responsibility to inform their province or territory and to register with their new province or territory. During the transition, they will be covered by their previous jurisdiction's health coverage for up to three months (see the *Supporting Mr. Woloshyn: Health Insurance Portability* box on page 30).
4. **Accessibility.** People can receive medically necessary services regardless of their income, age, health status, gender, or geographical location. Additional charges *(Privatization)* for insured services are not permitted.
5. **Public administration.** The insurance plan must be run by a public organization on a nonprofit basis. The public organization must be accountable to the citizens and the government of the province or territory.

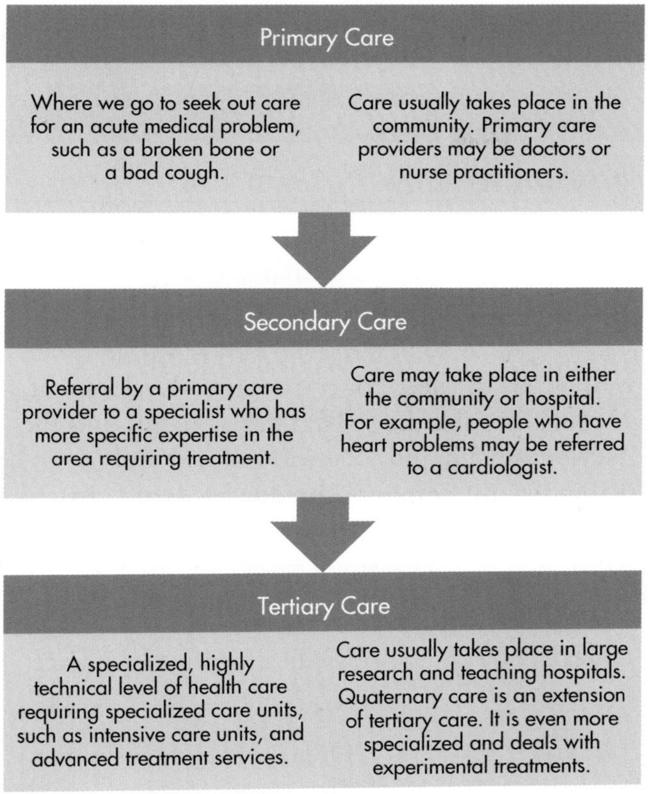

FIGURE 2–2 A Brief Comparison of Primary, Secondary, and Tertiary Levels of Health Care

Primary, Secondary, and Tertiary Health Care Delivery

In the past, most health care funding went to hospitals and equipment, and the focus of health care was to make people better *after* they became ill. The Canadian government has recognized that secondary or tertiary health care delivery, while still important, can be shortened or prevented altogether with adequate preventive measures taken in the primary health care delivery stage. Every province and territory provides primary, secondary, and tertiary health care (**FIGURE 2–2**).

Primary health care delivery is the first point of contact most people have with the health care system. It could be through a doctor, a nurse, or another health care provider or perhaps through phone-based or computer-based services. Primary health care delivery usually takes place in the community but can also take place within a hospital. Primary health care delivery offers a wide range of services, focusing mostly on health promotion, early diagnosis of disease or disability, and disease prevention.[6]

Examples of recent primary health care reforms in Canada include the establishment of more community primary health care centres that provide services throughout the day; the creation of primary health care teams that include family nurse practitioners; increased coordination and integration of comprehensive health services; improvements to the work environments of primary health care providers; and greater emphasis on promoting health, preventing illness and injury, and managing persistent diseases.

Coordinated primary health care teams include family doctors, nurses, nurse practitioners, and other health care providers. These team members can vary according to the needs of the community they serve and the provincial or territorial priorities. This team approach, along with the introduction of medical telephone call centres that provide advice and after-hours access to primary health care services (**Telehealth**), reduces the use of emergency care units.

Secondary health care delivery is assessment, diagnosis, treatment, and preventive services associated with more complex medical issues. It is generally provided by specialist physicians and other specialized health care providers. An example of secondary health care delivery would be a referral from a family doctor or nurse practitioner to a medical specialist for a specific medical issue that may require diagnosis and treatment. It can take place in the community (such as the specialist doctor's office) or in a hospital.[6]

Tertiary health care delivery is a specialized, highly technical level of health care that takes place in large research and teaching hospitals. Tertiary health care delivery usually takes place within specialized care units such as an intensive care unit and requires advanced diagnostic and treatment support services and highly specialized personnel. It is the most costly level of health care delivery. A new specialized section of tertiary health care delivery is called *quaternary care*, which includes experimental medicines or surgical procedures. Because it is so specialized, not every health care centre will offer quaternary care.

The Provincial or Territorial Role

Each province and territory is responsible for developing and administering its own health care insurance plan. The provincial or territorial government finances and plans its health care services, following the five basic principles outlined in the *Canada Health Act*. For example, provincial and territorial governments decide where hospitals or long-term care facilities will be located and organized; how many physicians, nurses, and other service providers will be needed; and how much money to spend on health care services. Provincial and territorial health insurance plans (TABLE 2–1) pay for hospital and physician costs.

TABLE 2–1 Provincial and Territorial Health Insurance Programs

Province/Territory	Name of Plan
Alberta	Alberta Health Care Insurance Plan
British Columbia	Medical Services Plan
Manitoba	Manitoba Health
New Brunswick	Medicare
Newfoundland and Labrador	Newfoundland and Labrador Medical Care Plan
Northwest Territories	NWT Health Care Insurance Plan
Nova Scotia	Medical Service Insurance
Nunavut	Nunavut Health Care Plan
Ontario	Ontario Health Insurance Plan
Prince Edward Island	Medicare
Quebec	Assurance maladie (Medicare)
Saskatchewan	Saskatchewan Medical Care Insurance Plan
Yukon	Yukon Health Care Insurance Plan

Source: Health Canada. (2015). *Provincial/territorial role in health*. Retrieved from http://healthycanadians.gc.ca/health-system-systeme-sante/cards-cartes/health-role-sante-eng.php.

HEALTH CARE CHALLENGES, SUPPLEMENTARY SERVICES, AND TRENDS

Challenges

The Canadian health care system has come under stress in recent years. Many factors challenge the country's ability to provide quality, universal health care, and these factors are expected to continue into the future.[4] They include:

- ***Worker shortages.*** Many rural and remote areas face severe shortages of physicians, nurses, and other health care workers. The growing trend of people moving to bigger cities leaves smaller communities in need of educated workers.
- ***Aging of the baby boomer generation (those born between 1945 and 1964).*** The Canadian society is aging. For the older-adult population to live safely and with dignity and independence, the costs of our health care system will rise.
- ***Aging of health care workers.*** Health care workers are also aging. Many studies are investigating the effects of different types of work on older bodies. One finding is that older workers have fewer injuries, but the injuries they have tend to be more severe.[7]
- ***Long waiting lists for surgeries, diagnostics, and medical procedures.*** Long wait times cause stress and a possible worsening of their condition for many clients in need of treatment.
- ***Long waiting times for admission to long-term care facilities.*** Clients who are ill and waiting for long-term care placement must often stay in an acute-care hospital because it is unsafe for them to live at home. Overcrowded hospital units and emergency departments have resulted. To remedy the situation, many hospitals have restructured their care delivery to include continuing care units, where these clients can await long-term care admission.
- ***The steadily rising cost of care.*** Of all the challenges facing the health care system, its rising cost is the greatest. Drugs and technology that help treat diseases and disabilities are better than ever before. However, these advances come at a high price due to the cost of developing them. Building

and labour costs, too, are always spiralling upward, and taxpayers bear the burden.

Additional (Supplementary) Services

Provinces and territories provide coverage to certain people (e.g., older adults, children, and recipients of social assistance) for services that are not generally covered under the publicly funded health care system. These supplementary health benefits often include prescription drugs, dental care, vision care, medical equipment and appliances (e.g., prostheses, wheelchairs), independent-living assistance, and the services of other health care providers such as chiropractors. The level of coverage varies across the country.[4] Additional health insurance, sometimes referred to as **benefits**, covers services that are not government funded, such as some of the costs of rehabilitation and extended care services.

Private Insurance

Those who do not qualify for supplementary benefits under government plans pay for these services with individual, out-of-pocket payments or through private health insurance plans. Many Canadians are covered by private health insurance, paid for by their employers or themselves. The level of service provided varies according to the plan purchased. Each company may provide its own unique plan. Exactly what is covered and by how much (e.g., ambulance services, drugs, home care) will differ according to the plan.

To help pay for services not covered by provincial or territorial insurance, people can buy extra health insurance policies. Some private insurance coverage is comprehensive; others cover very few services or only a percentage of the costs of services. Some people do not have any private insurance, so they receive no funding other than what is provided by their province or territory.

Health Care Trends

To reduce some of the pressures placed on our health care system, new ways of providing care have been introduced to Canadians, with the intent of providing quality care while avoiding needless spending. Instead of Canadians' relying on hospitals and doctors, there is a trend toward providing alternative care in clinics, in health care centres, and through home care. Many families now seek medical services not only from doctors but also from nurse practitioners. Medical advances have led to more surgical procedures being done through day surgery on an outpatient basis. Some procedures (such as elective cosmetic surgeries) are offered in private clinics. Post-acute services and hospital-alternative services are now more frequently provided in the home and community.[4]

As a result of health care delivery changes and redistribution of health care funding, the number of acute-care hospital beds has decreased. This decrease, however, has led to hospital overcrowding in some communities, where there are not yet sufficient community services.[8]

Most provinces and territories have tried to control costs and improve delivery by decentralizing decision making on health care delivery to the regional or local board level. Such regional authorities are managed by elected and appointed members who oversee hospitals, nursing homes, home care, and public health services in their areas. As part of these reforms, provincial and territorial governments are now focused on two areas:

- Health promotion and disease prevention
- Home care

Alternative Health Practices

Alternative health practices are health treatments that have not been taught or practised in traditional medical communities and offer therapies that differ from standard medical practice. They include massage therapies, homeopathy, herbal medicines, and acupuncture. These practices are gaining widespread acceptance by the same medical community (also known as *Western medicine*) that once disregarded them and are now often ordered by physicians and used in conjunction with traditional treatments. Many of these services are also now covered by some provincial and territorial health care plans.

Health Promotion and Disease Prevention

Traditionally, the purpose of a health care system has been to diagnose, treat, and cure illnesses. A more recent approach to health care, however, involves developing ways to promote health and prevent diseases. Preventing illness and injury, while keeping people healthy, is more effective and cheaper than providing treatments in hospitals. **Health promotion** refers to strategies that improve or maintain health and independence. **Disease prevention** refers to strategies that prevent the occurrence of disease or injury. Health promotion and disease prevention are now important functions of Canada's health care system.

Some sectors of government and industry have policies to promote health and prevent illness by improving the quality of people's lives. Examples of such policies include:

- Immunization programs
- Prenatal and parenting classes
- Information campaigns to reduce drinking during pregnancy, unsafe sex, and tobacco use and to encourage healthy eating and physical activity
- Efforts to improve housing, decrease poverty, monitor drinking water for safety, and protect the environment

Support workers contribute to health promotion and disease prevention and are needed more now than ever before since they provide nonmedical care and services that can help prevent major health problems. Take, for example, Mr. Lukovic, who has been on bed rest for a long time. He is at risk for pressure ulcers, pneumonia, and blood clots. To prevent these complications, you, as his support worker, help him keep his skin clean and dry, change his position in bed frequently, and help him perform range-of-motion exercises. By doing these important things for Mr. Lukovic, you can help improve his quality of life now and prevent him from developing illness or disability in the future.

Home Care

The Canadian health care system has seen a shift in focus from hospital care to home care. Traditionally, people entered the health care system through hospitals. However, over the past two decades, the role and structure of hospitals have changed dramatically. Operating a hospital requires a tremendous amount of money. Over a third of all health care spending goes into hospitals. Therefore, to cut costs, most provincial and territorial governments have reduced the number of hospitals. Hundreds of hospitals have closed, merged, or been converted into other types of care facilities.

Partly to save money and partly as a result of technological advances, clients are sent home sooner after hospital procedures. Each year, fewer clients stay in hospital overnight, and if they do stay overnight, they stay for shorter periods than they would have in the past. To support patients who leave hospitals early, governments have gradually increased spending on home care. **Home care** is health care and support services provided to people in their places of residence, including private homes, licensed residential care facilities, and assisted-living facilities (see Chapter 3). Home care is the most common of the community-based services.

Home care was first created to provide care for people who needed at-home assistance after hospital discharge. Today, home care provides community care and support to a range of people. Clients include older adults; families with children; people who have mental, physical, or developmental disabilities; people with short-term and long-term medical conditions; and people in the recovery, rehabilitative, or final stages of a life-ending disease. Home care services provide assistance to families who need help with a new baby. They enable people with disabilities to get up in the morning and get ready for school or work. They help people adjust to a disability or recover from an illness (**FIGURE 2–3**). They enable

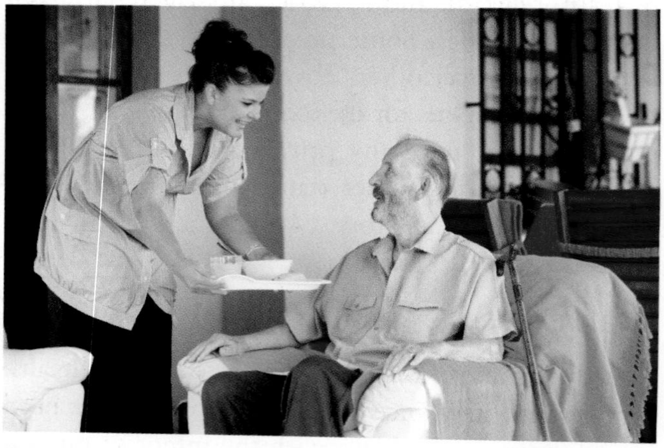

FIGURE 2–3 This man receives assistance through home care services so he can continue to live by himself at home. (**Source:** MANDY GODBEHEAR/Shutterstock.com)

people who are dying to remain at home rather than be admitted to hospital.

One major focus of home care is to enable people to remain in their homes, as healthy as possible and independent for as long as possible. For some people, home care replaces hospital or other facility care. For others, home care allows them to maintain their health and independence, thus delaying or preventing admission to a facility.

Services and Funding

Support workers provide most home care support services. In most provinces and territories, support services are provided by both public and private agencies that can be either for-profit or not-for-profit organizations. Every province and territory has a publicly funded home care program. In addition, Health Canada's First Nations and Inuit Health Branch uses contribution agreements with the Canadian government to provide funding for health programs and services for First Nations people on reserves and Inuit people in the North.[9]

The funding for the specific type of care that a client receives depends on his province's funding policies. Because the *Canada Health Act* does not say what services must be provided, each province and territory has defined and funded its own home care system; therefore, the services offered and how they are provided vary across the country (**BOX 2–4**).

All provinces and territories, however, offer the following:

- Client assessment—determining if the person is eligible for services
- Case coordination and management (see Chapter 5)
- Nursing services
- Support services for eligible clients

Eligibility and hours of services provided will also vary, depending on the province or territory. Some people may want home care services that are not funded by their province or for which they do not qualify. In such a case, they can hire a private agency and pay for these services themselves or with private insurance plans (see "Private Insurance" on p. 27).

Home care services are classified into the following categories:

- ***Personal care services.*** These nonmedical services offered through home care, often by support workers, include the following:
  - Assisting with activities of daily living (ADLs—e.g., bathing, feeding, mobility, and dressing)
  - Providing comfort care to clients who are dying
- ***Home support services.*** These services, often provided by support workers to clients who live at home, include the following:
  - Assisting with home management
  - Assisting with ADLs
  - Assisting with taking medications
- ***Nursing and professional services***. Therapies and treatments provided by the relevant health care providers include the following:
  - Nursing care
  - Physiotherapy
  - Occupational therapy
  - Speech therapy
  - Nutrition counselling

BOX 2–4 How Home Care Is Governed and Delivered

How home care is governed and delivered differs across provinces and territories. In all jurisdictions, the ministries or departments of health and social or community services are responsible for home care services. These departments monitor the services and decide on budgets, policies, and standards of care.

Service delivery involves:

- Assessing clients' needs
- Determining clients' eligibility for government-sponsored professional and support services
- Coordinating and monitoring home care services provided by private or not-for-profit agencies
- Providing information and referrals to other long-term care services (e.g., volunteer-based community services such as Meals on Wheels), some of which charge user fees to the client
- Providing placement services to assisted-living facilities and extended care facilities (known in some provinces as *long-term care facilities*)

- Social work
- Respiratory therapy
- ***Support for instrumental activities of daily living (IADLs).*** These services, often provided by support workers, include the following:
  - Shopping with a client
  - Assisting a client with banking
  - Teaching a client how to follow a recipe

Volunteer services such as Meals on Wheels (**FIGURE 2–4**) and friendly visiting can be provided by anyone who meets the volunteer criteria.

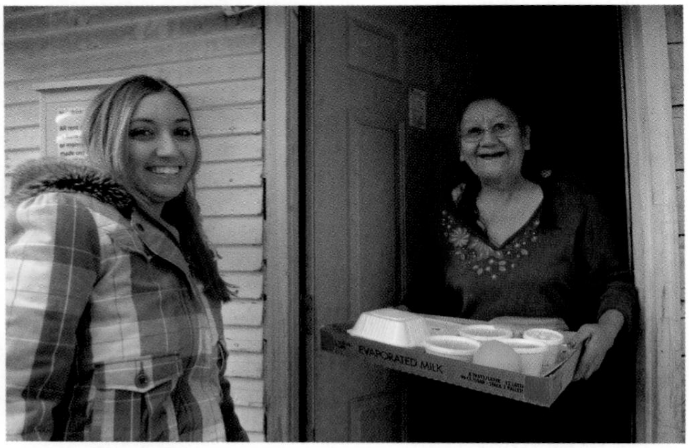

FIGURE 2–4 Delivery of hot meals to clients in their homes. (**Source:** U.S. Air Force photo/Airman 1st Class Katrina Heikkinen)

Supporting Mr. Woloshyn: Health Insurance Portability

Ivan Woloshyn is a 65-year-old widower who was seriously injured in an explosion in his factory about 6 months ago, just a few weeks before he was to retire. In the months since his accident, he has been cared for at home by nurses, physiotherapists, and occupational therapists for the severe burns he received to his face and right arm. Since he was also blinded in the accident, he requires support workers to assist him with taking a bus to his various appointments as well as with his banking and grocery shopping.

Mr. Woloshyn, who lives in Manitoba, has decided that he would like to move in with his married daughter, who lives in Ontario. He has been told that his private insurance, through his employer, would still cover his ongoing treatments and support after he moves. He is not sure, however, about what to do about his provincial insurance coverage. What can you tell him? How can he find out about switching coverage?

CHAPTER REVIEW

KEY POINTS

- Canada's publicly funded health care system is best described as an interlocking set of 10 provincial and 3 territorial health insurance plans.
- Medicare provides access to universal, comprehensive coverage for medically necessary hospital and physician services. These services are administered and delivered by the provincial and territorial governments and are provided at no additional cost to the client.
- To receive their full share of federal funding for health care, the provincial and territorial health insurance plans must meet the five criteria of the *Canada Health Act*—comprehensiveness, universality, portability, accessibility, and public administration.
- Health care delivery is divided into primary, secondary, and tertiary delivery categories. Primary care is aimed at preventing illness whenever possible. Tertiary health care delivery is the most expensive to deliver.
- Many factors challenge and stress the Canadian health care system. These factors include (1) severe shortages of physicians, nurses, and other health care workers in rural areas; (2) the aging of the baby boomer generation; (3) long waiting lists; and (4) the steadily rising cost of care and new technology, which is the greatest challenge.
- Supplementary health benefits often include prescription drugs, dental care, vision care, medical equipment and appliances, independent-living assistance, and the services of other health care providers, such as chiropractors. The level of coverage varies across the country.
- Residents may have private insurance plans that pay for these supplementary services.
- New trends in health care include (1) alternative care in clinics, (2) health care centres, and (3) home care programs.
- To control costs, provincial and territorial governments are focusing on (1) health promotion and disease prevention and (2) home care.
- Support workers provide most home care support services.
- In most provinces and territories, support services are provided by for-profit and not-for-profit public and private agencies. Every province and territory has a publicly funded home care program, but the funding per client will vary depending on the province's funding policies.
- Home care services are classified by (1) personal care services, (2) home support services, (3) nursing and professional services, and (4) support for IADLs.

CRITICAL THINKING IN PRACTICE

How do the following issues impact our Canadian health care system: (a) escalating costs of care, (b) privatization of services, (c) continuity of care, and (d) electronic health records?[10]

REVIEW QUESTIONS

Answers to these questions are at the bottom of p. 32.

Circle the BEST answer.

1. Canada's health care system is:
   A. Strictly a federal responsibility
   B. Delivered by government employees
   C. Funded by private insurance companies
   D. Publicly funded through provincial or territorial and federal taxes

2. Provincial and territorial governments are responsible for:
   A. Paying the full amount of all medical procedures
   B. Planning, financing, and delivering their own health care insurance plans
   C. Delivering health care services to Indigenous peoples and military personnel
   D. Delivering health care services to inmates of federal penitentiaries and to the RCMP

3. Which law ensures that every citizen has access to health care?
   A. The *Medical Care Act*
   B. The *Canada Health Act*
   C. The *Long-Term Care Facilities Act*
   D. The *Hospital Insurance and Diagnostic Services Act*

4. Canadians who travel to other parts of the country still maintain their provincial or territorial health care coverage. Which principle of medicare does this exemplify?
   A. Portability
   B. Universality
   C. Comprehensiveness
   D. Public administration

5. The most pressing cause of health care reform has been:
   A. The Great Depression
   B. Lack of accessibility
   C. Lack of available technology
   D. Rising costs of providing technology, drugs, and services

6. A recent trend in health care is to focus on:
   A. Cutting back on home care services
   B. Opening more hospitals in rural areas
   C. Cutting back on public health policies
   D. Public policy that promotes health and prevents disease

7. Immunization programs are an example of a:
   A. Medicare system
   B. Disease prevention program
   C. Home care service
   D. Facility-based treatment

8. One major focus of home care is to:
   A. Diagnose and treat disease
   B. Enable clients to remain in their own homes
   C. Provide accommodation for people with disabilities
   D. Provide accommodation for acutely ill people who do not want to go into the hospital

9. Home care services provided by support workers might include:
   A. Vacuuming and dusting
   B. Respiratory therapy
   C. Assisting the client with physiotherapy
   D. Assisting the client with banking

10. Which statement about Canadian home care programs is correct?
    A. All home care is free to Canadians.
    B. Provincial government funding is shifting to home care.
    C. Hospital care is a cheaper and better alternative for most people.
    D. All provinces and territories govern their programs in a similar manner.

11. In Canada's provinces and territories, support services are governed by:
    A. Regional health boards
    B. The federal government
    C. Private or not-for-profit agencies
    D. The provincial or territorial government

Answers: 1.D, 2.B, 3.B, 4.A, 5.D, 6.D, 7.B, 8.B, 9.A, 10.B, 11.D

Chapter opener image: xtock/Shutterstock.com

CHAPTER 3

Workplace Settings

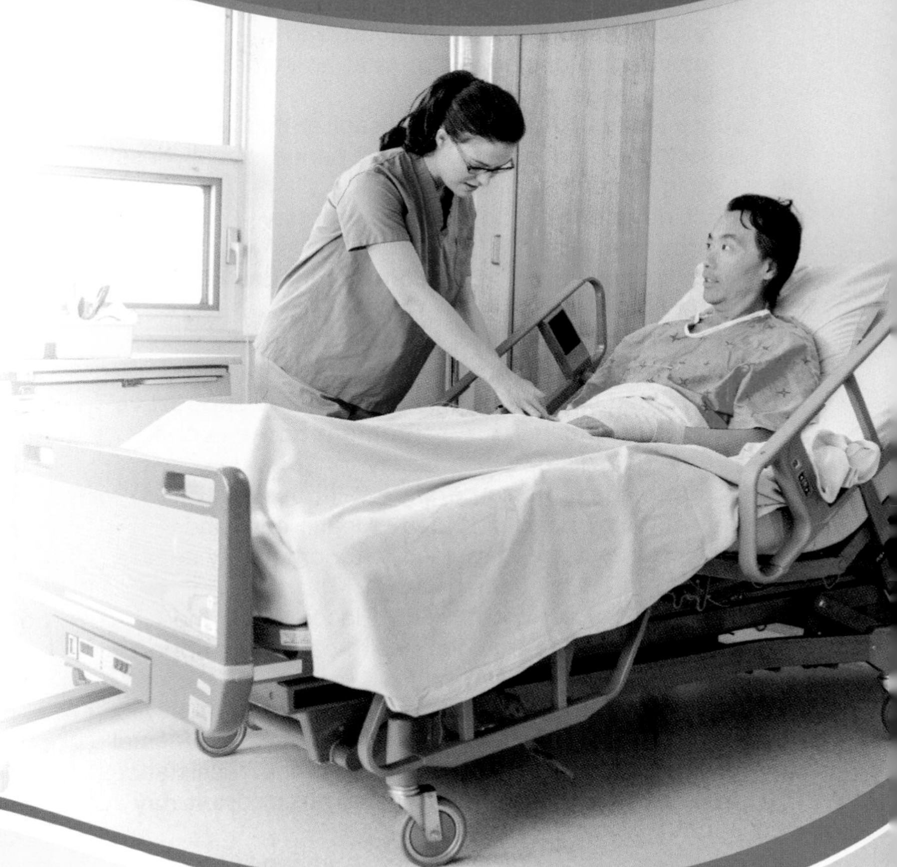

OBJECTIVES

After reading this chapter, the learner should be able to do the following:

- Differentiate between community-based care and facility-based care.
- List the work settings where support workers are employed.
- Differentiate between residential facilities and medical facilities.
- Describe the various types of residential facilities.
- Identify the issues and challenges support workers encounter in the workplace.

KEY TERMS

acute care Health care that is provided for a relatively short time (usually days to weeks) and is intended to diagnose and treat an immediate health issue. *p. 35*
acute illness An illness or disability that appears suddenly and lasts for a short period, usually less than 3 months. *p. 35*
adult day centre See **community day program**. *p. 40*
adult day program See **community day program**. *p. 40*
assisted-living facility A residential facility where residents live in their own apartments and are provided support services (also called **supportive housing facilities**). A **retirement home** is one type of assisted-living facility. *p. 36*
chronic illness See **persistent illness**. *p. 35*
community-based services Health care and support services provided in a community setting, not in a facility setting. *p. 36*
community-based settings Places within the community that provide health care and support services. *p. 36*
community day program A daytime community-based program for people with physical or mental health issues or older adults who need assistance. Also known as **adult day program** or **adult day centre**. *p. 40*
complex continuing care Comprehensive inpatient care provided to people who are recovering from surgery, injury, an acute illness, or an exacerbation of a disease process. Also known as **subacute care**, *convalescent care*, or *transitional care*. *p. 35*
end-of-life care See **palliative care**. *p. 35*
facility-based settings Workplaces that provide clients with accommodations, health care, and support services. *p. 37*
group home A residential facility in which a small number of people with physical or mental disabilities live together and are provided with supervision, care, and support services. *p. 39*
hospice A type of palliative care that provides home, residential, or inpatient care to a client who has a terminal diagnosis and is no longer seeking life-prolonging care. *p. 36*
hospital A facility for clients with acute illnesses or injuries who require admission and care on a relatively short-term basis, often not even overnight. *p. 37*
inpatient A client who is assigned a bed and is admitted to stay in a facility overnight or longer. *p. 41*
long-term care Medical, nursing, and support services provided over the course of months or years to people who cannot care for themselves. Also known as *chronic care* or *continuing care*. In some provinces, this is also known as **complex continuing care**. *p. 35*
long-term care facility A facility that provides accommodations, 24-hour nursing care, and support services to people who cannot care for themselves at home but who do not need hospital care. Also known as *chronic care facility* or *continuing care facility*. In some provinces, it is called a *complex care facility* or *nursing home*. *p. 37*
mental health care services Services provided to individuals and families confronting mental illness or disorders. Also known as **psychiatric care services**. *p. 36*
outpatient A client who does not stay overnight in a facility. *p. 41*
palliative care Services for clients (and their families) living with or dying from a progressive, life-threatening illness. Also known as **end-of-life care**. *p. 35*
persistent illness An ongoing illness or disability, slow or gradual in onset, that may or may not grow worse over time. Also known as *chronic illness*. *p. 35*
psychiatric care services See **mental health care services**. *p. 36*
rehabilitation services Methods, therapies, and educational programs used to restore or improve the client's independence and functional abilities. *p. 35*
respite care Temporary care of a person who requires a high level of support, care, and supervision; respite care gives caregivers a break from their duties. *p. 35*
restorative care Care that is aimed at re-establishing a client's sense of independence to its greatest potential. *p. 35*
retirement home A facility in which older adults who are independently mobile can live independently but receive hospitality services such as meals and housekeeping services (also known as an **assisted-living facility** or **supportive housing facility**). *p. 36*
subacute care See **complex continuing care**. *p. 35*
supportive housing facility See **assisted-living facility**. *p. 36*

This chapter describes common community-based and facility-based workplace settings for support workers. It also explores issues and challenges you may encounter in these settings. Wherever you work, you provide people with vital services that enable them to be as safe, comfortable, dignified, and independent as possible. ***In any work environment, you should be familiar with the scope of practice for support workers in your province, and you should always stay within this scope. Agreeing to perform tasks that are beyond your support worker role and scope of practice can possibly risk legal action against you or your employer.***

WORKPLACE SETTINGS AND SERVICES PROVIDED

Support workers provide care in many settings. Each setting has different goals and services. Each employer should have a specific and formalized job description for its support workers, and any task the support workers do should fall within this job description.

- **Acute care**—health care that is provided for a relatively short time (usually days to weeks) and is intended to diagnose and treat an immediate health issue. It is provided mainly in hospitals. An **acute illness** appears suddenly and lasts a short time, usually less than 3 months. Symptoms can be severe. Examples of acute illnesses are pneumonia and influenza.
- **Subacute care** (also known as *convalescent care* or **complex continuing care**)—health care or rehabilitation for people recovering from surgery or injury or being stabilized after a serious illness or health challenge. A client in subacute care is in stable condition but still needs care requiring complex equipment and procedures. Many hospitals provide subacute care. After a hip replacement, for example, a client may not be ready to go home because he or she needs frequent physiotherapy and dressing changes. Some hospitals have wards that are dedicated to providing subacute care. Eventually, the client is discharged home or to another level of care.
- **Long-term care**—health and support services provided over the course of months or years to people who cannot care for themselves. Many people who require long-term care have persistent illnesses. A **persistent illness** (also known as **chronic illness**) is an ongoing illness, slow or gradual in onset, that may or may not grow worse over time. Examples of persistent illnesses are diabetes, multiple sclerosis, and Alzheimer's disease. Because persistent illnesses cannot be cured, the focus of care is on preventing complications of the illness. These illnesses can sometimes be managed, and complications prevented. In some cases, long-term care is provided for the remainder of the client's life. The goal of long-term care is to help the resident cope with the challenges of living with a long-term illness or disability while maintaining a good quality of life. Some hospitals provide long-term care, but more often, long-term care is provided in a residential care setting, such as a long-term care facility, or through home care services.
- **Respite care**—temporary care of a person who requires a high level of support, care, and supervision. Respite care gives the person's caregivers a break from their duties. Respite care is often provided by support workers in the client's home. However, many hospitals and other facilities also offer respite care.
- **Rehabilitation and restorative care services**—therapies and educational programs designed to restore or improve the client's independence and functional abilities. These services are for people who are or have been ill, injured, or disabled. Hospitals, residential facilities, and clinics offer rehabilitation services. Services may include life skills training, occupational therapy and rehabilitation services, behavioural management, speech therapy, physiotherapy, job coaching, and family counselling. Support workers may assist the client with personal care or activities of daily living (ADLs) or assist with program delivery.
- **Palliative care**—care for clients with progressive, life-threatening illnesses or conditions. Also known as **end-of-life care**, palliative care includes services that aim to relieve or reduce uncomfortable symptoms, not to produce a cure. Palliative care is an approach to care that emphasizes client goals, relief of pain and suffering, and quality of life. Palliative care and hospice (below) often work together to help the client and the family during

the client's journey near the end of her life. End-of-life care is provided through an interdisciplinary approach.

- **Hospice**—an element of palliative care that provides home, residential, or inpatient care to a client who has a terminal diagnosis and is no longer seeking life-prolonging care. The philosophy of hospice is to provide support for the client's emotional, social, and spiritual needs, as well as medical needs, as part of treating the whole person. Hospice workers try to make the client's last days as painless, comfortable, and dignified as possible. Support workers assist with personal care and ADLs, as well as provide emotional support and encouragement to the client and family (see Chapter 46).
- **Mental health care services** (also known as **psychiatric care services**)—services for people with mental health disorders (such as schizophrenia, bipolar disorder, and addictions). Entire facilities, health care centres, and hospital units are devoted to caring for people with mental health disorders and offer both inpatient and outpatient services. Clients are usually encouraged to return to the community rather than stay in a hospital. Assessment and treatment programs enable these clients to function as independently as possible within the community, where they have access to community-based care and support services.

WORKING IN COMMUNITY-BASED SETTINGS

Community-based settings are places within the community that provide health care and support services. Examples of community-based settings include clients' homes, group homes, and retirement homes in which clients live as independently as possible. The most common community setting is the client's home (**FIGURE 3–1**). Support workers sometimes assist their clients with social integration, and they may teach their clients important skills such as doing laundry, shopping for groceries, managing their money, doing their own banking, taking a bus, or applying for a job.

As discussed in Chapter 2, the current trend within the Canadian health care system is to decrease hospital costs and to increase resources offered through community-based services. **Community-based services** include health care and support services provided in community settings, such as schools, community health centres, and doctors' offices. As part of this trend, the health ministries of all the provinces and territories have initiated more community-based programs to support clients in living longer and avoiding being hospitalized. The increase in home-based and community-based programs has created an ever-growing demand for support workers; in fact, community-based service providers are hiring more support workers than ever before. Home care agencies, residential facilities, group homes and retirement residences, day programs, and school boards are all community-based services that hire support workers.

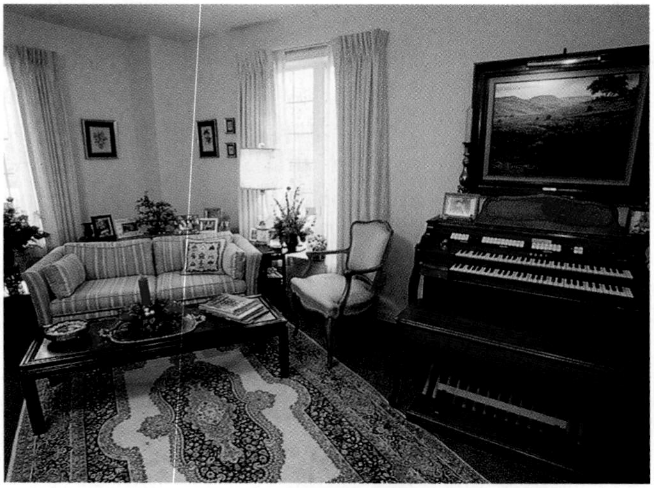

FIGURE 3–1 A room in a community-based setting. It is easy to see how the client has personalized this room, making it look homey and comfortable. (**Source:** Sorrentino, S.A., & Remmert, L. (2012). *Mosby's textbook for nursing assistants* (8th ed.). St. Louis, MO: Mosby.)

While the majority of support workers who work in private homes are employees of an agency, some are privately employed by the client or the client's family. Clients can live in a variety of settings, such as **retirement homes**—which may also be called **assisted-living facilities** or **supportive housing facilities**—group homes, or their own houses or apartments. A retirement home is a facility where older adults who are independently mobile can live independently but receive hospitality services such as meals and housekeeping services. Some may offer additional services such as bathing, dressing, or assistance with medication.[1]

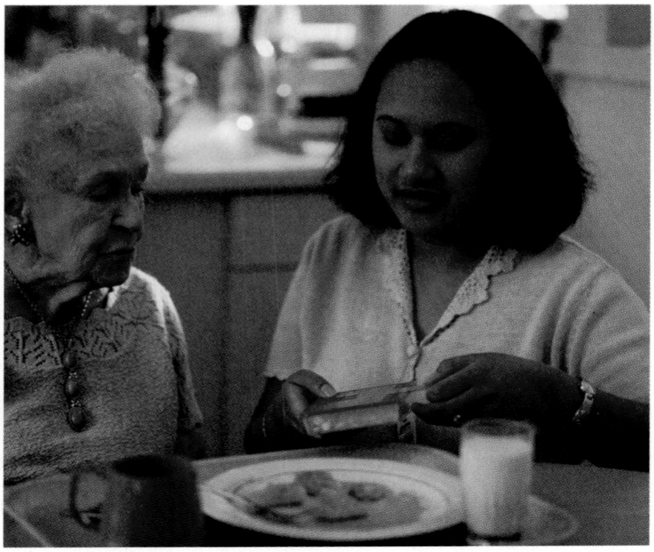

FIGURE 3–2 With the assistance of support workers, many clients are able to remain in their own homes. (**Source:** Keith Brofsky/Photodisc/Getty Images.)

Home Care

Home care is a vital part of Canada's health care system (see Chapter 2). Support workers have a central role within home care. It has been estimated that support workers are responsible for 80% of the total hours worked by all home care workers.[2] Support workers are responsible for providing a range of home care services, including assisting with personal care (**FIGURE 3–2**), ADLs, child care, transportation, and home management.

Support workers providing home care services are hired on a full-time, part-time, or casual basis and must follow their agency's policies and procedures. Some agencies offer further education, and many offer in-servicing, to keep staff up to date with new procedures. **BOX 3–1** describes some of the issues and challenges associated with working in home care (also see Chapter 7).

WORKING IN FACILITY-BASED SETTINGS

Facility-based settings are workplaces that provide clients with accommodations, health care, and support services. Several types of facilities, including hospitals and long-term care facilities, employ support workers. A **hospital** is a facility for clients with acute illnesses or injuries who require admission and care on a relatively short-term basis. Some clients require admission for procedures or rehabilitation on an outpatient basis only; these clients would generally not be required to stay overnight for care and observation. A chronic care, continuing care, or **long-term care facility** (**FIGURE 3–3**) is home to people who are not able to live independently or in their own homes and who require the availability of 24-hour nursing services to meet their personal care needs but do not need hospital care. In some provinces, long-term care facilities are called *complex care facilities* or *nursing homes.* Support workers also may be employed in mental health facilities, which admit and treat clients with acute or long-term mental health disorders.

Residential Facilities

A residential facility is a facility that provides living accommodations, care, and support services. These facilities vary in size and levels of care and support.

People using residential facilities are called *residents* because they reside, or live, in the facility. The facility is their temporary or permanent home. Therefore, these facilities provide care in a comfortable, homelike atmosphere (**FIGURE 3–4**) and ensure that they meet the social and emotional needs of the residents.

Clients need residential care when they require supervision and assistance with some or all of their ADLs but do not need acute medical care or high-level nursing care. Such clients include the following:

- Frail older adults
- Individuals of all ages who have physical disabilities, mental health challenges, or both
- Individuals with substance addiction

The type of residential facility appropriate for a client (e.g., assisted-living facility, retirement home, long-term care facility) depends on the individual's needs and level of independence. Note that the labels given to facilities vary across Canada.

Assisted-Living Facilities

Also called *supportive housing facilities,* **assisted-living facilities** are residential facilities where people live in their own apartments and receive support

BOX 3–1 Issues and Challenges Associated With Working in Home Care

- ***Working on your own.*** Many support workers prefer the variety of activities and the stimulation in a facility setting, whereas others like working one-on-one with a client by providing home care services. Some support workers miss the routines that are followed in facility settings, whereas others enjoy the independence that home care offers. However, not having a supervisor around may sometimes present a challenge. Although your supervisor can be reached by phone, you sometimes need to use your own judgement to solve problems.
- ***Taking direction from different health care providers.*** You may be expected to take direction from your supervisor as well as a number of other health care providers. For example, a client's physiotherapist visits during your shift and asks you to perform tasks that your supervisor has not requested you do. If you are asked to do tasks that are unfamiliar to you or not allowed by agency policy, always check with your supervisor before doing them.
- ***Maintaining professional boundaries.*** You often work closely with clients and their family members. However, it is never appropriate to become personally involved in the client's life decisions and family relationships. You should always be caring and compassionate but respect that a boundary exists in your relationship with clients and their families. Do not confuse professionalism and empathy with friendship. Clients and their families need your skills, services, and undivided attention. Do not discuss your personal problems or ask for advice, and do not pry into clients' problems or offer advice.
- ***Providing for client safety.*** Clients' homes may present many safety hazards (e.g., frayed electric cords and unsafe smoking practices). Discuss any safety concerns you have with the client and your supervisor.
- ***Providing for your personal safety.*** In home care, you do not have control over the environment that you will enter. You will travel to unfamiliar areas. You may have to drive in hazardous weather conditions. You may face abuse or violence in unfamiliar homes. At such times, you must look out for your own safety (see Chapter 22).

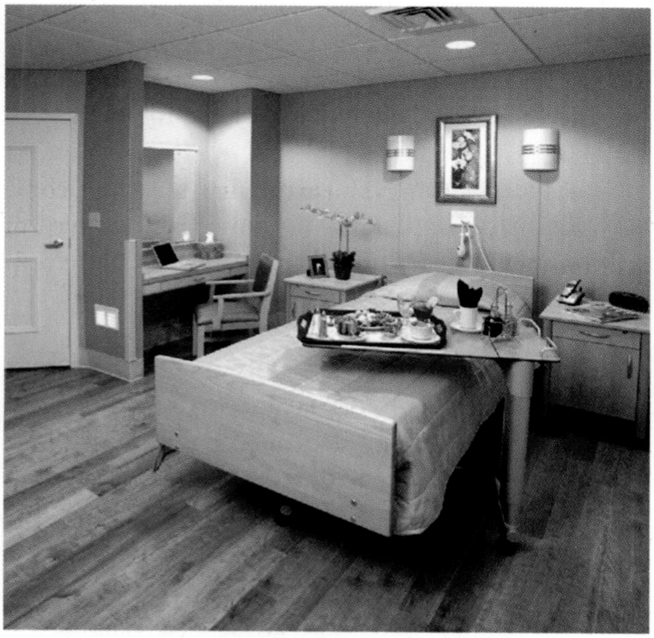

FIGURE 3–3 A room in a long-term care facility. Note how the desk and framed print can make it seem homier to the client residing there. (**Source:** Courtesy of Wingate Healthcare)

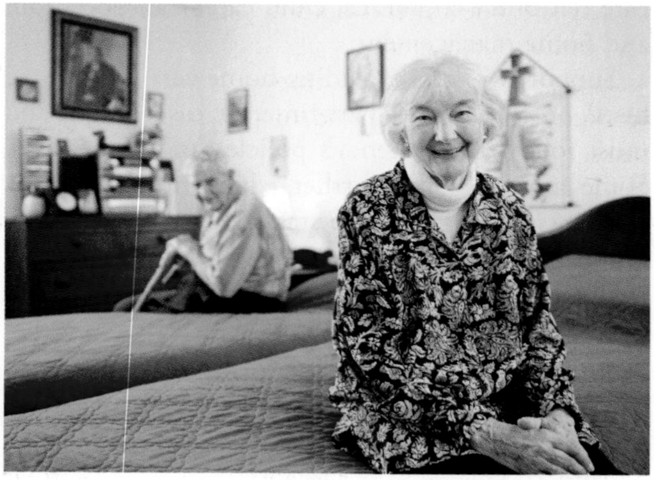

FIGURE 3–4 The atmosphere of a residential facility is made as homelike as possible. (**Source:** Radius Images / Alamy Stock Photo)

services. Because they are located in the community, assisted-living facilities are considered to be community-based services. Residents are usually older adults who require assistance with some of their ADLs and instrumental activities of daily living (IADLs). Usually constructed as multi-storey apartment buildings or condominium complexes, these facilities typically offer residents in-unit kitchens so they can cook their own meals. Many assisted-living facilities provide a common living area, an activity room, and a games room. Residents usually receive the following support services:

- 24-hour supervision and emergency response services
- Social and recreational programs
- One or two daily meals
- Housekeeping and laundry services

Not all residents need or want the same services. Some residents may purchase extra support services if needed, and some may qualify for home care.

All assisted-living facilities must be approved and licensed by the provincial or territorial government, which provides partial funding for the services offered. Public or private agencies manage the facility and hire and supervise support workers. A supervisor may be responsible for one or several assisted-living facilities. Some supervisors work onsite; others visit the facility only periodically. Because the level of assistance needed differs among residents, support workers are often required to perform a variety of tasks.

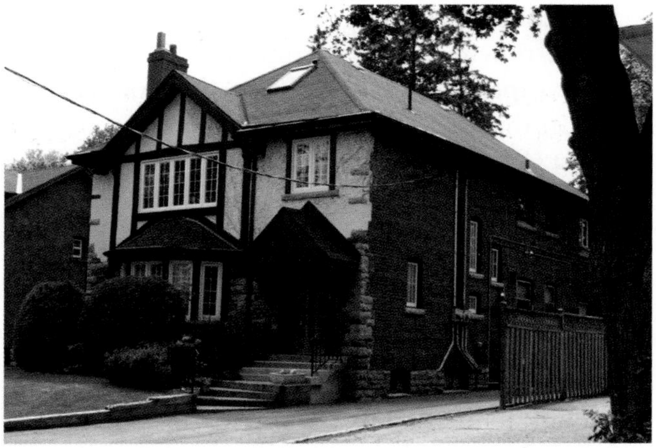

FIGURE 3–5 Group homes, another type of assisted-living facility, are usually situated in residential neighbourhoods. (**Source:** Dick Hemingway.)

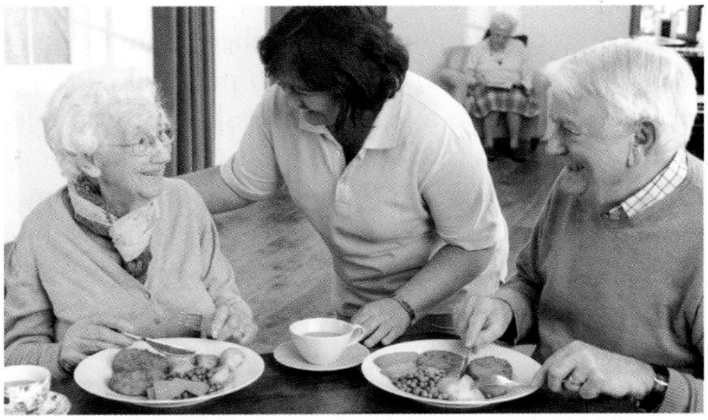

FIGURE 3–6 Residents living in retirement homes share common living and dining areas in a homelike environment. (**Source:** © Can Stock Photo Inc./monkeybusiness.)

Group Homes

Group homes also offer assisted-living services. A **group home** is a residential facility in which a small number of people with physical or mental disabilities live together and receive supervision, care, and support services. Rather than having their own apartments, residents share a house in a residential neighbourhood (**FIGURE 3–5**). Usually, residents have their own bedrooms but share bathrooms and living and dining areas. They receive 24-hour supervision, meals, housekeeping and laundry services, and assistance with personal care and ADLs.

Residents of group homes are often adolescents or young adults with disabilities, behavioural or conduct disorders, or mental impairment; older adults needing care; women leaving abusive situations; or people with substance abuse issues. The number and type of staff employed by a group home depend on the residents' needs.

Retirement Residences

A retirement residence (or *retirement home*) is a facility that provides accommodation and supervision for older adults. Residents have their own bedrooms and bathrooms but share common living and dining areas (**FIGURE 3–6**). They may need help with housekeeping but limited supervision and little to no assistance with personal care. The goal of a retirement residence is to allow older people to live as independently as possible while providing security, support services, and varying degrees of care, as needed.

Regulations governing retirement residences vary. In some provinces and territories, they are usually privately operated and not financed by the government. In this case, residents are required to pay the full cost. Standards, prices, and services differ from one facility to another. These facilities may be small, converted houses or high-rise apartment buildings.

Support workers are almost always hired directly by the facility or the resident. Support workers hired by a resident provide care for only that person. They perform functions such as running errands, providing transportation, assisting with activities or social and recreational events, and helping with tasks such as unpacking suitcases or arranging bedrooms. In some provinces, support workers may even be required to assist the residents with taking their medications, including insulin injections.

Residents in retirement homes do not have illnesses or disabilities that prevent them from meeting their own personal care needs, so personal care services are limited to a few simple tasks. For example, a support worker may help a client get in and out of a bathtub. Residents needing more than minimal daily care have to move to a long-term care facility. Some facilities house both a retirement residence and a long-term care facility; residents, therefore, do not have far to move once they need full-time access to nursing and personal care services.

Community Day Programs

An adult **community day program** (also called **adult day centre** or **adult day program**) is a daytime program for people with physical or mental health issues or for older adults who need assistance. Day programs aim to meet the client's needs and provide a break for family caregivers. These programs may be held in hospitals, nursing homes, community and recreational centres, adult day centres, church basements, or other settings. In some provinces, support workers are hired by school boards to assist with clients who are attending school instead of a day program.

Each day program is unique. Some programs offer rehabilitation to people with disabilities. Others offer counselling to people with mental impairment. Many day programs offer recreational activities (**FIGURE 3–7**), such as arts and crafts, social events, films, and board or card games.

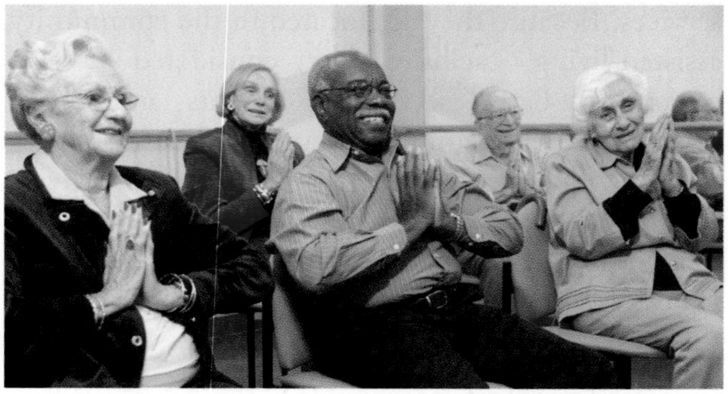

FIGURE 3–7 Community day programs provide recreational or other activities to clients during the day. (**Source:** © Can Stock Photo Inc./monkeybusiness.)

Some provinces hire support workers to work in community day programs, whereas other provinces do not. Support workers in a community day program provide personal care and assistance to people attending the program and may assist with hosting the recreational and social activities. As always, if you work with a community day program, make sure that you follow all employer policies and procedures. **BOX 3–2** lists common issues and challenges associated with working in a community day program.

Working Directly for Clients

A support worker may be hired by, supervised by, and work directly for a client or the client's family. Clients may hire their own support workers if they need a service that is not provided by local agencies or if their province provides funding assistance directly to them rather than to an agency for their care. **BOX 3–3** describes issues and challenges associated with working directly for clients.

WORKING IN A FACILITY

A health care facility is a building designed or established for the delivery of specific care, treatment, and support services. Such facilities provide a range of services.

Hospitals and Other Medical Facilities

Clients in hospitals usually have serious illnesses or injuries that require treatment in a timely manner, skilled professional care, and complex equipment.

BOX 3–2 Issues and Challenges Associated With Working in a Community Day Program

- ***Working closely with a team and a supervisor.*** In most community day programs, support workers work closely with a supervisor and other team members. This closeness can be either a challenge or a benefit. Teamwork can be a success if team members share a common goal and work well together. It can be difficult, though, if conflicts occur within the team. Effective communication skills are necessary (see Chapters 5 and 6).
- ***Working in a structured environment.*** Many day programs have highly structured environments, particularly programs that provide rehabilitation. People with conditions such as Alzheimer's disease usually benefit from a predictable routine. Working well in a structured environment requires strong organizational skills and sensitivity to clients' needs.
- ***Meeting multiple needs.*** Support workers may have to attend to the needs of many people. They must be able to focus on each person and quickly decide whose needs to address first. Good judgement and time management are essential.

BOX 3–3 Issues and Challenges Associated With Working Directly for Clients

- ***Clarifying the terms of employment.*** Some clients who employ a support worker may want to have a contract signed. Always read the contract carefully before signing it. Hours and pay for individual clients may change from week to week. Make sure you understand how many hours you are expected to work and what pay you can expect. If you are hired directly, your employer may be required to pay benefits, such as unemployment insurance.
- ***Establishing work limits.*** Before you begin working for the client, find out what exactly is expected of you and how your performance will be evaluated. Ask for this information in writing. Find out as much as you can about the client's preferences and standards.
- ***Knowing scope-of-practice limits and your role and responsibilities.*** A private employer may ask you to do something that is beyond your scope of practice (see Chapter 1). In this event, you may feel uneasy but may not know who to contact to confirm what you are allowed to do. It is therefore important that you inform your private employer of the scope of your role and that you know someone (a former teacher or employer, for example) who can answer your questions if such a situation ever arises.
- ***Needing to carry liability insurance.*** When you are self-employed, you are legally responsible for any injury or workplace mishap that might occur while you are providing care. In addition, without health insurance, you would not be compensated for lost wages if you were to become ill and miss time from work.

Not all hospitals hire support workers, but in those that do, support workers usually report to and are supervised by a nurse.

Depending on the region and the hospital's hiring policies, support workers may be employed in any unit in a hospital, including the critical care unit (CCU) and the emergency department (ED). Their role may be to provide basic care such as feeding, transporting people, taking specimens to the lab, or measuring vital signs. In some hospitals, they may assist nurses before, during, or after surgical or medical procedures. Support workers may perform other tasks, if requested and supervised by the nurse. They usually do not provide care to clients in unstable conditions but may assist the nurse in moving, turning, or bathing a client in such areas as the CCU or the ED.

Health care services are offered both to **inpatients** (patients who are assigned a bed and admitted to stay in the facility overnight or longer) and to **outpatients** (patients who do not stay overnight in the facility).

Hospitals and other medical facilities provide a variety of services, including acute care, subacute care, complex continuing care, respite care, rehabilitation services, palliative care, and mental health services. Not all hospitals provide all these services. In some cities and towns in Canada, these services are accessed through separate, specialized facilities. You may work in these or other medical facilities. Some of these facilities may require, and also provide, further education.

Long-Term Care Facilities

Long-term care facilities (also called *nursing homes, homes for the aged, long-term care homes,* and *special care homes*) offer higher levels of care than do retirement residences and assisted-living facilities. They provide accommodations, 24-hour professional nursing care, and support services to clients who cannot care for themselves at home but do not need hospital care. Most residents are frail older adults with many health issues. Some residents, though, are young or middle-aged adults who have severe, persistent health conditions or disabilities. The goals of these facilities are to maintain the residents' health and independence to the greatest extent possible and to meet their physical, emotional, social, intellectual, and spiritual needs.

Residents stay on a ward or in private or semi-private bedrooms. Usually, each room has a bathroom with a toilet and a sink. Tubs and showers are located in the common bathrooms. Besides nursing care, these facilities offer access to medical and rehabilitative care. They also provide assistance with personal care and ADLs, meals, laundry service, and recreational and social activities.

Long-term care facilities are licensed, regulated, and funded by the province or territory in which they are located. Medicare covers some costs, with the balance paid through a monthly fee by residents. Residents also must pay for personal clothing, toiletries, hairdresser services, special nail care services and other incidentals. Government or charitable organizations operate some facilities on a not-for-profit basis. Private facilities operate on a for-profit basis. Each facility hires its own staff.

Most long-term care facilities serve many residents with various physical or other disabilities. Therefore, to function efficiently, these facilities maintain highly structured work environments. Support workers are members of the health care team in a long-term facility and report to a nurse. Nurses plan and coordinate resident care. Support workers provide personal care and assist clients with various ADLs (**FIGURE 3–8**). They make important contributions to the clients' care plans, and during discussions in family conferences, they provide valuable feedback based on their observations of the client.

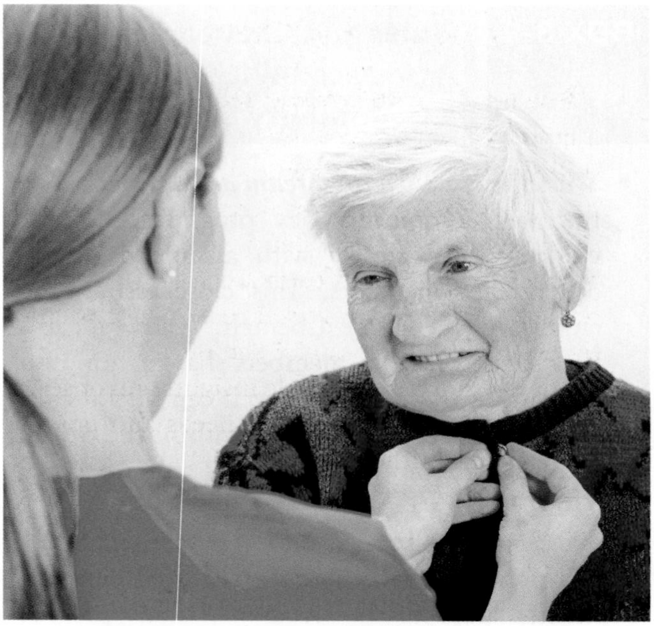

FIGURE 3–8 Residents in long-term care facilities may need support workers to assist them with activities of daily living. (**Source:** © Can Stock Photo Inc. / obencem)

Some long-term care facilities have subacute care units where a client may be admitted to convalesce after surgery if not yet able to go home. Some facilities also have special care units for residents with specific disabilities. For example, a facility may have a dementia care unit for people with Alzheimer's disease or other dementias. Respite care and palliative care units are also part of some long-term care facilities. Support workers may work in any of these units but may require extra training to do so.

Support workers may also work in a facility's recreation department, where they may help organize and carry out recreational outings and activities. Here, they would report to the recreation supervisor.

As with working in the community, working in a facility also presents issues and challenges for the support worker (**BOX 3–4**) (also see Chapter 7).

BOX 3–4 Issues and Challenges Associated With Working in a Facility

- ***Working in a structured team environment.*** Support workers work on a team with highly skilled professionals. Some may feel less confident in such an environment. Remember that you are a valuable member of the team and have much to contribute at team meetings. In residential facilities, support workers usually spend more time with the clients than the nurses and physicians do. You have valuable insights and observations about the client's daily needs and possible changes in health.
- ***Meeting multiple needs and demands.*** Support workers are required to respond to the many needs and demands of clients. It may not be possible to respond immediately to all demands, so, as a support worker, you should be able to prioritize clients' needs and manage your time. You must be flexible, diplomatic, and consistent. Effective organizational and communication skills are essential.
- ***Doing many tasks within a short period.*** Support workers must provide thorough, competent, and respectful care within a short time. This ability requires self-discipline, dedication, and efficiency.
- ***Respecting your role and scope of practice.*** Support workers work closely with nurses and may become familiar with many nursing procedures. You might sometimes be asked to perform a procedure that is beyond your scope of practice. Never attempt any procedure that you are not legally allowed to perform. Perform only those procedures allowed by law and facility policy. Also, never perform a procedure unless your supervisor is allowed to train you on that procedure and has given you sufficient training so that you are comfortable doing it. The facility will have written policies to guide you.
- ***Working in shifts.*** Most facilities are staffed through the entire day. You may have to work evening and night shifts, and your shifts may be 8 to 12 hours long, depending on the agency. Many support workers love the variety of working different shifts, whereas some have difficulty adjusting to the changes in sleep and lifestyle habits demanded by shift work. Those who have families may also find that it is a challenge to participate in their children's activities. In time, these workers usually get used to their varying sleep cycle and other routines in their lives.

Especially in Hospitals or Other Medical Facilities

- ***Dealing with people in distress.*** Clients admitted to hospital or other medical facilities may show signs of intense emotional or physical distress. They may be in pain, afraid, upset, or angry and not cooperate with their care providers. Remain calm and professional, no matter how these clients express themselves. Also, be sensitive to their feelings. Try to imagine how they are feeling. Sometimes, you can provide emotional support just by holding the client's hand or listening. In the case of palliative care, you need to be strong and supportive in the presence of intense suffering and emotions. If the client is facing a life-threatening illness, you need to be comfortable with your own feelings and attitude toward death. Otherwise, you may find it very difficult to care for the client.

Especially in Residential Facilities

- ***Making the facility feel like a home.*** A residential facility is, primarily, the resident's home. Treat the setting with as much respect as you would your own home. Be careful with the client's personal possessions. Make all areas of the facility cheerful, comfortable places. Every staff member must contribute to creating a positive, homelike environment.
- ***Respecting the client's privacy and dignity.*** In any work setting, support workers must respect their clients' privacy and dignity. Lack of privacy can result in loss of self-esteem, particularly during personal care. Remember to knock on the door and announce your presence before entering a client's room. Carefully screen off the area, and cover the client. This step may seem obvious, but

Continued

BOX 3–4 Issues and Challenges Associated With Working in a Facility—cont'd

sometimes, it is easy to focus more on getting the job done than on respecting the client's need for privacy. As in other care situations, respecting privacy also includes keeping discussions with co-workers about the client confidential and professional, respecting the client's property, and recognizing the client's right to express his preferences.

- ***Maintaining professional boundaries.*** Support workers may provide care to residents who have no close personal relationships. Working closely with clients may foster strong attachments. This aspect of the job may be one of the main attractions of support work. However, do not become too personally involved with clients and their families. Always be caring and supportive, but remember that your main responsibility is providing care and maintaining a professional attitude.

CASE STUDY Choosing a Place to Work

Therese LeCroix is a new support worker who has just graduated from a reputable support worker program. She was a highly motivated and interested student who enjoyed all of the placements that she was given during her support worker program. She is now looking for a permanent position but does not know where to begin. She has seen ads listed in her local newspaper, as well as online, for many jobs available in her town for support workers.

Therese has decided to ask her classmates where they are going to apply for jobs. She is amazed that many of them are fairly certain of what type of support work they prefer. Some love providing home care, and some others are interested in working in long-term care facilities. Other classmates have decided to apply for positions at the local hospitals that hire support workers. Finally, many of Therese's classmates say that they would love working in the community for agencies that offer day programs for special groups of clients.

Therese finally begins to understand why it is so difficult for her to decide: There are *many* opportunities for support workers in a variety of settings. She then decides that she should keep an open mind and apply to different agencies and settings that might *best work for her*, based on her family commitments, interests, and location in the city. Therese realizes that she is lucky to be in a line of work that offers such a variety of opportunities and in which the workers are so much in demand!

CHAPTER REVIEW

KEY POINTS

- Regardless of where you work, you should be familiar with the scope of practice for support workers in your province, and you should always stay within this scope. Agreeing to perform tasks that are beyond your support worker role and scope of practice can risk legal action.
- The current trend within the Canadian health care system is to decrease hospital costs and to increase its community-based services.
- With the increase of home- and community-based programs, there is an ever-growing demand for support workers.
- Community-based services include the health care and support services provided outside of a facility and in a community setting such as (1) school boards, (2) community health centres, (3) doctors' offices, (4) home care agencies, (5) day programs, and (6) residential facilities.
- You may work directly for a client or the client's family. Such clients select and supervise their own support workers. Clients may pay support workers from their own resources, or their province may provide funding assistance to them.
- Facility-based services include the health care and support services provided within facilities such as hospitals or long-term care facilities.
- There are positive aspects as well as issues and challenges associated with any type of service, regardless of the setting.

CRITICAL THINKING IN PRACTICE

It is 0900 hours. Set priorities for completing the assigned tasks below. What would you do if you were unsure of the correct order?

- Take Mr. Boyle's blood pressure and pulse before 1000 hours.
- Assist Ms. Wynn to the bathroom.
- Assist Ms. Warner and Mrs. Loy to the activity room. The activity begins at 1000 hours. Assist them back to their rooms at 1115 hours.
- Give Mr. Rollins a shower.
- Help Mr. Rollins to his son's car for lunch outside the centre at 1200 hours.

REVIEW QUESTIONS

Answers to these questions are at the bottom of p. 46.

Circle the BEST answer.

1. A current trend in the Canadian health care system is to:
   A. Increase public spending on hospitals
   B. Decrease spending on community-based services
   C. Focus on providing more community-based services
   D. Promote facility-based services over home care

2. Home care is an example of:
   A. A community-based service
   B. A facility-based service
   C. A community day program
   D. Palliative care

3. Which work setting provides acute care?
   A. Home care
   B. Long-term care facilities
   C. Assisted-living facilities
   D. Hospitals

4. Which work setting may provide subacute care?
   A. Retirement homes
   B. Long-term care facilities
   C. Group homes
   D. Hospices

5. What type of service aims to provide a temporary break to family caregivers?
   A. Acute care services
   B. Palliative care
   C. Respite services
   D. Outpatient services

6. Which of the following is an example of a residential facility?
   A. Hospital
   B. Methadone clinic
   C. Private residence
   D. Assisted-living facility

7. Residents in retirement facilities generally include:
A. People with mental impairment
B. Young adults with physical or other disabilities
C. Frail older adults with multiple health problems
D. Older adults with limited care needs

8. Residents in long-term care facilities generally require:
A. 24-hour nursing care and support services
B. Supervision and limited support services
C. Acute care
D. Housekeeping services, but not meal services

9. In which setting is maintaining a homelike atmosphere *especially* important?
A. Hospital
B. Doctor's office
C. Community day program
D. Long-term care facility

Answers: 1.C, 2.A, 3.D, 4.B, 5.C, 6.D, 7.D, 8.A, 9.D

CHAPTER 4

Health, Wellness, Illness, and Disability

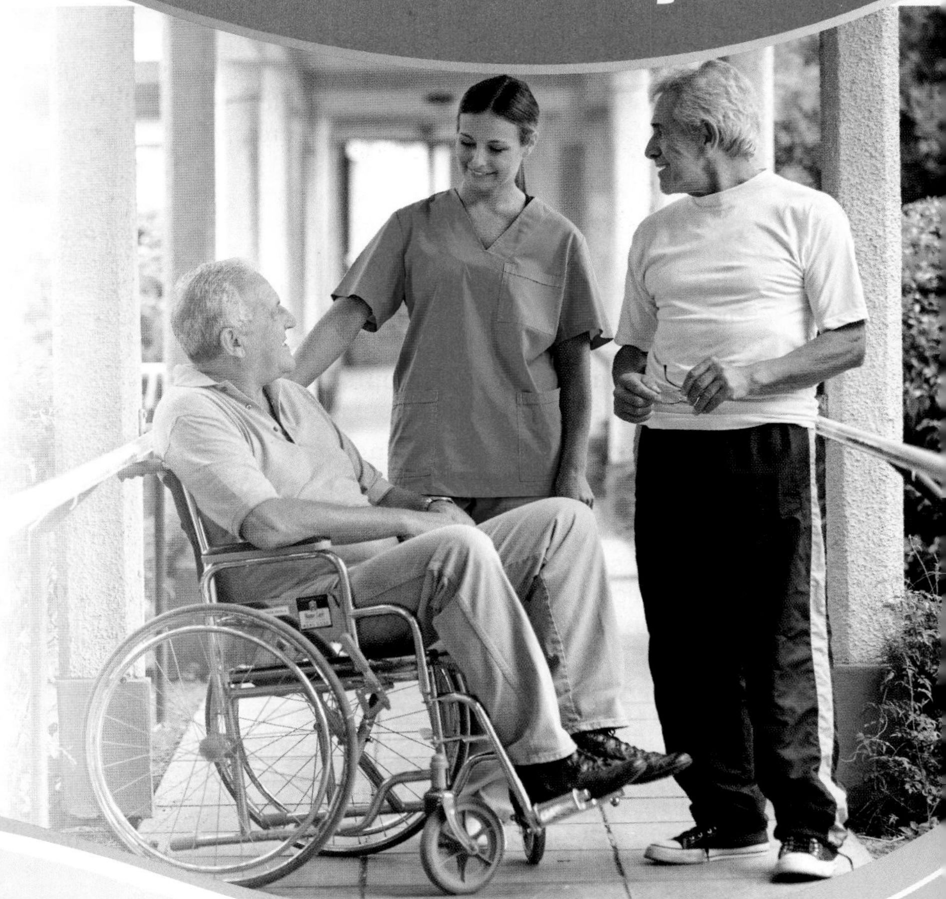

OBJECTIVES

After reading this chapter, the learner should be able to do the following:

- Differentiate between the current definition of *health* and the one used in the past.
- Describe the concept of holism and explain how it affects the role of a support worker.
- Explain the current concepts of health and wellness.
- Describe how health can be achieved in all dimensions of life.
- Explain the effects of culture, stigma, and discrimination on clients who have illnesses and disabilities.
- Describe personal factors that can influence health.
- Explain how people, families, or communities who follow good holistic health practices can still become very ill.
- Describe the 12 aspects of our health and environment that are beyond our immediate control (known as the *determinants of health*).
- Explain common reactions to illness and disability.
- Describe change and loss associated with illness and disability.

KEY TERMS

attitude A person's beliefs, values, or opinions toward engaging in healthy behaviours. *p. 53*

cognitive health Well-being in the intellectual dimension, achieved through an active, creative mind. *p. 51*

determinants of health The most important factors—such as lifestyle, environment, human biology, and health services—that determine health status in an individual or a community. *p. 54*

dimensions of health All aspects of a person's health: physical, emotional, social, spiritual, cognitive. Holistic health considers all of these aspects. *p. 49*

disability The loss of physical or mental function. *p. 56*

discrimination The unfair treatment of people on the basis of such aspects as their physical characteristics, health history, or group membership. *p. 60*

emotional health Well-being in the emotional dimension, achieved when people feel good about themselves. *p. 50*

environmental health According to the WHO, "all the physical, chemical, and biological factors external to a person and all the related factors impacting behaviours." *p. 55*

equitable Fair, reasonable, and just. *p. 55*

gender The roles, personality traits, attitudes, behaviours, values, and relative power and influence assigned to the sexes by society. *p. 56*

genetic endowment The genetic makeup that predisposes an individual to adopt certain behaviours that affect health status. *p. 56*

health A state of well-being in all dimensions of one's life. *p. 49*

holism A concept that considers the whole person; the whole person has physical, social, emotional, cognitive, and spiritual dimensions. *p. 49*

holistic health A state of well-being in all dimensions of one's life. *p. 49*

illness The loss of physical or mental health. *p. 56*

marginalize The act of excluding people who are not part of the majority culture. *p. 56*

optimal health State of achievable maximum well-being in each of the five dimensions: physical, emotional, social, cognitive, and spiritual. *p. 52*

personal empowerment Understanding and accepting that you can make your own healthy lifestyle choices, free from the influences of others. *p. 54*

physical health Well-being in the physical dimension, achieved when the body is strong, fit, and free from disease. *p. 49*

primary prevention strategies Strategies that are aimed at preventing a disease or illness by reducing its risk factors. *p. 56*

prognosis The expected course of recovery, which may range from full recovery to death, based on the usual outcome of the illness. *p. 57*

social health Well-being in the social dimension, achieved when people have stable and satisfying relationships. *p. 50*

social support system An informal group of people who help each other or others outside the group. *p. 50*

spiritual health Well-being in the spiritual dimension achieved through the belief in a purpose greater than the self. *p. 51*

stigma Social disgrace associated with a particular circumstance, quality, or person that causes one to feel shame or embarrassment—for example, "the stigma of being fired from a job." *p. 60*

wellness The achievement of the best health possible in all dimensions of one's life. *p. 52*

A support worker's job is to help clients achieve or maintain optimal health. But what exactly is "optimal" health? This chapter examines the concepts and experiences of health and wellness as well as illness and disability and tries to explain what optimal health is. A support worker providing supporting care to a client who lives with an illness or disability might be tempted to focus on the medical condition rather than on the *whole* person. However, by trying to understand what the person may be experiencing, support workers can provide better, more compassionate care and support.

As a support worker, you must focus your care and support on improving (or maximizing) a person's health potential, whatever that potential may be. All caregivers need to understand how health practices, lifestyle, and social status can influence a person's health.

"I realized back then that my biggest disability was my attitude."

—Rick Hansen, Canadian activist and athlete with spinal cord injury, on the days immediately following his spinal cord injury

HEALTH AND WELLNESS

Past Definitions of *Health*

The definition of the term **health** has changed over the years. At the end of the 1800s, *health* was defined by what it was not: Health was the state of *not* being sick. At that time, the leading causes of death were diseases that spread from one person to another. Pneumonia, tuberculosis, and influenza, for example, were frequent killers. Anyone lucky enough to avoid being infected during an outbreak was considered healthy. During the first half of the twentieth century, vaccinations, antibiotics, health education, and cleaner living conditions reduced the spread of diseases. People were living longer and getting sick less often. But were they *healthy*?

Modern Definitions of *Health*

During the latter part of the twentieth century, people started to realize that health is more than the absence of disease. As they recognized that health is affected by factors such as lifestyle and environment, liscussions of health began to focus more on the erson rather than on the absence or presence of sease. A *whole person* has physical, emotional, :ial, cognitive, and spiritual dimensions. **Holism** uses on all these **dimensions of health**. Each ıension relates to and depends on the others. rent views on health give importance to **holistic th**—a state of well-being in all dimensions of life (FIGURE 4–1). Providing holistic health care s caring for all dimensions of the person, not ıe physical.

idely accepted definition of health is that of orld Health Organization (WHO), which Health is a state of complete physical, mental, ial well-being and not merely the absence of disease or infirmity." In more recent years, the WHO has also recognized that health includes the ability to lead a "socially and economically productive life."[1]

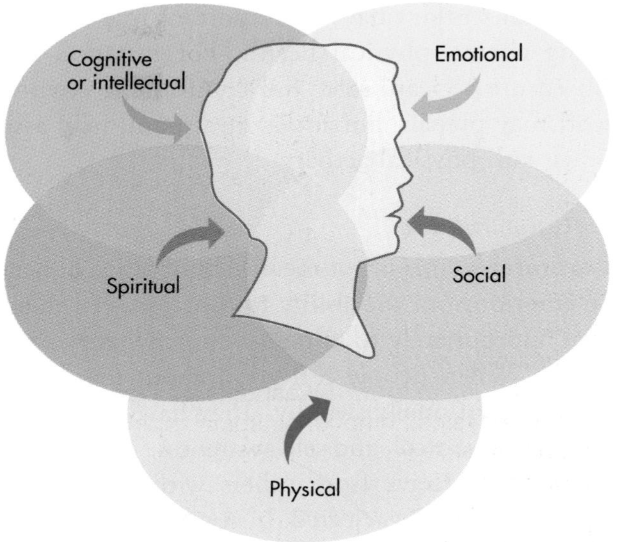

FIGURE 4–1 A whole person has physical, emotional, social, intellectual or cognitive, and spiritual dimensions. Optimal (or holistic) health is a state of achievable well-being in all dimensions.

Dimensions of Health

The five dimensions of health—physical, emotional, social, spiritual, and cognitive—all must be considered in a discussion of whole health. These elements are discussed below.

Physical Health

Influenced by genetics and lifestyle, **physical health** is achieved when the body is strong, fit, and free from disease. The following factors contribute to the physical health of all people, including caregivers:

- Following a nutritious diet according to *Canada's Food Guide* (see Chapter 28)
- Exercising regularly
- Living in a smoke-free environment
- Drinking alcohol moderately or not at all
- Having a good night's sleep
- Maintaining optimal body weight according to body mass index
- Following safety practices, such as using seat belts and bike helmets
- Seeking medical attention when needed

Support workers have an important role in maintaining clients' physical health. For instance, they help ensure a clean, safe, and comfortable environment; may prepare nutritious meals; and may assist clients with physical activity.

Emotional Health

Emotional health is not merely the absence of negative emotions but the ability to function well in and adapt appropriately to circumstances, whatever they may be. When people feel good about themselves, they are emotionally healthy. They have strong self-esteem, self-control, and self-awareness. They are able to give and receive from others without worrying about being hurt or rejected. In contrast, emotionally unhealthy people may be depressed or have intense feelings of insecurity. When upset, they may feel overwhelmed and become aggressive.

Emotional health varies throughout one's life. For example, Mr. Szabo was a confident and happy person and enjoyed many social relationships. However, at the age of 60, a series of tragedies destroyed his emotional health: His daughter died in a car accident, his grandson died from a drug overdose, and Mr. Szabo himself suffered a heart attack. While recovering from the heart attack, he experienced major depression. This example shows that even emotionally strong individuals cannot always withstand misfortune and suffering.

Support workers work with emotionally healthy as well as emotionally unhealthy individuals. The behaviours of some of these clients may be surprising. For instance, a client who is usually cheerful may sometimes be irritable. Avoid judging them. Instead, learn to read your clients' emotions so that you can respond in a caring manner.

Social Health

Social health is achieved through stable and satisfying relationships. Socially healthy people treat others with respect, warmth, and openness. They like and trust others. People with poor social health may show little regard for others and may use others for their own gain.

Few people enjoy strong social health all through life. Feelings of isolation and loneliness are common among older adults and people who have lost their partners, friends, or other social relationships. New immigrants are also at risk for poor social health. Being in an unfamiliar place and not speaking the local language can be very socially isolating.

Most people have friends and acquaintances who help them meet their needs. These needs may be practical, such as a ride to work. Others may be deeper, such as the need for:

- Companionship and a feeling of belonging
- Comfort, emotional support, and encouragement
- Reassurance of one's self-worth
- Help, guidance, and advice

A **social support system** is an informal group of people who help each other or others outside the group. Research has shown that social support systems help improve overall health. Indeed, social support may be as important to wellness as a nutritious diet, a smoke-free environment, and regular exercise. Social support systems can provide food, housing, financial aid, and emotional support during crises. They can make it possible for ill and frail people to continue to stay in their homes rather than move to a facility (FIGURE 4–2). Social supports may also help people who have dementia stay in their homes longer. Support workers may be key members

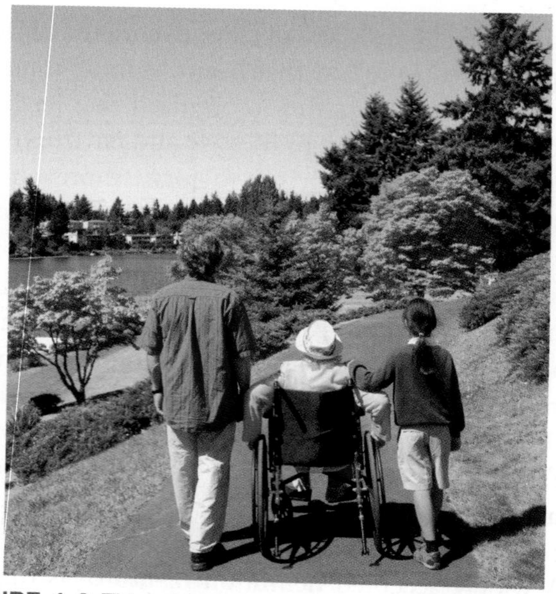

FIGURE 4–2 This older woman is able to stay in her own home because of her strong social support system. She has help from her son, her granddaughter, and support workers. (**Source:** © Big Cheese Photo/maXximages.com.)

of a client's social support system. As a support worker, you provide practical support such as help with activities of daily living (ADLs) and home management and emotional support by practising compassionate care.

Spiritual Health

Spiritual health is achieved through belief in a purpose greater than the self. It may or may not involve being a member of a formal religion or even believing in a higher being. People who are spiritually healthy have a clear understanding of what they believe to be right and wrong, and their behaviours reflect their beliefs. They feel their life has meaning. They are more concerned about personal fulfillment than about material things. Compassion, honesty, humility, forgiveness, and charity are elements of spiritual health.

For some people, spiritual health is closely linked to religion. Being able to attend regular religious worship may be very important for their spiritual health. Support workers must respect clients' expressions of their spirituality. If you work in a facility, you may be responsible for transporting clients to religious services conducted within the building (**FIGURE 4–3**). Make sure you are not late for this task. In a private home, you may see symbols of the person's faith, such as religious icons, displayed in many areas of the house. Always handle these items with respect. People of different cultures may express their spirituality in unique ways (see the *Respecting Diversity: Diversity, Health, and Spirituality* box).

Cognitive Health

Cognitive health is achieved by keeping the mind active and creative throughout life. Recall the last time you talked with a child. You may have marvelled at the curiosity the child showed as she asked

Respecting Diversity

Diversity, Health, and Spirituality

In traditional Indigenous culture, health and spirituality are closely connected. Illness may be prevented if the mind, body, and spirit are in harmony. Indigenous healers include herbalists, diagnosticians, and shamans. In the Cree culture, shamans have special powers to bring the Earth and the spirit world into harmony to aid in the healing process. Today, many Indigenous people combine traditional knowledge with modern health practices.

Source: Potter, P.A., Perry, A.G., Ross-Kerr, J.C., et al. (2010). *Canadian fundamentals of nursing* (rev. 4th ed., p. 129). Toronto, ON: Elsevier Canada.

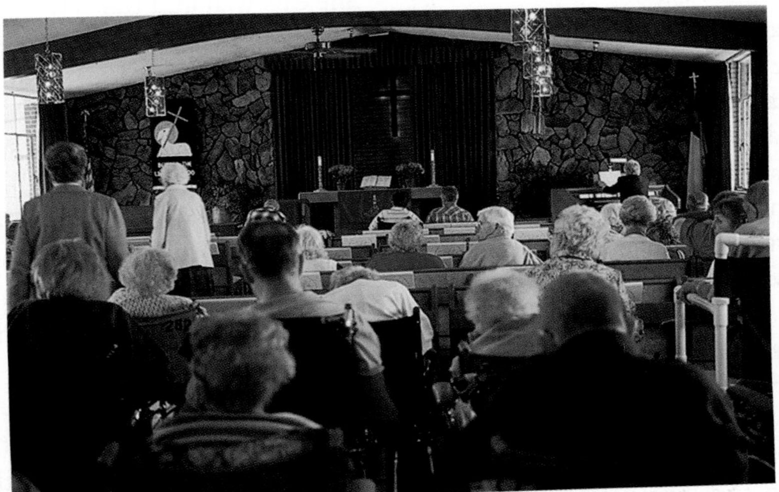

FIGURE 4–3 Residents attend a religious service in their own long-term care facility. (**Source:** Sorrentino, S.A., & Gorek, B. (2004). *Mosby's textbook for nursing assistants* (6th ed., p. 86). St. Louis, MO: Mosby.)

you endless questions. Cognitively healthy people maintain this curiosity throughout life. They are interested in what is going on around them. They analyze, reason, and solve problems. They are open-minded and eager to learn.

People who have cognitive health challenges may try to avoid participating in community and world events and avoid being involved in the lives of others. They may be embarrassed by their loss of ability to think, reason, or communicate as they once did or may suddenly find themselves confused by world events. They often suffer from poor overall health as well. It should be stressed that most people with cognitive health challenges experience these changes not as a result of their lifestyle but rather as a result of their declining overall health.

Many residential facilities have recreational programs and activities that promote cognitive and social health. Residents are encouraged to take part in games and outings that are organized for them. They are encouraged to continue to be intellectually active even when they are in their rooms. Activities such as reading, doing crossword puzzles, keeping indoor plants, doing crafts, and knitting challenge the mind and keep it active. As a support worker, you can promote your clients' cognitive health by encouraging them to perform all these activities and by talking with them about community and world events (**FIGURE 4–4**).

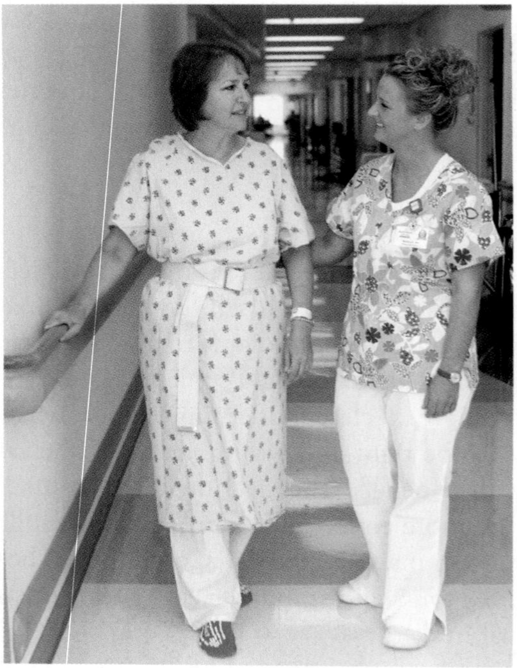

FIGURE 4–4 This support worker is ensuring that the client is walking safely while also providing companionship to the client. Note the support worker's body language. (**Source:** Potter, P.A., Perry, A.G., & Wood, M.J. (2009). *Canadian fundamentals of nursing* (rev. 4th ed., p. 306). Toronto, ON: Elsevier.)

Achieving Optimal Health

Optimal health, or **wellness**, is the achievement of the best health possible in all five dimensions of one's life. It is the perfect balance of body, mind, and spirit. A holistic approach to health care takes into account not only a client's physical health but also his or her psychological well-being and health. This approach, including Erikson's stages of psychosocial development and Maslow's hierarchy of needs, is discussed further in Chapter 12.

Although many people try to achieve wellness, few actually have it. It is difficult to be healthy in all areas of life all the time. At some point, everyone experiences ill health in one or more dimensions. Seeking wellness is a lifelong process. It involves continually making choices that improve quality of life. It also involves becoming one's best self in all areas of life, despite limitations. Therefore, even people with diseases or disabilities can have a high level of wellness.

Interestingly, even some individuals with excellent physical health may not achieve wellness. For example, Soo Hee is an athlete and in excellent shape. She eats well and trains daily. However, she does not make time for friends or family and suffers from loneliness and a lack of meaningful relationships. So she is not content with her life. To achieve wellness, she needs to improve the emotional and social dimensions of her life. Compare her with Josef, who has diabetes but manages his disease well, feels good about himself, and has strong relationships and an active mind. He feels he has a meaningful, productive life. Despite his illness, he has achieved a high level of wellness.

Health is a continuum (**FIGURE 4–5**). On one end is optimal (complete) health or wellness, and on the other end is extreme ill health. A person's place on the continuum shifts, depending on life's circumstances. Remember that health is not constant throughout life. Everyone experiences physical illness

Optimal (Complete) Health ←	Good Health	Average Health	Poor Health	→ Extreme Ill Health
Strong self-esteem/ability to meet life's demands				Severe emotional distress
Healthy lifestyle				Unhealthy lifestyle
Positive social relationships				Social isolation/ depression
Balance of mind, body, and spirit				Imbalance of mind, body, and spirit
Absence of disease				Severe mental or physical illness
Effective handling of disability				Severe mental or physical disability

FIGURE 4–5 We all aspire to optimal health (the far left column) on the continuum of health, but achieving it is rare.

and emotional stress during their lives, and, therefore, most people can be said to have only average health.

Culture and Health, Wellness, Illness, and Disability

Throughout history, some cultures have treated their old and sick members as important persons in need of the utmost care and respect; others cultures, however, have believed that people who cannot contribute to society should be segregated from those who can, in some cases even seeking to exterminate those who were chronically ill, mentally challenged, or otherwise deemed "unacceptable." However, here in Canada, one of our fundamental principles is to accept all people regardless of their differences. Chapter 10 deals in detail with diversity among clients.

Personal Factors That Can Influence Health

We all make choices that affect our health in one way ›r another. Some people eat the wrong foods or drink ›o much alcohol. Others may take drugs, engage in afe sex, or drink and drive. A person's attitude rd health is important since it influences the ›s that person makes. In this context, **attitude** can be defined as a person's beliefs, values, or opinions toward engaging in healthy behaviours.

A number of personal factors can influence our health, but the five main factors are (1) personal lifestyle choices, (2) stress, (3) personal beliefs about health care, (4) social relationships and belonging, and (5) a sense of control. They are described below.

1. Personal Lifestyle Choices

Some people make the wrong health choices for themselves or their family because they lack the knowledge or education to make the right choices. For example, some parents who are not aware of the importance of eating nutritious foods might demonstrate making poor nutritional choices to their children. These children then grow up with their parents' habits and lead their own children to make the same poor choices. This example illustrates the importance of teaching healthy lifestyle choices in Canadian schools.

As a health care worker, you should have healthy habits yourself in regard to drinking alcohol or using recreational drugs. For example, more than two alcoholic drinks a day is harmful for most people. Women who have more than 10 drinks a week have higher rates of cancer and other health problems compared with women who drink less. Men who have more than 15 drinks a week also have higher rates of alcohol-related health problems.[2]

2. Stress

We all must deal with stress in our lives. However, it is the manner in which we deal with our stresses that influences our health in the long term. For example, some people deal with their stresses by drinking excessive amounts of alcohol or by smoking cigarettes (unhealthy behaviours), whereas others choose to go jogging or to meditate (healthy behaviours).

3. Personal Beliefs About Health Care

Personal choices and beliefs can influence whether or not a person will seek medical treatment, take prescribed medications or herbal or nonmedicinal supplements, or even accept care from someone who is not a family member. Personal choices and beliefs can also influence when and how a person will accept care. For example, some people may view North American medicines as poisons and therefore distrust any advice from Western doctors, nurses, or support workers. (See "Culture," one of the determinants of health, on p. 56, as well as Chapter 10.)

Whereas mainstream psychology generally focuses on only one part of the person, such as the person's thinking, feeling, or behaviour, First Nations people include such values as balance, interconnectedness, nature, and spirituality into their view of the delicate balance of health, healing, and spirituality. They believe that interconnectedness is an important part of healing and that balance is important because illness occurs when a person lives in an unbalanced way. First Nations healing practices consider the individual in the context of the family, community, culture, and all of creation. Nature and spirituality, which play a prominent role in First Nations healing practices, have historically been almost nonexistent in mainstream therapies. However, with an ever-increasing understanding of the need for a balanced lifestyle in order to achieve health, mainstream health practitioners are now focusing on healing by incorporating the physical, emotional, mental, and spiritual aspects as important parts of the whole self.[3]

4. Social Relationships and Belonging

It is important to the majority of us to be loved and accepted by others. Some people will make unhealthy lifestyle choices to be accepted by others. For example, a teen may engage in sexual activity before she is emotionally ready because she does not want to "lose" her boyfriend. In another example, even though he knows he has a gambling addiction, a man may go to a casino after work because his friends are going.

5. Sense of Control

Some people make unhealthy lifestyle choices because they feel powerless to make the correct ones. For example, a teen may start smoking cigarettes because his friends pressure him to smoke. When educating about healthy behaviours, many health care workers teach people that they should make their own decisions and realize that they do not *have to be* influenced by the choices of others. This option is called **personal empowerment** and is an important step toward making healthy lifestyle choices.

Influences on Our Health Beyond Our Immediate Control: Determinants of Health

A person might follow good holistic health practices and encourage everyone in the family to do so as well but may still become very ill if he gets a genetic (inherited) health condition. Similarly, in spite of holistic health practices, people (or even an entire community) could become very ill if they live close to a toxic waste dump or are several hundred kilometres from the closest hospital and are unable to access health care.

In Canada, we know that achieving individual health is an important part of a community's health. To ensure the health of all Canadians, we need to improve not only the quality of health care that is available to Canadians but also their living conditions. Realizing that health may be influenced by factors beyond a person's immediate control, Health Canada has tried to identify those factors and to focus its efforts on addressing them. These factors are known as the **determinants of health**.[4] The 12 identified determinants of health focus on the "bigger picture" of where we live—that is, our environment—and how it impacts our health (see the *Case Study: Jason and His Determinants of Health* box). Although each of these factors is important in its own right, it is their *interrelationship* that is of particular importance.

CASE STUDY Jason and His Determinants of Health

This deceivingly simple story illustrates how Jason's environment and life situation (also known as his determinants of health) can affect his health. Every Canadian's health is influenced by his or her own determinants of health.

"Why is Jason in the hospital?"

"Because he has a bad infection in his leg."

"But why does he have an infection?"

"Because he has a cut on his leg, and it got infected."

"But why does he have a cut on his leg?"

"Because he was playing in the junkyard next to his apartment building, and there was some sharp, jagged steel there that he fell on."

"But why was he playing in a junkyard?"

"Because his neighbourhood is kind of run down. A lot of kids play there, and there is no one to supervise them."

"But why does he live in that neighbourhood?"

"Because his parents can't afford a nicer place to live."

"But why can't his parents afford a nicer place to live?"

"Because his Dad is unemployed and his Mom is sick."

"But why is his Dad unemployed?"

"Because he doesn't have much education and he can't find a job."

"But why ...?"

Source: *Towards a Healthy Future: Second report on the health of Canadians*. Public Health Agency of Canada, 1999. Adapted and reproduced with permission from the Minister of Health, 2016.

The 12 key determinants of health are described below:[5]

1. ***Income and social status***. Health status improves as you go up the ladder of income and social standing. High income determines living conditions, such as safe housing, and the ability to buy sufficient, nutritious food. The healthiest populations are those in societies that are prosperous and have an **equitable** distribution of wealth.
2. ***Social support networks***. Support from families, friends, and communities is associated with better health. Such social support networks can be very important in helping people deal with and solve problems as well as in maintaining a sense of control over the circumstances of their life. The caring and respect that occur in social relationships result in a sense of satisfaction and well-being and seem to provide protection against health problems.
3. ***Education and literacy***. Health status improves with level of education. Education is closely connected to socioeconomic status; effective education for children and lifelong learning for adults -e key contributors to the health and prosperity - only of individuals but also of the country as a whole. Education contributes to health and prosperity by equipping people with knowledge and skills for problem solving. It gives people a sense of mastery over their circumstances. It increases job opportunities, income security, and job satisfaction. Education improves people's ability to access and understand information that will help them maintain their health.
4. ***Employment and working conditions***. Unemployment, underemployment, and stressful or unsafe work are associated with poor health. People who have more control over their work circumstances and fewer stress-causing demands in their jobs are healthier and often live longer than those in more stressful or riskier jobs and activities.
5. ***Social supports.*** The importance of social support extends to the broader community. The strength of social networks within a community, region, province or territory, or country is reflected in the institutions, organizations, and practices that people create to share resources and build attachments with others.
6. ***Physical environments***. All aspects of the physical environment (both natural and man-made) directly affect our environmental health. The WHO defines **environmental health** as "all

the physical, chemical, and biological factors external to a person and all the related factors impacting behaviours."[6] It includes the assessment and control of those environmental factors that can potentially affect health. Some aspects of the physical environment include air quality, noise levels, soil and water conditions, climate, safety hazards, and presence of pests. When we can reduce or eliminate harmful influences on our bodies from our physical environment, people within our communities have a greater chance of being healthy.[7]

7. ***Personal health practices and coping skills***. Individuals can take actions to help prevent diseases and promote self-care, cope with challenges, develop self-reliance, solve problems, and make choices that enhance health. Personal health practices are not only the outcome of individual choices. There is a growing recognition that such life "choices" are greatly influenced by the socioeconomic environments in which people live, learn, work, and play. Environments should support and encourage a person to make healthy lifestyle choices in a world where many choices are possible.
8. ***Healthy child development***. A young person's development is greatly affected by his housing and neighbourhood, family income, the level of parents' education, access to nutritious foods and physical recreation, genetic makeup, and access to dental and medical care.
9. ***Biology and genetic endowment***. **Genetic endowment** is a person's tendency toward a wide range of individual responses that affect health status. It provides people with the potential for easy emotional adaptation to their individual situations. Although socioeconomic and environmental factors are important determinants of overall health, in some circumstances, genetic endowment appears to predispose certain individuals to particular diseases or health problems.
10. ***Health services***. Health services, particularly those designed to maintain and promote health, prevent disease, and restore health and function, contribute to population health. The WHO Constitution states that it is the *right* of everyone to have "access to timely, acceptable and affordable health care of appropriate quality."[8]
11. ***Gender***. **Gender** refers to the roles, personality traits, attitudes, behaviours, values, and relative power and influence assigned to the sexes by society. "Gendered" norms influence the health system's practices and priorities. Many health issues are a function of gender-based social status or roles.
12. ***Culture***. People or groups whose cultural practices differ from the dominant cultural practices and values within their socioeconomic environment may face additional health risks. Having different practices and values tends to **marginalize** these people or groups. This marginalization results in a loss or devaluation (lessening of the importance) of their language and culture and a lack of availability to culturally appropriate health care and services.

Disease and Illness Prevention Strategies

Primary prevention strategies aim to prevent disease by reducing risk factors that cause disease. For example, we may come to know that many children living in a particular community are developing a certain type of cancer, but until we make the effort to *prevent* the root cause of the problem—and not just *treat* the cancers—that community will continue to have serious health issues.

ILLNESS AND DISABILITY

Illness is the loss of physical or mental health, whereas **disability** is the loss of physical or mental function. Illness or disability may limit a person's ability to communicate, move, or perform ADLs without assistance. Although the symptoms of acute illnesses can be severe, acute illnesses (such as influenza) and disabilities (such as a broken arm) last for a relatively short period. On the other hand, a persistent, or chronic, illness (such as acquired immune deficiency syndrome [AIDS]) or disability (such as paraplegia) is ongoing, slow or gradual in onset, and may or may not grow worse over time. Because a persistent illness cannot be cured, the focus of care is on preventing the complications of the illness. Both acute and persistent illnesses are discussed further in Chapter 37.

It is important to remember that clients with illnesses and disabilities are whole persons with many

Supporting Mrs. Davidson: Maintaining Cognitive Function

Salman is a support worker at a long-term care facility. He works on the floor for residents with physical problems such as arthritis and osteoporosis. Mrs. Davidson, 92, is a resident on Salman's floor. Mrs. Davidson loves to read. She reads the newspaper every morning and listens to an audiobook in the afternoon. One day, Mrs. Davidson tells Salman that she misses talking about books with other people. Salman knows some other residents who also like to read and listen to stories. He wonders if there is a way to bring these clients together as a group.

Salman suggests to his supervisor that the facility start a book club. He explains that discussing books will help the residents maintain their cognitive function. Belonging to a book club will also help them develop friendships. Salman's supervisor likes his idea and speaks to the recreation director about it. By the end of the month, a weekly book club meeting is up and running, with Mrs. Davidson as its leader. The book club becomes so popular that within a year the members form two separate clubs—one for fiction and another for nonfiction.

dimensions. They are more than their medical conditions. As a support worker, while you help them achieve their best physical health possible, you must also consider their emotional, social, cognitive, and spiritual health (see the *Supporting Mrs. Davidson: Maintaining Cognitive Function* box).

SUPPORTING CLIENTS WITH ILLNESS AND DISABILITY

Illness and disability usually affect all aspects of a client's life. For example, Mr. Spinelli recently suffered severe vision loss. As a result, his cognitive health suffers because he can no longer read or pursue his other hobbies; his social health is affected because he can no longer travel to meet friends; his emotional health suffers because he is frustrated and depressed; and his spiritual life is affected because he is angry at God and no longer wants to attend church services.

No two clients will experience illness and disability in the same way. Some severely ill clients remain cheerful and calm throughout their illness; some who are not seriously ill complain constantly or grow easily sad or frustrated. Many clients with disabilities are not ill, and they do not consider themselves to be ill. Clients who are born with disabilities have never known life any other way, and many clients who get disabilities later in life learn to adjust to their situations and need no further medical care. Although clients' experiences vary, health care providers have identified some common reactions to a newly diagnosed illness or a recently acquired disability (**BOX 4–1**).

Factors affecting a client's experience of illness and disability include:

- The nature of the illness or condition
- The client's age
- The client's level of physical fitness
- The amount and degree of pain and discomfort the client experiences
- The **prognosis** (the expected course of recovery based on the usual outcome of the illness)
- The client's emotional, social, cognitive, and spiritual health
- The client's personality and ability to cope with difficulties
- The client's cultural background, which may influence how she views the illness, seeks treatment, and interacts with caregivers and health care workers (see Chapter 10)
- The presence of emotional, social, and financial support

Change and Loss Associated With Illness and Disability

Clients with a serious illness or a recently acquired disability must cope with change and loss. The following are just a few of the many changes these clients must face.

Change in Routine

During illness, daily routines almost always change. Time previously spent at work or with friends and

BOX 4–1 Common Reactions to Illness and Disability

- ***Fear and anxiety.*** When even minor illnesses can cause anxiety, it is understandable that clients with serious illnesses have many fears and anxieties—the effects of their illness on their family; how they will manage their daily responsibilities; financial issues; their families' future; and death. Some clients worry about any change in their role within the family unit. Clients with disabilities, disfigurements, or speech or memory impairments may worry about embarrassing themselves in front of others. Clients with mental health disorders often experience severe anxiety. Some of the fears of clients may make sense to you as a support worker; others may not. To the person experiencing the fear, however, it is real. Some clients will communicate their fear and anxiety to you, but many will not and may prefer to keep their concerns to themselves.
- ***Sadness and grief.*** Clients facing any kind of loss are usually sad. Those with serious illnesses and disabilities often deal with many kinds of losses—loss of position, loss of independence, loss of confidence. For some, there is loss of their dreams for the future. These losses can cause intense grief. These clients are grieving and need to mourn. Observe and listen to your clients so that you can understand their needs. Some clients may not want to talk about their feelings, whereas others may find it helpful to talk to an understanding, caring person.
- ***Depression.*** Fear, anxiety, sadness, and grief can cause anyone to feel depressed. This manifestation is called *reactive depression* (see Chapter 35). However, clients who are coping with serious illnesses, progressive disabilities, or, in the case of some older clients, the losses of lifelong friends and family members are at risk for more serious depression called *clinical depression*. Clients who are depressed are often tired, anxious, and uninterested in life. They may avoid contact with other people. Clients who are severely depressed may be suicidal. Observe closely for any changes in a client's mood, energy levels, and behaviour. Report these changes to your supervisor immediately (see Chapter 35).
- ***Denial.*** Denial is a refusal to recognize and admit the truth. Clients who are afraid that they might be seriously ill may downplay or deny symptoms. Even clients who know that they are seriously ill may deny their situation. For example, a teenager with diabetes may refuse to take her insulin or may demand foods that she should avoid. A middle-aged man with heart disease may continue to shovel his driveway in spite of his doctor's strict order not to do such heavy work. Their way of coping may be to deny that they have serious health problems. If you think a client is denying his or her condition, be understanding and show a positive attitude. If the person's denial may cause harm, let your supervisor know.
- ***Anger.*** Some clients may be angry because they resent their limitations, their illnesses, and their inability to have control over their lives. They may direct their anger toward their physician, family, friends, or caregivers. Some clients may direct their anger toward their support worker. If you become the target of a client's anger, you should remain calm, patient, and gentle with the client. Avoid becoming angry yourself. Reacting negatively will only make the situation worse. Try to understand the client's needs and problems. Imagine what life must be like for him. However, you do not have to accept abuse. See Chapters 16 and 35 to learn what to do when faced with an angry client.

Source: Potter, P.A., Griffin Perry, A., Ross-Kerr, J.C., et al. (2009). *Canadian fundamentals of nursing* (4th ed., p. 129). Toronto, ON: Elsevier Canada.

Supporting Mr. Vitale: The Effect of Serious Illness on Self-Esteem

On Wednesday, Tony Vitale felt on top of the world. He got up at 6:00 a.m., as usual, and ran for half an hour. Over breakfast, he reviewed the speech he was to give at his company's annual meeting. He was looking forward to announcing that profits were up. At the age of 46, he had achieved his life's goal of becoming the chief executive officer (CEO) of a major corporation.

Mr. Vitale never gave his speech. As he stepped up to the podium, he let out a short gasp and collapsed to the floor. When he awoke 10 hours later, he did not recognize his wife or his 2 children. He could not speak or understand anything that was said. He had suffered a severe stroke.

Within 4 months, it became clear that Mr. Vitale would never recover sufficiently to be able to return to his job. Although his memory eventually returned, his speech remained difficult for others to understand. He also had difficulty understanding others. The news that his position had been filled by a new CEO overwhelmed him with sadness and anger. Throughout his adult life, Mr. Vitale's job had given him the recognition, prestige, and status that he desired. Without it, he felt useless and depressed. He slowly began to be consumed by anger. He was angry at his body for "betraying" him and at his caregivers for not being able to "make him better." He shouted at his family each time they came to visit him. He was angry that they were able to survive without him.

During 8 months of therapy and rehabilitation, Mr. Vitale made impressive progress. Although he found long sentences difficult to comprehend, other people could now understand much of what he said. With the support of his family and a caring health care team, his depression was gradually reduced. He began to realize that he still had something to offer to the world. This realization also helped lift the anger that had pressed him down. He understood that his family loved him, and he began to feel pride that they were independent enough to survive without his financial support. He discovered that he enjoyed painting. He spent time volunteering with people who had sustained a brain injury. His newfound self-esteem came from the knowledge that he was making a useful contribution.

family is often now filled with doctors' appointments, tests, and treatments. For many clients, simple ADLs suddenly become challenges. Such routine matters as getting to the bathroom, making meals, eating, and controlling pain now become serious issues.

Change in Work Life

Many clients with serious illnesses or disabilities quit their jobs or limit their workloads. Clients who used to feel rewarded and fulfilled by their work may suddenly feel worthless when they can no longer do it (see the *Supporting Mr. Vitale: The Effect of Serious Illness on Self-Esteem* box). The loss of work may also result in financial problems and loss of social interactions.

Change in Family Life

Serious illness or disability almost always disrupts family life. When one family member is ill, often the lives of everyone in that person's home change greatly. Every family member must make adjustments to the new situation and take on new roles. For example, Mrs. Kim has survived a severe stroke. She can no longer be the sole provider and caregiver for her teenage children. Her role changes to that of a person who needs care. While she recovers, her children must take care of her, with help from professional caregivers. The children may have to give up after-school activities or time with their friends.

Changes and new roles often create stress. Sometimes the stress on family members is so severe that their own health suffers as a result (see Chapter 11).

Change in Sexual Function

Disability and illness often affect sexual function. The client may feel unfit for closeness and love and may lose interest in sex. Or the adverse effects of medications or the illness itself may render a client physically unable to have sex. Reproductive surgery, heart disease, stroke, spinal cord injuries, and nervous disorders are some of the conditions that can affect sexual function in men and women. Changes in sexual function can significantly affect clients and their partners. Fear, anger, worry, and depression are common but normal and expected reactions. Time, understanding, and a caring partner will be helpful to the client. Professional counselling may help the client and his or her partner adjust to the situation.

Loss of Independence

Independence is the state of being able to do things for oneself. Losing one's independence can be very hard. It is particularly distressing when the onset of the illness or disability is sudden and there is little or no hope for recovery. As the support worker, you must try at all times to enable your clients to be as independent as they can be.

Loss of Dignity

Independence and dignity are closely related. For some clients, loss of independence can lead to loss of dignity, particularly when they need help with personal care. It can be extremely difficult for some clients to have to depend on others to perform private functions, including bodily functions. Always be sensitive to your clients' need for dignity.

Change in Self-Image

Self-image is the individual's view of himself or herself. Changes to a person's body caused by illness may affect self-image. Clients who have lost body parts or have scars from surgery or accidents may feel that they are unattractive or even repulsive. Others who have conditions that negatively affect the way they look, move, walk, or speak may feel very self-conscious.

You can help clients with illnesses and disabilities by understanding how their condition affects various aspects of their lives. Do not make assumptions. Do not judge the person's behaviour or compare one client's reaction to illness with another's. Do everything you can to communicate warmth, acceptance, and respect to clients. Always keep in mind the goal of support work (DIPPS—see Chapter 1). (See the *Providing Compassionate Care: Caring for Clients With Illnesses or Disabilities* box.)

Attitudes of Others Toward Illness and Disability

Some people are uncomfortable or fearful when they encounter people who have illnesses or disabilities. Other people may stare or avoid eye contact. They may treat the person with an illness or disability differently from the way they treat people who are well and able-bodied.

Ms. Leblanc used a wheelchair after an injury to her spinal cord. She said that it was very hard getting used to the way some people treated her. "The first time my husband and I went out to dinner after the accident, the waiter asked my husband what I wanted for dinner. To the waiter, I was invisible. Since then I have met many people who ignore me or treat me like a child. I've learned to live with it, but it still hurts."

Some clients experience stigma and discrimination because of their illness or disability. **Stigma** is social disgrace associated with a particular circumstance, quality, or person that causes one to feel shame or embarrassment. One person describes her experience with stigma: "My arthritis was so bad that I wasn't able to type any longer. Because of that, I was fired from my job, and now, my former co-workers treat me differently. I can just feel it. I haven't been able to face any of them either because I am so ashamed." A person who is stigmatized by others is thought of as being different in a negative way. **Discrimination** is the unfair treatment of people on the basis of such aspects as physical characteristics, health history, or group membership. Some clients with AIDS, mental health disorders, or substance abuse disorders are likely to face discrimination. Sometimes, they are blamed for their conditions and they and their families are deprived of much-needed social support. Such rejection can lead to isolation, loneliness, and depression as well as feelings of self-blame and guilt.

The language that we use can also convey negative or demeaning images of people, especially those who have disabilities (see **BOX 4–2**). It is important to use language that is inclusive, respectful, and accurate at all times.

Providing Compassionate Care

Caring for Clients With Illnesses or Disabilities

- ***Dignity.*** Needing help with bathing, toileting, and other ADLs can be extremely embarrassing and can affect a client's dignity. Never expose a client's body unnecessarily. Be aware of your facial expressions and gestures while you are providing care, as they may reveal that you are disturbed by the client's disfigurement or body odours. Such a reaction will cause feelings of shame in the client.
- ***Independence***. Encourage clients to participate in their care. Tell them what you are about to do and ask if they can help. Clients may be able to carry out some of the steps in a procedure themselves. Also, let clients make decisions for themselves if they are able. For example, clients who are paralyzed may not be able to dress themselves, but they can decide what to wear.
- ***Preferences***. Ask clients how they want tasks done. You may have to ask for specific information. For example, ask them what is important to them, what they enjoy doing, what they are able to do, what they find easy, and what they find difficult.
- ***Privacy***. Clients may, in some situations, feel that their privacy has been violated. They may need to adjust to having caregivers around. Never snoop and look at your client's belongings when you are in a client's room or house. The following actions promote privacy: knocking before entering, drawing curtains and blinds, closing doors and windows, covering the client during personal care activities, and keeping client information confidential. Clients with illnesses or disabilities still have sexual needs, including the need for touching, caressing, and embracing. Allow privacy for clients to fulfill their sexual needs.
- ***Safety***. All clients need to feel safe from harm. Clients with illnesses or disabilities have special safety needs. Check with your supervisor and the care plan for specific safety measures for each client. Look at clients' rooms from their viewpoints and ask yourself if there is a safe passage to the bathroom or if any items could be in the way and cause falls or injuries. When you recognize signs and symptoms of tiredness or overexertion, allow the client time for rest. If you are not sure the client's safety needs are being met, talk to the client and to your supervisor. Follow the safety measures described in Chapter 22.

BOX 4–2 Suggested Guidelines for Language to Promote Positive Images of People With Disabilities

General Guidelines

It is important to remember that words have a precise meaning and are not interchangeable. The following guidelines suggest appropriate terminology to use when speaking or referring to people with disabilities.

- A disability is a functional limitation or restriction of an individual's ability to perform an activity. The word "disabled" is an adjective, not a noun. People are not conditions. It is therefore preferable not to use the term "the disabled" but rather "people with disabilities."
- Avoid categorizing people with disabilities as either super-achievers or tragic figures. Choose words that are non-judgmental, non-emotional, and are accurate descriptions. Avoid using "brave," "courageous," "inspirational," or other similar words to describe a person with a disability. Remember that the majority of people with disabilities have similar aspirations as the rest of the population, and that words and images should reflect their inclusion in society, except where social isolation is the focal point.
- Avoid references that cause discomfort, guilt, pity, or insult. Words like "suffers from," "stricken with," "afflicted by," "patient," "disease," or "sick" suggest constant pain and a sense of hopelessness. While this may be the case for some individuals, a disability is a condition that does not necessarily cause pain or require medical attention.
- Avoid words such as "burden," "incompetent," or "defective," which suggest that people with disabilities are inferior and should be excluded from activities generally available to people without disabilities.

People with disabilities are comfortable with the terminology used to describe daily living activities. People who use wheelchairs go for "walks," people with visual impairments "see" what you mean, and so on. A disability may just mean that some things are done in a different manner, but that doesn't mean the words used to describe the activity must be different.

Remember that, although some disabilities are not visible, it does not mean they are less real. Individuals with invisible disabilities such as epilepsy, hemophilia, and mental health and learning or developmental disabilities also encounter barriers and negative attitudes.

Focus on the issue rather than the disability. If the disability is not relevant to the context, it is not necessary to report it.

Appropriate Words

Instead of...	Please use...
Birth defect, congenital defect, deformity	Person born with a disability, person who has a congenital disability
Blind (the), visually impaired (the)	Person who is blind, person with a visual impairment
Confined to a wheelchair, wheelchair-bound	Person who uses a wheelchair, wheelchair user
Cripple, crippled, lame	Person with a disability, person with a mobility impairment, person who has a spinal cord injury, arthritis, etc.
Hard of hearing (the), hearing impaired	Person who is hard of hearing Note: These individuals are not deaf and may compensate for a hearing loss with an amplification device or system.

BOX 4–2 Suggested Guidelines for Language to Promote Positive Images of People With Disabilities—cont'd

Instead of...	Please use...
Deaf-mute, deaf and dumb	Person who is deaf Note: Culturally-linguistically deaf people (that is, sign language users) are properly identified as "the Deaf" (upper-case "D"). People who do not use sign language are properly referred to as "the deaf" (lower-case "d") or "persons who are deaf."
Epileptic (the)	Person who has epilepsy
Fit, attack, spell	Seizure
Handicapped (the)	Person with a disability
Handicapped parking, bathrooms	Accessible parking, accessible bathrooms
Inarticulate, incoherent	Person who has a speech disorder, person who has a speech disability
Insane (unsound mind), lunatic, maniac, mental patient, mentally diseased, mentally ill, neurotic, psychotic	Person with a mental health disability Note: The term "insane" (unsound mind) should only be used in a strictly legal sense. The expression "person with a mental health disability" is broad. If relevant to the story, you can specify the type of disability, for example, "person who has depression" or "person who has schizophrenia."
Invalid	Person with a disability
Learning disabled, learning disordered, dyslexic (the)	Person with a learning disability
Mentally retarded, defective, feeble minded, idiot, imbecile, moron, retarded, simple, mongoloid	Person with an intellectual disability Note: If relevant to the story, specify the type of disability.
Normal	Person without a disability
Person who has trouble...	Person who needs...
Physically challenged, physically handicapped, physically impaired	Person with a disability
Spastic	Person who has spasms
Suffers from, stricken with, afflicted by	Person with a disability Note: People with disabilities do not necessarily suffer.
Victim of cerebral palsy, multiple sclerosis, arthritis, etc.	Person who has cerebral palsy, multiple sclerosis, arthritis, etc. Person with a mobility impairment, person with a disability

Source: Title: *A Way with Words and Images, Suggestions for the portrayal of people with disabilities*, Human Resources and Skills Development Canada, © 2006, URL: http://www.esdc.gc.ca/eng/disability/arc/way_with_words.pdf. Employment and Social Development Canada, 2016. Reproduced with the permission of the Minister of Employment and Social Development Canada, 2016.

CHAPTER REVIEW

KEY POINTS

- A whole person has physical, emotional, social, cognitive, and spiritual dimensions.
- Holism involves considering all dimensions of health (physical, emotional, social, cognitive, and spiritual), and optimal (complete) health is a state of *achievable* maximum well-being in all of these dimensions.
- Health is a continuum with optimal health or wellness on one end and extreme ill health on the other end. A person's place on the continuum shifts, depending on life circumstances.
- Personal factors that can influence the dimensions of health are (1) personal life skills, (2) stress, (3) personal beliefs about health care, (4) social relationships and belonging, and (5) a sense of control.
- The influences on health that are beyond a person's immediate control are called *determinants of health*. The 12 determinants of health focus on the "bigger picture" of where we live—that is, our environment—and the way it affects our health.
- Illness is the loss of physical or mental health, whereas disability is the loss of physical or mental function.
- Illness or disability usually affects all aspects of a client's life, and no two clients will experience illness or disability in the same way.

CRITICAL THINKING IN PRACTICE

Mr. Jaynz has always eaten warm cereal for breakfast and before bedtime. Why are routines such as eating warm cereal important to people? How can varying his routine affect Mr. Jaynz?

REVIEW QUESTIONS

Answers to these questions are at the bottom of p. 65.

Circle the BEST answer.

1. In the 1800s, good health was considered to be:
   A. Well-being in all dimensions of life
   B. Optimal wellness
   C. The absence of disease
   D. Physical, emotional, and social well-being
2. A holistic approach to health is one that:
   A. Takes a realistic view of a person's health problems
   B. Takes into account the whole person
   C. Focuses on the person's illness or disability
   D. Focuses on the person's physical health
3. Which of the following is one of the five dimensions of health?
   A. Recreational health
   B. Income and social status
   C. Emotional health
   D. Education and literacy
4. Which of the following is one of the key determinants of health?
   A. Cognitive health
   B. Biology and genetic endowment
   C. Fear and anxiety
   D. Change in sexual functioning
5. Which factor *best* contributes to good physical health?
   A. A high-fat diet
   B. Smoking outside
   C. The regular use of seat belts
   D. Avoiding all animal protein
6. People with strong emotional health:
   A. Exhibit self-control
   B. Read the paper and are curious about life
   C. Can become angry easily when provoked
   D. Practise good eating habits

7. A *social support system* is:
- A. A group of people who volunteer in the community
- B. A system of social welfare
- C. An informal network of people who help each other or others
- D. Another term for a health care team

8. An acute illness:
- A. Appears suddenly and lasts for a short time
- B. Is a slow, progressive illness
- C. Results in disability
- D. Is another term for influenza

9. Which of the following is true of persistent illness?
- A. People usually recover.
- B. The symptoms often appear quickly.
- C. Most of us have a persistent illness.
- D. It is a slow, progressive illness.

10. Which of the following is a true statement?
- A. People respond to illness and disability in much the same way.
- B. People's responses to illness and disability vary.
- C. Almost all people with illnesses or disabilities are depressed.
- D. Most people with illnesses or disabilities are in denial.

11. The term *discrimination* means:
- A. Denial
- B. An artificial opening between the colon and the abdominal wall
- C. The unfair treatment of people on the basis of their physical characteristics, health history, or group membership
- D. A refusal to admit the truth

Answers: 1.C, 2.B, 3.C, 4.B, 5.C, 6.A, 7.C, 8.A, 9.D, 10.B, 11.C

Chapter opener image: Robert Kneschke/Shutterstock.com

CHAPTER 5

Interpersonal Communication

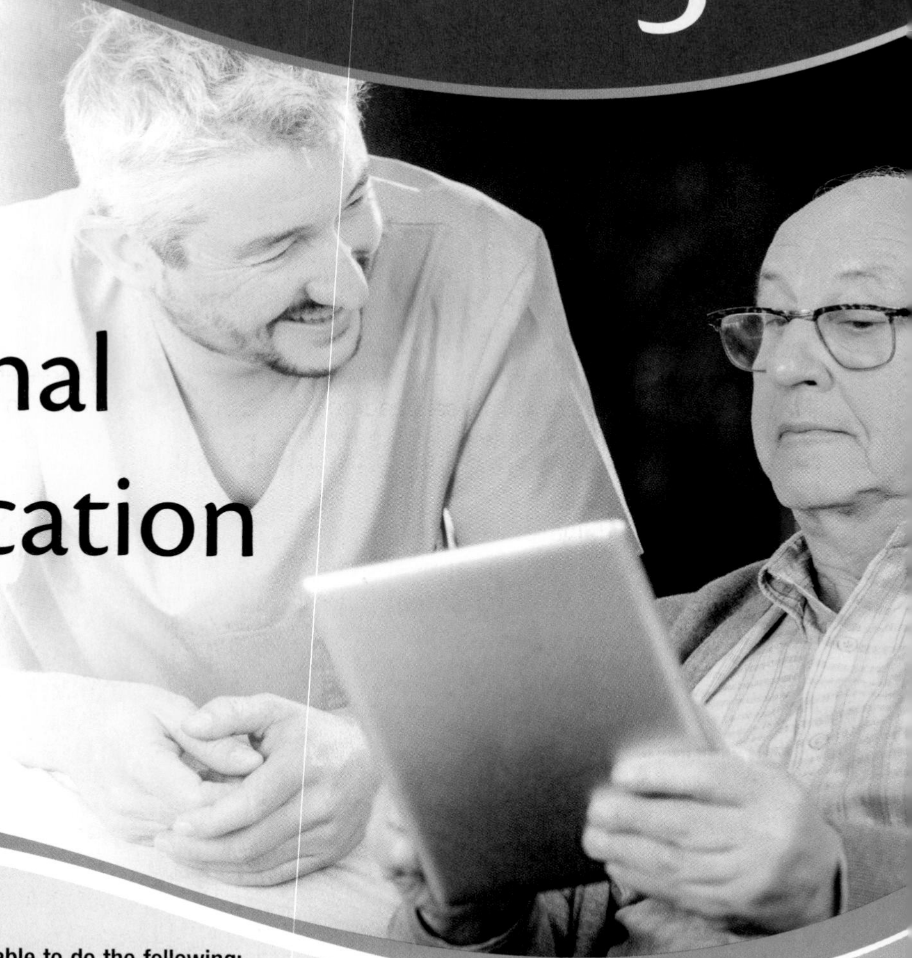

OBJECTIVES

After reading this chapter, the learner should be able to do the following:

- Describe the communication process.
- Describe verbal and nonverbal communication.
- List common defence mechanisms and explain how they can interfere with effective communication.
- Explain the methods of and barriers to effective communication.
- Explain how messages can be misinterpreted when conveyed electronically.
- Describe how to communicate with an angry client.
- Explain why assertive communication is important.
- Learn how to explain procedures and tasks to clients.
- Explain ways to effectively communicate with clients who have dementia.

KEY TERMS

active listening A nonjudgemental communication technique that focuses not only on understanding the content of what is being said but also on the underlying emotions and feelings conveyed by the sender. Active listeners concentrate fully on what is being said and pay attention to the client's nonverbal cues. *p. 71*

assertiveness A style of communication in which thoughts and feelings are expressed positively and directly, without offending others. *p. 79*

body language An important part of nonverbal communication that can reveal a person's physical, mental, or emotional state through powerful messages such as gestures, postures, and facial expressions. *p. 72*

closed questions Questions that are structured so that the response can be restricted to one word such as *yes* or *no* or to a few words. *p. 74*

defence mechanisms A subconscious practice intended to either delay—or avoid altogether—uncomfortable feelings such as anxiety, guilt, stress, or embarrassment. These practices include **denial**, **displacement**, **fantasizing**, **projection**, **rationalization**, **regression**, **repression**, **suppression**, **passive-aggressiveness**, and **submissiveness**. *p. 78*

denial An unwillingness to accept the truth or a certain reality. *p. 78*

displacement A transfer of feelings (usually of anger) onto another person or item instead of onto the person who is the source of the anger. *p. 78*

electronic communication The transfer of information through electronic media. *p. 69*

empathetic listening A nonjudgemental technique that requires the listener to be attentive to the sender's feelings. *p. 74*

fantasizing Daydreaming as an escape instead of dealing with reality. *p. 79*

focusing Limiting the conversation to a certain topic. *p. 76*

interpersonal communication The exchange of information between two people, usually face to face. *p. 68*

nonverbal communication Messages sent without words. *p. 71*

open-ended questions Questions that invite a person to share thoughts, feelings, or ideas. *p. 75*

paraphrasing Restating someone's message in one's own words. *p. 74*

passive-aggressiveness The practice of expressing negative emotions, resentment, or anger toward others through passive, indirect ways (such as through procrastination or manipulation) instead of by verbalizing feelings in an assertive manner. *p. 79*

projection Blaming someone else for one's own behaviour. *p. 79*

rationalization Justifying a behaviour or action by explaining it as being less harmful or hurtful than it really is. *p. 79*

regression A return to an earlier developmental stage as a way to escape from stress. *p. 79*

repression The involuntary action of blocking painful memories from the conscious mind. *p. 79*

social media Websites and applications through which users create virtual communities or networks to share information, ideas, personal messages, and other content. *p. 69*

submissiveness A show of obedience, meekness, and compliance in the face of conflict or a difference of opinion, instead of assertiveness. *p. 79*

suppression A conscious refusal to acknowledge a painful or upsetting situation. *p. 79*

verbal communication Messages sent through the spoken word. *p. 70*

workplace etiquette Professional, ethical, friendly, and respectful behaviour toward all staff and co-workers at all times. *p. 70*

Effective interpersonal communication leads to better relationships with clients, families, and co-workers. It is also necessary for providing safe and effective health care. Health care team members share information about what has been done for the client, what needs to be done for the client, and the client's response to care and treatment. Through your communication with clients, you find out about their needs, feelings, likes, and dislikes and also express your own thoughts and ideas. It is important to the communication process that you understand your personal communication experiences.

You will be taught the theory of communication in class, but in practice, your life experiences will affect your responses to clients. Remember that *what* you say and *how* you say it are of equal importance. Your words, expressions, or gestures can console or upset a client. As you develop your communication skills, your ability to communicate effectively with your friends, family, and clients will improve. You will learn how to interpret messages from your clients and how to respond effectively. You will also gain an understanding of how many people use defence mechanisms as a means of coping with—or avoiding—stressful situations. In this chapter, you will also learn the best way to communicate with a client who has dementia.

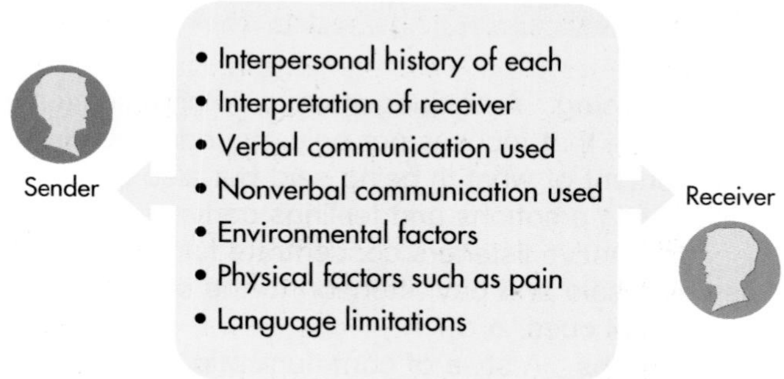

FIGURE 5–1 Communication is affected by the relationship between the sender and the receiver as well as by many other factors.

FACTORS THAT INFLUENCE COMMUNICATION

Interpersonal communication is the exchange of information between two people, usually face to face. A message is sent by one person (the *sender*) and is received and interpreted by another person (the *receiver*). Often, the receiver provides information in response to the message (*feedback*). During the exchange of information, each person usually acts as both a sender and a receiver.

Successful interpersonal communication occurs when the receiver understands the meaning of the message. However, sometimes, the receiver does not interpret the message in the way the sender intended, and mistakes and hurt feelings can occur. At times, the sender may not be aware that the receiver does not understand the message as intended. As well, there is a possibility that the receiver has hearing difficulty or a cognitive problem. The relationship between the sender and the receiver also affects their communication. Communication is easiest when the people involved understand and respect each other (**FIGURE 5–1**). Numerous factors can influence both the communication between members of the health care team, clients, and their family members and the interpretation of the message, such as the following:

- ***Perceptions.*** Perceptions are how a person views events and understands messages. They are based on an individual's culture, education, and personal background. As a support worker, you need to understand that your client's perceptions may be very different from yours and may require you to adjust your communication style.
- ***Experience and confidence.*** Clients can often tell when support workers feel hesitant or uncertain about what they are instructing their clients to do. As a result, the client may hesitate to cooperate with the support worker's instructions and be resistant to care. It is important to try to communicate in an assertive and professional manner at all times.
- ***Physical and mental health.*** Physical and mental conditions can affect not only your client's ability to communicate with you but also your ability to communicate with your client. Chapters 35 through 39 describe some of these conditions and how to better communicate with clients with these conditions.
- ***Mood and emotions.*** Many clients can perceive when their caregiver is angry or upset and will then be hesitant to ask for assistance. As a result, clients can injure themselves trying to do something they should ask for assistance with. As a support worker, you must try to keep your emotions under control at all times. It is also important to be prepared for changes in your client's emotions and respond with appropriate communication. Report and record your observations.
- ***Values.*** Your clients may have values that are different from your own, and these differences can affect their communication with you. As a professional, you must respect your client's methods of communication without making any reference to the difference in values.
- ***Beliefs and cultural influences.*** As a support worker, you will be working with clients from

different cultures. The health care team will need to research these cultures to be able to communicate appropriately with clients and to respect their dignity and their willingness to share information.

- ***Gender.*** Males and females communicate in different ways. Numerous books and other sources of information are available to help you understand the differences in communication styles between the genders. Males tend to use less verbal communication and are more likely to initiate conversations and address issues directly. Females tend to disclose more personal information, use more active listening (see p. 71), and respond in ways that encourage and maintain conversations.
- ***Age.*** People within an age group or culture may use expressions and terms that are not easily understood or may be misinterpreted by others who are not part of that group. For example, the word *dude* might mean "male" to a teenager, but an older adult who has not heard that expression used recently might think that the "dude" was a cowboy! In addition, the onset of hearing and vision loss may make it more difficult for the older person to communicate effectively (see Chapter 40).
- ***Electronic communication and social media.*** **Electronic communication** is the transfer of information through electronic media. **Social media** includes websites and applications through which users create virtual communities or networks to share information, ideas, personal messages and other content. More and more people use social media sites and personal cellphones as a means of communicating with others each day. However, an ever-increasing number of people send written messages to their friends rather than *speaking* to them. While the use of electronic communication has many benefits, messaging and social media sites generally do not require the sender to use body language or other nonverbal forms of communication. In addition, many people use "cyber-speak," which are abbreviations used when communicating electronically through text messages or social media. Not everybody understands these abbreviations, and some may think they have another meaning (**FIGURE 5–2**). As a result, the receiver may not be receiving the messages the sender intended to send.[1,2]

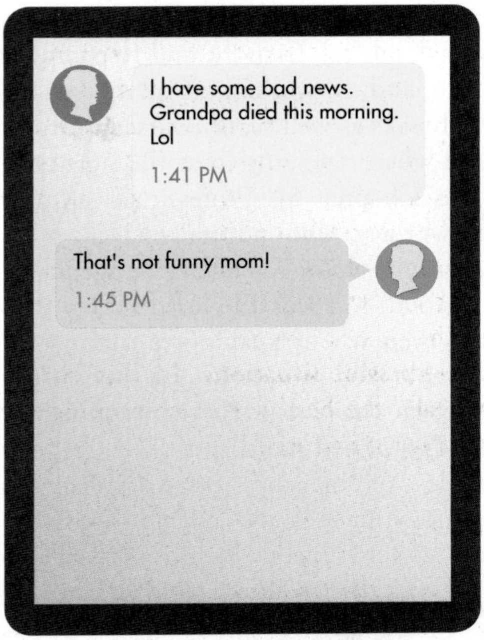

FIGURE 5–2 This exchange shows how the receiver may misinterpret the message that is being sent. The sender thought the abbreviation "LOL" meant "lots of love," while the receiver understood it to mean "laugh out loud."

To communicate effectively with clients, you need to understand, respect, and be sensitive to each client's unique situation and needs, including a client's culture and religion. You also must understand that stresses, problems, and frustrations can affect how a message is sent and received by both you and your client. Remember that clients are whole persons who are coping with illnesses or disabilities. They are physical, emotional, intellectual, social, and spiritual human beings. With this in mind, you must try to understand the real meaning behind their words. Effective communication also requires that your verbal and nonverbal cues do not conflict, that you use language the client can understand, and that you communicate in a professional, caring, and empathetic manner.

PROFESSIONAL COMMUNICATION

Support workers are valued members of the health care team that delivers necessary care to clients. It is therefore important that they act professionally at all times. An important part of professionalism involves professional communication. Avoiding slang terms and swear words and using professional behaviours and body language in the workplace are essential.

Workplace etiquette requires people to behave in a professional, ethical, friendly, and respectful manner to all staff and co-workers at all times, including while on breaks as well as, of course, at team conferences and when reporting in at the start and end of shifts (see Chapter 6). Professional etiquette also requires workers who normally speak a language other than English (or French, if the agency conducts care in French) to speak English in the workplace at all times, even when speaking to a co-worker who uses the same language. It is seen as disrespectful to use a language that excludes others in the room even if not talking directly to them.

Examples of breaches of workplace etiquette include gossiping about clients or other team members either verbally or through the Internet; breaching confidentiality; avoiding eye contact; making nonsupportive facial expressions, such as eye-rolling; speaking a language that others cannot understand; or texting on a cellphone while sitting with co-workers at breaks. Another breach of workplace etiquette is bullying (also sometimes called *horizontal violence*) (see Chapter 16).

Even outside the workplace, people who work in health care, as well as those in many other public-service fields, have to be careful in their communications. For example, it will be increasingly important for you, as a professional, to become more selective about what you post on social media sites. Employers may visit sites when considering you for employment (see Chapter 47). As well, breaches of confidentiality, whether spoken or written, and undesirable behaviours have a way of surfacing and may negatively affect a person's employment status.

When communicating with clients, their families, and the health care team, it is important to remain professional and to understand the difference between a professional relationship and a friendship. A friendship is a voluntary and informal bond between two individuals who share intimacies and seek to spend time together. In contrast, a professional relationship is essentially an assignment. Clients may start to consider support workers their friends as they share their thoughts and concerns. As a professional support worker, however, you should not share your thoughts, personal information, or worries with your client.

Other ways of showing professionalism and courtesy to clients include knocking on closed doors before entering, calling people by their names, and saying "please" and "thank you." You should always introduce yourself to the client before taking any action and explain what you will be doing. Initially, it is respectful to address clients by a courtesy title (e.g., Mr., Ms., Mrs.) and their last name until they ask you to call them by their first name. Using terms such as "honey," "dear," or "sweetheart" is not appropriate and is disrespectful to the client.

Confidentiality

Ensuring confidentiality is an important part of professional communication. In the course of your work, you will learn private and sensitive information about your clients, and this information should be protected. *Only pertinent information should be shared with other team members providing direct care to the client.*

Observing the need for confidentiality includes choosing where and when to discuss a client. For example, discussing a client with staff who are not involved in that client's care is breaching confidentiality. In addition, discussing clients in stairwells, in a lunchroom, or in the parking lot are examples of confidentiality breaches. Confidentiality must extend to your personal time. It is inappropriate, for example, to post pictures of clients or to discuss clients on a social media site or in a personal conversation, even if you avoid using their names.

VERBAL COMMUNICATION

In **verbal communication**, messages are sent through the spoken word. Sometimes, symbols substitute for spoken words; for example, sign language is used to converse with a person who cannot hear.

To effectively communicate with words, you need to do the following:

- ***Choose your words carefully.*** Words must have the same meaning for both you and the other person. Try to avoid words with more than one meaning. For example, the words *small*, *moderate*, and *large* mean different things to different people. Is "small" the size of a pea or the size of a walnut? Instead, use words that are specific and descriptive: Telling your supervisor that a client's temperature is 37.9°C is clearer than saying, "His temperature is up."

- ***Be aware that emotions can affect your communication.*** A person who is angry or upset can unintentionally convey these feelings when he communicates with others. This display of emotion may, in turn, confuse or upset the listener, who is not aware of the background context of why you are communicating in such manner. It is important to maintain a positive attitude at all times when speaking to clients, their families, or co-workers.
- ***Use simple, everyday language.*** You will become familiar with medical terminology as you study and gain experience in health care. However, do not use these medical terms when communicating with clients and their families because these terms may be unfamiliar to them. Also, use correct grammar, and avoid vulgar words and slang. Be aware that culture may influence people's choice of words and how they use them. By using certain words, you may insult or confuse a person from another culture.
- ***Speak clearly, slowly, and distinctly.*** Do not mumble or speak quickly. Move your lips as you speak, slow down your speech, and pause between sentences. Do not, however, slow down your speech so much that your client feels embarrassed by it. Ensure the room in which you are communicating is well lit and quiet so the client can see your facial expressions and body mannerisms. Do not shout or overexaggerate words; doing so will distort your speech.
- ***Use visual clues.*** Write your message down for clients who cannot hear but can read, and use objects or pictures to help them understand. For example, show the client the meals he or she can choose from.
- ***Control the volume and tone of your voice.*** How your voice sounds sends a message. Do not shout, because shouting can suggest irritation or anger. Similarly, do not talk in a harsh or abrupt manner. As well, avoid speaking to adults in high-pitched tones as you might when speaking to children.
- ***Be brief and concise.*** Do not add unrelated or unnecessary information. Focus on what you are saying, stay on the subject, and do not use too many words. Instructions that are too wordy may confuse the client and may reduce the possibility of the client understanding them. Speak in short sentences to emphasize your words, as short sentences are more clearly understood.
- ***Present information in a logical manner.*** Organize your thoughts before you speak, and present them in sequence (in the right order). Think about what has happened, or what is going to happen, step by step.
- ***Ask one question at a time.*** Give the client time to answer each question you ask, and do not rush him. Avoid providing the answer for the client.
- ***Determine understanding.*** Do not assume that the client understands what you are saying. Ask the client to repeat the message in her own words.
- ***Do not pretend to understand.*** If you do not understand what the client has said, ask him to restate or rephrase the message. Repeat the message, if needed, to indicate that you have understood it.

Humour

Humour is an important, but often underused, technique in communicating with clients and co-workers. Research has shown that laughter shared among clients, family members, and the support worker can reduce tension, increase trust, and promote bonding. When caring for clients whose first language is not the same as your own, however, you may not be able to use verbal humour, because it may be misunderstood or misinterpreted. Gauge whether the use of humour would be both comfortable for you as a support worker and appropriate for your client.

NONVERBAL COMMUNICATION

In **nonverbal communication**, messages are sent without words through body language, touch, and the use of silence. The meaning of messages sent through nonverbal communication varies, depending on the sender's age, gender, life experiences, and culture (see Chapter 10). Using active listening skills to observe your clients' body language can help you understand them better. **Active listening** is a nonjudgemental communication technique that focuses not only on understanding the content of what is being said but

Supporting Mr. Reyes: Verbal and Nonverbal Behaviours Send Differing Messages

Most older clients are aware of your body language

You have been giving support care to Jim Reyes in his home for several months. His physical condition has deteriorated, and he now requires 24-hour care. You are making your last home visit today and ask him how he is doing. Mr. Reyes says, "I am looking forward to moving to the nursing home. I am sure I will make some new friends." However, you see tears in his eyes and he looks away from you. His verbal communication suggests that he is happy, but his nonverbal communication shows sadness. How can you give him support and comfort?

Most older clients are aware of your body language

also on the underlying emotions and feelings conveyed by the sender. A person listens actively by concentrating fully on what is being said and paying attention to the client's nonverbal cues, as well as by conveying interest in the conversation by nodding, making eye contact, and responding when appropriate. This technique helps develop rapport and fosters a trusting relationship. For example, a slumped posture and a slow, shuffling walk may indicate that a client is not happy or is not feeling well. Sometimes, clients may say they feel fine, but their facial expressions may indicate that they are in pain. Nonverbal clues often reflect a person's true feelings, and because they are usually involuntary and unconscious, they may send messages more accurately than words can (see the *Supporting Mr. Reyes: Verbal and Nonverbal Behaviours Send Differing Messages* box).

Body Language

Body language includes the following:

- Posture
- Appearance (dress, hygiene, and adornments such as jewellery, perfume, visible tattoos, the presence of many piercings and obvious use of cosmetics)
- Facial expressions
- Body movements
- Eye contact
- Gestures

Body language greatly affects communication and can change the meaning of a verbal message. For example, someone can say, "Yes, I can do that" while either smiling in a friendly manner or rolling his eyes and sighing. In both cases, the body language sends a message. A person who says one thing with words but another with body language is sending *mixed messages*, which are confusing and unhelpful.

Just as you can learn from your client's body language, you need to be aware of the messages *you* send with your appearance and body language. Your facial expressions and how you stand, sit, walk, and look at a person all send messages. Your body language should show interest and enthusiasm for your work and caring and respect for your clients. For example, show respect to a client who is in a bed or wheelchair by sitting or squatting so that you are at eye level. Your general appearance also communicates information. Some clients and their families may assume that you will provide poor care if you show up in a wrinkled or soiled uniform. Visible tattoos, especially with images such as skulls, dragons, or weapons, and body piercings may startle, frighten, or intimidate some clients.

In some situations, you may need to consciously control your body language when providing care to clients. Do not react visibly, for example, to bodily odours; often such odours are beyond the control of clients. Your reaction is likely to increase a client's embarrassment and humiliation.

Touch

Touch is a very important form of nonverbal communication. It can convey warmth, comfort, concern, affection, trust, and reassurance. For example, holding a person's hand can provide comfort, and gently stroking a person's shoulder or back can promote rest and relaxation. The use of touch is very personal. While most people respond well to a touch on their hand because it helps them feel less lonely, not everyone would feel comfortable being hugged or patted on the head. Your touch should be gentle, not hurried or rushed, and should be restricted to

CASE STUDY Silence and Touch During Sad Times

How do you show your client that you care? Words may not be enough. You may have to be completely silent and comfort the client just with your touch if it is culturally allowed and the client gives permission. Often, holding the client's hand can provide more comfort than words can. Jessica, a support worker in a long-term care facility, relates this experience:

"Mrs. Robinson has lived in our facility for 3 years. She is severely disabled by osteoarthritis. She is a friendly, cheerful woman, who rarely complains. One morning, she didn't reply when I knocked on her door. After knocking three times, I opened the door. I was afraid that she was ill. She was sitting in her wheelchair. She looked very sad. I sensed that something was wrong.

"I sat down in a chair beside her and asked if I could help. When there was no reply, I placed my hand on hers. I didn't say anything. After a few minutes, she told me that her son had just called. Her grandson had been killed in a car accident. He was 19, and he had just finished his first year at university. I told Mrs. Robinson that I felt very sad for her. We sat there quietly, my hand on hers, for 5 minutes. I asked her if anyone else at the facility knew and if there was anything that I could do. She asked me to tell the nurse. Then she said, 'You are very kind to sit with me. I know how busy you are.'"

"public" areas of the body, such as the hands or shoulders. Your employer and the care plan will direct your care.

Touch can mean different things to different people. Pulling away or tensing of the body may indicate that the client does not want to be touched because she is in pain and it hurts to be touched. Or she may be uncomfortable with touch because of her cultural background. For some people who have experienced torture, spousal or child abuse (physical, sexual, or both), rape, or bullying, any touching from another person may be beyond uncomfortable. ***It is very important that you ask your client for permission each time you touch his body or possessions.***

Silence

The use of silence can convey messages of acceptance, rejection, fear, or the need for quiet and time to think. As a support worker, you may find it difficult to accept silence when you want to comfort your client. Sometimes, however, especially during sad times, you do not need to say anything; just being there shows that you care. Silence can give you and others time to organize thoughts and choose words. It is also useful when the client is making difficult decisions or is upset and is trying to regain control. In these situations, silence on your part shows respect and empathy for the client (see the *Case Study: Silence and Touch During Sad Times* box).

COMMUNICATION METHODS

Certain communication skills help you share information more effectively with others and result in better relationships with people.

Active Listening

As discussed on page 71, *active listening* means paying close attention to a client's verbal and nonverbal communication—listening to the content, the intent, and the feelings behind the words. Remember, nonverbal clues may reveal the client's true feelings. For example, Mrs. Gorecki tells you that her knees do not hurt today. However, you observe that she is rubbing her knees and grimacing. Her nonverbal behaviour indicates that she is in pain.

Active listening requires you to be interested in your client and to show that you care. The following are guidelines for active listening:

- ***Face the client.*** Your client will often need to see your facial expressions and body language to be assured that you are listening.
- ***Make eye contact.*** However, do consider cultural preferences in regards to eye contact.

- ***Lean toward the client.*** Do not sit back with your arms crossed. Crossed arms can be interpreted as an indication that you are not open to what the client is telling you.
- ***Respond to your client.*** Note, however, that sometimes your client just may not want to talk or may not respond to your normal communication style.
- ***Avoid communication barriers.*** See page 76.

Paraphrasing

Paraphrasing is restating another person's message in one's own words. A paraphrase usually uses fewer words than the original message. Paraphrasing serves three purposes:

1. It shows that you are listening.
2. It lets both you and the sender know that you understood the message.
3. It promotes further communication.

People usually respond well to a paraphrased statement. For example:

Mrs. Cummings: I was a keen reader when I could see. I miss books so much. Those talking books are hard to follow.

You: You love stories, but talking books are not as good as real books.

Mrs. Cummings: Exactly. I wish you had time to read to me.

When paraphrasing, try not to interpret the client's words. Guide the conversation in such a way that the client feels comfortable expressing thoughts or feelings. If you misinterpret a client's meaning, you could put an end to the conversation or cause offence (see the *Case Study: Using Paraphrasing and Questioning Skills* box for an example of effective paraphrasing).

Empathetic Listening

Empathetic listening requires being attentive to the speaker's feelings. *Empathy* means being open to and trying to understand the experiences and feelings of others. It involves acknowledging the other person's point of view without judging. Clients need to know that they are understood. Empathy can help reduce feelings of loneliness and sadness and can create bonds of trust between a support worker and the clients they support.

When paraphrasing, you acknowledge the other person's words. When empathizing, you acknowledge his feelings. To show empathy, follow the person's lead. While he speaks, listen quietly. Do not rush him or change the subject. Stay focused on him and not on your own opinions. For example, if the client mentions a difficult situation, you could say, "I can see you are upset. Do you want to talk about it?" This comment shows that you recognize and care about how he feels.

Avoid quick, thoughtless responses such as the following:

- "I know how you feel." (Nobody can ever know how another person feels.)
- "I feel sorry for you." (This implies pity.)
- "I wouldn't want to be in your shoes." (This suggests superiority and implies pity.)

Consider these two responses to a complaint:

Mr. Witowski: I can't believe they have made me move to this new room. I felt settled in the other room, and I liked the view of the lawn and the pond. Now all I see when I look out the window is an asphalt parking lot.

Jane: The move couldn't be helped, unfortunately. The old wing was falling apart.

Carlos: Being moved can be upsetting. Your old room had a lovely view. I can see why you miss it.

Jane's response is not empathetic—she focuses on facts, not on Mr. Witowski's feelings. Carlos's response is empathetic—he paraphrases Mr. Witowski's statement, which lets Mr. Witowski know Carlos has understood his message, and then he acknowledges his feelings about moving.

Asking Closed Questions

Closed questions focus on specific information, so use them when you need to learn something precise. Some closed questions require a yes or no answer. Others require a brief response. For example:

CASE STUDY Using Paraphrasing and Questioning Skills

Sophia provides personal care to 48-year-old Mr. Dupuis. He is severely disabled by multiple sclerosis. On her first visit, Sophia helped Mr. Dupuis shave and dress. On this second visit, she is to assist him with bathing and preparing breakfast.

Mr. Dupuis: Oh, it's you. I was still asleep. It's awfully early.

Sophia: A 7:30 start is a little early for you. You're not ready for me. *(paraphrasing)*

Mr. Dupuis: Yes, I've asked the case manager to start the morning care at 8:00 instead.

Sophia: Perhaps she is working on the schedule change. I will check with the agency.

Mr. Dupuis: Thanks.

Sophia: The care plan calls for a bath today. Would you like to rest in bed until I prepare your breakfast and then do your bath after you have had your breakfast? *(closed question)*

Mr. Dupuis: It doesn't matter much. I wish I didn't need to take a bath. Being bathed by someone else is not much fun.

Sophia: Can you tell me what you dislike about your bath? *(open-ended question)*

Mr. Dupuis: The lack of privacy really bothers me.

Sophia: We can work together on giving you privacy.

Mr. Dupuis: That would be a good idea. I don't think my last support worker cared much about my privacy.

Sophia: We will work on this, and I will try to provide you with more privacy.

Paraphrasing and questioning skills can help you improve the care you provide to your clients. In this case, Sophia listens to Mr. Dupuis and uses paraphrasing, closed questions, and open-ended questions in her responses. Sophia uses paraphrasing to show Mr. Dupuis she has understood his concern and to prompt him to provide more information. She asks a closed question when she needs specific information about Mr. Dupuis's preferences. She asks an open-ended question to encourage Mr. Dupuis to share his feelings about being given baths. Once Sophia understands Mr. Dupuis's worries about privacy, she can take steps to solve this problem.

You: Would you like butter on your toast this morning, Mrs. Cummings?

Mrs. Cummings: Yes, please.

You: Would you like strawberry jam or marmalade?

Mrs. Cummings: Marmalade, please.

Asking Open-Ended Questions

Open-ended questions invite a person to share thoughts, feelings, or ideas. Answers must be more than a yes or no. However, the person being questioned chooses and controls what is talked about and the information given. Consider these questions: "What was it like growing up in Scotland, Mrs. Cummings?" (open-ended question) and "Did you like living in Scotland?" (closed question). The first question encourages Mrs. Cummings to talk about herself. It shows her that you are interested in hearing about her life. The second question requires a yes or no answer. It does not encourage Mrs. Cummings to talk about herself, nor does it communicate as much interest in her life.

Use open-ended questions in combination with closed questions to find out about a client's needs and preferences and to find out if a client is satisfied with your care. For example, a closed question ("Are you comfortable?") can give you the necessary information. An open-ended question ("Is there anything I can do to make you more comfortable?") can encourage a client to express thoughts or feelings. The *Case Study: Using Paraphrasing and Questioning Skills* box shows an example of a support worker using both types of questions to improve a client's care.

Clarifying

Clarifying helps you make sure that you have understood a person's message. You can ask the person to repeat the message, say that you do not understand, or restate the message as a question. For example:

- "Could you say that again?"
- "I'm sorry, Mr. Hart. I don't understand what you mean."
- "Are you saying that you want to go home?"

Focusing

Focusing is limiting the conversation to a certain topic. It is useful when a client rambles or wanders in thought. Consider these examples:

- Mr. Reyes talks at length about his favourite foods and restaurants. You need to know why he did not feel like eating dinner. You focus the conversation on the subject of dinner by saying, "Let's talk about today's dinner. You said you didn't feel like eating."
- The care plan for Mrs. Hooda directs you to provide two choices when helping her dress. She becomes distracted by the pattern on one of the dresses. You guide the conversation back to the task of dressing by saying, "Would you like to wear the dress with the pretty pattern?"
- Mrs. Cummings has just told you that she does not want to go for a walk. She then reminisces about her early life. Your response encourages her to focus on her reason for not wanting to walk:

Mrs. Cummings: We used to walk for miles in the Lake District. It was usually raining. It rained constantly in Edinburgh, too.

You: There is no rain today, and the sun is shining. Let's go for a walk and not get wet.

COMMUNICATION BARRIERS

Communication barriers prevent the sending and receiving of messages, limiting communication or causing it to fail completely. Some barriers cannot be avoided, so they must be worked around. For example, some clients have hearing and vision problems that interfere with communication, and some clients have nervous system disorders that limit communication. As a support worker, you must learn special techniques to communicate effectively in these situations (**FIGURE 5–3**; see Chapters 39 and

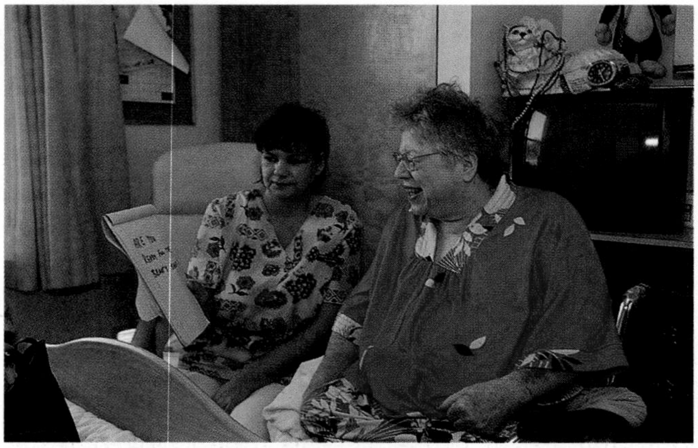

FIGURE 5–3 The support worker communicates with a client with impaired hearing by writing a note.

40). Cultural differences can also interfere with communication since clients may attach different meanings to verbal and nonverbal communication (see Chapter 10). Other barriers include factors in the environment, such as loud noises, lack of privacy, and distractions. As much as possible, try to ensure a calm, quiet setting when talking with a client.

Certain behaviours can also create communication barriers. Improve communication with clients by avoiding the following: interrupting, answering your own questions, giving advice, minimizing problems, using patronizing language, and failing to listen.

Interrupting

Interrupting a person stops communication. People usually interrupt others when they:

- Jump to conclusions about what the speaker is trying to say
- Become impatient with the speaker or the way the story is being told
- Become bored and wish to change the subject to something more interesting
- Wish to change the subject because the topic is upsetting
- Feel hurried or stressed
- Are focused on a task, not on the person

Answering Your Own Questions

Avoid answering your own questions. Some people do this in any conversation they have, and others do it only with people who take a long time to respond. Answering questions or completing thoughts for people discourages openness. Note the following different responses to the same question, phrased slightly differently:

You: How did you sleep last night? Okay? *(answer provided)*

Mrs. Cummings: Yes.

You: How did you sleep last night? *(answer not provided)*

Mrs. Cummings: I was pretty restless. It took me a long time to fall asleep. The last time I looked at the clock, it was 3:00 a.m.

Giving Advice

Avoid giving advice to clients and their family members. Let people express their feelings and concerns without offering your opinion. You could create confusion, anxiety, and resentment. Your advice could go against the family's wishes, the physician's orders, or the care plan. Even if a client asks for your advice, do not give it. You could instead suggest that the client speak to your supervisor or the case manager. In the following example, the support worker tactfully avoids giving advice to Mrs. Van Doorne:

Mrs. Van Doorne: I don't feel ready to leave my home, but I'm too much of a burden on my daughter. I just don't know what to do. Sometimes I feel that we'd all be better off if I moved into a nursing home. At other times I hate the thought of it. What do you think I should do?

Support worker: I can see what a difficult decision it is, Mrs. Van Doorne. I wish I could help, but it's not my role to give you advice. Is there anyone else you can talk to about this?

Mrs. Van Doorne: I've tried to talk to Anne (*her daughter*), but she would never admit that I'm a burden.

Support worker: What about talking to Mrs. Stainer *(the case manager)*? I'm sure she could help.

Mrs. Van Doorne: That's a good idea. I'll do that.

Minimizing Problems

Do not minimize a client's problems. Avoid making comments like these: "Everything will be fine," "Don't worry—it's really not that bad," "Look on the bright side," and "It could be worse." These comments block communication and imply that the client is complaining or exaggerating the problem. They also show that you are judging the client or the situation when you have no right to do so. Minimizing problems makes people feel that you are ridiculing their concerns, feelings, and fears. Clients could believe that you do not care about what they think or feel. Consider these two responses to a hospital client's concerns:

Mr. Lam: I'm so nervous about this operation. I've never even been in a hospital before.

Eduardo: Believe me, you have nothing to worry about. These surgeons could do this operation with their eyes closed. You will be just fine. *(Walks away.)*

Helga: Having surgery is frightening, especially when it's your first operation. The doctors and nurses will explain everything to you so that you know what to expect. *(Reports Mr. Lam's concerns immediately to the nurse, who reassures him about the surgery.)*

Eduardo's response minimizes Mr. Lam's worries about his surgery, whereas Helga's response is empathetic. She uses paraphrasing to let Mr. Lam know that she understands his concerns and also reassures him by expressing confidence in the health care team.

Using Patronizing Language

Sometimes, the words you use can make a person feel unimportant and inferior. These words are *patronizing*. They imply that you are better than the other person. To avoid using patronizing language:

- Do not address clients as "sweetie," "dude," "gramps," "love," "dear," "honey," or any other term of endearment (or "sweet talk").
- Do not use a client's first name without his permission.
- Do not use terms such as "good girl" or "good boy" or "you guys" with adults.
- Do not use the term "we" when you really mean "you."
- Do not use "baby talk" or expressions such as "There, there."
- Do not talk to co-workers or family members as if the client were not present.
- Do not correct a client's speech or language.

BOX 5–1 Avoiding Patronizing Language

Poor Communication Skills

Support worker: Hello, Doris. How are we feeling today, dear?

Mrs. Crossley: I'm feeling much better, thank you.

Support worker: Have you been doing your exercises?

Mrs. Crossley: Yes.

Support worker: Good girl!

Improved Communication Skills

Support worker: Hello, Mrs. Crossley. How are you feeling today?

Mrs. Crossley: I'm feeling much better, thank you.

Support worker: How have your exercises been going?

Mrs. Crossley: Very well, thank you. I'm up to half an hour a day now.

Support worker: That's excellent progress!

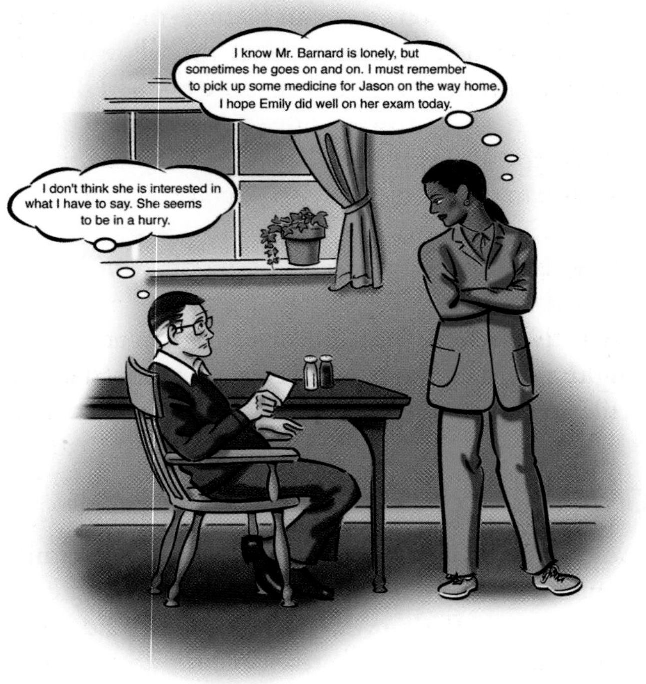
I know Mr. Barnard is lonely, but sometimes he goes on and on. I must remember to pick up some medicine for Jason on the way home. I hope Emily did well on her exam today.
I don't think she is interested in what I have to say. She seems to be in a hurry.

FIGURE 5–4 This client senses that his support worker is not listening to him.

Some health care workers mistakenly use patronizing language when intending to convey warmth and friendliness (BOX 5–1).

Failing to Listen

Communication is blocked if you fail to listen with interest and sincerity (FIGURE 5–4). Pretending to listen is often obvious to the speaker and conveys a lack of interest and caring. Equally problematic, not listening means you can miss important complaints of pain, discomfort, or other abnormal sensations that must be reported to your supervisor.

DEFENCE MECHANISMS

Defence mechanisms are used subconsciously in communications with others in order to delay—or avoid altogether—uncomfortable feelings such as anxiety, guilt, stress, or embarrassment.[3,4] Defence mechanisms may be used for a short term or long term and may be used in positive ways or negative ways as a coping means. For example, a client who is awaiting a big surgical procedure may use denial and tell others that "everything will be all right" in order to reduce his own presurgery anxiety. In this case, the client has used denial in a positive way. However, in another situation, someone may use denial to tell her family that she "is not a problem drinker." In this case, her denial may lead to unhealthy lifestyle choices and interfere with her acceptance of health teaching from her family and friends.

As a support worker, you may experience difficulty when trying to communicate effectively with a client who is using a defence mechanism instead of accepting reality or facing a painful truth. Some examples of defence mechanisms are the following:[4]

- **Denial**: An unwillingness to accept the truth or a certain reality. For example, a person who has a terminal illness refuses to believe that he is ill.
- **Displacement**: A transfer of feelings (usually of anger) onto another person or item instead of onto

the person who is the source of the anger. For example, a woman who is abused by her partner abuses her children instead of dealing with the conflict between her and her partner.

- **Fantasizing**: Daydreaming as an escape instead of dealing with reality. For example, a person who wishes to be a singer one day daydreams about his future singing successes instead of practising his singing.
- **Passive-aggressiveness**: The practice of expressing negative emotions, resentment, or anger toward others through passive, indirect ways (such as through procrastination or manipulation) instead of by verbalizing feelings in an assertive manner. For example, a student who is not happy with the role her project group assigns her submits her part of the project late, affecting the rest of her team's grades.
- **Projection**: Blaming someone else for one's own behaviour. For example, a student blames her bad test marks on her roommate's noise, when in reality, the student did not prepare adequately for her test.
- **Rationalization**: Justifying a behaviour or action by explaining it as being less harmful or hurtful than it really is. For example, a woman does not admit that her bad cough is a result of her heavy smoking but instead blames it on the dry air produced by the air conditioner.
- **Regression**: A return to an earlier developmental stage as a way to escape from stress. For example, a toddler who was already toilet-trained begins to wet her bed after a new sibling is born.
- **Repression**: The involuntary action of blocking painful memories from the conscious mind. It is not uncommon for people with repressed painful memories to suffer from depression or other mental health disorders. For example, a victim of an assault "forgets" that he was assaulted.
- **Submissiveness**: A show of obedience, meekness, and compliance in the face of conflict or a difference of opinion, instead of assertiveness.
- **Suppression**: A conscious refusal to acknowledge a painful or upsetting situation. For example, a teenager tells her friends that she "doesn't want to talk about it" after her boyfriend ends their relationship.

COMMUNICATING WITH ANGRY PEOPLE

Anger is a common response of both clients and family members to illness and disability (see Chapter 4). The many underlying causes of anger include frustration, anxiety, fear, and pain. Another common cause is hurt feelings—people may react with anger if they feel their self-esteem is being attacked. Loss of body function and of one's independence can also incite anger. People who are angry are often feeling helpless about a situation.

Anger also is a symptom of diseases that affect thinking and behaviour. For example, people who abuse alcohol or drugs can show anger. Some people are often angry or unhappy, and few things please them. There could be numerous reasons for their demeanour. Do not judge an angry client, but do report a client's angry behaviour to your supervisor. Provide these clients with the same high-quality, compassionate care that you give all your clients.

Anger can be communicated verbally or nonverbally. Verbal expressions of anger include outbursts, shouting, using a raised voice, and rapid speech. An angry client may tell you what to do or may threaten you. Some clients may remain silent when angry, whereas others become uncooperative and refuse to answer questions. Nonverbal signs of anger include rapid movements, pacing, clenched fists, and a reddened face or neck. The angry client may glare at you, get too close to you when speaking (see Chapters 9 and 36), or display violent behaviours. Effective communication is important to prevent and deal with anger. Follow the guidelines in **BOX 5–2** when communicating with an angry client.

COMMUNICATING ASSERTIVELY

Assertiveness is a style of communication in which thoughts and feelings are expressed positively and directly without offending others. An assertive person stands up for her rights while respecting the rights of others. When being assertive, a speaker conveys his opinion with the goal of ensuring that his needs are met. However, not all people will agree with that opinion, and the speaker must respect others' right to disagree.

BOX 5–2 Communicating With an Angry Client

- Recognize that the client is feeling frustrated or frightened. Put yourself in the client's situation. How would you feel? How would you want to be treated?
- Treat the client with respect and dignity.
- Answer the client's questions clearly and thoroughly. Tell the client that your supervisor will answer the questions that you cannot answer.
- Keep the client informed. Tell the client what you are going to do and when.
- Do not keep the client waiting for long periods. If you tell the client that you will do something for him, do it promptly.
- Stay calm and professional. Speak in a normal tone. Do not respond to a client's anger with your own anger. Try not to take the client's anger personally. The anger has more to do with the client's own feelings than with you or the care you give.
- Do not argue with the client.
- Listen and use silence. The client may feel better after expressing angry feelings.
- Protect yourself from violent behaviours. Leave the client, and call your supervisor if you think you are in danger (see Chapter 22).
- Report the client's behaviour to your supervisor. Discuss how you should deal with the client.
- There are courses available to teach you how to deal with angry clients. In most provinces, the course is called "Non-Violent Crisis Intervention." Other courses may also be available, depending on your area.

People who communicate assertively appear confident, calm, and composed. They speak gently, firmly, and positively. They do not hesitate or appear anxious. They are respectful.

Being assertive is different from being aggressive and from being passive. A person who communicates aggressively will appear upset, cold, or angry and may sound threatening. Aggressive communication is usually not respectful. A person who communicates passively will appear hesitant, apologetic, and timid. A passive person does not want to hurt or offend others. But passive behaviour can make others feel uncomfortable. Assertiveness rarely has this effect because people usually like direct, honest, and sincere communication.

Some people have trouble communicating assertively with people in authority. They feel intimidated. As a support worker, you will have regular contact with physicians, nurses, and other members of the health care team. You need to be confident and assertive when you communicate with them. Your observations are very important to ensuring that any changes in your client's condition are addressed. Remember that suggestions you make in a care conference can help improve the care your client receives.

The *Case Study: Communicating Assertively* box describes three responses to a situation that requires assertiveness.

EXPLAINING PROCEDURES AND TASKS

One of your responsibilities as a support worker is to explain procedures and tasks to clients, as some procedures may be unfamiliar or frightening to them. Some personal care activities may require staff who are strangers to the client touching his or her private body parts. ***It is a good practice to explain every task that you are doing, prior to and while doing it, regardless of how "routine" it might feel to you.*** For example, you might have assisted your client, Mrs. Jones, with toileting every day that week, but because she has dementia, she may not remember what you are doing and why you need to remove her clothing prior to toileting. Explain what you are doing step by step each time you toilet her. In the case of some procedures, you need to find out your client's preferences *before* you begin. Clients feel safer and more secure if they understand what is going to be done before the procedure is performed. They should know why the procedure is done, who will do it, how it will be done, and what sensations or feelings they can expect. They should also know which parts of the procedure (if any) they will participate in and which parts you, as the support worker, will perform. Then, as you are doing the procedure, you should tell the client what you are doing with each step. In addition, to reduce the client's anxiety, pay attention to

CASE STUDY Communicating Assertively

Kara just graduated as a support worker. Her first job is at a long-term care facility, where she was hired to replace Debbie. Mr. Beruti is a 28-year-old client, who has had both his arms amputated. While Kara is shaving him, he shouts, "Be careful! You almost nicked me. You obviously don't know what you're doing. The nurse told me this is your first job. You're not nearly as good as Debbie. If you don't get better at this, I'll report you."

Consider the following responses:

- "Report me if you like, Mr. Beruti. I wouldn't have been assigned to you if I were useless. You're just missing Debbie. I can assure you that I am just as qualified as she is. I won't tolerate your abuse." (*This response is aggressive and hostile. It makes a judgement by assuming that Mr. Beruti misses Debbie. It shows no empathy or respect, and it disregards his safety needs.)*
- "I'm so sorry, Mr. Beruti. I am so clumsy and rough. I'll try to do better." *(This response is passive. It suggests that Kara lacks confidence and also implies that Kara has doubts about her ability to provide safe and competent care.)*
- "It's hard when caregivers do things in different ways. I can assure you that your safety and comfort are important to me. Can you tell me how you like to be shaved?" *(This response is compassionate yet assertive. It should reassure Mr. Beruti. It shows that Kara is confident in her ability to adapt her shaving method and also that she is open to Mr. Beruti's preferences for care.)*

your tone of voice and your body language. By using a soothing, calm voice and by smiling, you may put a client at ease and may encourage the client to be more cooperative during the procedure.

You may help clients practise tasks they have been taught by other health care providers. For example, Mr. Krueger, 88, has osteoporosis. His physiotherapist has shown him how to perform muscle-strengthening exercises. The physiotherapist has also shown you how to help him with the exercises. As part of Mr. Krueger's care plan, you work with him daily on these exercises.

You may be expected to teach seemingly simple tasks to your clients. For example, Mrs. Ali has hemiplegia (paralysis on one side of her body) and needs to learn a new method for dressing herself. You have been taught a method for dressing clients with hemiplegia, and the care plan calls for you to teach this method to Mrs. Ali and to practise it with her until she is able to dress herself.

Whatever the situation, you must give clear, precise explanations and instructions that the client can understand. Organize your thoughts before you speak. Use simple, everyday language. Give your client the chance to discuss the task and to ask questions.

Most clients learn tasks best when they are shown how to do them. The following four-step teaching method works for most clients:

1. Describe to the client the steps in the task.
2. Show the client how to do each step.
3. Have the client try each step.
4. Review the client's success with each step.

Follow the guidelines in **BOX 5–3**.

COMMUNICATING WITH CLIENTS WHO HAVE DEMENTIA

It is especially important to pay attention to your verbal and nonverbal messages when communicating with people who have dementia. As clients lose their language skills, they rely more heavily on following the nonverbal cues of others, especially their caregivers. You can assist clients to maintain their sense of dignity and their identity as people by observing the tips in **BOX 5–4**.

BOX 5–3 Guidelines for Assisting Clients With Their Tasks

- ***Put the client at ease.*** Relax and smile. Do not give the impression that you are in a hurry. If the client senses you are tense or rushed, learning will be difficult.
- ***Start with small steps.*** Break the task into small steps. Focus the client's attention on one step at a time.
- ***Start with easy steps.*** Confidence increases with success. If possible, start with the steps the client is most likely to achieve.
- ***Observe and listen.*** Clients do not always tell you when they do not understand something. Or they may say they understand it when they actually do not. Watch body language, and listen actively. Be alert for signs of fatigue.
- ***Use positive statements.*** Positive statements are easier to follow than negative statements are. For example, saying "Bend your arm" is more effective than saying "Don't use a straight arm."
- ***Let the client set the pace.*** Be patient, and do not rush the client. Allow time for rest.
- ***Provide support and offer encouragement.*** Positive comments help the client feel successful and also encourage the client to continue trying. It is important to recognize what the client has achieved. Even small achievements deserve recognition and a positive comment.
- ***Give time for practice.*** Allow time for practising a task. Practice helps a client remember.

BOX 5–4 Tips for Communicating With Someone With Dementia

Before You Speak:

- When possible, if you are rushing or feeling stressed, try to take a moment to calm yourself.
- Consider what you are going to talk about. It may be useful to have an idea for a particular topic ready or to ask yourself what you want to achieve from the conversation.
- Make sure you have the person's full attention.
- Make sure that the person can see you clearly.
- Try to make eye contact. This will help the person focus on you.
- Minimize competing noises, such as the radio, TV, or other people's conversations.

How to Speak:

- Speak clearly and calmly.
- Speak at a slightly slower pace, allowing time between sentences for the person to process the information and to respond. This might seem like an uncomfortable pause to you, but it is important for supporting the person to communicate.
- Avoid speaking sharply or raising your voice, as this may distress the person.
- Use short, simple sentences.
- Don't talk about people with dementia as if they are not there or talk to them as you would to a young child—show respect and patience.
- Humour can help to bring you closer together and may relieve the pressure. Try to laugh together about misunderstandings and mistakes—it can help.
- Try to include the person in conversations with others. You may find this easier if you adapt the way you say things slightly. Being included in social groups can help people with dementia to preserve their sense of identity. It can also help to reduce feelings of exclusion and isolation.

What to Say:

- Try to be positive.
- Avoid asking too many direct questions. People with dementia can become frustrated if they can't find the answer. If you have to, ask questions one at a time, and phrase them in a way that allows for a "yes" or "no" answer.
- Try not to ask the person to make complicated decisions. Giving someone a choice is important

Continued

BOX 5–4 Tips for Communicating With Someone With Dementia—cont'd

when they can cope with it, but too many options can be confusing and frustrating.

- If the person doesn't understand what you are saying, try to get the message across in a different way rather than simply repeating the same thing. You could try breaking down complex explanations into smaller parts and perhaps also use written words or objects.
- As dementia progresses, the person may become confused about what is true and not true. If the person says something you know to be incorrect, try to find ways of steering the conversation around the subject rather than contradicting them directly. Try to see behind the content to the meaning or feelings they are sharing.

Listening:

- Listen carefully to what the person is saying, and give them plenty of encouragement.
- When you haven't understood fully, tell the person what you have understood and check with them to see if you are right.
- If the person has difficulty finding the right word or finishing a sentence, ask them to explain it in a different way. Listen for clues. Also pay attention to their body language. The expression on their face and the way they hold themselves and move about can give you clear signals about how they are feeling.
- If the person is feeling sad, let them express their feelings without trying to "jolly them along." Sometimes the best thing to do is to just listen and show that you care.
- Due to memory loss, some people won't remember things such as their medical history, family and friends. You will need to use your judgement and act appropriately around what they've said. For example, they might say that they have just eaten when you know they haven't.

Body Language and Physical Contact:

- A person with dementia will read your body language. Sudden movements or a tense facial expression may cause upset or distress and can make communication more difficult.
- Make sure that your body language and facial expression match what you are saying.
- Never stand too close or stand over someone to communicate: It can feel intimidating. Instead, respect the person's personal space and drop below their eye level. This will help the person to feel more in control of the situation.
- Use physical contact to communicate your care and affection and to provide reassurance—don't underestimate the reassurance you can give by holding or patting the person's hand or putting your arm around them if it feels right.

Source: Alzheimer's Society. (2016). *Communicating*. Retrieved from https://www.alzheimers.org.uk/site/scripts/documents_info.php?documentID=130.

KEY POINTS

- The communication process is the means by which people exchange information. Communication skills are used in all environments including at work, school, and home.
- Interpersonal communication is the exchange of information between two people, usually face to face.
- Messages sent are sometimes misunderstood by the receiver because factors such as perception, experience, physical and mental health, emotions, values, beliefs, culture, gender, and age can influence understanding.
- To communicate effectively with words, you need to choose your words carefully; use simple, everyday language; speak clearly, slowly, and distinctly; control the volume and tone of your voice; be concise; present information in a logical manner; ask one question at a time; determine understanding; and do not pretend to understand.
- Before starting and while doing a task, explain to the client what you are doing, regardless of how routine the task might feel to you.
- Professional communication requires being courteous and ensuring confidentiality at all times.
- Workplace etiquette requires support workers to behave in a professional, ethical, friendly, and respectful manner to co-workers at all times, including while on breaks.
- Nonverbal communications are messages sent without words through body language, touch, and the use of silence.
- Communication methods include active listening, paraphrasing, empathetic listening, asking closed questions, asking open-ended questions, clarifying, and focusing.
- Communication barriers include interrupting, answering one's own questions, giving advice, minimizing problems, using patronizing language, and failing to listen.
- People subconsciously use defence mechanisms to avoid uncomfortable feelings such as anxiety, guilt, stress, or embarrassment. Defence mechanisms include denial, displacement, fantasizing, projection, rationalization, regression, repression, and suppression.
- At times, support workers will be faced with angry clients. Effective communication is important to preventing and dealing with anger.
- Assertiveness is a style of communication in which thoughts and feelings are expressed positively and directly without offending others.
- When teaching clients new tasks, describe to the client the steps in the task, show the client how to do each step, have the client try each step, and review the client's success with each step.
- It is especially important to pay attention to your verbal and nonverbal messages when communicating with people who have dementia. As clients lose their language skills, they rely more heavily on following nonverbal cues.

CRITICAL THINKING IN PRACTICE

You are employed at a long-term care facility. A co-worker did not show up for work. You and the other staff members have extra work. How do you respond? Can you refuse to do the extra work assigned to you? Do you complain or keep silent about this situation, maintaining a positive attitude? How will you plan, prioritize, and manage the extra work?

REVIEW QUESTIONS

Answers to these questions are at the bottom of the *p. 85.*

Circle the BEST answer.

1. During an exchange of information, a message is sent:
   A. From a sender to a receiver
   B. From a receiver to a sender
   C. From a sender to a sender
   D. Without feedback

2. Which is true?
   A. Verbal communication does not involve the spoken word.
   B. Verbal communication is the truest reflection of a person's feelings.
   C. Messages can be sent by facial expressions, gestures, posture, body movements, appearance, and eye contact.
   D. All people like to be touched.

3. To communicate with your client, Mr. Lam, you should:
   A. Use medical words and phrases
   B. Listen to his concerns and report them to the supervisor, who can answer his questions
   C. Give your opinion when he is sharing fears and concerns
   D. Ask closed questions when you need specific information

4. When talking with Mr. Long, which of the following might indicate that you are listening?
   A. You continue making the bed with your back to him.
   B. You have direct eye contact with him.
   C. You cross your arms and look away.
   D. You roll your eyes at what he has said.

5. You and Ms. Jones are talking about her surgery. Which of the following is a closed question?
   A. "Do you feel better now?"
   B. "Tell me what your plans are for home."
   C. "What will you do when you fully recover?"
   D. "How long will you be off work?"

6. Your client tells you she is not happy that she has to use a walker. Which of the following responses shows empathy?
   A. You tell her about the time you had to use crutches.
   B. You suggest methods that might help her use her walker more efficiently.
   C. You quickly try to change the subject to something happier.
   D. You listen to her and acknowledge her feelings.

7. Focusing is a useful communication tool when:
   A. A person is rambling
   B. You want to make sure you understand the message
   C. You want the person to share thoughts and feelings
   D. You need information

8. Which statement will promote communication?
   A. "Don't worry."
   B. "Everything will be just fine."
   C. "This is a good facility."
   D. "I see you are upset. Do you want to talk about this?"

9. Which is a barrier to communication?
   A. Interrupting
   B. Repeating what the person says
   C. Giving advice
   D. A and C

10. A client is angry. Which of the following statements is true?
    A. The person probably has a disease that affects thinking and behaviour.
    B. Drug or alcohol abuse is likely.
    C. You should tell the person to calm down and that everything will be fine.
    D. Listening and using silence are important.

11. In regard to assertive communication, which of the following is true?
    A. You appear upset, cold, or angry.
    B. You appear confident, calm, and composed.
    C. You are usually not respectful.
    D. You appear hesitant, apologetic, and timid.

Answers: 1.A, 2.C, 3.B, 4.B, 5.A, 6.D, 7.A, 8.D, 9.D, 10.D, 11.B

Chapter opener image: Tyler Olson/Shutterstock.com

CHAPTER 6

Working With Others: Teamwork, Supervision, and Delegation

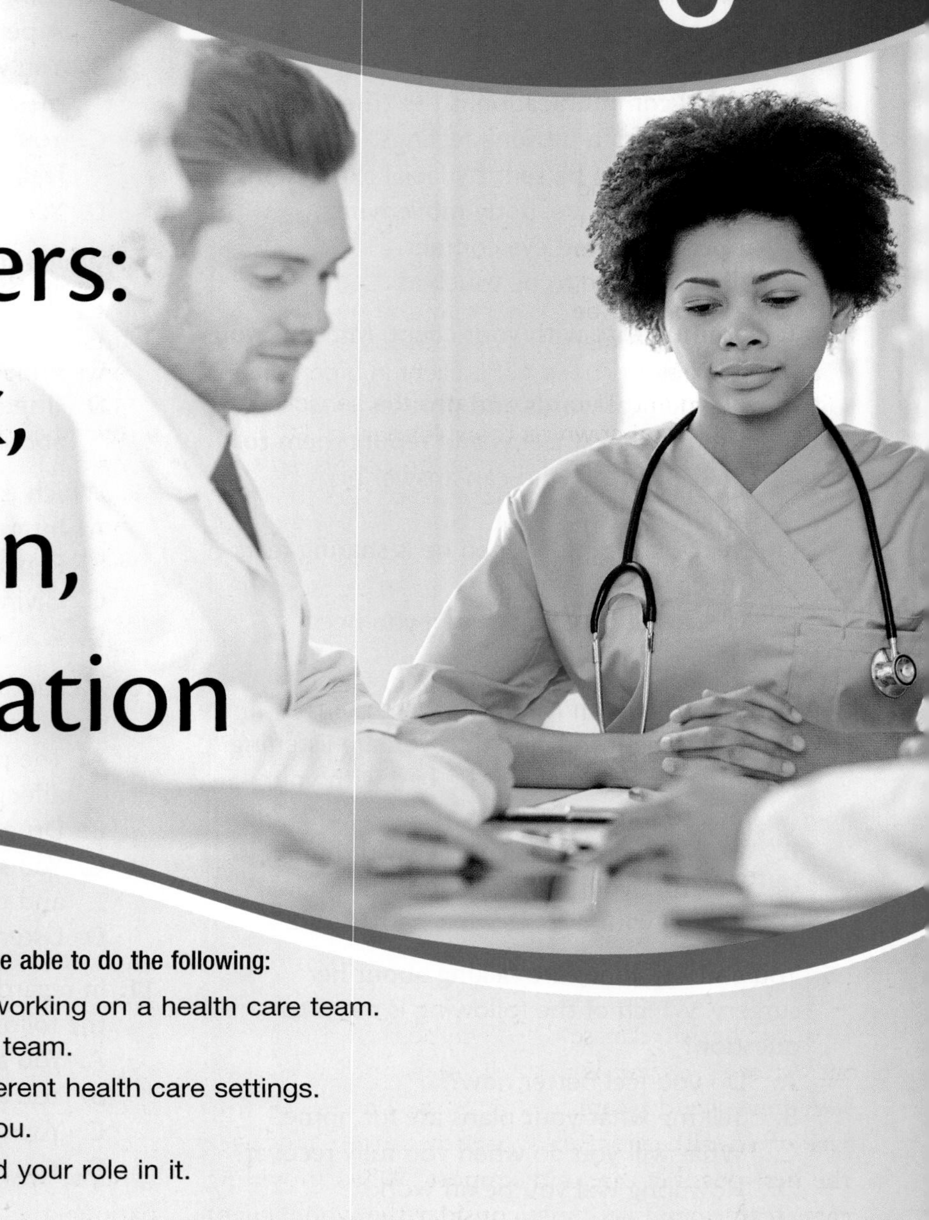

OBJECTIVES

After reading this chapter, the learner should be able to do the following:

- List the benefits and challenges of working on a health care team.
- Explain your role on the health care team.
- Describe how teams function in different health care settings.
- Explain how delegation applies to you.
- Describe the delegation process and your role in it.

KEY TERMS

accountability The willingness to accept responsibility and to explain one's actions, inactions or omissions, intentions, and decisions. *p. 91*

assigning Appointing someone to take on the responsibility to complete a task while providing client care or support. *p. 92*

authority The legal right to do something. *p. 92*

care conference See **family conference**. *p. 90*

case manager A manager who assesses, monitors, and evaluates the needs of a client in a community care setting and also coordinates the services of the team. Also known as **team leader**. *p. 91*

controlled acts Tasks that must be performed only by those authorized to perform them. Controlled acts are considered to be harmful if performed by unqualified individuals. *p. 92*

delegation A process by which a nurse authorizes another health care provider to perform certain tasks, including controlled acts. *p. 92*

family conference A meeting attended by the health care team and family members to discuss the client's care. Also called **care conference**. *p. 90*

interdisciplinary team A team of health care providers from a variety of backgrounds and specialties who work together to meet the client's needs. Also known as *intradisciplinary team, interprofessional team, interprofessional health care team, or multidisciplinary team. p. 90*

mentor A person who shares her expertise and knowledge to create a safe, encouraging learning environment for the learner. *p. 88*

supervising Being responsible for monitoring and overseeing the activities of others on the health care team. *p. 91*

task A function, procedure, or activity that a support worker assists with or performs for the client. *p. 92*

team leader See **case manager**. *p. 91*

transfer of function A process by which a nurse authorizes another health care provider to perform certain tasks. *p. 92*

THE HEALTH CARE TEAM

In most health care settings, support workers work on a team. A *team* is a group of people who work together toward a common goal (see Chapter 1). The goal of a health care team is to provide the client with the best possible care and support. When providing care, team members must consider the whole client and promote health in all five dimensions of the client's life: physical, emotional, social, cognitive, and spiritual (see Chapter 4). Health care team members depend on each other to perform their roles to the best of their abilities. It is also important that all members of the team conduct themselves professionally at all times and use correct terminology when reporting observations about the client (see Chapter 13).

In some situations, you and one other person—usually a nurse who is your supervisor—may be the only health care providers on the team. Depending on the setting, your supervisor may not be a nurse but will be another regulated health professional, such as a physiotherapist or occupational therapist. In other situations, you may be part of a larger team that includes health care providers from a variety of backgrounds and specialties who work together to meet the client's needs, such as physicians, nurses, support workers, dietitians, physiotherapists, occupational therapists, speech therapists, and others who are providing alternative care.

Members of effective teams support one another, understand each other's scope of practice, and communicate with each other effectively. The members of a health care team vary depending on the place of employment and the client's needs, and usually include the client unless he or she is not mentally capable of being involved in the teamwork or chooses not to participate. For example, Tom Brown, 15, has mental health issues. Tom, his parents, a nurse, a psychiatrist, a social worker, and a support worker work together as a team. Tom's team is different from Mrs. Darby's team. Mrs. Darby, 86, is recovering from hip surgery. She and her daughter are on a team that also includes a nurse, a social worker, a physiotherapist, and support workers.

Benefits of Working on a Team

There are many benefits to the team approach in health care. A group of people is more effective at making correct decisions and solving problems than one person is. The many benefits of a team approach to care include the following:

- ***Opportunities for collaboration.*** All team members are encouraged to *collaborate* (to work together toward a common goal). Successful collaboration creates a positive atmosphere that even the client can sense. Staff and clients both benefit when team members share information. For example, as a support worker, you may find a way to ease a client's discomfort during a bed bath. You share this information with the nurse and your co-workers in the appropriate manner. The nurse instructs other support workers to use your method by incorporating your information and suggestions into the client's care plan.
- ***Opportunities for communication.*** Team meetings provide the opportunity for all team members to share experiences, opinions, and ideas. Without the meetings, valuable ideas might be missed. **BOX 6–1** contains part of a dialogue from a team meeting. Note how each team member contributes to the complete picture of the client's health.
- ***Opportunities for mentorship.*** Many newly hired support workers depend on the mentorship of more experienced co-workers to assist them to become familiarized with the agency's clients and routine duties. A **mentor** is a person who shares her expertise and knowledge to create a safe, encouraging learning environment for the learner. Some people are assigned to be mentors to new employees, but many do so voluntarily.
- ***A wide range of abilities, skills, and perspectives.*** Teams are made up of individuals with a range of abilities, skills, training, and experience. Each team member, based on his or her scope of practice, brings ideas and viewpoints to the team. In **BOX 6–1**, note the support worker's contributions. Because she is the only person who has daily contact with Mrs. Darby, she is able to provide important information. The other team members know more about the health and medical conditions that are discussed; however, only the support worker is in a position to report daily observations about the client.
- ***Better decision making and problem solving.*** Many support workers have been taught how to perform certain tasks by following a specific sequence of steps. However, it may be necessary in some circumstances to vary the order of steps while performing a task, as long as the principles of safety, client dignity, and legislation are followed. For example, a co-worker who is assisting you while bathing Mrs. Jones suggests that you change your sequence of bathing steps to reduce the need to turn Mrs. Jones from side to side, something that she does not easily tolerate. When team members discuss issues, they are more likely to make sound decisions and find appropriate solutions to problems.
- ***A positive, trusting atmosphere.*** Trust develops when team members can be relied upon to do their jobs well, to respect each other, to mentor each other, and to share responsibility. The team leader or case manager is responsible for fostering a high level of trust. The leader should encourage team members to openly discuss problems. Team members also play a role in creating trust. They must not blame others for their own mistakes and should take responsibility for their own actions. An effective team provides support to each other during difficult emotional situations, such as the death of a client.

Just as there are many benefits to working on a team, there are also challenges:

- ***Recognizing role boundaries.*** In successful teams, team members understand one another's role and appreciate and value each person's role on the team. You will become familiar with tasks that support workers are not permitted to perform. You must be aware of your scope of practice and your employer's policies and procedures and never take on any task that you are not allowed to perform.

BOX 6–1 Contributions to a Team Meeting

A health care team in a long-term care facility is meeting to discuss a client's rehabilitation following her hip surgery. Mrs. Darby is 86 years old. The team consists of Mrs. Darby, her daughter, a nurse, two support workers, a social worker, and a physiotherapist. At the previous meeting, the physiotherapist had suggested exercises to help Mrs. Darby regain mobility. Since then, the physiotherapist has shown Mrs. Darby how to do the exercises, and a support worker has helped her practise the exercises. Mrs. Darby has chosen not to attend the team meeting. The following team members are at the meeting:

- The nurse, who is also the team leader
- The support worker (Meredith)
- The physiotherapist
- The social worker
- Mrs. Darby's daughter (Sandra)

Nurse: I understand that Mrs. Darby is having difficulty with some of her exercises. Meredith, could you please tell the team what you have observed?

Support worker: Well, Mrs. Darby has been having trouble with all the exercises. They give her great pain. She has such a grimace on her face when she attempts them. Let me tell you what she said on Tuesday morning. *(Checks notes.)* "I can't do these exercises. It feels like someone is boring holes in my hip."

Physiotherapist: Can you tell me how high she is able to lift her leg?

Support worker: About 5 cm off the bed.

Physiotherapist: Is she taking her pain medication?

Nurse: Yes, I help her with her medication. She takes it regularly. To me, Mrs. Darby seems much less cheerful than usual. Has anyone else noticed this?

Support worker: Yes, I've noticed that she is much less outgoing than usual. Also, she used to read the newspaper in the mornings. Now, she just sits in her chair. When I ask her how she is feeling, she says she is tired. She told me that she is not attending this meeting because she is very tired.

Nurse: Perhaps Mrs. Darby is depressed. Sandra, what do you think?

Daughter: I'd say that Mom is definitely feeling down. I just thought it was because of the broken hip and the surgery. Who wouldn't be down after what she has been through? She used to be so cheerful and outgoing. Perhaps Mom *is* depressed. I haven't heard her mention any of her friends lately.

Social worker: Didn't your mother tell you that she is worried about her roommate, Mrs. Martino, who has been in hospital for 2 weeks? Your mom is concerned that she might not be coming back here.

Daughter: No, she didn't mention it. That's odd. Gosh, she is very close to Mrs. Martino.

Nurse: I think someone needs to talk to Mrs. Darby to find out how she is feeling. Maybe she'll have some ideas about how we can help her. She might benefit from some outings and other social activities.

Social worker: I'll talk with Mrs. Darby. We may also need to discuss this with her family physician.

The discussion continues.

- ***Being flexible.*** Teams function best when members are flexible and willing to meet each other's needs. For example, you can help ensure quality client care at your agency by agreeing to switch to a different unit when that unit is short-staffed due to staff illness.
- ***Handling conflict.*** Within any group of people, there are bound to be disagreements. The way conflict is handled affects the whole team. The team leader or case manager plays a critical role in the resolution of conflict, and team members should feel comfortable discussing problems with their leader. It is always better to address conflict rather than hope it will go away. (See Chapter 5 for more information on conflict resolution.)
- ***Expressing your needs and views.*** Support workers may sometimes feel intimidated or less confident on a team that includes physicians and

other health care providers. You *are* a valuable team member and have a great deal to contribute to team meetings (see the *Supporting Mr. Rodriguez: How Team Input Can Make a Difference* box). You spend more time with the client than other team members do. Your day-to-day reporting of progress and concerns is heard by registered staff and reported to your supervisor.

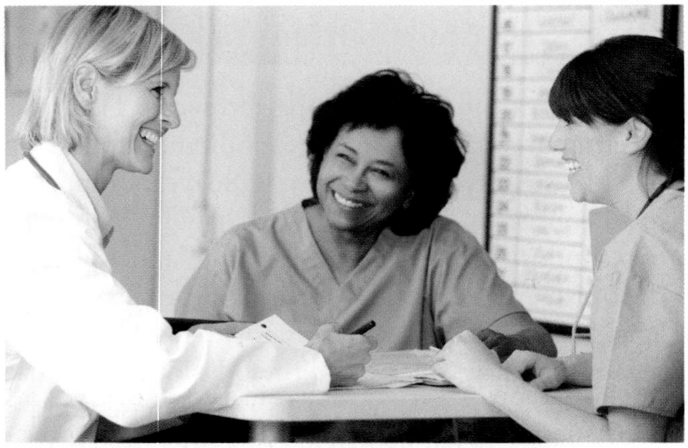

FIGURE 6–1 A team in a long-term care facility meets to discuss a client's care. (**Source:** © Monkey Business Images/Shutterstock.com)

Teamwork in Facilities

Teams in facilities vary as much as the settings themselves. For example, a team at a retirement home functions differently from a team at a hospital, and a hospital team functions differently from a team in a long-term care facility. However, most teams in facilities have one thing in common: Team members work in the same location, giving them many opportunities to meet and collaborate and making communication easy.

Hospitals

Team functions and members vary from hospital to hospital and department to department. Many departments use a multidisciplinary team approach. An **interdisciplinary team** (also called an *interprofessional health care team*) includes health care providers from a variety of backgrounds and specialties, as needed, who work together to meet the client's needs.

Long-Term Care Facilities

Teams in long-term care facilities include physicians, nurses, social workers, support workers, therapists, the client, and the client's family. In a large facility, teams may also include pharmacists, activity directors, dietitians, and other staff members. Often, one nurse is the team leader for all the clients, and the same team may provide care to all clients. In larger facilities, there may be a specific team for each unit. Support workers will have opportunities to work with many different health care providers (**FIGURE 6–1**).

Hospices and Palliative Care Units

A health care team in a hospice or palliative care unit may consist of nurses, support workers, physicians, social workers, volunteers, dietitians, the client, and his or her family members. Depending on the client's wishes, other individuals, such as a spiritual advisor, may also be on the team.

Although hospices and palliative care units are facilities, they are also considered community-based services. They have outreach programs that provide palliative care to people at home. Team members of such programs meet in the facility or in the client's home.

Support workers at hospices and in palliative care units are usually involved in family conferences. A **family conference** (also called a **care conference**) is a meeting attended by the health care team and family members to discuss the client's care. Family conferences are held regularly and whenever a difficult situation arises. Family members can ask questions, express feelings, and make difficult decisions. Family conferences are most common in hospice and community care settings but are also held in hospitals and other facilities.

Assisted-Living Facilities

Assisted-living facilities are community-based and are usually located in a single building. Being in one building makes communication easier. These facilities (which include group homes) usually have only a few staff members made up of professionals from various disciplines. The makeup of the team depends on the needs of clients. Teams usually include a supervisor (who may be a nurse, a social worker, or a qualified youth care worker) and one or two support workers. There may also be other assistive personnel.

Teamwork in Community Settings

Teams in community settings also vary in membership and function.

Home Care

The home care team usually includes the client, family members, the case manager, the family physician, nurses, and support workers and their supervisors. Social workers and therapists may also be on the team.

The **case manager** or **team leader** assesses, monitors, and evaluates the needs of a client in a community care setting and also coordinates the services of the team. A case manager could be a nurse, a social worker, or another regulated health care provider. Occasionally, the client chooses to be the case manager (see Chapter 3).

Home care teams do not always meet regularly. Team members may communicate with each other by telephone or written reports. The case manager schedules a team meeting when the need arises.

Community Day Programs

Teams in community day programs function differently from home care teams. A rehabilitative program team may include a supervisor (who is often a nurse or another health care provider), other professionals, and support workers. A recreational program team may include a supervisor (who is usually a recreational or occupational therapist) and support workers. As a support worker in a day program, you will probably work with the same team every day and have regular opportunities to discuss your clients' progress. You may meet before the program starts, after it is over, or once a week.

Supporting Mr. Rodriguez: How Team Input Can Make a Difference

Jingco Rodriguez is a 52-year-old client with your home care agency. You have been giving him support care for several weeks, ever since he was discharged from the hospital following his cerebrovascular accident (CVA, or stroke). You have been able to develop a good relationship with him because you speak his native language. In addition to the support services that you provide in his home, he goes for physiotherapy at the local hospital three times a week. To get there, he has to take a taxi.

On the day of your last visit, Mr. Rodriguez seemed sad. He tearfully confided in you that he used to work as a cement mason and was self-employed before his stroke. Now being out of work, it was financially hard on him and his family to pay for his taxi. Because of that, he had gone for his physiotherapy only once that week. He told you that he wanted to get better but could not afford to spend any more money in this way. You acknowledge his frustration during your conversation with him.

As a support worker, you knew that you had to report this information to your supervisor and the rest of the team at your weekly conference. After you reported this information, and with Mr. Rodriguez's permission, arrangements were made through a church volunteer group to drive Mr. Rodriguez to and from the hospital.

WORKING UNDER SUPERVISION

Support workers have a responsibility to their supervisor, client, and co-workers and are accountable to their supervisor. In facilities and agencies, the supervisor is usually a nurse. In some community care settings, the supervisor may be a nurse, a social worker, or another health care provider. **Supervising** means being responsible for monitoring and overseeing the activities of others on the health care team.

- ***Supervision in a facility.*** In many facilities, the team leader (usually a nurse) supervises the support workers. The team leader has overall responsibility and **accountability** for the client's care and the work of the other team members. However, the team leader may not be on duty when you are working. You would then report to the *charge nurse* (the nurse on duty for that shift). Depending on your provincial or territorial legislation, in some care homes, there may not be a nurse on duty on the night shift, but support workers would have a contact number for one.

- ***Supervision in a community setting.*** In a community setting, the support workers and supervisor work for an agency, which is accountable for the actions of all employees. The agency may be hired by a health district or community services organization. In this case, a case manager will arrange with the agency to provide care or support for the client. The case manager—usually, but not always, a nurse—communicates with the supervisor, who then gives you, the support worker, information and instructions about care for specific clients.

Sometimes, an agency's services may be paid for privately by the client or the client's family. In such a case, the client and the family will give your supervisor the overall instructions. Your supervisor will then give you information about the client and instructions about her care.

In some situations, clients hire a support worker directly. In these circumstances, there is no agency supervisor; rather, the client is the supervisor. If you work directly with clients, it is advisable to have a written contract outlining each person's responsibilities, rate of compensation, hours of work, and so on. The contract must be acceptable to both you and the client and should be signed by both of you. Both should also keep a copy of the contract to refer to if necessary. This contract would prevent unethical clients and their families from taking advantage of you. Do not hesitate to have the contract reviewed by a lawyer.

Respecting Your Supervisor and Employer

You must respect your supervisor and your employer. Avoid talking with others about your clients or co-workers. Try not to be negative, even if co-workers complain about a policy or a situation. Instead, if you are unhappy with a situation, talk to your supervisor. If you have difficulties communicating with your supervisor, try some of the strategies discussed in Chapters 5 and 7. If you remain unhappy, it might be best for you to find a position with a different agency.

Most important, do not discuss your work problems with your clients. You represent your employer, and the client trusts the facility or agency to provide quality care. A negative, disrespectful attitude could destroy this trust and harm your client's health.

ASSIGNING AND DELEGATION

Assigning means appointing someone to take on a task or responsibility of providing client care or support that is within that person's scope of practice or scope of employment. A **task** is a function, procedure, or activity that a person assists the client with or performs for the client. For example, your supervisor *assigns* your daily tasks. Your assigned tasks are listed on your assignment sheet. They will not require a nurse's education and professional judgement, as your tasks will be within the support worker's scope of practice. For example, you may be assigned to assist with or perform the following tasks:

- Activities of daily living (ADLs)—dressing, personal hygiene, mobility, feeding, toileting
- Instrumental activities of daily living (IADLs)—handling finances, managing medications, handling transportation, shopping, preparing meals, using a telephone or other communication devices, doing housework and basic home maintenance (see Chapter 1)
- Social and recreational activities
- Household management—housecleaning, meal preparation
- Basic support care tasks—measuring height, weight, and vital signs

Only regulated health care providers, such as nurses, have the **authority** (the legal right) to perform certain tasks because they have the skill, knowledge, and training to perform them. These tasks are called **controlled acts** and are considered to be harmful if they are performed by unqualified individuals. Examples of controlled acts include inserting catheters and giving insulin. In certain situations, controlled acts may be delegated to you. **Delegation** (also called **transfer of function**) is a process by which a nurse authorizes another health care provider to perform certain tasks. A controlled act procedure—normally performed only by a regulated health care provider—may be delegated to a member of the client's household, a family member, a support worker, or another unregulated care provider. However, specific conditions, called *exceptions*, must be met for delegation to be permitted to those *outside* of a regulated health profession.[1] It is important to remember that while the nurse maintains the authority to delegate to others, the support worker does not. Regulated health professions legislation states that if the controlled act is determined to be a routine ADL or IADL for a particular client, delegation can occur.[2]

Each client's situation is different. As part of the delegation process, the nurse must first determine if it is appropriate to delegate the task. The nurse must feel confident that the support worker (1) understands what the responsibilities are when performing the task; (2) knows when and who to ask for assistance; and (3) knows when, how, and to whom to report the outcome of the task. After training a support worker to do the task, the nurse then supervises and monitors the performance of the task to make sure it is being done correctly. Tasks that may be delegated to support workers must be routine ones with predictable outcomes that require little supervision, and they can be delegated for stable clients only. It is important to note that the *same* procedure may be a routine ADL in one situation but not in another. Tasks that you may be delegated to perform include suctioning of a permanent tracheotomy; in-and-out catheterization; and administering glucometers, dressings, tube feedings, and medication.

Only some nursing tasks can be delegated. Your employer's policies and guidelines, your job description, and provincial or territorial legislation determine what tasks can be delegated to you. They also determine when and how tasks can be delegated. Although there are many similarities across the country, each province and territory has its own rules for delegation (see examples in BOX 6–2). For example, in a home care agency in Ontario, a nurse can delegate to a support worker the task of giving Mr. Kupper his insulin since he is medically stable and his insulin injection is part of his IADLs. However, upon the client's admission into a long-term care (LTC) facility, a nurse must administer his insulin because Ontario does not permit delegation to support workers to administer insulin in an LTC facility or hospital.[3]

Who Can Delegate?

Depending on the legislation of each province and territory, delegation to support workers is the responsibility of a regulated health care provider, such as a registered nurse (RN), registered practical nurse (RPN), or licensed practical nurse (LPN). When making delegating decisions, the regulated health care provider must always protect the client's health and safety. The delegating regulated health care provider remains accountable for properly following all the steps involved in delegation. However, ***you are also accountable to the employer and to the client for your actions and to ensure the task is done correctly*** **(see BOX 6–3 on page 95).** ***You, therefore, must understand the regulations for delegation acts in your area and in your facility or agency.***

The Delegation Process

As a regulated health care provider, the nurse considers factors that are unique to the client's situation when delegating tasks to you. In some provinces, a task that has been delegated is not transferable to another client. This rule varies among provinces and territories. For example, you have been taught how to give an enema to Mr. Lau. Mr. Davis is also your client and requires an enema. You cannot give an enema to Mr. Davis without being taught again, as he is a new client. ***It cannot be stressed enough that guidelines for delegation acts vary, so you must know the laws in your province or territory.***

Delegated tasks must be within the legal limits of what you can do. Before delegating tasks to you, the nurse must know the following:

- What tasks your province or territory allows support workers to perform
- The tasks included in your job description
- What you were taught in your training program
- What skills you have learned and how they were evaluated
- Your work experience

BOX 6–2 Delegation in British Columbia, Alberta, and Ontario

All provinces and territories have legislation that guides nursing practice, usually called a *nursing act*. British Columbia, Alberta, and Ontario also have legislation that applies to all regulated health professions. This legislation prevents unqualified people from performing professional functions.

Regulated health professions legislation and nursing acts list tasks that only nurses are legally able (authorized) to perform. In British Columbia, these authorized tasks are called *reserved acts*, and delegation is known as *transfer of function*; in Alberta, they are known as *restricted activities*; and in Ontario, they are called *controlled acts*. Only nurses—and *not* support workers—are authorized to do the following:

- Perform a procedure below the skin or mucous membrane (e.g., cleaning and dressing an open wound)
- Administer a substance by injection or inhalation
- Insert an instrument, hand, or finger into a client's body openings, including the client's bladder, esophagus, trachea, nose, ears, bloodstream, or surgically created body openings (e.g., inserting urinary catheters and rectal tubes)

Unregulated health care workers (including support workers) are not normally allowed to perform authorized acts. However, unregulated workers may perform an authorized act if a nurse properly delegates it. In the delegation process, the nurse transfers authority to the unregulated health care worker. However, ***you can be delegated an authorized act only if it is allowed within your job description and employer policy.*** It remains the responsibility of the nurse to determine how and when an unregulated care provider can perform these acts.

Unregulated workers can be assigned authorized acts if the task is a routine activity of living. A routine activity of living is an activity that:

- The client needs done on a regular basis
- Has already been done for the client by a nurse, with consistent and safe results

For example, administering an enema is an authorized act. Take these examples: (1) Mr. Patel is paralyzed. He requires regular enemas to aid elimination. Because the procedure is a predictable and safe part of his routine, his support worker is assigned to perform the procedure. (2) Ms. Wolfe requires an enema before her surgery. She has never had an enema before. In her situation, the enema is not routine. Therefore, in some provinces and territories, a support worker is not legally allowed to administer it. In this case, only a nurse is authorized to give the enema. Support workers are not responsible for deciding when to do a task. You will be assigned or delegated the task, as appropriate.

Even if a task is in your job description and you have done it before, the nurse may decide not to assign or delegate it to you. The nurse makes delegation decisions after considering the questions in **BOX 6–3**. The circumstances, the client's needs, the task, and the support worker performing the task must all be right. If the client's needs and the task require the knowledge, judgement, and skill of a nurse, the nurse must perform the task. You may, however, be asked to assist.

Do not get offended or angry if you are not allowed to perform a task that is part of your job description and that you usually do. The nurse must make a decision that is best for the client at that time. This decision is also best for you at that time. You do not want to perform a task that requires a nurse's judgement and critical thinking skills. For example, you often care for Mrs. Mills. You provide personal care to her and assist her with walking. One weekend, she visits with her son. When she returns to the long-term care facility, she has bruises on her face and arms. She reports that she fell down the stairs. The nurse suspects abuse. Instead of assigning you the task of bathing Mrs. Mills, the nurse does it herself. The nurse wants to assess Mrs. Mills for other signs of abuse and to talk with her. Although you are able to give Mrs. Mills a bath, at this time, she needs the nurse's knowledge and judgement.

BOX 6–3 Factors Affecting Delegation Decisions for the Nurse

To make decisions about the effective, safe, and ethical delivery of care by a support worker, before delegating a task, the nurse will take the following into consideration:

1. Is it appropriate that a support worker perform this task considering the client's condition, associated risks, and environmental supports?
2. Will the support worker be performing the task frequently enough to maintain competence?
3. Can the support worker be adequately supervised in the setting?
4. Is a nurse available to help if the client's condition changes or problems arise?
5. Is this a task that can be delegated to a support worker, and is it included in her job description?

Source: College of Nurses of Ontario. (2013). *Working with unregulated care providers*. Pub. N. 41014. Retrieved from http://www.cno.org/globalassets/docs/prac/41014_workingucp.pdf.

The client's circumstances are central factors in making assignment and delegation decisions. These decisions should always result in the best care for the client. Poor decisions could place a client's health and safety at risk and result in serious legal problems.

A nurse who delegates a task is required to:

- Have the knowledge, skill, and judgement to perform the task competently.
- Have the additional knowledge, skill, and judgement to teach the task to others. The delegating nurse is responsible for providing all necessary teaching, but not everybody is able to teach others how to perform something. Good communication skills and patience are required.
- Accept responsibility for teaching the task to the support worker. The nurse must first determine the risks and benefits of teaching the task and be able to confidently predict its outcome.
- Assess your performance. The nurse must determine that you are able to perform the task correctly.
- Determine if the task that is taught can be performed for more than one client.[2] Each client is unique, and you can never assume that the task that you are being taught should ever be performed on another client. In some circumstances, however, the nurse can delegate the support worker to perform the task on more than one client. In this case, the rules for delegation apply to each of these clients.
- Monitor you over time to ensure you remain able to perform the task correctly and safely. Monitoring may be done in a number of ways, at the discretion of the nurse. There must be policies dictating when communication is necessary. There also has to be a means for timely communication between the nurse and the support worker whenever necessary.

Support workers cannot assign or delegate, so you cannot authorize someone to perform a task that has been assigned or delegated to you. A co-worker can help you with tasks that have been *assigned* to you. However, only *you* can perform a delegated act.

Delegation in the Community

In the community, your supervisor will be a nurse for health care needs. The nurse usually does not work in the same building, so as part of teaching you how to perform the controlled act, the nurse should provide you with written instructions on how to carry out the task, the predicted outcome, and what you need to record.

For example, you have a client who requires in-and-out catheterization (see Chapter 32). The nurse determines that this is a routine ADL by answering the questions in BOX 6–3. The nurse will teach you the task; assess your performance; and provide you with written instructions on how to do the task, when to ask for assistance, and what you need to record (e.g., the results of the in-and-out catheterization). The nurse will then monitor your performance regularly, and you must be able to seek assistance and receive it in a timely manner.

Some agencies provide educational programs or workshops for support workers. These programs educate workers about specific ADL tasks. For example, you might attend a program given by a nurse on how to do catheterizations for clients with paraplegia. You graduate from the program only after the nurse is satisfied that you can perform the task safely and competently. The agency is responsible for monitoring your performance over time.

In home settings, when no other health care providers are present, clients and caregivers may ask a support worker to do certain tasks. You must never perform a task that is beyond your scope of practice. Explain that you are not allowed to perform the task without the authorization of your supervisor, and then call your supervisor to discuss the situation.

Your Role in Delegation

Although the nurse is responsible for teaching, supervising, and monitoring your performance, you are responsible for your own actions. You have the choice when you are delegated a task to either *agree* or *refuse* to do the task. Before accepting a delegated task, ask yourself the questions listed in **BOX 6–4** and **BOX 6–5**.

It is also possible, especially in the community, that a professional who is not a nurse and not your supervisor will ask you to perform a task that you do not usually do. Before taking on the task, use your judgement, and consider your agency's policies. (If you need clarification of those policies, contact your supervisor). Usually, you can do a simple, noninvasive task that you have done for the client before. But in any of the following circumstances, tell the person who made the request that you cannot fulfill it:

- You have concerns about your ability to do the task.
- It is beyond your scope of practice.
- The client's condition changes.

BOX 6–4 The Five Rights of Delegation

The National Council of State Boards of Nursing in the United States identifies five rights of delegation. These rights are relevant in Canada as well:

1. ***The right task.*** Can the task be delegated? Does the provincial nursing act or regulated health professions act allow the nurse to delegate the task? Is the task in your job description? Have you been trained to do the task? A written job description and job routine for a particular shift should be available to support workers when they are hired and kept in the procedure manual for review.
2. ***The right circumstances.*** What are the client's physical, emotional, social, cognitive, and spiritual needs at this time? Do you understand the purpose of the task for the client? Do you have the equipment and supplies to perform the task? Do you know how to use the equipment and supplies?
3. ***The right person.*** Do you have the training and experience to safely perform the task for this client? Do you have concerns about performing the task?
4. ***The right directions and communication.*** Has the nurse provided clear directions and instructions? Has the nurse told you what to do, when to do it, what observations to make, and when to report back? Are the directions legal, ethical, and consistent with employer policies? Can you review the task with the nurse? Do you understand what the nurse expects?
5. ***The right supervision and evaluation.*** Is a nurse available to answer questions? Is a nurse available if the client's condition changes or if problems occur? After the task is completed, does the nurse assess how the task affected the client? Does the nurse discuss your performance with you, telling you what you did well and how you can improve your work?

Source: Texas Department of Aging and Disability Services. (2010). *The five rights of delegation*. Retrieved from https://www.bon.texas.gov/pdfs/delegation_pdfs/Delegation-fiverights.pdf.

BOX 6–5 Factors Affecting Delegation Decisions for the Support Worker

The support worker is responsible for taking the following into consideration:

1. Is this task included in my job description and posted in my agency's written policies for care?
2. Is this task a part of the client's ADLs or IADLs?
3. Am I aware of how the client *usually* responds when this task is performed? Would I be able to compare the usual response to today's response if I were to perform it now?
4. Is it appropriate for me to perform this task considering the client's *current* condition?
5. Am I aware of the risks associated with performing this task?
6. Is the client (or representative) able to direct his or her own care and allow me to perform this task?
7. *(If learning)* Will I be adequately supervised in this setting to ensure that the task is performed correctly and the client not harmed? Will I be performing the task frequently enough to maintain competence?
8. Is an appropriate health care provider available to help me if the client's condition changes or if problems arise?
9. *(If deemed competent to do this task in the past)* Do I remember all the steps necessary to *safely* perform this task now?
10. Am I able to refuse this task if I feel I am not competent enough to perform it now with the supervision that is available to me?

Your responsibilities when asked to perform dele-ated tasks are summarized in **BOX 6–5**.

cepting a Task

en you agree to perform a task, you are account- for your own actions. Remember, what you do il to do can harm the client. *You must complete sk safely.* Do not hesitate to ask for help if you nsure or if you have questions about a task. s report what you did and your observations.

ng a Task

ve the right to say no. If you have a good for not doing a task, refusing to do it is your d your duty. Use the five rights of delegation (**BOX 6–4**) as a guide, and protect clients and yourself by using common sense. Ask yourself if what you are doing is safe for the client.

That said, you must never ignore an order or request to do something. If you have concerns, communicate them to the delegating nurse. With good communication, you and the nurse should be able to solve the problem. If problems continue, talk to your supervisor, instructor, or another professional to help you sort them out (see Chapters 5 and 7).

You must not refuse a delegated task simply because you do not like or want to do the task. You must have sound reasons for your refusal. Otherwise, you could place the client at risk for harm. You also risk losing your job.

g

o

er

CHAPTER REVIEW

KEY POINTS

- As a support worker, you may work with different types of team members, depending on the setting in which you are employed.
- Benefits of working on a team include opportunities for collaboration; opportunities for communication; a wide range of abilities, skills, and perspectives from team members; opportunities for mentorship; better decision making and problem solving; and a positive, trusting atmosphere.
- Challenges of working on a team include recognizing role boundaries, being flexible, handling conflict, and expressing your needs and views.
- Delegated procedures or acts are legislated by each province and territory and are different across Canada. For your own protection, you must be aware of the legislation in your location and your agency or facility policies.
- The five rights of delegation that will determine the nurse's decision to delegate a task to a support worker include the right task, the right circumstances, the right person, the right directions and communication, and the right supervision and evaluation.

CRITICAL THINKING IN PRACTICE

The nurse supervising your work was supposed to return from a break 15 minutes ago. The nurse did not tell you who is supervising your work during the break. You have a question about a patient's care. What will you do? Who should you tell about the problem?

REVIEW QUESTIONS

Answers to these questions are at the bottom of p. 99.

Circle the BEST answer.

1. The membership of a health care team is determined by:
   A. The client's needs
   B. The nurse's needs
   C. The physician's needs
   D. The needs of the client's family
2. Which of the following is a benefit of the team approach to health care?
   A. Opportunities for confidentiality
   B. Opportunities for delegation
   C. Opportunities for collaboration
   D. Opportunities for assignment of tasks
3. The following statements are about health care teams and facilities. Which is true?
   A. Teams are often interdisciplinary.
   B. Family conferences do not include the client.
   C. Team members usually work in different locations.
   D. Team members have few opportunities to meet.
4. In a community setting, who usually assesses, monitors, and evaluates a client's needs and coordinates the services of the health care team?
   A. The family physician
   B. The case manager
   C. The occupational therapist
   D. The social worker
5. Delegation means:
   A. Giving someone responsibility for providing care
   B. Authorizing an unregulated care provider to perform a task
   C. Transferring responsibility to another work
   D. Giving the support worker the power to enforce an act

6. Which factor affects delegation decisions made by a nurse?
   A. Is the client's condition stable?
   B. Does legislation restrict who can perform this task?
   C. What tasks are included in the support worker's job description?
   D. All of the above.

7. If a nurse delegates a task to you, which of the following is true?
   A. The nurse is completely responsible for your actions; you are not responsible.
   B. The nurse has overall responsibility for your actions; you are also responsible.
   C. You are completely responsible for your actions; the nurse is not responsible.
   D. Neither you nor the nurse is responsible.

8. A procedure can be delegated to you:
   A. By any regulated health care provider
   B. By a physician
   C. By the client
   D. By a nurse only

9. A nurse delegates a task to you that you are not comfortable doing. Which of the following is a true statement?
   A. You must perform the task.
   B. You can refuse to perform the task.
   C. You cannot ask for further training on how to perform the task.
   D. You cannot ask the nurse to stay while you perform the task.

10. You are assisting Mr. Chiang with personal care in his home. Mrs. Chiang asks you to change her husband's dressing. Nurses have delegated dressing changes to you for other clients. What should you do?
    A. Tell Mrs. Chiang that you are not allowed to perform the procedure without the authorization of your supervisor. Call your supervisor.
    B. Tell Mrs. Chiang that you can change the dressing if her husband (your client) asks you to do it.
    C. Tell Mrs. Chiang that you can change the dressing if she stays in the room during the procedure.
    D. Tell Mrs. Chiang she has to obtain permission from your supervisor.

Answer: Answers: 1.A, 2.C, 3.A, 4.B, 5.B, 6.D, 7.B, 8.D, 9.B, 10.A

ener image: Syda Productions/Shutterstock.com

CHAPTER 7

Managing Stress, Time, and Problems

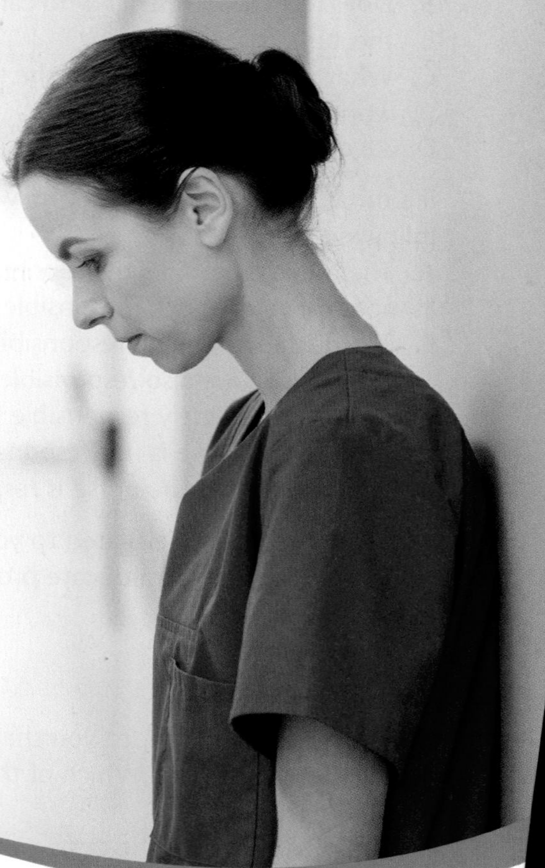

OBJECTIVES

After reading this chapter, the learner should be able to do the following:

- Describe how stress can affect all dimensions of life.
- List the signs of stress.
- Describe common stressors.
- Discuss how people use defence mechanisms to cope with stress.
- Recognize how stress can affect a person's health.
- Identify ways to support clients who are stressed.
- Define SMART goals.
- Describe positive ways to manage stress.
- Describe stress-reducing methods that may improve a person's decision-making and problem-solving abilities.
- Identify ways to deal with stress and conflict in the workplace.

KEY TERMS

acute stress A type of stress that is short in duration. *p. 101*
anxiety A vague, uneasy feeling, often including a sense of impending danger or harm. *p. 104*
burnout A state of physical, emotional, and mental exhaustion that results in feelings of discouragement, negativity, and powerlessness. *p. 101*
chronic stress Ongoing stress that can lead to burnout. *p. 101*
conflict A clash between opposing interests and ideas. *p. 103*
emotional pressure The feeling of being pushed beyond one's limits or abilities. *p. 102*
eustress A type of stressor that is healthy and gives one a feeling of fulfillment or other positive feelings. *p. 101*
stress The emotional, behavioural, or physical response to an event or situation. *p. 101*
stressor An event or situation that causes stress. *p. 101*
validate To acknowledge, recognize, or confirm the client's feelings. *p. 105*

This chapter deals with four key challenges support workers face: (1) handling stress, (2) managing time, (3) making decisions, and (4) solving problems. As a support worker, if you can manage time, make wise decisions, and solve problems, you will have less stress. Much of what is discussed in this chapter can be used to deal with issues in your personal as well as your professional life.

For example, Marissa became a support worker because she likes helping people. She feels great compassion for her clients. Most of the time, she likes her job, but she sometimes worries that she is not doing her best. She feels stressed and rushed and has trouble making decisions. She discusses her feelings with her supervisor, who encourages her to take a time-management course. Her supervisor also offers to help Marissa become a better decision maker and problem solver. As a result, she is able to recognize when clients are under stress, and she can try to help them reduce their stress.

STRESS

Stress is a normal part of life that everyone experiences at one time or another. **Stress** is the emotional, behavioural, or physical response to an event or situation. People face various types of stress in their lives, some positive and some negative. **Eustress** is a type of stress that is healthy and gives one a feeling of fulfillment or other positive feelings. **Acute stress** is short in duration, whereas **chronic stress** is ongoing.

Stress affects the whole person. It can have positive or negative effects in all dimensions—the physical, emotional, social, intellectual (cognitive), and spiritual (TABLE 7–1). Chronic stress can lead to **burnout**—a state of physical, emotional, and mental exhaustion. A person experiencing burnout feels discouraged, negative, and powerless. We discuss the topic of burnout in more detail on pages 106–107. For some individuals with underlying mental health issues, severe or prolonged stress may trigger the onset of mental health symptoms, especially if the client experiences changes in eating or sleeping, increases use of drugs or alcohol, or feels impulses to engage in reckless behaviour (also see Chapter 35).

Sources of Stress

Stress can be caused by various factors, called **stressors**. The more frequently the stressor occurs and the longer it lasts, the more likely it is to affect the person's health. Stressors that last for a few minutes to a few hours—for example, daily irritations—usually create only mild stress. Stressors that last for months or years, such as persistent illness, disability, or family relationship problems, can cause severe stress.

Some common stressors are discussed below.

Changes

Whether it is positive or negative, change is always a source of stress. Regardless of age, many people find change difficult, while others seem to embrace it

TABLE 7–1 Stress Can Affect All Dimensions

Dimension	Example of Stressor	Example of a Negative Effect	Example of a Positive Effect
Physical	Pneumonia	Death	Infection resolved
	Breast cancer	Loss of breast	Being fitted with a prosthesis
Emotional	Sexual assault by a man	Fear of men; depression	Finding fulfillment as a mentor for others at a sexual assault crisis centre
	Divorce	Anger, resentment, crying, inability to work	Seeking help through employment assistance program
Intellectual (Cognitive)	Diagnosis of cancer	Denying the presence of cancer and refusing to consider treatment	Learning about the disease to make informed decisions about care
	Final exam	Deciding not to continue to study	Planning a study schedule
Social	Alcoholism	Withdrawal from family and other social contacts	Participation in Alcoholics Anonymous support group
	Move to new city, knowing no one	Remaining isolated, becoming depressed	Joining a group that shares similar interests, (e.g., ski club) or taking a course
Spiritual	Injury	Feeling abandoned by God	Seeking counselling from spiritual advisor; finding comfort in faith
	Death of a family member	Abandoning faith	Seeking comfort from faith or from other people

Adapted from Potter, P.A., Perry, A.G., Ross-Kerr, J.C., et al. (2001). *Canadian fundamentals of nursing* (2nd ed., p. 647). Toronto, ON: Harcourt Canada.

without exhibiting signs of stress. For example, most older adults have lived through numerous changes and personal difficulties. Many of them are still able to adapt well to new changes in health status or to the loss of partners and friends. Meanwhile, some younger adults can be very negatively affected by life changes and personal loss. Common life changes include the following:

- Death of a loved one
- Divorce
- Loss of a job
- Increase in financial obligations
- Marriage
- Getting a promotion
- Move to a new home
- Chronic illness or injury
- Emotional problems (depression, anxiety, anger, grief, guilt, low self-esteem)
- Caring for a sick or aging family member
- A traumatic event, such as a natural disaster, theft, rape, or violence against the person or a loved one

Emotional Pressure

Emotional pressure is the feeling of being pushed beyond one's limits or abilities. People feel pressure for different reasons, including being rushed, having too many demands on them, and feeling unable to

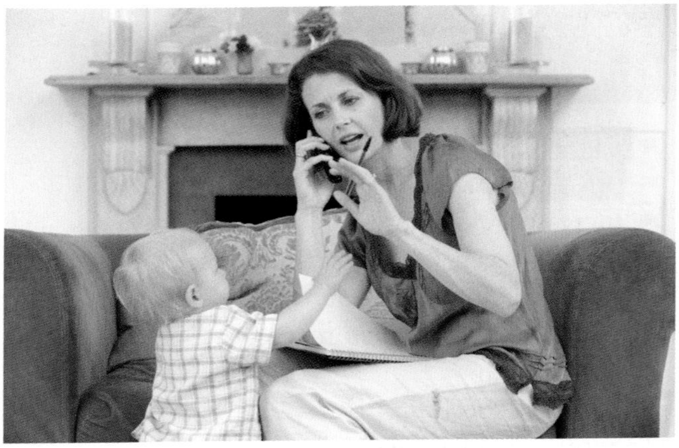

FIGURE 7–1 This woman feels pressured because she is unable to fulfill the demands made on her by both her children and her job. (**Source:** © Can Stock Photo Inc./ monkeybusiness.)

fulfill others' expectations (**FIGURE 7–1**). People sometimes put pressure on themselves by setting goals that are difficult or impossible to achieve. For example, Penelope is frustrated with herself because she fails to lose 15 pounds in 1 month, and, as a result, she feels stress. Clearly, her goal was too difficult to achieve.

Lack of Control

Some people experience stress when they feel they cannot control what happens to them and to the environment around them and they instead have to depend on someone else. For example, loss of work, economic hardship, violence, illness, discrimination, and death of a loved one all cause stress. Not being able to control one's own behaviour is also a stressor. For example, Ms. Kumar wants to quit smoking. She tries and fails, and she is angry at her apparent lack of self-control. As a result, she feels stress, to which he responds by smoking.

onflict

nflict is a clash between opposing interests and as. Conflicts with a partner, friend, child, co-worker, client are serious sources of stress. People also rience conflict within themselves when sorting heir problems or making decisions.

ol

nts often become stressed by heavy workloads gnments, tests, exams, and clinical placements. Many also face the demands of their family, as they are not only students but also partners, parents, children, employees, and so on, with responsibilities outside school. Families often have difficulty understanding that the student in the house may not be able to do everything he did before he returned to school.

Daily Frustrations

Frustrations can sometimes cause stress—for example, losing car keys, being stuck in traffic, or oversleeping. As a support worker, you may encounter frustrations such as having to manage with insufficient staff to complete all the required care or being sent to another floor, where the clients are unfamiliar, to cover for someone else. People's reactions to a frustrating situation vary. For some, any unexpected incident can cause stress.

Responses to Stress

People may respond differently to the same stressor. A person's responses to stressors are influenced by several factors, including (but not limited to) the following:

- Gender
- Perception of personal control and feelings of competence
- Availability of social supports
- Cognitive awareness
- Health
- Temperament or personality
- Past experiences with the same or similar stressors
- The number of other stressors being experienced
- The nature, severity, and duration of the stressor

People can display physical responses to stress (**BOX 7–1** and **BOX 7–2**) and emotional and behavioural responses (**BOX 7–3** on p. 105). Physical responses are the same for most people, but emotional and behavioural responses vary among individuals. Many people have their own way of coping with stress. Some behaviours—for example, crying and talking—relieve stress. Some other behaviours—for example, smoking and drinking—are unhealthy and may eventually increase rather than decrease stress.

FOCUS ON OLDER ADULTS

Stress

Some of the common stressors faced by older adults include the following:

- Loss of spouse, other family members, friends, and, unfortunately, sometimes grandchildren
- Health problems
- Economic worries, since a large number of older adults are on a limited, fixed income
- Increased dependency on another person to help with personal care, finances, or housekeeping
- Loneliness and isolation
- Decline in abilities because of the normal aging process

Although they may face numerous stressors, older adults can cope with stress equally well as other adults. Many older adults rely on their spirituality to cope with illness or severe stress.

Adapted from Potter, P.A., Perry, A.G., Ross-Kerr, J.C., et al. (2014). *Canadian fundamentals of nursing* (5th ed., pp. 384–387, 451). Toronto, ON: Harcourt Canada.

BOX 7–1 Physical Signs and Symptoms of Acute Stress

- Rapid pulse
- Rapid respirations
- Increased blood pressure
- Rapid speech, higher-pitched voice
- A "lump" in the throat
- "Butterflies" in the stomach
- Dry mouth
- Sweaty palms
- Sore muscles in neck, arms, and back
- Perspiration
- Nausea
- Diarrhea
- Urinary frequency
- Urinary urgency
- Difficulty sleeping
- Change in appetite
- Change in weight

FOCUS ON CHILDREN

Stress

Infants and children also react to stressors and may show the same signs of stress as adults do. For example, a child under stress might have stomach aches, irritability, changes in appetite, or changes in sleep patterns.

Children might not be able to communicate their feelings very well in words and are more likely to indicate how they feel with their actions. A child's behaviour that is out of the ordinary may be a sign of stress—for example, a normally content baby cries for an hour after being overstimulated; a fully toilet-trained 4-year-old suddenly begins to wet the bed after his mother becomes seriously ill; or a usually calm adolescent begins to engage in physical fights with peers after his parents' divorce.

BOX 7–2 Physical Signs and Symptoms of Chronic Stress

- Chronic headache
- Mood swings
- **Anxiety** (a vague, uneasy feeling, often including a sense of impending danger or harm)
- Substance abuse
- Memory disturbances
- Weakening of immune system function, which can result in frequent attacks of cold and flu
- Cardiovascular diseases ranging from heart attacks to strokes; increased blood pressure
- Bowel disorders
- Decreased sexual drive
- Sleeplessness

BOX 7–3 Emotional and Behavioural Signs and Symptoms of Stress

- Anxiety
- Depression
- Anger
- Worry
- Fear
- Burnout
- Irritability
- Loss of self-esteem
- Fatigue
- Dissatisfaction
- Forgetfulness
- Poor concentration
- Difficulty focusing or following directions
- Emotional outbursts, including yelling or crying
- Smoking
- Drinking
- Talking about the stressor

Defence Mechanisms in Times of Stress

Most people use defence mechanisms at one time or another, especially when they are under stress. Defence mechanisms are used to delay—or avoid altogether—uncomfortable feelings such as anxiety, guilt, stress, or embarrassment. In this way, they relieve stress by helping the person avoid facing a troubling reality (see Chapter 5). For example, a client in a facility is upset that her daughter is not able to visit her frequently. She blames the city bus system since she believes that if the buses were more reliable, her daughter would visit more often. Even though she focuses her anger on the bus system, she really is disappointed with her daughter.

When working with clients who are under stress, being able to recognize their defence mechanisms is useful. Understanding defence mechanisms gives you insight into what your clients may really be feeling. You can help them by being empathetic to their feelings, by trying to **validate** their feelings, and by providing compassionate care. *Validation* means to acknowledge, recognize, or confirm the client's feelings (see Chapter 36).

As a support worker, you must recognize the common responses to stress in your clients. Tell your supervisor when you notice a client showing signs of stress, such as loss of appetite or sleep, a change in behaviour or mood, or increased use of alcohol or other substances. Remember, your role is to observe and report, not to assess or diagnose. It is *not* within your scope of practice to diagnose clients by using defence mechanism terms; instead, you need to *describe* the client's behaviour when reporting it. It is important, however, to be familiar with these terms when they are used, as an understanding of them will help you when giving care to your client. For example, when a client complains of headache and nausea, do not assume that the client is suffering from stress, because these could also be symptoms of a physical condition. Rather, note and report your observations since professionals such as nurses and social workers can help clients cope with stress.

Managing Stress in Your Life

Stress is common among health care workers, particularly in support work, which can be very demanding. You may feel physical stress from all the lifting, moving, and carrying that you are required to do every day. You may feel cognitive stress while trying to do many things at the same time. For example, a client asks for the bedpan every time you walk by the room, and another needs to be turned and repositioned every 15 minutes. You may feel emotional stress from working with clients who are sick, lonely, frail, or dying. You may also work with clients or family members who are angry or distressed. For example, a wife who is the primary caregiver for her ill husband is angry with her boss for insisting that she always stay late at work. She may direct her anger toward you, or you might feel upset for her. Depending on how you react, such situations can cause severe stress.

Managing stress is essential, so do not ignore the signs of stress. Letting stress build can result in burnout or illness. Not dealing properly and immediately with stress can cause some support workers to take out their frustrations on their clients or someone in their personal lives, leading to abuse or neglect, which cannot be allowed to happen.

The following strategies can help in managing stress:

- ***Develop self-awareness.*** Know what causes your stress. Think about when you felt under stress. What was the source? Does it occur often? After determining your stressors, you need to decide how to eliminate them, avoid them, or cope with them. Avoid people who cause you stress.
- ***Take care of your needs.*** A healthy mind and body enable people to cope better with stress. Getting enough sleep is important. Mild irritations may seem like serious problems if you are sleep deprived. Exercising regularly and following a nutritious diet are also important. Do not ignore your social, cognitive, and spiritual needs. Often, the key to managing stress is finding ways to balance family, work, relaxation, and recreation. Keep track of how you spend your time. Which parts of your life get too much time? Which parts are neglected? How might you achieve a better balance? Make time for fun and relaxation.
- ***Think positively.*** A positive attitude can help you manage stress. Focus on what you do well and what you can control. Remember that every person perceives stress differently. Put the stressor into perspective—try not to let a minor stressor become a major one. Try to change your perspective to see how a stressor can create a positive outcome. Keeping a sense of humour also helps reduce tension. Look at the big picture. Ask yourself how important this stressful situation will be in the long run. Will it matter in a month or a year? If the answer is no, focus your time and energy elsewhere.
- ***Assert yourself.*** Nonassertive people say yes to things when they really want to say no. They take on tasks when they have no time for them. They also give in to the demands of others without considering their own needs. Never agree to do more than you can do safely (see Chapter 12).
- ***Ask others for help and support.*** To avoid stress, you have to accept that you cannot do everything yourself. Assert yourself at work and in your home life. If you need help with an assignment, tell your supervisor. At home, let your family know that you need their help and support. Discuss sharing household duties with your roommates, siblings, spouse, or children. Let them know what you need and expect, and take the time to explain to them how to do the activities you usually do. Be encouraging, and avoid being critical if things are not done to your standard.
- ***Practise calming exercises***. As soon as you feel the first sign of stress, find a way to calm yourself (**BOX 7–4**). Some people, for example, do daily meditation to cope with stress (**BOX 7–5**).
- ***Learn to accept the things you cannot change***. You cannot control the behaviour of other people. However, you can choose to change how you react to that behaviour.

BOX 7–4 Calming Yourself When Feeling Stress

- Close your eyes (if safe to do so), and take deep, slow breaths. Relax your stomach muscles. Breathe in through your nose and out through your mouth. Your stomach should rise about 3 cm (1 inch) as you breathe in. As you inhale, count slowly up to 4. As you exhale, count slowly back down to 1. Pause between breaths. Continue breathing slowly and rhythmically until you feel yourself relaxing.
- If you feel your muscles tensing, relax them. People tend to clench their jaws and tighten their necks and backs when they are under stress. Relax your muscles, from your face down to your feet.
- If possible, take a few minutes to yourself. Remove yourself from the stressful situation. ***However, never leave a client unless it is safe to do so.***

Job Burnout

Burnout is common among health care workers since these helping professions can be very demanding physically, emotionally, and mentally (see *Supporting Kathy: Support Workers Can Face Burnout Also*). As discussed earlier, severe or prolonged stress can lead to burnout, which is a state of physical, emotional, and mental exhaustion caused by long-term exposure to demanding work situations. Like stress, burnout can have negative consequences for your health, such

BOX 7–5 Meditation

- At home, sit in a comfortable position in a quiet place. Turn off the phone.
- Pick a word that can be repeated during meditation. Single-syllable words, such as "one," are very effective.
- Relax all muscle groups, beginning with the head and working progressively down to the feet.
- Breathe in slowly through the nose, and exhale slowly through the mouth.
- Silently repeat the chosen word while inhaling and exhaling.
- Focus your thoughts on this rhythmic chanting and breathing for 10 minutes.
- Allow images and thoughts to flow freely.

Based on Potter, P.A., Perry, A.G., Ross-Kerr, J.C., et al. (2001). *Canadian fundamentals of nursing* (2nd ed., p. 655). Toronto, ON: Harcourt Canada.

as insomnia, weight gain or loss, depression, anxiety, and other emotional difficulties (also see Chapters 5 and 35).

The following are some of the signs of burnout:

- Increasing criticism of others or sarcasm at work
- Changed sleep habits
- Changed appetite
- Fatigue—for example, having trouble getting the day started
- Less patience with clients and co-workers
- Self-medicating—using food, drugs, or alcohol to feel better

If you are showing signs of burnout, do not ignore them. Talk to your supervisor, doctor, or employee assistance program counsellor. Recovery can take time, but keep an open mind and consider all of your options.

Supporting Kathy: Support Workers Can Face Burnout Also

Kathy is a support worker, who has been working at the same continuing care facility for over 20 years. If asked if she likes her job, she would say, "It pays the bills." You have noticed that she arrives at work a few minutes late every day and takes longer breaks than the other employees do. When everyone else is getting up to go back to work after their break time ends, Kathy announces, "Well, I'm going to the bathroom." She then returns to the unit 5 to 10 minutes after everyone else. You suspect that she goes outside to have another cigarette because she usually smells strongly of tobacco upon her return.

You do not enjoy working with Kathy because she is opinionated and occasionally rude to you when you ask her questions. You have also seen her being abrupt with some of the more challenging or demanding residents. Kathy rarely smiles and hardly ever speaks to you. She usually talks only to the other senior staff.

Today, at change-of-shift report, the nurse reports that Mrs. Price—a client you liked very much—has died. Kathy says loudly, "Good. One less person I've got to toilet." Lately, you have been thinking about doing something to address Kathy's attitude but do not know where to begin. You do not want to quit because the facility is located conveniently just down the street from where you live. What should you do?

TIME MANAGEMENT

Time management, which is essential to reducing stress, is important in support work. You can use time-management strategies in all aspects of your life. If you reduce your overall stress levels, stress at work will also decrease.

To manage your time, you must identify your priorities. Doing so helps you stay focused on what is important to you. While you are at work, providing competent, compassionate care is a priority. To determine your priorities outside of work, ask yourself these questions:

- What do I value most in life?
- What gives me satisfaction?
- What principles do I want to live my life by?

Respecting Diversity

As a support worker, you must remember that some people may not value keeping strict adherence to time schedules. When working in the community, you could be scheduled to arrive in your client's home for 9:00 a.m. but then find that your client is not ready for your appointment and would like you to wait and chat until she is ready. Talk to your supervisor if adhering to the schedule is an ongoing problem with your client. In facilities, late starts could create a challenge for both workers and clients when a routine has to be followed.

You may identify a large number of priorities. Take some time to decide which ones are the most important. Assign a number to each, with 1 being the most important and 10 being the least important. Now you are ready to turn your priorities into goals.

Setting SMART Goals

Setting goals for yourself will help you manage time and stress. Your goals should give you direction and motivate you to take action. Start with your priority number 1, and work down the list to number 10. Do not set more than 10 goals, or you may lose your focus. Your goals should be SMART: **S**pecific, **M**easurable, **A**chievable, **R**ealistic, and **T**imely.[1]

- ***Specific.*** Goals must be clear. For example, "losing weight" is not a specific goal. The goal of "losing 5 kg by the end of March" is specific and gives direction and focus.
- ***Measurable.*** Measurable goals tell you if you are making progress. The goal stated above is measurable in two ways: "5 kg" and "by the end of March."
- ***Achievable.*** Goals should be challenging yet achievable. When setting goals, consider how much time and effort you can put into them. A goal may need two or more parts to be achievable. For example, to lose the weight, you are going to need to investigate a diet plan or an exercise plan and determine how much time will be needed to put your plan into action.
- ***Realistic.*** A realistic goal accounts for time, resources, and skills. For example, losing 5 kg in 3 months is realistic. It would not be realistic, however, if you were planning to take a vacation during this time.
- ***Timely.*** A target date for meeting goals increases commitment. Break goals into parts, and set schedules. As each part is achieved, you will gain confidence and be motivated to reach higher goals. For example, your goal can be broken down into losing 1.6 kilograms a month.

Planning Your Life and Your Work

Well-organized people have weekly and daily plans and include their personal and professional goals in their planning. Goals are easier to achieve when time is spent planning at the start of each week. For example, every Sunday, Raj, a busy support worker who has a wife and two children, plans his week. He is working the evening shift this week, which means his wife must pick up the children, make dinner, and take them to after-school activities. Since Raj's wife is going to be out of town on Thursday, Raj makes a note to arrange for his sister to look after the children that day. One of Raj's goals is to build a backyard hockey rink, as he promised his children. He decides to work on the rink each day before leaving for work. Raj reviews his work schedule for the week. His supervisor has asked him to coach a new support worker, which means he will be taking the new support worker on client visits. Since one of his clients may be uncomfortable with the presence of another support worker, his supervisor has asked him to call the client ahead to prepare him for the new worker. Raj makes a note to telephone this client on Monday.

Daily planning and scheduling are important to meeting goals. Review your assignment sheet and the care plan for each client, and decide how you will approach each task. If you prepare ahead of time (the night before or just before your shift), you will not have to spend the valuable time you have with clients scheduling tasks. However, just because you have prepared does not mean that you will never have to change a schedule once it has been set. You must stay

BOX 7–6 Tips to Save Time and Stay Organized

- Follow the assignment sheet or the care plan.
- Remember the client's needs and priorities.
- Know what tasks need to be done at a certain time.
- Set yourself time limits; work within those limits unless a client's needs are more pressing.
- Develop routines that work for you and for the client.
- Allow for more time than you need when possible.
- Remain flexible at all times.
- Start with the tasks that must get done.
- Remind yourself not to get sidetracked by non-essential things.
- Learn to say no—firmly, positively, and tactfully.
- Use a calendar to note down important dates and reminders.
- Make sure that you have the necessary equipment and supplies before you start a task.
- Put equipment and supplies back in their proper place after the task has been completed.

flexible and responsive to the needs of the client (see the *Supporting Mrs. Paget: Daily Planning* box).

Use your planning and scheduling time to think about problems that might arise. Review the tasks on your list. Plan how much time each task will take. To improve scheduling, ask yourself these questions:

- What are the client's needs and priorities?
- How much time will each task or activity require?
- When will I do each task or activity?
- Can I organize my time so that some of the tasks overlap?
- Have I allowed time for the unexpected?
- Is there anyone with whom I should coordinate these activities?

Giving each task a time limit will help you stay focused and complete a task on time. See **BOX 7–6** for ways to manage your time and stay organized. At the end of your workday, compare what you planned to do with what you actually did. Did you accomplish what you planned? If not, try to identify why. Did problems arise? Were there interruptions? Was it a poor schedule?

Supporting Mrs. Paget: Daily Planning

Chona is a support worker in a long-term care facility. Before her morning shift begins, she reviews her assignment sheet and the care plans for each of the clients she supports. The care plan notes that Mrs. Paget, a new client, requires assistance in making decisions for herself and that all care providers should help Mrs. Paget make decisions by providing choices.

Chona considers the choices that she could provide for Mrs. Paget during the day. She decides that she can offer Mrs. Paget two sets of clothes to wear for the day, two different items for breakfast, and two different items for lunch. As she provides morning care, Chona can familiarize Mrs. Paget with the activities that are available during the morning and offer Mrs. Paget her choices. After lunch, she can talk to her about activities available for the afternoon and again offer her choices. Planning these choices in advance will help Chona keep her day on schedule. There may be other opportunities during the day when Mrs. Paget can be given choices as situations occur. Chona will need to include in her plan time for completing flow charts and reporting to the charge nurse.

DECISION MAKING

As a support worker, you make numerous decisions in the course of your workday as you organize your time, make a schedule, and provide care to clients. For example, you decide:

- The order in which you are going to carry out tasks
- The equipment and supplies you need for each task

- The amount of time to spend with each client
- When a problem or an observation needs to be reported immediately
- Whether you need help to complete a task
- Whether you need to consult with your supervisor
- Whether you will accept or refuse a delegated task

Skills You Need to Make Decisions

Do you know anyone who always seems to make the right decisions? Such people are usually decisive and calm. The following skills will help improve your decision making:

- ***Focus***. Focus requires concentration, involvement, and commitment. Focus on the client and the task at hand to make the right decisions. Focusing includes asking questions and listening actively (FIGURE 7–2).
- ***Flexibility***. You need to be flexible and responsive. Involve clients in decisions that affect them, and be ready to adapt in response to a client's needs. Remember, each client is an individual with unique needs, which are affected by age, culture, and health status. For example, (1) Mr. Johnston, 91, lives in a facility and has no family or friends living nearby. He tells you he feels lonely. You decide to chat with him while helping him bathe; (2) Ms. Chow, 35, is recovering at home after surgery. She tells you she feels exhausted. Since listening and talking can be tiring, you remain quiet while helping Ms. Chow with her bath. You ask her if she would like to rest afterward, and she says yes. The same task is done differently because you responded to each client's unique needs.
- ***Decisiveness***. Stick to your decisions unless they are not working. Indecisiveness on your part can upset clients; they expect you to be confident and competent.

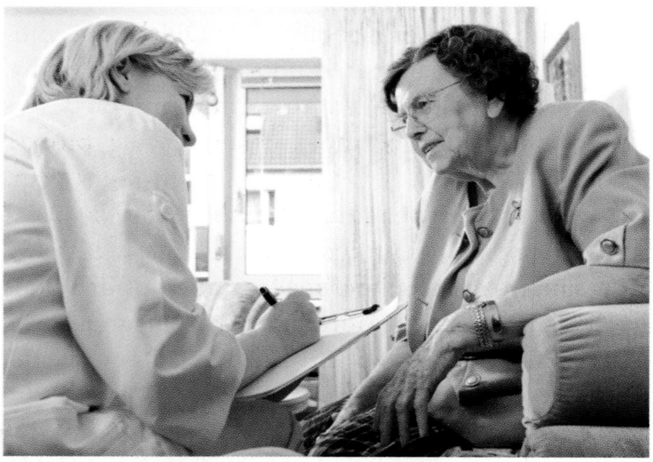

FIGURE 7–2 This support worker listens carefully to a client so she can make the right decision. (**Source:** © Can Stock Photo Inc./gajdamak.)

Decision Making in Different Health Care Settings

You will face similar kinds of decisions in most settings, even though some differences exist between facilities and private homes. In a facility, you care for several clients and also assist nurses, as needed. Sometimes you have to decide which person's needs are to be met first. For example, you see a client shouting angrily at her roommate. Another client needs to be shaved. You need to decide who should be helped first.

If working in home care, you must plan your time so that you can be punctual for the next client. Since your supervisor is not on site, you also have to make decisions on your own.

PROBLEM SOLVING

Problem solving is a process that requires identifying and analyzing a problem, finding a solution, and devising a plan to apply that solution.

Identify the Problem

You must first determine if you have a problem and what it is. Ask yourself the following questions:

- Is the situation or issue affecting you, a co-worker, your supervisor, or one of your clients?
- Should you be concerned about the situation?
- Can you influence or contribute to a positive outcome?
- Does the issue require immediate attention?

Consider the following two examples:

1. Miles helps Mr. Rossi, 85, get dressed in the mornings. Most days, Mr. Rossi chooses to wear the

same tattered sweater. Miles is tired of seeing it on him. He knows that Mr. Rossi has other sweaters. However, when Miles considers the above questions, he answers no to each. He knows that the sweater is clean, that Mr. Rossi enjoys wearing it, and that he has the right to choose what he wears. Miles decides that this situation is not a problem.

2. Cheryl assists Mr. McDonald, 88, with lunch in the dining room of a long-term care facility. He chooses tomato soup for lunch. After one spoonful, he refuses to eat. Cheryl is concerned. She knows that if Mr. McDonald does not eat, he tends to get dizzy and may fall. She knows this situation is a problem that requires her immediate attention.

Analyze the Problem

Once you know you have a problem, think about what kind of problem it is. Decide if it is one that you can solve on your own. Consult the assignment sheet or care plan to make sure you know what is expected of you. Remember to consult your supervisor when:

- There is an emergency
- You observe a change in the client's condition or normal functioning
- The client becomes ill—for example, the client vomits, has diarrhea, or develops a fever
- The client is in distress
- You believe the client's safety is at risk
- A problem involving medications exists
- The client complains about his condition or care
- The client asks you a question about her diagnosis, condition, or treatment plans
- The client or family member asks you to do something that goes against the care plan
- You have a conflict with a client or family member
- A question or problem arises and you need help to deal with it

Your supervisor is always available to provide guidance and help solve problems. Even in a community setting, your supervisor is just a phone call away.

Analyzing a problem involves communication. Ask the client questions about the problem, and listen attentively to the answers. Remember to pay attention to verbal as well as nonverbal messages (see the *Supporting Mrs. Kao: Asking, Listening, and Observing* box). Do not make assumptions about the cause of a problem.

For instance, in example 2 above, when Cheryl asks Mr. McDonald why he does not want to eat, he says that he has a sore on the inside of his cheek where he bit himself the other day. She can tell by his expression that his mouth hurts. Cheryl knows that Mr. McDonald's care plan does not specify a special diet. He is able to eat anything from the available menu. She therefore decides to try solving the problem by urging him to select softer foods until his mouth heals. She should notify her supervisor of her observations, as well as report and record Mr. McDonald's complaints. She should also notify her supervisor if his discomfort increases.

Find a Solution

Think of as many solutions as you can. Decide which is the most practical and helpful, but always be sure that it is safe. Try the solution to see if it works. For example, Cheryl thinks that the tomato soup may be too hot and acidic for Mr. McDonald's sore mouth. She suggests he try a cooler, blander meal. He chooses macaroni and cheese. He is able to eat it without discomfort. Cheryl later reports to her supervisor what she did to try to remedy Mr. McDonald's sore in his mouth and whether it was effective. She also needs to document this information in his chart (see Chapter 14).

Devise a Plan

The planning part of the problem-solving process may involve creativity. Do not be afraid to try a plan, as long as it is safe. Consider Ruth's creative solution to a problem: Ruth's client, Mrs. Klassen, is in the early stages of Alzheimer's disease. Mrs. Klassen is upset because she cannot remember her grandson's name. He will be visiting the next day, and she wants to be able to call him by his name. Ruth has the grandson's name listed on the care plan. She then gently suggests a way to help Mrs. Klassen remember it. They find a picture of her grandson and write his name on it. Ruth then tapes the picture to the wall

Supporting Mrs. Kao: Asking, Listening, and Observing

Emma, a support worker on a surgical ward in a hospital, is assigned to help Mrs. Kao do range-of-motion (ROM) exercises after her surgery. When Mrs. Kao refuses, Emma asks her why she does not want to do the exercises. Mrs. Kao says that her legs ache and she does not feel like moving them. Emma tries to encourage Mrs. Kao and asks her if the nurse explained why the exercises are important. Mrs. Kao says she knows why the exercises are important. Emma suggests that Mrs. Kao start by moving her toes, but when she does move her toes, Emma sees her grimace. She asks Mrs. Kao if she is in pain, and Mrs. Kao says, "No, I'm not in pain."

Emma realizes that there is nothing more that she can do or say. She has asked Mrs. Kao the right questions, listened to her responses, and observed her behaviour. It is not her job to assess or diagnose Mrs. Kao's problem. So she informs her supervisor of her conversation with Mrs. Kao and reports that Mrs. Kao grimaced when she moved her toes. She is careful to quote Mrs. Kao's exact words.

Supporting Mrs. Samuels: Creative Solutions

Josephine's client, Mrs. Samuels, 34, is a single mother who is receiving chemotherapy for ovarian cancer. Mrs. Samuels has 3 boys, aged 9 years, 5 years, and 20 months. Mrs. Samuels tells Josephine that ever since she became ill she does not feel that she is doing enough for her children.

Josephine asks Mrs. Samuels what sorts of things she misses doing for her children. Mrs. Samuels says that she wishes she could dress her two little boys in the morning. She also regrets not being able to drive her older boy to after-school activities. Josephine decides to look for opportunities to consult and involve Mrs. Samuels in the care of her children. As the 5-year-old gets ready for school the next morning, Josephine suggests to him that he ask his mother to zip up his jacket and help him put on his mittens and hat. Later, she asks Mrs. Samuels what she would like the baby to wear that day.

by the phone. Mrs. Klassen will have the picture handy when her grandson visits. Ruth records this event on the task sheet. At her next visit with Mrs. Klassen, she asks her if their solution worked (see the *Supporting Mrs. Samuels: Creative Solutions* box for another example of a support worker devising a plan to solve a problem).

DEALING WITH CONFLICT

Some problems can be resolved at once, but others take longer. Interpersonal problems, which are a common cause of stress, may take weeks to solve. People bring their own values, attitudes, opinions, experiences, and expectations to the work setting. Differences often lead to conflict, and disagreements, misunderstandings, arguments, and unrest can occur. Conflicts may arise over issues or events—for example, work schedules, absences, and the amount and quality of work performed. The problems must be worked out to avoid unkind words or actions. When the work environment becomes unpleasant, care of clients is affected.

You may occasionally experience conflict with clients or their families or with your co-workers or supervisors. In dealing with any conflict, remember that caring for the client's needs is always your first priority.

It is important for you to identify your usual response to conflict.

- Do you wait and avoid dealing with the problem, hoping it will go away?
- Are you agreeable and nonassertive even at the expense of your personal work ethics?
- Do you feel you must win at any cost?

Remember that clients and family members can respond differently to conflict. In a conflict situation, you need to step back and think about how you, your client, or a client's family member is responding to the conflict and talk to your supervisor about how to resolve it.

Conflict between you and a client could occur if a client is too tired, overstimulated, confused, or having difficulty communicating. For example, Mrs. Jones had been out to a doctor's appointment in the morning and is refusing to eat her lunch. You know it is important that she eat something. If you do not recognize that Mrs. Jones is too tired and you persist in trying to get her to eat, the conflict could escalate. Perhaps you should allow Mrs. Jones to rest first and eat later, and you should report this decision to your supervisor. Report all conflicts with clients to your supervisor, including ones that you have resolved. You can prevent conflict from escalating by remaining calm and respectful, understanding the client's needs and feelings, and recognizing the reason for the client's behaviour.

Conflict can also occur between you and the client's family members. It is important to remember that in most cases, they are only trying to ensure the best care for their family member who is ill. The conflict usually occurs because of a failure to understand the nursing care plan, the reasons for a change in the client's condition or treatment, or the policies of the facility or agency. You should listen to the family's concerns in a calm, nonjudgemental way. If your explanation does not satisfy them, contact your supervisor to ensure that the situation does not worsen. Even if you have made the situation better, you must still report the family members' concerns to your supervisor.

Conflict between co-workers can have a negative effect on the care of clients. Unresolved conflict causes stress and hinders communication and teamwork. To some extent, such conflict is unavoidable since you are not always going to agree with your supervisors or team members. Applying some of the principles outlined in **BOX 7–7** can help you resolve conflicts. You do not need to report conflicts with co-workers if they have been resolved. However, if you cannot resolve a conflict, discuss it with your supervisor. Communication and work ethics are essential in preventing and resolving conflicts. Identify and solve problems before they become major issues.

Respecting Diversity

Different People Deal With Conflict in Different Ways

Differences in communicating may be influenced by a person's culture, an individual's discomfort in dealing with conflict, or the way the person's family dealt with conflict. Some people value an indirect method of communication for reasons of face-saving, harmony, or long-term gains versus short-term gains.

At all times, when dealing with clients, families, co-workers, and supervisors, keep the following in mind:

- Depending on the culture, family, or specific situation, some people may simply deny that a problem exists (or may downplay the problem).
- Taking action could cause displeasure, so some people may choose not to address the conflict.
- Some may choose to blame others for the problem.
- Some people may not respond verbally at all.

Talk to your supervisor, who may have more knowledge of the background of your client or co-worker and may provide information and guidance.

BOX 7–7 Managing Conflict

- Approach the person with whom you have a conflict, and ask to talk with him privately.
- Be polite and professional in your approach.
- Agree on a time and place to talk.
- Talk in a private setting. Others should not see or hear you and another person having what might seem like an argument.
- Explain the problem and what is bothering you. Give facts, and describe specific behaviours. Focus on the problem, not on the person. For example, say, "I need to know when you cannot help me so that I can make other plans." Avoid criticizing the person—for example, saying, "You are always late and never call to let me know."
- Listen to the person's response. Do not interrupt.
- Identify ways to resolve the problem. Offer your own thoughts, and ask for the other person's ideas.
- Schedule a date and a time to review the situation.
- Thank the person for meeting with you.
- Implement the solutions.
- Review the situation, as needed.
- If you are unable to resolve the conflict, ask your supervisor for some time to talk privately. Explain the situation, and ask for advice in solving the problem. Give facts and specific examples.

Scenario: Your teacher has just handed back a major assignment, and you do not understand why you have received such a low mark. You face the choice of becoming very upset, complaining to other students about the teacher, becoming discouraged and dropping out of the program, or managing this conflict. To manage this conflict, you should do the following:

- Ask to talk privately with the teacher.
- Set a time and private place to talk.
- Explain the problem, and ask the teacher to review the assignment with you so that you can understand where you made errors or did not meet the required standards.
- Listen carefully to the teacher's explanation.
- Calmly explain why you feel your mark should be higher.
- Offer your ideas on how to resolve the problem, and ask for the teacher's ideas.
- Set a time to review the situation. Allow 10 days for a response.
- Thank the teacher for meeting with you.
- Implement the solution you have arrived at.

CHAPTER REVIEW

KEY POINTS

- Stress is the emotional, behavioural, or physical response to an event or situation.
- Stress can affect all aspects of a person's life, including physical, emotional, cognitive, social, and spiritual aspects.
- As a support worker, you need to recognize the signs of stress in yourself, your clients, and their families.
- Some common stressors affect us all: change, pressure, lack of control, conflict, school, and daily frustrations.
- Ways to manage stress include developing self-awareness, taking care of one's own needs, thinking positively, asserting oneself, asking others for help and support, practising calming exercises, and learning to accept the things that cannot be changed.
- We all have defence mechanisms to deal with stress (see Chapters 5 and 36).
- Setting SMART goals helps with managing time and stress. Goals should be **S**pecific, **M**easurable, **A**chievable, **R**ealistic, and **T**imely.
- Support workers make many decisions each day so must be focused, flexible, and decisive.
- As a support worker, you will need to be able to identify problems that you can solve yourself and ones you need your supervisor's help to solve. When faced with a problem, identify the problem, analyze the problem, find a solution, and then devise a plan.
- Conflict can occur between you and your co-workers, clients, or clients' families or within your own family. You need to be aware of how to deal with conflict in any of these situations.

CRITICAL THINKING IN PRACTICE

You are assisting a resident in the bathroom. The resident is not to be left alone while in the bathroom. ʼou hear another resident's chair alarm (see Chapter ` sound in the hallway outside the door. What will ·lo? If the chair alarm sounds repeatedly, how ·'s affect your job satisfaction?

REVIEW QUESTIONS

Answers to these questions are at the bottom of p. 116.

Circle the BEST answer.

1. Stress is:
   A. The way you cope with and adjust to everyday living
   B. The emotional, behavioural, or physical response to an event or situation
   C. A mental or emotional disorder
   D. A thought or an idea

2. A stressor is:
   A. An event or situation that causes stress
   B. A coping strategy
   C. A defence mechanism
   D. A reaction to stress

3. Which of the following influences a person's reaction to a stressor?
   A. Past experiences with the same stressor
   B. The person's gender
   C. The person's temperament or personality
   D. All of the above

4. Which of the following can be a physical sign of stress?
   A. Fatigue
   B. Depression
   C. Diarrhea
   D. Irritability
   E. All of the above
   F. A, B, and D

5. A defence mechanism is used to:
   A. Blame others
   B. Avoid facing reality
   C. Solve problems
   D. Make excuses for behaviour

6. Which of the following is a sign of burnout?
   A. Increased patience with clients and co-workers
   B. Improved appetite
   C. Increased use of sarcasm
   D. Getting enough sleep at night

7. Goals should be SMART. What does SMART stand for?
   A. Simple, monthly, allowable, reasonable, timely
   B. Specific, measurable, achievable, realistic, timely
   C. Simple, measurable, achievable, reasonable, topical
   D. Specific, monthly, allowable, realistic, topical

8. When trying to stay organized and save time, it is best to:
   A. Save the important tasks until last
   B. Not set yourself a time limit for each task
   C. Develop a routine that works for you and the client
   D. Remain inflexible

9. The first step in the problem-solving process is to:
   A. Call for help
   B. Learn to say no assertively
   C. Identify the problem
   D. Think of as many solutions as you can

10. What is an important part of resolving conflict?
   A. Communication and good work ethics
   B. Focusing on the person, not the problem
   C. Avoiding the person with whom you have a conflict
   D. Confronting the person with your supervisor for support

Answers: 1.B, 2.A, 3.D, 4.E, 5.B, 6.C, 7.B, 8.C, 9.C, 10.A

Chapter opener image: Syda Productions/Shutterstock.com

CHAPTER 8

Ethics

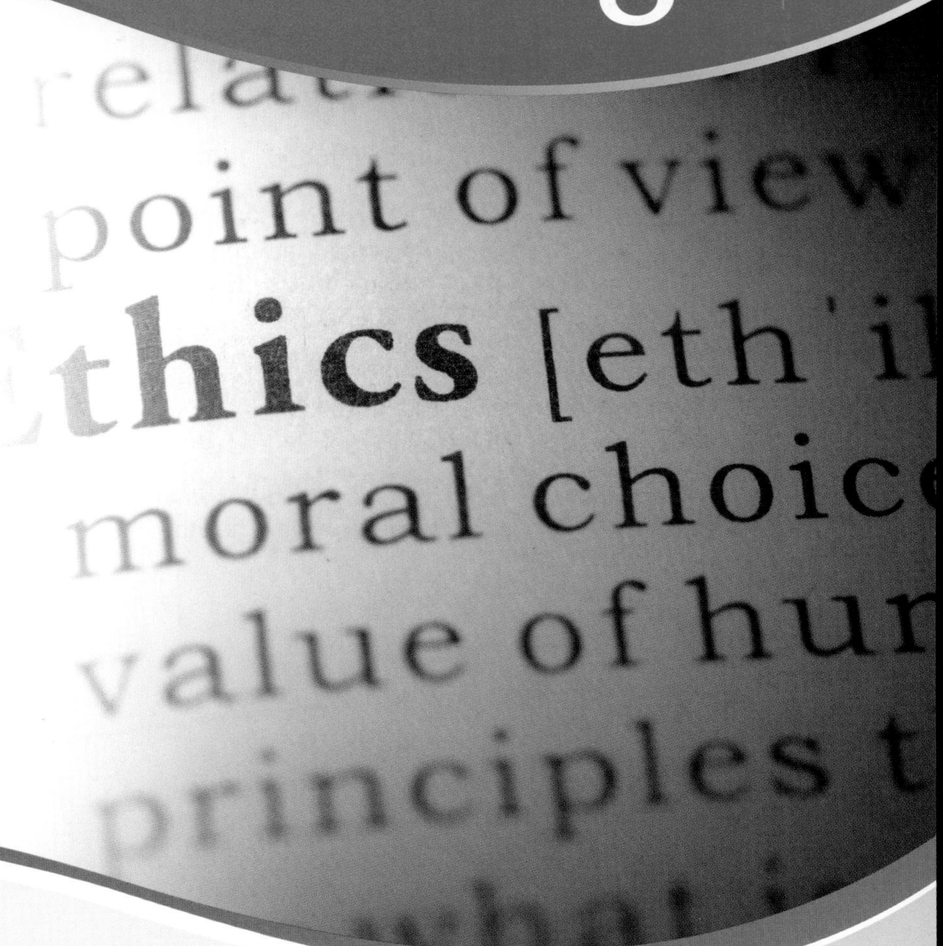

OBJECTIVES

After reading this chapter, the learner should be able to do the following:

- Explain the purpose of a code of ethics.
- Define *belief* and *values*.
- Differentiate between ethics and morals.
- Identify the basic principles of health care ethics.
- Describe how each of the principles applies to support work.
- Define the term *ethical dilemma*.
- Apply the principles to solve ethical dilemmas.

KEY TERMS

autonomy Having the freedom and choice to make decisions that affect one's life. Also known as **self-determination.** *p. 123*

belief Conviction that something is true. *p. 118*

beneficence Doing or promoting good. *p. 123*

conduct Personal behaviour. *p. 119*

ethical dilemma An apparent conflict between opposing moral choices; choosing one would result in going against another moral choice. *p. 121*

ethics The rules of conduct that guide us when deciding what is right and what is wrong, and what is good and what is bad. *p. 118*

health care ethics The philosophical study of what is morally right and wrong when providing health care services. *p. 121*

immoral Conflicting with traditionally held moral principles; often regarded as indecent or deviant (not normal). *p. 118*

justice Fair and equal treatment. *p. 123*

morals The fundamental principles of behaviour each person believes to be *right or wrong for him- or herself* without concern for legalities or customs. *p. 118*

nonmaleficence The ethical principle of doing no harm. *p. 124*

self-determination See **autonomy.** *p. 123*

unethical Not morally correct. *p. 118*

values What an individual considers to be worthwhile or desirable qualities in a person. *p. 118*

The term **ethics** refers to the rules of conduct that guide us when deciding what is right and what is wrong (**immoral**). These rules come from society's expectation of how people should conduct themselves. **Morals** are the fundamental principles of behaviour each person believes to be *right or wrong for him- or herself* without concern for legalities or customs. Support workers must be aware that people's culture and personal circumstances may influence their ethical beliefs, morals, and values, and all of these influence their actions. **Values** are what an individual considers to be worthwhile or desirable qualities in a person. A **belief** is a conviction that something is true. *Ethics* and *morals* are often incorrectly used to mean the same thing, and some people think of *morals* as focusing specifically on standards of behaviour related to sexual activity. Morals and ethics play a part in our everyday lives, and we apply them when making both big and small decisions. Whether we realize it or not, they have a great impact on our personal and professional relationships. As a support worker, when you have to make difficult choices or decisions, you will rely on your ethical beliefs, morals, and values to guide your conduct.

THE INFLUENCE OF CULTURE ON BELIEFS, VALUES, MORALS, AND ETHICS

Most people would probably agree that it would be wrong, or **unethical**, to kill another person. However, what if you were a soldier, fighting to protect your country from a foreign invader? If you were to learn that, in the past, a client had to kill or injure other people in self-defence, would you consider the client's act unethical?

As Canadians, we are obligated to obey the laws that govern us (addressed in Chapter 9). However, as support workers, we should understand that our clients' values, beliefs, morals, ethics, and behaviours may have been influenced by their cultures and life's circumstances (also refer to Chapter 10). (See the *Supporting Mr. Medvjed: How Past Experiences Can Affect One's Beliefs* box.)

CODES OF ETHICS

Members of the health care team have special responsibilities as they form professional helping relationships with clients who require care and services. To guide health care workers' interactions with clients, ethical standards have been established.

Regulated professionals (such as physicians and nurses) are guided by codes of ethics provided by their governing colleges. These codes describe the ideals of the profession as well as standards of conduct that group members must follow.

Support workers do not have a formal code of ethics. However, each agency or facility has its own code of ethics that describes the values and personal qualities that should guide its employees' work and **conduct**. Codes of ethics vary among employers, but most affirm the goals of support work that are identified in this text: being an advocate in promoting the client's dignity, independence, preferences, privacy, and safety, as well as honouring the client's right to confidentiality (also see Chapter 1). **BOX 8-1** illustrates a sample code of ethics for support workers.

Supporting Mr. Medvjed: How Past Experiences Can Affect One's Beliefs

Ibro Medvjed is a 55-year-old man receiving home support after he was hit by a drunk driver and left partially paralyzed. He is now at home, and Lisa, his support worker, assists him with his activities of daily living (ADLs) while his wife is at work.

During his care, Mr. Medvjed often discusses his life before coming to Canada 15 years ago. Last week, he told Lisa that as a youth, he survived a mass shooting by soldiers who tried to exterminate his entire peaceful and happy village. Today, he told Lisa that he thought that "all drunk drivers should be shot and killed." He told her that he believed that all lawbreakers should go to jail and that "rapists and drug dealers should also be shot and killed." This was upsetting to Lisa, who thought that Mr. Medvjed's sense of justice is much too harsh. She is uncertain about whether to ask Mr. Medvjed to elaborate on his feelings, so she spoke to her supervisor about it. What do you think Lisa's supervisor would say to her? What would you suggest to Lisa?

BOX 8–1 A Sample Code of Ethics for Support Workers

- ***Support workers provide high-quality personal care and support services. They work within their scope of practice.*** They promptly report to their supervisors any concerns and observations about clients' health and well-being. They perform only those tasks for which they have received the necessary education. They know and follow employer policies as well as federal and provincial or territorial laws. They work within the parameters of national and provincial or territorial laws at all times.
- ***The support worker needs to be aware of the policies and procedures for each area.*** If the support worker is employed for more than one client or agency, the required skills may vary. It should never be assumed that the skills allowed at one agency can be automatically transferred to another agency.
- ***Support workers provide compassionate care to all clients.*** They promote the client's physical, emotional, intellectual, social, and spiritual well-being. They encourage clients to maintain as much independence as possible during times of normal health and in situations of illness, injury, or disability or while dying. They respect and promote the family's roles and relationships.
- ***Support workers value the dignity and worth of all clients.*** They advocate for their client whenever necessary. They strive to treat all clients in an honest, fair, and just manner. They do not discriminate against a client on the basis of age, race or ethnicity, colour, religion, sexual orientation, or culture.
- ***Support workers respect their clients' choices about how they receive or participate in their care.*** They respect and promote the client's wishes

Continued

BOX 8–1 A Sample Code of Ethics for Support Workers—cont'd

and use discretion to avoid causing distress or embarrassment to a person (see the *Supporting Mrs. Glass: Recognizing the Need for Discretion* box).

- ***Support workers respect their clients' right to privacy and confidentiality.*** Information about the client learned while providing care is not shared with anyone outside the health care team.
- ***Support workers do not misuse their position of trust.*** They do not accept gifts or tips from their clients. They do not buy property from their clients, nor do they sell products to them. They do not try to impose their own religious or other beliefs on their clients. Their behaviour toward clients and co-workers is professional at all times (see the *Supporting Mr. Creishilo: Maintaining a Professional Relationship* box).
- ***Support workers are reliable.*** They arrive at work on time and complete all assignments. They are patient and courteous with clients. They notify their supervisor if they are going to be late or are unable to work, or if they are working in the community or in a home care setting, they inform their client. Their conduct is professional and based on ethical principles.
- ***Support workers promote and maintain their clients' safety.*** They report mistakes and unsafe situations immediately to their supervisors. They consider their clients' safety when performing all tasks and activities.

Supporting Mrs. Glass: Recognizing the Need for Discretion

Esther Glass is a 92-year-old woman who lives in a retirement home. She engages in a number of activities there and plays euchre, a card game, in the dining room with several other clients several times a week. One day, while the clients were playing cards, one of the support workers noticed a smell of feces coming from one of the clients. She told Safrikata, the student support worker, to check on the clients and to change the incontinence brief of the client who needed it.

Safrikata wanted to follow the instructions of the support worker. She walked up to the table and asked the clients, "Which one of you needs to go to the washroom?" Mrs. Glass was the one who had been incontinent, but she was very upset at Safrikata's lack of discretion. She said to Safrikata, "Go away!" Safrikata was surprised that Mrs. Glass refused to talk to her or to admit that she needed help with cleaning herself. How should Safrikata have handled this situation?

Supporting Mr. Creishilo: Maintaining a Professional Relationship

Sam Creishilo is a 32-year-old client to whom you have provided support care in his home for several months after he was injured at the factory where he works. Mr. Creishilo is a bachelor and lives alone. He has always been very pleasant to you, and you have developed a professional relationship with him. On your last visit, he asked if he could have your home phone number so that he could invite you "out for a coffee sometime." You do not know what your response to him should be. You are also wondering whether the fact that you are single and have no family responsibilities has any bearing on this situation.

THE PRINCIPLES OF HEALTH CARE ETHICS

Most codes of ethics are based on the principles of health care ethics. **Health care ethics** is the philosophical study of what is morally right and wrong when providing health care services. Ethical decisions are sometimes easy to make, such as assisting an unsteady but ambulatory client who requests your help with toileting. However, at other times, ethical decisions are more difficult. An **ethical dilemma** is a situation in which there is an apparent conflict between opposing moral choices, and choosing one would result in going against another moral choice. See BOX 8-2 for examples of ethical dilemmas.

The four basic principles of health care ethics are:

- Autonomy—respecting the client's right to make choices for himself or herself
- Justice—being fair
- Beneficence—doing good
- Nonmaleficence—doing no harm

Understanding the principles of health care ethics will help you think and behave ethically toward your clients and co-workers.

BOX 8–2 Ethical Dilemmas

Scenario 1

You are assigned to work for a family with a 2-year-old boy and newborn twins. You are responsible for helping with care of the 2-year-old. The mother mentions that since the birth of the twins, the toddler has been throwing temper tantrums around lunchtime. She wants to stop this problem behaviour and tells you that if the toddler throws a tantrum or misbehaves, he is to be sent to his room for 15 minutes, or longer if he has not settled down by the end of that time.

Discussion

Consider how applying the main principles of health care may cause conflict. What should you do?

Autonomy: The mother has the right to make parenting decisions.

Justice: Would it be fair to the child to leave him alone in his room for so long?

Beneficence: Will the disciplining help the child improve his behaviour? Can other actions improve his behaviour?

Nonmaleficence: Could leaving the child in his room cause harm?

Scenario 2

Miki works in a long-term care facility. Mr. Petrova is a resident on her resident care unit. Miki smells alcohol on Mr. Petrova's breath following his son's visit. She comments on this to Mr. Petrova, and he tells her that his son had brought him a bottle of liquor. Residents keeping alcohol in their rooms is against facility rules. Mr. Petrova says that alcohol eases his pain and asks Miki to promise not to tell anyone about the liquor.

Discussion

Telling her supervisor about the liquor would disregard Mr. Petrova's wishes and his autonomy. However, not telling her supervisor could harm Mr. Petrova. For example, alcohol may interfere with his medications or cause adverse effects. Not telling could also harm Miki. She could lose her job for knowing a resident has broken facility rules and not reporting it.

Miki explains to Mr. Petrova that she is ethically and legally obligated to tell her supervisor about the bottle of liquor in his room. She explains her reasons, but Mr. Petrova still gets upset. Miki, however, knows that she has followed the ethical principle of nonmaleficence. Also, she has avoided betraying Mr. Petrova's trust by refusing to make a promise she cannot keep.

Scenario 3

John's home care client is Mrs. Jessop, whose care plan states that she is not allowed sugary foods because she has diabetes. Today is Mrs. Jessop's birthday, and her neighbour brings her a cake. Mrs.

Continued

BOX 8–2 Ethical Dilemmas—cont'd

Jessop tells John that every year on her birthday she chooses to go off her diet. She asks him to cut her a piece of cake. Serving Mrs. Jessop a piece of cake would respect her autonomy. However, the cake could harm Mrs. Jessop's physical health.

Discussion

John decides not to serve the cake to Mrs. Jessop. He knows that she can serve herself or her neighbour can serve it to her. John says that he should perhaps call Mrs. Jessop's case manager about the situation, but Mrs. Jessop does not want John to make the call. She goes ahead and eats the cake. John observes her carefully for any ill effects but notices no change in her condition. Later, he telephones his supervisor to report the incident. His written notes also describe what happened exactly.

John upholds the principle of autonomy by allowing Mrs. Jessop to decide to eat the cake. He also upholds the principle of nonmaleficence by not serving her the cake and by advising that they consult her case manager before she eats a piece of cake. Because he has reported what happened, he has also followed the principle of beneficence.

Scenario 4

Tomas is a support worker in a long-term care facility. One afternoon, he observes that Mrs. O'Brian seems upset. He asks her if anything is wrong, and she starts to cry. She tells Tomas that her 17-year-old grandson has been arrested for drunk driving. She asks Tomas not to tell anyone because the family wants to keep the matter private. She also asks Tomas not to tell the nursing staff that she is upset.

Keeping the information confidential and telling no one about her emotional state would respect Mrs. O'Brian's privacy. However, Tomas is expected to report his observations about residents' emotional health. Not doing so could cause Mrs. O'Brian harm since she may suffer from the effects of stress.

Discussion

Tomas decides to tell the charge nurse that Mrs. O'Brian is upset about a private family matter. First, though, Tomas explains to Mrs. O'Brian that he is required to report his observations of his clients' emotional health. He also assures her that anything he reports will be kept confidential by the health care team.

Tomas's solution respects the ethical principles of autonomy and justice. It also upholds the principle of nonmaleficence. By reporting that Mrs. O'Brian is upset, Tomas ensures that someone with authority will take responsibility for Mrs. O'Brian's emotional health.

Scenario 5

P.J. is a support worker caring for Mrs. Osillo, an older woman who has a "G-tube" for feeding. As P.J.'s supervisor explained to him, this tube goes directly into Mrs. Osillo's stomach through an opening made in her abdomen, and all of her foods and nutrients are given through it. She cannot have anything to drink, as she has severe problems swallowing and any food or fluids would go into her lungs, resulting in respiratory problems and pneumonia. Mrs. Osillo has already been admitted to the hospital for pneumonia twice this year.

Mrs. Osillo complains that she feels thirsty all the time and begs P.J. to give her something to drink.

Discussion

P.J. cannot give Mrs. Osillo anything to drink because doing so would violate the principle of nonmaleficence. Anything that is taken orally can cause severe problems for Mrs. Osillo. P.J. decides that he should discuss this situation with the supervisor so that together they can come up with a solution that respects Mrs. Osillo's right to autonomy and that is in keeping with the principle of beneficence.

After a discussion with the supervisor and Mrs. Osillo's doctor, P.J. gives Mrs. Osillo ice chips to suck on several times a day. In between the ice chips, Mrs. Osillo is given mouthwashes to gargle and spit out and an oral spray, which keeps her oral membranes moist. Mrs. Osillo says that these solutions have helped get rid of the dry-mouth feeling that she had been experiencing all the time.

Autonomy

Autonomy (also called **self-determination**) means having the freedom and choice to make decisions that affect one's life. As long as a person is mentally competent, he or she has the right to make decisions about lifestyle and medical care and services. This concept is critical to health care ethics. Laws have been established to protect the client's right to autonomy (see Chapter 9). For example, physicians, facilities, and agencies must, by law, ensure that clients give informed consent before any procedure is performed on them. Clients, therefore, decide what kind of treatment they want or do not want.

As a support worker, you must always respect your clients' choices and preferences. The client has autonomy even in the case of routine tasks; for example, if a client asks you to use his own blue sheets to make his bed, it is important that you do so. Using other sheets shows a lack of respect for the client's choice. Even if a client wants a certain hairstyle that you think is unattractive, you must respect her choice. It would be unethical to ignore her preference and style her hair according to your own taste.

Respecting a client's autonomy becomes more complicated if you think his decisions are unsafe. The client has the right to make choices and to take risks. For example, an older client may refuse to use his cane in spite of knowing that he is at risk of falling. After explaining why he should use the cane, you must accept his decision, whatever it may be. Always consult with your supervisor if you have concerns about the client's safety.

Respecting your clients' autonomy also means that you do not judge their choices or lifestyles. While you base your judgements and opinions on your own values and standards, your clients may have values and standards different from yours. For example:

- A daughter decides that her mother needs nursing home care. In your culture, children usually take care of their aging parents at home. You do not understand why the daughter will not care for her mother at home.
- A client has multiple tattoos and body piercings. You disapprove of tattooing and body piercing.
- A client mentions to you that he has decided not to seek treatment for his cancer. You believe he should try everything possible to save his life.

You should set aside your biases and avoid judging your clients and their decisions on the basis of your values or standards. Do not give advice to clients, and never express your disapproval or opinions about their choices, preferences, politics, religion, or lifestyle.

Justice

The principle of **justice** means that all people should be treated in a fair and equal manner. Justice is an ideal that is central to Canada's universal health care system—all Canadians, regardless of their ability to pay, receive equal access to the same medical services. Unfortunately, this ideal is not a reality for all people across Canada. Clients who can afford it can buy services that are not readily available to everyone. Examples of such services include private clinics, medical tests and procedures (e.g., magnetic resonance imaging [MRI], hip replacement), and elective procedures (e.g., plastic surgery).

You can uphold the principle of justice by being concerned for all clients, regardless of their conditions or temperaments. For example, some people are easier to work with than others, so you may be tempted to spend less time with a client who is demanding and ungrateful. Or you may wish to avoid a client whose lifestyle is very different from your own. However, doing so would be unjust and unethical. Every client deserves your attention and care equally.

Treating people justly also means that you do not betray their trust. Clients trust that you will handle their possessions with care, respect their privacy, perform your services competently and skillfully, and keep all conversations and health information confidential. Do not snoop in clients' homes, pry into their personal lives, or gossip with your friends or co-workers about them, either in person or electronically. Share information about the client only with your supervisor and the health care team. Never speak about a client where others may overhear you—for example, in public areas such as dining rooms, lounges, locker rooms, and elevators. Confidentiality is a basic right. It is so important that laws have been passed to protect it (see Chapter 9).

Beneficence

Beneficence means doing or promoting good. The principle of beneficence is central to your work.

Support work is about promoting wellness, helping people in their daily lives, and supporting them during difficult times.

To apply the principle of beneficence in your work life, always consider meeting the client's needs to be your most important function. That means the client's needs come before those of his or her family. Consider the following: Mr. Mijovick lives with his son and daughter-in-law in their home and receives home care services. Marcia is assigned to give Mr. Mijovick a bed bath. His son, however, insists that Marcia not bathe Mr. Mijovick and instead finish early that day because he is expecting a visitor. When deciding what to do, Marcia focuses on Mr. Mijovick's needs, not on his son's. She calls her supervisor to report the situation and seek guidance.

The concept of beneficence and professionalism are closely related. To meet your clients' needs, stay within the boundaries of a professional helping relationship (see Chapter 5). Do not ask clients to do something that is in your interests rather than theirs. For example, if your child is selling chocolate bars to raise money for a school trip, do not ask your client to buy a chocolate bar. Avoid asking clients to do something for you, even if it aims to benefit others more than yourself or your family. For example, even if you are canvassing for United Way, do not ask your client to contribute to the campaign.

When caring for a client, avoid focusing on yourself or burdening the client with your problems and worries. Never take advantage of a client's compassion and generosity. If you tell a client your problems, he or she may try to help you. For example, if you tell a client you are having financial difficulties, the client may offer you money. ***Never ask for or accept money or loans from clients regardless of how long you have been working with them. To do so is unethical.***

Clients can become very attached to their support workers. If family relationships are strained, the client may see the relationship with a support worker as a substitute for the relationship with a family member. Never take advantage of strained family relationships or forget that your relationship with your clients is professional. Do not take sides with a client against a family member. Never flirt, date, or accept invitations from a client or a client's family member. When support workers become entangled in their clients' affairs, serious consequences can result. For example, a support worker's being named as a beneficiary in a client's will could lead to legal problems for that worker and the employer.

It may be necessary for you to advocate (see Chapter 1) for your client in order to do the most good for her. For example, you have observed that Mrs. Smith hates being showered but enjoys being bathed. It is important for you to share that observation with the health care team so that Mrs. Smith's care plan indicates her preference.

To do the most good for your clients, always give your best effort at work. Unless the person has unexpected problems or needs that require your attention, finish all your assigned tasks. Be careful, alert, and exact when following instructions. Also, be compassionate and empathetic. Self-discipline is essential, especially when working in home care. Avoid any temptation to use your work time for your own interests, including watching television, talking on the telephone, and stopping for an extra cup of coffee.

Nonmaleficence

Nonmaleficence means doing no harm. Harm can be intentional (abuse) or unintentional (accidental injury or negligence). To avoid harming a client, perform only tasks that you have been trained to do. By recognizing the limits of your role and knowledge, you are protecting your clients from the risk for harm. Clients or family members may ask you to perform functions that could be dangerous if not performed correctly. Most often, such requests are made innocently. The client may forget that you are not qualified to do certain tasks. Although this confidence in you as a support worker is to be appreciated, it is not safe or wise to take on tasks that you are not trained to do, even if you have the best of intentions.

Clients and their family members may also ask you for information about diagnoses or medical, surgical, or treatment plans. You must never reveal these details, whether or not you are asked. You could give the wrong information and cause harm or distress. Not only is giving or discussing medical information outside your scope of practice; it is also unethical. Refer all such questions to your supervisor.

To provide safe and effective care, you must keep your skills and knowledge current. Participate in educational programs offered by your employer. Consider enrolling in courses or workshops relevant to your work. Support work is continually changing. What you are trained to do this year may become outdated in a few years. The more knowledge and practice you get, the better and safer your skills will be.

You must keep clients as safe as possible. You can protect them from harm by practising infection control techniques (see Chapter 23) and by recognizing common safety hazards and knowing how to prevent accidents (see Chapter 22).

Dealing With Ethical Dilemmas

Codes of ethics provide only guidelines for ethical behaviour. They do not have the answers or rules for every situation. Occasionally, you may come across a situation that will involve a conflict between two opposing moral choices, and choosing one would result in going against the other. When confronted with such an ethical dilemma, you need to know how to decide on the right thing to do.

When making an ethical decision, carefully consider the four principles of health care ethics. Collect as much information about the situation as possible. Consider all possible options to resolve the dilemma. Ask yourself these questions about each option:

- Does the option respect the client's wishes and preferences?
- Does the option treat the client justly and fairly?
- Does the option provide the client with a short-term benefit or a long-term benefit?
- Could the option cause harm or increase the client's risk for harm?
- What are all of the possible consequences to the client, family, or others with this option?

Answers to these questions may contradict each other. For example, one option may benefit the client but go against his or her wishes. Another option may reflect the client's preferences but increase the risk for harm. Because you must protect the client from harm and also avoid serious legal problems for yourself and your employer, if any one option could harm the client, you must involve your supervisor in finding the solution.

See **BOX 8-2** for a discussion on how support workers deal with ethical dilemmas, and then read the *Supporting Mr. Adamson: Facing an Ethical Dilemma* box. What would you do in these situations? Remember to consider the four principles of health care ethics when making your decision.

Supporting Mr. Adamson: Facing an Ethical Dilemma

Mick Adamson is a 62-year-old man who has amyotrophic lateral sclerosis (ALS, also known as Lou Gehrig's disease). ALS is a devastating neurodegenerative disease that causes progressive paralysis in clients living with the disease as the upper and lower motor neurons in their brain and spinal cord begin to degenerate.[1] Mr. Adamson's family was told that 80% of people with ALS die within 2 to 5 years of diagnosis, gradually becoming unable to breathe or swallow.

Mr. Adamson's illness has progressed to a point at which he is unable to stand, turn himself in bed, or toilet himself. He is being cared for at home, and you are one of the support workers at the agency that has been contracted to provide care and support for him.

Today, Mr. Adamson has told your supervisor that he just "wants to die." During your work with him, he refuses both his food and his fluids whenever you try to feed him. While you empathize with Mr. Adamson, you do not want to merely watch and do nothing while he tries to starve himself to death. You feel frustrated by your inability to change Mr. Adamson's situation. You are also frightened by the thought that you might be assisting Mr. Adamson to die by suicide, something that you never imagined you could do and that you know is not within your scope of practice. How can you handle this ethical dilemma? Who do you turn to for support?

CHAPTER REVIEW

KEY POINTS

- The term *ethics* refers to the principles or values that guide us when differentiating right from wrong and good from bad.
- Morals are the fundamental principles of behaviour each person believes to be right or wrong for him- or herself without concern for legalities or customs.
- Support workers must be aware that culture and personal circumstances may influence ethical beliefs, morals, and values, and all of these influence one's actions.
- *Values* are qualities that an individual considers to be worthwhile or desirable in a person.
- A *belief* is a conviction that something is true.
- The principle of justice means that all people should be treated in a fair and equal manner.
- The principle of autonomy means having the freedom and choice to make decisions and to be independent enough to do so.
- The principle of beneficence means doing or promoting good.
- The principle of nonmaleficence is seeking to do no harm.
- To make an ethical decision, a support worker should carefully consider the four principles of health care ethics, collect as much information about the situation as possible, and consider all possible options.

CRITICAL THINKING IN PRACTICE

You are assisting a client in a residential facility with feeding. The client refuses to eat. The client's wife, who is concerned about his weight loss, has told you to "Force the food into him." What should you do? Does the client have the right to refuse to eat? Does the client's wife have a right to demand that her husband be force-fed? What is the agency's responsibility?

REVIEW QUESTIONS

Answers to these questions are at the bottom of p. 127.

Circle T if the answer is true, and circle F if the answer is false.

1. T F Ethics apply only to life-and-death situations.
2. T F Codes of ethics provide rules and answers to ethical dilemmas.
3. T F Ethics are a guide when deciding between right and wrong, and good and bad.
4. T F Keeping a resident's information confidential is ethical behaviour.
5. T F Any decision regarding a client's care is ethical if it does not harm the person.

Circle the BEST answer.

6. Providing a safe environment is an example of:
   A. Autonomy
   B. Justice
   C. Beneficence
   D. Nonmaleficence
7. Showing respect and protecting a client's dignity is an example of:
   A. Autonomy
   B. Justice
   C. Beneficence
   D. Nonmaleficence
8. Treating all clients with equal care and attention, regardless of their condition or temperament, is an example of:
   A. Autonomy
   B. Justice
   C. Beneficence
   D. Nonmaleficence

9. Respecting personal preferences is an example of:
A. Autonomy
B. Justice
C. Beneficence
D. Nonmaleficence

10. Which question is least helpful when deciding on an ethical solution to a problem?
A. Does the solution respect the client's wishes and stated preferences?
B. Does the solution treat the client justly and fairly?
C. Does the solution provide a short-term benefit or a long-term benefit to the client?
D. Does the solution benefit you?

11. Mr. Will, a client in a long-term care facility, refuses to be lifted into his chair for meals because he says being moved makes him too uncomfortable. As a result, he is developing pressure sores on his buttocks. You know that it is important to change positions frequently (see Chapter 26). Your supervisor has advised that he be "forced" out of bed, but you wish to respect his wishes. Which of the following should be done first to deal with this ethical dilemma?
A. Leave Mr. Will in his bed for meals.
B. Tell Mr. Will that he has to be moved but do it quickly so his pain is minimized.
C. Discuss your concerns with the other team members, Mr. Will, and his family to see if a compromise can be reached.
D. Ask for a different client to take care of.

Answer: 1.F, 2.F, 3.T, 4.T, 5.F, 6.D, 7.C, 8.B, 9.A, 10.D, 11.C

Chapter opener image: Feng Yu/Shutterstock.com

CHAPTER 9

Legislation: The Client's Rights and Your Rights

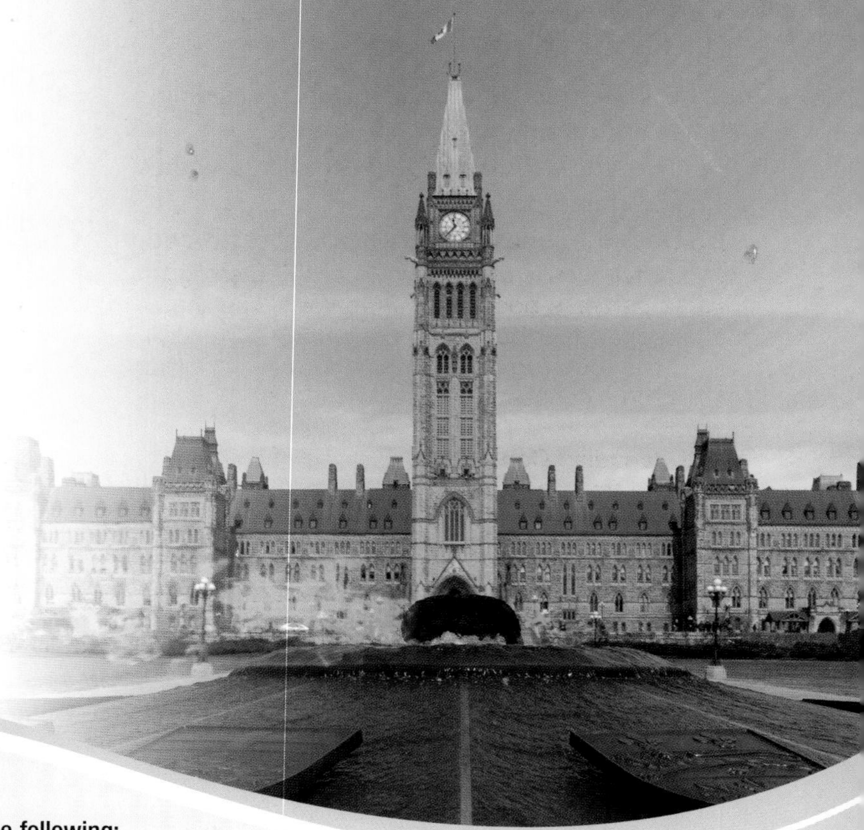

OBJECTIVES

After reading this chapter, you should be able to do the following:

- Explain the basic rights protected by the *Canadian Charter of Rights and Freedoms* and the provincial and territorial human rights codes.
- Describe client rights.
- Identify ways you can respect your client's rights.
- Describe the difference between criminal law and civil law.
- Describe how negligence, defamation, assault, battery, false imprisonment, and invasion of privacy apply to your job.
- Define electronic privacy and describe how confidentiality can be maintained electronically.
- List the types of legislation that address support workers' rights and duties.
- Apply the information in this chapter to your clinical practice properly.

KEY TERMS

act A specific law that has passed through the required legislative steps. *p. 131*
administrator The person appointed by the provincial courts to administer the estate of a client who has died without leaving a will. *p. 140*
advance care directive See **advance directive**. *p. 138*
advance directive A legal document in which a person states wishes about future health care, treatment, and personal care. Also known as an **advance care directive** or a **living will**. *p. 138*
assault Intentionally attempting to or threatening to touch a person's body without consent, causing the person to fear bodily harm. *p. 142*
battery The touching of a person's body without the person's consent. *p. 142*
Canadian Charter of Rights and Freedoms Part of the Canadian Constitution that lists the basic rights and freedoms to which all Canadians are entitled. *p. 130*
civil laws Laws that deal with relationships between people. *p. 140*
consent Agreement or approval—for example, to medical treatment, health care, or personal care services. *p. 137*
crime A violation of criminal law. *p. 140*
criminal laws Laws concerned with offences against the public and against society in general. *p. 140*
defamation The injuring of the name and reputation of a person by making false statements to a third person. *p. 143*
electronic privacy A person's right not to have his image, words, or character description or comments about his reputation made public by electronic means. *p. 136*
estate trustee The person chosen by the now-deceased person to deal with his or her possessions, as stated in the will. Also known as **guardian of property** or **executor** or **executrix**. *p. 139*
executor, executrix See **estate trustee**. *p. 140*
false imprisonment Unlawful restraint or restrictions of a person's freedom of movement. *p. 142*
guardian of property See **estate trustee**. *p. 139*
harassment Troubling, tormenting, offending, or worrying a person through one's behaviour or comments. *p. 143*
informed consent Consent obtained under the legal condition whereby a person is first given complete, accurate, and relevant information so as to fully understand the action or procedure and its potential implications. *p. 137*
invasion of privacy Violation of a person's right not to have his or her name, photograph, private affairs, health information, or any personal information made public without consent. *p. 142*
legislation A body of laws that govern the behaviour of a country's residents. *p. 130*
liable Legally responsible. *p. 140*
libel The making of false written statements that hurt the reputation of another person. *p. 143*
living will A document that lets the reader know one's preferences about care intended to sustain life. *p. 138*
negligence Failure to act in a careful or competent manner, resulting in harm to a person or damage to property. *p. 140*
oath of confidentiality A pledge that promises that the signer will respect and guard personal and private information about a client, family, or agency. *p. 136*
power of attorney See **substitute decision maker for health care**. *p. 138*
proxy See **substitute decision maker for health care**. *p. 138*
regulations Detailed rules that implement the requirements of a legislative act. *p. 131*
right Something to which a person is justly entitled. *p. 130*
slander The making of false verbal statements that hurt the reputation of a person. *p. 143*
substitute decision maker for health care A person authorized to make health care decisions on behalf of a living person who is unable to do so. Also called **power of attorney** for health care or **proxy**, depending on the province. *p. 138*
substitute decision maker for property The person who would represent an incapable person's interests regarding his or her belongings. *p. 139*
tort A wrongful act committed by an individual against another person or the person's property. *p. 140*
will A legal document stating a person's wishes concerning the distribution or disposal of his or her property. *p. 139*

The foundation of a good client–worker relationship is a basic understanding of the client's rights and the worker's rights and legal responsibilities. As a support worker, how you conduct yourself at work and how you relate to your clients are determined by:

- Your professional code of ethics (see Chapter 8)
- Your employer's policies
- Federal and provincial or territorial laws

Whereas ethics could be said to be rules of conduct that *guide* society when deciding what is right and what is wrong, and what is good and what is bad, legislation tells society what it *can* and *cannot do*. **Legislation** is a body of laws that govern the behaviour of a country's residents. In Canada, legislation helps to make sure that all health care clients receive safe and skillful care and enjoy the privacy that all people deserve. Enforced by the courts, legislation also protects clients' rights and health care providers' rights.

UNDERSTANDING RIGHTS

A **right** is something to which a person is justly entitled. Some rights, sometimes called *moral rights*, are based on a sense of fairness or ethics. For example, when you and a classmate arrange to study together, you have the right to expect that the classmate will show up and be prepared to work. In another example, if you discussed a personal matter with a friend, you have the right to expect that your friend will not repeat this information to others. These rights are not based on written laws. They are based on moral principles: Commitments should be honoured, and secrets should be kept.

Rights that are formally recognized in law are *legal rights* based on rules and principles outlined in the law and enforced by society. For example, various laws give you the rights to vote, to receive medical care, to own property, and to receive fair treatment if accused of a crime. Laws reflect the values of the society that created them. Canadians enjoy rights and freedoms that enable a life of equality and dignity.

BASIC HUMAN RIGHTS IN CANADA

The **Canadian Charter of Rights and Freedoms** is federal legislation that applies to all Canadians regardless of where they live. As part of the Canadian Constitution, the Charter applies at the federal level, so all provincial and territorial laws must be consistent with its rules. The Charter lists the basic rights and freedoms to which all Canadians are entitled. They include the following:

- Freedom of conscience and religion
- Freedom of thought, belief, opinion, and expression
- Freedom of peaceful assembly and association (usually these freedoms are associated with the right to form a union or engage in a strike)
- The right to vote
- The right to enter, stay in, or leave Canada
- The right to life, liberty, and security
- The right to equality before and under the law, without discrimination based on race, ethnic origin, colour, religion, gender, age, or mental or physical disability

(The Charter is also discussed in Chapters 10 and 16 as this legislation pertains to the topics discussed there.)

Each Canadian province and territory also has a human rights code. These codes reaffirm the principle that all people are entitled to equal rights and opportunities—such as the same type and quality of support services—without discrimination because of race, ethnicity, religion, gender, age, or disability.

BASIC RIGHTS OF PEOPLE RECEIVING HEALTH SERVICES

The *Human Rights Act* is provincial and territorial legislation based on the *Canadian Human Rights Act* and applies to its specific province or territory. Each *Human Rights Act* is intended to (1) prevent discrimination and (2) promote and advance human rights in that jurisdiction. Some of the issues addressed by the *Human Rights Act* of each province or territory include:

- Indigenous rights
- Age discrimination
- Disability
- Employment
- Gender identity

BOX 9–1 Some Complex-Care Facility Issues Controlled by Legislation (British Columbia)

- Bedroom requirements—space, furnishings, privacy, windows, and lighting
- Room temperature and water temperature
- Bathrooms and bathing facilities
- Safety requirements, including fire safety and call systems
- Mobility and access
- Dining area, lounges, recreation, and outside activity area
- Social activities and recreation programs
- Care and supervision; care plans
- Confidentiality and privacy
- Neglect and abuse
- Use of restraints
- Preparation and service of food
- Medication safety; administration of medication; medication records
- Access to health services; oral health

Source: Province of British Columbia. (2002). Bill 73: Community Care and Assisted Living Act, Adult Care Regulations. Copyright © Queen's Printer, Victoria, BC.

- Hiring practices
- Housing
- Pregnancy and breastfeeding
- Racism
- Religious rights
- Sexual harassment
- Sexual orientation

As well, all provinces and territories have legislation that addresses the rights and freedoms of people using health care services. Your clients, however, may be unable to exercise their rights because of illness or injury; physical, cognitive, or mental challenges; or ɔld age, if the client is frail, confused, or isolated.

The laws governing health care have different titles :ross the country and may differ in details. You ɔuld be aware of the acts that govern your province territory, which can easily be found on the Inter- Provincial and territorial governments constantly 'e health care legislation and introduce new laws otect the rights of people receiving care in facili- ıd in the community.

ılth care legislation consists of acts and regula- An **act** is another term for a law. **Regulations** ıiled rules that implement the requirements :ct. Most health care acts consist of general ıents for maintaining health, safety, and g. For example, British Columbia's *Com- 'are and Assisted Living Act* sets out general nts for the licensing, administration, oper- inspection of long-term care facilities and also sets out broad standards of care. The Residential Care Regulation, which accompanies the Act, sets out detailed rules for meeting those broad standards of care. **BOX 9–1** outlines some of the rules covered in British Columbia's Residential Care Regulation.

Some provincial and territorial governments do not have regulations that lay out detailed rules. Instead, they issue standards that expand on their legislation. For example, Alberta's long-term care legislation is accompanied by standards called Continuing Care Health Service Standards. Regardless of whether detailed rules are contained in regulations or standards, all residential facilities in a province or territory must abide by these rules. Not to do so could result in removal of their licences.

Bill of Rights

There is no single list of rights afforded to all Canadians receiving care in facilities and in the community. However, some provinces, such as Manitoba and Ontario, have created a bill of rights for clients, which is essentially a summary of the lengthy rules contained in regulations and standards. For example, consider Ontario's Residents' Bill of Rights for long-term care clients (see **BOX 9–2**) and Bill of Rights for community care clients (**BOX 9–3**).

Some facilities and agencies write their own bills of rights based on provincial or territorial laws. Clients must receive a written list of their rights. As a support worker, you must know your provincial or

ued

BOX 9–2 Ontario's Residents' Bill of Rights

1. Every resident has the right to be treated with courtesy and respect and in a way that fully recognizes the resident's individuality and respects the resident's dignity.
2. Every resident has the right to be protected from abuse.
3. Every resident has the right not to be neglected by the licensee or staff.
4. Every resident has the right to be properly sheltered, fed, clothed, groomed, and cared for in a manner consistent with his or her needs.
5. Every resident has the right to live in a safe and clean environment.
6. Every resident has the right to exercise the rights of a citizen.
7. Every resident has the right to be told who is responsible for and who is providing the resident's direct care.
8. Every resident has the right to be afforded privacy in treatment and in caring for his or her personal needs.
9. Every resident has the right to have his or her participation in decision making respected.
10. Every resident has the right to keep in his or her room and display personal possessions, pictures, and furnishings in keeping with safety requirements and rights of other residents of the home.
11. Every resident has the right to:
    i. participate fully in the development, implementation, review and revision of his or her plan of care;
    ii. give or refuse consent to treatment, care or services for which his or her consent is required by law and to be informed of the consequences of giving or refusing consent;
    iii. participate fully in making any decision concerning any aspect of his or her care, including any decision concerning his or her admission, discharge or transfer to or from a long-term care home or a secure unit and to obtain an independent opinion with regard to any of those matters; and
    iv. have his or her personal health information within the meaning of the *Personal Health Information Protection Act*, 2004 kept confidential in accordance with the Act, and to have access to his or her records of personal health information, including his or her plan of care, in accordance with that Act.
12. Every resident has the right to receive care and assistance toward independence based on a restorative care philosophy to maximize independence to the greatest extent possible.
13. Every resident has the right not to be restrained, except in the limited circumstances provided for under the [*Long-Term Care Homes*] *Act* and subject to the requirements provided for under this Act.
14. Every resident has the right to communicate in confidence, receive visitors of his or her choice, and consult in private with any client without interference.
15. Every resident who is dying or is very ill has the right to have family and friends present 24 hours per day.
16. Every resident has the right to designate a person to receive information concerning any transfer or any hospitalization of the resident and to have that person receive that information immediately.
17. Every resident has the right to raise concerns or recommend changes in policies and services on behalf of himself or herself or others to the following persons and organizations without interference and without fear of coercion, discrimination or reprisal, whether directed at the resident or anyone else:
    i. the Residents' Council
    ii. the Family Council,
    iii. the licensee, and, if the licensee is a corporation, the directors and officers of the corporation, and, in the case of a home approved under Part VIII, a member of the committee of management for the home under section 132 or of the board of management for the home under section 125 or 129,
    iv. staff members,

Contin

BOX 9–2 Ontario's Residents' Bill of Rights—cont'd

v. government officials,
vi. any other person inside or outside the long-term care home.

18. Every resident has the right to form friendships and relationships and to participate in the life of the long-term care home.
19. Every resident has the right to have his or her lifestyle and choices respected.
20. Every resident has the right to participate in the Residents' Council.
21. Every resident has the right to meet privately with his or her spouse or another person in a room that assures privacy.
22. Every resident has the right to share a room with another resident according to their mutual wishes, if appropriate accommodations are available.
23. Every resident has the right to pursue social, cultural, religious, and other interests, to develop his or her potential, and to be given reasonable provisions by the licensee to pursue these interests and to develop his or her potential.
24. Every resident has the right to be informed in writing of any law, rule, or policy affecting the services provided to the resident and of the procedures for initiating complaints.
25. Every resident has the right to manage his or her own financial affairs unless the resident lacks the legal capacity to do so.
26. Every resident has the right to be given access to protected outdoor areas in order to enjoy outdoor activity, unless the physical setting makes this impossible.
27. Every resident has the right to have any friend, family member, or other person of importance to the resident attend any meeting with the licensee or the staff of the home.

Source: Long-Term Care Homes Act, 2007. Retrieved from https://www.ontario.ca/laws/statute/07l08#BK5.

BOX 9–3 Ontario's Bill of Rights for Community Care Clients

Note: The term "service provider" refers to either an agency or a person paid to provide the community service; in other words, a support worker is a service provider.

1. A client receiving a community service has the right to be dealt with by the service provider in a courteous and respectful manner and to be free from mental, physical and financial abuse by the service provider.
2. A client receiving a community service has the right to be dealt with by the service provider in a manner that respects the client's dignity and privacy and that promotes the client's autonomy.
3. A client receiving a community service has the right to be dealt with by the service provider in a manner that recognizes the client's individuality and that is sensitive to and responds to the client's needs and preferences, including preferences based on ethnic, spiritual, linguistic, familial and cultural factors.
4. A client receiving a community service has the right to information about the community services provided to him or her and to be told who will be providing the community services.
5. A client applying for a community service has the right to participate in the service provider's assessment of his or her requirements, and a client who is determined under this Act to be eligible for a community service has the right to participate in the service provider's development of the client's plan of service, the service provider's review of the client's requirements and the service provider's evaluation and revision of the client's plan of service.

Continued

BOX 9–3 Ontario's Bill of Rights for Community Care Clients—cont'd

6. A client receiving a community service has the right to give or refuse consent to the provision of any community service.
7. A client receiving a community service has the right to raise concerns or recommend changes in connection with the community service provided to him or her and in connection with policies and decisions that affect his or her interests, to the service provider, government officials or any other client, without fear of interference, coercion, discrimination, or reprisal.
8. A client receiving a community service has the right to be informed of the laws, rules and policies affecting the operation of the service provider and to be informed in writing of the procedures for initiating complaints about the service provider.
9. A client receiving a community service has the right to have his or her records kept confidential in accordance with the law.

Source: Ontario's Long-Term Care Act, 1994, S.O. 1994, c. 26, s. 3(1). Part III: Bill of Rights (Consolidated as of January 1, 2005) (See https://www.ontario.ca/laws/statute/94l26#BK4, Part III).

territorial laws and your employer policy regarding client rights. Generally, all clients have the following rights, which are a combination of moral and legal rights:

- The right to be treated with dignity and respect
- The right to privacy and confidentiality
- The right to give or withhold informed consent
- The right to autonomy

The Aphasia Institute of Ontario introduced the first-ever pictographic version of the Ontario Residents' Bill of Rights in 2005 (**FIGURE 9–1**). In residential facilities, it must be posted near the text version of the Residents' Bill of Rights. This pictogram offers effective ways to communicate with clients who retain thinking and social skills but have difficulty expressing themselves when speaking, understanding the speech of others, and reading and writing.

The Right to Be Treated With Dignity and Respect

The right to dignity is both an ethical principle and a legal obligation throughout Canada. It is also a guiding principle of caregiving, as emphasized throughout this textbook under the acronym DIPPS (dignity, independence, preferences, privacy, and safety).

Most health care legislation aims to protect and promote the client's dignity. For example, British Columbia's *Community Care and Assisted Living Act* states that facilities must be operated "in a manner that will maintain the spirit, dignity, and individuality of the client being cared for."[1] Ontario's *Long-Term Care Act* states that the client has the right to be dealt with "in a courteous and respectful manner . . . that respects the client's dignity" and in a manner that "recognizes the client's individuality and that is sensitive to and responds to the client's needs and preferences, including preferences based on ethnic, spiritual, linguistic, familial and cultural factors."[2]

Respecting the client's dignity is a basic and important part of support work. For most people, dignity and independence go together. To respect your clients' dignity, encourage them to be independent, allowing them to do as much for themselves as possible (**FIGURE 9–2**). For example, if a frail older man can put on his shoes, let him do so. It may save you time to put his shoes on for him. However, letting him do it himself helps him maintain some independence.

Be careful not to make any assumptions about a client's abilities, interests, and limitations. By making assumptions, you may discourage him from doing

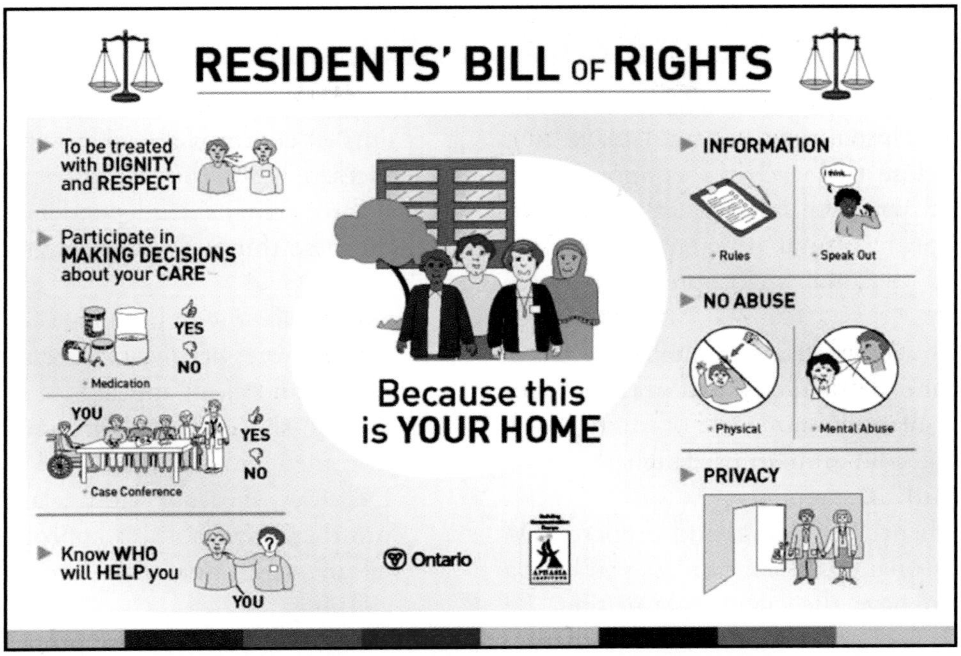

FIGURE 9–1 Pictographic version of the Residents' Bill of Rights. (**Source:** Aphasia Institute (2005). Residents' bill of rights: Pictograph. Toronto, ON. Retrieved from http://www.aphasia.ca/shop/ontario-residents-bill-of-rights/.)

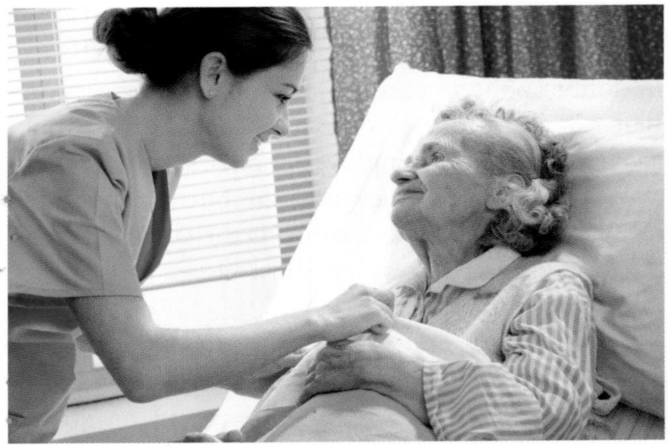

FIGURE 9–2 Support workers should treat their clients with dignity and respect. (**Source:** © Can Stock Photo Inc./gajdamak.)

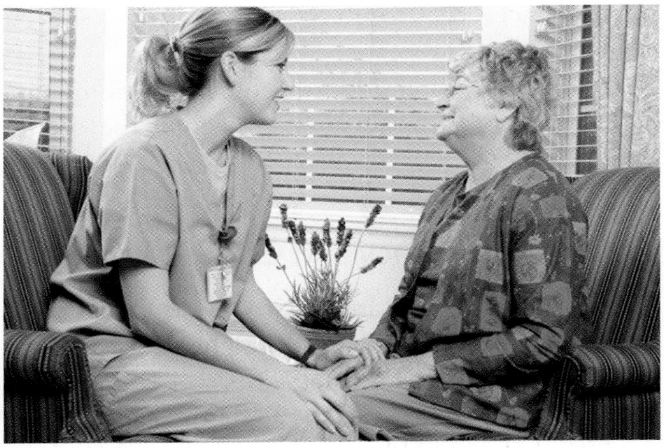

FIGURE 9–3 Listen to the client by facing her, maintaining appropriate eye contact, and leaning toward her. (**Source:** Sorrentino, S.A., & Remmert, L. (2012). *Mosby's textbook for nursing assistants* (8th ed., p. 98). St. Louis, MO: Mosby.)

tasks and activities that he *can* do. Observe what your client is capable of doing, and check the care plan. A client who is dependent in one area is not necessarily dependent in all areas. For example, Mrs. Mukherjee needs help getting out of a chair. However, she can feed herself. Mr. Simpson needs help shaving, but he can comb his hair and brush his teeth. Mrs. MacDonald can easily walk by herself, but because of Alzheimer's disease, she may wander off and therefore needs to be supported in a secure environment.

Respecting people's dignity means relating to them the way you would want to be related to if you were in their position. Speak respectfully to them, keeping in mind their hearing or sight limitations if they have any (FIGURE 9–3). In support work, how you relate to a client is just as important as the care you provide. Treating clients with dignity provides them with

BOX 9–4 Respecting the Client's Right to Dignity

- Make eye contact with the client if culturally appropriate, and listen attentively (see **FIGURE 9–3**).
- Stand or sit close to the client, as appropriate. Use touch if you are sure the client would approve. Respect cultural differences regarding touching and personal space preferences (see Chapter 10).
- Be patient. Provide kind and thoughtful care.
- Say "please" and "thank you," and practise other common acts of courtesy.
- Never yell at, scold, embarrass, laugh at, or be sarcastic toward the client.
- Respect the client's belongings and property. Do not touch personal possessions unless you have a reason to and have the client's permission. Be sure to put items back where you found them.
- Address an adult client by title and last name, unless the client tells you otherwise. Never call a client "honey," "sweetie," "dear," "grandma," "grandpa," or any other such term.
- Tell your supervisor about the client's complaints or concerns about the agency, facility, or services.
- Reinforce clients' independence by allowing them to do things for themselves. Avoid creating dependency.
- Assist the client with personal care and grooming whenever necessary. Make sure the client has:
  - A neat and clean appearance
  - A clean-shaven face or groomed beard
  - Trimmed and clean nails
  - Dentures, hearing aids, glasses, and other prostheses available, as appropriate
  - Clean and properly fitted and fastened clothing
  - Shoes and socks or hose properly applied and fastened
  - Extra clothing for warmth, as needed, such as a sweater or lap blanket

emotional support and greatly contributes to quality of life. **BOX 9–4** lists ways of respecting the client's dignity.

The Right to Privacy and Confidentiality

People using health care services have the right to personal privacy. They have the right to receive care in private and in a way that does not expose their bodies unnecessarily. Only staff members involved in the client's care should see, handle, or examine the client's body.

Information about the client's care, treatment, and condition is confidential (see Chapter 1). All provinces and territories have legislation that protects the privacy and confidentiality of clients' health information. This legislation is usually called a *privacy act*. Privacy acts provide guidelines to facilities and agencies on how to collect, use, and disclose personal health information. Most agencies require that all staff (and usually volunteers and students) sign an **oath of confidentiality**, a pledge that promises that the signer will respect and guard personal and private information about a client, family, or agency. When in doubt about whether or not to discuss something that you saw in regard to the client, you should always follow your employer's policies.

Providing for privacy and confidentiality shows respect for the client and protects the client's dignity. **BOX 9–5** lists measures that show respect for privacy and confidentiality.

Electronic Privacy

Almost everyone now uses some method of electronic communication—we routinely use our home computers, tablets, or cellphones to communicate with and send pictures to others. There are websites dedicated to allowing users to look at pictures or video clips of other people doing things, almost in real time. When a celebrity was photographed in compromising circumstances with a woman other than his wife, the image was shared worldwide and resulted in the celebrity's devastated wife filing for divorce immediately.

In today's age of electronic communication, people tend to forget that everyone has the right to privacy. In health care, **electronic privacy** could be defined

BOX 9–5 Respecting the Client's Right to Privacy

- Knock on the client's door and wait for permission to enter.
- Ask others in the room to leave before giving care to the client. To stay, they must have the client's permission.
- Close the door, and use curtains or screens when providing care or whenever the client requests it. Also, close drapes and window shades.
- Drape the client properly during personal care and procedures. Expose only the body part involved in the treatment or procedure.
- Keep the client covered when moving him through a facility's corridors and elevators.
- Close the bathroom door when the client is using the bathroom. If the client needs help, stay in the bathroom with the client, and keep the door closed.
- Do not open or read the client's mail or personal documents (**FIGURE 9–4**).
- Do not touch or examine the client's belongings without permission.
- Allow the client to visit with others in the facility and to use the telephone in private.
- Do not pry into the client's private life or ask for personal information that is not necessary for your work.
- Keep all personal and health care information about the client confidential.
- Do not discuss a client with your family, friends, or the client's family. Talk about the client only with your supervisor and members of the health care team who need to know.

as a person's right not to have his image, words, or character description or comments about his reputation made public by electronic means. (See Chapter 5 for more discussion on electronic communication.) It is wrong, both ethically and now legally in most provinces, to post pictures, names, or discussions about your clients, no matter how "nice" you think you are being to that client (see the *Supporting Mrs. Jones: Social Media Versus a Client's Right to Confidentiality* box for an example of how one client's privacy rights were violated).

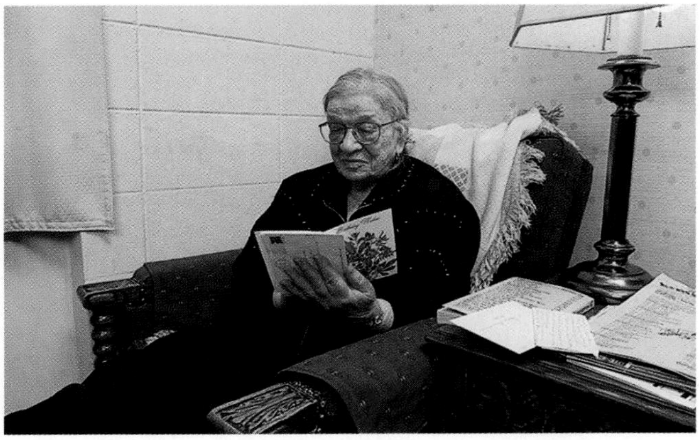

FIGURE 9–4 A client is reading her mail. Clients have a right to privacy, so never open or read their mail. (**Source:** Sorrentino, S.A. (2004). Assisting with patient care (2nd ed., p. 339). St. Louis, MO: Mosby.)

The Right to Give or Withhold Informed Consent

All people have the right to decide for themselves whether or not they agree to medical treatment, health care, or personal care services. Such agreement is called **consent**. ***All provinces and territories have legislation that describes when and how consent is to be obtained.***

For consent to be valid, it must be **informed consent**, which is based on having received accurate and complete information.[3] This information is provided to the client by the facility, agency, or physician.[3] Consent is informed when the client clearly understands the following:[3]

- The reason for the treatment or service
- What will be done
- How it will be done
- Who will be doing it
- The expected outcomes
- Potential risks and side effects of the treatment
- Other treatment options
- The likely consequences of not having the treatment

When a client enters a facility or hires an agency, he or she signs a form giving general consent to treatment (see "Advance Directive," below). Special

Supporting Mrs. Jones: Social Media Versus a Client's Right to Confidentiality

Jane (not her real name) was a student support worker who was really very fond of one particular client, Mrs. Jones, to whom she provided support care in her home. On the client's birthday, Jane took a picture of her on her cellphone and posted the picture on a social networking site. The picture showed Mrs. Jones smiling and wearing a hat with a cellophane bow that had been taken from the wrapping of a birthday present.

Mrs. Jones's teenage grandchildren, who live in another city, happened to come across this site, where they saw the picture of their grandmother. The grandchildren showed it to their parents, who were shocked and horrified that their mother (usually a very proper woman) was displayed in such an undignified manner. When they questioned their mother, she recalled that it was the student who took her picture. The client's children called the student's school and filed a formal complaint.

The school's lawyer agreed that the student violated the client's right to privacy by posting her picture on the Internet without her permission. The lawyer also reminded the school of its obligation to inform students that ***they must destroy any client information (printed or electronic) in such a way that it cannot be retrieved or reassembled.*** The student was eventually asked to leave her support worker program because her actions went against the oath of confidentiality that she had signed in the first week of her program.

consent forms, however, are required for surgery and other complex and invasive procedures. The physician is responsible for informing the client about all aspects of the surgery or procedure. ***The support worker is never responsible for obtaining written consent or giving medical information.*** As a support worker, you may or may not be allowed to witness clients' signatures on consent forms. Know your employer's policy.

Advance Directive

Advance directives (also known as **advance care directives**) are legal documents that allow clients to convey their decisions about their own end-of-life care. These documents are signed ahead of time, often when a client is admitted to an extended care facility, and are usually completed in consultation with the client, next of kin (usually the **substitute decision maker for health care**—called the **power of attorney** or **proxy** in some provinces), and the agency's director of care or administrator.[4]

Advance directives provide a way for clients to communicate their wishes to their families, friends, and health care providers and are intended to avoid confusion later on, when the clients are perhaps less cognitively aware of their surroundings.[4]

Living Will

Some people who are still living in their own home will want their family and friends to know whether or not they want care that is intended to sustain their life, and some may write these thoughts down in what is called a living will. In a **living will**, a person can state whether she wishes to accept or refuse medical care under certain circumstances. A living will can address such issues as the following:

- The use of dialysis and breathing machines
- Resuscitation if breathing or heartbeat stops
- Tube feeding
- Organ or tissue donation

A living will is ***not*** legally enforceable (see the *Supporting Mme. LeBrun: Is a Living Will Enforceable?* box) but is merely used to encourage family members to make decisions that respect the client's wishes.

Substitute Decision Makers for Personal Care or for Property

Clients under the legal age (usually 18 years) and clients who are unable to make informed decisions for themselves or their property need another person to provide consent on their behalf. The generally accepted legal term for this person in Canada is *substitute decision maker*. In most provinces, people refer

Supporting Mme. LeBrun: Is a Living Will Enforceable?

Mme. Violette LeBrun lives in a province that issues an organ donor section on her health card. Mme. LeBrun indicated that she would like her organs to be donated upon her death. She also instructed her friends and family that if anything happened, she did not want to be kept alive on life support. Mme. LeBrun even purchased over the Internet a "living will kit," filled it out, and gave it to her lawyer for safekeeping until the time came for her family to make this decision.

Later, Mme. LeBrun was involved in a head-on motor vehicle accident and was declared brain-dead by the emergency department doctor. She was placed on life support until her family could be notified. Her family immediately rushed to the emergency department and then were shown Mme. LeBrun's organ donor request on her health card that indicated her wish to donate her organs. Her family were then asked if they would give permission for Mme. LeBrun's organs to be taken from her body.

Mme. LeBrun's husband and daughter, both in a state of shock, refused to allow the doctors to retrieve any of Mme. LeBrun's organs. They decided that "Mom had been through enough pain" and asked for her to be taken off the life-support system. Her body was then sent to the funeral home that her family specified.

to the substitute decision maker as having *power of attorney*. (See Chapter 46 for more information about powers of attorney.)

Substitute Decision Maker for Personal Care

People with certain mental illnesses, confusion, dementia, or intellectual disabilities may not be able to give informed consent. In some situations, for example, an unconscious client cannot give consent for a procedure. Such situations require a substitute decision maker for health care. Depending on the province, the title *proxy* or *power of attorney for personal care* may be used instead.

The substitute decision maker for health care makes health care decisions, such as giving or withholding consent for treatments, if the client is unable to do so. Usually, the substitute decision maker is a husband, wife, daughter, son, or legal representative. As with consent given by the client, consent given by a substitute decision maker must be informed consent.

If your client has a substitute decision maker, this person will consult with the health care team to make decisions on the client's behalf. All provinces and territories have legislation that addresses substitute decision making.

Substitute Decision Maker for Property

As in situations that require a substitute decision maker for health care, in some cases, the client may be unable to make decisions regarding his belongings. In this case, the client's interests would be represented by a **substitute decision maker for property**. This person may or may not have been chosen by the client when he was able to make such decisions. A substitute decision maker for property cannot make personal care decisions unless a separate document is signed identifying that person also as the substitute decision maker for personal care.

If a client does not have a substitute decision maker for property, the provincial or territorial court may appoint someone to act as one. The appointed person would be legally bound to act in the client's best interests. Although terms may vary among jurisdictions, a generally accepted term in Canada for the person who acts on behalf of a client in regard to property is an **estate trustee** (or **guardian of property**).

Most adults have a **will**—a legal document that states one's wishes about where (or to whom) his or her property should go. It should be written while the client is cognitively intact, witnessed by a lawyer, and kept in the lawyer's office. Some people also keep copies of their wills in secure, fireproof places, such as a safe or a safety deposit box.

After the Client Dies

Upon the client's death, the substitute decision makers for health care or property cannot automatically decide what will happen to the deceased person's body. Decisions regarding releasing the client's body for funeral preparations or for burial must be made by the estate trustee who is named in the deceased person's will, by the deceased person's spouse or adult children, or by an **administrator**, the person appointed by the court if there are any conflicts. (If the client dies without leaving a will, the provincial or territorial court will appoint an administrator to divide up the client's property.) In most provinces and territories, the estate trustee is also known as an **executor** if the person is a man and an **executrix** if the person is a woman.

The Right to Autonomy

Autonomy, or self-determination, means having the freedom and choice to make decisions that affect one's life (see Chapter 8). People using health care services have a right to autonomy when making decisions about their care and lifestyle. Clients have the right to be involved in issues concerning their admission, discharge, or transfer to or from a facility (see the *Focus on Long-Term Care: Autonomy* box). They also have the right to participate fully in assessing and planning their own care and treatment, whether receiving care in a facility or at home.

FOCUS ON LONG-TERM CARE

Autonomy

Long-term care clients have the right to choose activities, schedules, and care based on personal preferences. They have the right to choose when to get up and go to bed, what to wear, how to spend their time, and what to eat (**FIGURE 9–5**). They are also free to form friendships and receive visitors inside and outside the facility. They have the right to share a room with their spouse or partner if they wish to and if a room is available. They also have the right to manage their own financial affairs or receive an accounting of transactions done on their behalf.

To have autonomy, people need (and have the right to) complete and accurate information about their health condition, care, and treatment. However, if clients ask you about their condition, their care, or your employer's policies, inform your supervisor, and he or she will provide the client with this information. Remember, you must not discuss diagnoses or health conditions with clients.

When you are providing client care, make sure your clients know your name and title, and remember to explain procedures before performing them.

Personal choice is important for quality of life, dignity, and self-respect, so respect for an individual's personal preference is emphasized throughout this book. As a support worker, you must allow your clients to make choices whenever it is safely possible.

UNDERSTANDING LEGAL ISSUES

Client rights are based on laws. Like all health care team members, you, as the support worker, must act in a legally appropriate manner. If you break the law or violate someone's rights, you are legally responsible (**liable**) for your actions and could be fined, sued, or even imprisoned.

You must obey both criminal laws and civil laws. **Criminal laws** are concerned with offences against the public and against society in general. A violation of criminal law is called a **crime**—for example, theft, murder, rape, or abuse—and a person found guilty of a crime is fined or sent to prison.

Civil laws deal with relationships between people. For example, laws relating to business disputes, divorce, or adoption are civil laws. A **tort** is a wrongful act committed by an individual against another person or the person's property. A person who commits such an act can be sued by the injured person. Torts may be intentional or unintentional. An example of an unintentional tort is negligence. Examples of intentional torts are assault, battery, false imprisonment, invasion of privacy, and defamation of character.

Negligence

Clients expect their health care providers to do their jobs competently and carefully. **Negligence** occurs when a person fails to act in a careful or competent manner and thereby harms the client or damages property. Negligence is an unintentional wrong because the person at fault did not intend to cause harm. He or she either failed to do what a reasonable and careful person would have done or did what a

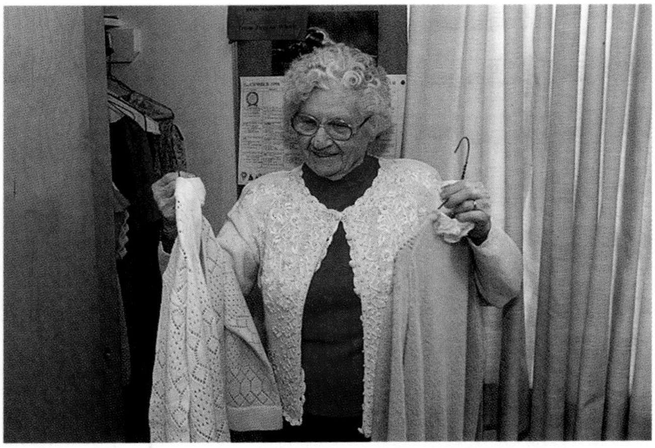

FIGURE 9–5 The client chooses what clothing to wear.

reasonable and careful person would not have done. The negligent individual may have to pay damages (a sum of money) to the injured person. The causes of negligence are given below.

- ***Not performing a task or procedure correctly.*** As a support worker, always perform your tasks and procedures exactly as you have been taught. Not following procedures can harm the client. For example, you are taught to keep a urinary drainage bag below the client's bladder level. If you keep it above the bladder level, urine will not drain, and the client could develop a urinary tract infection. Such negligence could harm the client, and charges could result.
- ***Performing a task or procedure that you are not qualified to do.*** You are legally allowed to do only those tasks and procedures that you are qualified to do. Do not do more than is allowed within your job description, your employer's policies, and legislation within your province or territory. You may be asked to do something beyond your scope of practice—for example, giving medications. Even if you are assured that you are not liable, you should remember that *you are responsible for your own actions*. In other words, you may, in fact, be liable. In such a situation, remember that refusing to follow through on a request that is beyond your scope of practice is your right and your duty.
- ***Making a mistake because of carelessness that causes harm to a client.*** Everyone makes mistakes sometimes, but a mistake that results from carelessness and causes harm is a negligent act. For example, if you do not mop up a spill, you could cause a client to slip and fall, and your carelessness could be considered negligence. **BOX 9–6** contains examples of negligent acts committed by support workers.

BOX 9–6 Examples of Negligent Acts Committed by Support Workers

- A support worker leaves the bed in the raised position. The client falls out of bed and breaks his hip.
- A support worker raises the bed rails when the care plan states that they should be left down. The client falls while trying to climb over the bed rails.
- A support worker does not raise the bed rails when the care plan states they should be raised. The client falls out of bed.
- A support worker does not check the temperature of the bath water. The client is burned.
- A support worker drops a client's dentures. The dentures break.
- A client complains to the support worker of chest pain and difficulty breathing. The support worker does not report the complaints to the supervisor. The client has a heart attack and dies.
- A client calls for help using the call bell. The support worker ignores the call. The client goes into shock because of sudden, severe bleeding.
- A support worker does not secure a client's garden gate. The client, who has Alzheimer's disease, wanders out onto the street and is hit by a car.

A client could be harmed even when you do your job competently and carefully. It is important to record every procedure accurately, following your employer's policy. What you record may later on protect you from charges of negligence. For example, a client confined to bed develops serious pressure sores. The family thinks she was left lying in the same position too long. Your charting shows that you repositioned her every hour, as stated in her care plan. This proves that you gave the required care and did not cause the pressure sores. If you had not recorded that you repositioned her every hour, it could have been presumed that you did not do it (see Chapter 14 for further discussion of recording).

Assault and Battery

Assault and battery may result in both civil and criminal charges. **Assault** is identified in Canada's Criminal Code and can be defined as intentionally attempting or threatening to touch a client's body without the client's consent, causing the client to fear bodily harm. Threatening to "tie down" an uncooperative client is an example of assault. **Battery** (which is part of tort law) is the actual intentional touching of a client's body without the client's consent. A battery can be committed without an intent to injure; just touching a client without his permission is battery. Force-feeding a client is an example of battery. Another is giving a treatment (such as a blood transfusion) to a person who has refused the treatment, even if the health care provider thinks the treatment will "help" the person.

You are not required to obtain written consent before you perform a task or procedure. However, you must always be aware of the client's wishes. Also, a client who has signed a consent form has the right to withdraw her consent at any time. Always explain the procedure and what you are going to do, and make sure the client agrees to it. Consent may be verbal ("yes" or "okay") or physical (a gesture such as a nod, turning over for a back rub, or holding out an arm for a blood pressure measurement). If the client objects to or declines your services, respect her wishes and stop the procedure or task, and immediately inform your supervisor since the client's decision may affect her well-being.

In some provinces and territories, registered health care providers may delegate to support workers duties that are beyond the scope of their practice (see Chapter 6, Chapter 43, and Chapter 44). If a support worker performs duties that are beyond the scope of his practice, and these duties were never delegated and taught by a registered staff member, the support worker is actually assaulting the client. It is the responsibility of the support worker to understand the responsibilities within his role and to safely act within these boundaries!

False Imprisonment

False imprisonment is the unlawful restraint or restrictions on a person's freedom of movement. For example, preventing a client from leaving a facility is false imprisonment. So is the unnecessary use of restraints (discussed in Chapter 22).

Invasion of Privacy

Every client has the right not to have her name, photograph, private affairs, health information, or any personal information made public without having given consent. Violating this right is an **invasion of privacy**, a term recognized in tort law. Your employer may require you to sign an oath of confidentiality, binding you to keep all dealings with clients and your employer confidential (see p. 136). This document may refer to the provincial or territorial privacy act that protects the privacy of individuals. Signing the document obliges you not to reveal information about clients obtained in the course of your work.

Freedom of Information

Canada is on the rapidly growing list of countries that have freedom of information and data protection legislation.[5] Federal laws have been passed to govern access to information and privacy, the two main laws being the Access to Information Act and the Privacy Act. In Canada, the Access to Information Act allows citizens to demand records from federal bodies. This law is enforced by the Information Commissioner of Canada.

The complementary Privacy Act was introduced in 1985. The Privacy Act's purpose is to (1) extend the present laws of Canada that protect the privacy of individuals with respect to personal information about themselves held by a federal government institution and (2) to provide individuals with the right of access to that information. Complaints about possible violations of the Privacy Act may be reported to the Privacy Commissioner of Canada.

The provinces and territories of Canada also have legislation governing access to government information; some acts also include privacy legislation. For example, the Freedom of Information and Protection of Privacy Act applies to Ontario's provincial ministries and agencies, boards, and most commissions, as well as community colleges and district health councils. In Quebec, the Freedom of Information and Protection of Privacy Act governs access to documents held by public bodies and the protection of personal information.

Defamation of Character

Defamation is injuring the name and reputation of a person by making false statements to a third person. **Libel** is a criminal offense when it is knowingly making false statements that harm a person's reputation in print, writing, or through pictures or drawings. In civil law, **slander** is making harmful false statements orally. As a support worker, protect yourself by never making false statements about a client, co-worker, or any other person. Examples of defamation include the following:

- Implying or suggesting that a client has a sexually transmitted disease
- Saying that a client is insane or mentally ill
- Implying or suggesting that a client is corrupt or dishonest

YOUR LEGAL RIGHTS

Federal, provincial, and territorial legislation ensures that Canadian workers receive fair wages and work in a fair and safe environment. Laws have been enacted to protect workers' rights and clarify their requirements and duties. These laws have different names across the country and vary in their details. In general, however, all provinces and territories have legislation that addresses human rights, occupational health and safety, employment, labour relations, workers' compensation, long-term care services, and community services.

Human Rights Legislation

Human rights codes protect workers' basic human rights. This legislation states that employers must treat all workers equally and not discriminate on the basis of a worker's race, colour, gender, sexual orientation, religion, age, or disability. Employers and employment agencies also cannot discriminate at the request of a client. Human rights legislation declares that workers have the right to be free from harassment in the workplace by the employer, the client, or a fellow worker. **Harassment** means troubling, tormenting, offending, or worrying a person through one's behaviour or comments.

Occupational Health and Safety Legislation

All provinces and territories have occupational health and safety (OH&S) legislation. This legislation outlines the rights and responsibilities of workers, employers, and supervisors in creating and maintaining a safe work environment. OH&S legislation, however, is not enforceable in a home care environment and does not protect support workers in home care.

Employers must "take every precaution reasonable in the circumstances for the protection of a worker."[6] Workers have a right to receive (and employers must provide) proper education, instruction, and supervision to ensure their safety. Employers who do not fulfill these duties may be fined. Workers have the right to refuse to work if the work poses a danger to themselves or others. In some provinces and territories, however, health care workers cannot refuse to work if by not working they endanger a client's health or safety.[7]

OH&S legislation also details how hazardous materials used in the workplace are to be identified and managed. WHMIS (Workplace Hazardous Materials Information System) is a national plan developed to provide information on the safe use and potential health risks of hazardous materials (see Chapter 22).

Employment Standards Legislation

Employment standards legislation states the minimum employment standards acceptable within the workplace. This legislation covers basic rules about issues such as minimum wage, how wages are paid, how many hours of work per day and per week are acceptable, what is fair overtime pay, how many holidays and vacation days should be given, and what situations qualify a worker for a leave of absence.

Labour Relations Legislation

Provinces and territories have legislation that addresses how employers and employees can resolve workplace issues. According to these laws, all employees have a basic right to form or join a trade union of their choice and to participate in lawful union activities. These unions can negotiate wages and other issues with the employer on behalf of all union members. Labour relations legislation sets out the rules for these negotiations (also called *collective bargaining*), identifies what obligations must be fulfilled before a legal strike can take place, and identifies unfair labour and employee conduct.

Workers' Compensation Legislation

The provinces and territories have workers' compensation legislation covering how workers are financially compensated for accidental injuries on the job. Generally, an employee is considered to be on the job from the time of reporting to work until the end of the shift. If travel is work related, accidents that happen while travelling may also be covered by workers' compensation. This legislation also discusses worker and employer rights when an injury occurs.

Long-Term Care Facilities Legislation

All long-term care facilities are regulated by provincial and territorial legislation. These laws address the basic rights of clients and describe requirements for the operation of the facility. Licensing and placement requirements, funding structures, accountability systems, guidelines about creating and maintaining health care records, and the level of training required of the staff are all listed as well.

Community Services Legislation

Community services legislation sets out the rules and procedures for accessing and providing community services, including support work. It defines the different types of community services and details how the services are to be provided.

CHAPTER REVIEW

KEY POINTS

- As a support worker, your conduct at work is determined by (1) your code of ethics, (2) your employer's policies, and (3) federal and provincial or territorial laws.
- The Canadian Charter of Rights and Freedoms lists the basic rights and freedoms to which all Canadians are entitled. All provincial and territorial laws must be consistent with its rules.
- All people have the right to be treated with respect and dignity, as reinforced throughout this book by the acronym DIPPS (dignity, independence, preferences, privacy, and safety).
- All people have a right to decide whether or not to agree to medical treatment or health care or personal care services—called *consent.* This right extends further in that people have a right to complete, accurate, and relevant information about the situation and the potential implications for consenting or refusing to consent—called *informed consent.*
- Wills are legal documents drawn up by people stating how they want their property distributed upon their death. A living will is a written statement that tells the person's wishes in regard to accepting or refusing medical care in the event that the person is unable to express such a decision. Living wills are not legally enforceable. Advance directives are legal documents that allow clients to communicate their decisions about their own end-of-life care.
- A substitute decision maker, or power of attorney, is a person appointed to make decisions for a client who is unable to make informed decisions about herself or her property. A substitute decision maker for health care (also known as a *proxy* in some provinces) makes informed health care decisions if the client is unable to do so. A substitute decision maker for property (known as an *estate trustee*) makes decisions regarding the client's belongings if the client is unable to do so.
- Criminal laws are concerned with offences against the public and against society in general (e.g., rape, murder). Civil laws deal with relationships between people. A tort is a wrongful act committed by one person against another person or his property.
- Negligence occurs when a person or his property is harmed due to another's failure to act carefully or competently.
- An assault is an intentional attempt or threat to touch a person's body without consent, causing the person to fear bodily harm. Battery is the actual touching of a person's body without consent.
- All clients have a right to privacy, including electronic privacy and confidentiality. Violating this right is an invasion of privacy and is punishable by law.
- As a worker, you have legal rights to receive fair wages and to work in a safe and fair environment.

CRITICAL THINKING IN PRACTICE

Mrs. Lopez has dementia (see Chapter 36) and weakness in her legs. She uses a wheelchair and often tries to get up without help. When you assist her with toileting, she occasionally tries to scratch you. How will you provide for her basic needs? Is she breaking the law by scratching you? As her support worker, what are your rights?

REVIEW QUESTIONS

Answers to these questions are at the bottom of p. 146.

Circle the BEST answer.

1. Which statement about the Canadian Charter of Rights and Freedoms is true?
   A. The Charter is still awaiting final passage in the courts.
   B. It lists the basic rights and freedoms to which all Canadians are entitled.
   C. It protects the right to equality of residents of Canada as long as they are citizens.
   D. It was made to protect all adults over the age of 18.

2. Provincial and territorial human rights codes promote:
   A. Freedom from poverty by reducing taxes
   B. Unequal treatment with respect to services and facilities
   C. The right to vote
   D. Equal treatment with respect to age, gender, and ethnicity

3. Which of the following is an example of treating a client with respect and dignity?
   A. Assuming that the client needs your help before he or she asks
   B. Forgetting to insert the hearing aids for the client
   C. Ordering the client's food at mealtime
   D. Being careful with the client's personal possessions

4. Which of the following is required to help a client give informed consent?
   A. Asking the client politely to hurry up and make a decision
   B. Ignoring details about the potential risks and side effects of the treatment
   C. Reassurance that the proposed treatment is the only option
   D. Information about the likely consequences of not having the treatment

5. Who decides the kind of recreation activities a long-term care client will do?
   A. The client's family
   B. The client's physician or nurse
   C. The facility
   D. The client

6. If a client complains to you about the home care agency's policy, you should:
   A. Inform your supervisor about the complaint
   B. Advise the client to speak to your supervisor
   C. Ignore the client's complaint
   D. Try to distract the client

7. Which of the following statements about negligence is true?
   A. It is an intentional tort.
   B. The client acted in a reasonable manner.
   C. Harm was caused to a client or a client's property.
   D. A prison term may result.

8. The intentional attempt or threat to touch a person's body without consent is:
   A. Assault
   B. Battery
   C. Defamation
   D. False imprisonment

9. The illegal restraint of a person's movement is:
   A. Assault
   B. Battery
   C. Defamation
   D. False imprisonment

10. Mr. Mohammed's photograph is made public on the Internet without his consent. This is:
   A. Battery
   B. Unintentional tort
   C. Invasion of privacy
   D. Libel

11. Informed consent is obtained by the:
   A. Client's family
   B. Registered staff
   C. Client's substitute decision maker
   D. Support worker

12. The basic rules about wages, work hours, and vacation days are covered in:
   A. Labour relations legislation
   B. Workers' compensation legislation
   C. Employment standards legislation
   D. Regulated health professions legislation

Answers: 1.B, 2.D, 3.D, 4.D, 5.D, 6.A, 7.C, 8.A, 9.D, 10.C, 11.B, 12.C

Chapter opener image: Martin Good/Shutterstock.com

CHAPTER 10

Caring About Culture and Diversity

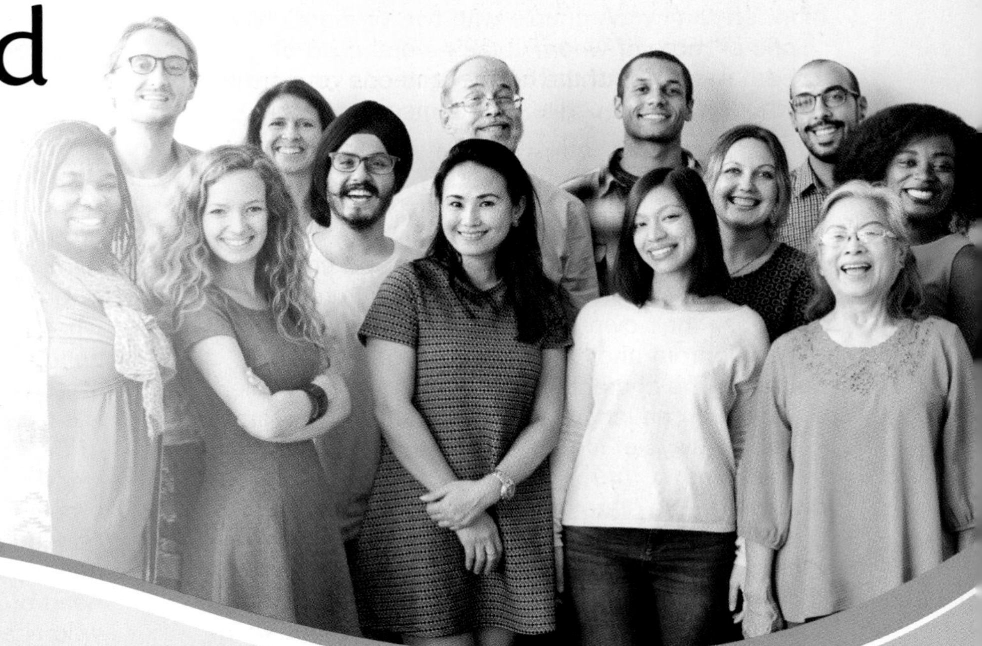

OBJECTIVES

After reading this chapter, the learner should be able to do the following:

- Distinguish among *race* (or *ethnicity*) and *culture*.
- Describe the factors that influence a person's culture.
- Summarize how culture influences a person's attitudes and behaviours.
- Describe how culture may affect communication, family organization, religious convictions, and perceptions about illness and health care.
- Analyze how your own cultural biases may affect your relationships with your clients.
- Apply the information in this chapter in your work by providing culturally sensitive care.

KEY TERMS

ageism Feelings of impatience, intolerance, or prejudice based on negative attitudes and stereotypes toward a person or group of people because of their age. *p. 151*

assimilate Adopt the traditions of the larger society. *p. 150*

bias A point of view that prevents a person from being impartial. *p. 150*

blended family A couple with two or more children, one or more of whom is the natural child of both members of the couple and one or more of whom is the stepchild of one member of the couple. *p. 154*

cultural competence The ability to interact effectively with people from different cultures or socioeconomic backgrounds. *p. 153*

cultural conflict Negative feelings and conduct that can result when people from one culture try to impose their own set of values and behaviours on people from another culture. *p. 152*

culture The characteristics of a group of people, including the language, values, beliefs, customs, habits, ways of life, rules for behaviour, music, and traditions. *p. 149*

diversity The state of different individuals and cultures coexisting. *p. 148*

ethnic identity The ethnic background a person feels a part of, based usually on similar language and customs. *p. 149*

ethnicity The sharing of a common history, language, geography, national origin, religion, or identity. *p. 149*

ethnocentrism The belief that one's own culture or ethnic group is better or more important than others'. *p. 149*

homophobia Negative attitudes toward or intolerance of homosexuality or people who are identified or perceived as being lesbian, gay, bisexual, transgender, or questioning their sexuality (**LGBTQ**). *p. 152*

LGBTQ An abbreviation that stands for the group of people who identify themselves as lesbian, gay, bisexual, transgender, or questioning their sexuality. *p. 152*

nuclear family A family consisting of a father, a mother, and children. *p. 154*

personal space The area immediately around one's body. *p. 156*

prejudice An attitude that forms an opinion about a person based on his or her membership in a group. *p. 150*

racism Feelings of superiority over, and intolerance or prejudice toward, a person or group of people who may have different physical appearances or cultural practices. *p. 149*

same-sex family A family in which both adults who live together in a loving, intimate relationship are of the same gender. *p. 154*

sexism Feelings of intolerance or prejudice toward a person or group of people because of their gender. *p. 152*

single-parent families Families in which the adult head of the household does not have a partner who shares the home. *p. 154*

stereotype An overly simple or exaggerated view of a group of people. *p. 151*

transgender A person's gender identity differing from that person's physical sex characteristics. *p. 152*

This chapter addresses one of the most important values that all support workers—and all caregivers, for that matter—must possess: respect for diversity. **Diversity** is the state of different individuals and cultures coexisting. During your career as a support worker, you will care for and work with people whose lifestyles, beliefs, customs, and rituals are different from your own. It is necessary that you are always respectful of a person's age, race, gender, occupation, sexual orientation, and lifestyle. ***Respect for diversity is a theme that will be repeated throughout this textbook and will be reinforced throughout your career as a support worker.***

Canada has a very diverse population, and Canadians are known for embracing this diversity and celebrating it. Unlike the American *melting pot*, which illustrates how all peoples and cultures are unified and blended within that country, Canada is known as a *cultural mosaic*, or a *cultural salad*, which illustrates a country of many distinct pieces. This reality was even enacted into federal laws. In 1971, Prime Minister Pierre Trudeau declared that Canada would adopt a multicultural policy, recognizing and respecting the diversity in languages, customs, religions, and practices of its people. Multiculturalism was recognized by Section 27 of the Canadian Charter of Rights and Freedoms (1982) and became law in 1988 in the *Canadian Multiculturalism Act*. This law declared equal rights to all Canadian citizens, ensured Aboriginal rights, and identified both French and English as the official languages of Canada, although other languages can be used. As a result, all Canadians are protected by law from discrimination based on the person's sex, gender, race, age, sexual orientation, language, religion, origin, caste or class, income or property, beliefs or opinions, and health or disability.[1]

Your client (or a co-worker) may be a third-generation Canadian, an Indigenous Canadian, or a new immigrant. Another client (or co-worker) may be in a same-sex relationship, and yet another may voice very different political or religious beliefs than you do. Each of us has a unique background and culture, and we all have a right to our own personal viewpoints. As a support worker, you must possess good listening skills and be both understanding and accepting of other peoples' differences and perspectives. You should also be aware of and respectful toward each client's cultural background in order to provide the best care possible. Your supportive care should never be less respectful for one client than it is for any other client for any reason. Lastly, when giving support care, you should never try to change the client to fit in with your care but rather adapt your care and support to fit the client.

DIVERSITY: ETHNICITY AND CULTURE

Two terms are often confused when discussing diversity—*ethnicity* and *culture*. Because many people find the word *race* insulting or misleading, this chapter will avoid this term and use *ethnicity* instead. While the authors agree that it is not a seamless replacement, it is the one that is usually used.

In nearly any part of Canada, you will notice people with different skin colours and facial features that show that they come from different ethnicities and backgrounds. This variety is an example of the ever-increasing diversity of our country. **Racism** results when people have feelings of intolerance or prejudice toward a person or group of people because of their racial or ethnic backgrounds. **Ethnocentrism**, the belief that one's own culture or ethnic group is better or more important than others', may be less obvious than racism, but neither racism nor ethnocentrism is in keeping with the spirit and intention of the Canadian Charter of Rights and Freedoms.

Ethnicity

Ethnicity refers to the sharing of a common history, language, geography, national origin, religion, or identity. Examples of ethnic groups include the Irish, the Inuit, and the Chinese. An ethnic group is not necessarily a nationality. For example, you may have been born in Canada, so your nationality is Canadian, but you may consider your **ethnic identity** to be Ukrainian because your family came from Ukraine and you still speak its language or practise many Ukrainian ethnic customs. Canada can be proud that it has many interesting ethnic groups within it.

Culture

Culture makes a society distinctive. **Culture** refers to the characteristics of a group of people—the language, values, beliefs, habits, ways of life, implied rules for behaviour, music, and traditions—that are shared or perhaps even passed from one generation to the next. Culture may be influenced by age, race, gender, occupation, sexual orientation, or lifestyle.

Cultural characteristics, which are learned by living within a group, influence a person's attitudes and behaviours. Examples of cultural groups include high school students (numerous subgroups exist within this main group!), farmers, and snowboarders. Everyone is part of a culture. Some people belong to more than one culture at the same time. For example, you might be a college student, belong to a religious organization, have parents with whom you speak another language, and go jogging with a set of friends regularly. Each of these groups of people that you associate with can have its own culture.

Ethnicity is an important influence on a person's culture, but it is not the only influence. A person might have come from China as a young child, spoken Chinese at home, and loved Chinese food and customs. Having grown up in Canada, however,

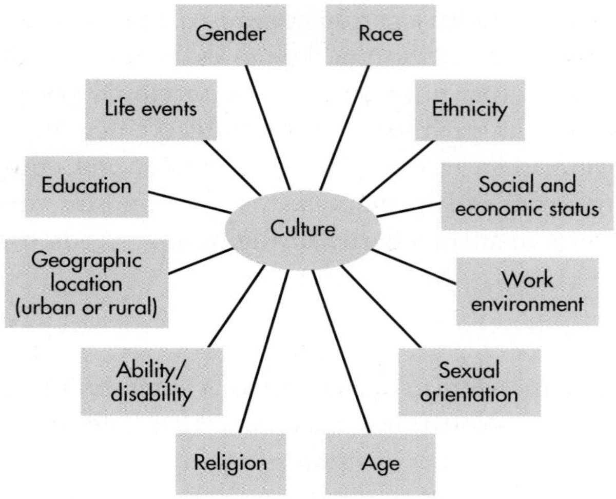

FIGURE 10–1 Culture is influenced by a number of factors.

she might be very different from her parents, who came to this country as adults. Her ethnicity has influenced her, but so has being schooled in Canada, having outside interests, and making friends from different social, cultural, and religious backgrounds. Because her experiences are different from her parents' experiences, she has been subject to different cultural influences than they have been.

Some people have chosen to **assimilate** their styles of dress, eating habits, or other behaviours when with people from another culture. Examples of assimilation are a Muslim woman who no longer wears a hijab or a First Nations person who changes eating habits (see the *Supporting Amy Longfeather: How Cultural Habits Can Influence Health* box).

FIGURE 10–1 shows some of the main factors that shape an individual's culture. As the figure depicts, every person reacts to the various cultural factors in her own way, and because of this, each person is culturally unique. A person's culture can change over time as the person leaves one group and joins another or encounters new life experiences.

Supporting Amy Longfeather: How Cultural Habits Can Influence Health

Growing up, Amy Longfeather ate different kinds of foods that her family hunted and gathered, such as moose, rabbit, and tea made from marsh roots. She also helped with hunting and gathering this food, activities that allowed her to become physically fit and healthy. Her diet was very high in protein and very low in fat and simple carbohydrates.

Several years ago, Amy moved to a big city to seek employment and, as a result, changed her lifestyle and diet. Amy now buys high-fat, prepackaged foods that she microwaves at mealtime in her staff lunchroom, as some of her co-workers do. In addition, she no longer engages in the same physical activities as she did at home, instead watching television for several hours every evening after supper with her roommate. As a result of this lifestyle change, Amy has gained a considerable amount of weight. Several months ago, she was diagnosed with insulin-dependent diabetes.

Last week, Amy fell and badly scraped her arms on her way home from work. Because of her diabetes, her arms have become infected. She is now getting home care from a nurse, who assists her with her insulin injections, as well as a support worker, who assists her to change her dressings and to wash her hair. Amy realizes that she needs to go back to her former healthier eating and lifestyle habits, but she likes the ease and convenience of her new lifestyle and diet. What should she do?

Adapted from Sandy Lake First Nation. (n.d.). *Traditions and culture*. Retrieved from http://www.sandylake.firstnation.ca/traditions-and-culture.

Prejudice and Discrimination

Unfortunately, prejudice and discrimination do still exist throughout the world. **Prejudice** is an attitude toward or opinion of a person based on his or her membership in a group. It is formed from the word *prejudge*, which implies that value assumptions regarding a person are formed before even meeting or knowing that person. Similarly, a **bias** occurs when a person is unable to impartially judge the issues at hand because of a preformed point of view.

Acting on one's prejudices results in *discrimination*, the unfair treatment of people on the basis of their physical characteristics, health history, or group membership. An example of discrimination is using the assumption that "All people who are _______ are lazy" to justify why a certain person is not hired.

Types of Prejudice

In an ethnically and culturally diverse society such as Canada's, prejudices and discrimination should not be tolerated. As a support worker, you will be caring for and supporting all types of people and must be prepared to give all your clients the same high quality of care, regardless of their differences.

Some people stereotype ethnic or cultural groups by assuming they are "all alike" or by believing that everyone in that group acts or behaves in a certain way. A **stereotype** is an overly simple or exaggerated view of a group of people. An example of a stereotype is "Women are shorter than men." While many women may be shorter than some men, this general statement is certainly not true.

Ageism refers to feelings of intolerance or prejudice toward others because of their age, based on negative attitudes, stereotypes, or impatience (see **BOX 10–1**). North American society has long fostered

BOX 10–1 Ageism and Age Discrimination (Fact Sheet)

The term *ageism* refers to two concepts: a socially constructed way of thinking about older persons based on negative attitudes and stereotypes about aging and a tendency to structure society based on an assumption that everyone is young, thereby failing to respond appropriately to the real needs of older persons.

Ageism is often a cause for individual acts of age discrimination and also discrimination that is more systemic in nature, such as in the design and implementation of services, programs and facilities. Age discrimination involves treating persons in an unequal fashion due to age in a way that is contrary to human rights law. The Ontario Human Rights Code prohibits age discrimination in employment, housing accommodation, goods, services and facilities, contracts, and membership in trade and vocational associations.

Age discrimination is often not taken as seriously as other forms of discrimination. However, it can have the same economic, social, and psychological impact as any other form of discrimination.

To combat ageism it is necessary to raise public awareness about its existence and to dispel common stereotypes and misperceptions about aging. Aging is a highly individual experience and it is not possible to generalize about the skills and abilities of an older person based on age, any more than it is possible to make assumptions about someone based on any other aspect of their identity. Human rights principles require people to be treated as individuals and assessed on their own merits, instead of on the basis of assumptions, and to be given the same opportunities and benefits as everyone else, regardless of age. It is important to recognize that older persons make significant contributions to our society and that we must not limit their potential.

At the same time, ageism can be combated through inclusive planning and design which reflects the circumstances of persons of all ages to the greatest extent possible. The Supreme Court of Canada has recently made it clear that it is no longer acceptable to structure systems in a way that assumes that everyone is young and then try to accommodate those who do not fit this assumption. Rather, the age diversity that exists in society should be reflected in design stages for policies, programs, services, facilities and so forth so that physical, attitudinal and systemic barriers are not created. Where barriers already exist, those responsible should identify them and take steps to remove them.

Finally, it is important to remember that the experience of ageism and age discrimination may differ based on other components of a person's identity. For example, certain groups of older persons may experience unique barriers because of their age combined with their gender, disability, sexual orientation, race, colour, ethnicity, religion, culture, and language.

Source: Ontario Human Rights Commission. *Ageism and age discrimination* (fact sheet). Retrieved from http://www.ohrc.on.ca/en/ageism-and-age-discrimination-fact-sheet. © Queen's Printer for Ontario, 2014. Reproduced with permission.

a desire to look young and "act young," and older people who are frail or have cognitive decline are often seen as less worthy of attention, less valuable to society, and less employable. In fact, even some academic health care programs focus only on the characteristics and health needs of young adults, instead of emphasizing the types and consequences of age-related bodily changes. As a result, some health care workers overlook serious symptoms in older adults, such as signs of fever, medication interactions, or urinary tract infections.

Sexism is feelings of intolerance or prejudice toward a person or group of people because of their gender. Many examples of sexism exist even today. For example, some people still believe that men make better politicians than women. In some workplaces, men are paid more than women who perform the same job. In some countries, couples who are trying to conceive a baby seek medical assistance to ensure a baby of a preferred gender.

Some people have **homophobia**, negative attitudes toward or an intolerance of homosexuality or people who identify themselves as part of the **LGBTQ** community, consisting of people who are lesbian, gay, bisexual, transgender, or questioning their sexuality. **Transgender** means that a person's gender identity is different from that person's physical sex characteristics (see *Supporting Jimmie: Respecting Diversity in Transgender Clients*). Although discrimination against people in the LGBTQ community is illegal, such discrimination exists. Of the children or youth in Canada who identify themselves as part of the LGBTQ community, more than half have reported being verbally harassed about their perceived gender or sexual orientation, and over 20% have been physically harassed or assaulted.[2]

Cultural Conflict

Cultural conflict occurs when a person tries to dictate to another person what his culture should be. Unfortunately, we often see examples of cultural conflict even in our multicultural society. For example, people may be forced by others not to wear anything

Supporting Jimmie: Respecting Diversity in Transgender Clients

Jimmie (not his real name) is a 75-year-old client who fell and broke his right hip and ulna after slipping on a patch of icy sidewalk. He was rushed by ambulance to an emergency department, and then undressed so the medical team could assess his injuries. It was at that time it was discovered he was not a man. In tears, Jimmie confided that his childhood name was Jocelyn. He had run away from home at a young age and broken ties with his family, who never accepted him as a man. For over 50 years, he lived as a man, binding his breasts and wearing baggy clothing to disguise his shape. Never married, he worked as an electrician until he retired.

Jimmie had to be admitted to the hospital because of the extent of his injuries. Because of his health care benefits, he was admitted to a four-bed ward of women, where the staff referred to him as Jocelyn in spite of his insistence that he be called Jimmie.

Discussion

Unfortunately, most hospitals, schools, and public buildings are not yet equipped to deal with the needs of the transgender community. In spite of this shortfall, health care workers can honour the DIPPS principles (dignity, independence, preferences, privacy, safety) in the following ways when caring for transgender clients:

- Address the client using the name the client prefers.
- When referring to the client, use the pronoun the client prefers, such as "he," "she," or "they." Never use "it," which is disrespectful.
- Realize that not all transgender clients have undergone sex-reassignment surgery.
- Do not assume that or ask about whether a transgender client is a homosexual or lesbian. Gender identity is different from *sexual orientation*.
- Advise your agency of the client's gender identity so that fair and respectful accommodations can be considered on behalf of all clients.[3]

CASE STUDY Cultural Conflict

Salvinia Di Silva is a 75-year-old widow receiving home care. She and her husband moved from Portugal to Canada in the 1960s with their three young children. For the next 30 years, Mr. Di Silva worked on the assembly line of an automobile factory, while Mrs. Di Silva worked as a dressmaker. They worked long hours to pay for their children's education. All three children now have successful careers and their own families.

Mrs. Di Silva's health began to decline after her husband died. Severe arthritis in her leg and hip progressed to the point that she could no longer walk. A family conference was held, and the children agreed that their mother no longer could care for herself, even with the aid of a support worker. They thought it was unsafe for her to live alone. None of the children felt that they could manage their mother's care and the demands of their own families and careers, so they told their mother that she should consider moving into a long-term care facility.

Her children's suggestion came as a great shock to Mrs. Di Silva. She and her husband had taken care of her mother years before, until her mother's death. Mrs. Di Silva had assumed that one of her children would do the same for her. In Portugal, it was common for children to take care of their older parents. Mrs. Di Silva felt as if she was being cast aside. The idea of leaving her home and moving into a facility with strangers depressed her greatly. Her depression, in turn, caused feelings of guilt and remorse among the Di Silva children, who deeply loved their mother. This situation is an example of conflict between two cultures. Mr. and Mrs. Di Silva had given their children opportunities to enter and succeed in a new culture. But because the children are now a part of the new culture, they, like others in their environment, are less willing to give up their lifestyles to care for their mother in their own homes. They see their friends' parents enjoying living in a retirement facility with other people their own age and hope their mother will also eventually settle in and feel at home there.

that reveals religious affiliation in certain environments. Or a caregiver might serve unfamiliar foods to a client because those foods are common in the caregiver's ethnic background, not the client's.

An individual living within different cultures at the same time can also have feelings of cultural conflict. A child raised in a very modest, religious family may experience cultural conflict when he grows up and moves out of the house to go to school. This person may struggle with trying to live by the family's rules, as expected by his parents, while trying to enjoy some newly found freedoms within his peer group. Refer to the *Case Study: Cultural Conflict* box for an example of cultural conflict experienced by an individual.

Cultural Competence

Cultural competence is the ability of a person to interact effectively with people from different cultures or socioeconomic backgrounds. In health care, it includes the ability to deliver care that is respectful and responsive to the health beliefs, practices, and linguistic (language) needs of clients. Cultural competence should be the goal of every health care worker in order to provide respectful, person-centred care. An essential element of cultural competence is learning about different cultures. In addition, it is respecting the client as part of a particular culture without attempting to change the client's values or beliefs. However, it is also important to understand that not everybody from a particular culture demonstrates identical health practices; part of cultural competence is refraining from prejudging a client's beliefs or behaviours.

THE EFFECT OF CULTURE

A person's culture affects how he or she deals with daily situations and problems. It is not possible to completely understand the beliefs and practices of all cultures. However, it is important to realize that culture affects a person's beliefs and behaviours toward such issues as:

- Family and social organization
- Religion and worship
- Health care practices and reactions to illness
- Communication

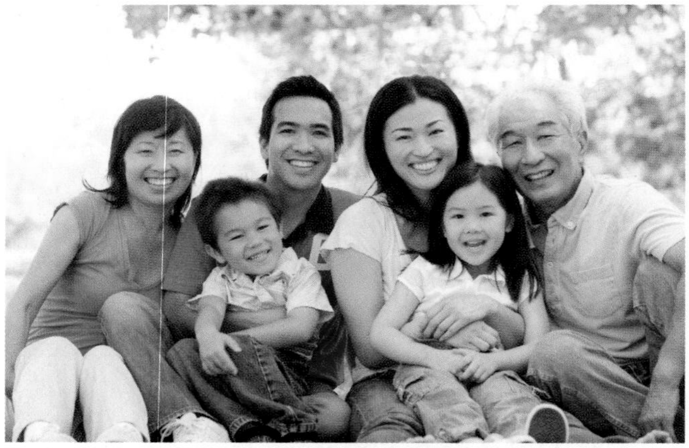

FIGURE 10–2 An extended family. (**Source:** Monkey Business Images/Shutterstock.com)

The Effect of Culture on the Family

In your career as a support worker, you will meet different kinds of families. Culture affects family structure, as well as the roles and responsibilities of various family members during times of illness. For example, in some cultures, adult children (especially daughters) are expected to care for their older parents.

Types of Families

In Western culture, the most common family structure is the traditional **nuclear family**, which consists of a mother, a father, and children. The family arrangement in today's Canada is very different, though, from what it was in previous generations. Now there is an increasing number of **single-parent families**, in which the adult head of the household does not have a partner who shares the home. Some families are **blended families**—that is, the family consists of a couple with two or more children, at least one of whom is the natural child of both members of the couple and at least one is the step-child of one of the partners. Another common family structure, the **same-sex family**, is one in which both partners living together in a loving, intimate relationship are of the same gender.

Western culture emphasizes self-reliance and independence. Children are usually encouraged to be self-sufficient, and most young adults leave the family home and live independently of their parents and siblings. Care of family members outside the nuclear family—such as that of grandparents, aunts, or uncles—is often entrusted to others outside the family.

In some cultures, such as Asian, South Asian, and Indigenous cultures, extended families (a couple, their children and parents, siblings, and siblings' children) commonly inhabit one household (FIGURE 10–2). In extended families, the needs of the entire family are more important than individual needs. Older adults and anyone who is unwell are often taken care of by family members. For example, in Vietnam and China, all family members are involved in the care of a member who has an illness.[4] Family members bathe, feed, and comfort the person with the illness. People from these and other such cultures continue this custom even in Canada, and those affected by illness are often surrounded by family during this time.

Sometimes children rebel against the culture of their parents. Children of first-generation immigrants often reject the roles and behaviours expected of them in favour of those of the new culture, causing great stress for the parents and family. The *Case Study* box on page 153 describes how cultural conflict affected one older person.

The Effect of Culture on Religion

In most cultures, religion is an extremely important influence. Religion relates to spiritual beliefs, needs, and practices and may promote beliefs and practices related to daily living habits, behaviours, relationships with others, diet, healing, days of worship, birth and birth control, medicine, and death.

Many people rely on religion for support and comfort during illness. They may want to pray and observe certain religious practices and may find it helpful to have a visit from a spiritual leader or advisor. If a client asks to see a religious leader, promptly report the request to your supervisor. Make sure the client's room is tidy for the visit. Ensure privacy during the visit.

Religions, including Christianity (Catholic and Protestant faiths), Judaism, Buddhism, Islam, Hinduism, Sikhism, and the Baha'i faith, among others, are practised by various groups within Canada. You will care for clients who have religious beliefs that are different from yours, and some clients may not follow any religion. Never try to convert your clients to your own belief system. You must always respect the client's beliefs, practices, and religious symbols and items (such as a rosary, yarmulke, prayer rug, or religious medal). Religious items should be treated with the greatest of respect and never touched or moved unless you are given permission to do so by the client.

The Effect of Culture on Perceptions of Health Care and Illness

Culture greatly affects how people view health care and illness and how they cope with the symptoms and stresses of being ill. Some cultures have certain beliefs about the causes of illnesses. In Western culture, the general belief is that disease and illness are caused by biological or environmental factors. Illness and disease can often be prevented, and people can be cared for or cured with scientifically proven methods. Some other cultures believe that illness is caused by supernatural forces, an imbalance with nature, or disharmony among mind, body, and spirit. People from these cultures may use charms, rituals, alternative medicines, or traditional or folk medicine that may include ancient remedies and rituals, passed down through generations. Some folk remedies involve herbs or a traditional healer, or shaman.

Folk remedies may help the person or may not have any effect on the person's health. If the practice does not harm the client and promotes her emotional well-being, the nurse or case manager would probably include it in the care plan. Some folk remedies, however, may interfere with the client's medical treatment. For example, some herbal medicines may interact with prescription drugs and produce harmful results. Often, clients try alternative therapies or cultural health care practices without telling their physician, nurse, or case manager.[5] The health care team must be aware of all health care practices to make sure they are not harmful to the client. Tell your supervisor if your client tells you that she is using alternative or folk remedies or if you observe a client using alternative or folk remedies.

The Effect of Culture on Communication

Communicating across cultures presents many challenges. Words and phrases may have different meanings to people from different cultures, even if they speak the same language! As a support worker, you must communicate with clients and their families in such a way that your message is clear and, in turn, the client understands your intended meaning. All communication should always adhere to the five principles of compassionate care (DIPPS: dignity, independence, preferences, privacy, and safety), which is the goal of support work.

The Use of Translators and Interpreters

Some of your clients may speak languages or dialects different from yours. Other clients may be deaf or hard of hearing and, therefore, unable to hear you. As a result, with some clients, you will work with an interpreter. Interpreters may be family members who are able to describe what the client is saying or trying to say and then translate back to the client what you would like to say to (or ask of) the client. In other cases, the interpreter may be a staff member who happens to speak the same language (or a similar language) as the client. Occasionally, a paid translator must be called in to interpret what a client is saying, especially if a legal consent is necessary. However, in certain situations, you may not have an interpreter handy when you need to communicate with clients who do not speak your language, and you must find a way to communicate with and understand the client (see the *Respecting Diversity: Communicating With Clients Who Speak a Language Different From Yours* box).

Body Language

Speaking the same language is only part of communicating. Information and messages are also sent using nonverbal cues, such as the use of touch, space, eye contact, and even silence. Body language, an

Respecting Diversity

Communicating With Clients Who Speak a Language Different From Yours

- Convey comfort to the client by your tone of voice and body language.
- Do not speak loudly or shout. It will not help the client understand English.
- Speak slowly and distinctly.
- Keep messages short and simple.
- Be alert to identify words the client seems to understand.
- Use gestures and pictures to convey your message.
- Repeat the message in different ways.
- Avoid using technical terms, abbreviations, and slang.
- Be certain that the client understands what is going to be done and consents to it before you begin a procedure. Be alert for signs that the client is only pretending to understand. For example, nodding and answering "yes" to all questions are signs that the client may not really understand what you are saying. You may need to clarify whether the client understands you by asking him to repeat what you have said (see Chapter 5).
- Learn a few useful phrases in the client's language. Key words such as "Toilet?," "Pain?," "Cold?," or "Hungry?" can assist you to communicate more easily with the client.

important part of nonverbal communication, is expressed through gestures, postures, and facial expressions, which can reveal a person's physical, mental, or emotional state. Support workers need to be aware, however, that nonverbal cues may mean different things to people of different cultures.

Touch

Touch is a very important form of nonverbal communication. It can convey comfort, caring, love, affection, interest, trust, concern, and reassurance. Clients are often comforted by being softly touched on their arms or having their hands held. However, cultural groups have different rules or expectations regarding who can touch, when touch can occur, and which parts of the body can be touched (**FIGURE 10–3**). Some cultures—for example, the Spanish, Italian, French, and South American cultures—are known to use touch freely.[6] People from some other cultures—for example, the English, German, and Chinese cultures—are embarrassed or uncomfortable with any casual touch by strangers and tend to avoid it.[7] People within cultures will also vary in their acceptance of being touched by caregivers. It is therefore very important to obtain consent each time you must touch a client to provide care.

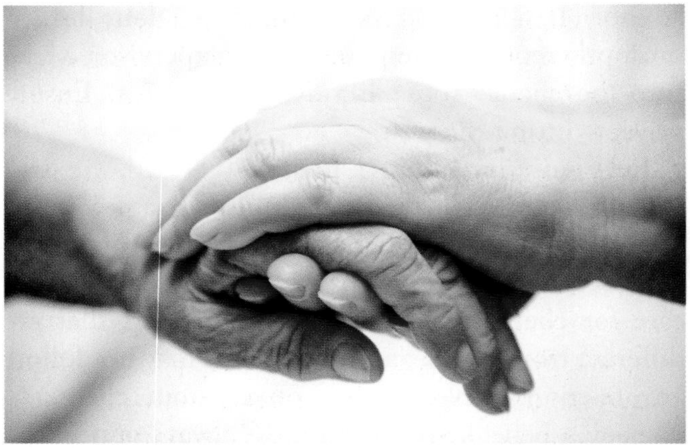

FIGURE 10–3 Culture may influence how a client responds to touch. (**Source:** Kuzma/Shutterstock.com)

Sometimes the cultural rules of touch depend on the person's gender. For example, in the Indian and Vietnamese cultures, men shake hands with other men but not with women.[7] You must be aware of what kind of touch and how much touch the client is comfortable with. Ask your supervisor for guidance, and watch how the client interacts with family members or with other people. ***Regardless of the situation, a support worker's touch should be gentle, not hurried or rough, and never sexual in nature.***

Personal Space

If someone stood too close to you, you would probably feel uncomfortable or anxious because your personal space was invaded. The same is true for your clients. **Personal space** is the area immediately around one's body. Everyone has personal space preferences, and it is not always dictated by culture.

Some people prefer more personal space than others do because of their own life experiences (see the *Supporting Donald Lundy: Respecting a Client's Sense of Personal Space* box).

The exact distance requirements vary among individuals and situations. However, people in the same cultural group tend to have similar personal space requirements.[8] In Western cultures, most people prefer to stand at a distance of about 90 cm (3 feet) to speak. People in other cultures may prefer to stand closer or farther away when interacting with others. When you are providing care, it is important not to invade your client's personal space. If the client steps back from you, does not face you directly, or pulls her chair away from you, she may be sending a message that you are too close.[9]

Eye Contact

Eye contact has different meanings within different cultures. In Western cultures, eye contact is usually a sign of positive self-concept, openness, interest in others, attention, and honesty, and it also communicates warmth. Lack of eye contact can communicate rudeness, guilt, dishonesty, shyness, or embarrassment. People from some other cultures, however, are not comfortable with direct eye contact. In some Asian and Indigenous cultures, eye contact is considered disrespectful and an invasion of privacy.[9] In the Indian culture, eye contact with people of a higher or lower social and economic class is usually avoided.[9]

Facial Expressions

Some facial expressions are universal. Expressions of pain, surprise, embarrassment, and happiness are similar around the world, but some cultures are more expressive than others are. It, therefore, may be hard to judge what others are feeling only on the basis of their facial expressions. For example, many Italian and Spanish people tend to use facial expressions and gestures often to communicate happiness, pain, or displeasure. In contrast, many Irish, English, and northern European people use fewer facial expressions, especially with strangers.[8] In some cultures, certain facial expressions may, in fact, suggest the opposite of what the person is really feeling. For example, in some Asian cultures, people may smile to hide negative emotions.[9]

Supporting Donald Lundy: Respecting a Client's Sense of Personal Space

Donald Lundy is an 82-year-old bachelor who lives by himself in his own house. He has always managed to care for himself and his pets until last week, when he fell while trying to clear the snow from the roof over his front porch, breaking several bones. Mr. Lundy now requires physiotherapy twice a week. Because he has no family or friends, his doctors decided that he would need a support worker to take him to and from the hospital for his therapy and to assist him with his personal hygiene and grooming.

You are Mr. Lundy's assigned support worker. Mr. Lundy is never willing to let you touch him or stand near him, even though he cannot manage his care on his own. You have noticed that Mr. Lundy shrugs, frowns, and turns away from you whenever you try to assist him with his personal care. Mr. Lundy has repeatedly told you that he is not used to having a person touch him or stand so close to him.

Today, you try something that your supervisor has suggested. You quietly put on gloves before providing any care for Mr. Lundy and avoid any direct skin-to-skin contact with him. You also make sure that you limit the time you spend on providing personal care for him and try not to stand close to him, whenever possible. Mr. Lundy seems less distressed because you respect his need for space and because you are wearing gloves. You are happy to report this outcome to your supervisor. What else could you have done to decrease Mr. Lundy's discomfort with being touched during his personal care and grooming?

Silence

Even the use of silence varies among cultural groups. In some cultures, such as the English and Arabic cultures, silence is usually used for privacy.[10] Among Russian, French, and Spanish cultures, silence usually indicates agreement between parties.[10] In some Asian cultures, silence is often used as a sign of respect, particularly in interactions with an older person.[10] In some Indigenous cultures, silence is considered a virtue: Speaking is reserved only for matters of extreme importance.[11] Among most Indigenous, Chinese, and Japanese people, silence is used as a communication aid. For example, if the person is speaking and suddenly stops, his silence may be intended to allow the listener to think about what has just been said before the speaker continues.[12]

PROVIDING CULTURALLY SENSITIVE CARE AND SUPPORT

Providing culturally sensitive care is important in support work. Remember that clients are unique individuals and respond to cultural influences in unique ways. Do not stereotype a person based on ethnicity, religion, or any other factor. ***You cannot apply the cultural behaviours of a given culture to all members of the group. Individuals may not follow every belief and practice of their culture and religion. Each person is unique.***

How to Care for Clients in a Nonjudgemental Way

Sometimes, people do not realize that they are prejudiced or that they discriminate against certain others. Remember that everyone has a culture (or more than one) and that attitudes and behaviours are shaped by culture. Some clients may react negatively or fearfully to cultural differences. You, as a support worker, however, must resist displaying such reactions and accept a client's differences. You do not have to agree with the client's beliefs and practices (see the *Supporting Mme. Couture: Respecting the Client's Personal Beliefs* box). However, you must be tolerant and not make judgements. To be tolerant and understanding of others, you need to understand how your own culture influences you.

Consider the following questions:

- Do you judge people by your own cultural standards?
- Do you have any prejudices or biases?
- Do you assume that if something works for you, it must work for others as well?
- Do you think there are "right" and "wrong" ways of doing things?
- Are you ever critical of another person's lifestyle because it is different from your own?
- Do you sometimes consider other people's lifestyles, religious beliefs, political viewpoints, superstitions, and beliefs silly or odd?
- Do you try to convert others to your religion or way of thinking and doing things?
- Do you believe that people from one ethnic group, culture, or religion should not marry people from another?
- Do you avoid trying new things?
- Do you draw conclusions too quickly?
- Do you respect people as individuals, or do stereotypes sometimes get in the way?
- Do you find yourself angry or revolted when you see people who dress in a way that identifies their affiliation with a specific religion?

To accept people of different cultures, you need to learn about them *from them*. Communicate with them, and listen to them attentively. Learn as much as possible about their thoughts, beliefs, and values. Respect and show interest in their traditions, foods, dress, and customs. Your clients will feel valued and respected.

DIPPS

The acronym DIPPS stands for dignity, independence, preferences, privacy, and safety. ***It is an important concept addressed throughout this textbook.*** Support workers must provide care and support that is free from all prejudice and discrimination. All clients have the right to compassionate care, which includes dignity, respect for their independence, respect for their own preferences, and respect for their need for privacy and for safety. Support workers who respect their clients' cultural and ethnic backgrounds practise the fundamental principles of DIPPS.

Supporting Mme. Couture: Respecting the Client's Personal Beliefs

Yvonne Couture is a client with a severe burn on the bottom of her foot. She mentions to her support worker, Nancy, that she has placed a medal of Saint John the Apostle under the top layer of bandage around her foot. Mme. Couture also explains that Saint John the Apostle is known for healing burns, and she believes that placing the medal in the dressing will help her wound heal quickly and safely.

Nancy knows that Mme. Couture has the right to make her own choices about her care. She also knows that Mme. Couture's strong spiritual beliefs may help her during her healing process. Nancy is concerned, however, that having the religious medal so close to the wound may be harmful. She calls her supervisor to report the conversation. The supervisor relates the message to the case manager, who is not aware of the situation. The case manager asks Mme. Couture's nurse to discuss the situation with her.

Based on College of Nurses of Ontario. (2005). *Practice guideline: Culturally sensitive care* (p. 11). Toronto, ON: College of Nurses of Ontario.

CHAPTER REVIEW

KEY POINTS

- Canada has a highly diverse population. To provide the best care possible, you should be aware of and respectful toward your client's cultural background.
- *Ethnicity* refers to the sharing of a common history, language, geography, national origin, religion, or identity.
- *Culture* refers to the characteristics—language, values, beliefs, habits, ways of life, implied rules of behaviour, music, and traditions—of a group of people that are shared and perhaps passed from one generation to the next. Culture is influenced by age, race, gender, occupation, sexual orientation, or lifestyle.
- Prejudice and discrimination are always wrong and often hurtful. There are various types of prejudice.
- A person's culture affects (1) family and social organization, (2) religion and worship, (3) health practices and reactions to illness, and (4) communication.
- It is important that support workers care for all clients in a nonjudgemental and supportive way.

CRITICAL THINKING IN PRACTICE

A resident, who does not speak English, uses his call light often. Some needs are urgent. Others are not. Since your shift began, he has called for help 15 times. You have noticed that the resident uses his call light more often at night, after family visits, and when he is not checked on regularly. How might this information be helpful in care planning? What are ways that you might be able to decrease the resident's anxiety?

REVIEW QUESTIONS

Answers to these questions are at the bottom of p. 161.

Circle T if the answer is true, and circle F if the answer is false.

1. T F Culture influences people's attitudes and beliefs but not their behaviours.
2. T F Believing that all members of a group share the same characteristics is an example of stereotyping.
3. T F Everyone has a culture.
4. T F Everyone within an ethnic group shares the same culture.
5. T F Each individual responds differently to cultural influences.
6. T F Everyone responds positively to a hug or to a pat on the back.
7. T F Although a person's experiences and situation may change over time, his culture never changes.

Circle the BEST answer.

8. Which of the following statements is true?
   A. Ethnicity refers to a group of people who share similar interests.
   B. A country usually has one ethnic group.
   C. A person's culture influences health and illness practices.
   D. People within an ethnic community always dress and think alike.
9. Which of the following statements is true?
   A. Culture rarely influences communication.
   B. Culture may affect roles and responsibilities within families.
   C. All people respond to cultural influences in the same way.
   D. Canadians view health care and illness usually in the same way.

10. Mr. Greene asks to see his spiritual advisor. You should:
   A. Report his request to your supervisor
   B. Question why he wants the meeting
   C. Offer to introduce him to your spiritual advisor
   D. Tell him to phone his spiritual advisor himself

11. Which statement is correct?
   A. We should all judge people on the basis of their group membership.
   B. In some situations, prejudice is acceptable.
   C. Prejudice frequently leads to respect.
   D. Stereotypes are often associated with prejudice.

12. Mr. Jones rides a motorcycle and refers to himself as a "biker." He likes to wear clothing that signifies membership in his motorcycle club, and he prefers to spend time with his other "biker" friends. This description is of a(n) __________ group.
   A. ethnic
   B. cultural
   C. religious
   D. racial

Answers: 1.F, 2.T, 3.T, 4.F, 5.T, 6.F, 7.F, 8.C, 9.B, 10.A, 11.D, 12.B

Chapter opener image: Rawpixel.com/Shutterstock.com

CHAPTER 11

Working With Clients and Their Families

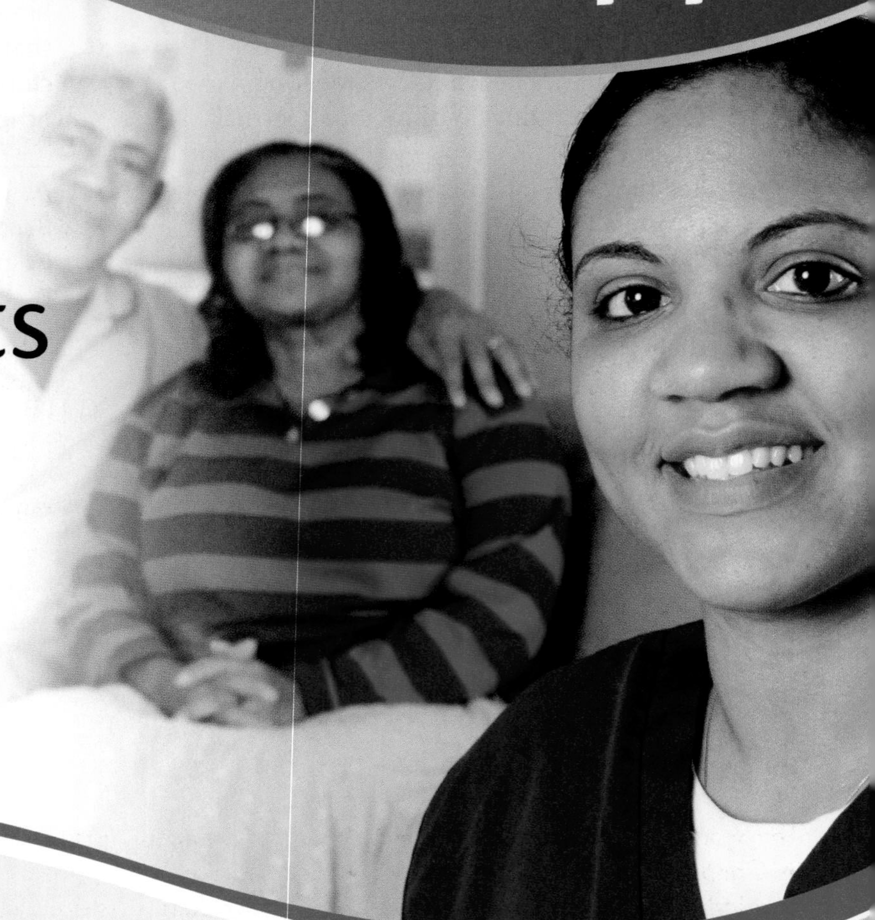

OBJECTIVES

After reading this chapter, the learner should be able to do the following:

- Explain the difference between a professional helping relationship and a friendship.
- Explain why it is necessary for a support worker to maintain a professional boundary.
- Describe common family patterns.
- Explain how the health care team assists the family.
- Explain independence, dependence, and interdependence.

KEY TERMS

compassion Awareness of the misfortune and suffering of another person and the desire to take action to reduce or eliminate the problem. *p. 165*

competence The ability to do a job well. *p. 165*

dependence The state of relying on others for support; being unable to manage without help. *p. 166*

family A biological, legal, or social network of people who provide support for one another. *p. 168*

independence The state of not relying on others for control or authority. *p. 166*

interdependence The state of relying on one another. *p. 166*

primary caregiver A person—usually a family member or close friend—who assumes the responsibilities of caring for a dependent person usually in the person's home. *p. 168*

professional boundaries Appropriate limitations on behaviour, meant to protect the vulnerable client from the caregiver who has access to private knowledge about him or her. *p. 163*

relationship The connection between two or more people, shaped by the roles, feelings, and interactions of those involved. *p. 163*

respect Acceptance and regard for another person. *p. 165*

self-awareness Understanding of one's own feelings, moods, attitudes, preferences, biases, qualities, and limitations. *p. 166*

self-esteem Thinking well of oneself and being well thought of by others. *p. 167*

sympathy Feeling compassion for or understanding the difficulties of another person. *p. 165*

The section entitled "Professional Communication" in Chapter 5 (p. 69) emphasized the need to communicate on a professional basis with both co-workers and supervisors. This chapter addresses the need to maintain a professional relationship with your clients. The client is usually part of a family, and your job as a support worker, in many circumstances, affects not only the client but also the client's family. It is therefore important to understand your role in the context of the family. You may get to know some members very well; however, your relationships with your clients and the family must remain professional at all times.

MAINTAINING A PROFESSIONAL RELATIONSHIP WITH THE CLIENT

Your relationship with your clients is a professional helping relationship that is established to benefit the client. It is different from a friendship, which is a personal social relationship that benefits both persons involved. A **relationship** is the connection between two or more people, and it is shaped by the roles, feelings, and interactions of those involved. Relationships can be either personal or professional. Mixing a professional relationship with a personal relationship is unethical.

Professional Boundaries[1]

As a support worker, you must remember that you are a professional and must maintain professional boundaries. **Professional boundaries** are appropriate limitations on behaviour, meant to protect the vulnerable client from the caregiver who has access to private knowledge about him or her. In any relationship in which one person is dependent on the other, the balance of power may not be equal. Being *aware* and trying to make allowances for potential imbalances of power in your relationships with your clients is an important aspect of maintaining a professional boundary. Another is maintaining confidentiality (see Chapter 1). As a support worker, you will be required to care for clients when they are at their most vulnerable (e.g., washing them after toileting). You may learn about their personal health history or financial situation. Some clients may wish to discuss private matters with you (see *Supporting*

Mrs. Chase: Maintaining Professional Boundaries), and they must feel confident that their information will remain private.

However, your clients or their family members may consider you to be a friend because of the intimate nature of the information they have disclosed to you, but you must not share your intimate information with them. Always remember to relate to a client as a professional helper, not as a friend. Friends share compassion, support, common experiences, problems, and advice and *choose* to spend time together. As a support worker, you are *assigned* the amount of time you will be providing care, although you may enjoy that time spent with your client. **BOX 11–1** compares professional helping relationships with friendships.

Supporting Mrs. Chase: Maintaining Professional Boundaries

Christina Chase is an older-adult home care client whom you have been assigned to help several times a week. Today, while you were assisting her to dress, she began to discuss her youth. She confided in you that, many years ago, she gave birth to several children with another man while she was separated from her husband. Her children were never told of this history, and after she reconciled with her husband, he agreed to raise the children as his own. To this day, her children do not know who their biological father really was.

Similarly, your sister had a baby with another man but later returned to her husband, who also agreed to raise the baby as his own. You are shocked at the similarities between the two situations and would like to discuss it with Mrs. Chase. Is it appropriate to do so? Does discussing your sister's situation with Mrs. Chase cross a professional boundary? Would it be wrong to discuss Mrs. Chase with your sister, even if you did not use Mrs. Chase's name? Do you have a right to discuss this information with Mrs. Chase's children?

BOX 11–1 Professional Helping Relationships Versus Friendships

Professional Helping Relationships	Friendships
Behaviour regulated by a code of ethics and professional standards; framed by agency policy	Behaviour guided by personal values and beliefs
Support worker paid to provide care to client	No payment for being in the relationship
Support worker provides care within a defined role and follows an established plan of care in meeting the client's needs	Pleasure- or interest-directed
Support worker has more power due to authority, knowledge, influence and access to privileged information about client	Relatively equal power in relationship
Support worker (not client) responsible for establishing and maintaining professional relationship	Equal responsibility for establishing and maintaining relationship
Support worker gives care within outlined hours of work	Personal choice regarding how much time is spent in the relationship

Adapted from College of Registered Nurses of British Columbia. (2016). *Professional versus personal relationships: Knowing the differences*. (https://www.crnbc.ca/Standards/resourcescasestudies/ethics/nurseclientrelationships/boundaries/Pages/PersonalVProfessional.aspx) originally adapted from Milgrom, J. (1992). Boundaries in professional relationships: a training manual. Minneapolis, MN: Walk-In Counseling Centre.

Although your professional relationship with a client and family is not friendship, you should still show that you care about them. Treat them with compassion and consideration, and recognize that each client is a unique individual. When working with clients and their families, demonstrate the following:

- ***Respect.*** Respect is showing acceptance and regard for another person. Accept your client's values, feelings, lifestyle, and decisions. When clients and their families are treated with respect, they feel valued and important, but when treated with disrespect, they feel ashamed, rejected, or hurt. Being respectful to clients means always being courteous and polite. For example, remember to say "please" and "thank you," as appropriate. On the other hand, being overly familiar with clients can be seen as lack of respect. Calling clients by their first names (or nicknames) without permission is an example of behaviour that shows a lack of respect. Failing to recognize a client's need for privacy and independence can also be seen as lack of respect. Respect your client's preferences for how tasks are done. As you perform the tasks, make sure that the client is comfortable, safe, and satisfied. Encourage clients to express preferences, make personal choices, and do as much as they can for themselves.
- ***Compassion.*** Compassion is characterized by a person's awareness of the misfortune and suffering of another and the desire to take action to reduce or eliminate the problem. Compassion requires an understanding that bad things can happen to people through no fault of their own. Compassion is not the same as pity. To pity someone may imply that you feel superior to that person. (See *Supporting Mark Vickers: Showing Compassion.*)

Supporting Mark Vickers: Showing Compassion

Mark Vickers, 16, has Down syndrome. His mother recently died of cancer, and since Mark's father abandoned the family long ago and Mark has no siblings or other family nearby, he has been moved into a group home.

Cynthia is a support worker in the group home. She notices that Mark sits all day in his room, staring at the wall. He refuses to join the other clients in the common room. Cynthia has great compassion for Mark. She tries to imagine what it must be like to lose the only person you had in the world and to be moved to a strange, new place. Cynthia recognizes that Mark needs time to deal with his grief and loneliness. She spends as much time as she can with Mark, sometimes simply sitting with him and holding his hand. Her quiet understanding of his sadness comforts Mark. After a few days, he begins to open up to Cynthia.

- ***Empathy.*** *Empathy* is the ability to recognize and understand another's emotions (see Chapter 1). Empathy involves being receptive to others and not being judgemental. Unless you have dealt with a similar situation, you can show only compassion; empathy means that you have faced a similar experience. Empathy may be felt in response to a full range of emotions. Eye contact and physical closeness can show empathy, so a smile, a kind word, or a gentle touch can be all that is needed to let your client know that you understand. An empathetic response can decrease a client's loneliness and create feelings of well-being and belonging.
- ***Sympathy.*** Sympathy differs from empathy and compassion. Whereas compassion involves listening and understanding, sympathy involves reacting. When you sympathize with your clients, you identify with their feelings to the point that you can feel their pain. Instead of merely listening as when using empathy, a sympathetic person can assist the client to find a solution to their concerns. Ensure that in your role, you know your agency or facility policy and the regulations of your province or territory as to who can provide the information the client needs to make informed decisions. Taking the problems of your clients on yourself, however, can leave you tense, tired, and anxious.
- ***Competence.*** Competence is the ability to do a job well. In support work, you must perform your tasks safely and skillfully; must be well-organized,

punctual, and reliable; and must know your scope of practice and personal limits. At the same time, you should be flexible and responsive to the client's needs. By being competent, you will earn the client's trust. Maintaining competence requires that you keep your knowledge up to date and continue to be able to perform your skills. To do so, you will need to seek and participate in lifelong learning opportunities (see Chapter 1).

- ***Self-awareness.*** Self-awareness is an understanding of one's own feelings, moods, attitudes, preferences, biases, qualities, and limitations. You must know yourself well to be genuine and nonjudgemental with others. To be self-aware, you must examine your own feelings and behaviours in an honest manner (see *Supporting Mr. Raftis: The Need for Self-Awareness*).

Supporting Mr. Raftis: The Need for Self-Awareness

Mr. Raftis requires assistance with self-care. Maia is the support worker who has been providing his care for the past 8 days. One morning, Mr. Raftis complains to Maia that she is too rough when shaving him. Maia feels that Mr. Raftis is questioning her competence and is hurt by his comment. She becomes quiet and withdrawn.

Later, Maia thinks about her reaction to Mr. Raftis's comment and feels upset with herself for having let the comment affect how she treated him. Mr. Raftis and Maia usually carry on a lively conversation while she provides care, but after his comment, she had barely said a word. She realizes now that her reaction may have had something to do with the fact that when she was a child, her father criticized her constantly, making her feel incompetent. Once she understands the reason for her hurt feelings, Maia understands that Mr. Raftis's comment was constructive rather than critical. The next day, she asks Mr. Raftis to explain how he would like to be shaved, and together they decide how she can make the task more comfortable for him.

Independence, Dependence, and Interdependence

Independence, dependence, and interdependence are fundamental concepts in professional helping relationships.

- **Independence** is the state of not relying on others for control or authority. People who are independent control and direct their own lives and can do things for themselves.
- **Dependence** is the state of relying on others for support and being unable to manage without help.
- **Interdependence** is the state of relying on one another. In most interdependent relationships, each person relies on the other for some things.

The above terms must be considered in relation to one another. No one is completely independent, and only infants, very young children, and unconscious people are completely dependent. Most people's relationships have elements of all three traits.

For example, Julie considers herself independent. She feels she is in control of her busy and rewarding life as a support worker, wife, and mother of two young boys. She works full time and drives her children to day care. Julie is independent because she is in control of her career and her home life. However, she also depends on others. Without reliable child care, she cannot work full time. Julie and her husband have an interdependent relationship—they rely on each other for emotional support and companionship and also for help with child rearing, housework, grocery shopping, and cooking.

An important goal of most clients' care is for the client to achieve or maintain as much independence as possible (**FIGURE 11–1**). Everyone makes choices about when to do things for themselves and when to rely on others. These choices coincide with setting goals and priorities. As a support worker, you must respect your client's choices to do some things independently and to accept help with other things, even though you may not fully understand the reasons for these choices.

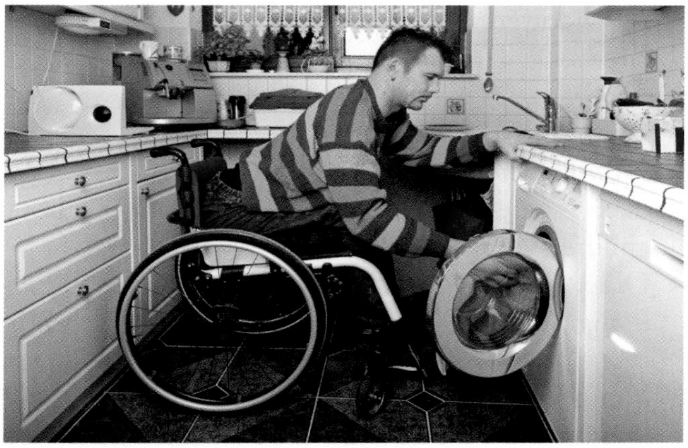

FIGURE 11–1 This client is able to function independently at home. (**Source:** Jenny Sturm/Shutterstock.com)

For example, Elena is hired to help Ms. Godin, 31, who has cerebral palsy. Elena's role is to help Ms. Godin get ready for work in the morning. Elena knows that Ms. Godin is capable of dressing, showering, and preparing breakfast without help. However, each task takes a long time for Ms. Godin. She chooses to put her energies into her work, not into getting ready for work. Elena respectfully accepts Ms. Godin's choices. Clients, like everyone else, make choices according to their wishes and capabilities and must never feel that you are judging their decisions.

Independence and Self-Esteem

What makes you feel good about yourself? Working hard at your job or school? Playing a sport? Caring for your family? How would you feel if you could no longer do these things? As children, we start to develop **self-esteem**, thinking well of ourselves, as we attain control over our bodies and our environments. Self-esteem generally strengthens when people feel that their lives have meaning for themselves and for others. Self-esteem is also closely associated with independence and can suffer when independence is limited or lost and when roles and identities change, as they do when a person is no longer in control of her life (see Chapter 4). You must be sensitive to how clients feel when they lose their independence because of illness or disability.

Clients who have lost their independence need to find ways to rebuild their self-esteem. Some clients cannot and, in turn, become frustrated or depressed, but others are able to find a new purpose in life. For example, at 17, Ricardo and two friends had been drinking at a party. On the way home, the driver lost control of the car and hit a telephone pole. Ricardo's two friends died at the scene, and Ricardo ended up with quadriplegia and was in the hospital for 7 months. After his accident, he lost much of the independence that he had taken for granted, such as for toileting and transferring. He became so depressed that he wished he had died with his friends in the accident. Then his high school principal asked him to speak to the students about the dangers of drinking and driving. Ricardo agreed, and since then, he has spoken to students at every school in his community, which has given him a purpose in life.

You can reinforce a client's self-esteem by offering encouragement and praising the client's successes. If the client is not successful yet, you should recognize the efforts made. You might say, "I can see how hard you are trying." Give the client honest, constructive feedback in a gentle, supportive fashion.

Independence and Balance of Power

Being aware of the balance of power in your relationships with your clients is important so that you avoid any controlling behaviour; it is easy to unconsciously become controlling. In some situations, controlling behaviour may lead to the stronger person abusing the dependent person (see Chapter 16). For example, Lynn's client, Mrs. Kerr, insists on wearing a blouse with 10 tiny buttons and doing them up herself. Mrs. Kerr takes 3 minutes to do up the first button. Lynn does not have 30 minutes to help Mrs. Kerr dress. She suggests to Mrs. Kerr that she wear something else, but Mrs. Kerr refuses. She is expecting visitors and wants to look good. Lynn undoes the button, removes the blouse, and hands Mrs. Kerr another garment, saying, "You will look just as nice in this sweater."

Instead of imposing your will on your clients, involve them in solving problems that may arise. For example, Lynn could have explained to Mrs. Kerr that her time was limited, and together they could have thought of a solution. Lynn might have suggested that they take turns doing up the buttons. Or she might have suggested that she carry on with doing other tasks (like tidying the room) while Mrs. Kerr dressed herself. Or Lynn could set some guidelines at the very beginning of the day's schedule: "Mrs. Kerr, I have 20 minutes today, and this is what we have to accomplish in that time frame."

THE CLIENT'S FAMILY

Close personal and family relationships are central to the lives of most people and involve some forms of dependency. Spouses depend on one another for emotional support, companionship, and financial support. Children depend on their parents to meet their physical, emotional, and financial needs. Older parents may depend on their adult children to help them with physical and emotional needs.

As a support worker, you will be working with all different types of families. There will be functional families that support your client and work as a team, and there will be dysfunctional families who are in conflict over many issues, some of which you may not be aware of. Every family has different dynamics that are influenced by culture, language, or role changes. In *patriarchal* families, the major decision maker in the home is the elder male, whereas in *matriarchal* families, it is the oldest female in the home who makes the family's decisions. It can be very stressful on these families when the head of the household becomes ill. The care plan that the health care team recommends for the client—and that you, as the support worker, need to follow—adds to the family's stress since having the health team in the client's house would interfere with the family's privacy. Be sensitive and aware that the family dynamics may go through changes when illness occurs. Communicate any concerns to your supervisor.

The **family** is a biological, legal, or social network of people who provide support for one another (see Chapter 10). Families can take many forms and may include people related by blood or marriage or unrelated people who have formed a close personal relationship. Examples of families include:

- A married couple with or without children or stepchildren
- An unmarried couple living together, with or without children
- A widowed grandmother raising two grandchildren
- A divorced parent living with a partner, who has children living elsewhere
- Two women or two men married or living together in a same-sex relationship, with or without children
- Older parents, adult children, and grandchildren living together

You may have different ideas about what a family is. However, as a support worker, you must always respect your client's definition of *family*. Your client will determine who she regards as family. Do not impose your values on the person.

Your Role in Assisting the Family

There are many situations in which you help families in your role as a support worker. You may care for new mothers and their babies. You may care for toddlers or older children when their parent is ill or unavailable. You may assist or provide needed respite for a **primary caregiver**, the person (usually a family member or a close friend) who assumes the responsibilities of caring for a person with an illness or a disability in the person's home (see the *Focus on Home Care: Assisting the Primary Caregiver* box). Whatever the situation, when working with a family, you indirectly support their relationships. By providing a family with basic care and support services, you enable family members to invest more time and energy in their relationships.

Chapter 4 discussed how roles change when illness or disability strikes a family. Very often, one family member becomes the primary caregiver for another family member. They form a different relationship, with new patterns of dependency, and this shift is rarely easy. The person with the illness or disability may feel angry about having to depend on the caregiver. The caregiver may feel burdened by the new responsibility in addition to other family and work demands.

Specific professionals on the health care team prepare family members to take on care responsibilities. When helping families cope, they consider the physical, emotional, social, spiritual, and intellectual health of all family members. They also consider

FOCUS ON HOME CARE

Assisting the Primary Caregiver

Sometimes you will work closely with the client's primary caregiver. For example, you assist Mrs. Kalopsis with housekeeping and meal preparation so that she can spend more time caring for her husband, who is ill.

Primary caregivers are often relieved to have assistance from the health care team. However, some may have mixed feelings about your presence in their homes. Some people may resent the interruption to their routines or may feel that you are invading their privacy. Some caregivers may also feel that they are failures for needing help or may regret that someone else is accomplishing tasks that they wish they had accomplished themselves.

Try to put the family caregivers at ease by showing that you are there to help, not to take over or judge their housekeeping or caregiving skills. Do not take on tasks that have not been assigned to you. As well, adapt your support work to suit the family's standards and preferences, not your own. Respect the family's routines, schedules, and ways of doing things. Consult with your supervisor if you think the family's wishes may affect safety.

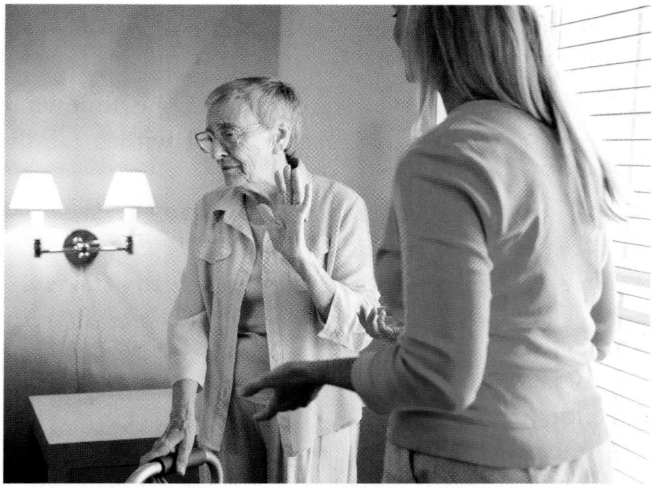

FIGURE 11–2 Tensions may erupt between the client and family members when forced to deal with the challenges of illness and disability. (**Source:** Golden Pixels LLC/Alamy Stock Photo.)

relationships within the family, including any conflict and potential for conflict. They may help the family deal with stress by working on improving the communication skills and problem-solving abilities of family members. Sometimes bringing them together in a family conference is needed to discuss how the caregiving can impact the entire family. As a support worker, you will be asked to attend such family conferences.

Families in Conflict

When illness or disability occurs, the stress on all family members may be great, and members may have to cope with conflict. Conflicts may take the form of expressions of irritation, anger, bickering, or arguments. Conflict may sometimes be hidden. Adult children may care for aging parents with whom they have unresolved conflicts. Siblings who have not spoken in years may be forced to see one another during a parent's illness. Sometimes, the health care team can help families resolve their difficulties in such situations. Members of palliative care teams are specially trained to help people resolve emotional problems that are causing them distress (see Chapter 7 for managing conflict).

When working with a family, try to be aware of family relationships and any conflicts, communication difficulties, and stressful situations (**FIGURE 11–2**). It is not part of your role to help families deal with their interpersonal problems, but there are some things you can do in a stressful situation. You could encourage communication without taking sides, or you could defuse (calm) a tense situation—for example, when angry words have been exchanged between the client and a family member, you may suggest to the family member to go out for a cup of coffee (see Chapter 7). Agencies and facilities have policies to guide you in dealing with conflicts you might encounter. You must observe and report on family interactions (see the *Case Study: Family Conflict* box) and also be alert for signs of abuse (see Chapter 16).

CASE STUDY Family Conflict

Mei is a support worker. She tells the following story about her experience working with a family in conflict:

"When I look back on the families I've worked with, one in particular stands out. Mr. Skala was an older man with cancer. His wife was his primary caregiver. They had a daughter living nearby, who had a family of her own. Just before Mr. Skala became ill, there had been a major argument over the family business. The result was that their daughter refused to speak to her parents. The Skalas' son-in-law brought their two young grandchildren to visit, but their daughter never came. She refused all attempts to resolve the conflict.

"Mrs. Skala found this situation extremely hard to bear. She asked me to talk to her daughter to try to mend the rift. I felt for Mrs. Skala and wanted to help, but I had to tell Mrs. Skala that it wasn't my role to get involved in the family's problems. The case manager arranged for a social worker to talk with them. Eventually, the daughter resolved her differences with her parents. In the last 3 weeks of Mr. Skala's life, the family spent meaningful time together."

CHAPTER REVIEW

KEY POINTS

- As a support worker, you need to know the boundaries between a professional relationship and a friendship.
- Independence, dependence, and interdependence are fundamental concepts in professional helping relationships.
- The family is a biological, legal, or social network of people who provide support for each other. Families can take many forms.
- When illness or disability occurs, the stress on all family members may be great, and they may have to cope with conflict.

CRITICAL THINKING IN PRACTICE

A client in your long-term care facility asks you to visit on your day off and wants you to bring your children. How will you respond? How do professional boundaries protect the person? Can bringing your children to meet a client affect professional boundaries?

REVIEW QUESTIONS

Answers to these questions are at the bottom of the page.

Circle the BEST answer.

1. Which of the following is true?
   A. Every client is a unique individual.
   B. Clients of the same age with the same condition are much the same.
   C. Support workers should focus only on the client's physical problems.
   D. People are not influenced by their genetics and their environments.
2. A professional helping relationship is established for the benefit of the:
   A. Client and the support worker
   B. Client, the support worker, and the health care team
   C. Client
   D. Client's family
3. A family is:
   A. A mother, father, and children who live together
   B. A biological, legal, or social network of people who provide support for one another
   C. Two or more people who are legally related to each other
   D. A group of people who live in the same house
4. Common courtesy is a sign of:
   A. Empathy
   B. Interdependence
   C. Respect
   D. Need
5. Independence is:
   A. Not depending on others for control or authority
   B. Being unable to manage without help
   C. Relying on others for support
   D. Showing acceptance for another person
6. When supporting clients from families in conflict, your supervisor expects you to:
   A. Help family members resolve the conflict
   B. Observe and report on family interactions
   C. Ignore any conflict you witness
   D. Take sides in family arguments

Circle T if the statement is true, and circle F if the statement is false.

7. T F Conflict in families may be hidden.
8. T F Part of your role is to help families deal with their interpersonal problems.
9. T F You should always take your client's side in a disagreement.

Answers: 1.A, 2.C, 3.B, 4.C, 5.A, 6.B, 7.T, 8.F, 9.F

Chapter opener image: Rob Marmion/Shutterstock.com

CHAPTER 12

Promoting Client Well-Being, Comfort, and Sleep

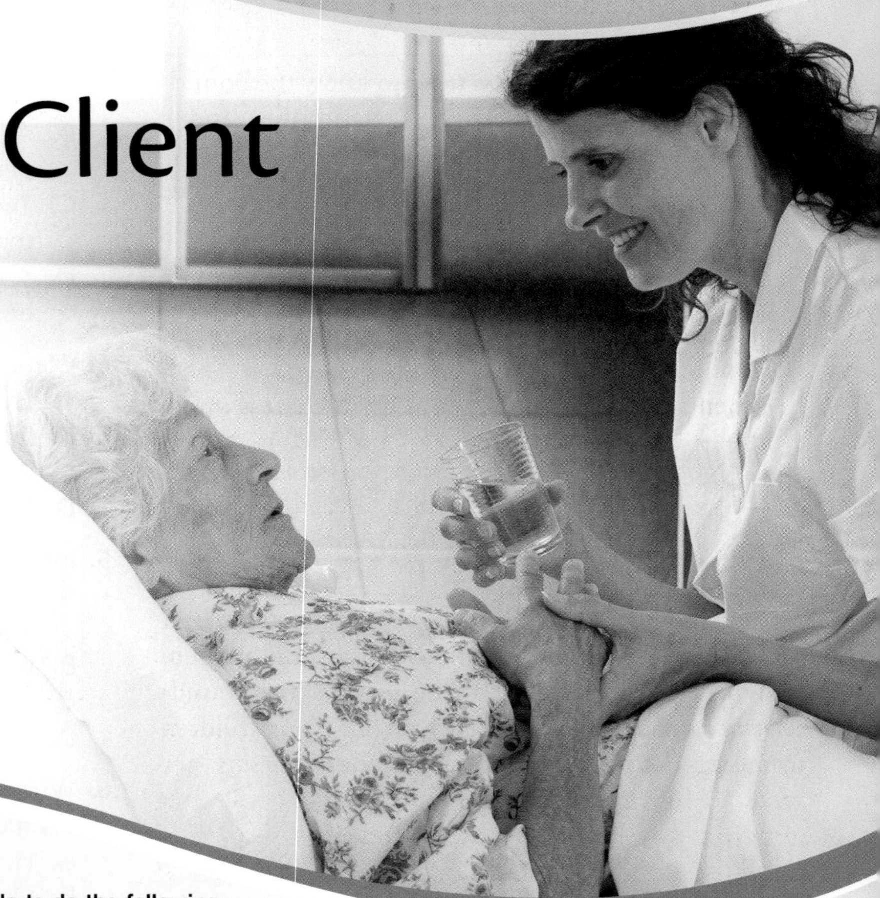

OBJECTIVES

After reading this chapter, the learner should be able to do the following:

- Recognize that each client is an individual and a whole person.
- Describe Erikson's developmental stages.
- Explain how understanding Maslow's hierarchy of needs applies to support work.
- Describe why comfort is important.
- Describe the types of pain.
- List the signs and symptoms of pain.
- List the care plan measures that relieve pain.
- Describe why rest and sleep are important.
- Describe the factors that affect sleep.
- Describe common sleep disorders.
- List care plan measures that promote sleep.

KEY TERMS

acute pain Sudden pain due to injury, disease, trauma, or surgery; it generally lasts less than 6 months. *p. 178*
chronic pain See **persistent pain**. *p. 178*
insomnia A persistent condition in which the person cannot go to sleep or stay asleep throughout the night. *p. 185*
need (basic human) Something necessary or desirable for maintaining life and psychosocial well-being. *p. 174*
nocturia The need to urinate (*uria*) during the night (*noct*). *p. 185*
persistent pain Pain that lasts longer than 6 months; it may be constant or occur off and on. Also known as **chronic pain**. p. *178*
phantom limb pain Pain felt in a body part that is no longer there. *p. 179*
psychosocial health Well-being in the social, emotional, intellectual, and spiritual dimensions of one's life. *p. 173*
radiating pain Pain that is felt not just at the site of tissue damage but extends to nearby areas. *p. 178*
referred pain Pain that is felt in a part of the body separate from the source of the pain. *p. 178*
self-actualization Realizing one's full potential. *p. 176*

Most clients of support workers have physical issues, but to provide good care, it is necessary to use a *holistic* approach to care. Every person is an individual shaped by a unique blend of genetics, environmental influences, and experiences. Considering only the physical part ignores the client's ability to think, make decisions, and interact with others. It also ignores the client's experiences, joys, sorrows, and needs. Support workers can play a key role in promoting the well-being of clients by understanding their psychosocial needs and knowing ways to help them feel safe, comfortable, and relaxed.

For example, Ms. Lalonde, 35, has a disorder that has caused paralysis. You help her to bathe and dress. You change her bed, do her laundry, and clean her house. You also position her in bed to make her more comfortable. She feels more relaxed and comfortable in fresh clothes and a clean environment. You also create an environment that is conducive to comfort, rest, and sleep.

PROMOTING CLIENT WELL-BEING AND PSYCHOSOCIAL HEALTH

A holistic approach to health care takes into account a client's physical health as well as his psychosocial well-being and health. **Psychosocial health** is well-being in the social, emotional, intellectual, and spiritual dimensions of one's life. Few people enjoy perfect psychosocial health throughout their lives.

Erikson's Stages of Psychosocial Development

One common theory that addresses a client's psychosocial health is Erikson's stages of psychosocial development. Erikson describes eight stages of psychosocial development (TABLE 12–1). Each stage involves a crisis of two opposing forces (e.g., trust versus mistrust). For example, if an infant has developed trust, she successfully moves on to the next psychosocial task. But if she has developed mistrust, this mistrust can influence her ability to form trusting, intimate relationships as she moves through the other psychosocial stages in her life. Another example is a toddler who is not allowed to learn by doing and thus develops a sense of doubt in his abilities. This doubt can complicate his later attempts at independence.

According to Erikson, factors that influence psychosocial health include the following:

- ***Personality.*** Personality is the blend of thought patterns, feelings, characteristics, and behaviours that makes a person unique.
- ***Family background.*** Children who grow up in caring, loving families are more likely to have good

TABLE 12–1 Erikson's Theory of Psychosocial Development, From Birth Through Old Age

Stage	Age (years)	Psychosocial Task	Description of Task
1	0–1	Trust versus mistrust	Babies learn to trust that their needs will be met, thereby beginning to believe that the world is a safe place.
2	1–3	Autonomy versus doubt	The toddler learns to become independent and develops self-confidence. Not learning independence creates feelings of shame and doubt.
3	3–6	Initiative versus guilt	The young child learns to initiate his or her activities. Accomplishing this task teaches the child to seek challenges later in life.
4	6–12	Competence versus inferiority	The child develops skill in physical, cognitive, and social areas. This task teaches independence and responsibility.
5	12–20	Identity versus role confusion	The adolescent tries out several roles and forms a single, unique identity.
6	20–40	Intimacy versus isolation	The young adult forms close, permanent relationships and makes career commitments.
7	40–65	Generativity versus stagnation	The person in middle adulthood helps younger people develop their lives.
8	65 on	Integrity versus despair	The older adult thinks back on life, experiencing satisfaction or disappointment.

Based on Matlin, M.W. (1999). *Psychology* (3rd ed., p. 370). Fort Worth, TX: Harcourt Brace.

psychosocial health than those who do not. On the other hand, those growing up in a family with serious problems may be harmed psychosocially through abuse, neglect, distrust, anger, and substance abuse. As they grow older, these children may have issues with trust and intimacy. They may repeat the patterns learned in childhood. Adults who were abused as children may abuse their own children. Likewise, children of substance abusers may develop their own substance abuse issues in adulthood.

- ***Environment.*** Experiences outside the family setting also strongly influence psychosocial health. For children and adolescents, such experiences include school, the influence of the media, and interactions with friends and acquaintances. For adults, they include experiences at work and in the community. Access to social support systems such as health care and social welfare can also influence psychosocial health.
- ***Life circumstances.*** Some people experience devastating losses or tragedies in their lives—for example, the death of a parent during one's childhood or the death of one's child. People who experience such losses may never enjoy strong psychosocial health afterward.

Maslow's Hierarchy of Needs

Abraham Maslow is another psychologist who has influenced ideas about psychosocial health. Maslow is best known for his theory of needs. A **need** is something that is necessary or desirable for maintaining life and psychosocial well-being. According to Maslow, certain basic needs must be met for a person to survive and function. These needs are

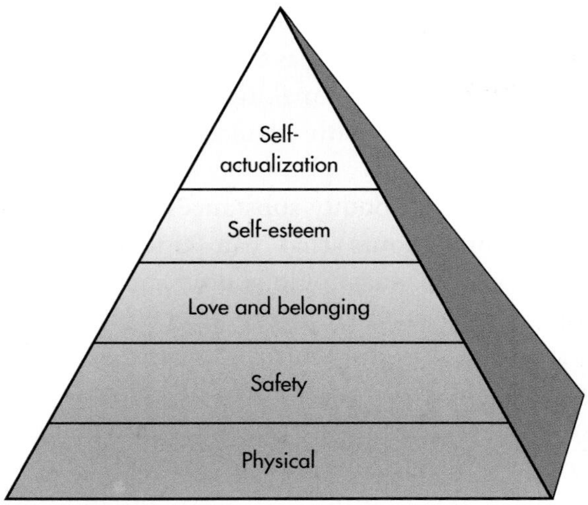

FIGURE 12–1 Maslow's hierarchy of needs. (**Source:** *Maslow, Abraham H.; Frager, Robert D.; Fadiman, James, Motivation and Personality*, 3rd Ed., ©1987. Reprinted by permission of Pearson Education, Inc., New York, New York.)

arranged in a *hierarchy*, or order of importance (FIGURE 12-1). Lower-level needs must be met before higher-level needs. These basic needs are, from the lowest level to the highest level, as follows:

- Physical needs (must be met first)
- The need for safety
- The need for love and belonging
- The need for self-esteem
- The need for self-actualization, or the fulfillment of one's potential (last need to be met)

Some people will deliberately ignore a particular need for a certain period to meet another need. For example, a person with addiction may choose to spend money on street drugs instead of spending it on food.

Physical Needs

The most basic needs in Maslow's hierarchy are physical needs. Oxygen, food, water, elimination, rest, and shelter are necessary for life, and since they are the most important for survival, they must be met before other needs. For example, people who are starving need food before they become concerned about their need for safety, self-esteem, and love.

Most adults are able to satisfy their own physical needs. However, children and adults with a serious illness or disability may depend on others to fulfill these needs. You, as the support worker, are often involved in meeting your clients' physical needs. For example, you feed clients who cannot feed themselves.

Safety Needs

Safety needs relate to protection from harm, danger, fear, and pain. Even minor illness and surgery can make people feel afraid. Most seriously ill clients feel extremely fearful. As well, many clients may be afraid of health care procedures, as many of them involve frightening equipment, require invasive techniques, and cause pain or discomfort. Clients feel safer and more secure when they are able to understand these procedures. Even in the case of a simple bed bath, clients should be informed about the following:

- Why the procedure is to be done
- Who will do it
- How it will be performed
- What sensations or feelings should be expected

Love and Belonging Needs

Love is a powerful human emotion that includes deep affection, tenderness, and devotion. Romantic love also involves physical desire. The need for belonging includes the need for a rightful place in society, in a peer group, and in a family. A peer group is a group of friends or acquaintances. Human beings are social creatures who need to be around others. When love and belonging needs are unfulfilled, people often feel lonely and rejected. Many cases have been reported of clients being slow to recover or dying because of lack of love and belonging. This risk is greatest among children and older adults.

Maslow believed that unfamiliar surroundings create a greater need for love and belonging. Clients in long-term care facilities have left their homes, friends, neighbours, pets, belongings, and familiar surroundings; as their support worker, you must be sensitive to the needs of those clients who are struggling with settling into their new environment.

Self-Esteem Needs

Esteem is the worth, value, or opinion one has of a person. *Self-esteem* is thinking well of oneself and being well thought of by others. When self-esteem needs are fulfilled, a person feels confident, adequate, and useful. Unmet self-esteem needs can result in feelings of inferiority, worthlessness, helplessness, and possibly depression. Clients often lose their self-esteem when they become ill or injured. Think about the following:

- How do ill parents feel when they cannot support or care for their children?
- Does a woman feel whole and attractive after a breast has been removed?
- Does a person who had a leg amputation feel complete, useful, and attractive?

You can help meet clients' self-esteem needs by being sensitive to their feelings and encouraging them to be as independent as possible.

Self-Actualization Needs

Self-actualization means realizing one's full potential. It involves learning, understanding, and creating to the best of one's ability. It is the highest need in the hierarchy and is rarely met. Most people constantly try to learn and understand more. However, the need for self-actualization can be postponed, and life will continue.

PROMOTING CLIENT COMFORT

Comfort is a feeling of contentment. A comfortable client is not in any physical or emotional pain and is calm and at peace. Age, illness, pain, and inactivity, as well as such factors as temperature, ventilation, odours, noise, and lighting affect comfort.

- ***Temperature.*** Most people are comfortable when the room temperature is between 20°C and 23°C (68°F–74°F). Infants, older adults, and people with illnesses generally need higher room temperatures for comfort. Government legislation in some provinces dictates minimum comfortable temperatures in long-term care facilities. In home care settings, clients set the temperature they want. Some clients, however, may be concerned with the cost of heating. You can help these clients keep warm by providing them with extra clothing or blankets.
- ***Ventilation.*** Stale room air affects comfort. Facilities have ventilation systems that ensure fresh air. In home care settings, you can open windows and doors and turn on fans, as the client desires. Protect clients from drafts by making sure they are dressed warmly, covered with blankets, and away from drafty areas.
- ***Odours.*** Many bodily substances and fluids have unpleasant odours that can embarrass clients. Body, breath, and smoking odours may also offend some. Some clients can experience great discomfort from perfumes worn by a caregiver. Do not wear perfumes or any scented products when you are at work. If you smoke, wash your hands and brush your teeth after you have smoked. If you do not have time to brush your teeth, use mouthwash or suck on a breath mint. A clean, fresh uniform must be worn for every shift. Never wear a uniform that has been exposed to cooking odours from your home, as those odours can cling to fabrics and be offensive to others. Good hygiene, housekeeping practices, and ventilation help eliminate odours. To reduce odours, do the following:
    - Empty and clean bedpans, urinals, commodes, and kidney basins promptly.
    - Change and dispose of soiled linens and clothing promptly.
    - Clean clients who are wet or soiled by urine, feces, vomit, or wound drainage.
    - Dispose of incontinence and ostomy products promptly.
    - Keep laundry containers closed.
    - Assist clients to maintain good personal hygiene.
- ***Noise.*** Ill clients are sensitive to noise. Health care facilities can be noisy places. The clanging of bedpans, the clatter of dishes, phones ringing, loud talking, and television sounds can disturb people. Answer phones promptly. Households, too, can be noisy, particularly when young children and teenagers live at home. Help control noise levels by talking quietly and handling equipment carefully. Some noises in facilities can be frightening, especially for new clients. Explain the source of the noise to help the client feel secure.
- ***Lighting.*** Glares, shadows, and dull lighting can cause falls, headaches, and eye strain. Dim light often helps clients rest better. Bright light is helpful when giving care, and it also helps clients feel cheerful and stimulated. Before adjusting lights, ask clients about their preferences. Make sure light switches are within reach. Some clients may

request a night light or the TV being left on all night.

Room Furniture and Equipment

Clients' rooms are furnished and equipped for comfort and safety:

- ***Bathrooms.*** Most facility bathrooms have a sink, call bell, mirror, and toilet with handrails (**FIGURE 12-2**), and some have showers. Toilets in some facilities are higher than regular toilets, which makes moving to and from wheelchairs easier for clients, especially for clients with joint problems. Some bathrooms are private, while others are shared. Most bathrooms in private homes do not have elevated toilets and handrails. In such cases, you must make sure the client's bathroom is clean and safe.
- ***Beds.*** For those who are confined to bed, comfort is especially important. Hospital beds have electric or manual controls that allow clients to sit up and lie down without effort. Many home care clients have regular beds. Use pillows to help clients sit comfortably in a regular bed (see Chapter 34).
- ***Overbed tables.*** Hospitals and many long-term care facilities have overbed tables. These tables can be positioned over the bed and the height adjusted for a client in bed or in a chair. The overbed table is used for placing meal trays, eating, reading, writing, and other activities. It is also used as a work area for bedside procedures. However, never place bedpans, urinals, or soiled linens on an overbed table. Always clean the table carefully after each use.
- ***Bedside furniture.*** Most hospitals and long-term care facilities have bedside stands for personal items (**FIGURE 12-3**). In private homes, bedside furniture varies—it could be a bedside stand or a small table—or there may be nothing at the bedside. Regardless of where the client is, furniture should be safely placed out of the client's pathway.
- ***Chairs.*** A hospital room usually has one or two chairs. Long-term care clients may bring their own chairs from home (**FIGURE 12-4**). Home care clients often have a favourite chair. Make sure that the chair is kept clean and free of food particles. Plump cushions regularly.
- ***Privacy curtains and screens.*** Standard in hospitals and long-term care facilities, privacy curtains

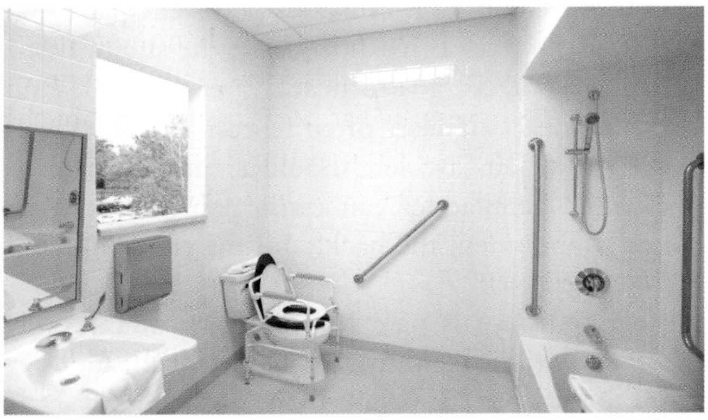

FIGURE 12–2 A facility bathroom. (**Source:** Brian Hillier.)

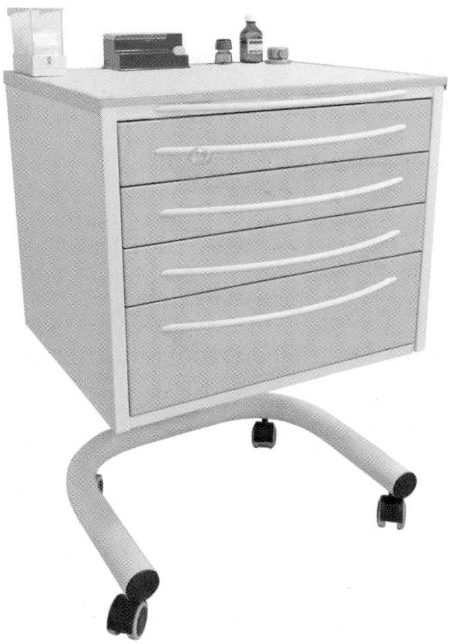

FIGURE 12–3 A bedside stand in a long-term care facility is used to store personal care items. (**Source:** © Can Stock Photo Inc./uatp1)

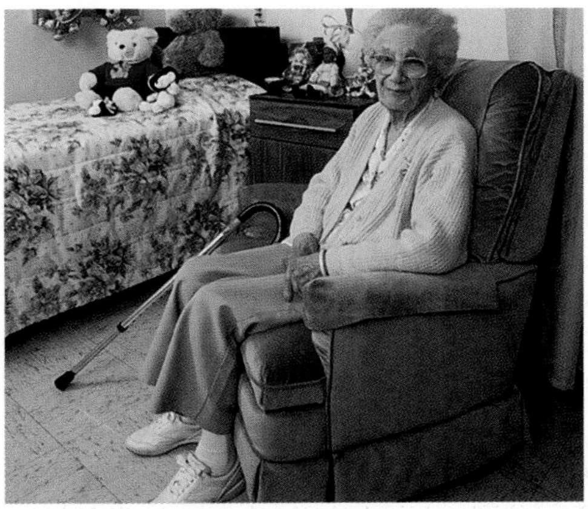

FIGURE 12–4 A client's room includes a chair and personal items from home.

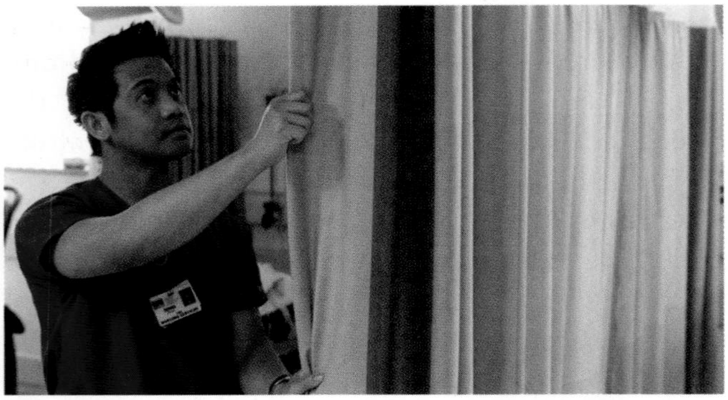

FIGURE 12–5 Curtains around the bed provide privacy in hospitals and long-term care facilities. (**Source:** Sorrentino, S.A. (2000). *Mosby's textbook for nursing assistants* (5th ed., p. 28). St. Louis, MO: Mosby.)

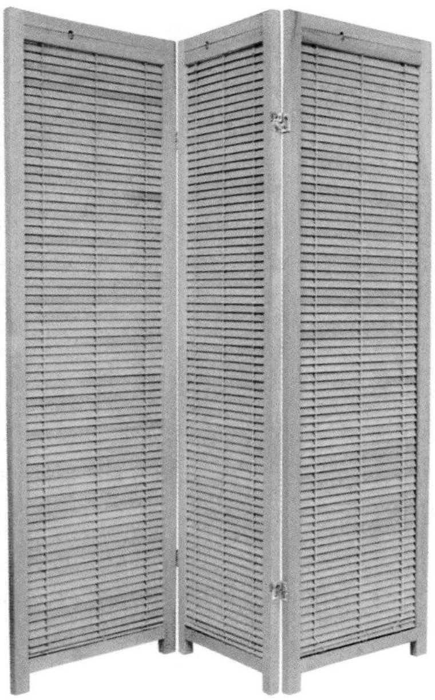

FIGURE 12–6 Portable screens provide privacy in the home. (Courtesy Orientalfurniture.com, Cambridge, Mass.)

are suspended from the ceiling and pulled around the bed before care (**FIGURE 12-5**). Privacy curtains prevent others from seeing the client, but they do not block sound or prevent conversations from being overheard. In home care settings, portable screens can be used for privacy (**FIGURE 12-6**).

- ***Closet and drawer space.*** Hospitals and long-term care facilities provide closet and drawer space for the client's clothing. Government legislation in some provinces states that long-term care clients must have easy access to the closet and its contents.

PAIN AND ITS IMPACT ON A CLIENT'S WELL-BEING

To have discomfort or pain means to ache, hurt, or be sore. Discomfort and pain are subjective. You cannot see, hear, touch, or smell a client's discomfort or pain. You must rely on what the client and the client's body language tell you. Report complaints and observations to your supervisor.

Pain is personal and differs for each client. What may be *hurt* to one client may be *ache* to another. What one client calls *sore*, another may call *burning*. If a client complains of pain or discomfort, the client *has* pain or discomfort, and you must believe the client. Remember, you cannot see, hear, feel, or smell the pain. Pain may signal tissue damage.

Pain is not only physical. Clients also feel emotional, social, and spiritual pain. When a person is suffering, the whole self feels the pain. Clients in pain may be sad, impatient, irritable, or angry. As a support worker, you must be especially kind and empathetic.

Older people may not report pain because they think it is a normal part of aging. Some clients have impairments that may affect their ability to recognize pain (e.g., Alzheimer's disease) or to report pain (e.g., aphasia).

Types of Pain

There are different types of pain.

- **Acute pain** is felt suddenly from injury, disease, trauma, or surgery, when tissue is damaged; it usually lasts less than 6 months and decreases with healing.
- **Persistent pain** lasts longer than 6 months. Pain is constant or occurs off and on. Arthritis and cancer are common causes of persistent pain.
- **Radiating pain** is felt not just at the site of tissue damage but extends to nearby areas as well. Pain from a heart attack is often felt on the left side of the chest, left jaw, left shoulder, and left arm. A diseased gallbladder can cause pain in the right upper abdomen, the back, and the right shoulder (**FIGURE 12-7**).
- **Referred pain** is pain felt in a part of the body separate from the source of the pain (e.g., a kidney stone may produce pain in the groin).

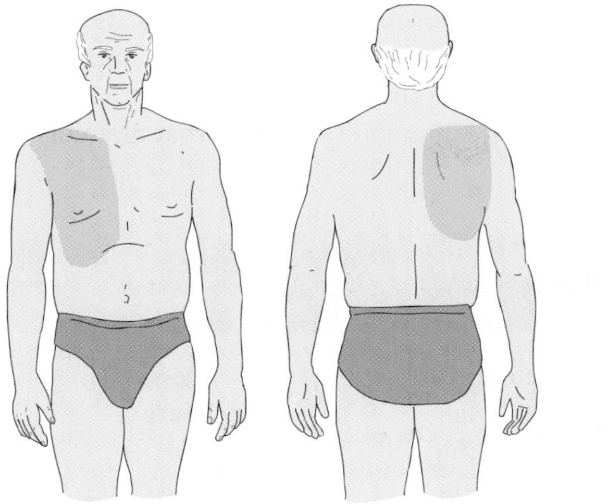

FIGURE 12–7 Gallbladder pain radiates to the right upper abdomen, the back, and the right shoulder.

- **Phantom limb pain** is felt in a body part that is no longer there; it occurs as a result of the disruption of nerve endings in the stump. A client who has had a leg amputated may still feel leg pain.

Factors Affecting Pain

Pain does not affect all clients the same way. Many factors affect reactions to pain.

- ***Past experience.*** A client may have had pain before. The severity of pain, its cause, how long it lasted, and whether relief occurred all affect the client's current response to pain. Knowing what to expect can help or hinder a client in handling pain. Clients who have never experienced pain may be fearful because they do not know what to expect.
- ***Anxiety.*** An anxious client feels troubled or threatened. Pain and anxiety are related—pain can cause anxiety, and anxiety can make the pain feel worse. Lessening anxiety, therefore, helps reduce pain. For example, the nurse explains to Mr. Schett that he will have pain after surgery and that he will receive medication for pain relief. When Mr. Schett feels pain after surgery, he knows what to expect—that medication will relieve it. This knowledge helps reduce his anxiety and, thus, the amount of pain he feels.
- ***Rest and sleep.*** Rest and sleep restore energy and help the body to repair itself. Ill and injured clients need more sleep than usual. Lack of rest and sleep affects how a client copes with pain. Pain seems worse when a client is tired or restless.
- ***Attention.*** The more a client thinks about the pain, the worse it can seem. Sometimes, pain is so severe that it is all a client thinks about. However, even mild pain can seem worse if a client dwells on it too much. Pain often seems worse at night when there are no distractions.
- ***The meaning of pain.*** Pain means different things to different people. Some see it as a sign of weakness or of a serious illness. Some clients ignore or deny their pain. Some clients may use their pain to avoid certain people or things, whereas some others use it to get attention.
- ***Support from others.*** Pain is easier to deal with when family and friends offer comfort and support. The presence of a friend or loved one can be very comforting. Clients who do not have caring family and friends must deal with their pain alone, a state that can increase fear, anxiety, and suffering. Be especially sensitive to clients who are suffering alone.
- ***Culture.*** Culture affects how a client responds to pain (see the *Respecting Diversity: Cultural Aspects of Pain* box). In some cultures, clients in pain show no reaction at all, whereas in other cultures, clients in pain display strong verbal and nonverbal reactions.
- ***Age.*** See the *Focus on Older Adults: Pain Reactions* box.

Signs and Symptoms of Pain

Your client may tell you about his pain, or body language and behaviour may indicate the pain. For example, Ms. Raj grimaces when she moves but denies having any pain. Report any information and observations about the client's pain to your supervisor, always using the client's exact words. Record and report the following:

- ***Location.*** Where is the pain? Ask the client to point to the area of pain (**FIGURE 12-8**). Remember, pain can radiate. Ask the person if the pain is anywhere else and to point to those areas, too.
- ***Onset and duration.*** When did the pain start? How long has the pain lasted?

- ***Intensity.*** Does the client complain of mild, moderate, or severe pain? Tools that can be used by clients to describe the intensity of pain include pain scales (**FIGURE 12-9**), the colour visual analogue scale (**FIGURE 12-10**), and the Oucher pain scale (**FIGURE 12-11**).
- ***Description.*** Ask the client to describe the pain. **BOX 12–1** lists some words used to describe pain. Write down what the client says, using the client's exact words.
- ***Factors causing pain.*** Factors causing pain may include moving or turning in bed, coughing or deep breathing, and exercise. Ask what the client was doing before the pain started and when it started.
- ***Vital signs.*** What are the client's pulse, respirations, and blood pressure? With the occurrence of pain often come increases in the readings of these vital signs.
- ***Other signs and symptoms.*** Does the client have other symptoms: dizziness, nausea, vomiting, weakness, numbness, tingling, or others? **BOX 12–2** lists the signs and symptoms that often occur with pain.

BOX 12–1 Words Used to Describe Pain

- Aching
- Burning
- Cramping
- Crushing
- Dull
- Gnawing
- Knifelike
- Piercing
- Pressing
- Sharp
- Sore
- Squeezing
- Stabbing
- Throbbing
- Viselike

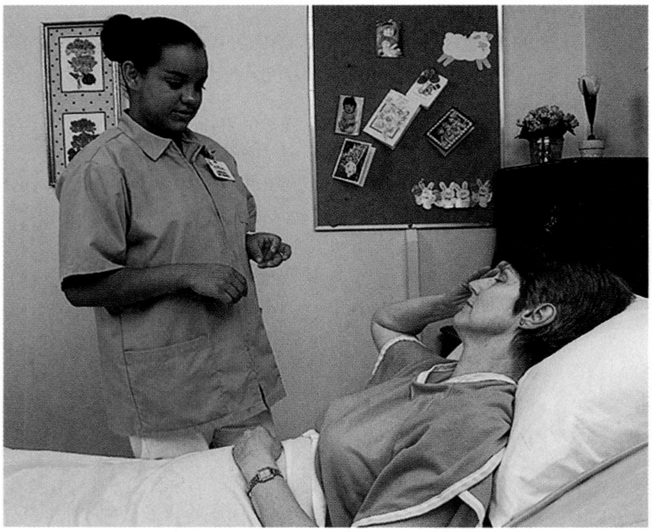

FIGURE 12–8 A client points to the area of pain.

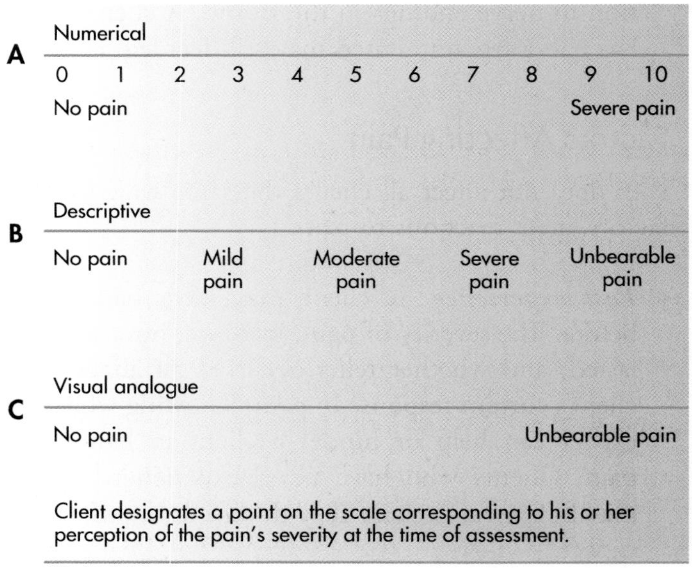

FIGURE 12–9 Sample pain scales. (**Source:** Potter, P.A., Perry, A.G., Ross-Kerr, J.C., et al. (2010). *Canadian fundamentals of nursing* (Revised 4th ed., p. 1023). Toronto, ON: Elsevier Canada.)

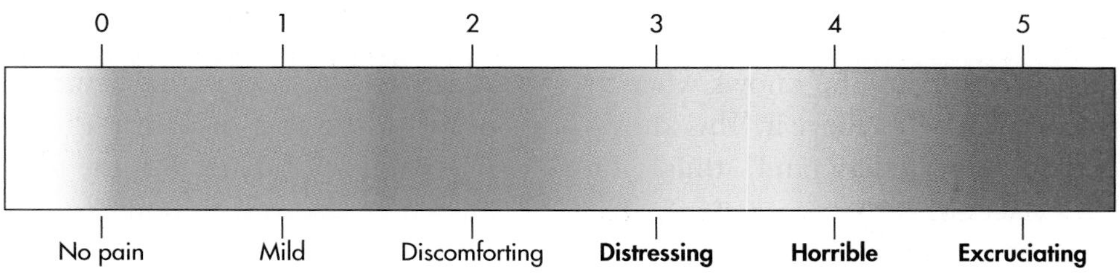

FIGURE 12–10 Colour visual analogue scale.

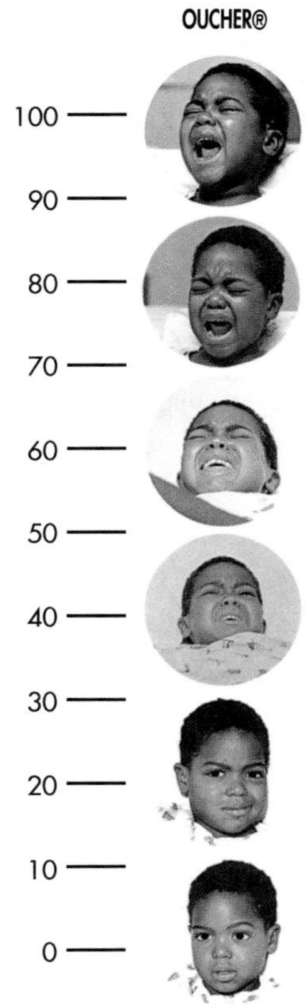

FIGURE 12–11 The Oucher pain scale. (**Source:** Potter, P.A., Perry, A.G., Ross-Kerr, J.C., et al. (2010). *Canadian fundamentals of nursing* (Revised 4th ed., p. 1024). Toronto, ON: Elsevier Canada.)

BOX 12–2 Signs and Symptoms of Pain

Body Responses

- Increased pulse, respirations, and blood pressure
- Nausea
- Pale skin (pallor)
- Sweating (diaphoresis)
- Vomiting

Behaviours

- Changes in speech: slow or rapid, loud or quiet
- Crying
- Gasping
- Grimacing
- Groaning
- Grunting
- Holding the affected body part (splinting)
- Being irritable
- Maintaining one position; refusing to move
- Moaning
- Being quiet
- Being restless
- Rubbing
- Screaming
- Rocking back and forth

Respecting Diversity

Cultural Aspects of Pain

Culturally acquired patterns of pain responses may also influence the neurophysiological and verbal responses to pain. A client's expectations concerning pain may influence how much pain can be tolerated. Response to pain may be limited by language used to describe or report pain. The degree of pain expression does not necessarily correlate with pain intensity. Preferences for pain-coping strategies are usually determined by culture; thus, nontraditional interventions to manage pain need to be explored with the client. How people view and respond to pain may influence your choice of interventions.

Implications for Support Workers

- Be aware of perceived causal factors of pain (fate, lifestyle, punishment, witchcraft).
- Emotional responses to pain (overt [obvious], stoic [bearing quietly]) vary among and within cultures.
- Words used to express pain vary among cultures (*hurt, ache, discomfort*).
- Personal and social meanings of pain and past pain experiences affect pain perception.
- Definitions of pain change the perception of pain intensity.
- Feelings about pain direct treatment.
- The health care professional's beliefs and expectations regarding pain expression sway pain-management strategies.
- Therapeutic goals of pain management are influenced by cultural beliefs.

Source: Potter, P.A., Perry A.G., Ross-Kerr, J.C., et al. (2014). *Canadian fundamentals of nursing* (5th ed., p. 1026). Toronto, ON: Elsevier Canada.

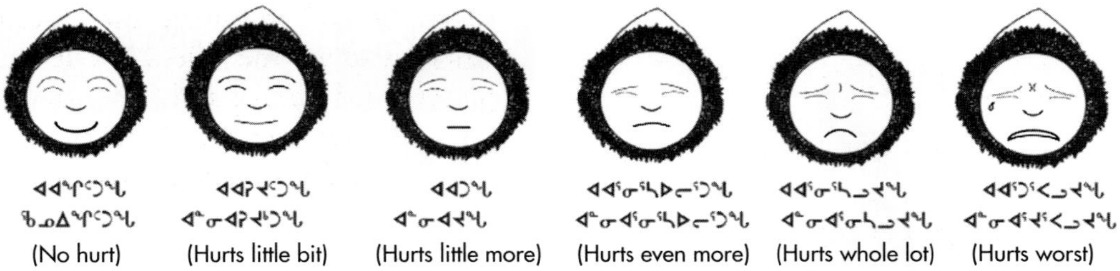

FIGURE 12–12 Northern Pain Scale. (**Source:** From Ellis, J.A., Ootoova, A., Blouin, R., et al. (2011). Establishing the psychometric properties and preferences for the Northern Pain Scale. *International Journal of Circumpolar Health, 70*(3), 274–285. Ellis/Ootoova is an adapted version of the Wong/Baker FACES ® Pain Rating Scale with special permission from the late Dr. Donna Wong. © 1983 Wong-Baker FACES Foundation. www.WongBakerFACES.org. Originally published in Whaley & Wong's *Nursing Care of Infants and Children*. © Elsevier Inc.)

Pain Reactions

Support workers may work with children who are dealing with pain because of their condition. Some children may not understand pain, as they have had few experiences with it. They do not know what to expect, how to deal with pain, or how to express their pain. They must, therefore, rely on adults for help to indicate the amount of pain they are suffering.

Caregivers, however, do not always know when children are in pain since toddlers and preschool children may not know the words to describe pain. Infants and toddlers who are crying and fussing can have many different problems, not just pain. Caregivers must, therefore, be alert for behaviours and situations that signal pain. One tool that can be used to assess pain in children is the Northern Pain Scale (see **FIGURE 12-12**), which uses six different faces ranging from a smiling, happy face to a very sad face. Children point to the face that indicates how much pain they are having.

FOCUS ON OLDER ADULTS

Pain Reactions

Some older adults have multiple health problems that cause pain, so they may think that a new pain is related to an existing health problem. Similarly, persistent pain that they are familiar with may mask new pain. In some cases, people may deny or ignore pain because of what it might mean. Without relief from pain, the older adult who is in pain experiences decreased appetite, changes in mentation (thought), or decreased mobility, which can lead to further health challenges.

Older adults may also have conditions (e.g., dementia) that affect their pain perception, or they may be unable to reliably recognize and report that they are in pain. This situation places them at greater risk for undetected disease or injury. Pain alerts a client to illness or injury, so if pain is not felt, the client may not realize the presence of a problem and not seek health care.

Some older adults have disorders that affect their thinking and reasoning, and some cannot communicate verbally. ***The only indication of pain in such cases will be changes in behaviour, so report any changes in a client's behaviour to your supervisor.***

Measures to Relieve Pain

Nurses and case managers use the care-planning process to promote comfort and relieve pain. **BOX 12-3** lists measures that are often part of the care plan. Medications ordered by a physician provide pain relief, but some can cause drowsiness, dizziness, and lack of coordination. Clients on pain relief medications must be protected from injury. Follow the care plan for safety practices.

Measures other than medications that control pain include distraction, relaxation, and guided imagery. Nurses and therapists teach clients these techniques, and you may be trained to assist with some of them.

- ***Distraction*** involves a change in a client's focus of attention. Attention is directed away from the

BOX 12–3 Measures to Promote Comfort and Relieve Pain

- Wait 30 minutes after administration of pain medication before giving care.
- Position the client in good body alignment. Use pillows for support.
- Keep bed linens tight and wrinkle-free.
- Make sure the client is not lying on drainage tubes.
- Assist with elimination needs.
- Provide blankets for warmth and to prevent chilling.
- Use correct lifting, moving, and turning procedures.
- Provide extra support for painful areas during movement. Use your hands or a pillow, if appropriate.
- Give a back massage.
- Provide soft music to distract the client.
- Use touch to provide comfort.
- Allow family and friends to visit, if requested by the client.
- Avoid sudden or jarring movements.
- Handle the client gently.
- Practise these safety measures if the client is receiving strong pain medication or sedatives:
  - If the client is in a hospital bed, keep the bed in the lowest position.
  - Follow the care plan for bed rail use.
  - Check on the client every 10 to 15 minutes.
  - Provide assistance when the client is up.
  - Provide heat or cold applications, as directed.
  - Provide a calm, quiet, darkened environment.

pain through distractions such as conversation, music, television, games, and needlepoint.

- ***Relaxation*** means absence of mental or physical stress. A relaxed state reduces pain and anxiety. The nurse or therapist teaches the client to breathe deeply and slowly and to contract and relax muscle groups. A comfortable position and a quiet room are important to achieve relaxation.
- ***Guided imagery*** involves creating an image in the mind and focusing on it. The client is asked to think of a pleasant scene—for example, a warm, sunny beach. The nurse uses a calm, soft voice when helping the client focus on the mental picture of the scene and also coaches the client to do relaxation exercises. Soft music, a blanket for warmth, and a darkened room may help.

REST AND SLEEP

To be rested means to be calm, at ease, relaxed, and free from anxiety and stress. Rest involves physical inactivity, but some people choose to do calming or relaxing activities while resting—for example, reading, listening to music, or watching television.

A comfortable position and good body alignment are important for rest. A quiet setting and a clean, dry, and wrinkle-free bed promote rest as well. Some clients rest easier in a clean, neat, and uncluttered room. Many clients spend a great deal of time in bed, so it is important for a support worker to know the different types of beds and how to position them for the client's comfort (see Chapter 34). Clients may sleep in very different ways. Some may not have slept in a bed for most of their lives, perhaps for cultural reasons. Some may want to sleep sitting in a chair for ease of breathing; for example, a client with chronic obstructive pulmonary disease (COPD) would find it easier to breathe in the sitting position. The client's personal preference is very important when promoting rest and sleep; for example, clients should choose the number of blankets they want on the bed.

Basic needs must be met for clients to rest. Thirst, hunger, elimination needs, pain, discomfort, anxiety, and fear, as well as unmet needs for love and belonging, can affect rest. You can promote rest by meeting clients' needs. For clients living in a facility or living alone, visits or telephone calls from family and friends may promote relaxation. (See the *Providing Compassionate Care: Helping Clients to Rest* box).

You must plan and organize care so that clients can rest without interruptions. Some clients feel refreshed after resting for 15 or 20 minutes, whereas others need more time. Health care routines usually allow time for an afternoon rest.

Clients with illnesses or injuries need to rest often. Some need to rest during or after care. For example, a bath tires Mr. Rajan, so to gather the energy to dress, he must rest in a chair. Some clients need up

Providing Compassionate Care
Helping Clients to Rest

- ***Dignity***. Protecting a client's dignity can promote rest. Some clients may find hospital gowns embarrassing and may rest better wearing their own gowns or pyjamas. Many clients feel better about themselves when they are clean and well groomed. Help clients with their personal hygiene and grooming before rest.
- ***Independence***. Many clients follow rituals or routines before resting—for example, going to the bathroom, brushing teeth, having a snack or beverage, praying, locking doors, and making sure loved ones are safe at home. Some clients have a favourite blanket. Ask clients about their preferences, and help them follow their rituals and routines, when possible.
- ***Preferences***. Allow clients to do as much as possible without assistance. Clients decide when and where they want to rest. Provide a restful environment according to their wishes.
- ***Privacy***. Lack of privacy can make rest impossible, so close the door and privacy curtains, if the client so desires.
- ***Safety***. The client's safety needs must be met (see Chapter 22) to achieve a good rest. Clients trying to rest must feel that they are safe from falls or other injuries. In facilities, the call bell must be within reach. Understanding the reasons for their treatments and knowing how procedures are done can also help clients feel safe, so make sure you explain procedures before they are performed.

to a few hours to complete oral hygiene, bathing, grooming, and dressing. Others need to rest after meals. Do not rush clients. Allow rest periods, as needed.

The physician may order bed rest for a client (see Chapter 26 for a discussion on bed rest, its complications, and advice on preventing complications). Sleep is a basic physical need. It saves the body energy, lets the mind and body rest, and allows body functions to slow down. During sleep, vital signs fall and tissue heals and repairs itself. Sleep lowers stress, tension, and anxiety. After sleep, a person usually feels refreshed, more energetic, and mentally alert. During sleep, the normal adult passes through four to six cycles of NREM and REM phases—four levels of nonrapid eye movement (NREM) and one level of rapid eye movement (REM) in each cycle. Children and infants sleep more deeply, whereas older adults sleep more lightly.

The amount of sleep required varies for each age group and declines with age (TABLE 12–2). Clients may require more sleep when they are sick or recovering from illness or injury (see the *Focus on Older Adults: Sleep* box).

TABLE 12–2 Average Sleep Requirements

Age Group	Hours Per Day
Newborns (birth to 4 weeks)	14–18
Infants (4 weeks to 1 year)	12–14
Toddlers/preschoolers (1 to 6 years)	11–12
Middle/late childhood (6 to 12 years)	10–11
Adolescents (12 to 18 years)	8–9
Young adults (18 to 40 years)	7–8
Middle-aged adults (40 to 65 years)	7
Late adulthood (65 years and older)	5–7

Source: Potter, P.A., Perry A.G., Ross-Kerr, J.C., et al. (2014). *Canadian fundamentals of nursing* (5th ed., pp. 1000–1001). Toronto, ON: Elsevier Canada.

Several factors affect the amount of sleep a person needs and the quality of sleep a person gets. *Quality* refers to how well a person sleeps. Does she sleep soundly and feel refreshed in the morning? Or is she restless and wakeful during sleep?

- ***Illness.*** Discomfort, pain, nausea, and coughing can affect sleep. Also, clients may be awakened frequently for treatment or medication.
- ***Nutrition.*** Certain foods and drinks can affect sleep—for example, those containing caffeine (such as coffee, chocolate, tea, and colas). A protein found in milk, cheese, and beef can promote sleep.
- ***Exercise.*** Exercise makes people tired and helps them sleep. However, it is also a stimulant. Exercising before bed may disrupt sleep. Allow at least 2 hours between exercise and bedtime.
- ***Environment.*** Most people sleep better in their own beds and in familiar surroundings. Any change in the environment, as well as noise and light, can affect sleep. Promote a quiet environment with the amount of light preferred by the client.
- ***Medications.*** Sleeping pills promote sleep. Medications for anxiety, depression, and pain can cause drowsiness and can also interfere with sleep. The person may not feel mentally alert or refreshed the next day.
- ***Alcohol.*** Alcohol disrupts normal sleep patterns. The person may wake up and have difficulty falling asleep again.
- ***Change and stress.*** Change disrupts sleep. Change can range from small variances in one's routine, such as staying up late to watch a game on television, to stressful life events such as a new job or a divorce.
- ***Emotional problems.*** Fear, worry, anxiety, and depression affect sleep. People in emotional distress may have difficulty falling asleep, or they may wake up often and have problems falling asleep again.
- ***Nocturia.*** **Nocturia**, the need to urinate during the night, disrupts sleep. With advancing age, bladder tone is reduced, increasing the need to void frequently.

FOCUS ON OLDER ADULTS

Sleep

Older adults have less energy than younger people do. They may nap at certain times or on and off during the day. Organize care so that naps are not disturbed. Avoid waking an older client from a nap.

Long-term care clients are allowed to choose when they nap and sleep. They also have the right to choose measures that help promote comfort, rest, and sleep for them. Follow the care plan and the client's wishes.

Clients are sometimes prepared for bed as early as 6:00 p.m. They may not be ready to sleep at this time but may want to watch television, listen to the radio, or read.

Source: Potter, P.A., Perry A.G., Ross-Kerr, J.C., et al. (2014). *Canadian fundamentals of nursing* (5th ed., p. 1001). Toronto, ON: Elsevier Canada.

Sleep Disorders

Sleep disorders are persistent problems that affect the amount and quality of sleep and can cause fatigue, irritability, poor judgement, and other problems. Signs and symptoms of sleep disorders are listed in **BOX 12–4**. Routines in many facilities do not accommodate residents' individual sleep-and-wake cycles. Frequent sleep interruptions during the night or early awakenings in the morning can cause sleep deprivation. Some facilities have adopted care philosophies such as GentleCare or Supportive Pathways, which include allowing clients to awaken themselves in the morning if appropriate.[1] Better incontinence products and mattresses in some facilities make it possible for clients to sleep better. Some facilities are changing their night routines to decrease the interruptions to their clients' sleep.

Insomnia

Insomnia is a persistent condition in which the person affected cannot go to sleep or stay asleep throughout the night. The person may also wake early and be unable to fall asleep again. Clients with illnesses or injuries often suffer from insomnia because they may be depressed or anxious, may be feeling pain and discomfort, or may be afraid of dying during sleep.

BOX 12–4 Signs and Symptoms of Sleep Disorders

- Hand tremors
- Slowed response to questions, conversations, or situations
- Difficulty finding the right word
- Decreased attention
- Decreased reasoning and judgement
- Irregular pulse
- Red, puffy eyes with dark circles
- Moodiness; mood swings
- Disorientation
- Fatigue, sleepiness, or both
- Restlessness, agitation, or both
- Irritability
- Hallucinations (see Chapter 35)
- Coordination problems
- Slurred speech

Source: Potter, P.A., Perry A.G., Ross-Kerr, J.C., et al. (2014). *Canadian fundamentals of nursing* (5th ed., p. 996). Toronto, ON: Elsevier Canada.

BOX 12–5 Sleep Deprivation Symptoms

Physiological Symptoms

- Drooping eyelids, blurred vision
- Fine motor clumsiness
- Slowed reflexes
- Slowed response time
- Decreased reasoning and judgement
- Decreased auditory and visual alertness
- Cardiac arrhythmias

Psychological Symptoms

- Confusion and disorientation
- Increased sensitivity to pain
- Being irritable, withdrawn, apathetic
- Excessive sleepiness
- Agitation
- Hyperactivity
- Decreased motivation

Source: Potter, P.A., Perry A.G., Ross-Kerr, J.C., et al. (2014). *Canadian fundamentals of nursing* (5th ed., p. 997). Toronto, ON: Elsevier Canada.

Sleep Deprivation

In sleep-deprived people, the amount and quality of sleep decline. Illness and hospital care are common causes of sleep deprivation in clients. The light and sound during nighttime care can interfere with sleep. Health care providers also often suffer from sleep deprivation because of rotating shifts. Symptoms of sleep deprivation can be both physiological and psychological (**BOX 12–5**).

Sleepwalking

Sleepwalkers walk about while they are sleeping, often for several minutes. They are not aware that they are sleepwalking and have no memory of doing so on awakening. Children sleepwalk more than adults do. Stress, fatigue, and some medications can cause sleepwalking. The risk of falling during sleepwalking is great. Clients with illnesses may trip or pull out tubes and catheters. Guide sleepwalking clients back to their beds. Awaken them gently, as they can startle easily.

Your Role in Promoting Rest and Sleep

If required, measures to promote sleep are included in the client's care plan (**BOX 12–6**). Check the care plan to make sure you are giving correct care. Observe the client closely, and report any of the signs and symptoms of sleep deprivation listed in **BOX 12–5**.

As mentioned earlier, many clients have rituals and routines before bedtime—such as having a bedtime snack, watching a television program, or reading a book. Some long-term care clients may like to check on friends and loved ones before going to bed. Whatever the routine, it is important to the client, and you must help with it as much as possible.

Sleep disturbances are common with some types of dementia. In clients with dementia, confusion and restlessness often increase at night, and night wandering is common. Night wandering in a safe and supervised setting can be helpful for some clients (see Chapter 36).

BOX 12–6 Measures to Promote Sleep

- Organize care to allow for uninterrupted rest.
- Encourage the client to avoid physical activity before bedtime.
- Discourage the client from tending to business or family matters before bedtime.
- Allow flexible bedtimes. Bedtime is whenever the client is ready to sleep.
- Ensure a comfortable room temperature.
- Help the client take a warm bath or shower.
- Provide a bedtime snack, if needed.
- Have the client avoid caffeine and alcohol.
- Have the client void before going to bed. Make sure incontinent clients are clean and dry.
- Follow the client's bedtime rituals.
- Make sure the client wears loose-fitting nightwear.
- Provide for warmth (blankets, socks).
- Make sure linens are clean, dry, and wrinkle-free.
- Allow the client to read, listen to music, or watch television if he so desires.
- Stay and talk with the client.
- Reduce noise.
- Darken the room: close shades, blinds, and curtains. Shut off or dim the lights in the room and hallway.
- Position the client in good body alignment. Support body parts, as ordered.
- Implement measures to relieve pain.
- Give a back massage, if ordered.
- Assist with relaxation exercises, as ordered.

CHAPTER REVIEW

KEY POINTS

- Psychosocial health is well-being in the social, emotional, intellectual, and spiritual dimensions of one's life.
- Factors that influence psychosocial health include personality, family background, environment, and life's circumstances.
- Two common theories that addresses a client's psychosocial health are Erikson's theory of psychosocial development and Maslow's hierarchy of needs.
- Pain can be acute, persistent, radiating, referred, or phantom limb. The signs and symptoms of pain will be different in every client.
- The care plan will identify the pain relief measures that have worked with your client, but inform your supervisor about whether these measures are giving relief.
- Rest and sleep are important to everyone. Many factors determine the amount of sleep individuals need, including age and physical condition.
- Insomnia, sleep deprivation, and sleepwalking are the most common persistent sleeping disorders.
- If required, measures to promote sleep are included in the care plan. Each client will have different routines to prepare for sleeping.

CRITICAL THINKING IN PRACTICE

Mr. Hawn is a new resident. He was admitted to the centre last month after his wife died. He could not care for himself at home. Mr. Hawn is withdrawn and angry toward the staff. He is impatient and agitated when his needs are not met right away. He does not sleep well and does not want the lights turned off in his room. Explain possible reasons for his behaviours. How can you provide quality care?

REVIEW QUESTIONS

Answers to these questions are at the bottom of page 189.

Circle T if the answer is true, and circle F if the answer is false.

1. T F *Psychosocial health* refers to a person's well-being in the social, emotional, intellectual, and spiritual dimensions of one's life.
2. T F Environmental experiences outside the family setting strongly influence psychosocial health.
3. T F *Self-actualization* means realizing one's full potential.
4. T F Pain affects all people in the same way.
5. T F Moderate exercise such as walking is considered rest.

Circle the BEST answer.

6. Spiritual health is the achievement of:
   A. Belief in a purpose greater than the self
   B. Secure, intimate love relationships
   C. Good physical health
   D. Strong social bonds in the community
7. Which of the following is part of Erikson's theory of psychosocial development?
   A. People must successfully complete a task in each stage before moving on to the next.
   B. Babies do not learn to trust that their needs will be met.
   C. People do not need to move through a series of stages throughout their lives.
   D. Moving to unfamiliar surroundings creates love and belonging needs.
8. Maslow's hierarchy of needs can best be described as:
   A. Another term for psychosocial health
   B. A system that arranges human needs into categories
   C. Physiological and safety needs
   D. Love and belonging needs

9. Which of the following is part of Maslow's hierarchy of needs?
   A. Financial needs
   B. Trust needs
   C. Intimacy needs
   D. Physical needs

10. Most long-term care facilities:
    A. Discourage clients from bringing personal items from home
    B. Have strict rules about the appearance of residents' rooms
    C. Encourage residents to make their rooms homelike
    D. Allow residents to bring only one piece of furniture from home

11. A client complains of pain on the left side of the chest, up into the left jaw, and down to the left shoulder and left arm. This is:
    A. Acute pain
    B. Chronic pain
    C. Radiating pain
    D. Phantom pain

12. The nurse gives Mr. Smith a medication for pain. A procedure is scheduled for 9:30 a.m. You should:
    A. Perform the procedure before the medication is given
    B. Perform the procedure right after the medication is given
    C. Wait 30 minutes to let the medication take effect
    D. Omit the procedure for the day

13. You must protect Mr. Smith from injury after he is given medication. You should do the following:
    A. Keep the bed in the lowest position
    B. Follow the care plan for bed rail use
    C. A and B
    D. Let him get out of bed on his own

14. Which measure is an example of a distraction?
    A. Avoiding talking with the client
    B. Keeping the room dark
    C. Turning off the radio
    D. Giving a back massage

15. Mr. Smith tires very easily. His morning care includes a bath, hair care, and getting dressed. His bed is made after he is dressed. When should he rest?
    A. After morning care is completed
    B. After his bath and before hair care
    C. After you make the bed
    D. Whenever he needs to

Answers: 1.T, 2.T, 3.T, 4.F, 5.F, 6.A, 7.A, 8.B, 9.D, 10.C, 11.C, 12.C, 13.C, 14.D, 15.D

Chapter opener image: JPC-PROD/Shutterstock.com

CHAPTER 13

Medical Terminology

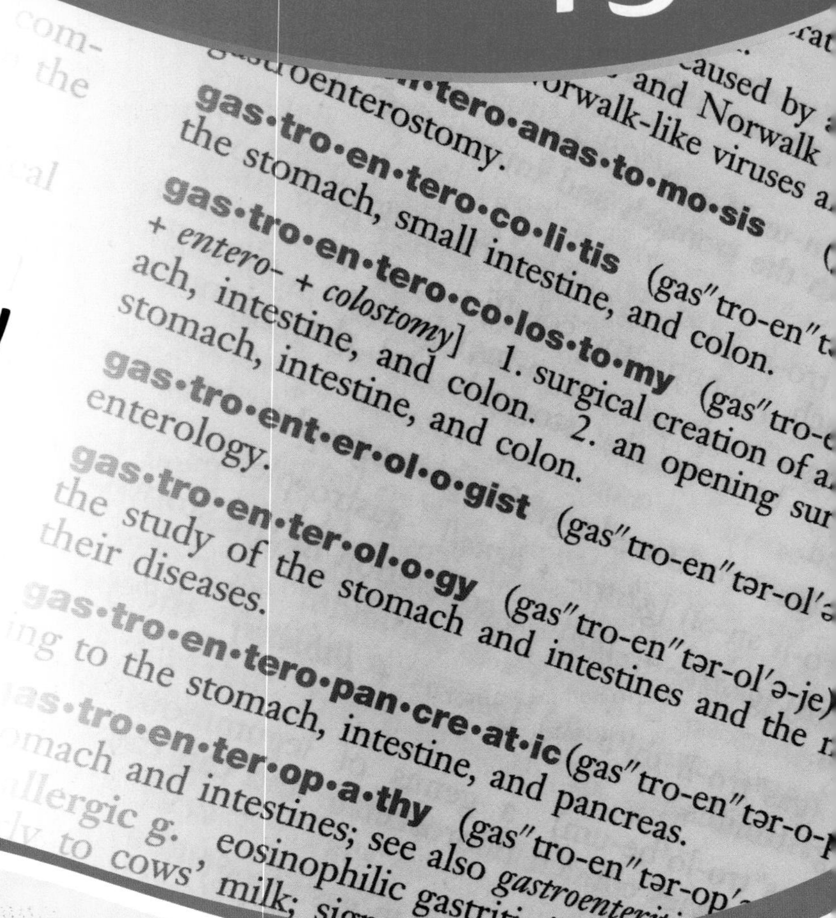

OBJECTIVES

After reading this chapter, the learner should be able to do the following:

- Identify the word elements used in medical terms.
- Know the meanings of common Greek and Latin prefixes, roots, and suffixes on which most medical terms are based.
- Combine word elements into medical terms.
- Know the meanings of common medical terms.
- Identify the abdominal regions.
- Define the directional terms that describe the positions of the body in relation to other body parts.
- Identify and define some of the abbreviations used in health care.

KEY TERMS

abbreviation A shortened form of a word or phrase. *p. 196*
anterior Located at or toward the front of the body or body part. Also called **ventral**. *p. 195*
combining vowel A vowel added between two roots or between a root and a suffix to make pronunciation easier. *p. 193*
distal The part farthest from the centre or from the point of attachment. *p. 195*
dorsal See **posterior**. *p. 196*
lateral The farthest away from the midline of the body. *p. 195*
medial The closest to the midline of the body. *p. 195*
posterior The back surface of the body—often used to indicate the position of one structure in relation to another. Also called **dorsal**. *p. 196*
prefix A word element placed at the beginning of a word to change the meaning of the word. *p. 191*
proximal Nearest to the trunk of the body or the point of origin. *p. 196*
root A word element containing the basic meaning of the word. *p. 193*
suffix A word element placed at the end of a root to change the meaning of the word. *p. 194*
ventral See **anterior**. *p. 195*
word element A part of a word. *p. 191*

Medical language can seem mysterious—the private code of physicians and nurses—and yet every day people outside the health care industry use medical terms, such as *flu*, *diarrhea*, *cancer*, *appendectomy*, *cardiac*, and *pneumonia*. Because health and medicine get a lot of attention in the media, these and many other medical terms are understood by most people.

Knowing medical terminology is important in your work as a support worker. As you gain more knowledge and experience, you will understand and use medical terms often and with ease. In Chapter 17, you will learn about the major organ systems in the human body, and medical terms will be used to describe each system. Other medical terms will be used throughout the text. Learning medical terms for illnesses, diseases, and common conditions such as bruises, baldness, or a "runny nose" can be fun and useful. This chapter introduces medical terminology and the common abbreviations used in health care. It is very important that you use correct terms and abbreviations for creating clear charts. There could be legal consequences if incorrect terms are used, as charts are legal documents.

You should also be aware that the use of certain abbreviations or symbols can change since some may be misinterpreted or involved in medication errors. TABLE 13–1 on page 192 offers a list of abbreviations, symbols, and dose designations that have been found to be dangerously misinterpreted in Canada and are therefore not to be used. It is also important to use ONLY the abbreviations that are approved at your agency. Some agencies may use their own abbreviations (such as "HOB" for "head of bed"), but since those are not official abbreviations, they are not listed here. ***If you are unsure of an abbreviation, it is important that you clarify the abbreviation with your supervisor. Note that all abbreviations must be policy-approved by your agency!***

WORD ELEMENTS

Like all words, medical terms are made up of parts, or **word elements**, that are combined in various ways. A term is translated by separating the word into its elements. Important word elements are prefixes, roots, and suffixes, which are all based in the Greek and Latin languages.

Prefixes

A **prefix** is a word element placed at the beginning of a word that changes the meaning of the word. The prefix *olig* (scant, small amount) is placed before the word *uria* (urine) to make *oliguria*—meaning a small amount of urine. Prefixes are always combined with other word elements. They are never used alone. You

TABLE 13–1 List of Abbreviations and Symbols That Should Never Be Used in Canada

Abbreviation	Intended Meaning	Problem	Correction
U	unit	Mistaken for "0" (zero), "4" (four), or cc.	Use "unit".
IU	international unit	Mistaken for "IV" (intravenous) or "10" (ten).	Use "unit".
Abbreviations for drug names		Misinterpreted because of similar abbreviations for multiple drugs; e.g., MS, MSO4 (morphine sulphate), MgSO4 (magnesium sulphate) may be confused for one another.	Do not abbreviate drug names.
QD QOD	Every day Every other day	QD and QOD have been mistaken for each other, or as "qid". The Q has also been misinterpreted as "2" (two).	Use "daily" and "every other day".
OD	Every day	Mistaken for "right eye" (OD = oculus dextra).	Use "daily".
OS OD OU	Left eye right eye both eyes	May be confused with one another.	Use "left eye", "right eye", or "both eyes".
D/C	Discharge	Interpreted as "discontinue whatever medications follow" (typically discharge medications).	Use "discharge".
cc	cubic centimetre	Mistaken for "u" (units).	Use "mL" or "millilitre".
µg	microgram	Mistaken for "mg" (milligram) resulting in one thousand-fold overdose.	Use "mcg".
Symbol	**Intended Meaning**	**Potential Problem**	**Correction**
@	at	Mistaken for "2" (two) or "5" (five).	Use "at".
> <	Greater than Less than	Mistaken for "7"(seven) or the letter "L". Confused with each other.	Use "greater than"/"more than" or "less than"/ "lower than".
Dose Designation	**Intended Meaning**	**Potential Problem**	**Correction**
Trailing zero	*X*.0 mg	Decimal point is overlooked resulting in 10-fold dose error.	Never use a zero by itself after a decimal point. Use "*X* mg".
Lack of leading zero	. *X* mg	Decimal point is overlooked resulting in 10-fold dose error.	Always use a zero before a decimal point. Use "0.*X* mg".

Source: Institute of Safe Medication Practices Canada. (2006). Retrieved from https://www.ismp-canada.org/download/ISMPCanadaListOfDangerousAbbreviations.pdf. Reprinted with permission from ISMP Canada.

need to learn the following prefixes to begin understanding medical terminology:

Prefix	Meaning
a-, an-	without, not, lack of
ab-	away from
ad-	to, toward, near
ante-	before, forward, in front of
anti-	against
auto-	self
bi-	double, two, twice
brady-	slow
circum-	around
contra-	against, opposite
de-	down, from
dia-	across, through, apart
dis-	apart, free from
dys-	difficult, abnormal
ecto-	outer, outside
en-	in, into, within
endo-	inner, inside
epi-	over, on, upon
eryth-	red
eu-	normal, good, well, healthy
ex-	out, out of, from, away from
hemi-	half
hyper-	excessive, too much, high
hypo-	under, decreased, less than normal
in-	in, into, within, not
infra-	within
inter-	between
intra-	into, within
leuk-	white
macro-	large
mal-	illness, disease
meg-	large
micro-	small
mono-	one, single
muco-	mucous
neo-	new
non-	not
olig-	small, scant
para-	beside, beyond, after
per-	by, through
peri-	around
poly-	many, much
post-	after, behind
pre-	before, in front of, prior to
pro-	before, in front of
re-	again, backward
retro-	backward, behind
sang-	blood
semi-	half
sero-	thin, watery fluid
sub-	under, beneath
super-	above, over, excess
supra-	above, over
tachy-	fast, rapid
trans-	across, over
uni-	one

Roots

The **root** contains the basic meaning of the word. It is combined with another root, with prefixes, and with suffixes in various combinations to form a medical term.

A vowel is often added when two roots are combined or when a suffix is added to a root. The vowel, usually an *o*, is called a **combining vowel**. An *i* is sometimes used when there is no vowel between the two combined roots or between the root and the suffix. A combining vowel makes pronunciation easier.

The most common roots and their combining vowels, in parentheses, are listed here. Their plural form, if other than an *s*, is indicated:

Root (Combining Vowel)	Meaning
abdomin(o)	abdomen
aden(o)	gland
adren(o)	adrenal gland
angi(o)	vessel
arteri(o)	artery (plural: *arteries*)
arthr(o)	joint
bronch(o)	bronchus (plural: *bronchi*)
card, cardi(o)	heart
cephal(o)	head
chole, chol(o)	bile (plural: *bile*)
chondr(o)	cartilage
col(o)	colon, large intestine
cost(o)	rib
crani(o)	skull
cyan(o)	blue

Continued

Root (Combining Vowel)	Meaning
cyst(o)	bladder, cyst
cyt(o)	cell
dent(o)	tooth (plural: *teeth*)
derma	skin (plural: *skin*)
duoden(o)	duodenum
encephal(o)	brain
enter(o)	intestines
fibr(o)	fibre, fibrous
gastr(o)	stomach
gloss(o)	tongue
gluc(o)	sweetness, glucose
glyc(o)	sugar
gyn, gyne, gynec(o)	woman (plural: *women*)
hem, hema, hemo, hemat(o)	blood
hepat(o)	liver
hydr(o)	water (plural: *water*)
hyster(o)	uterus
ile(o), ili(o)	ileum (plural: *ilea*)
lapar(o)	abdomen, loin, or flank
laryng(o)	larynx
lith(o)	stone
mamm(o)	breast, mammary gland
mast(o)	mammary gland, breast
men(o)	menstruation
my(o)	muscle
myel(o)	spinal cord, bone marrow
necr(o)	death
nephr(o)	kidney
neur(o)	nerve
ocul(o)	eye
oophor(o)	ovary (plural: *ovaries*)
ophthalm(o)	eye
orth(o)	straight, normal, correct
oste(o)	bone
ot(o)	ear
ped(o)	child (plural: *children*), foot (plural: *feet*)
pharyng(o)	pharynx
phleb(o)	vein
pnea	breathing, respiration
pneum(o)	lung, air, gas
proct(o)	rectum
psych(o)	mind
pulm(o)	lung

Root (Combining Vowel)	Meaning
py(o)	pus (plural: *pus*)
rect(o)	rectum
rhin(o)	nose
salping(o)	fallopian or uterine tube
splen(o)	spleen
sten(o)	narrow, constriction
stern(o)	sternum
stomat(o)	mouth
therm(o)	heat
thorac(o)	chest
thromb(o)	clot, thrombus (plural: *thrombi*)
thyr(o)	thyroid
tox(o)	poison
toxic(o)	poison, poisonous
trache(o)	trachea
ur(o)	urine, urinary tract, urination
urethr(o)	urethra
urin(o)	urine (plural: *urine*)
uter(o)	uterus
vas(o)	blood vessel, vas deferens
ven(o)	vein
vertebr(o)	spine, vertebrae

Suffixes

A **suffix** is placed at the end of a root to change the meaning of the word, but it is not used alone. For example, *nephritis* means inflammation of the kidney. It is formed by combining *nephro* (kidney) and *itis* (inflammation).

You need to learn the suffixes listed below:

Suffix	Meaning
-algia	pain
-asis	condition, usually abnormal
-cele	hernia, herniation, pouching
-centesis	puncture and aspiration of
-cyte	cell
-duction	make something happen
-ectasis	dilation, stretching
-ectomy	excision, removal of

Suffix	Meaning
-emia	blood condition
-genesis	development, production, creation
-genic	producing, causing
-gram	record
-graph	a diagram, a recording instrument
-graphy	making a recording
-iasis	condition of
-ism	a condition
-itis	inflammation
-logy	the study of
-lysis	destruction of, decomposition
-megaly	enlargement
-meter	measuring instrument
-metry	measurement
-oma	tumour
-osis	condition
-pathy	disease
-penia	lack, deficiency
-phasia	speaking
-phobia	an exaggerated fear
-plasty	surgical repair or reshaping
-plegia	paralysis
-ptosis	falling, sagging, dropping, down
-rrhage, -rrhagia	excessive flow
-rrhaphy	stitching, suturing
-rrhea	profuse flow, discharge
-scope	examination instrument
-scopy	examination using a scope
-stasis	maintenance, maintaining a constant level
-stomy, -ostomy	creation of an opening
-tomy, -otomy	incision, cutting into
-uria	condition of the urine

COMBINING WORD ELEMENTS

Medical terms are formed by combining word elements. A root can be combined with prefixes, other roots, or suffixes. The prefix *dys* (difficult) can be combined with the root *pnea* (breathing) to form the term *dyspnea*, meaning "difficulty in breathing." Similarly, the root *mast* (breast) combined with the suffix *ectomy* (excision or removal) forms the term *mastectomy*, which means "removal of a breast." Combining a prefix, root, and suffix is another way to form medical terms. *Endocarditis* (meaning "inflammation of the inner part of the heart") consists of the prefix *endo* (inner), the root *card* (heart), and the suffix *itis* (inflammation).

More complex combinations of prefixes, roots, and suffixes can be created:

- Two prefixes, a root, and a suffix
- A prefix, two roots, and a suffix
- Two roots and a suffix

The important things to remember are that (1) prefixes always come *before* roots and (2) suffixes always come *after* roots. You can practise forming medical terms by combining the word elements listed in this chapter.

ABDOMINAL REGIONS

The abdomen is divided into regions (**FIGURE 13–1**) to help describe the location of body structures, pain, or discomfort. The regions are as follows:

- Right upper quadrant (RUQ)
- Left upper quadrant (LUQ)
- Right lower quadrant (RLQ)
- Left lower quadrant (LLQ)

DIRECTIONAL TERMS

Certain terms describe the position of one body part in relation to another. These terms indicate the direction of the body part when a person is standing and facing forward. The following directional terms come from some of the prefixes listed earlier in this chapter:

- **Anterior (ventral)**—located at or toward the front of the body or body part
- **Distal**—the part farthest from the centre or from the point of attachment; for example, the foot is distal to the knee
- **Lateral**—the farthest away from the midline of the body
- **Medial**—the closest to the midline of the body

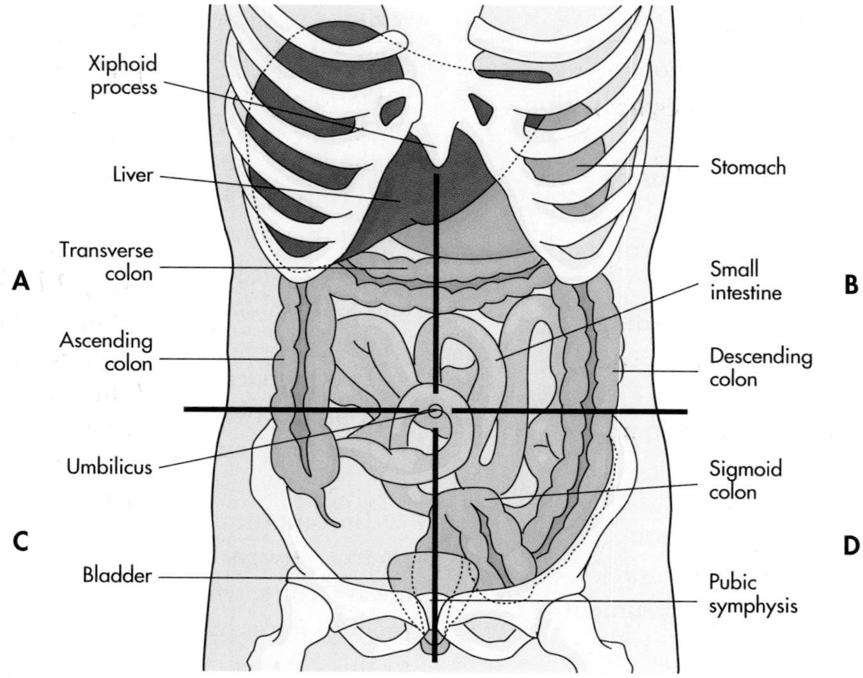

FIGURE 13–1 The four regions of the abdomen. **A,** Right upper quadrant. **B,** Left upper quadrant. **C,** Right lower quadrant. **D,** Left lower quadrant.

- **Posterior** (**dorsal**)—the back surface of the body—often used to indicate the position of one structure to another
- **Proximal**—nearest to the trunk of the body or the point of origin

ABBREVIATIONS

Abbreviations are shortened forms of words or phrases that help save time and space in written communication (see the table that follows). Each employer has a list of accepted abbreviations, which you should obtain when you are hired as a support worker. Use only the abbreviations accepted by your employer. If you are not sure an abbreviation is acceptable, write the term out in full to communicate accurately.

Common Abbreviations

Abbreviation	Meaning
abd	abdomen
ac	before meals
ADL	activities of daily living
ad lib	as desired
A.M., a.m.	morning
amb	ambulatory
amt	amount
bid	twice a day
BM, bm	bowel movement
BP, b/p, B/P	blood pressure
BRP	bathroom privileges
$\bar{c}$	with
C	centigrade
CA	cancer
cath	catheter
CBC	complete blood count
CBR	complete bed rest
c/o	complains of
CO_2	carbon dioxide
CPR	cardiopulmonary resuscitation
Dc, d/c	discontinue (NEVER used for "discharge")
DOA	dead on arrival
DON	director of nursing
Dx	diagnosis
ECG, EKG	electrocardiogram

Abbreviation	Meaning
EEG	electroencephalogram
ED	emergency department
°F	degrees Fahrenheit
FBS	fasting blood sugar
gal	gallon
GI	gastrointestinal
h, hr	hour
H_2O	water
HS, hs	hour of sleep; bedtime
ht	height
I&O	intake and output
in.	inch
IV	intravenous
lab	laboratory
LLQ	left lower quadrant
LPN	licensed practical nurse or licensed psychiatric nurse (in most provinces except Ontario)
LUQ	left upper quadrant
LVN	licensed vocational nurse
meds	medications
min	minute
mL	millilitre
neg	negative
NPO, npo	nothing by mouth
O_2	oxygen
OB	obstetrics
OR	operating room
OT	occupational therapy
pc	after meals
peds	pediatrics
per	by, through
P.M., p.m.	after noon
po (per os)	by mouth
Postop, post op	postoperative

Abbreviation	Meaning
Preop, pre op	preoperative
prep	preparation
prn	when necessary
Pt (pt)	patient
PT	physiotherapy
qh	every hour
q2h, q3h, etc.	every 2 hours, every 3 hours, and so on
qhs	every night at bedtime
qid	four times a day
R	rectal temperature; respiration; right
RBC	red blood cell; red blood count
RLQ	right lower quadrant
RN	registered nurse
ROM	range of motion
RPN	registered practical nurse; registered psychiatric nurse
RUQ	right upper quadrant
$\bar{s}$	without
SOB	shortness of breath
stat	at once, immediately
tbsp	tablespoon
tid	three times a day
TLC	tender loving care
TPR	temperature, pulse, and respirations
tsp	teaspoon
U/a (U/A, u/a)	urinalysis
V/S (vs)	vital signs
WBC	white blood cell; white blood count
w/c	wheelchair
wt	weight

mar medication administration
cc cubic centimeter
gtt drop
ungt ointment
SL sublingual - under the tongue

pv per vagina
pr per rectum
supp suppository
spec specimen
I+O intake and output
drsg dressing
qd every day

CHAPTER REVIEW

KEY POINTS

- Medical terms are formed by combining prefixes, roots, and suffixes, which come mostly from Greek and Latin. Understanding how medical words are formed will help you understand them better.
- The root contains the basic meaning of the word; a prefix comes before the root; a suffix comes after a root. Prefixes and suffixes always change the basic meaning of a word and are never used alone.
- The abdominal regions are the right upper quadrant, the left upper quadrant, the right lower quadrant, and the left lower quadrant.
- The terms that describe the position of one body part in relation to another include *anterior* (*ventral*), *distal*, *lateral*, *medial*, *posterior* (*dorsal*), and *proximal*.
- Each agency, facility, or province or territory will have a list of acceptable abbreviations. As a support worker, you must ask your employer for the list of abbreviations you are expected to use when charting and never use any abbreviations not on the list.

CRITICAL THINKING IN PRACTICE

You are a recently graduated support worker and were just hired at a home care agency. During your orientation, you were given the list of the only acceptable abbreviations allowed when documenting. Today, you notice the following documentation on your client's progress note: "Slept OK with HOB up o2p. c/o n&v but ø seen." You are unable to understand this documentation. What should you do? Why is it important to use acceptable abbreviations only?

REVIEW QUESTIONS

Answers to these questions are on page 200.

Fill in the blanks:

1. Word elements used in medical terminology are:
   A. Prefix
   B. Root
   C. Suffix
2. A Prefix ________ is placed at the beginning of a word to change the meaning of the word.
3. A Suffix ________ is placed at the end of a word to change the meaning of the word.
4. The four regions of the abdomen are:
   A. RUQ
   B. LUQ
   C. RLQ
   D. LLQ

Match the item in column A with its meaning in column B:

Column A	Column B
5. Distal	A. The part nearest to the centre or point of origin
6. Proximal	B. Relating to or located at the side of the body or body part
7. Anterior (ventral)	C. Located at or toward the front part of the body or body part
8. Medial	D. The part farthest from the centre or point of attachment
9. Posterior (dorsal)	E. Located at or toward the back of the body or body part
10. Lateral	F. Relating to or located at or near the middle or the midline of the body or body part

Write the definitions of the following prefixes:

11. a- without, not, lack of
12. dys- difficult, abnormal
13. bi- double, two, twice

14. ab- away from
15. trans- across, over
16. post- after, behind
17. olig- small, scant
18. hyper- excessive, too much, high
19. per- by, through
20. hemi- half
21. hypo- under, decreased, less than normal
22. ad- to, toward, near

Write the definitions of the following suffixes:

23. -algia pain
24. -itis inflammation
25. -ostomy creation of an opening
26. -ectomy excision, removal of
27. -emia blood condition
28. -osis condition
29. -rrhage excessive flow
30. -penia lack, deficiency
31. -pathy disease
32. -otomy incision, cutting into
33. -rrhea profuse flow, discharge
34. -plasty surgical repair or reshaping

Write the definitions of the following roots:

35. crani(o) skull
36. cardi(o) heart
37. mamm(o) breast, mammary gland
38. ven(o) vein
39. urin(o) urine
40. pnea breathing, respiration
41. cyan(o) blue
42. arteri(o) artery
43. col(o) colon, large intestine
44. arthr(o) joint
45. lith(o) stone
46. gastr(o) stomach
47. encephal(o) brain
48. gluc(o) sweetness, glucose
49. hem(o) blood
50. hyster(o) uterus
51. hepat(o) liver
52. my(o) muscle
53. nephr(o) kidney
54. phleb(o) vein
55. ocul(o) eye
56. oste(o) bone
57. neur(o) nerve
58. pneum(o) lung, air, gas
59. toxic(o) poison, poisonous
60. psych(o) mind
61. thorac(o) chest

Match the item in Column A with the item in Column B.

Column A	Column B
62. Intravenous	A. Inflammation of a joint
63. Apnea	B. Blood in the urine
64. Hemiplegia	C. Excessive flow of blood
65. Thoracotomy	D. Paralysis on one side
66. Arthritis	E. Surgical removal of the uterus
67. Bronchitis	F. No breathing
68. Anuria	G. Inflammation of the bronchi
69. Hematuria	H. Incision into the chest
70. Hysterectomy	I. No urine
71. Hemorrhage	J. Within a vein

Write the abbreviations for the following terms:

72. Bathroom privileges BRP

73. As desired ad lib

74. Complains of C/O

75. Twice a day bid

76. Hour of sleep HS, hs

77. Intake and output I&O

78. Nothing by mouth NPO, npo

79. When necessary prn

80. Postoperative postop, post op

81. Wheelchair W/c

82. At once, immediately Stat

Answers:

1. A. Prefix, B. Root, C. Suffix
2. Prefix
3. Suffix
4. A. Right upper quadrant, B. Left upper quadrant, C. Right lower quadrant, D. Left lower quadrant
5. D
6. A
7. C
8. F
9. E
10. B
11. Without, not, lack of
12. Difficult, abnormal
13. Double, two, twice
14. Away from
15. Across, over
16. After, behind
17. Scant, small
18. Excessive, too much, high
19. By, through
20. Half
21. Under, decreased, less than normal
22. To, toward, near
23. Pain
24. Inflammation
25. Creation of an opening
26. Removal of, excision
27. Blood condition
28. Condition
29. Excessive flow
30. Lack, deficiency
31. Disease
32. Incision, cutting into
33. Profuse flow, discharge
34. Surgical repair or reshaping
35. Skull
36. Heart
37. Breast
38. Vein
39. Urine
40. Breathing, respiration
41. Blue
42. Artery
43. Colon, large intestine
44. Joint
45. Stone
46. Stomach
47. Brain
48. Glucose, sweetness
49. Blood
50. Uterus
51. Liver
52. Muscle
53. Kidney
54. Vein
55. Eye
56. Bone
57. Nerve
58. Lung
59. Poison
60. Mind
61. Chest
62. J
63. F
64. D
65. H
66. A
67. G
68. I
69. B
70. E
71. C
72. BRP
73. Ad lib
74. c/o
75. bid
76. HS (hs)
77. I&O
78. NPO (npo)
79. prn
80. postop (post op)
81. w/c
82. stat

CHAPTER 14

Client Care: Planning, Processes, Reporting, and Recording

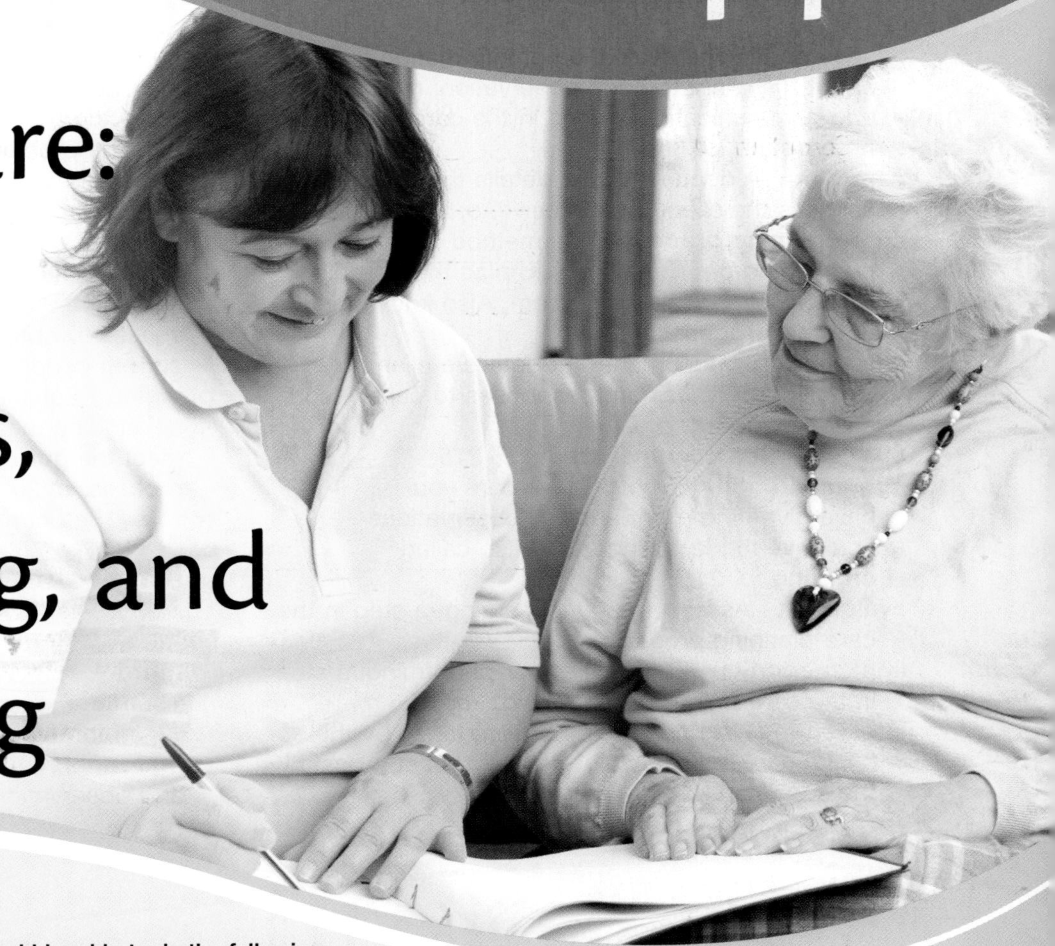

OBJECTIVES

After reading this chapter, the learner should be able to do the following:

- Explain the steps in the care-planning process in facilities.
- Explain the steps in the care-planning process in the community.
- Explain the function of the care plan.
- Describe the support worker's role in the care-planning process.
- Explain why observation is an important part of the support worker's role.
- Describe the difference between objective data and subjective data.
- Explain what makes an observation effective.
- Describe how reporting differs between a facility and a community setting.
- List the functions of a client's chart.
- Identify the types of documents found in a client's chart.
- List the basic rules for recording.
- List the basic rules for electronic documentation.
- Use the 24-hour clock.
- Explain why confidentiality is important in all aspects of the client's care.
- Describe how computers have affected the care-planning process.

KEY TERMS

assessment The evaluation of information collected about the client through observation, reflection, and communication; a step in the care-planning process. *p. 202*

care plan A document that details the care and services the client must receive. *p. 204*

care-planning process The method used by nurses and case managers to plan the client's care with the health care team. Also known as the **nursing process**. *p. 202*

chart A legal document that details a client's condition or illness and responses to care. Also called a **record**. *p. 210*

charting See **documentation**. *p. 215*

documentation Record of the care you have given the client and the observations you have made during care. Also called **charting**. *p. 215*

evaluation Assessing and measuring; a step in the care-planning process. *p. 205*

implementation Carrying out or performing; a step in the care-planning process. *p. 205*

intervention An action or measure taken by the health care team to help the client meet a goal in the care plan. *p. 204*

medical diagnosis The identification of a disease or condition by a physician. *p. 203*

nursing diagnosis A statement describing a health problem that is treated by nursing measures. *p. 203*

nursing process See **care-planning process**. *p. 202*

objective data See **signs**. *p. 207*

observation The active process of using the senses to obtain information about the client's current condition. *p. 203*

planning Establishing priorities and goals and developing measures or actions to help the client meet the goals; a step in the care-planning process. *p. 203*

record See **chart**. *p. 210*

signs Information about a client's health gained through observation and the use of other senses. Also known as **objective data**. *p. 207*

subjective data See **symptoms**. *p. 207*

symptoms Information reported by a client that cannot be directly observed by others. Also known as **subjective data**. *p. 207*

verbal report A spoken account of care provided and observations made. *p. 209*

Safe and effective care requires careful planning and coordination. It does not just happen. Facilities and agencies put systems and processes in place to protect clients from harm and to ensure high-quality care. This chapter discusses systems and processes you need to know as a support worker, including care planning, reporting, and recording.

THE CARE-PLANNING PROCESS IN FACILITIES

Nurses in facilities use a method called the **care-planning process** (also known as the **nursing process**) to plan and deliver care to clients. Its purpose is to meet the client's need for care and support. The care-planning process in facilities has the following steps:

1. Assessment
2. Nursing diagnosis
3. Planning
4. Implementation
5. Evaluation

Assessment

Assessment occurs through the evaluation of information collected about the client through observation, reflection, and communication. In some facilities, the team leader assesses the client's emotional, social, intellectual, and spiritual health. However, only a nurse or a physician can do a physical assessment of a client. The team leader—a nurse, social worker, or caseworker, depending on the facility or agency—gathers as much information as possible from various sources, including other health care providers on the team. Once the assessment has been completed, team members, including the client and the client's family, gather to set goals to meet the needs of the client.

Some facilities and agencies have adopted a client-centred approach that involves the client to a greater degree and also other health care providers, including support workers. This collaborative approach occurs at all stages of the care-planning process.

Nursing Diagnosis

The nurse uses information gathered from the assessment to make a nursing diagnosis. The support worker's **observations** are very important and must be reported so that the nurse has as much information as possible to determine a care plan.

The client may have a specific health problem or may be at risk for developing a health problem. Some clients may have more than one health problem and nursing diagnosis. A nursing diagnosis and a medical diagnosis are different. A **medical diagnosis** is made by a physician and is the identification of a disease or condition—for example, cancer, pneumonia, bipolar disorder, stroke, heart attack, acquired immune deficiency syndrome (AIDS), or diabetes. Medications, therapies, and surgery are ordered only by physicians to treat diseases or other medical conditions.

A **nursing diagnosis** is a statement describing a health problem that is treated by nursing measures. Nursing diagnoses take into account the whole client and are made only by nurses. Nurses regard all aspects of the client's health to be important. An example of a nursing diagnosis may be *low self-esteem*, *social isolation*, or *spiritual distress*. Most Canadian nurses use nursing diagnoses from the list established by the North American Nursing Diagnosis Association (NANDA) or from similar lists of diagnoses (see **BOX 14–1**, which contains a partial list).

BOX 14–1 Examples of NANDA International Nursing Diagnoses

1. BREATH:
   Decreased cardiac output
   Impaired gas exchange
   Ineffective airways cleaning
   Ineffective respiratory pattern
   Difficulty maintaining spontaneous ventilation
   Respiratory dysfunctional response to weaning
   High risk of asphyxia
   High risk of aspiration
2. FOOD/HYDRATION
   Nutrition, altered: excess
   Nutrition, altered: by default
   Nutrition, potential alterations: excess
   Liquids, excess volume
   Liquids, volume deficit
   Liquids, high risk of volume deficit
   Self-care, deficit: feeding
   Swallowing, impaired
   Ineffective breastfeeding
   Interrupted breastfeeding
   Effective breastfeeding
   Infant feeding ineffective pattern

(**Source:** Herdman, T.H. & Kamitsuru, H. (Eds.) Nursing Diagnoses—Definitions and Classification 2015–17. Copyright © 2014, 1994–2014 NANDA International. Used by arrangement with John Wiley & Sons, Inc. In order to make safe and effective judgments using NANDA-I nursing diagnoses it is essential that nurses refer to the definitions and defining characteristics of the diagnoses listed in this work.)

Planning

Planning involves establishing priorities and goals and developing measures or actions to help the client meet these goals.

Establishing Priorities

The client, the nurse, the family (or loved ones, if involved), and the health care team, including support workers, will discuss the client's needs and then decide on the client's priorities. They may use Maslow's hierarchy of needs to set priorities (see Chapter 12).

Setting Goals

After the client, the family, the case manager, and the health care team all agree on the priorities, they will discuss the goals for the client's care. In some situations, this discussion may involve only the client and the health care team. Goals are practical, achievable, and measurable and are time specific for evaluating the results (**FIGURE 14–1**). If a client does not achieve a goal by the date set by her and the team, the client must be the first person consulted in establishing a

Nursing diagnosis	Goal	Intervention
Constipation related to lack of privacy	Resident will have regular bowel movement by 6/30.	Ask resident to use call bell when urge to have bowel movement is felt. Answer call promptly. Assist resident to bathroom. Close bathroom door for privacy. Leave room if resident can be alone; tell resident you are leaving and that you will return if the call bell is turned on.
Sleep pattern disturbance related to noisy environment	Resident will report a restful sleep by 6/29.	Perform necessary care measures before bedtime. Close door to resident's room. Turn off television or keep volume low if the resident prefers. Ask staff to avoid talking outside the resident's room. Ask staff to speak in low voices. Turn off unneeded equipment.

FIGURE 14–1 Partial client care plan in a long-term care facility. Each nursing diagnosis has a goal, with nursing measures for each goal. The support worker is among those responsible for following the care plan.

more realistic goal. The team should then meet to develop a plan to help her meet this goal.

Determining Interventions

After setting the goals, the team will discuss interventions. An **intervention** is an action or measure taken by the health care team to help the client meet a goal. An intervention does not need a physician's order but may come from a physician's order. For example, if a physician orders that Mrs. Jacob walk 100 metres twice a day, the nurse will include this order in the care plan.

Establishing the Care Plan

Across Canada, various recording methods are used to provide you, as a support worker, with the information you will need to care for your client. Some facilities are still using a Kardex or paper system, although most now provide a computer-generated care plan. The **care plan** is a document that details the care and services the client must receive during each shift. The plan contains the client's diagnosis, goals, and the interventions required to achieve each goal. The care plan has several important functions:

- It lists the care and services the client must receive.
- It ensures that the client's care is consistent, no matter who provides the care. For example, Mr. Sayeed's care plan details methods for helping him overcome swallowing difficulties. Each care provider uses the same methods.
- It enables the health care team to effectively communicate details about the client's care. For example, as a support worker, when you start your shift in a long-term care facility, you see on the care plan that Mrs. Desormo has achieved the goal of dressing herself.

The care plan is not a finished document. It is continually reviewed and revised, depending on the client's needs, condition, and progress. For example, Mrs. Atkins's care plan is modified when she does not achieve the goal of bathing herself by May 20.

Usually, only the case manager, who has the overall responsibility for the client's care, makes changes to

Health care teams meet together and discuss the care plan.

the care plan. A support worker's input regarding any changes in the client is very important, as this information will assist the case manager in managing the plan. The support worker's observations of the abilities and needs of the client can alert the case manager to further assess him and change the care plan, as required.

Implementation

Implementation means carrying out or performing, and the actions listed in the care plan take place at this stage of the process. The nurse in charge of the client's care assigns or delegates tasks to the members of the health care team. As the support worker, you are only assigned or delegated tasks that are within the legal limits of your role and job description. The nurse will communicate the tasks assigned or delegated to you according to the facility or agency policy. This communication tells you what tasks you need to perform for each client.

The implementation process has four main functions:

- Providing the care
- Observing the client during the care
- Reporting and recording that the care has been completed
- Reporting and recording the observations made during the care

Observing the client is an important part of the implementation process. After care has been completed, support workers must report and record their actions and observations, according to employer policy.

Evaluation

Evaluation means assessing and measuring the progress a client has made toward meeting the goals that a team has agreed upon. Goals may be met totally, partly, or not at all. The nurse assesses the reasons a client may have made no progress or only partial progress toward reaching a goal. Your input of your observations will help the nurse change the interventions, complete further assessments, and alter the care plan, as required. Changes to the care plan are made in consultation with the client, family members, and other members of the health care team. Team meetings occur routinely, according to facility or agency policy. These meetings are held to share information, to set and modify goals, and to suggest ideas for modifying a client's care to meet her needs. You are an important part of the team, as you are the one spending the most time with your client (see Chapters 1, 6, and 11).

THE CARE-PLANNING PROCESS IN COMMUNITY SETTINGS

Case managers coordinate and manage client care. The care-planning process used by case managers in community settings usually involves four steps: assessment, planning, implementation, and evaluation.

Assessment

The case manager meets with the client and family members to identify the client's issues and needs. Usually, the meeting takes place in the client's home. If the client is coming home from the hospital, the case manager uses information from the hospital record or information obtained through a referral sent to the case manager's agency. The referral information may, in some cases, have been completed by a hospital case manager or the discharge planner.

The family is very important to the assessment process in community care settings. Serious illnesses and disabilities greatly affect family life (see Chapter 4). Family members take on new roles, including the role of caregiver to the client with an illness or disability. The case manager considers the needs, health, and well-being of the entire family. He also considers whether family members need help adjusting to the situation or training to help them care for the client. Together, the case manager, the client, and family members decide what care and services are needed. For example, they consider nursing and personal care needs and services, such as Meals on Wheels, housekeeping, and transportation, as well as the need for special equipment, such as for oxygen therapy.

The case manager also considers whether the client's home is a safe environment. For example, the home must be reasonably clean, be free of infestations, and have handwashing facilities and adequate heating and cooling systems. The case manager assesses whether the home needs modifications to accommodate the client's safety needs. For example, the home may need grab bars installed in the bathroom or a mechanical lifting device in the bedroom. Often, further safety assessments by other specialists are needed. For example, an occupational therapist may assess a home for wheelchair accessibility (see Chapter 27). Assessment tools such as the Resident Assessment Instrument (RIA) are available to team members.

Planning

In community care settings, the planning stage can be lengthy and complicated. First, the case manager, the client, and family members establish priorities, set goals, and determine available resources. Then, the case manager develops a master care plan based on the goals and puts together a health care team.

The case manager and family members consider the resources available for care. The case manager determines how much publicly funded home care the client and the family are eligible for. The family may choose to pay for additional care and services from a private agency.

The care plan includes the care and services provided by both family members and outside professionals and agencies. These professionals and agencies often develop their own care plans, but the case manager is in charge of the master plan. For example, the nursing care plan may be one part of the master care plan.

The case manager schedules all outside services and arranges financing for them. If the client needs help from a support worker, the case manager contacts an agency. A supervisor assigns a support worker to provide care or support to the client. The assignment may be communicated to the support worker by phone or on an assignment sheet.

When clients have multiple needs, several agencies may be involved. For example, Mr. Tremblay is recovering from a stroke. His wife is his primary caregiver. He needs 4 hours of nursing care a week as well as visits from respiratory, occupational, speech, and physical therapists. A support worker is also needed to help Mr. Tremblay prepare for bed when his wife is at work. Arrangements are made for Meals on Wheels so that Mrs. Tremblay does not have to prepare every meal.

Some clients in the community choose to coordinate and manage their own care. They may develop their own written care plan, or they may not write anything down. If there are no written directions for you, as the support worker, you will have to ask for detailed instructions from the client. You must ensure that you know exactly what you are allowed to do according to your employer's policies and what you must do if the client's expectations are beyond your scope of practice. If you are hired privately, you must decide whether you can or cannot provide the care requested based on your education since you are directly liable for legal actions.

Implementation

Agency staff provides care and services on the dates and times arranged by the case manager. If any unforeseen needs arise, the client or a family member calls the case manager. After assessing the situation, the case manager may ask the agency for an unscheduled visit. For example, Mrs. Tremblay feels too ill to care for her husband one morning. She calls her case manager, who contacts the agency for a support worker to care for Mr. Tremblay.

Evaluation

Evaluation in a home care setting is an ongoing process, so the case manager periodically meets with the client and the family to assess progress. The case manager also meets with and receives reports from the care providers and service providers, who continually monitor and evaluate their own care plans.

YOUR ROLE IN THE CARE-PLANNING PROCESS

In any health care setting, you, as the support worker, have an important role in the care-planning process. You make observations and relate these observations to the team members. You also provide feedback in response to the rest of the team's questions about the client and document the care you provide so that others on the team can use this information when reassessing the client's progress, revising client goals, and modifying the care plan.

Developing Observation Skills

Support workers generally spend more time with clients than other health care providers do. The support worker, therefore, may be the first to notice a change in a client's condition and observe the client's preferences and reactions to interventions. As a support worker, you are expected to make careful and accurate reports of these observations, which will be used in the care-planning process.

Objective Data

The information you gather using your senses is called **objective data** or **signs**. You need to use your senses of sight, hearing, touch, and smell. You may see the way the client shows discomfort when lying down, sitting, or walking, or you may observe flushed or pale skin and reddened or swollen areas on the client's body. You may hear abnormal sounds in the client's chest during respiration. You could feel by touch any changes in your client's skin temperature. With your sense of smell, you can detect any body, wound, and breath odours and unusual odours from urine and feces.

Subjective Data

Subjective data (or **symptoms**) consist of information reported by a client but not directly observed by others. The following statements are examples of subjective data:

- "I hardly slept last night. I lay awake from 1:00 a.m. until the sun came up."
- "With George gone, I just don't feel like living anymore. I feel so hopeless."
- "The pain is worse when I move. It is a sharp pain that goes up from my ankle to my hip. Thankfully, it comes and goes. I couldn't stand it if I felt it all the time."

When you report or record subjective data, do not interpret the client's comments. Use the client's exact words.

BOX 14–2 is a guide for making observations. It contains some basic observations, but you may observe other conditions and situations. Be alert to changes in your client's condition or behaviour.

BOX 14–2 Basic Observations

Ability to Respond

- Is the client easy or difficult to rouse?
- Can the client tell you his name, the time, and where he is?
- Does the client answer questions correctly?
- Does the client speak clearly?
- Does the client follow instructions correctly?
- Is the client calm, restless, or excited?
- Is the client conversing, quiet, or talking a lot?

Movement

Your initial observations should include the client's ability to perform any of the following tasks. These observations are important to note so that any progress in your client's condition can be documented.

- Can the client squeeze your fingers with either hand?
- Can the client walk?
- Can the client move her arms and legs?
- Are the client's movements shaky or jerky?
- Does the client complain of stiff or painful joints?

Pain or Discomfort

- Where is the pain located? (Ask the client to point to the area of pain.)
- Does the pain go anywhere else?
- When did the pain begin?
- What was the client doing when the pain began?
- How long does the pain last?
- How does the client describe the pain?
    - Sharp
    - Severe
    - Knifelike
    - Dull
    - Burning
    - Aching
    - Comes and goes
    - Depends on position
- Has the client felt this pain before?

Continued

BOX 14–2 Basic Observations—cont'd

- If the client has felt this pain before, what helped relieve the pain?
- Was medication given?
- Did the medication help relieve the pain? Is the pain still present?
- Is the client able to sleep and rest?
- What is the position of comfort?

Skin

- Is the skin pale or flushed?
- Is the skin cool, warm, or hot?
- Is the skin moist or dry?
- What colour are the lips and nails?
- Is the skin intact? Are there broken areas? If so, where?
- Are sores or reddened areas present?
- Are bruises present? Where are they located?
- Does the client complain of itching?

Eyes, Ears, Nose, and Mouth

- Is there drainage from the eyes? What colour is the drainage?
- Are the eyelids closed?
- Are the eyes reddened?
- Does the client complain of spots, flashes, or blurring?
- Is the client sensitive to bright lights?
- Is there drainage from the ears? What colour is the drainage?
- Can the client hear? Is it necessary to repeat questions? Are questions answered appropriately?
- Is there drainage from the nose? What colour is the drainage?
- Can the client breathe through the nose?
- Is there breath odour?
- Does the client complain of a bad taste in the mouth?
- Does the client complain of painful gums or teeth?

Respirations

- Do both sides of the client's chest rise and fall with respirations?
- Is breathing noisy?
- Does the client complain of difficulty breathing?
- What is the amount and colour of the sputum (saliva mixed with mucus, often coughed up)?
- What is the frequency of the client's cough? Is it dry or productive?

Bowels and Bladder

- Is the abdomen firm or soft?
- Does the client complain of gas (flatulence)?
- What are the amount, colour, and consistency of feces?
- What is the frequency of bowel movements?
- Can the client control bowel movements?
- Does the client have pain or difficulty urinating?
- What is the amount and colour of urine?
- Is urine clear or cloudy?
- Does urine have a foul smell?
- Can the client control the passage of urine?
- What is the frequency of urination?

Appetite

- Does the client like the diet?
- How much of the meal is eaten?
- What are the client's food preferences?
- Can the client chew food?
- How much liquid was taken?
- What are the client's liquid preferences?
- How often does the client drink liquids?
- Can the client swallow food and fluids?
- Does the client complain of nausea?
- If the client has vomited, what is the amount and colour of material vomited?
- Does the client have hiccups?
- Is the client belching?

Activities of Daily Living

- Can the client perform personal care without help?
  - Bathing?
  - Brushing teeth?
  - Combing and brushing hair?
  - Shaving?
- Does the client use the toilet, commode, bedpan, or urinal?
- Does the client feed herself?
- Can the client walk?
- What amount and kind of assistance are needed?

Focus your observations on the client's physical, mental, emotional, and social condition. Look for the following:

- Changes in physical condition—for example, the client's skin is red and blistering
- Changes in mental condition—for example, the client forgets how to use a toothbrush
- Changes in emotional states—for example, the client is crying
- Changes in social condition—for example, the client's friend does not visit at the usual time
- New conditions that you observe—for example, the client develops diarrhea

Describing Your Observations

Your observations are critical to the care-planning process since nurses and case managers use them for the assessment and evaluation steps. Remember these points when describing your observations:

- ***Be precise and accurate.*** Provide details of what you actually see, hear, touch, and smell. Measurements, calculations, and times must be accurate. When describing subjective data, report or record the client's exact words.
- ***Do not interpret or make assumptions.*** In most cases, your observations are sufficient, and you do not need to interpret them. Do not make assumptions. An *assumption* is a guess, usually based on insufficient evidence. When you make assumptions, you may be making a wrong or hasty conclusion.

BOX 14–3 contains some examples of ineffective as well as effective reporting of observations. Note that the support worker provides precise, accurate details but does not make any assumptions. The social worker and the nurse use the support worker's observations to make a judgement about the client's mental health.

VERBAL REPORTING

As a support worker, you need to report and record your actions and observations. A **verbal report** is the spoken account of care provided and observations made. Employers use different methods for verbal reporting, and all have policies about how often to report and what to report, so you need to know those policies. In certain circumstances, listed in **BOX 14–4**, you must always contact your supervisor. Verbal reports allow for quick, up-to-date information sharing. However, they lack a permanent record of what is reported.

Remember that information about a client is confidential. Be careful when communicating client information to other members of the health care team. Choose a quiet area where you will not be overheard by others. Do not discuss a client in his room or in a common area. Keep all your conversations about clients professional. When making reports by phone to your supervisor from your own home, make sure no one in your home can hear you.

Verbal Reporting in a Facility

In a facility, support workers report actions and observations to the charge nurse or to the supervisor. Reports must be prompt, thorough, and accurate.

- Always include the client's name, the room and bed number, and the time you made the observation or gave the care.
- Report only what you observed or performed.
- Prioritize items—start your report with the most important points.
- Give reports as often as the client's condition requires or as often as requested by the nurse.
- Immediately report any changes in the client's previously reported condition.

At the end of a shift, the charge nurse gives a report (called the *end-of-shift report*) to the incoming charge nurse. This report includes information about each client's condition, the care given, and the care that must be given on the next shift. Some facilities expect all team members to hear the end-of-shift report as they come on duty.

Verbal Reporting in a Community Setting

Employers have their own policies for verbal reports. Most employers in the community do not require support workers to make daily verbal reports.

BOX 14–3 Ineffective and Effective Observations Made by Support Workers

Ineffective Observation	Reasons the Observation Is Ineffective	Effective Observation	Reasons the Observation Is Effective
Mrs. Demarco is having trouble going to the bathroom this morning.	Correct terminology is not used. The statement is vague. No details are provided.	Mrs. Demarco urinated 3 times between 0900 and 0920. She said, "I feel a burning pain when I try to go to the bathroom, and only a trickle of urine is coming out."	Correct terminology and the client's exact words are used. The statement is a direct, precise observation. Both objective and subjective data are provided.
Mr. Quennell is having trouble remembering things.	The statement is an assumption. There is no supporting evidence.	Mr. Quennell did not remember eating his breakfast. He asked me to make breakfast 30 minutes after he had eaten. I told him he had already had breakfast. He said, "I don't remember."	The statement is an observation supported by detailed examples. Both objective and subjective data are provided.
Mrs. Rehman seems under the weather today.	Correct terminology is not used, and not everyone understands this expression. There is also no supporting evidence for this statement.	Mrs. Rehman did not play bridge today. She took only two bites of her lunch (a turkey sandwich). She said, "I'm not hungry. I feel tired, and I don't feel like doing anything."	The statement about Mrs. Rehman's behaviour and condition are observations supported by evidence. Mrs. Rehman's words are quoted exactly.

However, call your supervisor immediately if something unexpected happens. Follow employer policy and the guidelines in **BOX 14–4** and **BOX 14–5**.

CLIENT RECORDS OR CHARTS

A **chart** (also known as a **record**) is a permanent and legal document required to record a client's condition, signs and symptoms of any illness, the care and treatment given to the client, and the client's responses to care. This record documents the care provided from admission to discharge or death and is filed and kept (in Ontario, for a minimum of 5 years). It is used as a reference for future health care treatment, and it could be subpoenaed (ordered) for a court case involving malpractice.

In this age of technology, most facilities and agencies have implemented computerized reporting systems, but some employers are still using paper-based reports for some forms. This chapter will show you some of the forms that are used in the authors' area, but your facilities and agencies will have their own. Your employer will, as part of your orientation, ensure that you know what documentation it requires.

- ***Communication.*** Health care teams rely on reports to communicate information about their

BOX 14–4 When to Contact Your Supervisor

Contact your supervisor in any of the following cases:

- There is an emergency, such as finding your client lying unconscious on the floor.
- You observe a change in the client's condition or normal functioning.
- The client becomes ill; for example, the client vomits, has diarrhea, or develops a fever.
- The client is in distress, either physical or emotional.
- You believe the client's safety is at risk.
- A problem arises involving medications.
- The client complains about her condition or care.
- The client asks you a question about his diagnosis, condition, or treatment plans.
- The client or family member asks you to do something that contradicts the care plan.
- You have a conflict with a client or a family member.
- A question or problem arises, and you need help to sort it out.

BOX 14–5 Guidelines for Making Telephone Reports to Your Supervisor

- Keep agency phone numbers and extension numbers handy.
- Make sure you have a pen and paper handy.
- Identify yourself, the date, and the time of your call.
- Give a concise, accurate, and descriptive report. For example, say what you observed ("Client has an abrasion 5 cm by 3 cm on his buttocks"), when you made the observation ("I saw it when bathing the client"), and what the client said ("I fell down the stairs last night").
- Use the client's exact words.
- Speak clearly and slowly. Pause between sentences.
- Write down the instructions from your supervisor.
- Repeat the instructions back to your supervisor.
- Write the instructions on the appropriate document in the client's chart.
- Remember that the client's information is confidential. It is shared only with the health care team members involved in the client's care. Follow the rules outlined in the *Personal Information Protection and Electronic Documents Act (PIPEDA)*, available online. Legislation may vary between provinces and territories, so you must develop a working knowledge of the legislation that applies in your area.

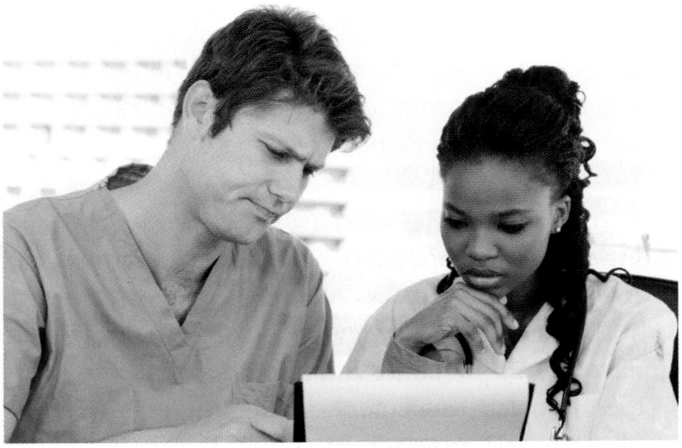

FIGURE 14–2 The nurse and respiratory therapist review a client's report. (**Source:** wavebreakmedia/Shutterstock.com)

clients (**FIGURE 14–2**). All team members must be informed about the client's condition and care during each shift. The report is a method to ensure that all members of the team are aware of the care the client has received. Recording is an accurate way to communicate information about the client. The care plan is one part of the report.

- ***Planning client care.*** The client record documents how the client tolerated a procedure or type of care. This information helps the health care team plan future interventions that would be best tolerated by the client.
- ***Currency.*** Care plans change as the client's needs, preferences, and condition change. Reports enable team members to keep the client's information up to date. Other areas of the report are also kept up

to date—for example, with the latest reports of laboratory tests and doctors' orders.

- ***Accountability.*** Printed charts are signed and dated by members of the health care team. Computerized charts offer automatic tracking. Ensure that you keep track of all printed charts and emails since all team members are accountable for their own words and actions. ***In a legal case, you may need to testify about what you wrote on the chart. Computer reports are traceable, as you would have used your log-in to update your reports, and are legally binding.***
- ***Continuity of care.*** Written documentation contains information on the client's past health issues and treatments. This information enables health care providers to detect patterns and changes in the client's condition. Because team members change over time, without a written record, care might become fragmented or uneven and unreliable.
- ***Quality assurance.*** Knowing that all care and interventions must be documented helps ensure that best practices are performed by all team members, the care plan is individualized for the client, and care delivery is consistent.
- ***Education and research.*** Client observations and responses to treatment inform future interventions. Data in client records may be used in future scholarly peer-reviewed articles so that findings can be shared with other health care providers.
- ***Funding.*** Based on the client records, the acuity (severity of illness) of the clients can influence staffing and equipment needs for the agency.

Documents Used in Charts

Most facilities, agencies, and acute-care settings now use computer programs for their documentation. Different programs are available, and, since most employers design their own documents, charts tend to vary from employer to employer. This section describes some common documents contained in a client's chart and offers some examples.

- ***Data forms*** include details about long-term care clients' physical, emotional, social, and cognitive health. Activities, interests, medications, treatments, and therapies are examples of information that is recorded.
- ***Assessment forms*** are used by nurses and case managers to record a client's health issues and needs. Assessments are based on information from the data form and other sources, including observations made by members of the health care team (FIGURE 14–3).
- ***Home assessment forms*** document the changes that need to be made to the client's home during rehabilitation (see BOX 27–2 on page 560).
- ***Care plans*** contain goals and interventions (action plan) based on the assessment. Sometimes the assessment and the care plan are on the same form.
- ***Progress notes (narrative notes)*** record information about the care given, the client's response to care, observations, the client's activities, special treatments, and medications. Progress notes also contain areas to record date, time, and initials (FIGURE 14–4 on page 214). Health care team members from various disciplines may or may not record care and treatment on the same set of notes. In some circumstances, progress notes may be separated into disciplines (for example, a section for nursing, a section for physiotherapy, and so on). This separation enables health care providers to easily access information for their own disciplines or to learn about the client's progress in a certain area of the client's health goals. Whether or not you record information on progress notes depends on your employer's policy.
- ***Graphic sheets*** record measurements and observations made on every shift, or three to four times per day. Information may include the client's blood pressure, temperature, pulse, respirations, height, and weight. Some graphic sheets have places to chart intake and output, routine care, bowel movements, and physician's visits (FIGURE 14–5 on page 214).
- ***Activities-of-daily-living (ADLs) checklists and flow sheets*** record actions relating to hygiene, food and fluids, elimination, rest and sleep, mobility, activity, and social interactions. ADL checklists (sometimes called *tick sheets*) require you to place check marks in boxes, whereas ADL flow sheets use codes for actions—for example, "I" for *independent* and "A" for *assist*. Both provide little

7 Day Observation Record – St Joseph's at Fleming

Resident Name ______________________

Dates of 7 Day Assessment **From:** ____________ **To:** ____________

PLEASE USE TICK MARKS UNLESS OTHERWISE INDICATED

*INDICATE THE **MOST** ASSISTANCE THE RESIDENT REQUIRED FOR EACH SHIFT*

	0			1			2			3			4			5			6			7		
Date:																								
Code Section: Shift:	N	D	E	N	D	E	N	D	E	N	D	E	N	D	E	N	D	E	N	D	E	N	D	E
G1 (c) - Walking in Room																								
Independent; requires no help																								
Staff cue resident only; requires no physical assistance																								
Guided maneuvering *(e.g. staff holds resident's hand)*																								
Weight-bearing assistance required *(# of staff?)*																								
Resident does not walk in room																								
Initials:																								
G1 (d) – Walking in Corridor																								
Independent; requires no help																								
Staff cue resident only: requires no physical assistance																								
Guided maneuvering *(e.g. staff holds resident's hand)*																								
Weight-bearing assistance required *(# of staff?)*																								
Resident does not walk in corridor																								
Initials:																								
G1 (e) – Locomotion on Unit by Wheelchair																								
Independent; requires no help																								
Staff cue resident only; requires no physical assistance																								
Guided maneuvering																								
Weight-bearing assistance required *(# of staff?)*																								
Not applicable																								
Initials:																								
G1(g) – Dressing																								
Self; no staff help required																								
Staff cue resident only; requires no physical assistance																								
Guided maneuvering																								
Staff do up buttons, zippers, tie laces etc.																								
Weight-bearing assistance required *(e.g. lift arm or lift leg to Apply KED stockings or prosthesis)*																								
Total assist																								
Number of staff required																								
Initials:																								

Form #

7 Day Observation Record – St Joseph's at Fleming

Resident Name: ______________________

Dates of 7 Day Assessment **From:** ____________ **To:** ____________

PLEASE USE TICK MARKS UNLESS OTHERWISE INDICATED

*INDICATE THE **MOST** ASSISTANCE THE RESIDENT REQUIRED FOR EACH SHIFT*

	0			1			2			3			4			5			6			7		
Date:																								
Code Section: Shift:	N	D	E	N	D	E	N	D	E	N	D	E	N	D	E	N	D	E	N	D	E	N	D	E
G1(h) – Eating ***(How resident eats or drinks, regardless of skill)***																								
Supervision only																								
Guided maneuvering of food or utensil to mouth																								
Weight-bearing assistance *(e.g. staff lifts resident's arm or hand To mouth)*																								
Total assist																								
Initials:																								
G1 (i) – Toileting ***(includes transfers on/off toilet)***																								
Independent; requires no help																								
Staff supervise/cue resident only; no physical assistance																								
Guided maneuvering of limbs, non weight-bearing help																								
Some weight-bearing assistance required *(# of staff?)*																								
Mechanical Lift/ Total assist (# of staff?)																								
Activity did not occur																								
Initials:																								
G1 (j) – Personal Hygiene ***(excludes baths or showers)***																								
Independent																								
Supervision or cueing or set-up required																								
Guided maneuvering of limbs, non weight-bearing help,																								
Weight-bearing assistance *(e.g. staff lift arm so resident can Brush hair or teeth)*																								
Total dependence																								
Resident refused hygiene care																								
Initials:																								

Form #

FIGURE 14–3 Example of an assessment form that may be used by support workers in a long-term care facility. Many agencies are replacing handwritten notes with similar electronic forms of documentation. (Courtesy of St. Joseph's at Fleming, Peterborough, ON.)

NNR – NARRATIVE NOTES – Client: ______________

TIME	DATE (D/M/Y):

Supplied by Nightingale Nursing

FIGURE 14–4 An example of narrative notes from a community agency. Many agencies are replacing handwritten notes with similar electronic forms of documentation. (Courtesy of Nightingale Nursing Registry, Peterborough, ON.)

or no space for writing details. Some of the items in an ADL flow sheet are shown in FIGURE 14–6.

- ***Task sheets*** are used by some employers in community settings to record care and services provided. The form has boxes for each day and sections for documenting care and support activities. You check the box for the day you provided the care or service (FIGURE 14–7 on page 216).
- ***Other flow sheets*** record frequent measurements and observations. Some record blood pressure, pulse, and respirations every 15 minutes or more often. Others record intake and output. Flow sheets are used to monitor the conditions of clients with serious illnesses.
- ***Summary reports*** summarize care and service provided over a period. These reports are used in community settings and by some long-term care facilities to provide summaries of the client's condition monthly or every second or third month.
- ***Incident reports*** are written accounts made after an accident, error, or unexpected event. In the community, these reports are commonly called *occurrence reports* (see Chapter 22).
- ***Kardex*** is a card file that summarizes information in the chart. It usually includes the client's current diagnosis, medications, treatments, any special

SALUS ET SPES
The Credit Valley Hospital

VITAL SIGNS FLOWSHEET

Signature/Status	Initials	Signature/Status	Initials

	Date :												
	Time :												
Temperature (C°)	: 40												
	39												
	38												
	37												
	36												
	35												
Pulse :													
Respirations :													
B.P. :	Lying :												
	Sitting :												
	Standing :												
Weight :													
	Initials												

FIGURE 14–5 Graphic sheet. (Courtesy of Credit Valley Hospital, Mississauga, ON. Reprinted with permission.)

Activities of Daily Living Flow Sheet

JAN FEB (MAR) APR MAY JUN JUL AUG SEP OCT NOV DEC

ORDER/INSTRUCTION	TIME	1	2	3	4	5	6	7	8	9	10	11	12	13	14	15	16	17	18	19	20	21	22	23	24	25	26	27	28	29	30	31
Bowel Movements L = Large M = Medium S = Small IC = Incontinent	11-7	M																														
	7-3			L																												
	3-11																															
Bladder Elimination I = Independent IC = Incontinent FC = Foley catheter	11-7	I	I	I	I																											
	7-3	I	I	I	I																											
	3-11	I	IC	I	I																											
Weight-Bearing Status TT = Toe touch AT = As tolerated P = Partial F = Full NWB = No weight bearing	11-7	AT	AT	AT	AT																											
	7-3	AT	AT	AT	AT																											
	3-11	AT	AT	AT	AT																											
Transfer Status ML = Medilift SBA = Stand by assist; A = Assist (of 1 or 2)	11-7	SBA	SBA	SBA	SBA																											
	7-3	SBA	SBA	SBA	SBA																											
	3-11	SBA	SBA	SBA	A-1																											
Activity A = Ambulate GC = Gerichair T = Turn every 2 hrs. W/C = Wheelchair	11-7	T	T	T	T																											
	7-3	A	A	A	A																											
	3-11	A	A	A	A																											
Safety LT = Lap tray SR = Side rails BA = Bed alarm SB = Seat belt	11-7																															
	7-3																															
	3-11																															
Feeding Status I = Independent S = Set up F = Staff feed SP = Swallow precautions TL = Thickened liquids	Breakfast	S	S	S	S																											
	Lunch	S	S	S	S																											
	Supper	S	S	S	S																											
Amount of food taken in %	Breakfast	75	100	100	75																											
	Lunch	75	75	100	75																											
	Supper	50	50	50	75																											

FIGURE 14–6 Some of the items in an activities-of-daily-living flow sheet. (Courtesy of Nightingale Nursing Registry, Peterborough, ON.)

equipment needs, and routine care measures. The Kardex system provides a quick source of current information and can be updated frequently to reflect changes. The Kardex system is used in some facilities but is rarely used in community settings.

Documentation

Documentation (also called **charting**) is a record of the care you have given the client and the observations you have made during care. Documentation is a legal requirement for health care providers. Support workers working in the community or the home care setting are required to document the care they provide. In facilities, support workers may or may not document care, depending on the agency's policy. Employers have their own policies for recording, including when to record, how often to record, what to record, and who should record. Policies address such issues as how to abbreviate, what colour of ink to use (if using a written report), and how to make corrections. When recording, focus on the following:

- What you observed, including symptoms the client reported to you
- What you did
- When you did it
- The client's response

Electronic Documentation

Both written reports and electronic reports have advantages as well as disadvantages. Written reports provide a permanent record, but they are time-consuming and can be difficult to read if the handwriting is not clear. Electronic reports are fast and efficient, but confidentiality can be more difficult to maintain because of the risk for data being accessed by unauthorized people. Use the guidelines in **BOX 14–6** and follow your employer's policies.

Hospitals, long-term care facilities, and community agencies are increasingly using electronic

LOG NOTES

Client: ______________________

Date: ______________________

PSW: ______________________

Activity/Task	3 pm–11 pm	7 am–3 pm	11 pm–7 am	Comments
Personal Care				
Awake				
Asleep				
Napping/In Bed				
Bed/Sponge Bath				
Shower				
Spa Tub				
Transfer to Wheelchair (specify times)				
Transfer to Bed (specify times)				
White Board on Tray				
Personal Hygiene				
Teeth				
Hair				
Nose				
Ears				
Deodorant				
Cut nails				
Other				
Pericare				
Dressing				

Meals and Snacks				
Meals/Snacks/Flush, etc.:				
11:00 am Meal and Flush				
4:00 pm Juice				
10:00 pm Meal and Flush				
1:15 am Meal and Flush				

Medical/Health/Safety				
Report from Previous Shift (5 min)				
Read Log Notes (5–10 min)				
Location and Condition (arrival)				
Location and Condition (departure)				
Check on client (every 15 minutes if				
not around client specify times)				
Meds:				
9:30 am				
3:00 pm–5:00 pm				
9:00 pm–11:00 pm				

FIGURE 14–7 An agency client care task sheet. Many agencies are replacing handwritten notes with similar electronic forms of documentation. (Courtesy of Nightingale Nursing Registry, Peterborough, ON.)

BOX 14–6 Guidelines for Electronic Documentation

- Log on using only your own personal identification number (PIN). Never share your PIN with anyone, and ensure that, when you are logging on, no one can see your numbers.
- As with all documentation, document only what *you* have observed, been told, or done. Never document as a favour for another person.
- Use only employer-approved abbreviations.
- Use correct spelling, grammar, and punctuation at all times.
- Be familiar with the electronic documentation software used in your agency and where you should document. Attend all training classes that are offered.
- Computers, smartphones, and electronic tablets are expensive so must be taken care of. Never consume food or beverages while around them to avoid accidentally spilling on them. Do not drop handheld devices. Do not leave them in a car, where they can be stolen or overheated.
- Confidentiality must be maintained. When typing on a monitor that can be seen by others, angle the screen away from their view.

charting. Some facilities have computers outside each client's room, and support workers are required to enter the care given, the amount of time it took to provide the care, and how much the client was able to help with the care. In some provinces, these data help determine how much funding facilities will receive. Other hospitals and long-term care facilities have computers at the nursing stations, where support workers enter data. Some community agencies are now using handheld digital devices to ensure that the recorded information regarding their clients is current.

Need for Consistency and Accuracy

Whether recording on paper or by computer, it is important for the support worker to communicate clearly and thoroughly. Make sure that measurements and numbers recorded are accurate. If there is a space for observations, be precise in your recording of them, and record everything that is relevant. You should avoid using the third person (*he*, *she*, *they*, or client's name) and focus specifically on the facts—for example, "Abrasion, 5 cm by 3 cm, noted on left knee" rather than "I saw an abrasion on Mrs. Smith's left knee." Appropriate reporting that follows standardized documentation guidelines is very important because more and more frequently, Canadians are suing care facilities and their staff for malpractice, neglect, and so on. Remember that your charting is part of a legal document. Use the guidelines in **BOX 14–7**, and follow your employer's policies.[1]

Recording Time

The 24-hour clock is used to document care. It uses a four-digit number for time (**FIGURE 14–8**). The first two digits are for the hour: 0100 = 1:00 a.m.; 1300 = 1:00 p.m. The last two digits are for minutes: 0110 = 1:10 a.m. The abbreviations "a.m." and "p.m." are not used, but sometimes the abbreviation *h* or *hr* is used. Follow your employer's policies. As **BOX 14–8** (on page 219) shows, morning hours are the same in the 24-hour clock as they are in the conventional clock. For "p.m." times, add 12 to the first two digits (the hours) of clock time. For example, if it is 2:00 p.m., add 12 to 2 to make 1400. For 8:35 p.m., add 12 to 8 to make 2035. The 24-hour clock helps make communication more accurate. Since health care team members do not have to write "a.m." or "p.m.," the risk of confusion is reduced.

Terminology and Abbreviations

In health care, medical terminology and abbreviations are used to communicate effectively and clearly (see Chapter 13). If a member of your health care team uses a word that you do not understand, ask the person what the word means. It is a good idea to keep a medical dictionary at hand so you can look up the meanings of unfamiliar words. All members of the health care team must use only terms and abbreviations approved by employer policy to ensure correct interpretations by everyone on the health care team.

Methods of Charting

Agencies and facilities use a variety of methods for charting. Some examples include progress (narrative)

BOX 14–7 Documentation Guidelines

For Documentation in Writing:

- Always use ink. Follow employer policy in regard to the colour of ink to be used.
- Make sure that your writing is legible and neat.
- Include the date and the time whenever a recording is made. Use conventional time (a.m. or p.m.) or 24-hour clock time, according to employer policy.
- Never erase or use correction fluid if you make an error. Draw a single line through the error. Write "error" or "mistaken entry" above it, and sign your initials. Then rewrite that part. Follow any other employer's policies for correcting errors.
- Sign all entries, and include your title, as required by your employer's policy.
- Do not skip lines. Draw a line through the blank space of a partially completed line or to the end of a page. This technique prevents others from recording in a space that has your signature.
- Make sure each form is stamped with the client's name and other identifying information.

For All Documentation:

- Use only employer-approved abbreviations.
- Use correct spelling, grammar, and punctuation.
- Record only what *you* observed and performed.
- Never chart a procedure or treatment until after its completion.
- Be accurate, concise, and factual. Do not record assumptions or opinions.
- Record in a logical manner and in the order in which tasks and procedures occurred.
- Be descriptive. Avoid terms with more than one meaning.
- Use the client's exact words. Use quotation marks to show that the statement is a direct quote.
- Report any changes in the client's previously reported condition. Also, report that you informed your supervisor and the time you made the report.
- Do not omit any information.
- Record all safety measures used, such as assisting a client when she is up or reminding a client not to get out of bed. This documentation will help protect you from legal action if the client has a fall. Remember that every record you submit, whether on the computer or on a paper chart, is a legal document and can be used in legal proceedings against you or your employer.

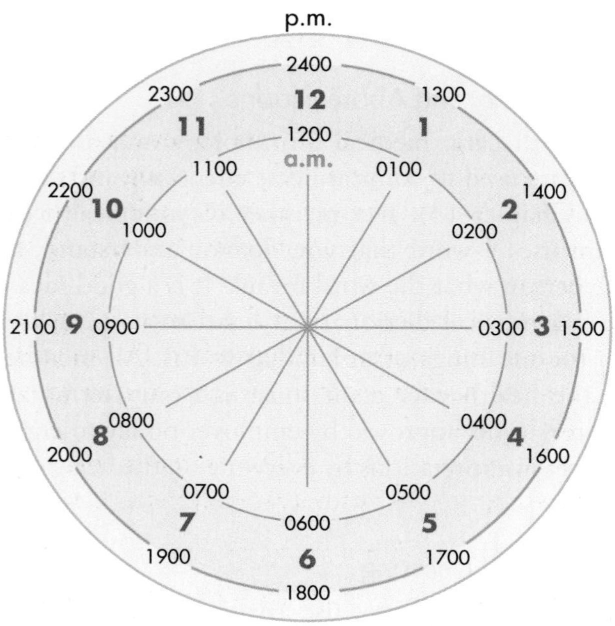

FIGURE 14–8 The 24-hour clock.

notes, SOAP charting, PIE charting, and focus (DAR) charting (**BOX 14–9**).

Narrative charting records information about the client and client care in chronological order. The content resembles a log of the client's day.

SOAP charting uses four essential components in recording. The components are:

S—subjective data
O—objective data
A—analysis, or assessment, of the data
P—plan of care

PIE charting uses three essential components in recording. The components are:

P—problem
I—intervention

BOX 14–8 24-Hour Clock

Conventional Time	24-Hour Clock	Conventional Time	24-Hour Clock
1:00 a.m.	0100	1:00 p.m.	1300
2:00 a.m.	0200	2:00 p.m.	1400
3:00 a.m.	0300	3:00 p.m.	1500
4:00 a.m.	0400	4:00 p.m.	1600
5:00 a.m.	0500	5:00 p.m.	1700
6:00 a.m.	0600	6:00 p.m.	1800
7:00 a.m.	0700	7:00 p.m.	1900
8:00 a.m.	0800	8:00 p.m.	2000
9:00 a.m.	0900	9:00 p.m.	2100
10:00 a.m.	1000	10:00 p.m.	2200
11:00 a.m.	1100	11:00 p.m.	2300
12:00 noon	1200	12:00 midnight	2400 or 0000

BOX 14–9 Examples of Progress Notes Written in Different Formats

SOAP (Subjective – Objective – Analysis – Plan)

1/19/16 Knowledge deficit related to inexperience regarding surgery 1630

S "I'm so worried about what it will be like after surgery."

O Client asking frequent questions about surgery. Has had no previous experience with surgery. Wife present; acts as a support person.

A Knowledge deficit regarding surgery related to inexperience. Client also expressing anxiety.

P Explain routine preoperative preparation. Demonstrate and explain rationale for turning, coughing, and deep breathing (TCDB) exercises. Provide explanation and teaching booklet on postoperative nursing care.
S. Lazarus, RPN

ADPIE (Analysis – Diagnosis – Problem – Intervention – Evaluation)

A Stated, "I don't know anything about this surgery"

D Knowledge deficit regarding surgery related to inexperience.

P Explain preoperative care to client and assess for understanding.

I Explained to client normal preoperative preparations for surgery. Demonstrated TCDB exercises. Provided booklet to client on postoperative nursing care.

E Client demonstrates TCDB exercises correctly. Needs review of postoperative nursing care.
S. Lazarus, RPN

Focus Charting (Data – Analysis & Action – Response)*

D Client states, "I'm so worried about what it will be like after surgery." Client asking frequent questions about surgery. Has no previous experience with surgery. Wife present; acts as a support person.

A Explained to client normal preoperative preparations for surgery. Demonstrated TCDB exercises. Provided booklet to client on postoperative nursing care.

R Client demonstrates TCDB exercises correctly. Needs review of postoperative nursing care.

*Note: Some agencies also add P (Plan).
Source: SOAP, PIE, and DAR information adapted from Potter, P.A., & Perry, A.G. (2014). *Canadian fundamentals of nursing* (5th ed., p. 209). Toronto, ON: Elsevier Canada. Updated "PIE" to "ADPIE" by author.

E—evaluation
ADPIE adds two additional components to PIE:
A—analysis
D—diagnosis
DAR charting also uses three essential components in recording. The components are:
D—data (or *diagnosis*)
A—analysis & action
R—response

Other methods of charting are being used across Canada. Your instructor will train you on the charting method commonly used in your area.

Recording in a Facility

In most acute-care settings, you will be required to document your care electronically using a computer program (see **FIGURE 14–9** and **FIGURE 14–10**). However, computers are not always available, so you may be required to record your care in writing.

In long-term care settings, you may document your care electronically, on ADL checklists, or on flow sheets. You may be expected to give summary reports on care provided to clients.

Recording in the Community

Agencies and case managers keep the bulk of client charts in their organizations; however, some parts of a client's chart are usually, but not always, kept in the client's home, often in a binder. The forms in the binder will vary according to agency policy and the client's condition and needs. Among other documents, the binder usually contains the care plan, progress notes, ADL checklists, flow sheets, and task sheets. Some agencies use smartphones or tablets that the support worker would document on.

Agency policies differ—some do not allow support workers to enter anything on the documents in the client record, whereas others *expect* support workers to accurately record tasks and observations in the appropriate manner. Most agencies have forms (or entry sections in electronic documentation systems) called *client care task sheets* that you carry with you to every assignment (see **FIGURE 14–6** on p. 215). You start a new task sheet for each client, and as you complete tasks, you check off the relevant areas of the form.

Most task sheets contain space to record special circumstances or observations. You may be expected to note whether the client performed activities independently, dependently, or with some assistance. As mentioned, any changes you observe in a client's normal functioning or condition should be reported by phone to your supervisor. Record on the task sheet any verbal reports that you make as well as phone instructions received from your supervisor.

You hand in your task sheets or download the gathered information monthly or weekly, depending on agency policy, along with forms that track work

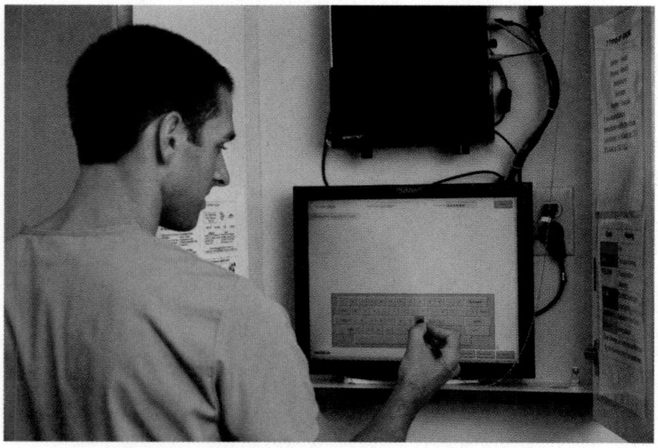

FIGURE 14–9 An electronic medical record.

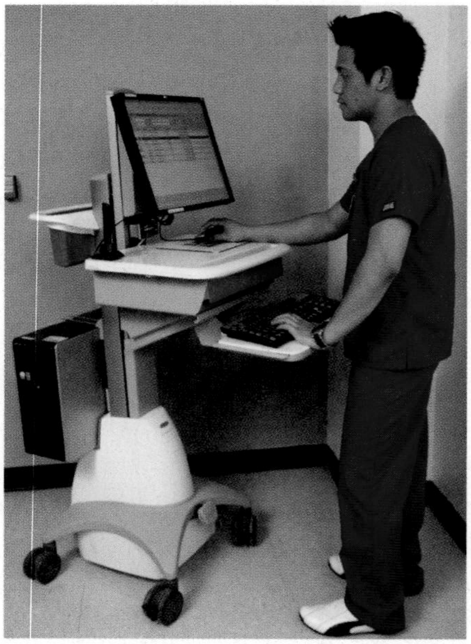

FIGURE 14–10 This support worker is recording client observations electronically on a portable computer station.

expenses such as mileage for your vehicle if you use one for your work. Your supervisor may use your task sheets to prepare a report on each client. For this report, you may be asked for additional information about some of your clients.

Confidentiality

You are ethically and legally bound to keep client information confidential, including any information about the client that you record in the client chart, whether by hand or on an electronic device. All employers have strict guidelines about the confidentiality of records and client information. You must be particularly careful to observe guidelines on accessing, reporting, and transporting information, depending on the regulations of your province or territory. The federal government has very strict guidelines to protect an individual's rights to privacy.

Only health care team members who are directly involved in the client's care have access to confidential information. Those not directly involved usually are not allowed access to the client's records. Housekeeping staff, kitchen staff, and office clerks, for example, do not need to see the records or hear any confidential details about a client. In a home care setting, only certain family members have access to these details. Your supervisor will tell you who is allowed to look at the record.

You may transport a document from a central file area to a client's room or other location in a facility, or, in a community setting, you may carry with you confidential information about a client. Be very careful when transporting confidential documents. Concentrate on what you are doing, and remind yourself of the importance of your task. If you become distracted, you could easily leave the documents in an inappropriate place.

Impact of Electronic Communication on Health Care and Recording

Electronic communication has opened the door to many changes in the way health care is researched, provided, and documented. For example, many clients research their health needs and get health questions answered by simply searching on the Internet. However, Internet search engines do not screen the available information for accuracy and reliability. To better inform the public, there are government websites and telephone services that can reliably answer a client (or family member's) questions on health care.

In many remote areas of the country, health care may be difficult to access, a situation that is especially problematic if the client's condition requires the services of a medical or nursing specialist. To assist clients in such areas, health care workers may send health data about the client electronically to a nurse practitioner, doctor, or health team many kilometres away. Electronic health records are easy to read and respond to and are helping to bridge this distance.

CHAPTER REVIEW

KEY POINTS

- Most facilities, agencies, and acute-care settings now record everyday care electronically. Some facilities require all client care to be documented electronically, whereas others are still using handwritten forms and documentation. If you are required to use electronic documentation, you will be trained in the reporting system used by your employer.
- In long-term care facilities and community agencies, nurses use a method called the *care-planning process* (or *nursing process*), which includes assessment, nursing diagnosis, planning, implementation, and evaluation. Nurses use information from support workers to adjust the care plan to meet the client's needs.
- In some provinces or territories, the funding an employer receives is based on the recorded information regarding the care given, the amount of time taken to provide the care, and the amount of assistance the client needs. Accurate reporting is essential.
- You need to understand your employer's policy regarding verbal reports. In care facilities, you must make sure your conversations are confidential, and in the community, you must ensure no one can overhear any conversation about your client.

CRITICAL THINKING IN PRACTICE

You are working from 0700 hours to 1500 hours. Mrs. Ryder is one of your assigned clients. Plan and prioritize Mrs. Ryder's care from the following tasks included on your assignment sheet:

- Assist her to physical therapy at 1000 hours.
- Assist her with breakfast in the dining room at 0800 hours.
- Help her to her daughter's car at 1200 hours for lunch outside the centre.
- Take her blood pressure and pulse before 1000 hours.
- Provide morning care, including oral care, combing her hair, and dressing.
- Change her bed linens.
- Help her to the bathroom before meals and to physical therapy as needed.
- Assist her to her chair to rest after physical therapy and after lunch.

What if you are unsure of the correct order in which to complete the tasks? How would you report and record your observations?

REVIEW QUESTIONS

Answers to these questions are at the bottom of page 223.

Circle the BEST answer.

1. Assessment involves:
   A. Collecting information about the client
   B. Carrying out or performing the elements of the care plan
   C. Implementing the care plan
   D. Evaluating and measuring the effectiveness of the care plan
2. The statement "Urinary elimination, impaired" is on a care plan. This statement is a(n):
   A. Nursing diagnosis
   B. Assessment
   C. Evaluation
   D. Medical diagnosis
3. Mrs. Muryama says, "I didn't sleep at all last night because of the pain in my back." This statement is:
   A. A nursing diagnosis
   B. Subjective data
   C. An intervention
   D. Objective data
4. You record the following: "Mr. Munro was better today." What is wrong with this observation?
   A. It does not say better than what.
   B. It is an assumption.
   C. It is an assessment.
   D. Nothing is wrong with this observation.

5. Which statement is false?
A. A chart is discarded after the client is discharged from hospital.
B. A chart is a permanent, legal document.
C. A chart is updated as a client's needs and condition change.
D. A chart provides a record of the accountability of health care providers.

6. A graphic sheet:
A. Records a client's activities of daily living (ADLs)
B. Is used to record measurements and observations made three to four times per day
C. Contains information about the care given, the client's responses to care, and observations about the client's condition
D. Summarizes a client's care and services over a period

7. A data form:
A. Is used in long-term care settings to detail a person's physical, emotional, social, and intellectual health
B. Is used in home care settings to assess changes that may be needed to the home
C. Includes boxes that are checked for the day on which care or service was provided
D. Is another name for Kardex

8. In 24-hour time, 1330 is:
A. 3:30 p.m.
B. 3:30 a.m.
C. 1:30 p.m.
D. 1:30 a.m.

9. If you make an error when recording, you should:
A. Put an X through the error, and write "error" over it
B. Erase the error
C. Draw a single line through the error, and write "error" over it
D. Use correction fluid

10. In a long-term care facility, who has access to clients' charts?
A. All staff members
B. Only the office staff and the nursing staff
C. Nurses, support workers, physiotherapists, occupational therapists, and dietitians
D. It depends on facility policy and procedures.

Answers: 1.A, 2.A, 3.B, 4.B, 5.A, 6.B, 7.A, 8.C, 9.C, 10.D

Chapter opener image: Monkey Business Images/Shutterstock.com

CHAPTER 15

Measuring Height, Weight, and Vital Signs

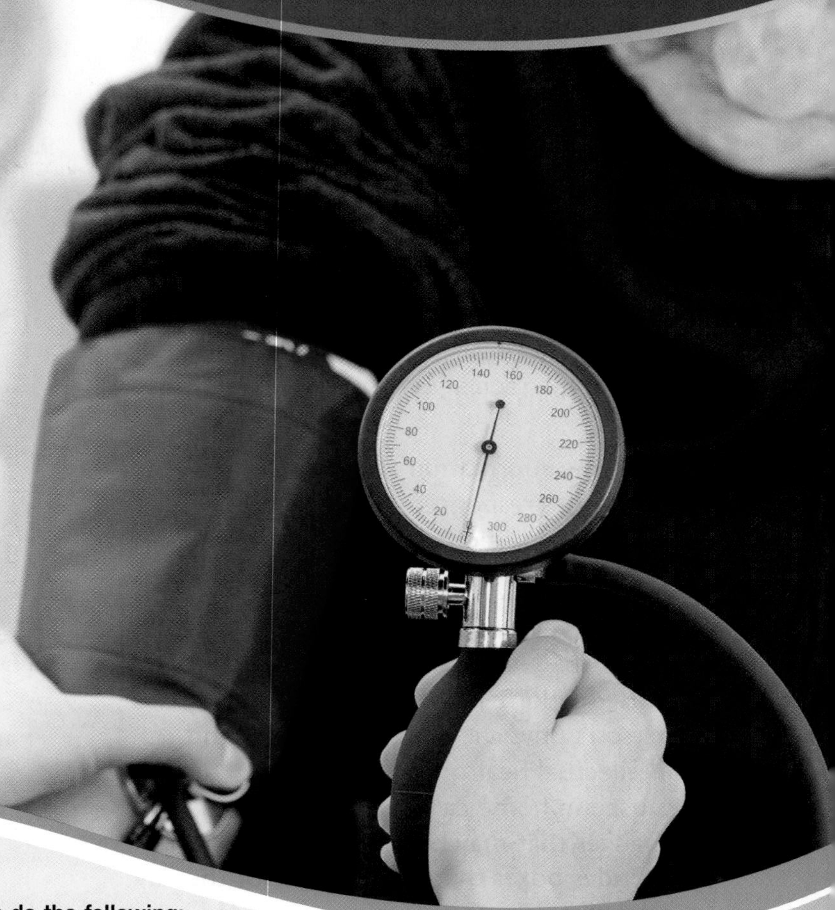

OBJECTIVES

After reading this chapter, the learner should be able to do the following:

- Explain how to measure height and weight.
- Explain why vital signs are measured.
- List factors that affect vital signs.
- Identify the normal ranges for temperature sites.
- Know when to use each temperature site.
- Identify why the older adult's normal body temperature range may be lower than a younger adult's range.
- Identify the sites for taking a pulse.
- Describe what a pulse oximeter does.
- Describe the correct manner of using a pulse oximeter.
- Describe normal respirations.
- Describe factors that affect blood pressure.
- Describe the practices to follow when measuring blood pressure.
- Know the vital sign ranges for different age groups.
- Perform the procedures described in this chapter.

KEY TERMS

blood pressure The amount of force exerted by the blood against the walls of an artery. *p. 241*

body temperature The amount of heat in the body; a balance between the amount of heat produced and the amount lost by the body. *p. 230*

bradycardia A slow (*brady*) heart rate (*cardia*); a rate less than 60 beats per minute. *p. 237*

diastole The period of heart muscle relaxation. *p. 241*

diastolic pressure The pressure in the arteries when the heart is at rest. *p. 241*

dysrhythmia An irregular rhythm of the pulse; beats may be unevenly spaced or skipped. *p. 237*

hypertension Persistent blood pressure measurements above the normal systolic (140 mm Hg) or diastolic (90 mm Hg) pressures. *p. 242*

hypotension A condition in which the systolic blood pressure is below 90 mm Hg and the diastolic pressure is below 60 mm Hg. *p. 242*

pulse The beat of the heart felt at an artery as a wave of blood passes through the artery. *p. 236*

pulse oximeter A device that measures both a client's pulse rate and the oxygen level in the blood. *p. 239*

pulse rate The number of heartbeats or pulses felt in 1 minute. *p. 236*

respiration The act of breathing air into (inhalation) and out of (exhalation) the lungs. *p. 240*

sphygmomanometer The instrument used to measure blood pressure. *p. 243*

SpO_2 Peripheral capillary oxygen saturation; the reading given by a pulse oximeter for the percentage of oxygen-saturated hemoglobin that is dissolved in the blood. *p. 239*

stethoscope An instrument used to listen to the sounds produced by the heart, lungs, and other body organs. *p. 244*

systole The period of heart muscle contraction. *p. 241*

systolic pressure The amount of force required to pump blood out of the heart and into the arterial circulation. *p. 241*

tachycardia A rapid (*tachy*) heart rate (*cardia*); a rate over 100 beats per minute in an adult. *p. 237*

vital signs Temperature, pulse, respirations, and blood pressure (and SpO_2 if possible). *p. 225*

The four **vital signs** of body function are temperature, pulse, respirations, and blood pressure. It may also include oxygen saturation levels (SpO_2), which will require special training by your employer. Vital signs reflect the function of three body processes essential for life: (1) regulation of body temperature, (2) breathing, and (3) heart function. Measuring and recording vital signs, as well as height and weight, provide important information for the care-planning process.

Your job description will tell you the vital signs you are approved to perform on your client. Usually, support workers can measure and record temperature, pulse, and respirations, and, in some agencies or facilities, oxygen saturation levels (SpO_2). It is very important that you report any changes in your client's vital signs to your supervisor immediately.

MEASURING HEIGHT AND WEIGHT

Height and weight are measured when a client is admitted to a facility and sometimes daily, weekly, or monthly. Some clients may be weighed daily when there is concern about fluid retention (e.g., in congestive heart failure) and to monitor weight gain or loss. Weigh the client at the same time of day for daily, weekly, or monthly measurements, and use the same scale. Before breakfast is the best time, as food and fluids add weight.

The client should wear only a gown or pyjamas when being weighed, as clothes add weight. Shoes or slippers add to the weight and the height. Also, have the client void (urinate) before being weighed, as a full bladder affects the weight measurement. If a urine specimen is needed, collect it at this time.

There are balance beam scales, chair scales, lift scales, wheelchair weigh scales, and digital scales (**FIGURE 15–1**). The most common weigh scale used in facilities is the weigh scale in the bathtub lift chair. Balance beam scales are used for clients who are able to stand, and chair and lift scales are used for those who are unable to stand. Wheelchair scales are used for clients in wheelchairs. Follow the manufacturer's instructions and employer policy when using scales. You must ensure that you weigh your client with the same clothing, at the same time of the day, and on the same scale (see the *Measuring Height and Weight* and *Measuring Height: The Client in Bed* procedures).

Digital scales have LED (light-emitting diode) displays that show the weight. Make sure the LED reads zero before weighing the client.

In the community, clients may have scales that still have imperial units (pounds). To convert to metric units, divide the pounds by 2.2 to get the weight in kilograms (e.g., 10 lb=4.5 kg, 160 lb=72.7 kg).

A B C D

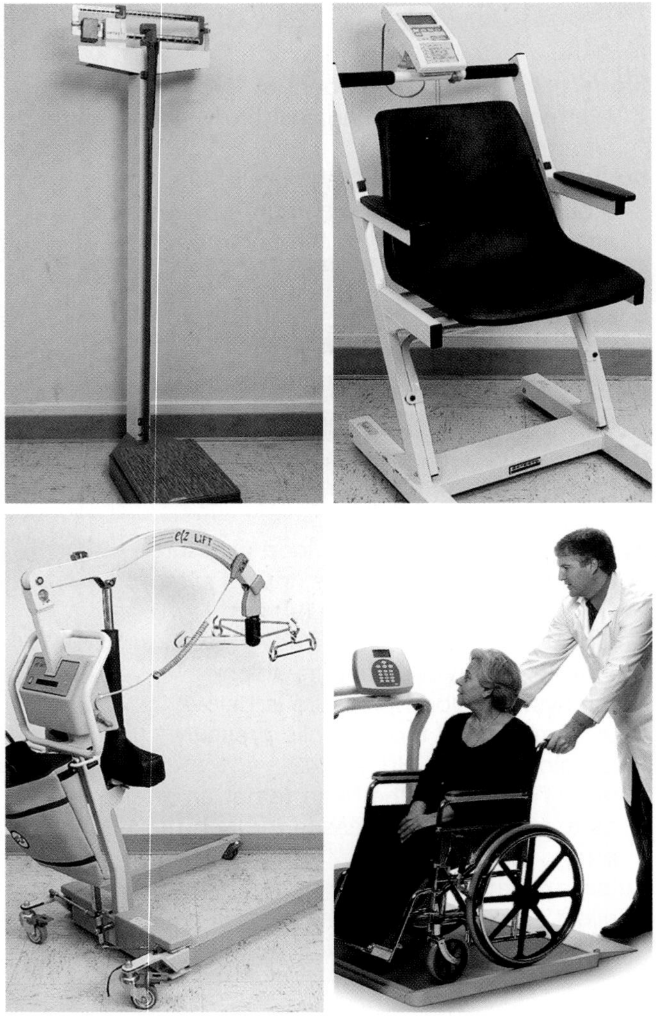

FIGURE 15–1 Types of scales. **A,** Balance beam scale. **B,** Chair scale. **C,** Lift scale. **D,** Wheelchair weigh scale. (**Source** (for *D*): Courtesy Pelstar LLC/Health o meter® Professional Scales, Alsip, IL 60803 USA.)

Measuring Height and Weight

Advocate on Behalf of the Client's Quality of Life by Promoting:

Dignity • Independence • Preferences • Privacy • Safety *(see BOX 1–4, on p. 17)*

PRE-PROCEDURE

1 Identify the client, according to employer policy.
2 Explain the procedure to the client.
3 Ask the client to void (see Chapter 32).
A full bladder affects the weight measurement.
4 Perform hand hygiene.
5 Collect the following supplies:
☐ **Scale**
☐ **Paper towels**
6 Provide for privacy.

Continued

Measuring Height and Weight—cont'd

PROCEDURE

7 *Balance beam scale (mechanical):*

a Perform hand hygiene.

b Disinfect the scale platform, according to employer policy. Dry it with paper towels.
This decreases the risk of pathogen spread.

c Raise the height rod before the client stands on the scale.
This prevents the client from accidental injury.

d Move the weights to zero (0). The pointer should be in the middle.
This ensures accurate reading.

e Have the client remove the robe and footwear. Assist as needed.
Clothing and footwear can add to the weight.

f Help the client stand on the scale platform. Arms should be at the sides.
If the client holds on to anything, it can affect the measurement of weight.

g Move the weights until the balance pointer is in the middle (**FIGURE 15–2**).
This ensures an accurate reading.

h Record the weight on your notepad or assignment sheet.
This ensures accurate recording of the weight on the client's record and prevents you from relying on your memory.

i Ask the client to stand very straight.
This ensures the client's weight is balanced on both feet.

j Lower the height rod until it rests on the client's head (**FIGURE 15–3**).
If the rod only touches the client's hair, the reading can be inaccurate.

k Record the height on your notepad or assignment sheet.

l Disinfect the scale platform after use, according to employer policy.

8 *Chair scale (mechanical):*

a Help the client transfer from the wheelchair to the chair scale (see the *Transferring the Client to a Chair or Wheelchair* procedure in Chapter 25). Ask for assistance if necessary.
This reduces the chance of the client falling.

A

B

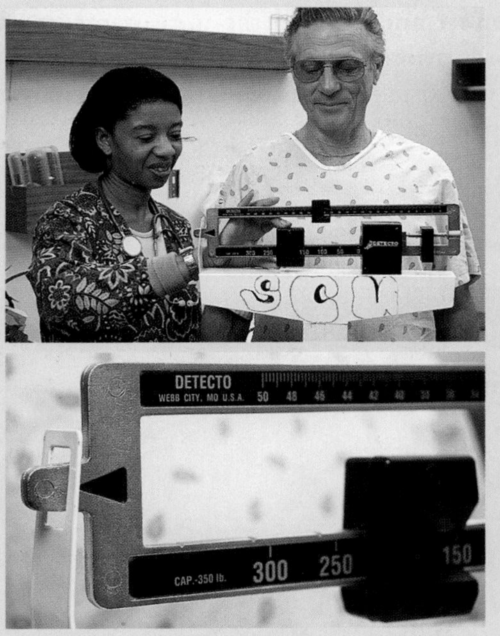

FIGURE 15–2 Using a mechanical scale. **A,** Adjust the weights. **B,** Read the weight when the balance pointer is in the middle.

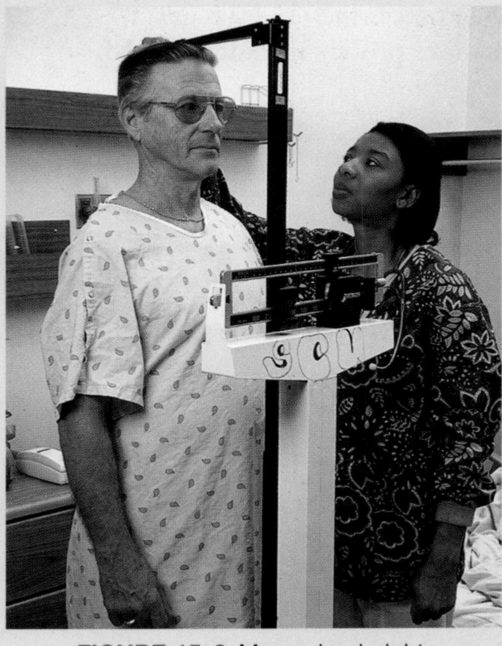

FIGURE 15–3 Measuring height.

Continued

Measuring Height and Weight—cont'd

- **b** Place the client's feet on the foot platform.
  This ensures an accurate reading.
- **c** Move the weights until the balance pointer is in the middle.
  If the scales are not balanced, the reading will not be accurate.
- **d** Record the weight on your notepad or assignment sheet

9 *Lift scale (mechanical):*

- **a** Attach the sling to the lift. Follow the manufacturer's instruction.
  This ensures the client's safety.
- **b** Place both weights on zero (0).
- **c** Level and balance the scale. Follow the manufacturer's instructions.
- **d** Remove the sling from the scale.
  This facilitates putting the sling on your client.
- **e** Place the client on the sling, and attach the sling to the lift. Raise the client about 10 cm (4 in.) off the bed (see the *Using a Mechanical Lift to Move a Client* procedure in Chapter 25).
  Raising the sling too high can increase your client's risk for injury in the case of a fall.
- **f** Move the weights until the balance pointer is in the middle.
  This ensures an accurate reading.
- **g** Record the weight on your notepad or assignment sheet.
- **h** Lower the client to the bed.
  The sling can be uncomfortable for the client.
- **i** Remove the sling.

10 Help the client dress if the client is up, or help the client back to bed.

POST-PROCEDURE

11 Provide for safety and comfort.

12 Place the call bell within reach.*
This provides an easy, safe way for the client to contact the staff if necessary.

13 If the client stays in bed, follow the care plan for bed rail use.*
This reduces the risk for a fall.

14 Remove privacy measures if used.

15 Return the scale to its proper place.
This makes it easier to find the next time it is needed.

16 Perform hand hygiene.

Report and Record the measurements and your observations, according to employer policy. Report any unusual measurements immediately to your supervisor.

*Steps marked with an asterisk may not apply in community settings.

Measuring Height: The Client in Bed

123

Advocate on Behalf of the Client's Quality of Life by Promoting:

Dignity • **I**ndependence • **P**references • **P**rivacy • **S**afety *(see BOX 1–4, on p. 17)*

PRE-PROCEDURE

1 Identify the client, according to employer policy.
This eliminates the possibility of mistaking one client for another.

2 Explain the procedure to the client.

3 Perform hand hygiene.

4 Collect the following supplies:

- ☐ **Measuring tape**
- ☐ **Ruler**

5 Ask for assistance. This procedure requires two people to obtain accurate measurements.

6 Provide for privacy.

Continued

Measuring Height: The Client in Bed—cont'd

PROCEDURE

7 Perform hand hygiene.
8 Have the client take the supine position if this position is allowed.
This ensures an accurate reading.
9 Have your helper hold the end of the measuring tape at the client's heel.
This ensures an accurate reading.
10 Pull the measuring tape alongside the client's body until it extends past the head (**FIGURE 15–4**).
This helps measure the client's height as if the person were standing.
11 Place the ruler flat across the top of the client's head. It should extend from the client's head to the measuring tape. Make sure the ruler is level.
If the ruler is not flat, the measurement will not be accurate.
12 Record the height on your notepad or assignment sheet.
This ensures accurate recording of the height when transferring the information to the client's record.

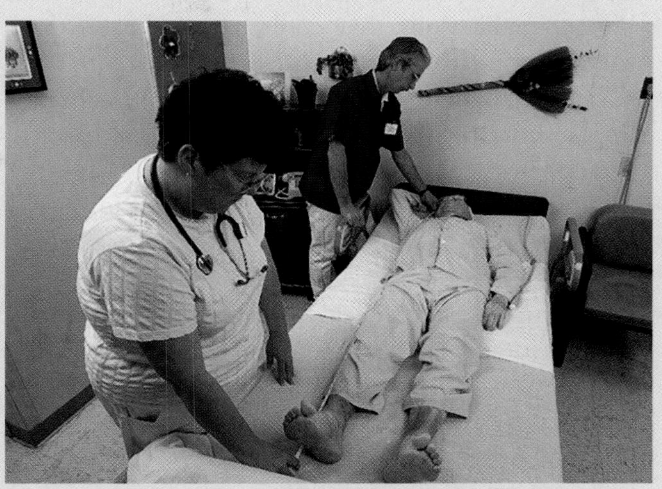

FIGURE 15–4 Measuring the height of a client in bed.

POST-PROCEDURE

13 Provide for safety and comfort.
14 Place the call bell within reach.*
This provides an easy, safe way for the client to contact the staff if necessary.
15 If the client stays in bed, follow the care plan for bed rail use.*
This reduces the risk for a fall.
16 Remove privacy measures if used.
17 Return the equipment to its proper location.
18 Perform hand hygiene.

Report and Record the height and your observations, according to employer policy. Report any abnormal reading immediately to your supervisor.

*Steps marked with an asterisk may not apply in community settings.

MEASURING AND REPORTING VITAL SIGNS

A person's vital signs can vary within certain limits, and they can be affected by medications, pain, illness, activity, exercise, sleep, foods, fluids, smoking, and emotions (e.g., excitement, anger, fear, and anxiety).

Vital signs are measured to detect changes in normal body function. They can indicate response to treatment and signal life-threatening events. Vital signs are part of the assessment process and are measured:

- During physical examinations
- When a client is admitted to a facility
- Several times a day for hospital clients and clients in subacute care units
- Before and after surgery

- Before and after complex procedures or diagnostic tests
- After certain care measures such as ambulation
- After a fall or other injury
- When medications that could affect the respiratory or circulatory system are taken
- Whenever the client complains of pain, dizziness, light-headedness, shortness of breath, rapid heart rate, or not feeling well
- As often as dictated by the client's condition
- As ordered by the doctor
- As stated on the care plan (usually daily or weekly)
- As instructed after the client has been given medication to relieve a fever

Vital signs reveal even minor changes in a client's condition. Accuracy is essential when you measure, record, and report vital signs. If you are unsure of the accuracy of your measurements, promptly ask your supervisor to take them again. Unless otherwise ordered, take vital signs with the client at rest and when the client is lying down or sitting. You should always compare any readings to the client's baseline reading. Immediately report:

- Any vital sign that is changed from a previous measurement
- Vital signs above the normal range
- Vital signs below the normal range

Employers have their own methods of recording vital signs. Some use graphic flow sheets, where the vital signs are graphed in red and blue inks. Some use books with pages divided into columns, where the information is recorded. Others record on the computer. Whatever system your employer uses, the following information must be clearly and accurately recorded:

- Client's name
- Date
- Time the vital sign was measured
- Vital sign measurement

Some employers require that changed or abnormal vital signs be circled in red or highlighted in some way. The nurse or physician compares current and previous measurements.

Vital signs recorded previously can help nurses and doctors compare current measurements.

BODY TEMPERATURE

Body temperature is the amount of heat in the body. It is a balance between the amount of heat produced from the client's metabolic rate and the amount of heat lost by the body. It remains within a normal, safe range when a person is healthy. Temperature normally changes slightly throughout the day and in response to different factors such as age, weather, exercise, pregnancy, the menstrual cycle, emotions, and stress. It is lower in the morning and higher in the afternoon and evening. Illness also affects body temperature, and temperatures above or below the normal range signal illness or health problems.

Temperature Sites

Temperature is measured using Centigrade/Celsius (°C). In the community setting, you may find that some clients have thermometers that show the temperature in Fahrenheit. To convert Fahrenheit to Celsius, subtract 32 from the Fahrenheit reading and then divide by 1.8 (e.g., 97.2°F=36.2°C). To convert Celsius to Fahrenheit, multiply the Celsius reading by 1.8 and then add 32.

Common sites for measuring temperature are as follows:

- Mouth (oral temperature)
- Underarm (axillary temperature—*axilla* means "underarm")
- Ear (tympanic temperature)

See the procedure *Taking Temperature With an Electronic Thermometer* on page 232 for direction on how to take oral, axillary, and tympanic temperature.

Body temperature can also be measured in the rectum (*rectal temperature*), but this site is rarely used. If a rectal temperature is required, a nurse or other regulated health care provider performs the procedure. Since taking a rectal temperature involves inserting an instrument into a body cavity, ***support workers are not authorized to take rectal temperatures.*** If you are delegated the procedure, you need to be properly trained and supervised.

Each body site has a normal range of temperature (TABLE 15–1), so check with your supervisor and the care plan to find out which site to use.

TABLE 15–1 Normal Body Temperature

Site	Average Temperature	Normal Range
Mouth (oral temperature)	37.0°C (98.6°F)	36°C–37.5°C (96.8°F–99.5°F)
Ear (tympanic temperature)	37.4°C (99.3°F)	35.8°C–38.0°C (96.4°F–100.4°F)
Underarm (axillary temperature)	36.5°C (97.7°F)	34.7°C–37.3°C (94.5°F–99.1°F)
Rectum (rectal temperature)	37.5°C (99.5°F)	35.5°C–38°C (95.9°F–100.4°F)

Older adults have lower body temperatures compared with younger people. A certain temperature may indicate fever in an older adult but may be a normal body temperature in a younger person. Always report temperatures that are not within the client's normal range. If a client demonstrates signs of a cold or infection (such as a runny nose, a congested cough, or a change in energy level), report these symptoms even if the client's body temperature seems to be normal.

Taking Oral Temperature

Oral temperature is *not* taken if the client:

- Is unconscious
- Has had surgery or an injury to the face, neck, nose, or mouth
- Has a nasogastric tube
- Is delirious, restless, confused, or disoriented
- Is paralyzed on one side of the body
- Has a sore mouth
- Has a convulsive disorder
- Is receiving oxygen therapy
- Breathes through the mouth and therefore does not close lips around the thermometer long enough for the temperature to register

Some activities can temporarily affect a client's temperature reading. Before taking an oral temperature, make sure the client has not done any of these activities within the previous 20 minutes:

- Eating hot or cold foods
- Drinking hot or cold fluids
- Smoking
- Chewing gum

Wait 15 to 20 minutes before taking temperature if resident has smoked

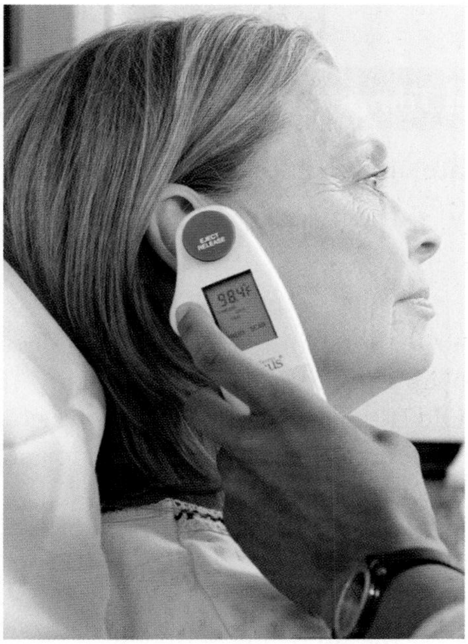

FIGURE 15–5 A tympanic thermometer. (**Source:** Sorrentino, S.A., & Gorek, B. (2011). *Mosby's textbook for long-term care nursing assistants* (6th ed., p. 480). St. Louis, MO: Mosby Elsevier.)

Taking Tympanic Temperature

If oral temperature cannot be taken, tympanic temperature is usually the next choice. Special thermometers are used for the ear (**FIGURE 15–5**). The temperature is measured in 1 to 3 seconds. Because temperature can be measured quickly and easily, tympanic temperature is often ordered for children and for clients with dementia (see the *Focus on Children: Taking Tympanic Temperature* box). Tympanic temperature is not taken if there is any drainage from the ear or if the client has complained of pain in that ear.

FOCUS ON CHILDREN

Taking Tympanic Temperature

The shape of a child's ear canal is different from that of an adult's. When taking tympanic temperature on a child, gently pull the child's ear down and forward, and insert the probe.

Taking Axillary Temperature

Using the axillary site is safe and noninvasive. It can be used in newborns and unconscious or uncooperative clients. Axillary temperature is less reliable than temperature taken by mouth or ear, so it is taken only when the other sites cannot be used. The axilla (underarm) must be dry. Do not use this site when the client has just had a bath. Axillary temperature is often taken on infants, very young children, and older adults (see the *Taking Temperature With an Electronic Thermometer* procedure).

Taking Temperature With an Electronic Thermometer 123

Advocate on Behalf of the Client's Quality of Life by Promoting:

Dignity • Independence • Preferences • Privacy • Safety *(see BOX 1–4, on p. 17)*

PRE-PROCEDURE

1 Identify the client, according to employer policy.

2 Explain the procedure to the client. The client should not have had anything to eat (including chewing gum), drink, or smoke for at least 20 minutes before the procedure.
Any of these activities may temporarily affect oral temperature reading.

3 Perform hand hygiene.

4 Collect the following supplies:
- ☐ **Electronic or digital thermometer**
- ☐ **Probe, if used—make sure you use the correct probe for the site**
- ☐ **Disposable plastic cover for thermometer or probe**
- ☐ **Tissues**
- ☐ **Towel (for axillary temperature)**

By collecting all the necessary equipment beforehand, you will not have to leave your client's side and can eliminate wasting time and energy in obtaining the forgotten equipment.

5 Plug the probe (if used) into the thermometer.

6 Provide for privacy.

PROCEDURE

7 Perform hand hygiene.

8 Position the client for oral, axillary, or tympanic temperature.
This ensures client comfort.

9 Insert the probe or thermometer tip into a disposable cover.
This decreases the risk of pathogen spread.

10 *For oral temperature:*

a Ask the client to open the mouth and raise the tongue. The thermometer will be placed under the tongue.

b Place the tip of the thermometer or probe at the base of the tongue (see **FIGURE 15–6**).
This is the warmest place in the mouth.

c Ask the client to lower the tongue and close the mouth. The mouth must remain closed. Remind the client not to talk or bite down on the thermometer or probe or talk while it is in place.
Breathing through the mouth can affect the accuracy of the reading. Biting down on the thermometer could break the thermometer.

Continued

Taking Temperature With an Electronic Thermometer—cont'd

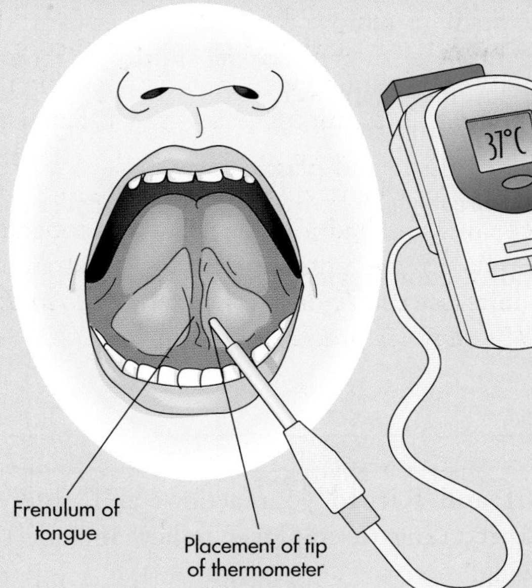

FIGURE 15–6 Place the thermometer at the base of the tongue.

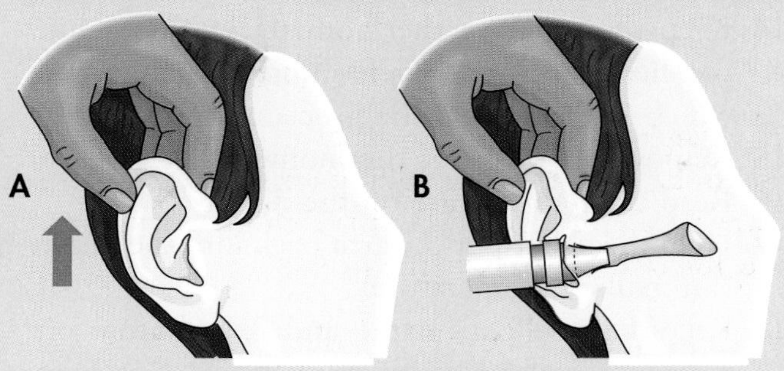

FIGURE 15–7 Taking an adult's tympanic temperature. **A,** Pull the ear up and back. **B,** Gently insert the probe into the ear canal.

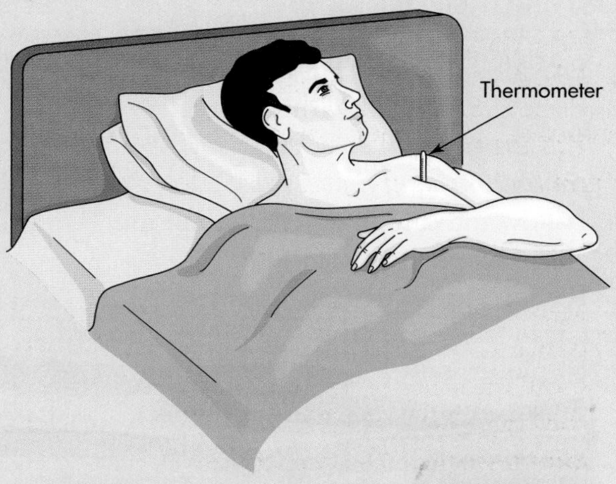

FIGURE 15–8 Taking the axillary temperature.

11 *For tympanic temperature:*

a Ask the client to turn the head so that the ear is in front of you. You need to be able to see the ear canal. If the client complains of a sore ear, do not insert the thermometer into that ear.
Inserting a thermometer into a sore ear can cause more discomfort to the client.

b Pull the ear up and back to straighten the ear canal (**FIGURE 15–7**). (In the case of children, pull the ear down and forward.)
The probe needs to be inserted into the ear canal.

c Insert the probe gently to avoid damaging the ear canal. The probe should seal the ear canal.

12 *For axillary temperature:*

a Help the client remove the arm from the sleeve. Do not expose the client.

b Dry the axilla with the towel.
This removes perspiration, which can interfere with the reading.

c Place the tip of the thermometer or probe in the centre of the axilla, pointing upward. Make sure the tip of the probe is in contact with the client's skin.
Contact is needed to ensure an accurate reading.

d Ask the client to place the arm over the chest to hold the thermometer or probe in place (**FIGURE 15–8**). Hold the arm in place if the client cannot do it. With children, it may be helpful to hold the child while taking the temperature, both to keep the thermometer in place and to comfort the child.
Moving the probe around can affect the reading accuracy.

13 Turn on the thermometer.

Continued

Taking Temperature With an Electronic Thermometer—cont'd

14 Keep the probe or thermometer in place until you hear a tone or see a flashing or steady light, which indicates that the procedure is finished.
15 Remove the probe or thermometer.
16 Read the temperature on the display.
17 Help the client put the arm back into the sleeve (for axillary temperature).
18 Record the client's name and temperature on your notepad or assignment sheet. Note the temperature site.
19 Use tissue to remove the plastic cover from the thermometer, or press the eject button to remove the plastic probe cover.
This decreases the risk of pathogen spread.
20 Discard tissue and plastic cover.
It is more hygienic to use a new plastic cover each time.
21 Perform hand hygiene.

POST-PROCEDURE

22 Provide for safety and comfort.
23 Place the call bell within reach.*
This provides an easy, safe way for the client to contact the staff if necessary.
24 Follow the care plan for bed rail use.*
This reduces the risk for a fall.
25 Remove privacy measures if used.
26 Clean and store the equipment, according to employer policy. Return electronic thermometer to the battery charging unit.
This keeps the battery charged for the next time it is needed.
27 Perform hand hygiene.

Report and Record your actions and observations, according to employer policy. Include the following:

- ☐ Temperature (note: Abnormal temperatures should be reported immediately.)
This could indicate an illness or another health issue.
- ☐ Site (*A* for axillary, *T* for tympanic, *O* for oral)
The ranges of normal readings are different for each site.

*Steps marked with an asterisk may not apply in community settings.

Thermometers

A variety of thermometers are available. Most facilities and agencies use electronic thermometers as well as disposable ones. Dot matrix thermometers and temperature-sensitive tape are also used. Glass thermometers are considered safety hazards and are now rarely used in any setting.

Thermometers can spread microbes, so protective disposable plastic covers are usually applied over the thermometer before use (**FIGURE 15–9**). Thermometers must always be cleaned, dried, and stored according to employer policy and the manufacturer's recommendations. Some employers require that thermometers be cleaned with a disinfectant such as alcohol before and after use. Always follow medical

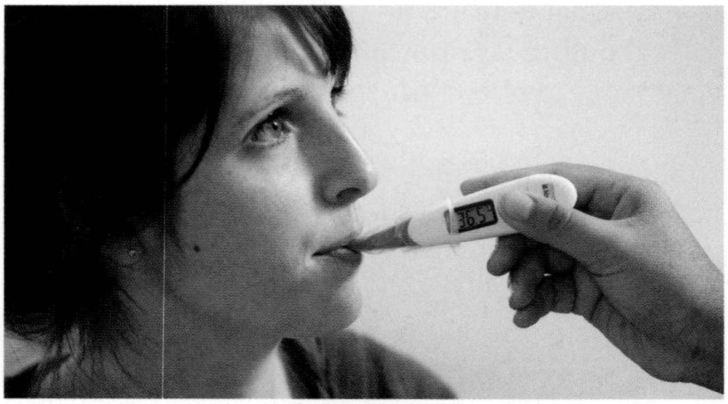

FIGURE 15–9 A disposable plastic cover over the thermometer probe helps prevent the spread of microbes. A fresh cover must be used for each client. (Courtesy of Brian Hillier.)

asepsis and Standards of Nursing Practice when using thermometers. Special thermometers are used for patients in isolation. Follow your employer's policies.

Electronic Thermometers

Electronic thermometers are battery operated. They measure temperature within 20 to 50 seconds and display a digital readout of the temperature. Some electronic thermometers consist of a handheld unit and a probe that is inserted into the unit (**FIGURE 15–10**). An electronic thermometer that has a low battery charge will not record temperature accurately. After using an electronic thermometer, replace it securely in the battery charging unit. Make sure the battery charging unit is plugged into an electrical outlet.

Electronic thermometers with probes can be used for any site, and the probes may be changed, depending on the site. Tympanic thermometers are electronic thermometers with probes made to fit in the ear canal (see **FIGURE 15–5,** on p. 231).

Electronic thermometers emit a tone or flashing light when the temperature reading is complete.

Electronic thermometers that are one-piece devices are called *digital thermometers*. They have a temperature-sensitive tip on one end and an on/off button on the other end. They display a digital readout of the temperature. Some have a memory mechanism that recalls the last temperature reading. The battery is not rechargeable, but the device shuts off after about 10 minutes. These thermometers may be used to take oral or axillary temperature. They are inserted into covers before use (**FIGURE 15–11**). Digital thermometers are used more in home care settings than in facilities (see the *Focus on Children: Special Thermometers* box).

Dot Matrix Thermometers

Dot matrix thermometers are thin plastic strips with small chemical dots on one end (**FIGURE 15–12**). The dots change colour when heated by the body. Each dot must be heated to a certain temperature before it changes colour. These thermometers are useful to measure oral and axillary temperature and are not for

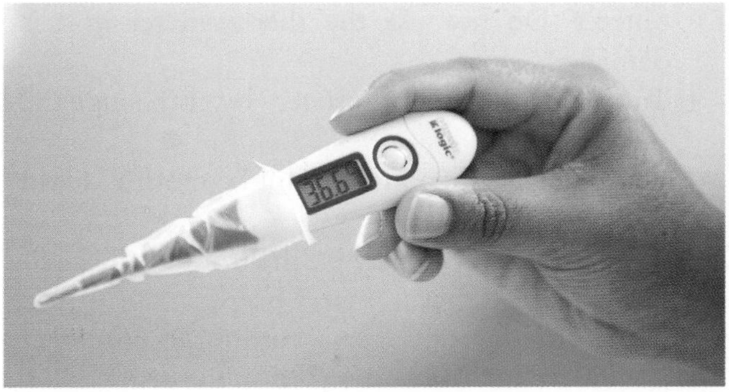

FIGURE 15–11 A digital thermometer. (Courtesy of Brian Hillier.)

A

B

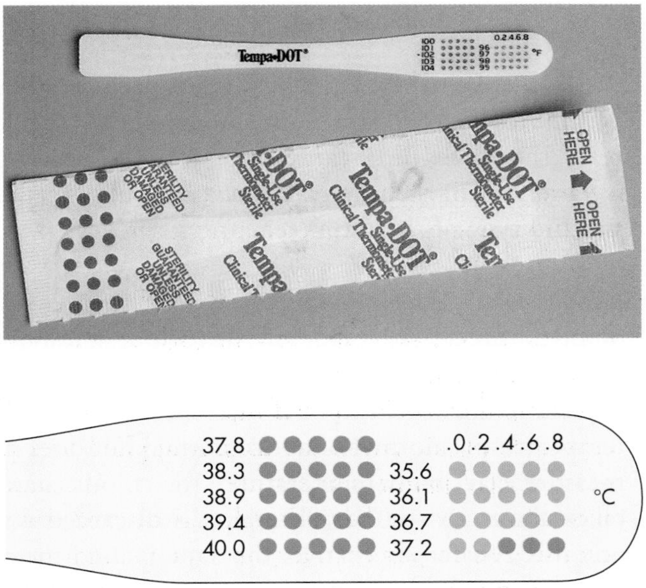

FIGURE 15–12 A, Single-use dot matrix thermometer with chemical dots. **B,** The dots change colour when the temperature is taken.

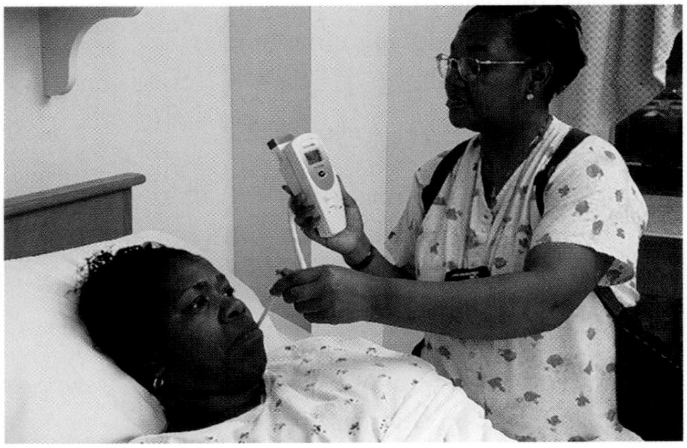

FIGURE 15–10 An electronic thermometer with a handheld unit and probe.

FOCUS ON CHILDREN

Special Thermometers

Pacifier thermometers are a type of electronic thermometer used for infants and toddlers. They are available in stores for home use. The pacifier thermometer has four parts: (1) a storage cover, (2) a nipple with a sensor, (3) a digital display, and (4) an on/off switch. Temperature is measured in about 5 minutes.

To use the thermometer:

- Remove it from the storage case.
- Check the pacifier for cracks or holes. These can occur if the child bites or chews on the thermometer. Do not use the thermometer if it is damaged.
- Turn on the thermometer by pressing the switch.
- Place the pacifier in the child's mouth. Hold and cuddle the child.
- Read the digital display on the front of the pacifier when the thermometer beeps.
- Clean the thermometer according to employer policy. Do not use boiling water, the dishwasher, or a sterilizer to clean the thermometer.
- Wipe the thermometer dry.
- Return it to the storage case.

use in the ear. They must be left in place for about 3 minutes before an accurate temperature can be read. They must be discarded after one use. This type is used when the caregiver has difficulty reading another type of thermometer.

Temperature-Sensitive Tape

Temperature-sensitive tape changes colour in response to body heat (**FIGURE 15–13**). When the tape is applied to the forehead or abdomen, it shows if the temperature is normal or above normal but does not measure exact body temperature. The colour change takes about 15 seconds. The tape is discarded after one use. A safer alternative, this tape is used mostly on young children who are unable to follow instructions.

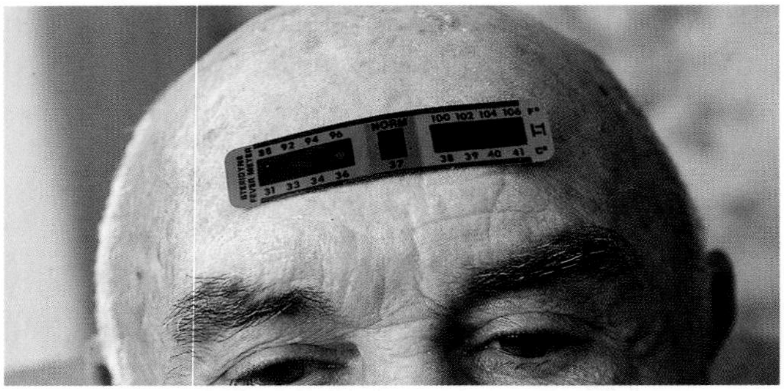

FIGURE 15–13 Temperature-sensitive tape.

PULSE

Pulse is the beat of the heart felt at an artery as a wave of blood passes through the artery. The pulse is felt every time the heart beats (see Chapter 17 for information about the structure and function of the heart and blood vessels.)

Sites for Taking the Pulse

You can feel the pulse by placing your fingertips over certain sites on the body. The temporal, carotid, brachial, radial, femoral, popliteal, dorsalis pedis (pedal), and posterior tibial pulses are felt on both sides of the body (**FIGURE 15–14**). The pulse is easy to feel at these sites because the arteries are close to the body's surface and lie over a bone.

To take the pulse, support workers often use the radial site because it is easy to reach and find and because the pulse can be taken without disturbing or exposing the client. The carotid pulse (in adults and children) and the brachial pulse or apical pulse (in infants) are taken during emergencies.

Rate and Rhythm of the Pulse

Pulse rate is the number of heartbeats or pulses felt in 1 minute. The rate varies for each age group (TABLE 15–2) and is affected by many factors, including the following:

- Elevated body temperature (caused by fever or exposure to hot environments)
- Exercise

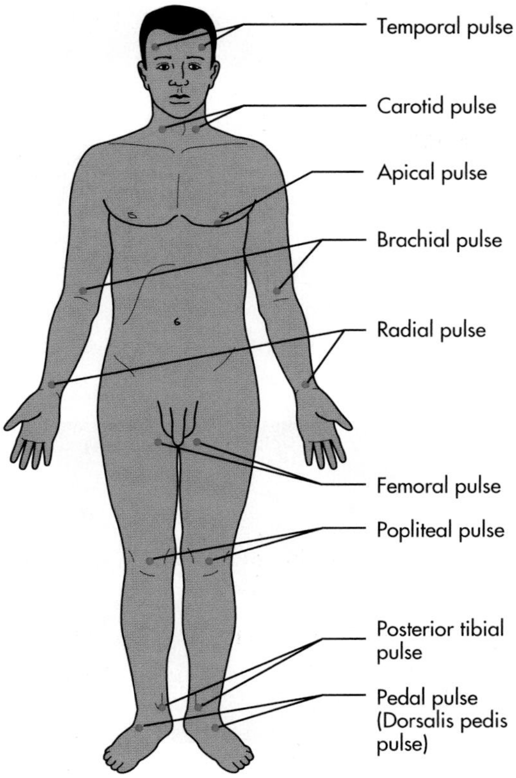

FIGURE 15–14 The pulse sites.

TABLE 15–2 Pulse Ranges According to Age

Age	Pulse Rate (Beats Per Minute)
Infant	120–160
Toddler	90–140
Preschooler	80–110
School-aged child	75–100
Adolescent	60–100
Adult	60–100

- Pain
- Position change (pulse rate temporarily increases when a client sits or stands after lying down)
- Caffeine
- Emotions (excitement, fear, anger, anxiety)
- Medications (can speed up or slow down the pulse)

The rhythm of the pulse should be regular; that is, the pulse should be felt in a pattern, and the same interval should be felt between beats. An irregular pulse occurs when the beats are unevenly spaced or beats are skipped. An abnormal rhythm—called **dysrhythmia**—must be reported at once.

A rate of less than the low end or more than the high end is not normal. Report abnormal rates and rhythms at once:

- **Tachycardia** is a rapid (*tachy*) heart rate (*cardia*). For example, the heart rate is over 100 beats per minute in an adult.
- **Bradycardia** is a slow (*brady*) heart rate (*cardia*). For example, the heart rate is less than 60 beats per minute in an adult.
- Irregular pulse rates will vary in pulse pattern or depth from beat to beat. If the client's pulse is irregular, it is important to take the pulse for a full 60 seconds and to record and report the pulse as irregular.

You need to know the client's normal pulse range. Immediately report pulse rates that are higher or lower than normal for that client or irregular.

Force of the Pulse

The force of the pulse relates to its strength. A forceful pulse is easy to feel and is described as *strong*, *full*, or *bounding*. The hard-to-feel pulse is described as *weak*, *thready*, or *feeble*.

Electronic blood pressure equipment (see p. 243) can also count the beats and shows the pulse rate along with blood pressure. However, it does *not* give information about pulse rhythm and force, which can be determined only by feeling the pulse.

Taking the Radial Pulse

The radial pulse is one of the routine vital signs you will have to take (see the *Taking the Radial Pulse* procedure).

Taking the Radial Pulse

123

Advocate on Behalf of the Client's Quality of Life by Promoting:

Dignity • Independence • Preferences • Privacy • Safety

(see BOX 1–4, on p. 17)

PRE-PROCEDURE

1 Identify the client, according to employer policy.
2 Explain the procedure to the client.
3 Perform hand hygiene.
4 Provide for privacy.

PROCEDURE

5 Have the client sit or lie down.
The heart works a bit harder when the client is standing.

6 Locate the radial pulse by placing your first two or three middle fingers against the client's radial artery, which is on the thumb side of the client's wrist (see **FIGURE 15–15**).
Your thumb has a pulse; by using your middle fingers to locate the client's pulse, you will not mistake your pulse for the client's.

7 Using a watch or clock with a second hand, count the beats for 30 seconds. Multiply the number obtained by two. Or count the beats for 1 minute if required by employer policy.
The length of time you take the pulse depends on agency policy.

8 Count the beats for 1 minute if the pulse is irregular.
This ensures a more accurate reading than taking it for 30 seconds.

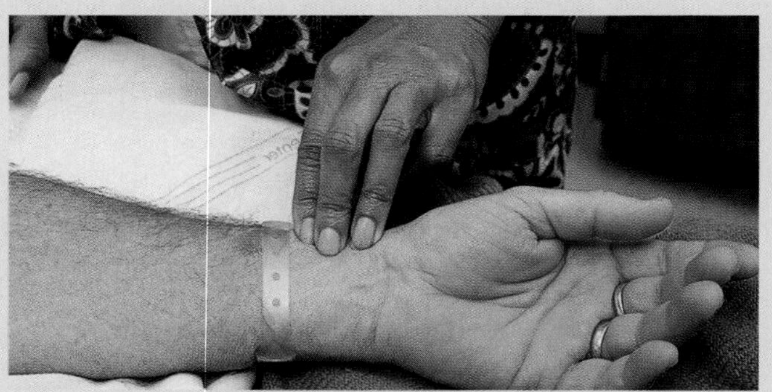

FIGURE 15–15 Taking the radial pulse.

9 Record the client's name and pulse rate on your notepad or assignment sheet. Note the strength of the pulse. Note if it was regular or irregular.
This will help ensure accurate information is reported on the client's record and avoid your forgetting some of the details.

POST-PROCEDURE

10 Provide for safety and comfort.
11 Place the call bell within reach.*
This provides an easy, safe way for the client to contact the staff if necessary.
12 Remove privacy measures if used.
13 Perform hand hygiene.

Report and Record the pulse rate (beats per minute), pulse force (strong, full, bounding, weak, thready, or feeble), pulse rhythm (regular or irregular), the time of day you took the pulse, and your observations, according to employer policy. ***Report immediately to your supervisor if the pulse is less than 60 or more than 100 beats per minute for an adult client, or if it is higher or lower than normal for the client.***

*Steps marked with an asterisk may not apply in community settings.

Using a Pulse Oximeter

A **pulse oximeter** (**FIGURE 15–16**) is a device that measures both a client's pulse rate and the oxygen level in the blood. The device is held in place on a client's index finger using a clothespin-like hinge clip (see the *Measuring the Pulse and Oxygen Concentration Using a Pulse Oximeter* procedure). It works by shining a light beam through the skin to the blood vessels below. The oxygen level in the client's blood is expressed as the percent (%) of oxygen saturation, or **SpO_2**. A 100% reading means that the red blood cells visible in the pulse oximeter's light are fully loaded with oxygen from the lungs. *SpO_2* stands for "peripheral capillary oxygen saturation."

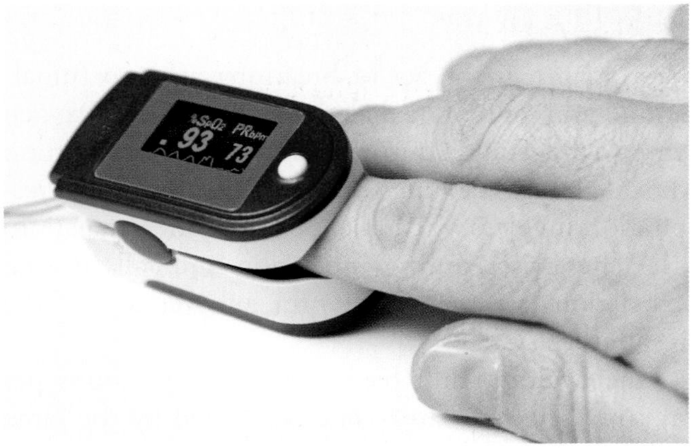

FIGURE 15–16 A pulse oximeter placed with the sensor over the client's index fingernail. (**Source:** Juan R. Velasco/ Shutterstock.com)

Measuring the Pulse and Oxygen Concentration Using a Pulse Oximeter 123

Advocate on Behalf of the Client's Quality of Life by Promoting:

Dignity • Independence • Preferences • Privacy • Safety *(see BOX 1–4, on p. 17)*

PRE-PROCEDURE

1 Identify the client, according to employer policy.
2 Explain the procedure to the client.
3 Perform hand hygiene.
4 Provide for privacy.
5 Ensure the client does not have nail polish or acrylic nail enhancements.
The use of nail polish or acrylic nail enhancements can cause inaccurate readings.

PROCEDURE

6 Have the client sit or lie down.
The heart works a bit harder when the client is standing.
7 Turn the pulse oximeter unit on. Clip the pulse oximeter over the client's index finger with the sensor centred over the client's fingernail (see **FIGURE 15–16**).
Do not place the pulse oximeter over the client's thumbnail, because the readings are less reliable with that digit.
8 Observe both the pulse reading (indicated in beats per minute, or bpm) and the client's oxygen level (indicated in percentage).

POST-PROCEDURE

9 Provide for safety and comfort.
10 Place the call bell within reach.*
This provides an easy, safe way for the client to contact the staff if necessary.
11 Remove privacy measures if used.
12 Perform hand hygiene.

Report and Record the pulse rate and the blood concentration level, the time of day you took these, and your observations, according to employer policy. You need to know the client's normal pulse rate, as you need to report a higher or lower rate immediately. ***Any blood concentration level reading below 95% should be reported to the supervisor.***

*Steps marked with an asterisk may not apply in community settings.

RESPIRATIONS

Respiration is the act of breathing air into (inhalation) and out of (exhalation) the lungs. Oxygen enters the lungs during inhalation, and carbon dioxide leaves the lungs during exhalation. Each respiration involves one inhalation and one exhalation. The chest rises during inhalation and falls during exhalation (see Chapter 17 for an overview of the respiratory system).

The healthy adult has 12 to 20 respirations per minute. The respiratory rate is affected by the same factors that affect temperature and pulse. For example, infections, heart disease, and respiratory diseases usually increase the respiratory rate.

Respirations are normally quiet, effortless, and regular. Both sides of the chest rise and fall in a uniform manner. If the chest barely moves during respiration, the breathing is described as shallow. Deep breathing occurs when the chest rises and falls significantly with every breath (see Chapter 41 and Chapter 46 for a description of abnormal respiratory patterns).

Count respirations when the client is at rest. Position the client so that you can see the chest rise and fall. To a certain extent, a client can control the depth and rate of breathing. Clients tend to change breathing patterns when they know their respirations are being counted, so try to count respirations without making the client aware of what you are doing.

Respirations are counted right after taking the pulse (see the *Counting Respirations* procedure). Keep your fingers over the pulse site and maintain the pressure so that the client believes you are still taking the pulse. To count respirations, watch the chest rise and fall. Count how many times the chest rises and falls in 30 seconds. Remember, the rise *and* fall of the chest together is counted as one respiration. Multiply the number by two for the number of respirations in 1 minute. If an abnormal pattern is noted, count the respirations for 1 minute.

Respiratory rates vary according to age (TABLE 15–3). Infants and children have higher respiratory rates than adults do. Count an infant's respiratory rate for 1 minute.

TABLE 15–3 Normal Respiratory Rates by Age

Age	Respirations per Minute
Newborn	30–60
Infant	25–50
Toddler	25–32
Child and preadolescent	20–30
Adolescent	16–19
Adult	12–20

Source: Potter, P.A., Perry, A.G., Stockert, P.A., et al. (2014). *Canadian fundamentals of nursing* (5th ed., p. 490). Toronto, ON: Reed Elsevier.

Counting Respirations 123

Advocate on Behalf of the Client's Quality of Life by Promoting:

Dignity • Independence • Preferences • Privacy • Safety *(see BOX 1–4, on p. 17)*

PROCEDURE

1 Continue to hold the client's wrist after taking the radial pulse.
This ensures a smooth transition from taking the pulse to counting respirations without alerting the client.

2 Do not tell the client you are counting respirations.
A client who is aware that respirations are being counted may begin to change her breathing pattern, which can affect the accuracy of the count.

Continued

Counting Respirations—cont'd

3 Begin each count when the chest rises and end when the chest falls. Count each rise and fall of the chest as one respiration.
Counting an inhalation and an exhalation as two respirations will result in a false count.

4 Note the following:
- ☐ If respirations are regular
- ☐ If both sides of the chest rise uniformly
- ☐ The depth of the respirations
- ☐ If the client has pain or difficulty breathing

Any irregularities in these observations could indicate illness or health problems for your client, so report them immediately to your supervisor.

5 Count the respirations for 30 seconds. Multiply the number by two. Follow your employer's policy.
If the respirations are regular, they do not change after 30 seconds.

6 Count respirations for 1 minute if they are abnormal or irregular.
This ensures a more accurate reading.

7 Record respiratory rate and other observations on your notepad or assignment sheet.
This ensures accurate recording of information on the client's record.

POST-PROCEDURE

8 Provide for safety and comfort.
9 Place the call bell within reach.*
10 Perform hand hygiene.

Report and Record your actions, the time of day you took the respirations, and your observations, according to employer policy.
Actions and observations should be recorded and reported for legal reasons and to keep the rest of the health care team informed.

*Steps marked with an asterisk may not apply in community settings.

Report and record the following observations after counting respirations:

- Respiratory rate
- Uniformity and depth of respirations (shallow, normal, or deep)
- Respiratory rhythm—regular or irregular
- Pain or difficulty breathing
- Any respiratory noises
- Any abnormal respiratory patterns (see Chapter 41)

BLOOD PRESSURE

Blood pressure is the amount of force exerted by the blood against the walls of an artery. Blood pressure is controlled by:

- The force of heart contractions
- The amount of blood pumped with each heartbeat
- How easily the blood flows through the blood vessels

The period of heart muscle contraction is called **systole**, and the period of heart muscle relaxation is called **diastole**.

Both the systolic and diastolic pressures are measured. The **systolic pressure**, which is the higher pressure, represents the amount of force needed to pump blood out of the heart into the arterial circulation. The **diastolic pressure**, which is the lower pressure, reflects the pressure in the arteries when the heart is at rest.

Blood pressure is measured in millimetres (mm) of mercury (Hg). The systolic pressure is recorded over the diastolic pressure. The average adult has a systolic pressure of 120 mm Hg and a diastolic pressure of 80 mm Hg. This reading is written as 120/80 mm Hg.

The role of the support worker in taking blood pressure can vary from employer to employer and

average 120/80 normal 100-140/60-90

BOX 15–1 Factors Affecting Blood Pressure

- ***Age.*** Blood pressure increases with age. It is lowest in infancy and childhood and highest in adulthood.
- ***Gender.*** Women usually have lower blood pressures compared with men, but blood pressures tend to rise in women after menopause.
- ***Blood volume.*** *Blood volume* is the amount of blood in the system. Severe bleeding lowers the blood volume and thus the blood pressure. Giving intravenous (IV) fluids rapidly increases the blood volume, raising the blood pressure as a result.
- ***Stress.*** Stress, including anxiety, fear, and other emotions, can increase blood pressure as the body responds.
- ***Pain.*** Generally, pain increases blood pressure. However, severe pain can cause shock, which can seriously lower blood pressure (see Chapters 12 and 37).
- ***Exercise.*** Physical activity increases blood pressure; therefore, blood pressure should not be measured immediately after exercise.
- ***Weight.*** Blood pressure is higher in overweight people and is lowered by weight loss.
- ***Ethnicity.*** Blood pressure tends to be higher among Canadians of South Asian, Indigenous, or African descent.
- ***Diet.*** A high-sodium diet increases the amount of water in the body, and the extra fluid volume, in turn, increases blood pressure.
- ***Medications.*** Medications can be given to raise or lower blood pressure. Other medications can cause high or low blood pressure as an adverse effect.
- ***Position.*** In clients who are on blood pressure medication, blood pressure may be lower when lying down and higher when standing. Sudden position changes can cause sudden changes in blood pressure (*orthostatic hypotension*). When a person stands suddenly, a rapid drop in blood pressure can occur, causing dizziness and fainting (see Chapter 26).
- ***Smoking.*** Smoking increases blood pressure. The nicotine in cigarettes causes blood vessels to narrow, making the heart work harder to pump blood through narrowed vessels.
- ***Alcohol.*** Excessive alcohol intake can raise blood pressure.

province to province. Ensure you are aware of your employer's policy.

Factors Affecting Blood Pressure

Blood pressure can change from minute to minute and can be affected by a number of factors (BOX 15–1). Because blood pressure can vary so easily, normal blood pressure has been assigned a range of values:

- Systolic pressure—normal range is between 100 and 140 mm Hg
- Diastolic pressure—normal range is between 60 and 90 mm Hg

Persistent measurements above the normal ranges of systolic and diastolic pressures are considered abnormal, and the condition is referred to as **hypertension** (see Chapter 37). According to the Heart and Stroke Foundation of Canada, blood pressure that is consistently more than 140/90 mm Hg is considered high, but in clients with diabetes, 130/80 mm Hg is considered high. Normal blood pressure is below 120/80 mm Hg. In young and middle-aged adults, report any systolic pressure above 140 mm Hg at once. Also, report if the diastolic pressure is above 90 mm Hg. Likewise, systolic pressure below 90 mm Hg and diastolic pressure below 60 mm Hg must be reported, as low readings can be a condition referred to as **hypotension**. Low blood pressure may be normal in some clients, but hypotension may be a sign of a life-threatening problem (see the *Focus on Children: Blood Pressure* and *Focus on Older Adults: Blood Pressure* boxes.)

Equipment

A sphygmomanometer and stethoscope are used to measure blood pressure. Before using any equipment, make sure you have been properly trained to use it. Follow the manufacturer's instructions and employer policy.

Sphygmomanometer

A **sphygmomanometer** is an instrument used to measure blood pressure. It consists of a blood pressure cuff and a measuring device (*manometer*). In some provinces and territories, support workers are allowed to use only electronic blood pressure machines. There are three types of manometers:

- ***Aneroid manometer***—has a round dial and a needle that points to the calibrations (see **FIGURE 15–17, *A***). These may be used in all settings. Many hospitals have wall-mounted mercury manometers in patient rooms.
- ***Mercury manometer***—has a column of mercury within a calibrated tube (see **FIGURE 15–17, *B***). Some settings use portable mercury manometers because they are easy to read; however, mercury is a hazardous substance. If a mercury manometer breaks, call for your supervisor at once. Do not touch the mercury, and do not let the client touch it. If possible, remove the client from the area. The facility or agency must follow special procedures for handling all hazardous materials (see Chapter 22).

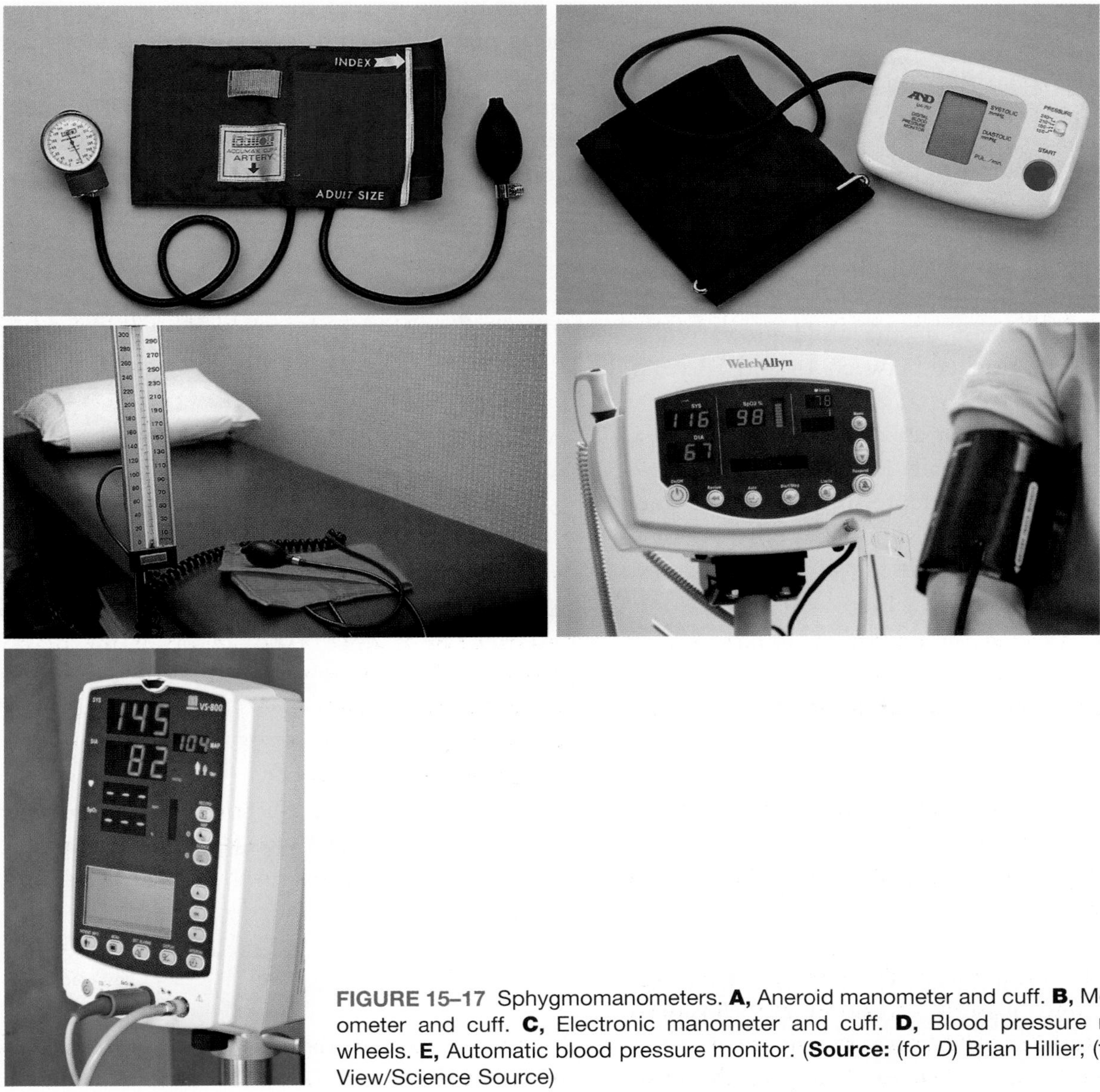

A B C D E

FIGURE 15–17 Sphygmomanometers. **A,** Aneroid manometer and cuff. **B,** Mercury manometer and cuff. **C,** Electronic manometer and cuff. **D,** Blood pressure machine on wheels. **E,** Automatic blood pressure monitor. (**Source:** (for *D*) Brian Hillier; (for *E*) Life in View/Science Source)

- ***Electronic manometer***—automatically displays the blood pressure measurement on the front of the device (see **FIGURE 15–17, *C***). The pulse rate is usually also displayed. The cuff automatically inflates and deflates on some models; some have only automatic deflation. Electronic manometers are common in facilities, and they are also available for home use. (**FIGURE 15–17, *D***, shows a blood pressure machine on wheels.)

The blood pressure cuff is wrapped around the upper arm of the client. A tube connects the cuff to the manometer, and another tube connects the cuff to a small handheld bulb. A valve on the bulb is turned so that the cuff inflates as the bulb is squeezed. The inflated cuff causes pressure over the brachial artery. The valve is turned the other way for cuff deflation, and blood pressure is measured as the cuff is deflated.

The right cuff size is important for accuracy. Children and clients with very small arms may need pediatric blood pressure cuffs, and those with very large arms may need extra-large cuffs.

Stethoscope

A **stethoscope**—an instrument used to listen to the sounds produced by the heart, lungs, and other body organs (**FIGURE 15–18**)—amplifies the sounds for easy hearing.

One of the uses of the stethoscope is to measure blood pressure. Sounds are produced as blood flows through the arteries, and the stethoscope is used to listen to these sounds in the brachial artery as the cuff is deflated. Stethoscopes are not needed with electronic sphygmomanometers.

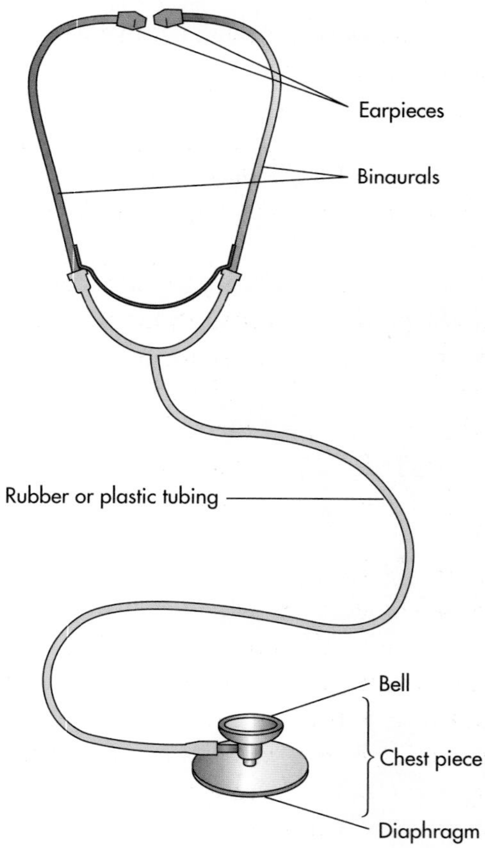

FIGURE 15–18 Parts of a stethoscope.

FOCUS ON CHILDREN

Blood Pressure

Infants and children normally have lower blood pressure values compared with adults (as is the case with other vital signs). A newborn's blood pressure is usually about 70/55 mm Hg. By 1 year of age, blood pressure increases to 90/55 mm Hg and continues to increase as the child grows older. Adult levels are reached between 14 and 18 years of age.

Taking an infant's or child's blood pressure is a complex task, as it usually involves special equipment. Measuring blood pressure in infants and children is, therefore, beyond a support worker's scope of practice, and the task should be the responsibility of a nurse.

FOCUS ON OLDER ADULTS

Blood Pressure

With aging, arteries narrow and lose their elasticity, so the heart has to work harder to pump blood through the vessels. As a result, both the systolic and diastolic pressures are higher in older adults—a blood pressure of 160/90 mm Hg is considered normal for most older adults. It should be noted that older adults are at risk for orthostatic hypotension (see Chapter 26).

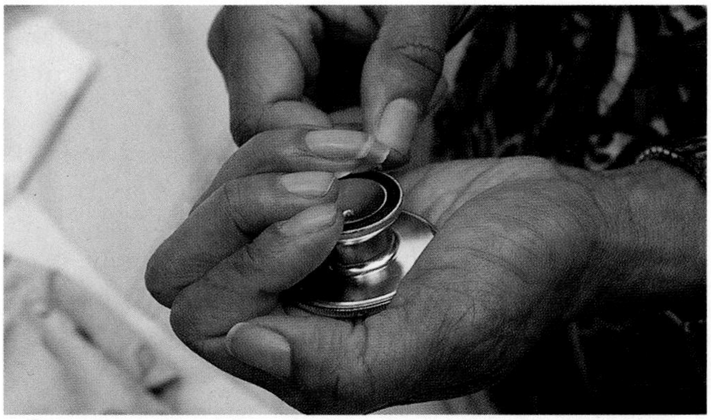

FIGURE 15–19 Warm the diaphragm of the stethoscope in the palm of your hand.

Stethoscopes come in contact with the skin of many clients and health care team members during use, so infection control is important. To prevent the spread of microbes, the earpieces and diaphragm must be cleaned before and after each use using disinfectant wipes or products recommended by your facility or agency. If you will routinely use a stethoscope, purchase your own device and keep it solely for your personal use.

Follow these measures when using a stethoscope to measure blood pressure:

- Wipe the earpieces and diaphragm with antiseptic wipes before and after each use.
- Warm the diaphragm in your hand before touching the client with it (FIGURE 15–19).
- Place the earpiece tips in your ears. The bend of the tips should point forward. Earpieces should fit snugly to block out external noises. They should not cause pain or discomfort. Note: Some people find they hear better if they adjust the stethoscope ear tip angle by raising the tubing or by lowering their chin with the ear tips inserted in the ear canals.
- Place the diaphragm over the client's brachial artery, and hold it in place (see FIGURE 15–20, C).
- Prevent noise. Do not let anything touch the tubing. Ask the client to remain silent while the blood pressure is being measured.
- If the tubing of the stethoscope has touched anything, it should be thoroughly cleaned with a disinfectant wipe before it is returned to its proper storage place.

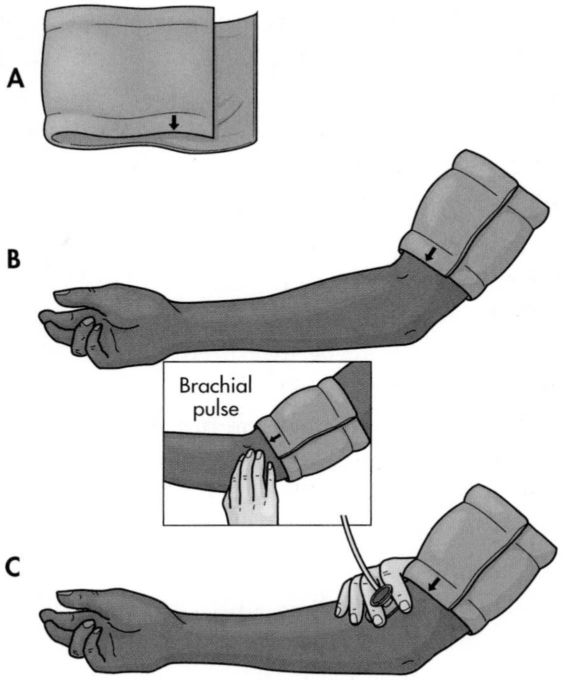

FIGURE 15–20 Measuring blood pressure using a stethoscope and sphygmomanometer. **A,** An arrow on the cuff marks the cuff's placement in relation to the brachial artery. **B,** Apply the cuff over the brachial artery. **C,** Place the diaphragm of the stethoscope over the brachial artery.

Measuring Blood Pressure

Measuring blood pressure is a delegated act in some provinces, territories, agencies, and facilities. Whenever you are asked to measure a client's blood pressure, it is very important to be accurate. Any change in blood pressure will affect the care plan for your client. If your care plan includes taking blood pressure, ensure the following:

- Your employer allows you to perform this procedure.
- The procedure is in your job description.
- You have received special training.
- You have reviewed the procedure with a nurse.
- A nurse is available to answer questions and to supervise you.

As mentioned earlier, blood pressure is normally measured in the brachial artery. BOX 15–2 lists the guidelines for measuring blood pressure (see also the *Measuring Blood Pressure Using a Stethoscope and Sphygmomanometer* and *Measuring Blood Pressure Using an Electronic Blood Pressure Machine* procedures).

BOX 15–2 Guidelines for Measuring Blood Pressure

- Do not take blood pressure on an arm with an intravenous (IV) infusion, a cast, or a dialysis access site. If a client has had breast surgery, do not take blood pressure on that side. Avoid taking blood pressure on an injured arm.
- Allow the client to rest for 10 to 20 minutes before measuring blood pressure.
- Measure blood pressure with the client sitting or lying down, unless the physician has ordered blood pressure to be measured with the client in the standing position.
- Use the correct-sized blood pressure cuff for each client. For example, use a pediatric cuff for a very small arm.
- Apply the cuff to the bare upper arm. Remove any clothing that can affect the measurement.
- Make sure the cuff is snug, as loose cuffs can cause inaccurate readings.
- Place the diaphragm of the stethoscope firmly over the artery. The entire diaphragm must be in contact with the skin.
- Make sure the room is quiet. Talking, TV, radio, and sounds from the hallway can affect an accurate measurement.
- Ensure that the manometer is clearly visible.
- Measure the systolic and diastolic pressures. Expect to hear the first blood pressure sound at the point where you last felt the radial or brachial pulse. The first sound is the systolic pressure, and the point where the sound disappears is the diastolic pressure (see **FIGURE 15-21**).
- Take the blood pressure again if you are not sure of an accurate measurement. Wait 30 to 60 seconds before repeating the measurement.
- Notify your supervisor at once if you cannot "hear" the blood pressure.
- Know the normal blood pressure ranges for the client. Immediately report any blood pressure measurement above or below the client's normal range.

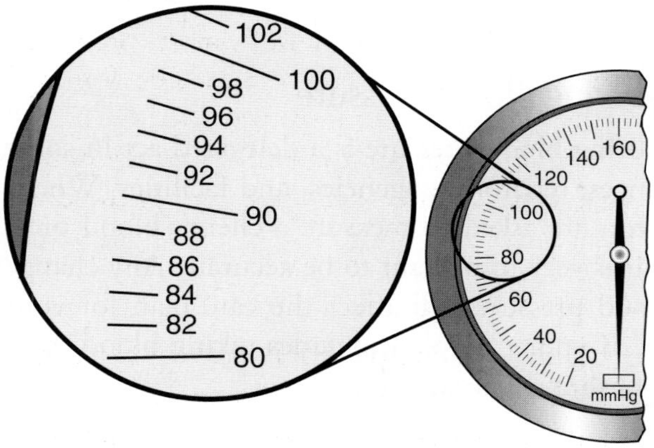

FIGURE 15–21 Reading the manometer. Long lines mark 10 mm Hg values. Short lines mark 2 mm Hg values.

Measuring Blood Pressure Using a Stethoscope and Sphygmomanometer 123

Advocate on Behalf of the Client's Quality of Life by Promoting:

Dignity • Independence • Preferences • Privacy • Safety *(see BOX 1–4, on p. 17)*

PRE-PROCEDURE

1 Identify the client, according to employer policy.
2 Explain the procedure to the client.
3 Perform hand hygiene.
4 Collect the following supplies:
- ☐ **Sphygmomanometer (blood pressure cuff)**
- ☐ **Stethoscope**
- ☐ **Antiseptic wipes**

By collecting all the necessary equipment beforehand, you will not to have leave your client's side and can eliminate wasting time and energy in obtaining the forgotten equipment.

5 Provide for privacy.
6 Perform hand hygiene.

Continued

Measuring Blood Pressure Using a Stethoscope and Sphygmomanometer—cont'd

PROCEDURE

7 Clean the stethoscope earpieces and diaphragm with antiseptic wipes.

8 Have the client sit or lie down. Ensure the client's legs are not crossed. Make sure the room is quiet and relaxing. Ask the client not to speak while you measure the blood pressure.
To get an accurate reading, ensure that your client is as relaxed as possible and that you are able to hear the pulse.

9 Choose the client's nondominant arm for taking the blood pressure unless this arm has been injured or has an intravenous inserted into it. Position the client's arm level with the heart. The palm should be face up.
This is most comfortable for the client and the best position for an accurate reading.

10 Stand no more than 1 m (3 ft) away from the manometer. A mercury model must be vertical, on a flat surface, and at eye level. The aneroid type must be directly in front of you.
You will need to have a clear view of the reading.

11 Expose the client's upper arm.
This is where you will place the cuff.

12 Squeeze the cuff to expel any remaining air. Close the valve on the bulb.
Not expelling all the air can affect the reading.

13 Find the brachial artery at the inner aspect of the elbow.
This is the usual site for taking blood pressure.

14 Place the arrow on the cuff over the brachial artery. Wrap the cuff around the upper arm at least 2.5 cm (1 in.) above the elbow. It should be even and snug (see **FIGURE 15–20**).
If the cuff is uneven or loose, the reading will not be accurate.

15 ***Follow your employer's policies.***

a Place the stethoscope earpieces in your ears.

b Locate the radial or brachial pulse.
These arteries are the most accurate sites to measure blood pressure.

c Inflate the cuff until you can no longer feel the pulse.
This ensures that you will get an accurate reading.

d Inflate the cuff 30 mm Hg beyond the point where you last felt the pulse.
This ensures that you will hear the first pulse beat as you deflate the cuff.

e Deflate the cuff slowly. Note the point when you feel the pulse.
If you deflate too quickly, you may miss noting when you first feel the pulse.

f Note the point where you hear the first sound. This is the systolic reading. It should be near the point where the radial pulse disappeared (see **FIGURE 15-21**).

g If the readings are different from the previous readings for the client, report this finding immediately to your supervisor.

h Continue to deflate the cuff. Note the point where the sound disappears. This is the diastolic reading.
Deflate the cuff slowly so that you do not miss the sound.

16 Deflate the cuff completely. Remove it from the client's arm. Remove the stethoscope.

17 Record the client's name and blood pressure on your notepad or assignment sheet.
Actions and observations should be recorded and reported for legal reasons and to keep the rest of the health care team informed.

18 Return the cuff to the case or wall holder.
This keeps the equipment safe and makes it easier to find the next time it is needed.

Continued

Measuring Blood Pressure Using a Stethoscope and Sphygmomanometer—cont'd

POST-PROCEDURE

19 Provide for safety and comfort.
20 Place the call bell within reach.*
21 Remove privacy measures if used.
22 Clean the earpieces and diaphragm with the wipes.
23 Return the rest of the equipment to its proper place.
24 Perform hand hygiene.

Report and Record the blood pressure, the time of day you took the blood pressure, and your observations, according to employer policy.
Other members of your team will need to be aware of the time you took the blood pressure, as it is important to take it at the same time every day unless your supervisor has requested a change. Your team members will need to compare their readings with yours.

*Steps marked with an asterisk may not apply in community settings.

Measuring Blood Pressure Using an Electronic Blood Pressure Machine 123

Advocate on Behalf of the Client's Quality of Life by Promoting:
Dignity • Independence • Preferences • Privacy • Safety (see BOX 1–4, on p. 17)

PRE-PROCEDURE

1 Identify the client, according to employer policy.
2 Explain the procedure to the client.
3 Perform hand hygiene.
4 Collect the following:
☐ **Blood pressure machine** (FIGURE 15–22)
☐ **Antiseptic wipes, as per agency policy**
By collecting all the necessary equipment beforehand, you will not to have leave your client's side and can eliminate wasting time and energy in obtaining the forgotten equipment.
5 Provide for privacy.

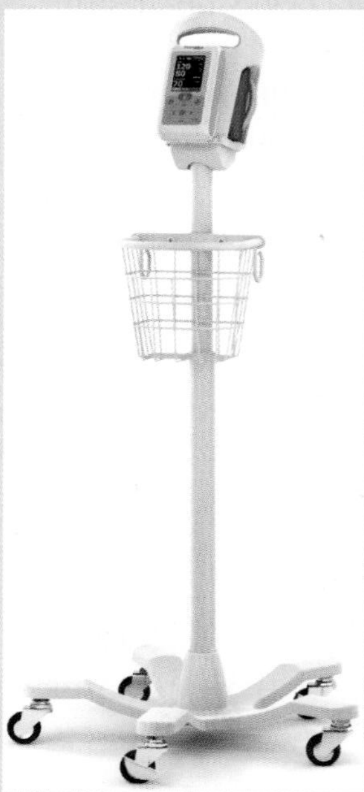

FIGURE 15–22 A blood pressure machine. (**Source:** Potter, P.A., & Perry, A.G., Stockert, P.A., et al. (2014). *Canadian fundamentals of nursing* (5th ed., p. 531). Toronto, ON: Reed Elsevier.)

Continued

Measuring Blood Pressure Using an Electronic Blood Pressure Machine—cont'd

PROCEDURE

6 Clean the surface of the cuff that will be placed next to the client's skin.
7 Perform hand hygiene.
8 Have the client sit or lie down. Make sure the room is quiet and relaxing. Ask the client not to speak while you measure the blood pressure.
To get an accurate reading, ensure that your client is as relaxed as possible and that you are able to hear the pulse.
9 Choose the client's nondominant arm for taking the blood pressure unless this arm has been injured or has an intravenous inserted into it. Position the client's arm level with the heart. The palm should face up.
This is most comfortable for the client and the best position for an accurate reading.
10 Stand close to the client (no more than 1 m [3 ft] away from the blood pressure machine).
You will need to have a clear view of the reading.
11 Expose the client's upper arm.
This is where you will be placing the cuff. Placing the cuff over clothing can give an inaccurate reading.
12 Find the brachial artery at the inner aspect of the elbow.
This is the usual site for taking blood pressure.
13 Place the arrow on the cuff over the brachial artery (see **FIGURE 15–20**, on p. 245). Wrap the cuff around the upper arm at least 2.5 cm (1 in.) above the elbow. It should be even and snug.
If the cuff is uneven or loose, the reading will not be accurate. These arteries are the most accurate sites to measure blood pressure.
14 Instruct the client to relax the arm. Press the On button on the blood pressure machine.
15 Wait for the entire cycle to occur. The finished blood pressure reading will appear on the screen.
16 Remove the cuff from the client's arm.
17 Offer to gently massage the client's arm.
The inflated cuff temporarily interferes with blood return to the heart. The client's arm may temporarily feel tingly or sore.
18 Record the client's name and blood pressure on your notepad or assignment sheet. If the readings are different from the previous readings for the client, report this finding immediately to your supervisor.
Actions and observations should be recorded and reported for legal reasons and to keep the rest of the health care team informed.
19 Return the cuff to the case or wall holder.
This keeps the equipment safe and makes it easier to find the next time it is needed.

POST-PROCEDURE

20 Provide for safety and comfort.
21 Place the call bell within reach.*
22 Remove privacy measures if used.
23 Clean the stethoscope's earpieces and diaphragm with the wipes.
24 Return the rest of the equipment to its proper place.
25 Perform hand hygiene.

Report and Record the blood pressure, the time you took the blood pressure, and your observations, according to employer policy.
Other members of your team will need to be aware of the time you took the blood pressure, as it is important to take it at the same time every day unless your supervisor has requested a change. Your team members will need to compare their readings with yours.

*Steps marked with an asterisk may not apply in community settings.

CHAPTER REVIEW

KEY POINTS

- Vital signs are measured to detect changes in normal body functions. They can indicate response to treatment and signal life-threatening events.
- Vital signs reveal even minor changes in a client's condition. Accuracy is essential when you measure, record, and report vital signs.
- Body temperature normally changes slightly throughout the day. Temperatures above or below your client's normal reading can indicate illness or other health problems.
- A variety of thermometers are available. Agencies will determine the type to use for each client.
- Pulse rate is the number of heartbeats heard in 1 minute. It varies with age and can be affected by a number of factors. The force of the pulse relates to its strength.
- To take the pulse, support workers often use the radial site. Any irregular pulse should be counted for 1 full minute to obtain the most accurate reading.
- Support workers may use a pulse oximeter to measure both a client's pulse rate and the oxygen level in the blood.
- Respirations are normally quiet, effortless, and regular. Normal respiratory rates vary with age. Abnormal rates can indicate illness or health issues in all ages.
- Blood pressure is the amount of force exerted by the blood against the walls of an artery. Blood pressure can change from minute to minute and can be affected by a number of factors.
- The period of heart contraction is called *systole*, and the period of heart muscle relaxation is called *diastole*. Measuring blood pressure is a delegated act in many areas. Ensure you know your scope of practice and your employer's policies.

CRITICAL THINKING IN PRACTICE

You measure an adult patient's vital signs. The pulse is 110. The respiratory rate is 24. The oral temperature is 38°C. You think you heard the blood pressure at 86/52. You are unsure of the measurement. What will you do? Which, if any, of these vital signs are abnormal? What must you do?

REVIEW QUESTIONS

Answers to these questions are at the bottom of page 251.

Circle the BEST answer.

1. The following statements are about measuring weight. Which one is true?
   A. Before lunch is the best time to weigh the client.
   (B.) Chair and lift scales are used to weigh clients who cannot stand.
   C. A digital scale should read "12" before the client is weighed.
   D. A full bladder does not affect weight measurement.

2. Which of the following statements is true?
   A. The vital signs are temperature, pulse, respirations, blood pressure, and SpO_2s.
   B. Vital signs cannot indicate changes in body function.
   C. Vital signs change only during illness.
   D. Sleep, exercise, medications, emotions, and noise do not affect vital signs.
   E. None of the above.

3. Which of the following should you report at once?
   A. An oral temperature of 37.4°C
   B. A tympanic temperature of 38.2°C
   C. An axillary temperature of 36.1°C
   D. An oral temperature of 36.6°C

4. You must take an infant's temperature. The care plan will likely tell you to take:
   A. An oral temperature with a glass thermometer
   B. A rectal temperature
   C. An oral temperature with a tympanic thermometer
   D. An axillary temperature

5. Which thermometer is rarely used in health care settings?
   A. Digital
   B. Glass
   C. Electronic
   D. Dot matrix

6. Which pulse location is generally used to take a pulse?
   A. The radial site
   B. The apical–radial site
   C. The apical site
   D. The brachial site

7. Which of the following must be reported to your supervisor at once?
   A. An adult has a pulse rate of 120 beats per minute.
   B. An infant has a pulse rate of 130 beats per minute.
   C. An adult has a pulse rate of 80 beats per minute.
   D. An adult has a pulse rate of 64 beats per minute.

8. The following describe normal adult respirations. Which one is true?
   A. There are between 8 and 12 per minute.
   B. They are quiet and effortless.
   C. They are irregular with both sides of the chest rising and falling uniformly.
   D. Noises occur on inhalation.

9. Respirations are usually counted:
   A. After taking the temperature
   B. After taking the pulse
   C. Before taking the pulse
   D. After taking the blood pressure

10. Which blood pressure is normal for an adult?
    A. 88/54 mm Hg
    B. 210/100 mm Hg
    C. 130/82 mm Hg
    D. 152/90 mm Hg

11. When taking the blood pressure, you should:
    A. Use the arm with an intravenous (IV) infusion
    B. Apply the cuff to a bare upper arm
    C. Turn on the TV or radio
    D. Locate the aortic artery

12. Which is the systolic blood pressure?
    A. The point where the pulse is no longer felt
    B. The point where the first sound is heard
    C. The point where the last sound is heard
    D. The point 30 mm Hg above where the pulse was felt

Answers: 1.B, 2.A, 3.B, 4.D, 5.B, 6.A, 7.A, 8.B, 9.B, 10.C, 11.B, 12.B

Chapter opener image: bikeriderlondon/Shutterstock.com

CHAPTER 16

Abuse Awareness

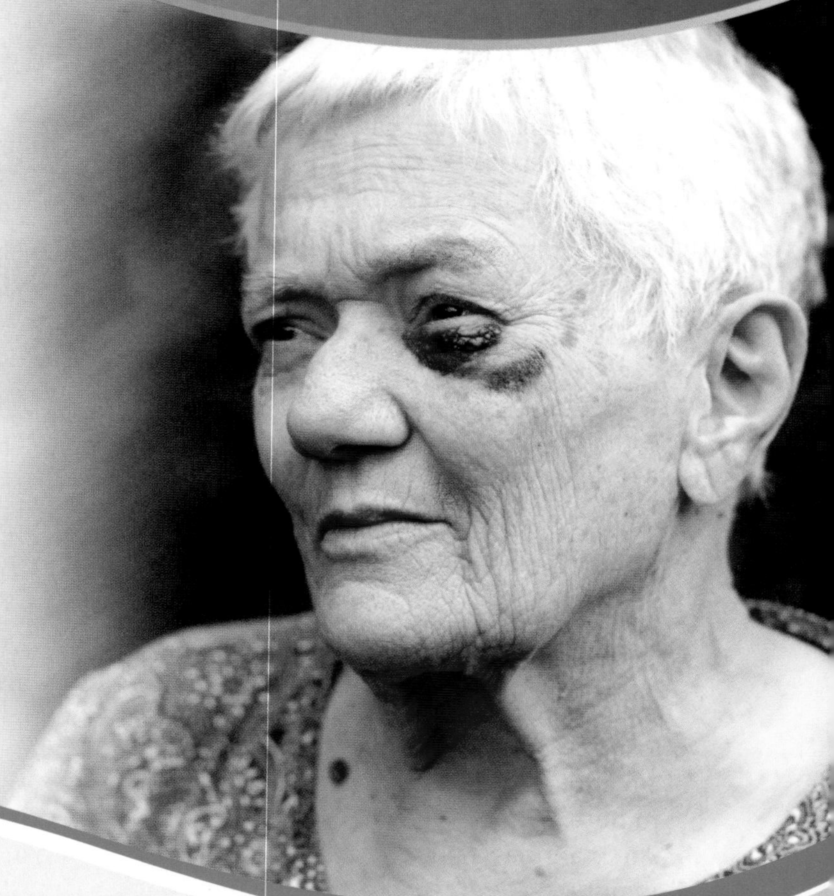

OBJECTIVES

After reading this chapter, the learner should be able to do the following:

- Identify the legal act that is meant to protect all Canadians, new immigrants, and visitors from abuse.
- Describe the types of abuse.
- Describe the cycle of abuse.
- Describe spousal abuse, child abuse, and abuse of older adults.
- Describe how clients and health care workers can be abused.
- Explain what to do if you have an abusive client.
- Identify signs of abuse.
- Explain your legal responsibilities when reporting abuse.
- Describe what to do if a client tells you about being abused.
- Apply the information in this chapter to your clinical practice properly.

KEY TERMS

abuse Physical or mental harm caused by someone in a position of trust. p. 253
child abuse Mistreatment or neglect of a child by a parent, guardian, or caregiver. p. 259
child neglect Failure by a child's parents or other caregivers to meet the child's basic needs for emotional, psychological, and physical development. p. 260
emotional abuse Words or actions that cause mental harm, especially on a person's self-esteem. Also known as **psychological abuse**. p. 254
emotional neglect Failure to meet a person's need to feel loved, wanted, safe, and worthy. p. 260
failure to thrive A term to describe infants, babies, or children who are below the norms for body weight, growth, or cognitive development. p. 260
financial abuse The misuse of a person's money or property. p. 254
marginalized Prevented from having any power or control over one's life or health care because of language, life circumstances, or role in society, resulting in being shunned from mainstream society. p. 257
neglect The state of being uncared for physically, emotionally, or psychologically. p. 254
physical abuse The deliberate application of force to any part of another person's body, which may result in a nonaccidental injury and sometimes death. p. 259
physical neglect Failure to adequately meet a dependant's need for food, clothing, shelter, cleanliness, medical care, and protection from harm. p. 260
psychological abuse See **emotional abuse**. p. 254
sexual abuse Any nonconsensual sexual act (including touching) that results from a threat, coercion, or force. p. 254
sexual harassment Any conduct, comment, gesture, threat, or suggestion that is sexual in nature; a form of **sexual abuse**. p. 254
spousal abuse Abuse of a partner by a partner in an intimate relationship such as a marriage or common-law relationship. p. 256
workplace bullying Acts or verbal comments that could mentally "hurt" or isolate a person in the workplace. p. 267

The Canadian government has enacted laws to protect people from abuse and discrimination of any kind. In Chapter 10, we discussed each person's right to be treated with respect and the need to accept people's differences at all times. Showing respect for all clients is especially important in the field of support work. It is an unfortunate truth, however, that some support workers do not recognize that ***all clients have the right to safe, respectful treatment***. When clients' rights are ignored, the clients become victims of abuse.

Abuse results when physical or mental harm is caused by someone in a position of trust, such as a family member, partner, or caregiver. Unlike random acts of violence, which take place in all societies, *abuse* implies a relationship between the abuser and the abused. The abuser has power and control over the abused, and often, the victim is physically, emotionally, or financially dependent on the abuser. Abuse occurs in all age groups, at all social levels, in all cultures, and in all races. It can occur in community settings and in health care facilities. As a support worker, you must know how to recognize and report suspected abuse.

In this chapter, we will discuss the Canadian Charter of Rights and Freedoms, which is the foundation for all of the country's laws that make abuse illegal. We will also discuss (1) the types of abuses, (2) persons who are at highest risk for abuse, and (3) ways to recognize and to report abuse.

CANADIAN CHARTER OF RIGHTS AND FREEDOMS

The basic human rights of Canadians, immigrants, and even visitors to Canada are protected by law. Since 1982, the most important protection has been the Canadian Charter of Rights and Freedoms, which states that Canada values equality and diversity and that no one should be abused and no one has the right to treat others unfairly. Knowingly failing to comply with the Charter is illegal and can be considered abuse.

The Charter also requires everyone—including government, the police, the courts, and all Canadians—to respect the basic human rights of others.

Because of the Charter, people living in Canada have many basic rights and freedoms (**BOX 16–1**).

TYPES OF ABUSE

There are many ways in which people can abuse others, and more than one type of abuse can occur at the same time. The different types of abuse are as follows:

- ***Physical abuse*** is force or violence that causes pain, injury, and sometimes death. Physical abuse includes pinching, hair pulling, pushing, slapping, hitting, shaking, choking, biting, or kicking. It also includes burning, poisoning, using weapons, or throwing things (e.g., a chair or a hammer) at someone.
- **Sexual abuse** is unwanted sexual activity such as rape and attempted rape. Unwanted touching, fondling, kissing, and exposure (i.e., the abuser showing his or her genitals to the victim) are also considered sexual abuse. **Sexual harassment**—another form of sexual abuse—is any conduct, comment, gesture, threat, or suggestion that is sexual in nature.
- **Emotional abuse** (**psychological abuse**) occurs through words or actions that cause mental harm. It usually involves an attack on a person's self-esteem—for example, constantly insulting, humiliating, or rejecting a person, or saying that she is "stupid" or "bad." All of these can harm the person's sense of worth and self-confidence. Emotional abuse can happen to infants, children, teens, adults, and older adults.
- Emotional abuse lessens the victim's dignity and self-worth because he or she is called names, yelled at, insulted, mocked, threatened, or sworn at. The victim may be ignored for long periods or may not be allowed to do preferred activities or visit with family, friends, or others. Threatening to harm someone or something that the victim loves (such as a child or a pet) is another example of emotional abuse.
- **Financial abuse** is the misuse of a person's money or property, usually for the abuser's financial gain. Financial abuse includes stealing, forging signatures, selling property or possessions without permission, and persuading or tricking victims to change their wills or give up control of their finances. Some abusers do not allow their victims access to their own money.
- **Neglect** is failure to meet the basic needs of a dependent person. Victims of neglect are usually children, people with disabilities, and frail older adults. Neglect occurs when a clean, comfortable, and safe environment is not provided. In some cases, the caregiver may even withhold or deny basic needs such as food, water, or clothing. Personal care, medical care, education, and attention and love may also be denied or withheld. The caregiver may knowingly neglect the victim or unintentionally neglect the person because of an inability to provide adequate care.

THE CYCLE OF ABUSE

Abuse usually occurs over and over again, as the abuser tries to dominate the victim with power and control. It often follows a pattern, known as the cycle of abuse (**FIGURE 16–1**). There are three phases in the cycle.

1. ***The tension-building phase.*** Tension starts to build between the abuser and the victim. Everyday events and comments irritate and anger the abuser. As the abuser becomes more angry and stressed, he grows more aggressive. The victim may try to calm, soothe, and please the abuser, stay out of the abuser's way, or try not to say or do anything that might anger or upset the abuser.
2. ***The abusive phase.*** Tension explodes into an abusive event. The abuse may involve neglect or physical, sexual, emotional, or financial abuse. Often, the abuse is triggered by an event unrelated to the victim's behaviour.
3. ***The honeymoon phase.*** The abuser feels ashamed or sorry. He apologizes and promises never to do it again. He may offer gifts or be very loving and attentive. At this stage, the abuser and victim may both believe that the abuser can change.

If specific measures are not taken to stop the cycle of abuse, it continues. There may be days, weeks, months, or years between abusive events. Usually, the

BOX 16–1 The Rights and Freedoms of All Canadians

The Canadian Charter of Rights and Freedoms (1982) ensures that all Canadians, new immigrants, and visitors to Canada have the following rights:

- ***Fundamental Freedoms.*** This section includes the rights to freedom of conscience and religion; freedom of thought, belief, opinion, and expression, including freedom of the press and other media of communications; and freedom of peaceful assembly and association.

  Therefore, Canadians, new immigrants, and visitors to Canada have the right to practise the religion of their choice and express their views without fear of being punished in any way. They can also voice their opinions in print (e.g., in a newspaper or pamphlet), in person, or on the Internet, radio, or television. We all have the right to choose who we want to communicate with (or not), and we can join together in a *peaceful* manner to express our opinions (e.g., to go on strike or to demonstrate in front of a building by holding up placards).
- ***Equality Rights.*** This section includes the rights to equal treatment before and under the law and equal benefit and protection of the law without discrimination based on race, national or ethnic origin, colour, religion, gender, age, and mental or physical disability. Other grounds of discrimination that were not specifically set out in the Charter, such as sexual orientation and marital status, were recognized in 1985.

  We are all considered equal, and nobody can get poorer (or special) treatment because of their differences.
- ***Democratic Rights.*** These sections contain the right to vote, the right to run for public office, and the maximum duration of legislative bodies.
- ***Mobility.*** This section ensures the right to move from place to place within Canada and ensures that Canadian citizens are free to enter and leave Canada as they please. It also gives citizens and permanent residents the right to move to and live in any province.
- ***Legal Rights.*** These sections set out the rights that protect us in our dealings with the justice system. These rights ensure that individuals who are involved in legal proceedings are treated fairly, especially those charged with criminal offences, and include the rights:
  - To have life, liberty, and security of the person
  - To be secure from unreasonable search and seizure
  - To be free from unnecessary detention or imprisonment
  - To be informed promptly of reasons for any arrest or detention
  - To retain and instruct counsel on arrest or detention
  - To be tried within a reasonable time by an impartial tribunal
  - To be presumed innocent
  - To have protection against self-incrimination
  - To be free from cruel and unusual treatment or punishment
  - To have the assistance of an interpreter
- ***Language Rights.*** These sections confirm that English and French are the official languages of Canada and assert the equality of the French and English languages in particular situations. The language rights include the right to use English or French in Parliament and in any court established by Parliament, including the Supreme Court of Canada. Federal laws must be published in both English and French.
- ***Minority Language Education Rights.*** This section establishes that provincial governments must provide certain English- or French-language minority rights. Minority language education applies when there is a sufficient number of eligible children to justify providing schooling in that language.

Source: Canadian Charter of Rights and Freedoms, s. 2, Part I of the Constitution Act, 1982, being Schedule B to the Canada Act 1982 (UK), 1982, c 11.

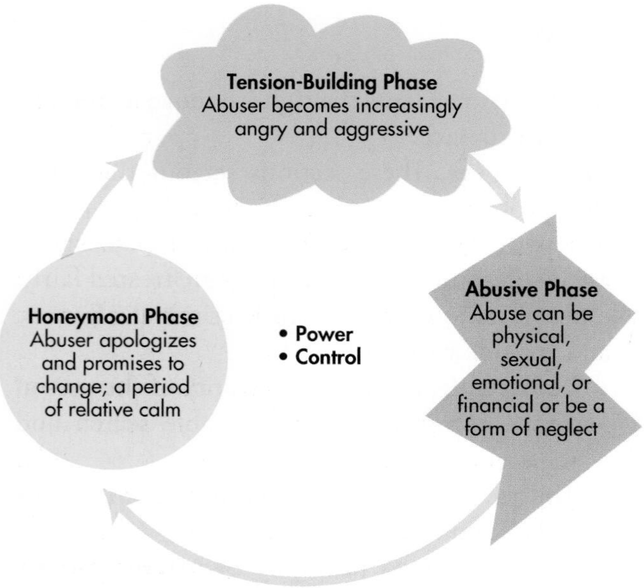

FIGURE 16–1 The cycle of abuse.

time between episodes gradually shortens, and the abuse becomes more frequent and more intense. It is important for the victim and abuser to recognize the problem and get help to stop the cycle.

RECOGNIZING THE SIGNS OF ABUSE

As a support worker, you are responsible for recognizing the signs of abuse. These signs generally apply to all abusive relationships in all settings. However, you are not qualified to judge whether or not your client is being abused. You may think you recognize one or some of the signs (see the *Think About Safety: Signs and Symptoms of Abuse* box), but such signs do not always mean that abuse has occurred. These signs might, however, suggest that abuse is a possibility.

Watch for signs of abuse or neglect in the course of your daily work with your clients. Immediately report any suspicions or observations to your supervisor. Your supervisor will ensure that the situation is investigated. Know your employer's procedures on reporting observations or suspicions.

ABUSIVE RELATIONSHIPS

Abuse can occur in many different kinds of relationships. An abuser can be a caregiver, such as a parent, child, grandparent, step-parent, or relative. Sometimes, the abuser is a nonrelative who is close to the person, such as a family friend or a parent's or adult child's partner. All age groups are at risk and are equally likely to be victims. Abuse occurs in all types of families: rich and poor, educated and uneducated. Both women and men can be abused by their spouses or partners; children can be abused by their parents; older adults can be abused by their adult children; clients can be abused by health care workers; and health care workers can be abused by their clients (**BOX 16–2**).

Abusive relationships are complex, and there is usually no single cause for the abuse. In most cases of abuse by the caregiver, the abuse has been triggered when the abuser felt overwhelmed and felt that no help was available to care for their physically or mentally challenged child or dependent parent. However, in all relationships, a person is more likely to be abusive if he or she:

- Has problems with alcohol or drugs
- Has a mental illness (for example, major depression) or severe personality flaws (for example, an explosive temper, inability to control impulses, or lack of empathy for others)
- Was abused as a child
- Is going through a period of high stress, such as divorce, unemployment, poverty, or illness

Spousal Abuse

Spousal abuse is abuse that occurs between intimate partners in a marriage or common-law relationship and may be physical, sexual, emotional, or financial. Usually, more than one type of abuse is present in the relationship. Spousal abuse is abuse in any love-partner relationship, including same-sex relationships.

Both women and men can be abused by their partners. However, women are usually more severely injured than men are. The incidence of male abuse in a man–woman relationship is not as well known, because in many cases, the male is less likely to report this abuse. Domestic violence rates among intimate couples usually increase when the woman is pregnant or caring for an infant.[1]

Why Do They Stay?

People who are abused by their partner often deny the abuse. They also often choose to stay with their

BOX 16–2 Persons at Highest Risk for Abuse

Even though potentially anybody could be abused (or, for that matter, be an abuser, given the right circumstances), there are certain groups of people that are *especially* at risk for being abused. Abuse may damage such persons' sense of self-worth and dignity and increase their social isolation, making them even more vulnerable to abuse. Also, abused persons may be unable to access (or not know about) support systems that are available. These people include:

- ***Marginalized persons (especially women).*** Those who (1) do not speak an official language, (2) belong to a visible-minority group, (3) are geographically isolated, (4) have a physical or intellectual disability, (5) have a mental health disorder, (6) have (or had) a substance abuse problem, or (7) work in the sex trade are considered to be **marginalized**; that is, they are prevented from having any power or control—because of their language (one other than English or French), their life circumstances (including poverty), or their role in society—and are shunned by mainstream society because of it.

  People who are marginalized are usually treated as though they were "invisible," and they often feel powerless to report abuse, or they may not be understood or believed, in which case authorities may not give as much attention to their reports as to other people's reports.
- ***Children.*** Children are usually dependent on the person who is caring for them. They are too young to know how to defend or protect themselves. Some parents or caregivers think that they have the right to "discipline" their children using abusive force or words. Others are overwhelmed with the stress and responsibilities of being a parent or guardian, or they very likely were abused themselves in their childhood.
- ***Socially or geographically isolated older adults.*** Older adults who cannot get out of the places where they live may not have an opportunity to tell anyone that they are abused. Bruises and other obvious physical signs might also go unnoticed if these older adults are prevented from having contact with others. Older adults may not know how to escape from an abuser or may lack the strength to seek safety and shelter.
- ***Older adults with reduced cognitive capacity.*** These people may not know or remember that they have been abused. They may no longer have control over their finances, so they may not know that their money or belongings are being taken.
- ***Dependent older adults with disabilities.*** If older adults do not have opportunities to interact with others, abuses can often go unrecognized. In the case of physical abuse, bruises are often explained away by the abuser as being caused by the disability, age, or general health condition of the older adult.
- ***Older adults cared for by people with substance abuse problems.*** People with substance abuse problems may lack impulse control—that is, the ability to control their angry outbursts or to deal with the older adult's challenging behaviours in a nonviolent manner. Others may have financial problems and steal from the older adult they care for to support their own substance addiction.

Source: Government of Canada, Department of Justice. (2011). *Elder abuse is wrong.* Retrieved from http://www.justice.gc.ca/eng/rp-pr/cj-jp/fv-vf/eaw-mai/pdf/eaw-mai.pdf.

partners in spite of serious physical violence. Some victims may stay because they are afraid of leaving their abuser, who may have threatened them with harm, death, or denial of child custody. In some circumstances, the victim may stay so that the children can continue to have the financial and other comforts of a two-parent home. Some victims stay because they do not know where to go or how to get help. Some others may believe that they are responsible for the abuse, that no one will believe them, or that the abuser will change and the relationship will work.

Think About Safety

Signs and Symptoms of Abuse

Victims of abuse can be subjected to one or more of the following types of abuse:

Physical Abuse

- Physical injuries (such as burns, bumps, bruises, scratches, cuts, or fractures) that frequently go untreated and either are unexplained or have unlikely explanations
- New injuries that appear while older injuries are still healing
- Frequent injuries (such as burns, bruises, welts, or cuts) on the face, neck, inner arms, back, upper arms, and inner thighs (people who are abused often try to hide their injuries under clothing or makeup)
- Welts, bruises, or burns that have the shape of the object that caused the injury; for example, the shape may be of a handprint, belt, or wooden spoon
- Unexplained missing or loose teeth
- A very groggy or overly sedated client

Sexual Abuse

- Irritation or injury (such as cuts and bruises or scarring) of the thighs, perineum, or breasts
- Intense fear of bathing or perineal care
- Torn, stained, or bloody underwear
- Vaginal discharge, genital odour, and painful urination
- Difficulty walking or sitting
- Avoidance of touching (see the *Supporting Emmy Lou: One Abuse Survivor's Struggle* box)

Emotional Abuse

- A change in behaviour, especially if the client seems depressed or unusually quiet or withdrawn
- Fearful behaviour, especially in the presence of the suspected abuser; for example, the client cowers, avoids eye contact, or trembles
- Unwillingness to talk or answer questions
- Change in behaviour when the suspected abuser enters and leaves the room
- Withholding of permission to socialize with family or friends or client's withdrawal from contacts
- Private conversations not allowed—the suspected abuser insists on being present or within hearing distance of all conversations
- Change in the behaviour of the suspected abuser (who may be the caregiver)—for example, on one occasion she is pleasant and cooperative and, on another, is defensive or hostile
- Caregiver's failure to show any affection toward the person in his or her care, or shows of affection seem strained or insincere
- Frequent statements by the caregiver that the person in his or her care is difficult or demanding

Financial Abuse

- Caregiver's refusal to spend money on caring for the person
- Unpaid bills (such as utilities, telephone, or rent) or bounced cheques, even though client has money
- Lack of adequate food, clothing, personal care items, or furnishings, even though client can afford them
- Suspected abuser's greater concern is the cost, rather than the quality, of the care
- Missing personal belongings, with no explanation
- Suspected abuser does not have a job and is secretive about his or her source of income
- Client has to ask for permission to write cheques or spend money

Neglect

- Unsafe, unclean, or inadequate living conditions
- Lack of personal hygiene; for example, a neglected client may have ingrown nails, decayed teeth, untreated sores, matted hair, body odour, or dirty clothing
- Signs of poor nutrition and fluid intake, such as weight loss; extreme thirst; a thin, bony appearance; sunken eyes or cheeks; and a dry, papery feeling to the skin
- Pressure sores
- Medications not purchased
- Lack of supervision or attention for prolonged periods

Continued

Think About Safety—cont'd

Infants and Children

All of the above as well as the following are signs of abuse or neglect in children and infants:

- Sudden behaviour changes—for example, bed-wetting, loss of bladder or bowel control during the day, or loss of appetite
- Prolonged vomiting or diarrhea
- Developmental delays, such as not gaining weight or not reaching developmental milestones (e.g., sitting or standing)
- Lack of energy in infants, shown by lack of interest in the surroundings, infrequent crying, and generally an undemanding disposition

Sources: Boyack, V. (1997). *Golden years—hidden fears: Elder abuse. A handbook for front-line helpers working with seniors* (p. 7). Calgary, AB: Kerby Centre; Quinn, M.J., & Tomita, S.K. (1997). *Elder abuse and neglect: Causes, diagnosis, and intervention strategies* (2nd ed., pp. 55, 76). New York, NY: Springer; Government of Canada, Department of Justice. (2011). *Elder abuse is wrong.* Retrieved from http://www.justice.gc.ca/eng/rp-pr/cj-jp/fv-vf/eaw-mai/pdf/eaw-mai.pdf.

Supporting Emmy Lou: One Abuse Survivor's Struggle

Emmy Lou is a 32-year-old woman who grew up in a loving family. One night, when Emmy Lou was in high school, she was babysitting her neighbour's two children, as she often did. She was upstairs putting the children to bed and did not hear the children's father come into the house and up the stairs. She greeted him when she walked out of the children's bedroom and asked him where his wife was. He explained that she was going to be late coming home from their meeting. At that point, Emmy Lou said that she should go home, as it was a school night and she had to get up early the next day for school.

The neighbour prevented her from going down the stairs, and he forced her to the floor in the hallway and sexually assaulted her. Later, Emmy Lou ran home and showered. She always blamed herself for what had happened and has never told anyone about that night. Since that incident, Emmy Lou has always hated being touched or having anybody stand close to her.

Last month, Emmy Lou was injured in a head-on collision caused by a drunk driver and became permanently paralyzed from her neck down (quadriplegia). As a support worker, you are assigned to provide basic care to her now that she is out of the hospital and at home with her parents. One day, when you are providing personal care to her, Emmy Lou begins to tear up. She shakes her head, and her lips are quivering. How would you proceed?

Child Abuse

Child abuse occurs when a parent, guardian, or caregiver mistreats or neglects a child, which may result in the following:

- Significant emotional or psychological harm
- Serious risk of harm to the child

Child abuse is a gross misuse of a caregiver's position of trust and authority over a child. Children who are abused tend to experience more social problems and perform less well in school than other children. As a result, as adults, they can remain poorly adjusted socially and lack success in life. Additionally, victims of childhood abuse are at greater risk for becoming violent abusers and criminals themselves. Child abuse can take many different forms:

- **Physical abuse**—the deliberate application of force on any part of a child's body, which may result in a nonaccidental injury. Physical abuse also includes behaviours such as shaking, choking, biting, kicking, burning, or poisoning a child, holding a child under water, or any other harmful or dangerous use of force or restraint. Some people confuse punishment with physical abuse.

- ***Emotional abuse***—(see general description of emotional abuse on p. 258). Other forms of emotionally abusive treatment include forcing a child into social isolation or intimidating, exploiting, terrorizing, or routinely making unreasonable demands on a child. Emotional abuse is often part of a pattern of family stress and dysfunctional parenting. In fact, some provinces in Canada now include exposure of a child to violence between the parents as a form of emotional abuse.[2] A recent study of wife assault found that children witness violence against their mothers in almost 40% of violent marriages.[3]

  Children who are both emotionally and physically abused exhibit the greatest degree of aggression, delinquency, and interpersonal problems. Women who were abused in childhood are more likely to suffer from depression, low self-esteem, and suicidal thoughts. While physical abuse will put a child in immediate danger of injury, psychological or emotional abuse can have even more negative and long-term consequences for the child.
- ***Sexual abuse***—the use of a child for sexual purposes by an adult or adolescent. Exposing a child to any sexual activity or behaviour constitutes sexual abuse. It may involve fondling, inviting a child to touch or be touched sexually, or even engaging the child in sexual intercourse, juvenile prostitution, or sexual exploitation through pornography. Sexual abuse is also considered a form of emotional abuse.
- **Child neglect**—failure by a parent or other caregiver to meet a child's basic needs for emotional, psychological, and physical development. **Physical neglect** occurs when a child's needs for food, clothing, shelter, cleanliness, medical care, and protection from harm are not adequately met. **Emotional neglect** occurs when a child's need to feel loved, wanted, safe, and worthy is not met. Emotional neglect can range from the context of the abuser's simply being unavailable to the abuser's open rejection of the child. Physical assaults are more likely to be reported, but neglect can have equally serious consequences for a child.
- ***If you witness or suspect child abuse, you are legally required to report it!***

Situations That Increase the Risk for Child Abuse

- ***Family crisis.*** Divorce, unemployment, moving, poverty, and crowded living conditions all cause stress. Stress can lead to abuse (see the *Supporting Taylor: Understanding Contributing Abuse Factors* box).
- ***Nonbiological or transient caregivers in the home.*** Children are more likely to be abused if they live in a household in which the biological parent shares parenting responsibilities with a partner (or partners) who does not have a committed and loving relationship with the children. The risk increases if either the partner or parent was abused or neglected as a child.[4]
- ***Isolation.*** Parents who mistreat or abuse their children are more likely to experience feelings of isolation, loneliness, and less social support as compared to other parents.[5]
- ***Caring for children with special needs.*** Children with physical or mental disabilities or chronic illness are especially at risk for abuse. Children with personalities or behaviours that the abuser considers "different" or unacceptable also face greater risk.

Failure to Thrive

Failure to thrive is a term that describes infants, babies, or children who are below the norms for body weight, growth, or cognitive development. One of the many known causes for failure to thrive is caregiver neglect. In extreme cases, it can lead to permanent developmental delays and even the death of the child. Many of the mothers of these infants were themselves likely abused as children.

What Can Be Done to Prevent Child Abuse?

Most abusive parents do not consciously set out to harm their children. If there are more and better efforts to assist troubled families, parents at risk for abusing may be reached and helped before they resort to violence. Prevention is a good investment, in terms of both the personal and social costs that can be

Supporting Taylor: Understanding Contributing Abuse Factors

Taylor is a 6-year-old boy who was born with fetal alcohol syndrome (see Chapter 38). His weight is below the average for a child his age, and he has hearing and vision difficulties as well as behavioural problems. You have been assigned to Taylor as his support worker, to assist him with bathing, toileting, and eating. Because of Taylor's frequent verbal outbursts and his tendency to bite, kick, and scratch, his mother has decided to home-school Taylor.

You arrive for your first visit with Taylor in his home, and his mother, a nicely dressed woman, greets you at the door. The house is clean, neat, and stylishly furnished. Her breath smells of alcohol, and there is an open bottle of vodka on the kitchen counter. In the course of your conversation, Taylor's mother tells you that she is a lawyer, and because of Taylor's situation, she plans on practising law from her home. During this initial visit, while she is showing you around the house, she repeatedly blames her ex-husband for Taylor's condition; she says her ex-husband had a "terrible drinking problem."

When you meet Taylor, he gives you a big hug and asks you if you can stay all day. He then turns on the television; because of his hearing and vision difficulties, he needs to sit very close to it, with the volume turned up. Taylor's mother yells at Taylor, telling him, "Turn the (*uses a swear word*) TV down!" Taylor does so but begins to cry. His mother then asks you to make sure that Taylor keeps quiet while you are with him.

Can you identify the factors that might contribute to Taylor's possible mistreatment at home?

saved. There are many ways to prevent abuse, including the following:[6]

- ***Parenting education***. With education, parents can better understand normal child development and how to have a more nurturing and enjoyable relationship with their children. Positive approaches to parenting can help parents deal with children of any age.
- ***Child abuse prevention programs***. Abused children tend to repeat the pattern of abuse when they become adults, so identification of potential abusers and prevention are the most effective means to stop the cycle of violence.
- ***Supportiveness***. If a child tells you, the support worker, about an abusive situation or experience, you need to show the child that you believe her and ensure that the information is promptly reported to the appropriate authorities.
- ***Education.*** Children should know how to recognize and say no to abusive or exploitative behaviour and be taught that they have the right to be free from abuse. As a support worker, you can help children and adults find information and assistance to prevent an abusive or neglectful pattern from developing.

Abuse of Older Adults

Older adults are at risk for all types of abuse—physical, sexual, emotional, and financial—as well as neglect. Financial and emotional abuses are most commonly reported by older adults. Abusers are usually family members such as adult children or grandchildren. Often, the abuser is the older adult's primary caregiver. Most abusers of older adults depend on their victims for financial help or housing[7]—for example, an adult son who moves in with his parent after losing his job.

Abused older adults sometimes choose not to complain about the abuse. Like abused spouses, they may fear the abuser or may not know where or how to get help. They may fear being forced to move into a long-term care facility if they report their caregiver. Some older adults are not able to report abuse, as they may have physical or mental disabilities. Victims of neglect especially are often unable to report their situation (see **BOX 16–2**).

In addition to the factors identified earlier in this chapter, some other factors that might increase an older person's risk for being abused include the following:

- ***Stress.*** Family caregivers are more likely to be abusive when they resent their role. Taking care of an older adult can be extremely stressful, especially when the person receiving care is physically or mentally disabled. If the caregiver is unprepared or unable to fulfill the duties, she can feel overwhelmed.
- ***Ageism.*** Ageism is another cause of abuse (see Chapter 21). Ageism is bias and discrimination against older adults. Caregivers who do not respect the dignity or abilities of older adults are more likely to be abusive. For example, a caregiver who thinks that older adults are incapable of managing money may take control of the person's finances without permission (financial abuse).
- ***Vulnerability.*** Many of the factors that increase older adults' vulnerability to abuse may also compound the effects of the abuse. According to the Department of Justice for the Government of Canada, older adults are vulnerable to abuse because the following factors may exist:[8]
  - Poor living conditions (inadequate housing, geographical isolation)
  - Unemployment (not employed or retired from an employer)
  - Dislocation (new to the area)
  - Racism (prejudice because of skin colour)
  - Homophobia (prejudice because of sexual orientation)
  - Disability (physical, mental, or developmental limitations)
  - Economic vulnerability (few financial resources or poverty)
  - Social isolation, lack of language or literacy skills (isolated because of geographical location, inability to speak, read, or write the local language)
  - Lack of access to community and health services
  - Lack of access to housing or long-term care facilities
  - Lack of access to the justice system

Abuse of Clients by Health Care Workers

Abuse of clients can happen in a facility or home care setting, and clients can be abused by any member of the health care team. In facilities, they can be abused by visitors or a member of the staff. Clients are at risk for all types of abuse—physical, sexual, emotional, and financial—as well as neglect. Abusive situations include using restraints inappropriately, handling the client roughly, isolating the client in his or her room, stealing from the client, not reviewing the care plan regularly, not responding to a call for help, not checking on the client for long periods, and leaving the client lying in soiled linen or clothes. ***Violating a client's rights is another form of abuse***—for example, providing care against the person's wishes, failing to provide privacy, failing to keep personal or medical information confidential, and not letting residents visit or use the phone in private.

Abuse can be very obvious, such as roughly handling or force-feeding a client. Or it can be very subtle (not obvious); for example, staff can demean or belittle clients by calling them "grandma" or "slugger" or by referring to their incontinence briefs as "diapers." These comments are embarrassing for the client and violate the DIPPS principles.

Stress Can Trigger Client Abuse

As with all abusive relationships, stress sometimes leads to or triggers the abuse of clients (see the *Supporting Mrs. Finnie: Witnessing Client Abuse* box). Some workers may not have received enough training or education to cope with the situations they are put in, or some may have too much work because of too few workers. As well, some clients can be uncooperative or abusive toward the staff—for example, they may hit or yell at the worker. Some workers respond to abusive clients by being abusive to them in return.

All agencies have policies about what to do in the case of client abuse. Examples of abusive behaviours from a health care worker to a client include the following:

- Threatening to harm the client or trying to scare the client

- Denying meal breaks, drinking water, bathroom use, or handwashing facilities
- Swearing, name calling, and using racial or cultural slurs
- Inappropriate touching
- Sexually assaulting or harassing

However, there is no excuse for abusive behaviour from a support worker. Sometimes, you will work with difficult clients in stressful situations, and you must recognize when you are feeling stressed. Take time out if you begin to lose your temper. Always treat your clients gently and with respect, even when they resist your care.

To prevent your behaviour from becoming abusive, immediately discuss difficult or aggressive clients with your supervisor. Your supervisor will help you decide how to handle them. If necessary, you can ask for a change of assignment (see Chapter 7 for a discussion on how to manage stress).

WHAT TO DO WHEN CLIENTS SPEAK OF ABUSE

You should be prepared for the possibility of a client or child telling you about being abused. In such situations, it is important that you support the person and know how to offer immediate help. Follow your employer's guidelines and policies. The following are some general guidelines on how to be supportive:

- Listen attentively. Let your clients tell you what happened in their own words. Recognize their feelings.
- Reassure the clients that you believe what they have said. Stay calm and do not show anger or

Supporting Mrs. Finnie: Witnessing Client Abuse

Evelyn Finnie is a 65-year-old woman who is a resident in an extended care facility. She has periods of confusion, but she is reasonably coherent most days. She has been in a wheelchair ever since she had a severe stroke 15 years ago and is dependent on supportive care for all of her basic needs. She is often described by the staff that you work with as "demanding" and "manipulative," and you have noticed that she does have specific preferences for how she is bathed, dressed, and fed.

This is your first time working evenings at this very busy agency. The nurse in charge seems nice and has asked you to talk to her whenever you have any questions; however, you are expected to be busy assisting the other support workers. You are told by the other support workers that h.s. (bedtime) care begins at 1830 hours (6:30 p.m.). You are shocked that it begins at such an early hour but decide to go along with the staff. Your co-worker Jane, whom you have been partnered with, has been working on evening shifts for the past 25 years. She tells you that Mrs. Finnie should be the first resident prepared for bed so that she can "get out of your hair." Jane tells you that she is just waiting to retire from her job and that she likes to get everyone in bed early so she can have a "decent break."

Jane advises you to put an incontinence brief on Mrs. Finnie instead of assisting her with toileting (which would require a mechanical lift). Mrs. Finnie gets very upset and says loudly that she wants to "go in the toilet." Jane steps in and completes putting the brief on Mrs. Finnie, telling her that she could just "let it go in her diaper all night." When Mrs. Finnie tries to wiggle during the application of her incontinence brief, Jane holds her down and says in a loud voice, "Who do you think you are? I am so tired of your acting like a queen. Now stay still, or this will really hurt!"

All the other residents who would normally be toileted by mechanical lifts have incontinence briefs applied to them as well, although none of the other residents complain. Jane is nice to some of the residents but seems impatient with some others. When you ask her about her behaviour toward them, she says, "I remember who gave me a hard time and who didn't!"

You are shocked and very disturbed by the evening's events but really do not know what to do. What should you have done? What would you do differently next time? Who should you tell?

disgust. Do not deny or ignore the problem. Do not ask what they did to make their abusers angry. Such questions only make the victims think that the abuse was their fault.

- Assure your clients that you will do what you can to help. Notify your supervisor at once. Your employer's guidelines and policies will note what should be provided to people who are living with abuse. Helpful community resources include the police, women's shelters, counselling services, telephone helplines, and legal clinics.
- Provide emotional support to your clients no matter what they decide to do. Remember, you cannot force adults to make a certain decision or take a particular action. People who are capable of making their own informed decisions have the right to decide for themselves whether to live with the abuse or to accept help. Some people choose not to accept help; this choice is their right, and you must accept their decision. People who are not capable of making informed decisions must get the help of a professional.

YOUR LEGAL RESPONSIBILITIES IN REPORTING ABUSE

Every Canadian province and territory has legislation that imposes a duty on members of the public and professional organizations to report cases in which they have reasonable grounds to suspect that a child, a person with physical or mental challenges, or an older adult is being abused by a parent, adult child, caregiver, or guardian. As a support worker, you have this obligation as well.

Some people think that abuse is a private family matter, and it should remain behind closed doors. Others believe that they cannot do anything about it, so they should not even try. Neither belief is true. If you have reasonable grounds to suspect that someone is being abused or neglected, promptly report your concerns to the child welfare agency, the provincial or territorial social services department, or the police force in your community. If necessary, the report can be made anonymously.

Reporting is not difficult or time-consuming. In all cases, the person reporting is protected from any kind of legal action, provided the report is not falsely made and motivated by malice.

Suspected Child Abuse

If you witness or even suspect child abuse, you must report it directly to child-protection authorities. (Look up your local child welfare agency or social service agency online.) Your name will be kept confidential. Do not rely on your supervisor to make the report for you. However, consult with your supervisor and get advice before making your report. In some provinces, ***failing to report child abuse can result in fines or imprisonment***.

Suspected Older-Adult Abuse

All provinces and territories have laws that require health care workers to report witnessed or suspected abuse of older adults or those with disabilities within facilities. In these provinces, workers must report abuse directly to a public authority. Even if your province or territory does not require public reporting, inform your supervisor about any cases or suspicions of abuse. Be sure to write down your observations, including as many details as you can, and keep this information in a safe place. It will help you remember details, if needed, in the future. Know your employer's policy and provincial or territorial law concerning the reporting of abuse within a facility.

In Canada, the Department of Justice has a fact sheet that describes what constitutes abuse of older adults. It is understood that mentally capable adults can make their own choices and decisions about seeking help. However, immediately report your suspicions to your supervisor, according to your employer's policies.

HOW TO REPORT ABUSE

Your employer will have specific rules regarding how to report your observations. It is very important to record all your observations and make your reports in writing. Keep all your notes in case you are asked to remember details later on. In general, when you report abuse—whether to your supervisor or to a public authority—you should record the following:

- The alleged victim's name, address, phone number, age, and gender

- The alleged abuser's name, address, phone number, and relationship to the victim
- Description of abuse or neglect, suspicions, and evidence obtained to date; the date, time, and place; only the facts that you know or were told by the victim—do not make assumptions

Whenever you report your suspicions, it is essential that you respect and protect your client's right to privacy. Tell only those who need to know. Do not gossip or tell anyone who is not directly involved.

Where to Go for Services

Contact these local organizations when abuse is suspected or recognized:

- Child welfare agency
- Social services agency
- Police department
- Hospital
- Mental health centre
- Distress centre
- Other community service organization that provides counselling and support to children and families

Many of these organizations are listed online or among the emergency telephone numbers on or near the first page of a local telephone directory.

Children who want help can also directly ***call the Kids Help Phone at 1-800-668-6868***.

ABUSE OF HEALTH CARE WORKERS

Sometimes, health care workers, including support workers, are abused while on the job. You are at risk for physical or verbal abuse from your clients, your clients' family members, or other members of the health care team.

Abuse of Health Care Workers by Clients

Health care workers are especially at risk for abuse when they work with clients who have a mental health disorder or a condition that affects behaviour, such as schizophrenia or dementia (see Chapters 35 and 36). Clients who are addicted to drugs or alcohol, who have a history of abusive behaviour, or who are being placed in restraints are also more likely to be abusive toward you.

Some clients are cognitively impaired and no longer have the ability to verbalize their feelings. Those clients may become aggressive because they are cold, uncomfortable, or ill (see Chapter 36). They are demonstrating responsive behaviours to how they are feeling when they are unable to tell you.

Staff abuse by clients should never be ignored or accepted as "part of the job." Your employer will have policies on dealing with abusive clients. The *Think About Safety: What to Do When a Client Is Abusive* box lists general safety measures to follow when dealing with abusive clients.

Examples of abusive behaviours by the cognitively aware client include the following:

- Swearing, name calling, and using racial or cultural slurs
- Hitting, pushing, kicking, spitting, biting, pinching, or other physical attacks
- Inappropriate touching
- Following you home or finding out your phone number and calling you at home

The Sexually Aggressive Client

Some clients want the health care team members to help meet their sexual needs, so they may flirt or make sexual advances or comments. Some may even expose themselves to, masturbate in front of, or inappropriately touch health care workers. Often, there are reasons for such behaviours, and they may be more common among clients who are cognitively impaired. Understanding the reasons behind the actions helps you deal with the problem (see Chapter 36).

Changes in a client's mental condition can reduce the social "filtering" that usually stops a person from acting on sexual urges in public. Sexual behaviour in a client is usually not intended to be abusive, but it still must be dealt with, and you must notify your supervisor if a client makes sexual advances toward you.

Clients who are cognitively aware and displaying aggressive or sexually aggressive behaviours can embarrass or even anger the support worker. Sometimes, clients do not have any mental or physical

Think About Safety

What to Do When a Client Is Abusive

- Stay calm.
- Stand up so that the client is not in a dominant position. Stand far enough away from the client, about 2 m (6 ft.), so that the client cannot hit or kick you.
- Position yourself close to a door in case you have to escape quickly.
- Note the locations of call bells, alarms, closed-circuit monitors, and other security devices.
- Keep your hands free. Do not touch the client.
- Listen to the client. Restate what the client says in your own words.
- Talk to the client calmly. Do not raise your voice or argue, scold, or interrupt the client. Be polite and positive. Avoid such comments as "Calm down" or "You have no reason to be mad at me." Instead, acknowledge the client's frustrations, and tell the client you will get your supervisor to intervene.
- Watch the client's body language, including shaking or clenching fists or a change in posture. Body language may indicate that the client is ready to hit or push.
- If you are in a facility, tell the client that you will get a nurse to intervene. Make sure that the client is safe, and quickly leave the room. Tell the nurse or the security officer about the situation. If you cannot leave and you suspect the client is going to lose control, sound a call bell, alarm, or other security device.
- If you are in a client's home, leave the house if you think you are in danger. Go to a safe place and immediately call your supervisor. If you cannot leave the house and you feel threatened, call the police by dialing 9-1-1.
- Complete an incident report after an abusive encounter (see Chapter 22 for an example of an incident report). In Chapter 36, the *Think About Safety: ABCDs of Managing Responsive or Challenging Behaviours* box has examples of different types of disruptive behaviours and ways to de-escalate most situations.

problems that cause sexual aggression but behave aggressively for other reasons. They may touch their health care workers because they have unmet needs for love and belonging or self-esteem and are feeling lonely or unloved. For example, a divorced client may behave sexually toward you because he wants to prove that he is attractive and can perform sexually. Remember that you must be professional in these situations:

- Ask the client not to touch you, telling him where you were touched.
- Tell the client that you will not do what he wants.
- Tell the client that his behaviour makes you uncomfortable. Politely ask the client not to act in that way.
- If you feel your safety is at risk, leave the client's room or house. Call your supervisor.
- Tell your supervisor about what happened. He can help you decide if further action is necessary. If you are uncomfortable being with the client, you have the right to ask to be assigned to another client.

Sexual Harassment

Sexual harassment—a form of sexual abuse—happens in the workplace when clients, their families, or co-workers make sexual comments, gestures, threats, or suggestions. If another person's behaviour offends you or makes you uncomfortable while you are at work, it is harassment. Sexual harassment is not only directed toward women; it can also be directed toward men, especially in a female-dominated workplace.

If a co-worker's comments make you uncomfortable, you must remember that it is *your* responsibility to firmly but politely explain to the person that her conduct is unwelcome and unacceptable. Never assume that she knows that you do not approve of this behaviour. Be assertive but never rude. Most people stop the harassing behaviour once they realize it is unacceptable.

Try to have a reliable witness when you make your objections, and always make a note of the details—when and where it happened and what was said. Keep this documentation in a safe place so that you will have a record if it ever happens again. If the harassment continues, tell your supervisor about it. In Canada, employers are legally required to prevent sexual harassment at work. All employers have policies on how to deal with sexual aggression and harassment.

Workplace Bullying

In Chapter 5, workplace etiquette was defined as "professional, ethical, friendly, and respectful behaviour toward all staff and co-workers at all times." While many workplaces strive to create a friendly and respectful atmosphere, other workplaces have allowed staff members to bully and be disrespectful, rude, and hurtful toward some of their co-workers. **Workplace bullying** manifests as acts or verbal comments that could mentally "hurt" or isolate a person in the workplace.[9] Sometimes bullying is obvious, but other times, it can be very subtle.

In Canada, it is the duty of employers to protect employees from risks at work. These risks include harm from both physical and mental health aspects (**BOX 16–3**). It should be remembered that it is not just the character of the incidents but the number, frequency, and especially the pattern that can reveal bullying or harassment. Health care workers' feeling bullied may also compromise client safety.[10]

If you feel that you are being bullied, discriminated against, victimized, or subjected to any form of harassment, you need to *firmly* tell the person that her behaviour is not acceptable and ask her to stop. You can ask a supervisor or union member to be with you when you approach the person. Other important actions include the following:[9]

- Keep a factual journal of daily events. Record the date, time, and event in as much detail as possible, including the effect the event had on you. You also need to include the names of witnesses.
- Keep copies of any letters, memos, emails, faxes, and so on received from the person.
- Report the harassment to the person identified in your workplace policy, your supervisor, or a delegated manager. If your concerns are minimized, proceed to the next level of management.
- ***Do not retaliate.*** You may end up looking like the perpetrator and will most certainly cause confusion for those responsible for evaluating and responding to the situation.

BOX 16–3 Effects of Bullying in the Workplace

People who are the targets of bullying may experience a range of effects, including:

- Anger
- Feelings of frustration or helplessness
- Increased sense of vulnerability
- Loss of confidence
- Physical symptoms such as loss of sleep or appetite
- Psychosomatic symptoms such as stomach pains or headaches
- Panic or anxiety, especially about going to work
- Family tension and stress
- Inability to concentrate
- Low morale and productivity

Bullying can affect the entire workplace and can lead to the following:

- Increased absenteeism
- Increased turnover
- Increased stress
- Increased costs for employee assistance programs, recruitment, and so on
- Increased risk for accidents and incidents
- Decreased motivation and staff morale
- Decreased quality of client care

Source: Excerpted from Canadian Centre for Occupational Health and Safety. (2014). *Bullying in the workplace.* Retrieved from http://www.ccohs.ca/oshanswers/psychosocial/bullying.html.

CHAPTER REVIEW

KEY POINTS

- All clients have the right to safe, respectful care.
- Abuse results when physical or mental harm is caused by someone in a position of trust, such as a family member, a partner, or a caregiver. The main types of abuse include (1) physical, (2) sexual, (3) emotional, (4) financial, and (5) neglect.
- Abuse occurs repeatedly, as the abuser tries to dominate the victim.
- The three phases in the cycle of abuse are (1) the tension-building phase, (2) the abusive phase, and (3) the honeymoon phase.
- All health care workers should be aware of the signs and symptoms of abuse in both adults and children (see pp. 258 to 259).
- People at highest risk for abuse are (1) marginalized people, especially women; (2) children; (3) older adults; (4) socially or geographically isolated older adults; (5) older adults with reduced cognitive capacity; (6) dependent older adults with disabilities; and (7) older adults cared for by people with substance abuse problems.
- Situations that increase the risk for child abuse include (1) family crisis, (2) presence of nonbiological or transient parental partners, (3) isolation, and (4) caring for children with special needs.
- All health care workers should be aware of what to do if they suspect that one of their clients has been abused or if a client admits to being abused: (1) follow your employer's rules on how to report your observations; (2) record all your observations and make your reports in writing; and (3) keep all notes in case you are asked to remember details in the future.
- When reporting abuse, record only the facts you know or were told by the alleged victim—do not make assumptions. Record the following: (1) the alleged victim's name, address, phone number, age, and gender; (2) the alleged abuser's name, address, phone number, and relationship to the victim; (3) your description of abuse or neglect, suspicions, and evidence obtained; (4) the date, time, and place of the abuse.
- When reporting abuse, it is essential to respect and protect your client's right to privacy. Tell only those who need to know. Do not gossip or tell anyone who is not directly involved.
- Health care workers should be aware of how to reduce the chances of being injured in an abusive situation involving a client (see pp. 265 to 266).
- Bullying in the workplace can have very negative effects on staff. It is the employer's duty to protect employees from risks at work.

CRITICAL THINKING IN PRACTICE

Ms. Hild has experienced urinary incontinence and chewing and swallowing problems since her stroke. When speaking to Ms. Hild, a co-worker uses the term "diaper" to describe her incontinence product and "bib" for her clothing protector. The same co-worker wipes spilled food from Ms. Hild's face with a spoon and threatens to withhold privileges if she does not finish meals.

How will you respond to your co-worker's statements and actions? What are your responsibilities if you witness this behaviour? Explain why it is important to treat the person as an adult and not a child.

REVIEW QUESTIONS

Answers to these questions are at the bottom of page 270.

Circle the BEST answer.

1. The Canadian Charter of Rights and Freedoms applies to:
   A. Citizens of Canada
   B. Visitors to Canada
   C. New immigrants
   D. All of the above
2. The Canadian Charter of Rights and Freedoms states that:
   A. Canada values equality and diversity
   B. No one should be abused or has the right to treat others unfairly
   C. People who are in jail have no rights
   D. A and B

3. Which example of abuse is considered to be physical abuse?
   A. Calling the person worthless
   B. Taking away access to banking information
   C. Not allowing the thermostat to be turned up on very cold days
   D. Withholding affection

4. In which phase during the cycle of abuse does the abuser seem loving and attentive?
   A. Honeymoon phase
   B. Resolution phase
   C. Tension-building phase
   D. Abusive incident

5. Who are more likely to be abusive?
   A. Women
   B. Men
   C. People who have a problem with alcohol or drugs
   D. Parents with close family and social relationships

6. Which statement about spousal abuse is true?
   A. You are obligated to press charges against your abusive spouse.
   B. Abuse involves only violence.
   C. Women and men can be abused.
   D. Only one type of abuse is usually present.

7. Which statement about child abuse is true?
   A. You must have proof that abuse has occurred before you report it.
   B. All victims of child abuse are girls.
   C. You must report any suspicions of child abuse directly to the child-protection authorities.
   D. Infants are not at risk for child abuse.

8. Children who are both physically and emotionally abused exhibit:
   A. More delinquency
   B. Greater resilience with their problems
   C. Fewer emotional problems
   D. Better grades and school attendance

9. A parent's not providing adequate medical or dental care is called:
   A. Emotional abuse
   B. Emotional neglect
   C. Physical abuse
   D. Physical neglect

10. You suspect that a child client is being abused. What should you do?
   A. Report your concerns to your supervisor.
   B. Tell your best friend.
   C. Tell the child's parents.
   D. Report your concerns to the Kids Help Phone.

11. Which of the following is an example of abuse of a client?
   A. Inappropriate use of restraints
   B. Reviewing the care plan regularly
   C. Responding to a call bell before taking a coffee break
   D. Asking clients to try to wash their faces themselves

12. When confronted by an abusive client, you should:
   A. Stand next to the person
   B. Stand about 1 m (3 ft) away from the person
   C. Sharply tell the person to stop
   D. Quickly leave the room or house if you think you are in danger

13. Which is a sign of physical abuse?
   A. Stiff and sore joints
   B. Old bruises and new bruises
   C. Fresh fruit in the fridge
   D. Confusion and dementia

14. Intense fear of bathing or perineal care may be a sign of:
   A. Physical abuse
   B. Emotional abuse
   C. Sexual abuse
   D. Neglect

15. Which of the following is a sign of emotional abuse?
- A. Isolation from family and friends
- B. Bills that are not paid
- C. Taking the older adult to the doctor
- D. Pressure sores

16. Mr. Deol states, "My daughter won't give me food until I give her my pension cheque." This is a sign of:
- A. Financial abuse
- B. Emotional abuse
- C. Neglect
- D. Physical abuse

17. You suspect an adult client is being abused. What should you do?
- A. Call the police
- B. Tell the family
- C. Tell your supervisor
- D. Ask the person if he or she is being abused

Answers: 1.D, 2.D, 3.C, 4.A, 5.C, 6.C, 7.C, 8.A, 9.D, 10.A, 11.A, 12.D, 13.B, 14.C, 15.A, 16.A, 17.C

CHAPTER 17

Body Structure and Function

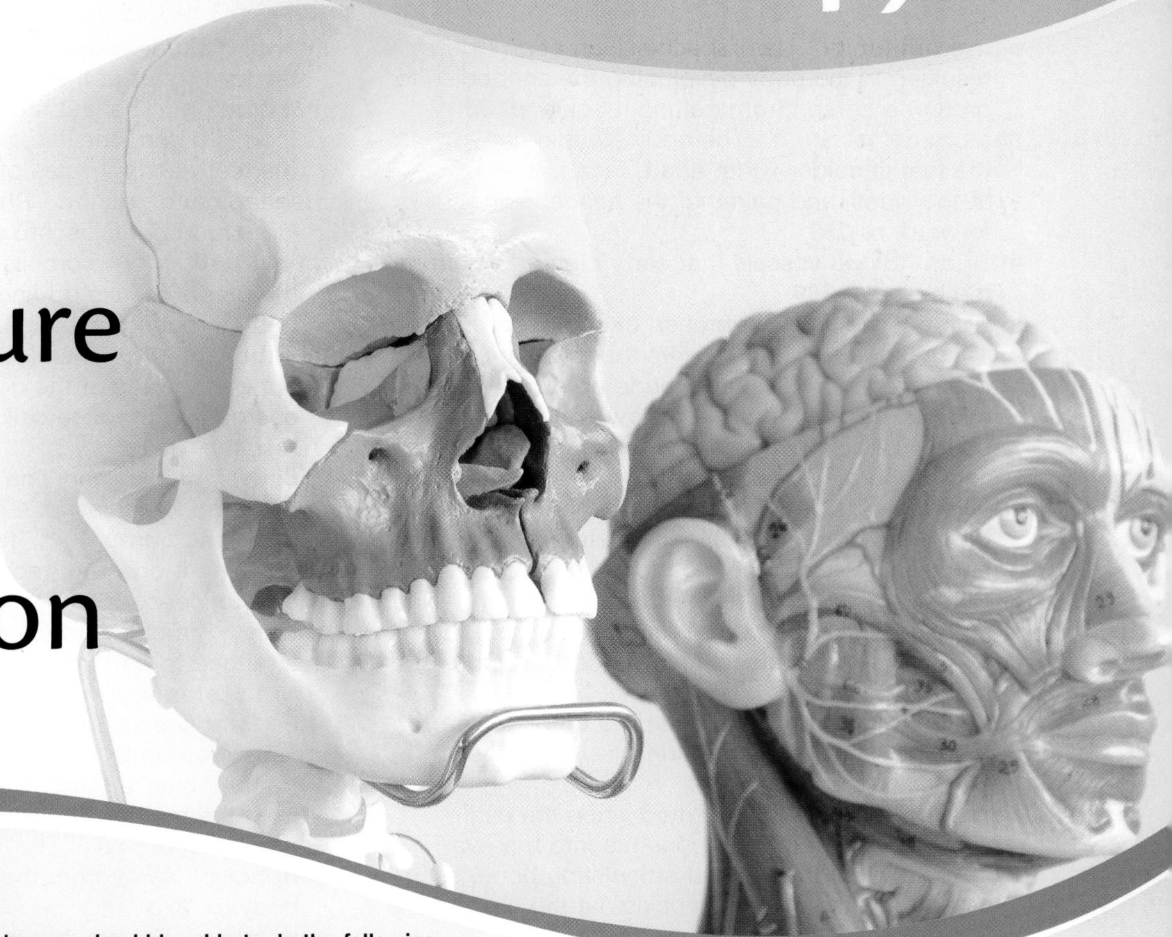

OBJECTIVES

After reading this chapter, the learner should be able to do the following:

- Identify the basic structures of the cell and explain how cells divide.
- Describe the different types of tissue.
- Identify the structures of each body system.
- Describe the functions of each body system.

KEY TERMS

active immunity Natural acquisition of an illness, resulting in the body developing the antibodies to protect a person from getting it again. *p. 300*

anatomical position The body standing erect, with the feet shoulder-width apart, face forward, arms at the sides, and palms of the hands facing forward. *p. 273*

arteries Blood vessels that carry blood away from the heart. *p. 289*

arteriole The smallest branch of an artery. *p. 289*

ball-and-socket joints Joints that allow movement in all directions. They are made up of the rounded end of one bone and the hollow end of another bone. The rounded end of one fits into the hollow end of the other. *p. 279*

capillaries The smallest form of blood vessels and the site of nutrient, gas, and waste exchange between cells and the bloodstream. *p. 289*

cartilage Connective tissue that cushions the joint so that bone ends do not rub together. *p. 279*

cell The basic functional unit of body structure and function. *p. 273*

chemical digestion The chemical breakdown of food into small nutrient parts that the body can absorb and utilize. *p. 294*

condyloid joint A joint formed when the oval articular surface of one bone fits into the oval depression of the second articulating bone, such as at the wrist and the knuckles at the base of the fingers. *p. 280*

deep Away from the surface or further into the body. *p. 273*

digestion The process of physically and chemically breaking down food into nutrients that can be absorbed for use by the cells. *p. 292*

gliding joint A joint formed by the interaction of the flat surfaces of the articulating bones, allowing for limited but complex gliding movements, such as in the wrist, ankle joints, and the vertebral column. *p. 280*

hemoglobin The substance in red blood cells that carries oxygen and gives blood its colour. *p. 287*

hinge joints Joints that allow movement in one direction around a single axis (e.g., elbow joint). *p. 279*

homeostasis A steady state or stable internal environment maintained when all of the organ systems in the human body work together. *p. 275*

hormone A chemical substance produced by the cells of specialized glands and secreted into the bloodstream. *p. 298*

immunity Protection against a disease or condition. *p. 300*

inferior Situated below another structure or toward the lower part of the body. *p. 273*

mastication The first step of digestion in which food is bitten, chewed, crushed, and ground by the teeth and muscles of the jaw. *p. 293*

mechanical digestion Physically breaking down large food particles into smaller pieces. *p. 293*

menstruation The process in which the lining of the uterus breaks up and is discharged from the body through the vagina. *p. 298*

metabolism The chemical processes carried out by the cells of the body that create and use energy and produce cellular waste products as a result. *p. 299*

midline An imaginary line that divides the body into right and left sides. *p. 273*

nonspecific immunity The body's reaction to anything it does not recognize as a normal body substance. *p. 300*

organs Structures made of different tissues that are arranged to perform a specialized function. *p. 275*

organ systems Organs that work together to perform special functions. *p. 275*

passive immunity A short-lived immunity passed from mother to fetus through the placenta and from the mother to the baby through breast milk. *p. 300*

peripheral Away from the centre of the body. *p. 273*

peristalsis The smooth muscle contraction that involuntarily pushes food forward in the digestive tract in one direction in a wavelike motion. *p. 293*

pivot joints Joints that allow turning from side to side. *p. 280*

saddle joint Joints that allow for a wide range of motion between two articulating saddle-shaped bones, such as at the base of the thumb. *p. 280*

specific immunity The ability of an organism to resist or overcome an infection or illness against a *certain* disease or infection caused by a pathogen or antigenic substance. *p. 300*

superficial Near the surface of the body. *p. 273*

superior Situated above another structure or toward the upper part of the body. *p. 273*

tissue A group of similar cells with a common function. *p. 274*

veins Blood vessels that carry blood back to the heart. *p. 289*

venules The smallest form of veins. The venules drain blood from the capillaries and come together to form the veins. *p. 289*

In your role as a support worker, you will help clients meet their basic needs since their bodies are not working at peak efficiency due to disability, illness, disease, or injury. To provide care to promote comfort, healing, and recovery to clients, you need a basic understanding of the body's normal structure and function—that is, anatomy and physiology. *Anatomy* is the study of body structures, and *physiology* is the study of how the body structures work. Understanding the normal functioning of the body will help you understand and identify changes in the body. See Chapter 21 for changes in body structure and functions that occur with aging.

ANATOMICAL TERMS

The terms used in the study of anatomy relate to the body in its **anatomical position**. In this position, the body is standing erect, with the face forward, the arms at the sides, and the toes and palms of the hands facing forward (**FIGURE 17–1**). The medical community uses specific terms to describe the position of body parts, areas of pain, and regions of the body (**BOX 17–1**).

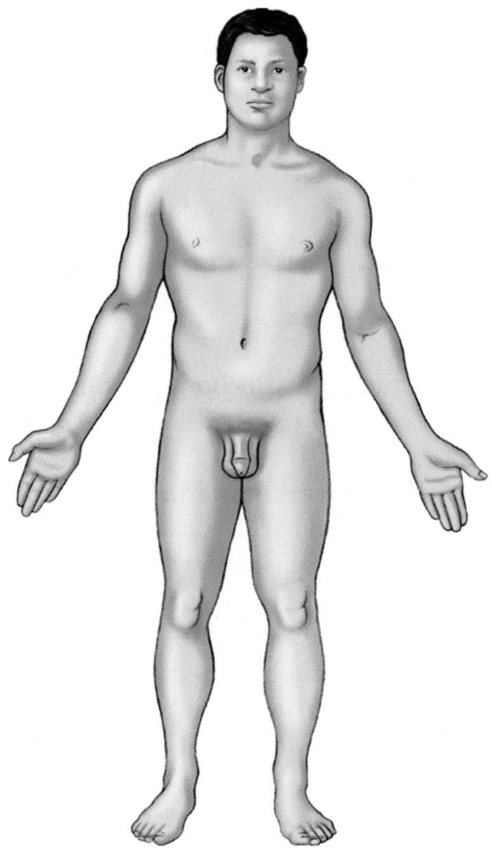

FIGURE 17–1 Anatomical position. (**Source:** Herlihy, B. (2014). *The human body in health and illness* (5th ed., p. 7). Philadelphia, PA: Elsevier/Saunders.)

CELLS, TISSUES, ORGANS, BODY CAVITIES, AND ORGAN SYSTEMS

Cells

The basic functional unit of body structure is the **cell**. Each cell has the same basic structure, but the function, size, and shape of cells may be different. Cells are so small that you need a microscope to see them. Cells need nutrients, water, and oxygen to live and to perform their functions.

The cell and its basic structures are shown in **FIGURE 17–2**. The *cell membrane* is the outer covering that encloses the cell and helps it hold its shape. The cell membrane also controls the movement of

BOX 17–1 Anatomical Terms Related to Position

Superior—situated above another structure; the upper part of the body
Inferior—situated below another structure; the lower part of the body
Anterior*—the front surface of the body; often used to indicate the position of one structure in relation to another
Posterior*—the back surface of the body; often used to indicate the position of one structure in relation to another
Midline—an imaginary line that divides the body into left and right sides
Medial*—closest to the midline of the body
Lateral*—farthest from the midline of the body
Proximal*—nearest the trunk of the body or the point of origin
Distal*—farthest from the trunk of the body or the point of origin
Superficial—near the surface of the body
Deep—away from the surface or farther into the body (e.g., bones are deep to the skin)
Peripheral—away from the centre of the body

*This term appears in Chapter 13's Key Terms.

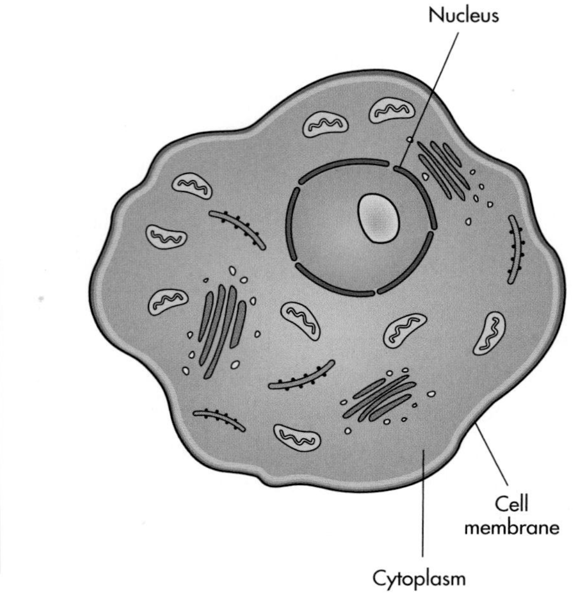

FIGURE 17–2 Parts of a cell.

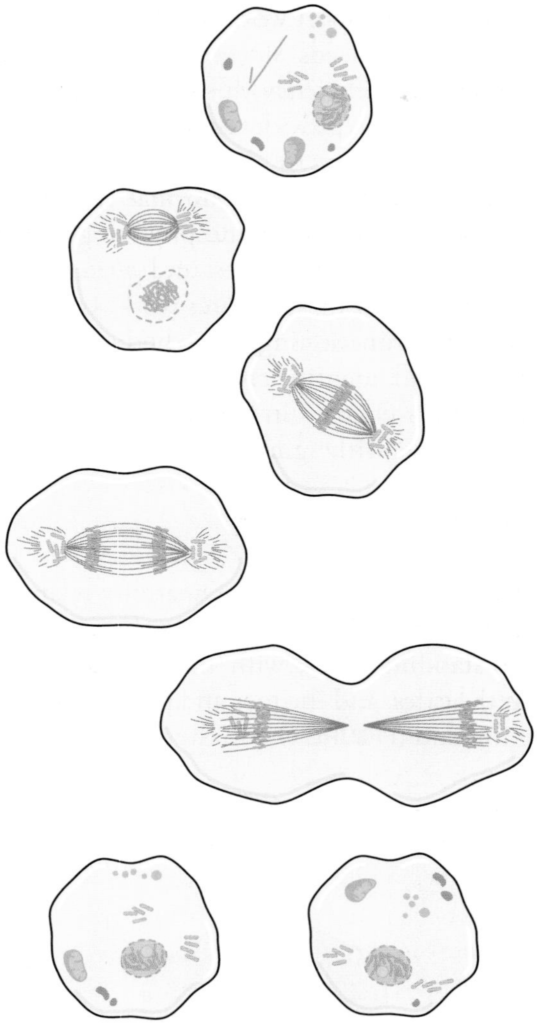

FIGURE 17–3 Cell division.

substances in and out of the cell. The *nucleus*—the control centre of the cell—directs the cell's activities and contains the cell's chromosomes (DNA, or deoxyribonucleic acid). The *cytoplasm* is a fluid that supports the cell's internal structures including the nucleus. There are small structures within the cell's cytoplasm called *organelles*, which work together to perform cell functions.

Chromosomes are threadlike structures within the nucleus that carry the cell's "instructions" that direct all cell processes. Each cell has 46 chromosomes that contain *genes*, which are passed on to new cells during reproduction. Genes determine the physical and chemical traits inherited by children from their parents. Inherited traits include height, eye colour, skin colour, and many other characteristics.

Besides controlling the cell's activities, the nucleus is responsible for cell reproduction. Cells reproduce by dividing in half and each half becoming a new cell. The process of cell division, called *mitosis*, is needed for the growth and repair of body tissues. The chromosomes replicate (or duplicate) and are pulled apart, and then the cell divides so that each new cell is identical, each with 46 chromosomes (**FIGURE 17–3**).

Tissues

The cells are the body's building blocks. **Tissue** is a group of cells that are similar to each other in structure and function. The body has four basic types of tissue:

- ***Epithelial tissue*** covers internal and external body surfaces. Epithelial tissue is classified according to the shape of the cells and the number of layers within each. The shape of epithelial cells is described as *squamous* (thin and flat, like fish scales), *cuboidal* (cube-shaped, like dice), and *columnar* (tall and narrow, like columns).

  Epithelial tissue forms the thin outer layer of the skin that lines the cavities that open to the outside in the nose, mouth, respiratory tract, stomach, urethra, vagina, and intestines. Many glands are also epithelial tissue. The function of epithelial tissue is to aid in protection, absorption, secretion, and filtration. Epithelial tissue has no blood supply of its own, so it depends on the blood supply of the underlying connective tissue for nourishment. Because it is composed almost entirely of cells and because it is so well nourished from the underlying connective tissue, it can repair or replace itself quickly. Epithelial tissue does contain sensory cells, so it is able to perceive sensations such as pain and pressure.

- ***Connective tissue*** anchors, connects, and supports other body tissues. Connective tissue is found in every part of the body. The types of connective tissue are *connective tissue proper*, made up of loose irregular cells in a viscous (thickened) fluid base or of dense irregular tissues, such as in joint capsules, and *specialized connective tissue,* which includes the following:
  1. Adipose tissue (fat), which supplies energy to surrounding cells, aids in body temperature regulation, and acts both as a cushion and a support to surrounding structures
  2. *Dense fibrous* connective tissue such as tendons (which attach muscles to bones) and ligaments (which connect bones and support joints)
  3. *Cartilage* connective tissue, which supports, protects, and cushions joints and provides framework
  4. *Bone* tissue, which can protect organs such as the brain and supports the weight of the body for moving
  5. *Blood*, which transports nutrients, hormones, and respiratory gases such as oxygen and carbon dioxide and waste materials
  6. *Lymph*, which drains interstitial fluids and is involved in the body's immune response
- ***Muscle tissue*** is responsible for almost all body movements through contraction. There are three types of muscle tissue (see pp. 280–281).
- ***Nerve tissue*** is the major tissue of the nervous system. It is the main component of the brain, spinal cord, and all the nerves in the body. It is responsible for relaying information to and from the brain and throughout the body.

Organs and Body Cavities

Organs are structures made of different tissues that are arranged to perform a specialized function. An organ performs one or more functions. Examples of organs are the heart, brain, liver, lungs, and kidneys.

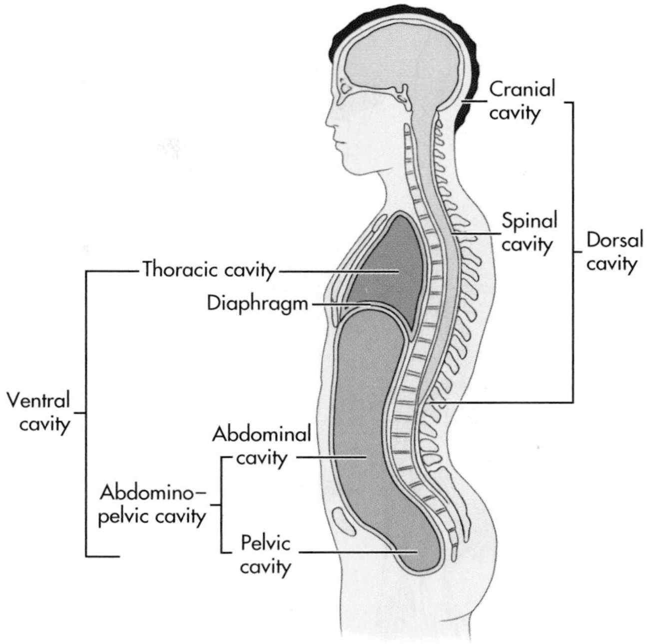

FIGURE 17–4 Major body cavities.

Organs are usually located within body cavities, but skin is also considered an organ. The two major cavities where organs are located are the dorsal cavity and the ventral cavity. The *dorsal cavity* has two cavities—the *cranial cavity* and the *spinal cavity*.

The *ventral cavity* consists of the *thoracic cavity*, the *abdominal cavity*, and the *pelvic cavity* (**FIGURE 17–4**).

Organ Systems

Cells, tissues, organs, and organ system

Organ systems are formed by organs that work together to perform special functions (**FIGURE 17–5**). **Homeostasis** is a steady state or stable internal environment maintained when all of the organ systems in the human body work together. For example, if the external temperature drops, our bodies start to shiver, and this action creates warmth and helps keep our internal temperature at the normal level.

We will discuss the major organ systems in this chapter: integumentary, musculo-skeletal, nervous (including the senses), circulatory (containing the

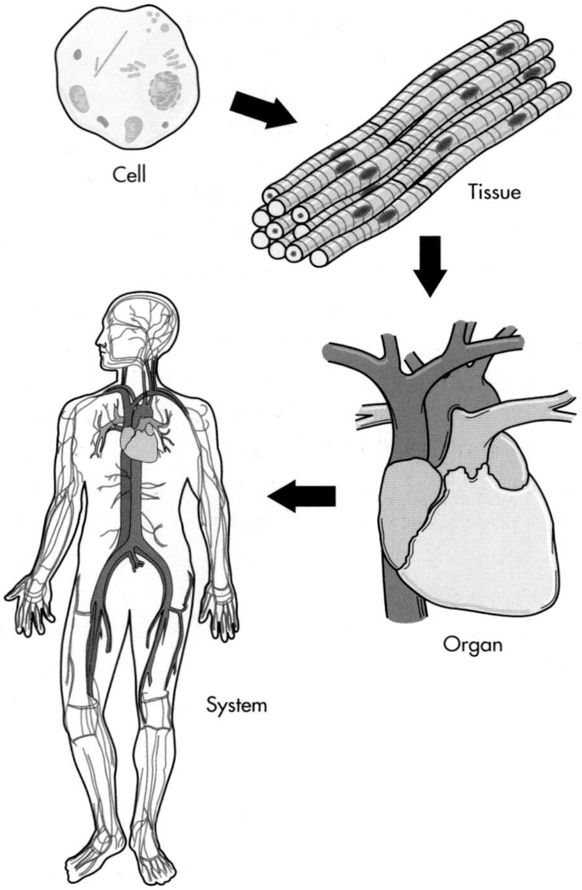

FIGURE 17–5 Organization of the body. (**Source:** Herlihy, B. (2014). *The human body in health and illness* (5th ed., p. 10). Philadelphia, PA: Elsevier/Saunders.)

cardiovascular and lymphatic), respiratory, digestive, urinary, reproductive, endocrine, and immune.

THE INTEGUMENTARY SYSTEM

The *integumentary system* consists of skin and its appendages—hair, nails, and sweat and oil glands. (A *gland* is a group of cells that produces and secretes a substance. The glands in skin produce and secrete sweat and oil.) The integumentary system is the largest system of the body since the skin is considered to be the largest organ by mass.

Integument means "covering." Skin is the body's natural covering, and it consists of all four types of tissue working together. There are two skin layers—the epidermis and the dermis (**FIGURE 17–6**). The *dermis* is the inner layer of skin and is made up of connective tissue. Blood vessels, nerves, sweat and oil glands, and hair roots are found in the dermis. The *epidermis* is the outer layer and contains living and dead cells arranged in specific layers. As the cells divide, creating newer cells, the older cells are pushed toward the surface, where they eventually die. Dead cells constantly flake off and are replaced by living cells. The living cells of the epidermis contain *pigment*, which gives skin its colour. The

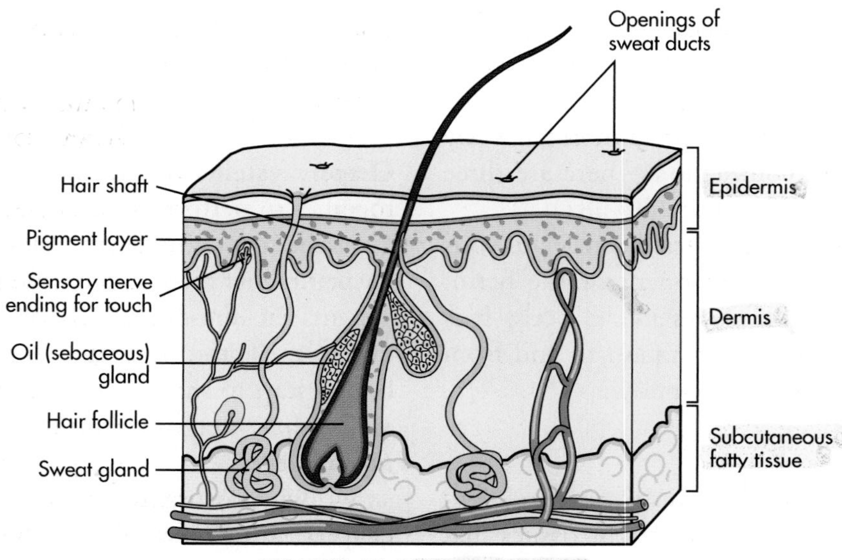

FIGURE 17–6 Layers of skin.

epidermis has no blood vessels, so it depends on blood vessels in the dermis for its nutrients and oxygen, but it does contain sensory cells and a few nerve endings, which perceive sensations like pain and pressure. Skin has four important functions:

1. It is the protective covering of the body. It prevents bacteria and other substances from entering the body, prevents excessive amounts of water from leaving the body, and protects organs from injury. The glands in the skin also produce and secrete substances that provide chemical protection against bacteria, viruses, and other potentially dangerous substances.
2. The nerve endings in skin protect the body by sensing heat, cold, pain, touch, and pressure stimulations. There are nerve endings over the entire body, and they are able to detect both pleasant and unpleasant stimulations.
3. Skin helps regulate body temperature. Blood vessels dilate (widen) when the temperature outside the body is high or when the temperature inside the body is high—for example, during a fever. More blood is brought to the body surface to be cooled during evaporation of sweat. During exercise, blood vessels dilate so that more blood reaches the skin to be cooled so as to cool the body. When we are cold and our body temperature is in danger of dropping, blood vessels constrict (narrow), and the body retains heat because less blood reaches the skin.
4. Like the urinary bladder and large intestine, the skin is an organ of elimination. Through perspiration, the skin eliminates cellular metabolism waste materials such as urea and other unwanted chemicals that may have accumulated in the perspiration.

Observing the condition of the client's skin can tell you several things about the client. The colour of skin can indicate a physical condition. For example, your client's skin or nails having a bluish (or grey–blue) tone could indicate a circulation problem. The client's skin being very dry could indicate dehydration.

The entire body, except the palms of the hands and the soles of the feet, is covered with hair. Hair in the nose, eyes, and ears protects these organs from dust, insects, and other foreign objects. Hair also helps retain heat, especially on body parts where it is plentiful (such as the head).

Nails protect the tips of fingers and toes and help fingers pick up and handle small objects. A client's general state of health and nutritional status can be reflected by the condition of the nails. Nail beds are generally pink, so a bluish tinge to the nail beds can indicate poor oxygenation (the amount of oxygen in tissues). Clubbing of the fingernails—the fingertips' being enlarged and the nails' curving down—can be caused by chronic lung disease and heart disease.

Sweat glands help the body regulate temperature. Sweat consists of water, salt, and a small amount of waste. Sweat is secreted through the pores in skin, and the body is cooled as sweat evaporates. Oil glands lie near hair shafts, and they secrete an oily substance into the space near the hair shaft. Oil travels to the skin's surface, helping keep hair and skin soft and shiny and also inhibiting the growth of bacteria on the surface of skin.

THE MUSCULO-SKELETAL SYSTEM

The *musculo-skeletal system* provides the framework for the body and allows the body to move. This system also protects the body and gives it shape. Besides bones and muscles, the system consists of ligaments, tendons, and cartilage.

Bones

Bones are hard, rigid structures that are made up of living cells surrounded by minerals that have been deposited by the living cells. A thin but strong membrane, called the *periosteum*, covers the entire surface of every bone in the body and merges with the ligaments and tendons that attach to the bones. Since the bones are living tissue, they require blood vessels to provide oxygen and nutrients; these vessels are found within the structure of the bones. The hard, dense layer of bone that forms the surface of every bone is called *compact bone*. It surrounds a softer, less dense form of bone called *spongy bone* (*trabecular bone*), which has many tiny hollow spaces (like a sponge). Inside these hollow spaces is a substance called *bone marrow*. Blood cells are manufactured in the bone marrow.

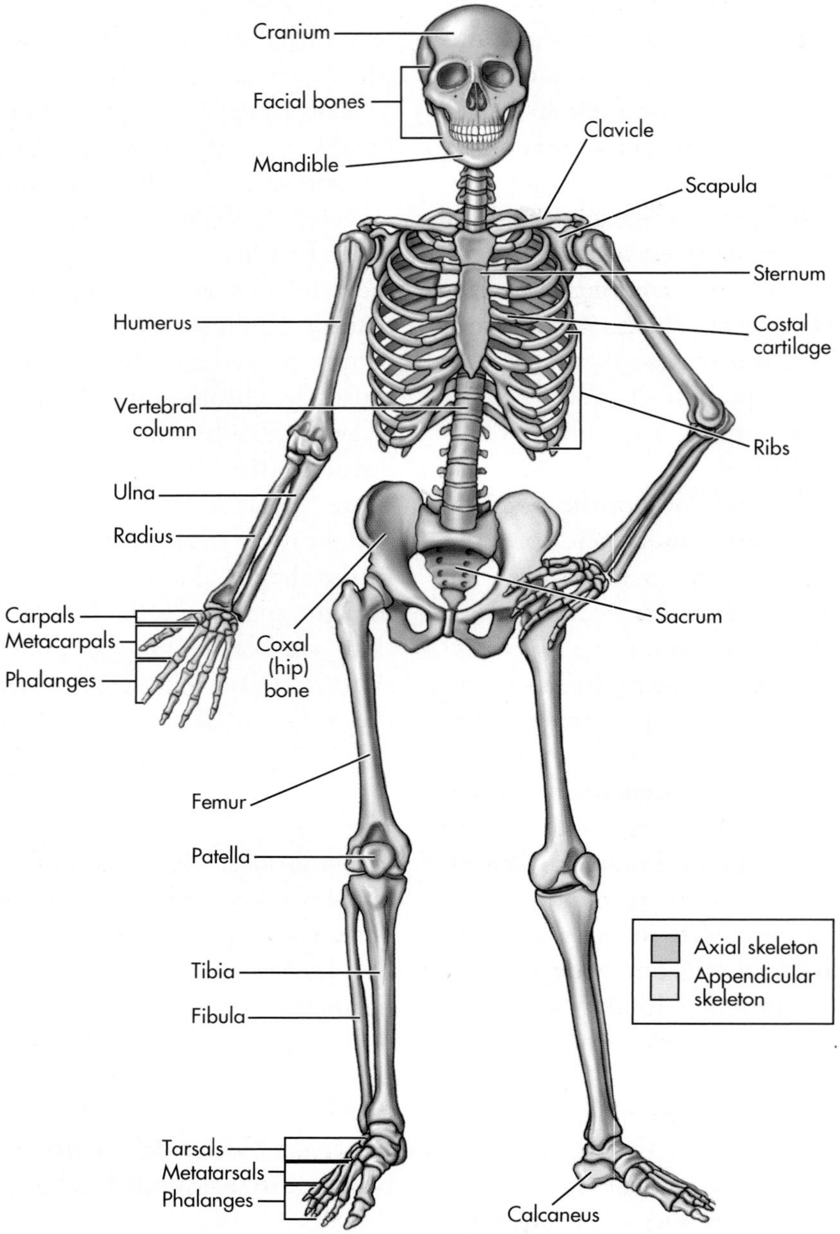

FIGURE 17–7 Bones of the body. (**Source:** Herlihy, B. (2014). *The human body in health and illness* (5th ed., p. 112). Philadelphia, PA: Elsevier/Saunders.)

The human body has 206 bones (**FIGURE 17–7**), consisting of five types:

1. ***Long bones*** are hard and dense bones that provide strength, structure, and mobility. They are longer than they are wide. Long bone structure is most recognizable in the bones of the arms (humerus, radius, and ulna) and legs (femur, tibia, and fibula) but also includes the metacarpals of the palms, the metatarsals of the feet, and the phalanges of the fingers and toes.
2. ***Short bones*** allow skill and ease in movement. The bones in the wrists and ankles are short bones. Short bones are cube-shaped.
3. ***Flat bones*** are thin, flat, and curved bones that protect the organs. Such bones include the ribs and sternum (breastbone), the skull, pelvic bones, and scapulae (shoulder blades).

4. ***Irregular bones*** are irregularly shaped bones with various bony projections and features that interact with other bones. These bones provide sites for muscle attachment and allow various degrees of movement and flexibility, along with some support. They include the hip bones, vertebrae in the spinal column, and various bones in the skull.
5. ***Sesamoid bones*** are usually short or irregular bones that are imbedded in a tendon and protect the tendon. These bones include the patella (knee cap), which is connected to the quadriceps tendon.

Joints

A *joint* is the point at which two or more bones meet. Joints allow movement (see Chapter 26). Cartilage is connective tissue that cushions the joint so that bone ends do not rub together. The *synovial membrane* lines the joint and secretes *synovial fluid*, which acts as a lubricant so that the joint can move smoothly. Bones are held together at the joint by strong bands of connective tissue called *ligaments*.

Joints can be classified into three groups according to the amount of movement: *fibrous*, or *immovable* (such as the sutures in the skull bound by fibrous connective tissue); *cartilaginous*, or *slightly movable* (such as the movement achieved in the spinal column between the cartilaginous intervertebral discs); and *synovial*, or *freely movable* (which provides much more flexibility and movement than the other two types of joints). A typical synovial joint is more complex than the other types of joints and includes the following structures:

- ***Articular cartilage***—which lines the articulating surface of each of the two bones, forming a smooth surface within the joint
- ***Joint capsule***—made up of fibrous connective tissue, enclosing the joint in a strong sleevelike covering
- ***Synovial membrane***—lines the joint capsule and secretes lubricating synovial fluid into the joint cavity
- ***Synovial fluid***—lubricates the bones in the joint and decreases the friction within the joint
- ***Bursae*** (singular: *bursa*)—small sacs of synovial fluid that function as a cushion and gliding surface between the joint and the tendons that cross over the joint (excessive use of the joint may cause a painful inflammation of the bursae, known as *bursitis*)

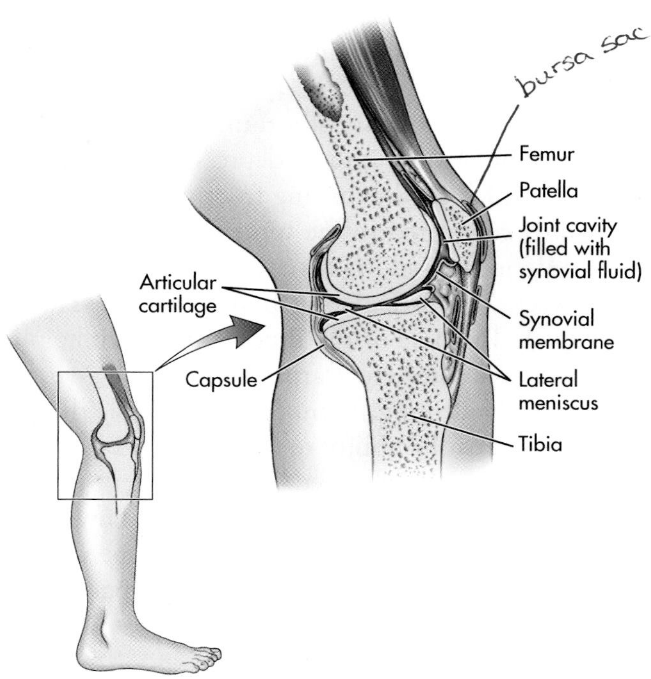

FIGURE 17–8 Freely movable, or synovial, joint structure (knee) and contents. (**Source:** Herlihy, B. (2014). *The human body in health and illness* (5th ed., p. 134). Philadelphia, PA: Elsevier/Saunders.)

Moving Synovial Joints

The body contains many types of freely movable synovial joints. The types of motion and the degree of flexibility vary with each type of joint. There are six types of movable synovial joints, classified by the type of movement allowed by the joint (see **FIGURE 17–8**).

- Ball-and-socket joint—allows movement in all directions. It is made up of the rounded end of one bone and a hollow cavity or depression in another bone. The rounded end of one fits into the cavity of the other. The joints of the hips and shoulders are ball-and-socket joints. Although the ball-and-socket joint allows for a wide range of movement, it also predisposes the joint to easy displacement. For example, a fall can cause the shoulder to dislocate.
- Hinge joint—allows movement in one direction around a single axis. The structure of these joints

is very similar to a hinge that you might find on a door. Hinge joints include elbows, knees, and fingers.

- **Pivot joint**—consists of a rounded projection on one bone fitting into a depression on another bone, which allows turning from side to side. The skull is connected to the spine by a pivot joint.
- **Saddle joint**—allows for a wide range of motion between two articulating bones that are saddle-shaped. The base of the thumb has a saddle joint known as a carpometacarpal joint, which gives the thumb a wide range of motion (opposable thumb) and gives us the ability to firmly grasp objects.
- **Gliding joint**—is formed by the interaction of the flat surfaces of the articulating bones, allowing for limited but complex gliding movements. Gliding joints are found in the wrist (intercarpal joints), ankles (intertarsal joints), and the vertebral column.
- **Condyloid joint**—is formed when the oval articular surface of one bone fits into the oval depression of the second articulating bone. The wrist (radiocarpal joint) and the knuckles at the base of the fingers (metacarpophalangeal joints) are examples.

Muscles

There are more than 600 muscles in the human body (**FIGURES 17–9 through 17–11**). Muscle tissue is categorized as forming *skeletal* (striated) muscles, *smooth* muscles, or *cardiac* muscles.

Skeletal muscles, the muscles attached to bones, are *striated*; that is, they look striped or streaked.

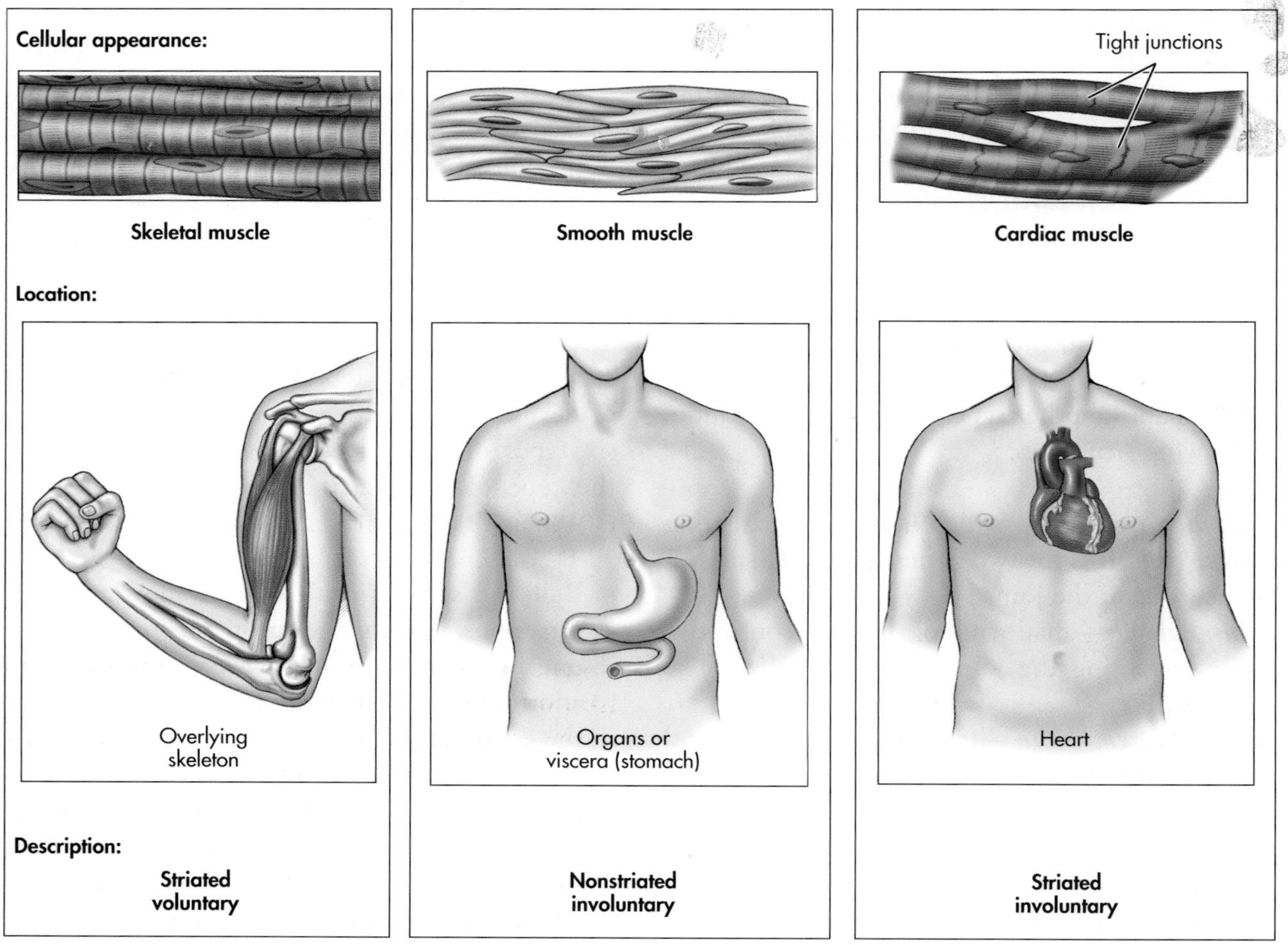

FIGURE 17–9 Three types of muscles. (**Source:** Herlihy, B. (2014). *The human body in health and illness* (5th ed., p. 143). Philadelphia, PA: Elsevier/Saunders.)

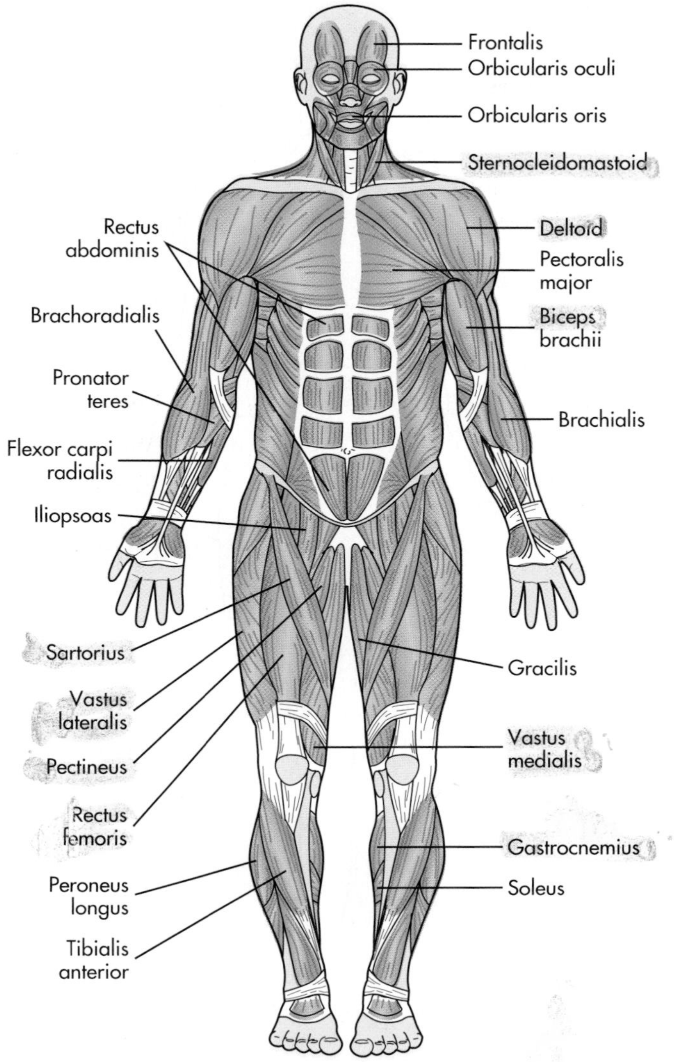

FIGURE 17–10 Anterior (front) view of the muscles of the body.

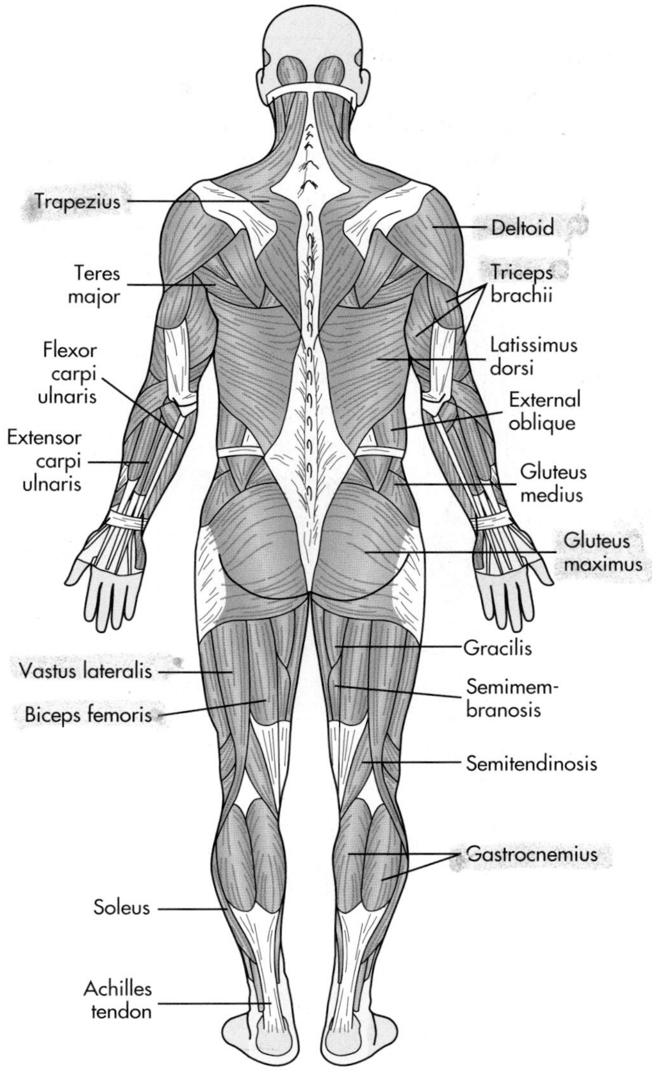

FIGURE 17–11 Posterior (back) view of the muscles of the body.

They are also *voluntary*, meaning they can be consciously controlled. Arm muscles or leg muscles do not work unless you move your arm or your leg.

Smooth muscles can be identified by their smooth appearance (they are not streaked or striped). Smooth muscles are *involuntary*, which means they work automatically and cannot be consciously controlled. Smooth muscles are present in the stomach, intestines, blood vessels, and other body organs.

Cardiac muscle is found only in the heart. Although it appears striated like skeletal muscle, it is involuntary muscle.

Muscles can do only two things: contract and relax. Most muscles contract and relax quickly. Muscles perform three important body functions:

1. Movement of body parts
2. Maintenance of posture
3. Production of body heat

Strong, tough connective tissues called *tendons* connect muscles to bones. When muscles contract (shorten), tendons at each end of the muscle cause the bone to move. The body has numerous tendons; the Achilles tendon is shown in **FIGURE 17–11**.

Some muscles constantly contract to maintain the body's posture. When muscles contract, they must metabolize nutrients to generate energy, resulting in the production of heat. The greater the muscular activity, the greater the amount of heat produced in the body. As a result, we get warm when we exercise.

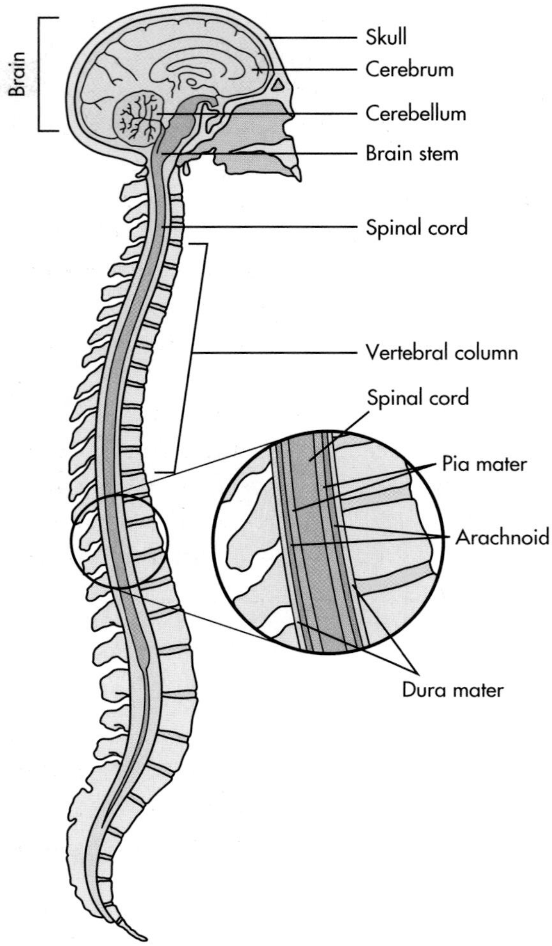

FIGURE 17–12 The central nervous system. (**Source:** Herlihy, B. (2014). *The human body in health and illness* (5th ed., p. 173). Philadelphia, PA: Elsevier/Saunders.)

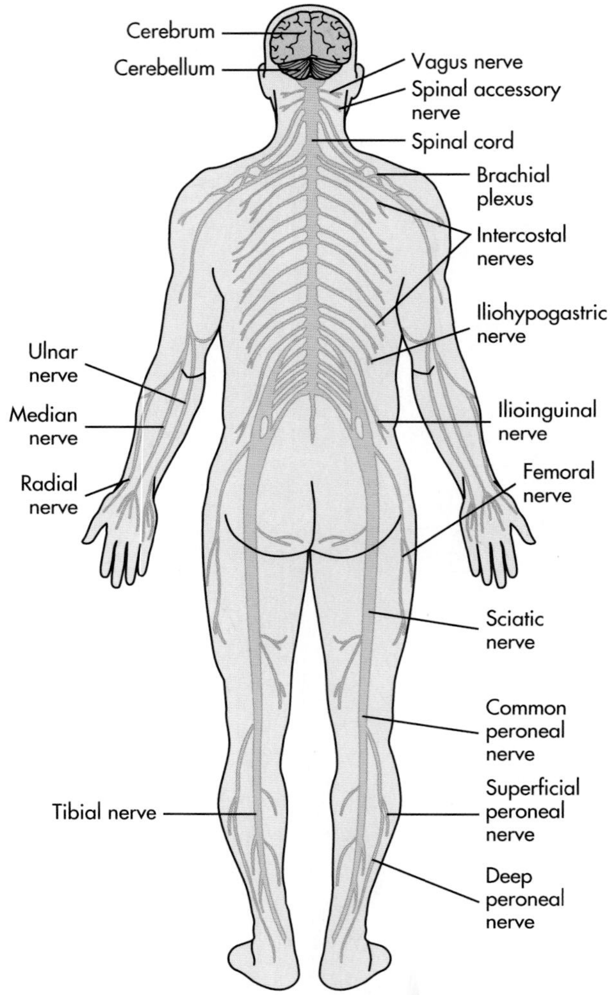

FIGURE 17–13 The peripheral nervous system.

Shivering is a way the body produces heat when exposed to cold. The shivering sensation arises from rapid, general muscle contractions.

THE NERVOUS SYSTEM

The nervous system controls, directs, and coordinates body functions. The two main divisions of the nervous system are the *central nervous system* (CNS) and the *peripheral nervous system* (PNS). The CNS consists of the *brain* and the *spinal cord* (**FIGURE 17–12**), and the PNS consists of the *nerves* throughout the body (**FIGURE 17–13**), which carry messages or impulses to and from the brain. All the nerves in the body are connected to either the spinal cord (through the spinal nerves) or the brain and brain stem (through cranial nerves). Nerve tissue is composed of two types of cells:

1. *Neuroglia*, which nourish, protect, and insulate neurons
2. *Neurons*, which transmit information in the form of electrical nerve impulses

A *nerve impulse* is a signal that is transmitted along the membrane of the neuron, starting at the point where the impulse was applied. Nerve impulses pass, chain-like, from one cell to another.

Each neuron is composed of three parts (**FIGURE 17–14**), through which these electrical nerve impulses pass:

1. The *dendrite*, which contains receptors that receive stimuli directly for sensations such as pain, cold, pressure, and heat. The dendrite transmits this information to the cell body from within the terminal ends of sensory neuron dendrites.

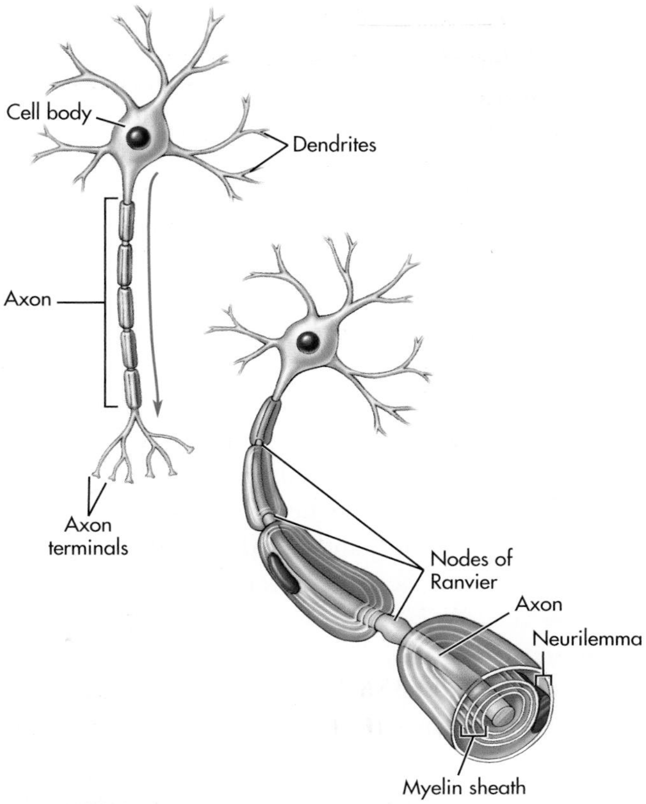

FIGURE 17–14 The structure of a neuron.

Dendrites usually (although not always) branch from the neuron cell body.

2. The *cell body*, which contains the organelles (smaller parts), including the nucleus. The electrical nerve impulse passes through the cell body.
3. The *axon*, which carries information away from the cell to the axon *terminals* (ends).

Nerve impulses have both electrical and chemical traits. Electrical impulses transmit a signal *within* a neuron, whereas chemical processes transmit the signal from one neuron to another or to a muscle cell. The electrical impulse may then be transmitted across the *synapse* (the gap between neurons) to the next dendrite. When a nerve signal, or impulse, reaches the ends of its axon, it has travelled as an *action potential* (a pulse of electricity, or temporary reversal of the polarity of the cell).[1]

While there is no cellular continuity between neurons because of the synapses, neurons form a network of electrical activities and, therefore, have to be interconnected in some way. A chemical process of interaction between neurons and *effector* (target) cells occurs at the end of the axon in the synapse.[1] The axon terminals produce and store chemical substances called *neurotransmitters*. The neurotransmitters are released by the *presynaptic* (before the synapse) membrane and seep across the gap to receptors on the receiving neuron's *postsynaptic* (after the synapse) membrane. The neurotransmitters bind to these receptors, causing changes to the membrane that can slow or speed up the impulse and also allows *ions* (charged particles) to pass in and out of the receiving cell.[1]

Nervous tissue is easily damaged and has a limited capacity for regeneration. Some nerve fibres have a protective covering called a *myelin sheath*, which also insulates the nerve fibre. Nerve fibres covered with myelin can conduct impulses faster than those fibres without the protective covering.

The Central Nervous System

The CNS consists of the brain and the spinal cord. The brain is contained in and protected by the skull. The three main parts of the brain are the *cerebrum*, the *cerebellum*, and the *brain stem* (see **FIGURE 17–12**).

The cerebrum is the largest part of the brain and is the centre of thought and intelligence. The cerebrum is divided into two halves called the right and left *hemispheres*. The right hemisphere controls movement and activities on the body's left side. The left hemisphere controls the body's right side. The outermost layer of the cerebrum is called the *cerebral cortex*, and it consists of billions of *unmyelinated neurons* (grey matter) (**FIGURE 17–15**). The cerebral cortex controls the highest functions of the brain: reasoning, memory, consciousness, speech, voluntary muscle movement, vision, hearing, sensation, and other activities.

The cerebellum regulates and coordinates body movements. The smooth movements of voluntary muscles and the body's balance are possible because of their control by the cerebellum. Injury to the cerebellum results in jerky movements, loss of coordination, and muscle weakness.

The brain stem connects the cerebrum to the spinal cord. Within the brain stem are important structures including the *midbrain*, the *pons*, and the *medulla*. The midbrain and the pons relay messages

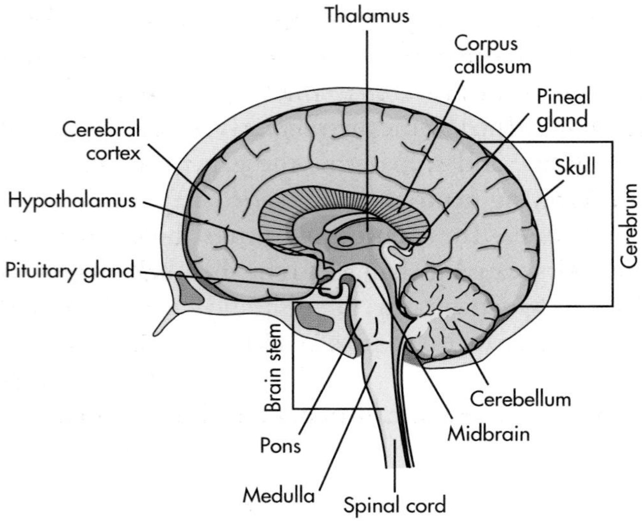

FIGURE 17–15 The brain.

between the medulla and the cerebrum. The medulla is directly below the pons. The medulla controls heart rate, breathing, blood vessel size, swallowing, coughing, and vomiting. The brain connects to the spinal cord at the lower end of the medulla.

The spinal cord lies within and is protected by the spinal column. The cord is about 45 cm (18 inches) long. It contains pathways that conduct messages to and from the brain and the spinal nerves.

The brain and the spinal cord are covered and protected by three layers of connective tissue called *meninges*. The outer layer, a tough covering called the *dura mater*, lies next to the skull and partially protects the brain from movement. The middle layer is called the *arachnoid*, and the inner layer is the *pia mater*, which adheres to the brain directly and contains the blood vessels surrounding the brain. The space between the middle and inner layers is the *arachnoid space*, and this space is filled with a fluid called *cerebrospinal fluid* that circulates around the brain and the spinal cord. The cerebrospinal fluid protects the CNS and cushions shocks that could easily injure the structures of the brain and the spinal cord.

The Peripheral Nervous System

The PNS has 12 pairs of *cranial nerves* and 31 pairs of *spinal nerves*. Cranial nerves conduct impulses between the brain and the head, neck, chest, and abdomen and thus the impulses for smell, vision, hearing, pain, touch, temperature, pressure, and voluntary and involuntary muscle control. The *vagus nerve* is the only cranial nerve that has extensive association with the entire body. Sensations including touch, pain, temperature, pressure, as well as the control of muscle activity are handled by the various spinal nerves associated with each region of the body. Spinal nerves carry impulses from skin, extremities (a limb of the body, especially a hand or a foot), and the internal body structures not supplied by cranial nerves.

Peripheral nerves with special functions form the *autonomic nervous system*. This system controls involuntary muscles and certain body functions that occur "automatically," including heartbeat, blood pressure, intestinal contractions, and glandular secretions.

The autonomic nervous system is divided into the *sympathetic nervous system* and the *parasympathetic nervous system*. These divisions balance each other. The sympathetic nervous system is responsible for what we refer to as the "fight or flight" response and generally (but not always) tends to speed up functions. The parasympathetic nervous system is responsible for maintaining our normal or "relaxed" condition with respect to body function and generally makes processes such as digestion and normal cell metabolism a priority (energy conservation). When you are angry, frightened, or excited, the sympathetic nervous system is stimulated. The parasympathetic system is more active during the remainder of the time or when the sympathetic system has been stimulated for too long.

THE SENSE ORGANS

The five senses are sight, hearing, taste, smell, and touch. Receptors for taste are located in the tongue and are called *taste buds*. Receptors for smell are located in the nose. Touch receptors are found in the dermis of skin in varying numbers throughout the body, with particularly large numbers in the fingertips, toes, and lips.

The Eye and the Sense of Sight

Receptors for vision are located in the eyes. The eye is easily injured. Bones of the skull, eyelids, eyelashes, and tears all protect the eyes from injury. Eye structures are shown in **FIGURE 17–16**. The eye has three layers:

- The *sclera*, the white of the eye, is the outer layer except for its anterior one sixth, which is the cornea. The sclera is made of tough connective tissue.
- The *choroid* is the second layer. Blood vessels, the *ciliary muscle*, and the *iris* make up the choroid. The iris gives the eye its colour. The opening in the middle of the iris is the *pupil*. Pupil size varies with the amount of light entering the eye. The pupil contracts (narrows) in bright light and dilates (widens) in dim or dark places.
- The *retina* is the inner layer of the eye. It contains receptors for vision and the nerve fibres of the optic nerve.

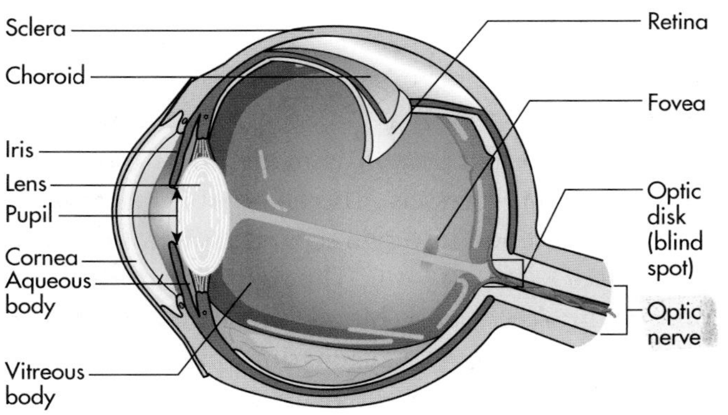

FIGURE 17–16 The eye.

Light enters the eye through the *cornea*. The cornea is the transparent part of the outer layer that lies over the eye. Light rays pass to the *lens*, which lies behind the pupil. The light is then reflected to the retina and carried to the brain by the *optic nerve* for its interpretation of what is being seen.

The *aqueous chamber* separates the cornea from the lens. The chamber is filled with a fluid called *aqueous humor*. The fluid helps the cornea keep its shape and position. The *vitreous humor* is found behind the lens. The vitreous body is a gelatin-like substance that supports the retina and maintains the eye's shape.

The Ear and the Sense of Hearing

The ear is a sense organ that functions for hearing and balance. The ear is divided into the *external ear, middle ear*, and *inner ear*. Ear structures are shown in **FIGURE 17–17**.

The external ear (outer part) is called the *pinna* or *auricle*. Sound waves are guided through the external ear into the *auditory canal*. Glands in the auditory canal secrete a waxy substance called *cerumen*, which catches particles that enter the ear. The auditory canal extends about 2.5 cm (1 in.) to the *eardrum*. The eardrum (*tympanic membrane*) separates the external ear and the middle ear.

The Eustachian tube (also called the auditory tube), which opens into the middle ear, connects the middle ear and the throat. Air enters the Eustachian

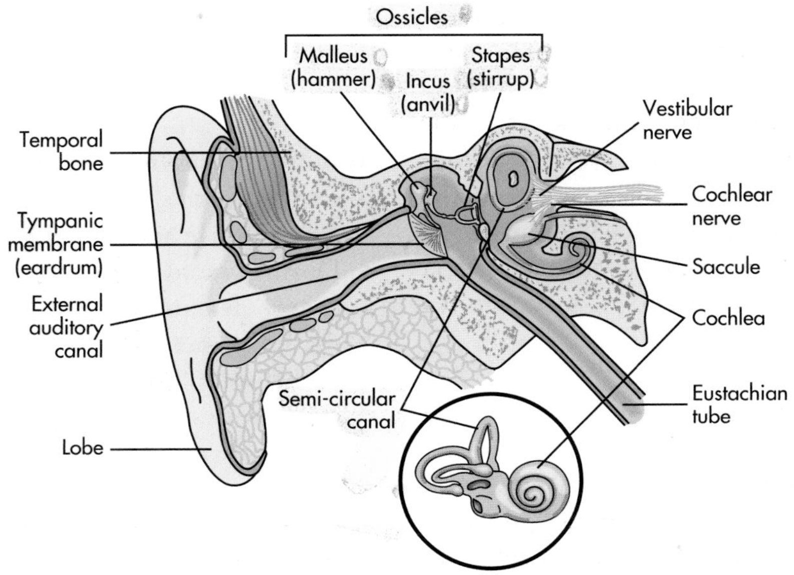

FIGURE 17–17 The ear.

tube from the throat so that the pressure is equal on both sides of the eardrum. The middle ear is a small space that contains three small bones called *ossicles*. The ossicles amplify sound received from the eardrum and transmit the sound to the inner ear. The three ossicles are as follows:

1. The *malleus*, which looks like a hammer
2. The *incus*, which resembles an anvil
3. The *stapes*, which is shaped like a stirrup

The inner ear consists of the *cochlea* and *semi-circular canals*. The cochlea, which looks like a snail shell, contains fluid. The fluid carries sound waves received from the middle ear to the *auditory nerve*. The *auditory nerve* then carries the message to the brain for interpretation of what is being heard.

The three semi-circular canals are involved in maintaining balance. They sense the head's position and any changes in position and send messages to the brain.

The Tongue and the Sense of Taste

The *taste buds* contain the receptors for taste. They are located around the small structures on the upper surface of the tongue, the soft palate, the upper esophagus, and the epiglottis. They relay sensations of different tastes to the brain for interpretation. The four basic taste sensations are salty, sweet, sour, and bitter. The receptors for each sensation are located on a particular area of the tongue. The anterior two-thirds of the tongue is controlled by the *facial nerve* (CN VII). Sweet sensation receptors are on the tip of the tongue. Salty receptors are on the sides near the front. Sour receptors are located on the sides near the back, and bitter sensation receptors are across the back of the tongue. The posterior third of the tongue is controlled by the *glossopharyngeal nerve* (CN IX).

The Nose and the Sense of Smell

Receptors for smell are located on the roof of the nasal cavity. These are called *olfactory receptors*, and sense of smell is controlled by the *olfactory nerve* (CN I). These receptors are stimulated by the fluid in the mucous membrane in the nose. The impulses are sent to the brain, where they are interpreted as smell. Smell and taste are very connected. When we have a cold and our noses are congested ("stuffed"), we find that foods often do not taste the same.

THE CIRCULATORY SYSTEM

The circulatory system is an organ system that transports and exchanges nutrients (amino acids, glucose, fatty acids), gases (oxygen and carbon dioxide), hormones, blood cells, and wastes to and from cells in the body to maintain normal cell processes and keep cells alive.

Two types of fluids move through the circulatory system: blood and lymph. Blood, the heart, and blood vessels form the *cardiovascular system*. The lymph, lymph nodes, and lymph vessels form the *lymphatic system*. The cardiovascular system and the lymphatic system together make up the *circulatory system*.

The Cardiovascular System

The cardiovascular system is made up of blood, the heart, and blood vessels. The heart works as a pump to transport blood into two separate systems of blood vessels (see **FIGURE 17–18**). The right side of the heart pumps unoxygenated blood (normally shown as blue) to the lungs for oxygenation (*pulmonary circulation*). The left side of the heart receives oxygenated blood (normally shown as red) from the lungs and pumps it to all of the tissues and organs of the body (*systemic circulation*).

The cardiovascular system has numerous important functions:

- Blood carries nutrients, oxygen, and other substances to the cells throughout the body so that they can live and function.
- During exercise or physical activity, increased energy demands of organs and muscles are automatically met through increased blood flow.
- To help stop bleeding and to promote healing, the circulatory system sends clotting cells and proteins to the site of injury or bleeding.
- Blood removes waste products from cells.
- Blood and blood vessels help regulate body temperature. Heat from muscle activity is carried by blood to other body parts. Blood vessels in skin

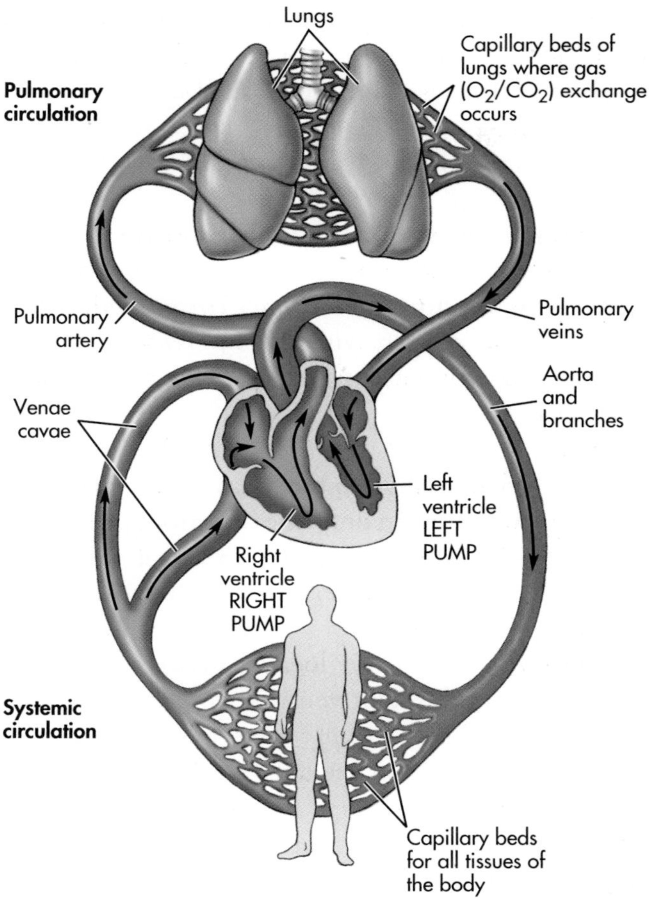

FIGURE 17–18 Pulmonary and systemic circulations. (**Source:** Herlihy, B. (2014). *The human body in health and illness* (5th ed., p. 311). Philadelphia, PA: Elsevier/Saunders.)

dilate if the body needs to be cooled. They constrict if heat needs to be kept in the body.

- The cardiovascular system also produces and carries white blood cells and antibodies that defend the body from disease-causing microorganisms.

Blood

Blood consists of blood cells and a liquid portion called *plasma*, which is approximately 90% water. Blood composition is approximately 55% plasma and 45% cells. Plasma carries blood cells to other body cells. It also carries other substances needed by cells for proper functioning. Nutrients (proteins, fats, and carbohydrates), hormones, chemicals, and waste products are some of the substances carried in the plasma.

Red blood cells are called *erythrocytes* and they give blood its red colour because of a substance in the blood cell called **hemoglobin**. As red blood cells circulate through the capillaries in the lungs, hemoglobin picks up oxygen from inhaled air and carries it to cells. When hemoglobin in red blood cells is saturated (filled) with oxygen, the blood appears bright red. As blood circulates to the tissues and organs, oxygen is released from the hemoglobin and is given to cells. It is the lack of oxygen that makes the colour of the blood change from bright red to "bluish-red." Cells release carbon dioxide (a waste product), which is picked up by the blood and transported back to the lungs, where it can be released and "exhaled" during ventilation.

There are about 25 trillion (25 000 000 000 000) red blood cells (*erythrocytes*) in the body. In a cubic millimetre of blood (the size of a tiny drop), there are about 4.5 to 5 million cells. These cells live for approximately 120 days, and as they wear out, they are destroyed by the liver and the spleen and replaced with new erythrocytes. Red bone marrow produces new red blood cells at a rate of about two million every second.

White blood cells, called *leukocytes*, are colourless. They protect the body against infection. There are 5 000 to 10 000 white blood cells in a cubic millimetre of blood. At the first sign of infection, white blood cells rush to the site of the infection and begin to multiply rapidly to kill the invading microorganisms to fight the infection. The number of white blood cells increases when there is an infection in the body. White blood cells are also produced by the bone marrow and live for approximately 9 days.

Platelets (*thrombocytes*) are necessary for the clotting of blood. They are also produced by the bone marrow. There are about 200 000 to 400 000 platelets in a cubic millimetre of blood. A platelet lives for approximately 4 days.

The Heart

The heart is a hollow, muscular organ that lies in the middle to lower part of the chest cavity and tilts slightly toward the left side (**FIGURE 17–19**). The chambers, major vessels, valves, and circulation pathways of the heart are shown in **FIGURE 17–20.**

The heart has three layers:

1. The *pericardium* is the outer layer. It is a thin sac surrounding the heart that forms a fluid-filled

peri
(outside)

space (pericardial fluid) around the heart called the pericardial space.

myo (muscle)

2. The *myocardium* is the second layer. This layer is the thick, muscular portion of the heart.
3. The *endocardium* is the inner layer. The endocardium is the membrane lining the inner chambers of the heart.

endo (inside)

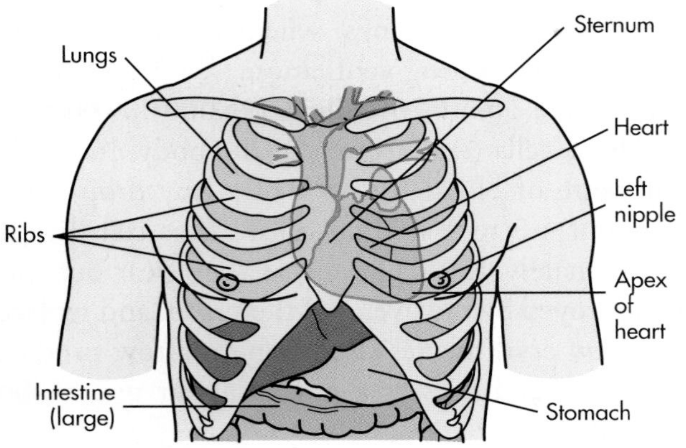

FIGURE 17–19 Location of the heart in the chest cavity.

The heart has four chambers:

- The two upper chambers—called *atria* (singular, *atrium*)—receive blood. The *right atrium* receives blood from body tissues, and the *left atrium* receives blood from the lungs.
- The two lower chambers—called *ventricles*—pump blood out of the heart. The *right ventricle* pumps blood to the lungs (*pulmonary circulation*), where it picks up oxygen, and the *left ventricle* pumps blood to all parts of the body (*systemic circulation*).

Valves, located between the atria and the ventricles, allow blood to flow in only one direction, preventing it from flowing back into the atria from the ventricles. The four valves are shown in **FIGURE 17–20**.

1. The *tricuspid valve* is located between the right atrium and the right ventricle.
2. The *mitral valve* (*bicuspid valve*) is located between the left atrium and the left ventricle.

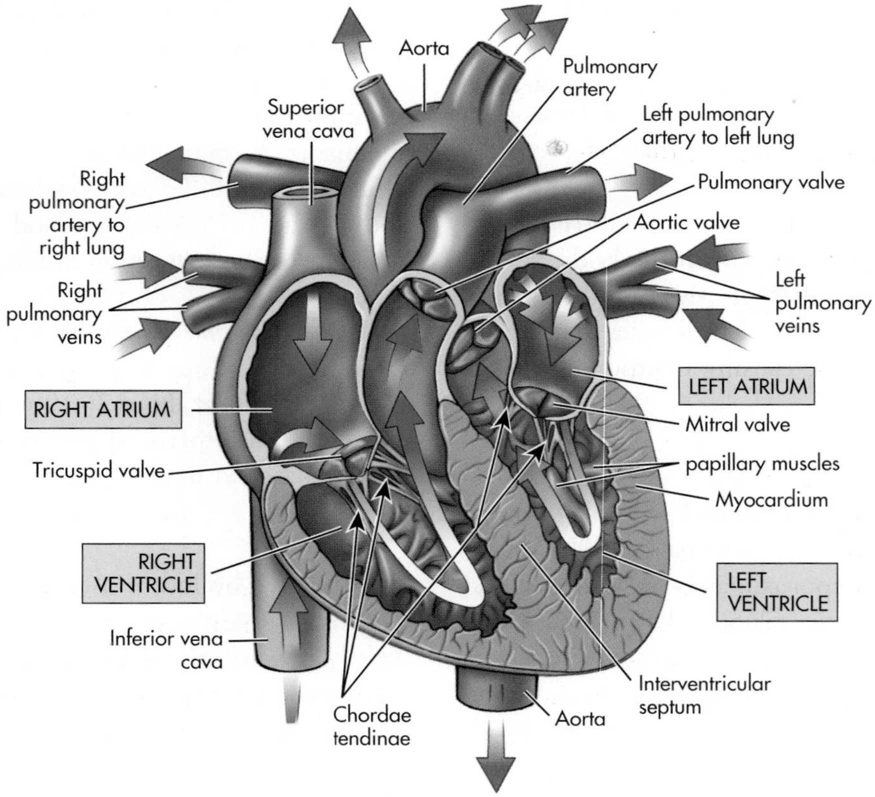

FIGURE 17–20 Structures and circulation pathways of the heart. (Adapted from Herlihy, B. (2014). *The human body in health and illness* (5th ed., p. 311). Philadelphia, PA: Elsevier/Saunders.)

arteries - leaving
veins - coming to

3. The *pulmonary valve* is located between the pulmonary artery and the right ventricle.
4. The *aortic valve* is located between the aorta and the left ventricle.

There are two phases of heart action. During *diastole*, the resting phase, heart chambers fill with blood. During *systole*, the working phase, the heart contracts. Blood is pumped through the major arteries exiting the heart to the blood vessels when the heart contracts.

The rate at which the heart beats (heart rate) can differ for various reasons. Generally, the larger the body size, the slower the rate is—men, therefore, have slower heart rates than women do. As well, heart rate generally slows with age. Disease, fever, exercise, and some medications can also influence heart rate. The *pulse* may be used to measure heart rate (refer to Chapter 15 for more information on pulse rate).

Blood Vessels

Blood flows to body tissues and cells through *blood vessels*. Blood vessels vary in size, structure, and function, and there are several types, including arteries, arterioles, capillaries, veins, and venules. **FIGURE 17–21** shows some of the major arteries and veins in the body.

Arteries carry blood away from the heart.

- *Systemic arteries* carry blood from the heart to the vessels that supply the tissues of the body. The *aorta* is the largest systemic artery and exits the heart directly from the left ventricle. The aorta branches into other arteries that carry oxygenated blood to all parts of the body, and these arteries, in turn, branch into various other vessels supplying all regions of the body.
- *Pulmonary arteries* carry blood from the heart to the vessels of the lungs, where gas exchange takes place. The *pulmonary trunk* is the largest pulmonary artery and exits the heart from the right ventricle. This pulmonary trunk branches into the right pulmonary artery, which goes to the right lung, and the left pulmonary artery, which goes to the left lung.

The smallest branch of an artery is an **arteriole**. Arterioles connect with blood vessels called

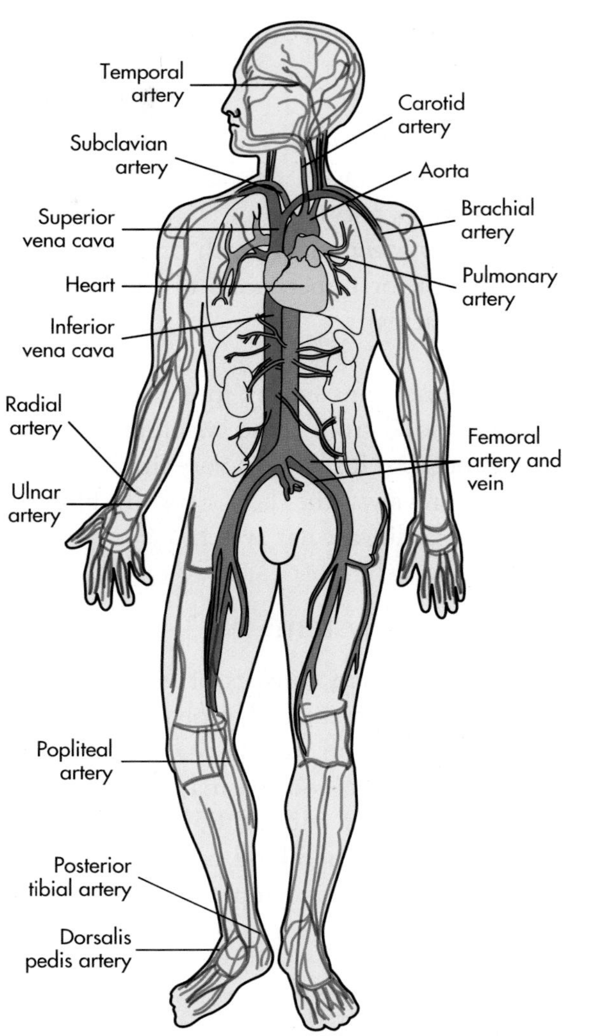

FIGURE 17–21 Some of the major arteries and veins in the body.

capillaries, which are tiny, thin-walled vessels. Nutrients, oxygen, and other substances pass from capillaries into cells, and waste products, including carbon dioxide, pass from cells into the bloodstream.

Veins return blood to the heart.

- *Systemic veins* collect blood from the vessels that drain the capillaries of the tissues in the body.
- *Pulmonary veins* carry blood back to the heart from the lungs after gas exchange has taken place in the pulmonary capillaries.

Venules are microscopic and the smallest form of veins. They drain blood from the capillaries and come together with the numerous branches of systemic veins near the heart to form two main veins:

1. The *inferior vena cava,* which drains blood from the inferior, or lower, areas of the body (abdominal structures and legs)
2. The *superior vena cava,* which drains blood from the superior, or upper, areas of the body (head, neck, and arms)

Both of these veins empty into the right atrium. The venous blood from these systemic veins is dark bluish-red because it contains very little oxygen.

BOX 17–2 reviews the key steps in blood flow through the cardiovascular system.

The Lymphatic System

The lymphatic system consists of lymphoid organs, lymph nodes, lymph ducts, lymphatic tissue, lymph capillaries, and lymph vessels. As blood circulates through capillaries, blood plasma leaks out into the spaces between cells. About 85% of the fluid is absorbed back into the blood capillaries. The other 15% drains into the lymphatic capillaries that surround the blood capillaries. This fluid is called *lymph* and is composed primarily of water, electrolytes, waste from metabolizing cells, and some protein. The lymphatic capillaries empty into larger lymph vessels.

Lymphatic vessels are distributed around the entire body and run beside veins. The lymph flows through larger and larger vessels until it reaches lymph ducts. These ducts drain into the veins below the collarbone, called *subclavian veins.*

Blood moves because it is pumped by the heart, but lymph depends on other means for movement. Lymph moves in response to contraction of skeletal muscles, the movement of the chest during respiration, and contraction of smooth muscles.

Lymphoid organs include lymph nodes, tonsils, the thymus gland, and the spleen.

Lymph nodes are small pea-shaped patches of lymphatic tissue. Cervical lymph nodes drain and filter lymph from the head and neck area. Axillary lymph nodes drain and cleanse lymph from the upper extremities, shoulders, and breasts. Inguinal lymph nodes are located in the groin and drain and cleanse lymph from the lower extremities and external genitalia (**FIGURE 17–22**).

BOX 17–2 Blood Flow Through the Cardiovascular System

1. The inferior vena cava and the superior vena cava empty the venous blood, which is high in carbon dioxide and poor in oxygen, into the right atrium.
2. From the right atrium, blood flows through the tricuspid valve and into the right ventricle.
3. The right ventricle pumps this blood through the pulmonary semi-lunar valve into the pulmonary arteries (right and left) and into the right or left lung. It is here that needed inhaled oxygen will be exchanged for carbon dioxide.
4. Oxygen diffuses into the capillary beds of the lungs for delivery to the tissues, and waste carbon dioxide is diffused from the blood into the lungs for excretion.
5. The oxygen-rich blood from the right or left lung empties from the right and left pulmonary veins into the left atrium.
6. This blood passes from the left atrium through the mitral valve (bicuspid valve) into the left ventricle.
7. The left ventricle pumps blood to the aorta, which branches off to form other arteries throughout the body.
8. The arterial blood is carried to all of the body's tissues by arterioles and then to cells by capillaries.
9. The cells receive oxygen and nutrients from capillaries in exchange for carbon dioxide and waste products.
10. Capillaries connect with venules.
11. Venules carry blood that contains carbon dioxide and waste products.
12. Venules form veins.
13. Veins return blood to the heart, into the right atrium.

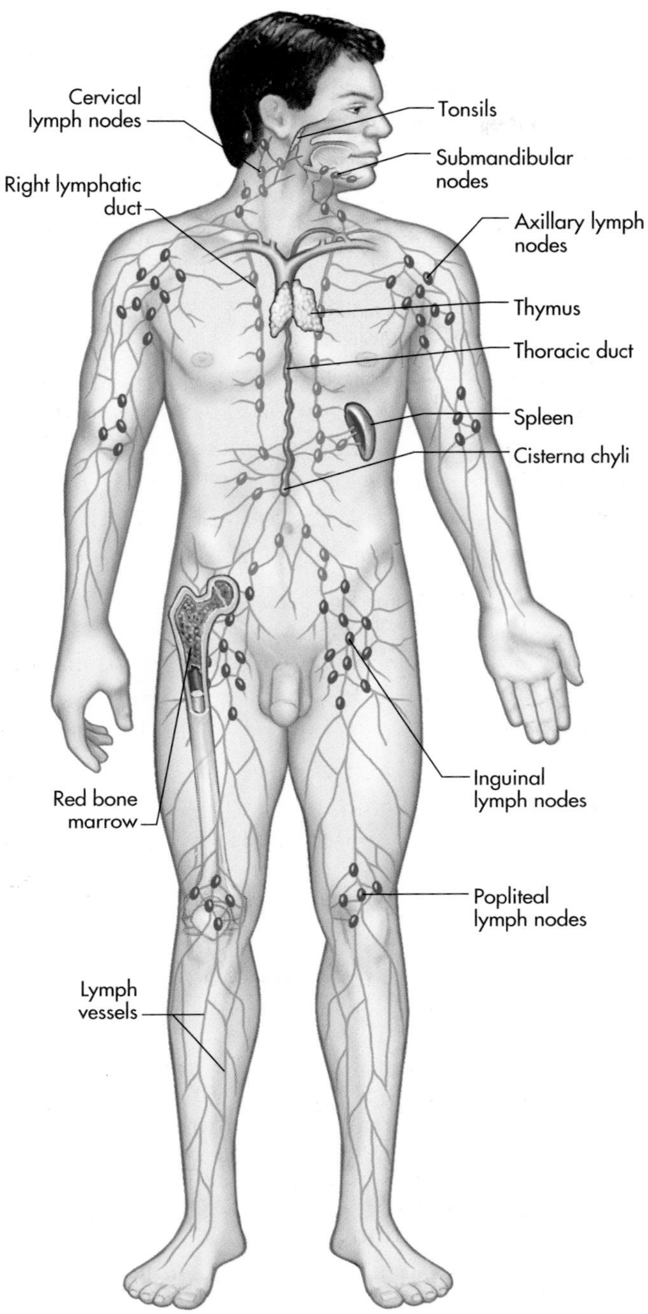

FIGURE 17–22 The distribution of lymph nodes. (**Source:** Thibodeau, G.A., & Patton, K.T. (2010). *The human body in health and disease* (5th ed.). St. Louis, MO: Mosby.)

Tonsils, which are located in the throat, filter tissue fluid contaminated by pathogens that enter the body through the nose, the mouth, or both.

The *thymus gland* is located in the thoracic cavity (see **FIGURE 17–4**). It plays a crucial role in the development of the immune system before birth and in the first few months after birth. After puberty, the gland shrinks but remains active. It secretes a hormone that aids the immune system.

The *spleen* filters blood rather than lymph. It cleanses blood and destroys microorganisms. The spleen also produces disease-preventing cells such as lymphocytes and macrophages.

THE RESPIRATORY SYSTEM

Since oxygen is necessary for survival, every cell needs oxygen. Air contains about 21% oxygen—enough to meet the needs of the body under normal conditions. The respiratory system (**FIGURE 17–23**) brings oxygen into the lungs and eliminates carbon dioxide. *Respiration* is the process of supplying oxygen to cells and removing carbon dioxide from them. It involves *inhalation* (breathing in) and *exhalation* (breathing out). The terms *inspiration* (breathing in) and *expiration* (breathing out) are also used; together, the process is referred to as *ventilation*. The respiratory system is divided into the *upper respiratory tract* and the *lower respiratory tract*. The upper respiratory tract includes the nose and nasal cavities, the pharynx, and the larynx. The lower respiratory tract includes the trachea, bronchi, bronchioles, and alveoli.

Air enters the body through the *nose* and passes into the *pharynx* (throat), a tube-shaped passageway for both air and nutrients. It then passes from the pharynx into the *larynx* (which contains the vocal cords or "voice box"). A piece of cartilage called the *epiglottis* acts like a lid over the larynx and prevents food and liquids from entering the airway during swallowing. During inhalation, the epiglottis lifts up so that air passes over the larynx and into the *trachea* (the windpipe).

The trachea divides at its lower end into the *right bronchus* and the *left bronchus*. Each bronchus enters a lung and further divides several times into smaller branches called *bronchioles*. Eventually, the bronchioles subdivide and end in tiny air sacs called alveoli, which are composed of a very thin membrane, only one cell layer thick.

Alveoli look like small clusters of grapes. They are surrounded by large numbers of pulmonary capillaries. Oxygen and carbon dioxide are exchanged between alveoli and capillaries. Blood in capillaries picks up oxygen from alveoli and is returned to the

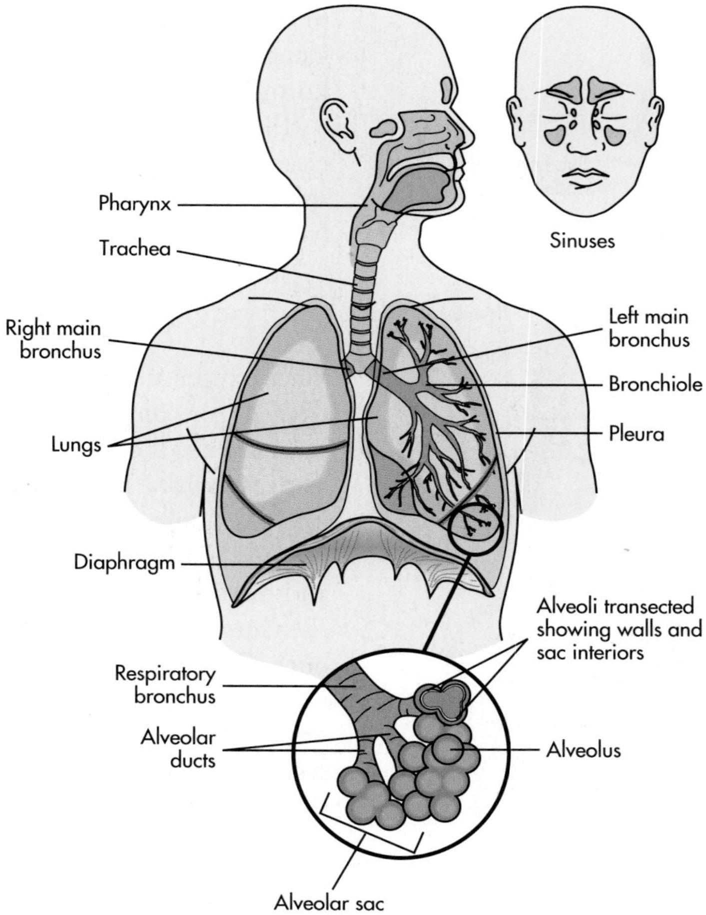

FIGURE 17–23 The respiratory system.

left side of the heart and is then pumped to the rest of the body. Alveoli pick up carbon dioxide from capillaries, and the carbon dioxide is then breathed out.

Lungs are spongy tissues filled with alveoli, blood vessels, connective tissue, and a few nerves. Each lung is divided into sections called lobes. The right lung has three lobes; the left lung has two. The lungs and airways are located in the thoracic cavity, which is separated from the abdominal cavity by a muscle called the *diaphragm*. The lungs contain no actual skeletal muscle tissue and, therefore, cannot move by themselves, so it is the movement of this diaphragm muscle that is the driving force for ventilation.

Each lung is covered by a two-layered sac called the *pleura*. One layer is attached to the lung, and the other to the chest wall. The pleura secretes a very thin fluid that fills the space between the layers. The fluid prevents the layers from rubbing together during inhalation and exhalation.

THE DIGESTIVE SYSTEM

The digestive system, also called the *gastrointestinal system* (*GI system*), breaks down nutrients physically and chemically so that they can be absorbed for use by cells—a process called **digestion**—and also eliminates solid wastes from the body.

The digestive system consists of the *alimentary canal* (*GI tract*) and the accessory organs of digestion (**FIGURE 17–24**). The alimentary canal is a long tube extending from the mouth to the anus. Its major parts are the mouth, the pharynx, the esophagus, the stomach, the small intestine, and the large intestine. The accessory organs of digestion are the teeth, tongue, salivary glands, liver, gallbladder, and pancreas.

Structure of the Digestive Tract Wall

Although modified for specific functions in different organs, the wall of the digestive tract has a similar

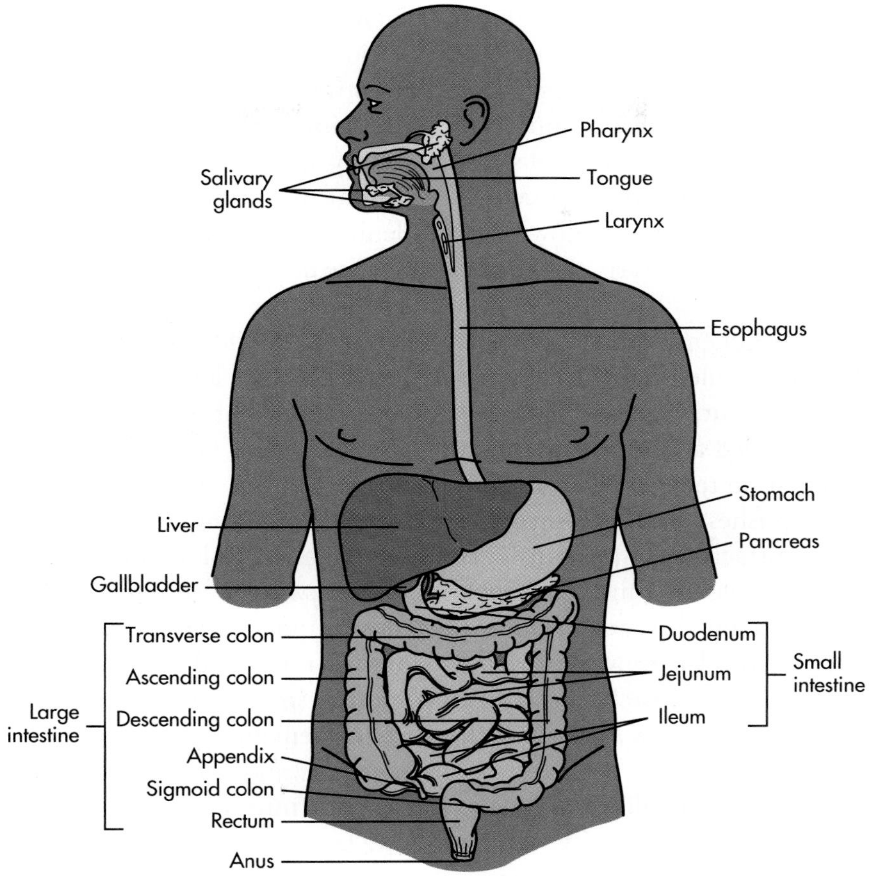

FIGURE 17–24 The digestive system.

structure throughout its length. The innermost layer of the digestive tract is the *mucosa*, which contains *glands* (which secrete mucus, digestive enzymes, and hormones) and *ducts* (which connect glands that empty into the digestive tract).

The middle layer of the GI tract is called the *submucosa*. It is composed of loose connective tissue containing blood vessels, nerves, glands, and lymphatic vessels.

The third and most superficial layer (the outermost layer) is called the *muscularis* or *muscle layer* and consists of two layers of smooth muscles. These muscles are responsible for two types of muscle movements in the digestive tract that aid in digestion. The first movement is a repeated relaxation and contraction of the stomach muscles, which mixes digestive juices with the food to digest the food mechanically in a "swishing" or back-and-forth motion. The second is called **peristalsis**, which is smooth-muscle (involuntary) contraction that pushes food forward in the digestive tract in one direction in a wavelike motion—similar to the way that toothpaste is squeezed through a tube.

The Process of Digestion

Food enters the *mouth*—also called the *oral cavity*—which receives nutrients and prepares them for digestion. The first step of digestion is called **mastication**. During this process, food is bitten, positioned by the *tongue* and cheeks, and then chewed, crushed, and ground by the *teeth* in order to increase the food's surface area. Physically breaking down large food particles into smaller pieces is called **mechanical digestion**. *Taste buds* are on the tongue's surface and on the soft palate, the upper esophagus, and the epiglottis; they contain nerve endings and allow sweet, sour, bitter, and salty tastes to be sensed (see p. 284). Taste buds and olfactory nerve stimulation trigger *saliva* to be secreted from *salivary glands* in the mouth. *Saliva* is a substance composed mostly of water (99%), with the remainder consisting of digestive enzymes, mucous, electrolytes, glycoproteins, and antibacterial chemicals. During mastication, the saliva moistens the food and aids in mixing and swallowing it. The saliva also contains enzymes such as *salivary amylase*, an enzyme that breaks down the carbohydrates within the food and starts the chemical digestion process.

Chemical digestion is the chemical breakdown of food into small nutrient molecules that the cells can absorb and utilize. At this point, the food has been altered into a moist ball (called a *bolus*) and is then swallowed for further digestion to take place. During swallowing, the tongue pushes nutrients into the pharynx. The pharynx contracts, pushing nutrients into the esophagus. The esophagus, a muscular tube about 25 cm (10 inches) long, extends from the pharynx to the stomach. Peristalsis moves nutrients down the esophagus into the stomach through a muscular valve called the *cardiac sphincter*, which controls the entrance to the stomach.

The *stomach* is a muscular, pouchlike sac in the upper left portion of the abdominal cavity. Strong stomach muscles stir and churn nutrients to break them up into even smaller particles. The stomach is lined with a mucous membrane, which contains glands that secrete *gastric juices*. Gastric juices contain strong acids that kill most microorganisms in the nutrients that have been eaten. The partially digested food is mixed and churned with gastric juices to form a semi-liquid substance called *chyme*. In addition to the gastric juice, other cells secrete both thicker mucus and bicarbonate that adhere closely to the stomach and small intestine lining and prevent the acidic gastric juices from digesting the body's own tissue! This chyme is very acidic, foul-smelling, and watery. Through peristalsis, the chyme is pushed from the stomach into the small intestine through another muscular valve called the *pyloric sphincter*.

The *small intestine* is about 6 m (20 ft.) long and has three parts. The first part is the *duodenum*, where more digestive juices are added to the chyme, along with a bicarbonate solution from the pancreas to reduce the acidity of the chyme. The enzymes in the digestive juices chemically break down the nutrients so that they can be absorbed. Peristalsis moves the chyme through the two remaining portions of the small intestine: the *jejunum* and the *ileum*. Tiny projections called *villi* (singular, *villus*) line the small intestine. Villi greatly increase the surface area of the small intestine so that digested nutrients can be efficiently absorbed into capillaries. Most of the absorption of nutrients takes place in the jejunum and the ileum.

One of the digestive juices is *bile*, which is a greenish liquid produced by the liver and stored in the *gallbladder*. Bile aids not only in the digestion of fat but also in the absorption of fat-soluble vitamins. It gives stool its brownish colour. The liver has important functions: (1) metabolizing fats, proteins, and carbohydrates; (2) detoxifying substances from blood; (3) storing fat-soluble vitamins; and (4) producing bile, cholesterol, and bilirubin.

The *pancreas* secretes the enzymes that are the most important of all the digestive enzymes because of their role to aid digestion. Juices from the pancreas and the small intestine are added to the chyme.

The remaining chyme along with any undigested nutrients and waste products passes from the small intestine into the *large intestine* (*large bowel* or *colon*). The large intestine has four functions:

1. It absorbs much of the water and electrolytes from the chyme.
2. It contains certain beneficial bacteria that aid in the production and metabolism of substances such as Vitamin K, Vitamin B12, and thiamine (Vitamin B1).
3. It temporarily stores *feces* (the remaining semi-solid material, consisting of water, solid wastes, and some mucus and microorganisms).
4. It aids in the elimination of feces through *defecation* (bowel movement).

Through peristalsis, feces pass through the colon into the *rectum*, where it can be temporarily stored. *Defecation* is the process of excreting feces from the rectum through the anus. The term *stool* refers to excreted feces.

THE URINARY SYSTEM

Waste products are removed from the body through the respiratory system, the digestive system, the integumentary system (skin), and the urinary system.

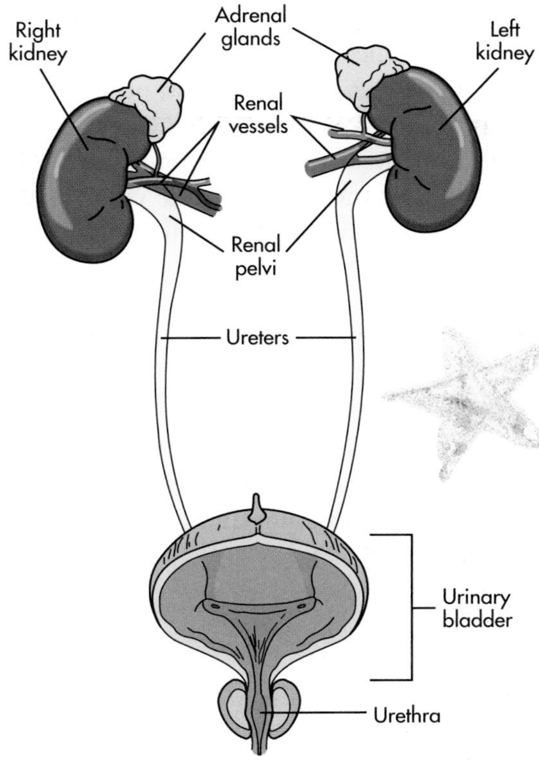

FIGURE 17–25 The urinary system.

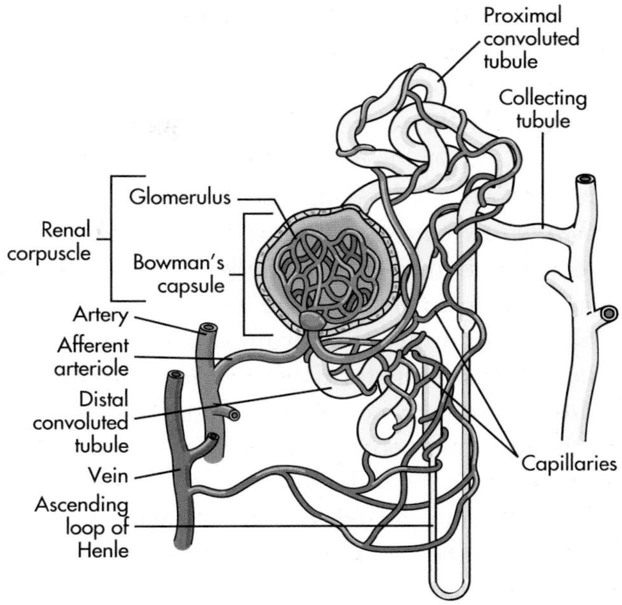

FIGURE 17–26 A nephron.

The digestive system rids the body of solid wastes; lungs rid the body of carbon dioxide; water and other substances are excreted in sweat through the skin. There are other waste products in blood as a result of body cells burning nutrients for energy, particularly proteins. The functions of the urinary system are to remove waste products from blood and to maintain water and electrolyte balance and acid–base balance within the body. The structures of the urinary system are shown in **FIGURE 17–25**. Note the relation of the bladder, urethra, and kidneys to the other pelvic structures shown in **FIGURES 17–26 and 17–27**.

The *kidneys* are two bean-shaped organs located just posterior to the abdominal cavity. They lie against the muscles of the back on each side of the spine and are protected by the lower edge of the rib cage. The kidneys perform the following six tasks:

1. Act as a filtration system for blood by removing waste products such as urea, uric acid, ammonia, and creatinine (all waste products from protein metabolism) from the blood
2. Regulate blood volume by determining the amount of water that is excreted
3. Help to regulate the electrolyte content of the blood and body fluids
4. Play a major role in the regulation of the body's acid–base balance (blood pH) by controlling the excretion of hydrogen ions
5. Help in the long-term regulation of blood pressure
6. Produce a hormone (*erythropoietin*) that stimulates the production and regulation of red blood cells

Each kidney has about a million tiny *nephrons*, which are the filtering units of the kidney (**FIGURE 17–26**). The nephrons' job is to regulate the concentration of water and soluble (dissolvable) substances by filtering the blood. Nephrons separate the nutrients and minerals in blood (water, sodium, amino acids, glucose) from toxins and waste products and produce urine as a waste product. The actual production of urine is a process known as *diuresis*, which consists of three major steps:

1. *Glomular filtration*. Every nephron has a *renal* (*convoluted*) *tubule* that ends in a *Bowman's capsule*. A cluster of capillaries, called the *glomerulus*, is contained in this capsule. Blood moves through the capillaries of the glomerulus, and the liquid portion of the blood (mostly water) is filtered out into the Bowman's capsule along with waste products as

well as valuable nutrients, minerals, and any substances small enough to cross the membrane.

2. *Tubular reabsorption.* The filtered fluid runs through a series of tubules, where most of the water and other necessary substances are reabsorbed by blood and recirculated in the body.
3. *Tubular secretion.* Additional substances are secreted into the urine from the blood, making final small adjustments to the composition of the blood and urine. Toxins and waste products stay in the tubules and form *urine*. Urine flows through the tubule to a collecting tubule, which drains into the renal pelvis in the kidney.

Urine is transported from the kidneys to the *bladder* through the *ureters* by muscular peristalsis. The two ureters are narrow tubes, each about 25 to 30 cm (10 to 12 in.) long. They run from the renal pelvis of each kidney to the urinary bladder. The bladder is a hollow, muscular sac situated toward the front in the lower part of the abdominal cavity.

Urine is stored in the bladder until the urge to urinate is felt, usually when there is about 250 ml (8 oz., or half a pint) of urine in the bladder. Urine passes from the bladder through the urethra. The opening at the end of the urethra is the meatus. Urine passes from the body through the meatus. In the adult male, the urethra is about 20 cm (8 in.) long and provides an exit for urine as well as semen during ejaculation. In the adult female, the urethra is about 3 cm (approximately 1.2 in.); its only purpose is to provide a means of urine to pass from the bladder to the urinary meatus. The differences in the length of the urethra and the relative anatomical positions of the urethra between males and females explain why females are more prone to urinary tract infections than men (see **BOX 32–3**, on page 693).

Urine is a clear, yellowish fluid. The amount of urine eliminated over a 24-hour period should be close to the amount of fluid consumed. The average output of urine is 1 500 ml per 24 hours (see Chapter 32).

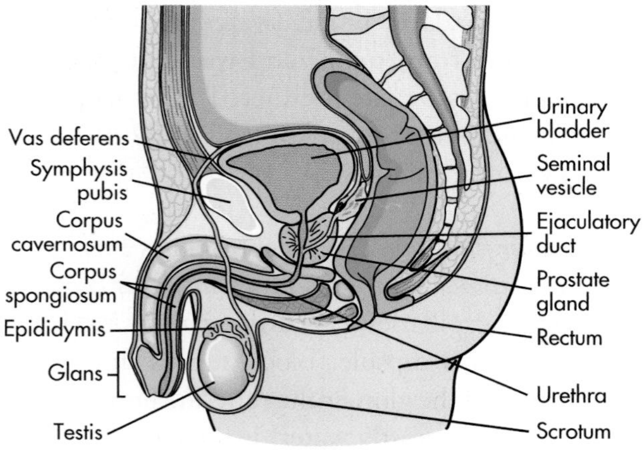

FIGURE 17–27 The male reproductive system.

THE REPRODUCTIVE SYSTEM

Human reproduction results from the union of a female sex cell and a male sex cell. The differing structures of the male reproductive system and the female reproductive system allow for the process of reproduction.

The Male Reproductive System

The structures of the male reproductive system are shown in **FIGURE 17–27**. The *testes* (*testicles*) are the male sex glands, also called *gonads*. The two testes, oval- or almond-shaped glands, are where the male sex cells, called *sperm*, are produced. *Testosterone*, the male hormone, is also produced in the testes. This hormone is needed for the functioning of the reproductive organs and for the development of the male secondary sex characteristics (see Chapter 18). The testes are suspended between the thighs at the base of the penis in a sac called the *scrotum*, which is made of skin and muscle.

Sperm travel from each testis to the *epididymis*, a coiled tube (6 m or 20 ft. in length) on the top and to the side of the testis. From the epididymis, sperm travel through a tube called the *vas deferens*. Eventually, each vas deferens joins a *seminal vesicle*. The two seminal vesicles store sperm and produce *semen*, a fluid that carries sperm from the male reproductive tract. The ducts of the seminal vesicles unite to form the *ejaculatory duct*, which passes through the prostate gland.

The *prostate gland*, shaped like a doughnut, lies just below the bladder and secretes fluid into the semen. This fluid plays a role in increasing the mobility of sperm. As the ejaculatory ducts leave the prostate, they join into the *urethra*, which also runs through the prostate. The urethra, contained within the penis, is the outlet for both urine and semen.

The *penis* is outside of the body and contains *erectile* tissue. When a man becomes sexually aroused, blood fills the erectile tissue, causing the penis to become enlarged, hard, and erect. The erect penis can enter the vagina of the female reproductive tract. The semen, which contains sperm, is then released into the female vagina during the act of sexual intercourse.

The Female Reproductive System

The structures of the female reproductive system are shown in **FIGURE 17–28**. The female gonads are two almond-shaped glands called *ovaries*. Ovaries are situated on each side of the uterus in the pelvic cavity and contain *ova*, or eggs, which are the female sex cells. During the woman's reproductive years, one ovum (egg) is released monthly, which is called *ovulation*. The ovaries also secrete the female hormones *estrogen* and *progesterone*. These hormones are needed for the functioning of the reproductive system and the development of secondary sex characteristics in the female (see Chapter 18).

When an ovum is released from an ovary, it travels through the *fallopian tube*, which is situated on either side of the *uterus* and attached to it at one end. The uterus is a hollow, muscular organ shaped like a pear and located in the centre of the pelvic cavity behind the bladder and in front of the rectum. The main part of the uterus is the *fundus*. The neck, or narrow section, of the uterus is the *cervix*. Tissue lining the uterus is called the *endometrium*. There are numerous blood vessels in the endometrium. If the sex cells from the male and the female (semen and ovum) unite into one cell, that cell implants itself into the endometrium, where it develops into a baby. The uterus serves as a place for the developing baby (*fetus*) to receive nourishment and grow.

The cervix of the uterus projects into a muscular canal called the *vagina*. The vagina opens to the outside of the body and is located just behind the urethra. The vagina receives the penis during sexual intercourse and also serves as part of the birth canal. Glands in the vaginal wall keep it moistened with secretions. In young girls, the external vaginal opening is partially closed by a membrane called the *hymen*, which can break for various reasons.

The external genitalia of the female are referred to as the *vulva* (**FIGURE 17–29**). The *mons pubis* is a rounded, fatty pad over a bone called the *symphysis pubis* and is covered with hair in the adult female. The *labia majora* and the *labia minora* are two folds of tissue on either side of the vaginal opening. The *clitoris* is a small, sensitive organ composed of erectile tissue and becomes hard when sexually stimulated.

The *mammary glands* are contained in the female breasts and produce and secrete milk after childbirth. They are made up of glandular tissue and fat (**FIGURE 17–30**). The milk drains into ducts that open into the nipple.

Menstruation

The endometrium is rich in blood to nourish the cell that grows into the fetus. If pregnancy does not occur, the endometrium breaks down and is discharged out of the body through the vagina. This

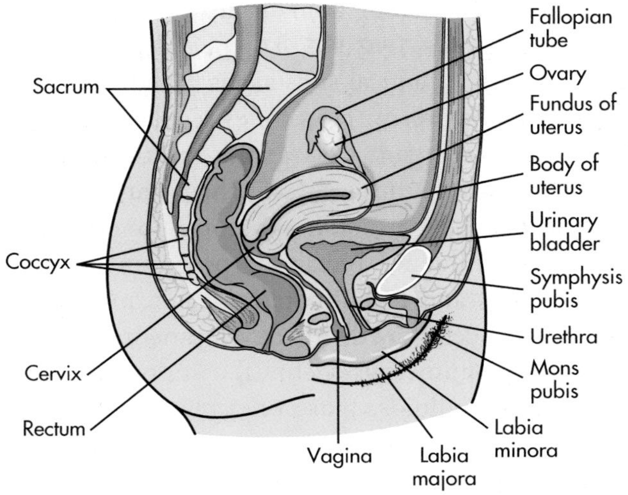

FIGURE 17–28 The female reproductive system.

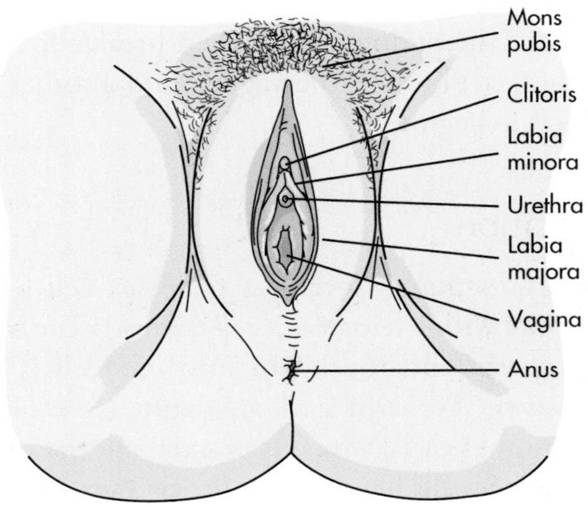

FIGURE 17–29 External female genitalia.

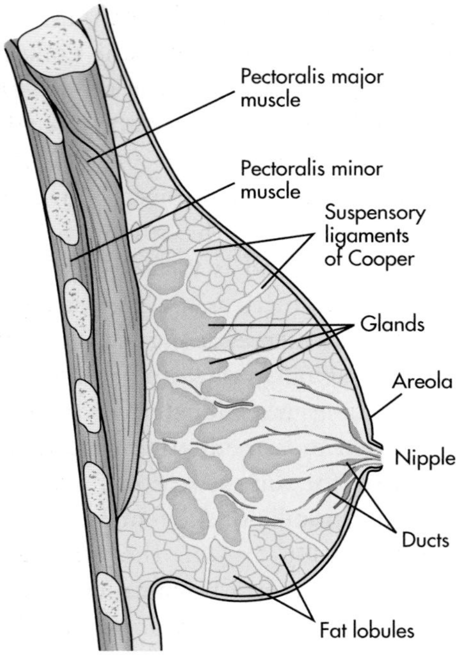

FIGURE 17–30 The female breast.

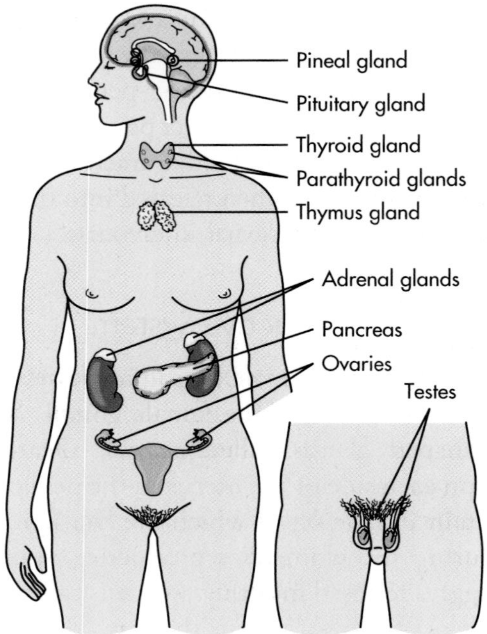

FIGURE 17–31 The endocrine system.

process, called **menstruation**, occurs about every 28 days and is therefore called the *menstrual cycle*.

The first day of the cycle begins with menstruation. Blood flows out from the uterus through the vaginal opening, usually lasting 3 to 7 days. During the next phase—ovulation—which occurs usually on or about day 14 of the cycle, an ovum matures in an ovary and is released.

Meanwhile, estrogen and progesterone (the female hormones) are secreted by the ovaries. These hormones cause the endometrium to thicken in preparation for possible pregnancy. If pregnancy does not occur, the hormones decrease in amount, and, because of this, blood supply to the endometrium decreases. The endometrium then breaks down and is discharged through the vagina, and another menstrual cycle begins.

Fertilization

For reproduction to occur, a male sex cell (sperm) must unite with a female sex cell (ovum). The uniting of the sperm and the ovum into one cell is called *fertilization*. A sperm and an ovum have only 23 chromosomes each, which is exactly half the number that all other cells have. When the two sex cells unite, the fertilized cell has 46 chromosomes.

During intercourse, millions of sperm are deposited in the vagina. Sperm travel up the cervix, through the uterus, and into the fallopian tubes. If a sperm and an ovum unite in the fallopian tube, fertilization occurs and may result in pregnancy. The fertilized ovum then travels down the fallopian tube to the uterus. After a short time, the fertilized cell implants itself in the thick endometrium and grows during pregnancy.

THE ENDOCRINE SYSTEM

The endocrine system is made up of glands called *endocrine glands* (**FIGURE 17–31**). The endocrine glands secrete chemical substances called **hormones** into the bloodstream. Hormones regulate the activities of other organs and glands in the body by binding to the receptor sites of their "target" tissue, similar to a key fitting in its corresponding lock. Hormones influence metabolic processes involving fat, proteins, and carbohydrates; water and electrolyte balance; cell growth and development; and regulation of the numerous chemical components in our cells and body fluids. Hormones play an important role in growth and reproduction.

The *pituitary gland* is also called the *master gland*. About the size of a cherry, it is located at the base of the brain behind the eyes. The pituitary gland is divided into the *anterior pituitary lobe* and the *posterior pituitary lobe*. The anterior pituitary lobe secretes the following:

- ***Growth hormone***—needed for the growth of muscles, bones, and other organs. It is needed throughout life to maintain normal-size bones and muscles. Growth is stunted if a baby is born with deficient amounts of growth hormone. Too much of the hormone causes excessive growth. More information about this hormone will become available from research being conducted in Canada and elsewhere.
- ***Thyroid-stimulating hormone*** (TSH)—needed for thyroid gland function.
- ***Adrenocorticotropic hormone*** (ACTH)—stimulates the adrenal glands.
- ***Reproductive hormones***—regulate growth, development, and function of the male and female reproductive systems.

The posterior pituitary lobe secretes *antidiuretic hormone* (ADH) and *oxytocin*. ADH prevents the kidneys from excreting excessive amounts of water. Oxytocin causes the uterine muscles to contract during childbirth. These two hormones are produced in a nearby structure in the brain called the *hypothalamus*. The hypothalamus is part of the brain, but it secretes several hormones, and so it is also considered part of the endocrine system. The hormones produced in the hypothalamus control or inhibit the release of other hormones.

The *thyroid gland*, shaped like a butterfly, is situated in the neck in front of the larynx and secretes two types of *thyroid hormones—thyroxine* (T_4) and *triiodothyronine* (T_3)—as well as a hormone called *calcitonin*. Thyroid hormones regulate **metabolism**, which is the burning of nutrients by the cells to produce heat and energy. The thyroid hormones T_3 and T_4 are responsible for the proper functioning of all other hormones, the maturation of the nervous system, and normal growth and development. Calcitonin, a hormone produced in the C cells of the thyroid, helps to regulate calcium levels in the body by lowering the amount of calcium in the blood plasma and increasing bone calcium content.

Too little of the thyroid hormones T_3 and T_4 results in slowed body processes, slowed movements, and weight gain. Too much of them causes increased metabolism, excess energy, and weight loss. If a baby is born with deficient amounts of thyroid hormone, physical and mental growth will be stunted.

The parathyroid glands are four small collections of cells, two on each side of the thyroid gland, and they secrete parathormone. Parathormone also regulates the body's use of calcium by increasing the amount of calcium available in the blood plasma. Calcium is needed for the proper functioning of nerves, contraction of muscles, bone development, and blood clotting. Insufficient amounts of calcium cause tetany—a state of severe muscle contraction and spasm—which, if untreated, can result in death.

There are two *adrenal glands*, one on the top of each kidney. The adrenal gland has two parts: the *adrenal medulla* and the *adrenal cortex*. The adrenal medulla secretes *epinephrine* and *norepinephrine*. These hormones stimulate the body to quickly produce energy during emergencies so that heart rate, blood pressure, muscle power, and energy all increase. The adrenal cortex secretes three groups of hormones that are essential for life: (1) *glucocorticoids*, which regulate the metabolism of carbohydrates and control the body's response to stress and inflammation; (2) *mineralocorticoids*, which regulate the amount of salt and water absorbed and lost by the kidneys; and (3) small amounts of male and female sex hormones.

The *pancreas* secretes both *insulin* and *glucagon*, which regulate the amount of glucose (sugar) in the blood available for use by cells. Insulin is needed for sugar to enter cells. If there is too little insulin, sugar cannot enter cells, resulting in excess amounts of sugar building up in blood. *Insulin* and *glucagon* are *antagonistic* hormones, which means that they result in opposite actions occurring in the body and can, therefore, "balance" one another. The actions of hormones such as insulin and glucagon are good examples of negative feedback mechanisms in the body that help maintain homeostasis.

The *gonads* are the glands of human reproduction. Male sex glands (testes) secrete *testosterone*. Female sex glands (ovaries) secrete *estrogen* and *progesterone* (see p. 297).

THE IMMUNE SYSTEM

The immune system defends the body against threats from inside and outside. Some of these threats include pollens, toxins, bacteria, viruses, and our own cells that have become abnormal (cancer). **Immunity** means that a person has protection against a disease or condition—the person will not get or be affected by the disease. There are two types of defence mechanisms, or immunity, classified as *nonspecific immunity* and *specific immunity*.

Nonspecific immunity is the body's reaction to anything it does not recognize as a normal body substance. There are two lines of defence in fighting threats.

The first line of defence includes the following:

- ***Mechanical barriers***—for example, intact skin and mucous membranes
- ***Chemical barriers***—for example, tears, stomach acids, saliva, perspiration
- ***Reflexes***—for example, coughing, sneezing, vomiting, and diarrhea

The second line of defence includes the following:

- ***Phagocytes***—white blood cells that digest and destroy microorganisms and other unwanted substances
- ***Inflammation***—the release of *histamine* to an injured or irritated area, causing blood vessels to dilate and bring more blood to the area (histamine causes redness, heat, and fluid leakage of the blood, which leads to swelling)
- ***Fever***—stimulates *phagocytosis* (ingesting or engulfing other cells) and decreases the ability of certain pathogens to multiply

Specific immunity is the ability of the body to resist or overcome an infection or illness against a *certain* disease or infection caused by a foreign agent such as a pathogen or antigenic substance. Special cells and substances provide immunity.

- ***Antibodies***—normal body substances that recognize abnormal or unwanted substances and attack and destroy such substances
- ***Antigens***—abnormal or unwanted substances (usually proteins) that cause the body to produce antibodies, which attack and destroy the antigens
- ***Lymphocytes***—white blood cells that produce antibodies, the production of which increases as the body responds to an infection
- ***B lymphocytes (B cells)***—cells that cause the production of antibodies that circulate in the plasma
- ***T lymphocytes (T cells)***—cells that destroy invading cells (*killer T cells* produce toxic substances near the invading cells; some T cells attract other cells that destroy the invaders)

When the body senses an antigen (an unwanted substance), the immune system is activated, and phagocyte and lymphocyte production increases. Phagocytes destroy the invaders through digestion, and lymphocytes produce antibodies that attack and destroy unwanted substances. Antibodies, produced by B cells, react to specific antigens.

Immunity to diseases can be classified as *genetic immunity* and *acquired immunity*. Genetic immunity protects a member of one species from diseases that afflict other species; for example, your cat will not catch chicken pox from you.

A person can get *acquired immunity* either naturally or artificially. Natural immunity can be acquired in two ways:

1. **Active immunity**. By naturally acquiring an illness (such as chicken pox), your body develops the antibodies to protect you from getting it again.
2. **Passive immunity**. Passive immunity is short-lived and passed from mother to fetus through the placenta and from the mother to the baby through breast milk. This protection lasts for about the first 6 months after birth.

Artificially acquired immunity is achieved by injection of a *vaccine* or *immune globulin* (*immunoglobulin*). A vaccine is a small amount of an antigen-bearing substance (*pathogen*) that is injected into a person to stimulate the production of antibodies. Immune globulin is obtained from a donor who already has the antibodies and is injected into a person to provide *passive immunity*.

CHAPTER REVIEW

KEY POINTS

- Anatomical positions are terms used in the study of anatomy related to the body.
- Cells are the basic unit of body structures. Groups of cells with similar functions combine to form tissues.
- Organs are groups of tissues that work together to perform a special function. Organ systems are formed by organs that work together to perform special functions.
- The major organ systems in the body include the following:
  - The *integumentary system*, which contains skin and its appendages—hair, nails, and sweat and oil glands
  - The *musculo-skeletal system*, which provides the framework for the body and allows the body to move
  - The *nervous system*, which controls, directs, and coordinates body functions, including the central nervous system, the peripheral nervous system, and the sense organs
  - The *circulatory system*, which is made up of the cardiovascular system (consisting of blood, the heart, and blood vessels) and the lymphatic system (consisting of lymph, lymph nodes, and lymph vessels)
  - The *respiratory system*, which brings air into the lungs by inspiration (inhalation), which is a process of ventilation, and allows the transfer of oxygen into the blood and the transfer of carbon dioxide out of the blood; the carbon dioxide is eliminated by expiration (exhalation), which is a process of ventilation
  - The *digestive system*, which breaks down food physically and chemically into basic nutrients so that they can be absorbed for use by cells
  - The *urinary system*, which removes waste from blood and maintains water and electrolyte balance
  - The *reproductive system*, which allows for the processes of development and reproduction
  - The *endocrine system*, which is made up of glands called *endocrine glands*, which secrete hormones into the bloodstream, to regulate the activities of other organs and glands in the body; the metabolic processes involving fats, proteins, and carbohydrates; water and electrolyte balance; cell growth and development; and numerous chemical components in our cells and body fluids
  - The *immune system*, which defends the body against threats from inside and outside

CRITICAL THINKING IN PRACTICE

A patient has a disorder that affects the immune system. How does such a disorder affect body function? How will you provide care in a way that protects the person?

REVIEW QUESTIONS

Answers to these questions are at the bottom of page 302.

Circle the BEST answer.

1. The basic unit of body structure is the:
   A. Cell
   B. Neuron
   C. Nephron
   D. Ovum

2. The outer layer of the skin is called the:
   A. Dermis
   B. Epidermis
   C. Integument
   D. Myelin

3. Which parts allow body movement?
   A. Bone marrow and periosteum
   B. Synovial membrane and tendons
   C. Joints
   D. Ligaments

4. Skeletal muscles:
   A. Are under involuntary control
   B. Appear smooth
   C. Are always under voluntary control
   D. Appear striped under a microscope

5. The highest functions of the brain take place in the:
A. Cerebral cortex
B. Medulla
C. Brain stem
D. Spinal nerves

6. Besides hearing, the ear is involved in:
A. Regulating body movements
B. Balance
C. Smoothness of body movements
D. Controlling involuntary muscles

7. The liquid part of blood is (are):
A. Hemoglobin
B. Red blood cells
C. Plasma
D. Alveolus

8. Which part of the heart pumps blood to the body?
A. Right atrium
B. Right ventricle
C. Left atrium
D. Left ventricle

9. Which of the following carry blood away from the heart?
A. Capillaries
B. Veins
C. Venules
D. Arteries

10. Oxygen and carbon dioxide are exchanged:
A. In bronchi
B. Between alveoli and capillaries
C. Between lungs and the pleura
D. In the trachea

11. The process of digestion begins in the:
A. Mouth
B. Stomach
C. Small intestine
D. Colon

12. Most nutrient absorption takes place in the:
A. Stomach
B. Small intestine
C. Colon
D. Large intestine

13. Urine is formed by the:
A. Jejunum
B. Kidneys
C. Bladder
D. Liver

14. The male sex gland is called the:
A. Penis
B. Semen
C. Testis
D. Scrotum

15. The endocrine glands secrete substances called:
A. Hormones
B. Mucus
C. Semen
D. Insulin

16. The immune system protects the body from:
A. Low blood sugar
B. Disease and infection
C. Falling and loss of balance
D. Stunted growth and loss of fluid

Answers: 1.A, 2.B, 3.C, 4.D, 5.A, 6.B, 7.C, 8.D, 9.D, 10.B, 11.A, 12.B, 13.B, 14.C, 15.A, 16.B

Chapter opener image: Tinydevil/Shutterstock.com

CHAPTER 18

Growth and Development

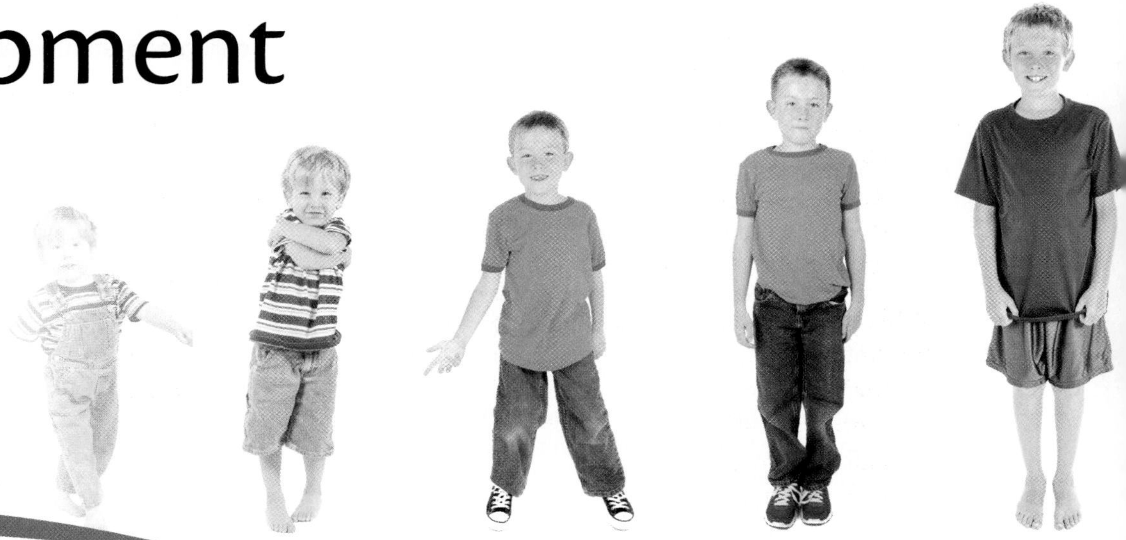

OBJECTIVES

After reading this chapter, the learner should be able to do the following:

- Understand the principles of growth and development.
- Identify the stages of growth and development and the normal age ranges for each stage.
- Identify the developmental tasks for each age group.
- Describe the normal and typical growth and development for each age group.

KEY TERMS

adolescence Ages approximately 12 to 18—the time between puberty and adulthood; a time of rapid growth and physical, sexual, psychological, and social maturity. *p. 312*

development The maturation toward adulthood; usually characterized by physical changes and increased ability and functionality. *p. 305*

developmental task An activity that must be mastered during a stage of development. *p. 305*

growth Increase in physical size and weight that occurs in a slow and steady manner. *p. 305*

infancy The first year of life, during which the body undergoes rapid physical, psychological, and social growth and development. *p. 305*

late adulthood Begins approximately at the age of 65 years. This stage is characterized by adjusting to decreased physical strength and loss of health, retirement, and reduced income; coping with the death of a partner; developing new friends and relationships; and preparing for one's own death. *p. 316*

late childhood Ages 9 to 12 years; characterized by becoming independent of adults; developing and keeping friendships with peers; understanding the physical, psychological, and social roles of one's identified gender; developing moral and ethical behaviour; developing greater muscular strength, coordination, and balance; and learning how to study. *p. 311*

menarche The time when menstruation first begins. *p. 312*

menopause The time when menstruation stops. *p. 315*

middle adulthood Ages approximately 40 to 65 years. This stage is characterized by seeing children growing up and moving away from home, adjusting to physical changes, developing leisure activities, and relating to aging parents. *p. 315*

middle childhood Ages 6 to 8 years; characterized by developing the social and physical skills needed for playing games; learning to get along with peers; learning behaviours and attitudes normative to one's gender; learning basic reading, writing, and arithmetic skills; developing a conscience and morals; and developing a good feeling and attitude about oneself. *p. 310*

newborn A baby, up to 28 days after birth; also called a *neonate*. *p. 305*

preschool Ages 3 to 5 years; characterized by gaining an increasing ability to communicate and understand others, becoming able to perform self-care activities, learning the differences between the genders, learning to distinguish right from wrong, learning to play with others, and developing family relationships. *p. 308*

puberty The period when the reproductive organs begin to function and secondary sex characteristics appear. *p. 312*

reflex An involuntary movement in response to a stimulus. *p. 306*

toddlerhood Ages 1 to 3 years; characterized by tolerating separation from the primary caregiver, gaining control of bowel and bladder functions, using words to communicate, and starting to assert independence. *p. 307*

young adulthood Ages approximately 18 to 40 years; characterized by choosing an education and an occupation, selecting and learning to live with a partner, becoming a parent and raising children, and developing a satisfactory sex life. *p. 314*

As a support worker, you will care for clients in different stages of their development. Having a basic understanding of human growth and development will help you better understand the client's needs and, therefore, give better care. This chapter presents the basic changes that occur in normal, healthy people from birth through old age.

Human growth and development are presented in nine stages; for each stage, the age ranges and typical characteristics are outlined. The stages overlap, so it is hard to see clear-cut endings and beginnings of each. Also, people vary in their rate of growth and development.

One area of understanding around human growth and development that is being challenged in modern Western society is that of gender differences—specifically, what society dictates versus what a child feels his or her personal gender affiliation to be. As researchers understand more about society's influences on gender role assignments, our definitions of these may change and evolve.

Children grow and develop within the structure of the family. In Canadian society, the family can take many forms (see Chapter 11). Sometimes, when parents are unable to raise their children, another person—for example, a grandparent, aunt, uncle, or court-appointed guardian—takes on the parental role.

In this chapter, the term *primary caregiver* refers to the person who is most responsible for providing for the child's basic needs. The primary caregiver may be a parent or another person assuming the parental role.

PRINCIPLES

Growth refers to the physical changes a person experiences that can be measured and that occur in a steady and orderly manner. Growth is measured by changes in height and weight, as well as by changes in physical appearance and body functions.

Development refers to changes in psychological and social functioning. A person behaves and thinks in certain ways at different stages of development. A 2-year-old thinks in simple terms and needs a primary caregiver for meeting many basic needs. A 40-year-old thinks in complex ways and meets most of his own basic needs without help from others.

- Growth and development occur from the moment of fertilization until death.
- The process goes from the simple to the complex. A baby learns to sit before standing, to stand before walking, and to walk before running. An adolescent learns to develop from dependence to independence.
- Growth and development occur in certain directions:
  - From the head to the foot—babies learn to hold up their heads before they learn to sit. After learning to sit, they learn to stand.
  - From the centre of the body outward—babies learn to control shoulder movements before they can control hand movements.
- Growth and development occur in a sequence and pattern. Certain **developmental tasks** must be completed during each stage, and no stage can be skipped, as each stage lays the foundation for the next stage. Children all over the world, whatever their culture or living conditions, must go through each stage of development before they can progress to the next task.
- The rate of growth and development is uneven—it does not occur at a set pace. Growth is more rapid during infancy. Also, children have growth spurts: Some children grow rapidly, whereas some others grow slowly. The rates of development is also uneven. Each stage of growth and development has its own characteristics and developmental tasks.
- Not all people fit into the developmental "norm" for each age category. The rate of development is determined by many things, including quality of stimulation, nutritional diet, and environment. Developmental stages are more like *guidelines* than *rules*.

INFANCY (BIRTH TO 1 YEAR)

Infancy is the first year of life, when rapid physical, psychological, and social growth and development occur. The developmental tasks of infancy are the following:

- Learning to walk
- Learning to eat solid foods
- Beginning to talk and communicate with others
- Beginning to have emotional relationships with primary caregivers, brothers, and sisters
- Developing stable sleep and feeding patterns

The *neonatal period* of infancy is the first 28 days after birth, and during this time, a baby is called a *neonate* or a **newborn**.

The average newborn is 48 to 53 cm (19 to 21 in.) long and weighs 3 200 to 3 600 g (7 to 8 lb.) at birth. ***However, genetics and ethnicity are important determinants for the differences in birth weight, length, and head circumference among babies.*** Birth weight usually doubles by the age of 5 to 6 months and triples by the first birthday.

The newborn's head is large compared with the rest of the body, and the skin is wrinkled. Arms and legs seem short compared with the trunk. The abdomen

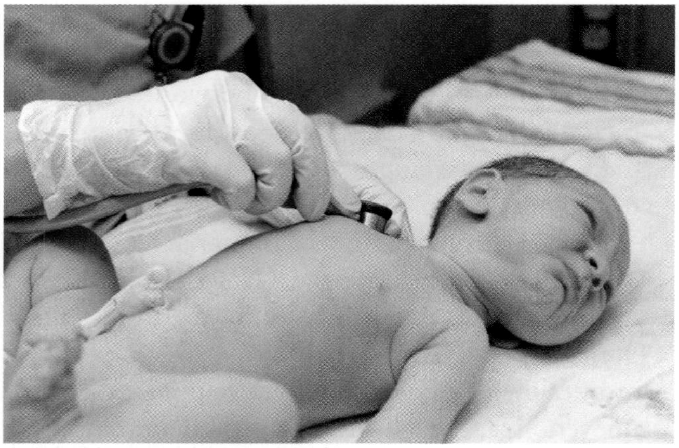

FIGURE 18–1 A newborn. (**Source:** © Can Stock Photo Inc./CarolinaSmith.)

is large and round. Skin and eye colour vary, depending on the baby's genetic background, and may change during the first year. The newborn has fat, pudgy cheeks; a flat nose; and a receding chin (**FIGURE 18–1**).

The infant's central nervous system is not well developed. Movements are uncoordinated and lack purpose. Infants can see at birth, although vision is not clear. They seem attracted to patterns, and as they develop, they prefer colours. Infants can hear well—they are startled by loud noises and soothed by soft sounds. They respond more often to female (higher-pitched) voices than to male (lower-pitched) voices. Infants react to touch, and the senses of smell and taste are well developed.

Newborns have certain **reflexes** (involuntary movements in response to a stimulus). These reflexes decline and then disappear as the central nervous system develops:

- The *Moro reflex (startle reflex)* occurs when an infant is frightened by a loud noise or a sudden movement. The arms are thrown apart, the legs extend, and the head is thrown back.
- The *rooting reflex* is stimulated when the infant's cheek is touched at or near the mouth. The infant's head turns toward the touch. The rooting reflex is necessary for feeding; it helps guide the infant's mouth to the nipple.
- The *sucking reflex* is produced by touching the cheeks or the sides of the lips.
- The *grasping reflex* occurs when the infant's palm is stimulated, causing the fingers to close around the object. This reflex begins to decline around the second month and disappears by the third month.

Infants sleep most of the time during the first few weeks of life. They wake up when hungry and fall asleep right after eating. The time between feedings lengthens as infants grow and develop. They stay awake more and sleep less as growth and development occur.

Body movements are initially uncoordinated, without purpose, and generally involuntary. As the central nervous system and muscular system develop, infants develop specific, voluntary, and coordinated movements. Newborns cannot hold their heads up. At 1 month, infants can hold their heads up when held and can lift and turn their heads when lying on their stomachs. At 2 months, they can smile and follow the movements of objects with their eyes. Three-month-old infants can raise their heads and shoulders when lying on their stomachs. They can sit, supported, for a short period and can hold a rattle. Infants 4 months of age are usually able to roll over and sit up, if supported. They may also sleep through the night by this time. The Moro and rooting reflexes disappear at this stage. Infants can hold objects with both hands, put objects into their mouths, and babble when spoken to. At 5 months, infants can grasp objects and play with their toes. Teeth start to appear.

Six-month-old infants usually have two lower front teeth and start to chew and bite finger foods. They can hold a bottle for feeding and can sit alone for a short time. At 7 months, upper teeth start to erupt. Infants at this age respond to their names, can say "dada" and "mama," and fear strangers. At 8 months, infants may be able to stand when holding on to something. They respond to the word "no." Infants at this age often do not like to be dressed or have diapers changed. Nine-month-old infants usually crawl, and more upper teeth appear. At 10 months, most infants can walk around while holding on to furniture (**FIGURE 18–2**). They can understand a number of words but can say only a few, and they indicate what they want by pointing or gesturing. They smile when looking into a mirror. Infants may begin to take a few steps at 11 months.

At 1 year of age, many start to walk and can hold a cup for drinking. One-year-olds know more words

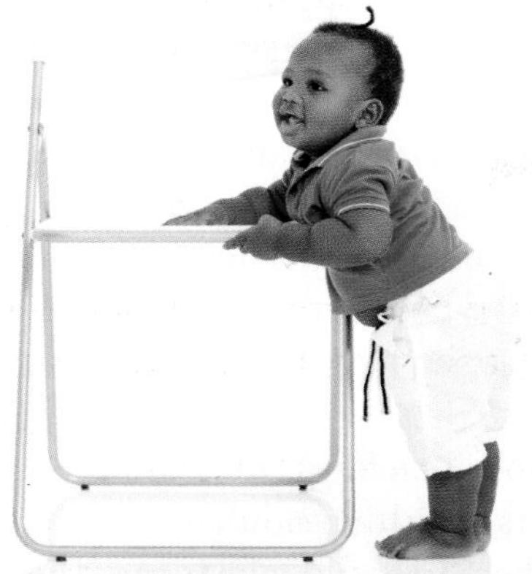

FIGURE 18–2 A 10-month-old infant can walk while holding on to furniture. (**Source:** © Can Stock Photo Inc./ michaeljung)

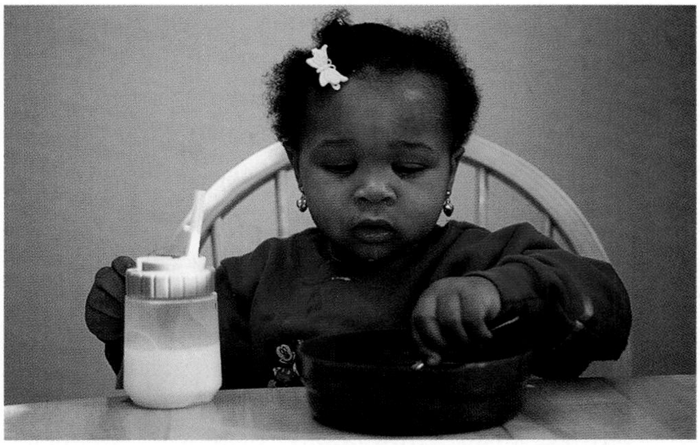

FIGURE 18–3 A toddler is able to use a spoon to eat food.

and can say "no" and shake their heads for "no." They try to imitate words spoken by adults around them. At this stage, infants usually play by themselves with their own toys; this is commonly called *solitary play*.

During the first 6 months, the infant's diet is mainly breast or formula milk. Solid foods (strained fruits and vegetables) are usually added to their diet at 5 to 7 months. The doctor or a nurse will advise dietary changes. Finely chopped foods are added during the ninth and tenth months, and a 1-year-old can eat table foods.

TODDLERHOOD (1 TO 3 YEARS)

Physical growth during the second year of life is not as rapid as during infancy. The developmental tasks during **toddlerhood** are as follows:

- Tolerating separation from the primary caregiver
- Gaining control of bowel and bladder functions
- Using words to communicate with others
- Becoming less dependent on the primary caregiver

Toddlers have the need to assert independence. With their increasing ability to move about and walk, plus their avid curiosity, toddlers get into everything: They touch, smell, and taste anything within reach. As toddlers become more coordinated, they start to climb onto things, and their new and increasing skills allow them to explore the environment. The child begins to learn that some things can be done without the help of the primary caregiver. By 3 years, the toddler can run, jump, climb, ride a tricycle, and walk up and down stairs.

Increased hand coordination gives toddlers new skills. Their need to feel, smell, and taste things is shown in their increasing ability to feed themselves. They progress from eating with fingers to using a spoon (FIGURE 18–3). Toddlers can drink from cups. They can scribble, build towers with blocks, string beads, and turn book pages. Right- or left-handedness is seen during the second year.

Toilet training is a major developmental task for toddlers. Since bowel control and bladder control are related to central nervous system development, children must be psychologically and physically ready for toilet training. The process starts with bowel control, which is easier because bowel movements are less frequent in a day than urination. Bowel training may be completed at about 2.5 years of age. Bladder control during the day is achieved before bladder control at night. Bladder training may be completed around 3 years of age.

Speech and language skills increase: Speech is clearer, and vocabulary increases. Words are learned by imitating others. Toddlers understand more words than they use. They are capable of forming two- or three-word sentences. By 3 years of age, children should be able to speak in short sentences.

Play ability increases. The 2-year-old plays alongside other children but does not usually play with them; this is commonly called *parallel play*. The toddler is very possessive and does not understand the concept of sharing; the word "mine" is often used.

Temper tantrums and saying "no" are common during this stage. When disciplined, the toddler may kick and scream. The temper tantrum is the child's way of objecting to having her independence challenged. It can frustrate the primary caregivers. The toddler years have many such power struggles between caregiver and child and are commonly referred to as the "terrible twos."

Another developmental task for toddlers is tolerating separation from the primary caregiver. As toddlers start to explore their environments, they tend to venture away from their primary caregivers. However, when they experience discomfort, frustration, or injury, they quickly return to their primary caregivers or cry for their attention. If the primary caregiver is consistently present whenever needed, a child learns to feel secure and to tolerate brief periods of separation.

PRESCHOOL (3 TO 6 YEARS)

Ages 3 to 6 years are considered the **preschool** years (early childhood). At this stage, children grow taller but gain little weight. Preschoolers are thinner, more coordinated, and more graceful than toddlers. The developmental tasks of the preschool years include the following:

- Being better able to communicate and understand others
- Performing self-care activities
- Learning the differences between the genders
- Learning to distinguish right from wrong and good from bad
- Learning to play with others
- Developing family relationships

The 3-Year-Old

Three-year-olds are more coordinated and can walk on tiptoe, balance on one foot for a few seconds, and run, jump, and climb with ease. Personal care skills increase—they can put on their shoes, dress themselves, manage buttons, wash their hands, and brush their teeth with help. They can feed themselves, pour from a bottle, and help set the table without breaking the dishes. Hand skills also include drawing circles and crosses.

Most 3-year-olds know roughly 1 000 words, imitate new words, and talk and ask questions constantly. A favourite question repeated many times a day is "Why?" Sentences are brief—usually three or four words long. Three-year-olds can name body parts, family members, friends, and animals.

Play is important at this stage, and 3-year-olds are able to play *with* other children and not just *beside* them. Because they are developing an understanding that others have feelings, they are more cooperative than toddlers. With an adult's encouragement, they are able to share toys and take turns. They play simple games and can follow simple rules. They enjoy using colouring books and crayons, doing crafts with child-safe scissors and paper, doing age-appropriate puzzles, and participating in role-playing games such as "house" and "dress-up" (**FIGURE 18–4**).

Three-year-olds have vivid imaginations and often play make-believe games. Imaginary friends are common at this age. They may be so involved in their make-believe worlds that they sometimes confuse fantasy and reality. For example, a child may believe that a character in a picture book is real. Their developing imaginations may cause some children at this age to have nightmares or daytime fears and insecurities. Some may need a night light by their beds.

At 3 years, children know that there are two genders and begin to identify with their own gender. During role-playing games, some children will often pretend to be women (such as a mom or a princess), and others will pretend to be men (such as a dad or

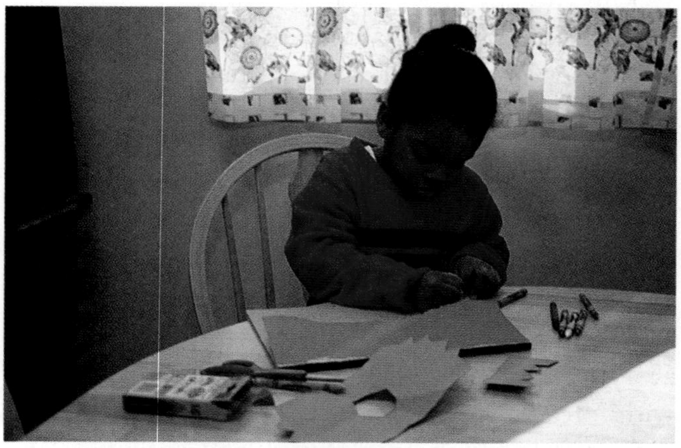

FIGURE 18–4 Three-year-olds have increased coordination. Many enjoy doing crafts such as cutting paper and using colouring books and crayons.

a cowboy). This type of play is their way of exploring the gender differences seen in their families and in the world around them (such as in books, television, and videos).

The concept of time develops, and 3-year-olds may speak of the past, present, and future. However, the words *yesterday* and *tomorrow* are still confusing to them.

Three-year-olds are less fearful of strangers and can tolerate separation from primary caregivers for short periods. They are less jealous of a new baby than toddlers are. They show that they want to please their primary caregivers.

The 4-Year-Old

Four-year-olds can hop, skip, and throw and catch a ball. They can draw faces, copy a square, and try to print letters. They can bathe with some help and usually tend to their own toileting needs with help.

Vocabulary increases to about 1 500 words, and the 4-year-old can sing simple songs, repeat four numbers, count to three, and name a few colours. The child continues to ask many questions and tends to exaggerate when telling stories. Many 4-year-olds can tell long and complex stories. Their constant chatter shows that they are learning the power of words. Sometimes, they may seem bossy as they use their developing language skills to tease, tattle, or tell others (including caregivers) what to do.

A 4-year-old's hand and finger coordination are well developed. They like to make crafts, build with blocks, and try to "write" with a pencil or pen. Children in this age group still enjoy playing "dress-up" and imitating adults (**FIGURE 18–5**). They still have vivid imaginations but are now better able to differentiate between reality and fantasy. They are more social than they were at 3 years of age and usually enjoy playing in groups of two or three. They also begin to develop close friendships and may try to be like their friends or show off to impress them.

At this age, many children express curiosity about sexuality. They may ask persistent questions about how babies are made and why boys' and girls' genitals are different. Playing "doctor and nurse" is common as curiosity about sexuality continues.

Four-year-olds may show a strong preference for the parent of the opposite gender to how they identify themselves. They show rivalries with their brothers and sisters, especially when they take their possessions or when the older children have more and different privileges.

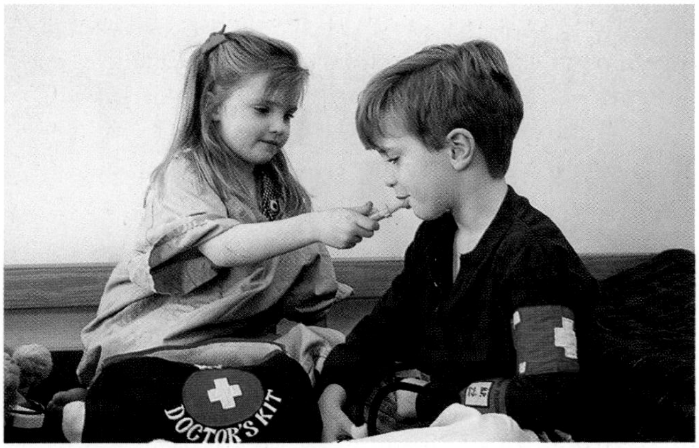

FIGURE 18–5 Four-year-olds play "dress-up" and imitate adults.

The 5-Year-Old

Coordination continues to develop, and 5-year-olds can jump rope, skate, tie shoelaces, dress, and bathe. They can use a pencil and copy diamond and triangle shapes. They can print a few letters and numbers and their first names. Drawings of people include the body, head, arms, legs, and feet.

Communication skills also increase. Vocabulary consists of about 14 000 words, and sentences have six to eight words. Five-year-olds ask fewer questions than they did when younger, but now the questions have more meaning. They want definitions for unknown terms and wish to take part in conversations. They can name four or more colours, coins, days of the week, and months. They can identify the objects that they draw and give detailed descriptions of the drawings.

Five-year-olds are generally responsible and truthful, and they quarrel less than when younger. There is greater awareness of rules and an eagerness to do things the right way, and they are proud of their accomplishments. They want to please others, especially teachers and caregivers, and display good manners. They are independent and can be trusted within limits. Five-year-olds have fewer fears but may continue to have nightmares.

Many 5-year-olds enjoy simple number and word games. Although they may cheat to win, they like

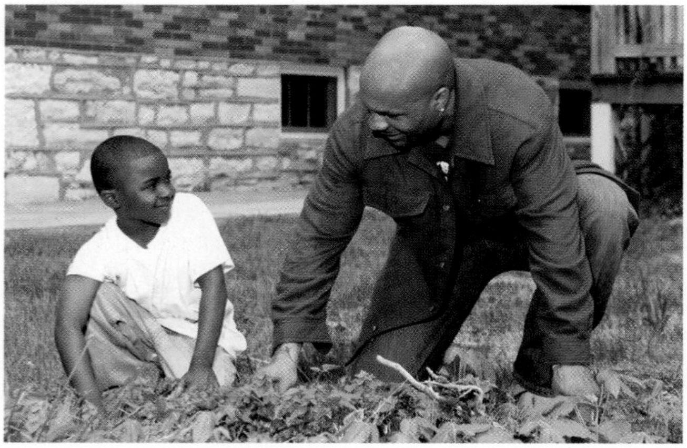

FIGURE 18–6 Five-year-olds enjoy doing things with the parent of their same perceived gender. [**Source:** Sorrentino, S.A. *Mosby's Textbook for Nursing Assistants* (8th ed., Fig. 10-16).]

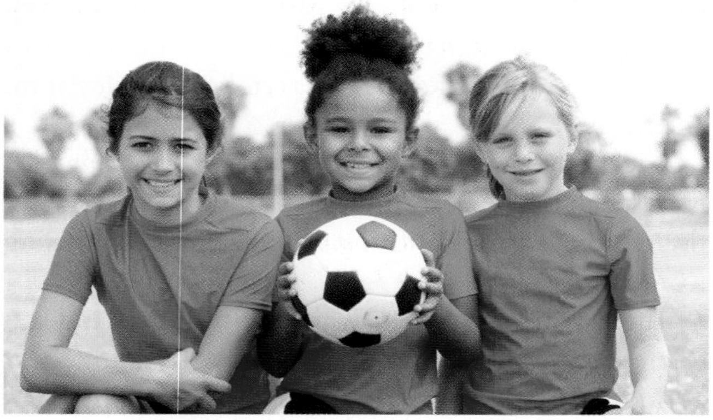

FIGURE 18–7 In middle childhood, belonging to a peer group is important. Children usually prefer playing with peers of the same gender they identify with. (**Source:** © Can Stock Photo Inc./monkeybusiness.)

having rules and try to follow them. They imitate adults during play and show a greater interest in watching television. They also enjoy activities with the primary caregiver of the same gender (**FIGURE 18–6**). Such activities include cooking, housecleaning, shopping, yardwork, and sports. Children at this age tolerate their brothers and sisters well. Although they consider younger children to be a nuisance, 5-year-olds usually are protective of them and enjoy playing with them.

MIDDLE CHILDHOOD (6 TO 8 YEARS)

Preschoolers often have nursery school and kindergarten experiences. However, **middle childhood** is the time school experiences begin in earnest. Children enter the world of peer groups, games, and learning.

The developmental tasks of middle childhood are the following:

- Developing the social and physical skills needed for playing games
- Learning to get along with other children of the same age and background (peers)
- Learning behaviours and attitudes normative to one's gender
- Learning basic reading, writing, and arithmetic skills
- Developing a conscience and morals
- Developing a good feeling and attitude about oneself

The 6-Year-Old

Between the sixth and seventh birthdays, a child will grow about 5 cm (2 in.) and gain 1 to 3 kg (2.5 to 6.5 lb.). Baby teeth are lost, and permanent teeth begin to erupt. Children at this stage are very active—they are skilled at running, jumping, skipping, hopping, and riding a bicycle and seem to be constantly on the go. They are content to sit only for a short time.

Six-year-olds enter Grade 1 and the world of school, activities, and interactions with other children. Children this age are often described as bossy, opinionated, charming, argumentative, and "know-it-alls." They have set ways of doing things and like to have their own way, so when they are frustrated, they may have temper tantrums. Six-year-olds play well with children of both genders. However, most begin to prefer playing with children of the same gender (**FIGURE 18–7**). They share more with others and may have a "best friend." They may cheat to win or may leave a game before it is over to avoid losing. Tattling is common at this stage.

Six-year-olds have a vocabulary of about 16 500 words. They know the alphabet and begin to read and spell. They have an improving ability to communicate thoughts and feelings.

Play interests range from rough play to quiet activities such as playing with cards, paints, and clay or playing computer games. They start collections of odds and ends rather than specific things such as stamps, rocks, or butterflies. More active play includes tag, hide-and-seek, playing with balls, skating, and playing in mud or sand.

The 7-Year-Old

Seven-year-olds grow about 5 cm (2 in.) in height during the year. The average 7-year-old weighs about 22 to 25 kg (49 to 55 lb.) and is 119 to 124 cm (47 to 49 in.) tall. Hand coordination increases, so they are able to do cursive writing and not just print. They are quieter than 6-year-olds and spend more time alone. They are more serious, less stubborn, and more concerned about being well liked by others. Seven-year-olds are more aware of themselves, their bodies, and the reactions of others. They do not like being teased or criticized and are sensitive about how others treat them. They usually like going to school, learning, and reading but may worry about marks and what the teacher thinks of them. Reading skills increase, and they can tell time.

Play includes swimming, biking, collecting and trading objects, playing ball and other games with rules, working on puzzles, and playing video games, usually in groups. In the case of children who have no personal gender-conflict issues, boys tend to prefer to play with boys, and girls tend to prefer to play with girls.

The 8-Year-Old

The 8-year-old enters Grade 3. Increases in height and weight continue, and more permanent teeth appear. Movements are faster and more graceful.

Peer-group activities and opinions are important at this stage in development. Being accepted and included in peer groups is vital for the fulfillment of the needs for love, belonging, and self-esteem. Children this age get along with adults, but they give more importance to peer-group fads, opinions, and activities. Boys and girls typically continue to play separately, and their interests relate to group games, collections, television, and movies.

Eight-year-olds are sometimes described as defensive, opinionated, practical, and outgoing.

They give advice freely to others but do not accept criticism well. They are able to help with many household tasks such as vacuuming, cooking, and yardwork but also expect more privileges than those given to younger brothers and sisters.

Learning continues, and these children are curious about science, history, and places and countries other than their own. School provides social opportunities with peers. Eight-year-olds are more daring in the classroom and may pass notes to or talk with others when they think the teacher is not looking. However, they are usually well mannered, relate well to adults, take part in adult conversations, and are friendly and affectionate.

LATE CHILDHOOD (9 TO 12 YEARS)

Late childhood (preadolescence) is the stage between leaving childhood, with its dependency on others, and entering adolescence. Developmental tasks at this stage are similar to those of middle childhood. However, a preadolescent is expected to show more refinement and maturity in achieving the following tasks:

- Becoming independent of adults and learning to depend on oneself
- Developing and keeping friendships with peers
- Understanding the physical, psychological, and social roles of one's identified gender
- Developing moral and ethical behaviour
- Developing greater muscular strength, coordination, and balance
- Learning how to study

Boys grow about 2.5 cm (1 in.) per year. Girls grow about 5 cm (2 in.) per year. Boys gain weight of about 1.8 kg (4 lb.) each year. Girls gain weight of about 2.3 kg (5 lb.) each year. Girls are usually taller than boys during late preadolescence. Most permanent teeth have erupted by this age.

Body movements are more graceful and coordinated (**FIGURE 18–8**). Muscular strength and physical skills increase. Skill in team sports is often important to the child.

Body changes begin to occur as the onset of puberty nears. In girls, the pelvis becomes broader, fat appears on the hips and chest, and the budding of breasts occurs. Boys show fewer signs of maturing sexually during this time, but genital organs begin to grow.

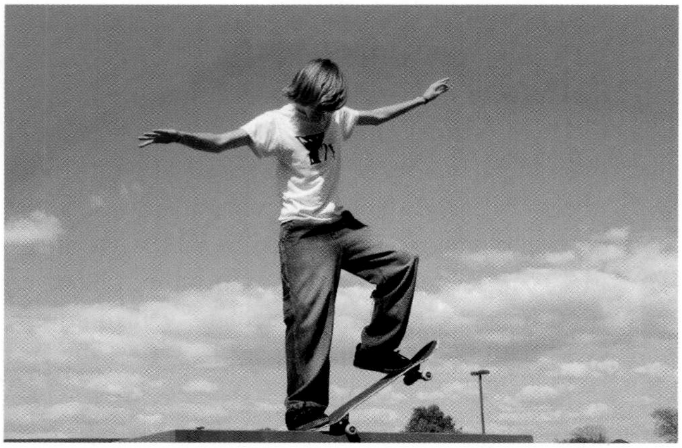

FIGURE 18–8 Movements are smooth and graceful in late childhood. (**Source:** © Can Stock Photo Inc./rhphoto.)

Children of this age must be given factual sex education. Information that is shared among friends about sex is often incomplete and inaccurate. Parents and children may be uncomfortable discussing sex with each other and may avoid the subject. When children do ask questions, with the parent's permission, you can give honest and complete answers in terms that the children can understand.

Peer groups, which are central to preadolescent activities, begin to affect the child's attitudes and behaviour. Preference for companions of the same self-identified gender continues. In most instances, boys need to show their strength and toughness and may give each other nicknames. Arguments between boys and girls are common, and they often tease each other.

At this stage, preadolescents are more aware of the mistakes and weaknesses of adults. They do not accept adult standards and rules without question, and rebellion against adults is common. Disagreements between parents and children increase, although parents continue to be important for the child's development.

ADOLESCENCE (12 TO 18 YEARS)

Adolescence is a time of rapid growth and psychological and social maturity. The stage begins with puberty. **Puberty** is the period during which the reproductive organs begin to function and secondary sex characteristics appear. Girls experience puberty between the ages of 10 and 14. Most boys reach puberty between the ages of 12 and 16. Knowing or questioning sexual orientation usually occurs at this stage of development.

Because the age of puberty varies, adolescence ranges from the ages of 12 to 18 years. The developmental tasks of adolescence include the following:

- Accepting changes in the body and appearance
- Developing relationships with others of the same age
- Accepting the role normative for one's age and identified gender
- Becoming independent from parents and adults
- Developing morals, attitudes, and values needed for functioning in society
- Increased use of social media and electronic communication devices for communicating with peers.

Menarche, the beginning of menstruation, marks the onset of puberty in girls and the appearance of secondary sex characteristics, which include the following:

- Increase in breast size
- Appearance of pubic and axillary (underarm) hair
- Slight deepening of the voice
- Widening and rounding of the hips

During late childhood, male sex organs begin to increase in size. This growth continues during adolescence. *Ejaculation* (the release of semen) signals the onset of puberty in boys, and involuntary *nocturnal emissions* ("wet dreams") occur: During sleep *(nocturnal)*, the penis becomes erect, and semen is released *(emission)*. The following secondary sex characteristics also appear:

- Appearance of facial hair
- Pubic and axillary (underarm) hair
- Hair on the arms, chest, and legs
- Deepening of the voice
- Increases in neck and shoulder size

A growth spurt occurs during adolescence. Boys grow about 10 to 41 cm (4 to 16 in.) and gain 7 to 27 kg (15 to 60 lb.) in weight. They usually stop growing between the ages of 18 and 21 years. Some continue to grow until about 25 years. Girls grow about 5 to 23 cm (2 to 9 in.) and gain between 7 and 23 kg (15 and 50 lb.) in weight. They usually stop growing between the ages of 17 and 18 years, but some girls continue to grow until about 21 years.

Adolescence is described as the "awkward stage." Awkwardness and clumsiness are caused by the uneven growth of muscles and bones. Coordination and graceful body movements eventually develop as muscle growth and bone growth even out.

Children at this stage often find changes in physical appearance hard to accept. Some girls are embarrassed about breast development, especially about very large or small breast size, and some boys may be concerned about genital size. Height may cause concern in both boys and girls—boys do not like being much shorter than their peers, and tall girls may feel embarrassed about being taller than other girls and boys. Many adolescents, especially girls, worry about their weight, and, thinking that they weigh too much, some try to diet and may develop eating disorders.

Teenagers often feel intense emotions, and their emotional conditions vary from high to low. Adolescents can be happy one moment and sad the next, so predicting their reaction to a comment or event can be difficult. Teenagers can control their emotions better later in this stage. Older adolescents (15- to 18-year-olds) can still become sad and depressed, but they can better control the time and place of their emotional reactions.

Adolescents need to become independent of adults, especially their parents. They must learn to function, make decisions, and act in a responsible manner without adult supervision. Many teenagers work toward developing this independence by looking for part-time jobs, babysitting, going to dances and parties, dating, taking part in school clubs and organizations, shopping without an adult, and staying home alone (**FIGURE 18–9**).

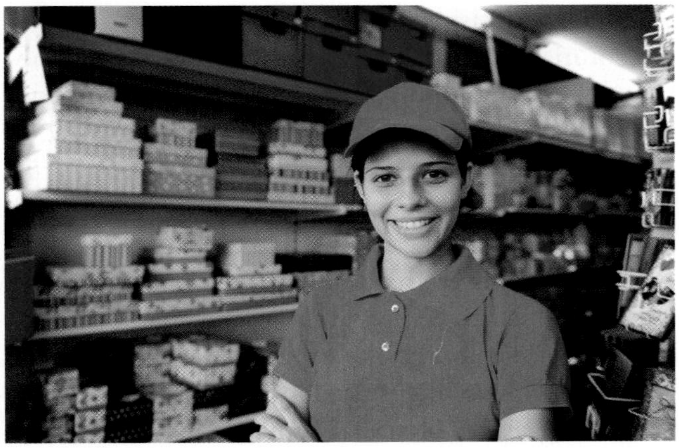

FIGURE 18–9 This teenager has a part-time job. (**Source:** © Can Stock Photo Inc./mangostock.)

Adolescents become increasingly able to use logic and reasoning, and they often form passionate opinions on many issues. However, their judgement and reasoning are not always sound. Guidance, discipline, and emotional and financial support from parents are still needed. Disagreements with parents are common, especially about behaviour and activity restrictions and limits. Adolescents would rather be with peers than do things with parents and other family members. Similarly, they tend to confide in and seek advice from peers or from adults other than their parents.

Teenage interests and activities reflect the need to become independent and to develop intimate relationships. All genders are often interested in parties, dances, and other social activities. Clothing, makeup, and hairstyles are often important to teenagers of all genders because their appearance enables them to define their identity and fit in with a group. Parents and teenagers often disagree about clothing and hairstyles. Teenagers may spend a lot of time with friends or converse with them through email, text messaging, or social media or on the phone. They also spend time participating in sports or in club activities, listening to music, or playing video games.

Dating begins during adolescence, and although the age of its onset varies from individual to individual, there is usually a dating pattern. "Crowd" dates are common in Grades 7 and 8. They are usually related to school activities such as dances or basketball games. The same group of girls just happens to be with the same group of boys during these social events. In Grade 9, pairing off between people who are attracted to each other is common during crowd dating. In Grade 10, couples go to social events together and then join other couples. Double dating occurs in Grade 11. In Grade 12, dates usually involve only one couple, although there is some double dating occasionally.

Difficult decisions and conflicts result as the adolescent matures physically, psychologically, and emotionally. Parents and teenagers often disagree about dating because parents worry that dating may lead to sexual activities, pregnancies, and sexually transmitted infections. Teenagers usually do not understand or appreciate these concerns. "Going steady" helps the teenager meet the needs for security, love and belonging, self-esteem, and, for some, gender identification or exploration. Teenagers sometimes have difficulty controlling sexual urges and considering the consequences of sexual activity.

Adolescents begin to think about careers and what to do after high school graduation. Interests, skills, and talents are some of the factors that influence the choice of further education or a job. Adolescents also need to develop morals, values, and attitudes for living in society. They need to develop a sense about what is good and bad, right and wrong, and important and unimportant. Parents, peers, culture, religion, television, school, and movies are some of the factors that influence teenagers. Drug abuse, unwanted pregnancy, alcoholism, and criminal acts are common problems among troubled adolescents.

YOUNG ADULTHOOD (18 TO 40 YEARS)

Psychological and social development continues during **young adulthood**. There is little physical growth because adult height has already been reached by this time, and body systems are fully developed. Developmental tasks of young adulthood include the following:

- Choosing further education and a career
- Selecting a partner
- Learning to live with a partner
- Becoming a parent and raising children
- Developing a satisfactory sex life

Education and occupation are so closely related that they can rarely be separated. Most jobs require specific knowledge and skills, so the amount and kind of education needed depend on a person's career choice. Most adults find that their job choices are greater with adequate educational preparation and that employment is necessary for economic independence and for supporting a family.

At this stage of development, young adults may choose to marry their partner, remain single, or live in a common-law relationship. Some of the reasons for marriage or common-law relationship are being in love, wanting emotional security, wanting a family, having a sexual relationship, wanting to leave an unhappy home life, looking for a certain social status, wanting companionship, and sharing financial security. Some marry to feel wanted, needed, and desirable. Factors such as age, religion, interests, education, race, personality, and love affect the selection of a spouse. Some marriages are happy and successful, whereas some others are not. There are no guarantees that a marriage will work, so the couple must work together to build a marriage based on trust, respect, caring, and friendship.

Partners (married or unmarried) must learn to live with each other, which may require habits, routines, household management, meal preparation, and leisure activities to be changed or adjusted to "fit" each other's needs. They must learn to solve problems, make decisions together, and work toward the same goals. Open and honest communication is essential to a successful partnership (**FIGURE 18–10**).

Young adults also need to develop a satisfactory sex life. Frequency of sex, desires, practices, and preferences vary among couples. Understanding and accepting a partner's needs are necessary for a satisfying and intimate relationship.

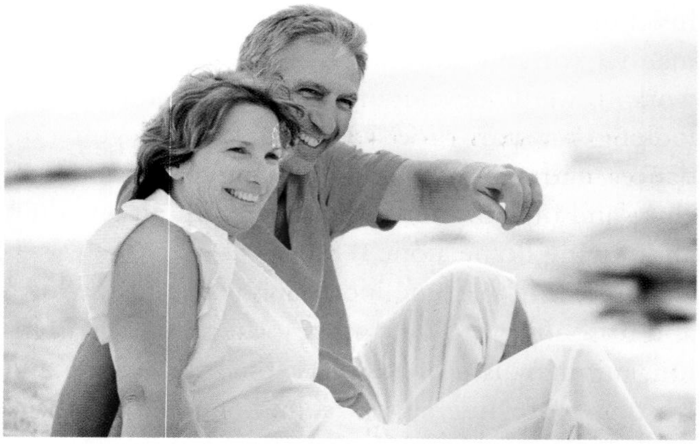

FIGURE 18–10 Communication is necessary for a successful partnership and a satisfactory sex life. (**Source:** © Can Stock Photo Inc./hannamonika.)

Statistically, most heterosexual couples decide to have children, and modern birth control methods allow them to plan how many children they want to have and when to have them. However, some pregnancies are unplanned. Many couples have a child during the first few years of marriage or partnership; some wait several years before starting a family. Some couples decide not to have children at all. Today, couples of any gender who wish to have children but may be unable to become pregnant, or experience difficulty having children, may choose to adopt a child, have *in vitro* (medically assisted) fertilization (sometimes with donor sperm), or arrange to have a surrogate carry the child. The availability of surrogacy and evolving adoption laws have enabled couples to choose the option that best fits their family. In these cases, there may be costly legal costs involved. Those couples deciding to have children must agree on methods of child rearing and discipline and must adjust to the children and the children's need for time, energy, and parental attention.

MIDDLE ADULTHOOD (40 TO 65 YEARS)

For some adults, **middle adulthood** is a stable and comfortable stage of development, a time when children have grown up and moved away and partners are able to spend time alone with each other, enjoy financial security, and have fewer worries about children. However, some adults in this stage have to deal with divorce, ailing parents, children moving back home or not moving out at all, and caring for grandchildren. The developmental tasks of middle adulthood include the following:

- Adjusting to physical changes
- Having grown-up children
- Developing leisure activities
- Relating to aging parents

Of the physical changes that occur in this period, several are gradual and go unnoticed, whereas some others become obvious early in this stage. People in their early forties may feel energetic and able to function as they did in their twenties. However, energy and endurance begin to decrease. People in this age group can develop any number of diseases and illnesses, which may be chronic or life-threatening. Weight control becomes a problem as metabolism and physical activities slow down. Facial wrinkles and grey hair appear (although grey hair can also naturally occur in people in their twenties). The need for eyeglasses is common at this stage, and there may be hearing loss or deterioration. In women, menstruation stops between the ages of 42 and 55, as **menopause** sets in. The ovaries stop producing eggs and secreting hormones, meaning the woman can no longer become pregnant.

Children leave home to pursue higher education, marry, move to homes of their own, and start their own families. Middle-aged adults have to cope with letting children go, being in-laws, and becoming grandparents. Parents must let their adult children lead their own lives while also remaining available to their children for emotional support in times of need.

Middle-aged adults often discover that they have a lot more spare time once the demands of parenthood have decreased significantly. Hobbies and leisure activities such as gardening, fishing, painting, golfing, volunteer work, and membership in clubs and organizations are sources of pleasure (**FIGURE 18–11**). These activities become even more important after retirement and during late adulthood.

Some middle-aged adults have parents who are very old and experiencing poor health; they take on the responsibility for their parents' care and often have to deal with the death of parents.

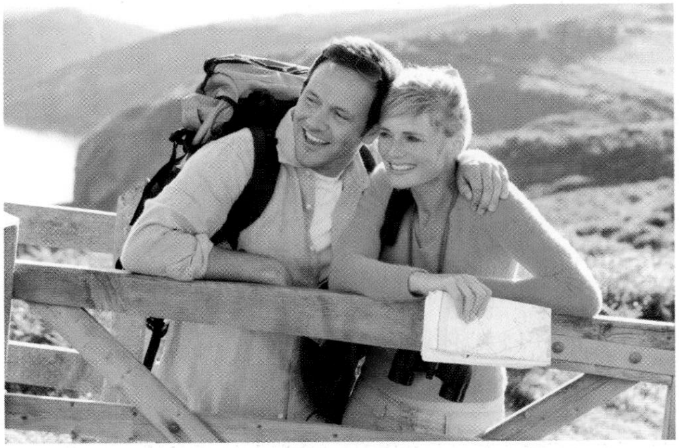

FIGURE 18–11 Middle-aged adults usually have more time for hobbies. (**Source:** © Can Stock Photo Inc./ monkeybusiness.)

LATE ADULTHOOD (65 YEARS AND OLDER)

Certain physical changes are a normal part of aging and occur in everyone in **late adulthood** (see **BOX 21–2** on p. 375). The rate and degree of change vary with each person. Some of these changes are a result of lifestyle choices including diet, general health, exercise, stress, environment, and heredity. Normal aging does not mean loss of health, so quality of life does not have to change with aging.

The developmental tasks of this stage are as follows:

- Adjusting to decreased physical strength and loss of health
- Adjusting to retirement and reduced income
- Coping with the death of one's partner
- Developing new friends and relationships
- Preparing for one's own death

See Chapter 21 for a detailed discussion of the numerous physical, psychological, and social changes that occur during late adulthood, as well as the specific care that older adults may need.

CHAPTER REVIEW

KEY POINTS

- Growth and development are ongoing from the moment of fertilization until death. They occur in a sequence, order, and pattern. Certain developmental tasks must be completed during each stage, and no stage can be skipped, as each stage lays the foundation for the next stage.
- Infant stage (birth to 1 year): Rapid physical, psychological, and social growth and development occur. Birth weight usually doubles by the age of 5 to 6 months and triples by the first birthday. Newborns have certain reflexes (Moro, rooting, sucking, and grasping) that are present at birth and disappear as the central nervous system develops. Developmental tasks for infancy are learning to walk, talk, and communicate with others.
- Toddlers (1 to 3 years): Physical growth during the second year of life is not as rapid as during infancy. Developmental tasks for toddlers are tolerating separation from the primary caregiver, gaining control of bowel and bladder functions, using words to communicate with others, and becoming less dependent on the primary caregiver.
- Preschool (3 to 6 years): Children grow taller but gain little weight. They are more coordinated than toddlers. Developmental tasks for toddlers are improving the ability to communicate with and understand others, performing self-care activities, learning about the differences between the genders and identifying with a gender, distinguishing right from wrong, learning to play with others, and developing family relationships.
- Middle childhood (6 to 8 years): Children usually grow 5 cm each year during this stage; weight gain will vary, depending on such factors as level of activity. Developmental tasks include acquiring the social and physical skills needed for physical games; a conscience and morals; a good feeling and attitude about self; the ability to get along with other children; behaviours and attitudes normative to one's gender; basic reading, writing, and arithmetic skills.
- Late childhood (9 to 12 years): Boys grow about 2.5 cm and gain 1.8 kg of weight per year. Girls grow about 5 cm and gain 2.3 kg of weight per year. Body changes begin to occur. Developmental tasks are developing moral and ethical behaviour; developing and keeping friendships; becoming independent of adults and learning to depend on oneself; understanding the physical, psychological, and social roles of one's identified gender; learning how to study; and developing greater muscular strength, coordination, and balance.
- Adolescence (12 to 18 years): Rapid growth and psychological and social maturing occur. Boys grow about 10 to 41 cm and gain 7 to 27 kg in weight. Girls grow about 5 to 23 cm and gain 7 to 23 kg in weight. Developmental tasks are accepting changes in one's body and appearance; developing relationships with others of the same age; accepting the role normative for one's age and identified gender; becoming independent from parents and adults; and developing morals, attitudes, and values needed for functioning in society.
- Young adulthood (18 to 40 years): Adult height has been reached, and body systems are fully developed. Developmental tasks include choosing further education and a career; selecting a partner; becoming a parent and raising children; and developing a satisfactory sex life. Individuals will make choices depending on their goals.
- Middle adulthood (40 to 65 years): Of the physical changes that occur, some are gradual and go unnoticed at first, whereas others may be more obvious—for example, grey hair, wrinkles, and a decrease in energy. Developmental tasks include adjusting to physical changes, having grown-up children, developing leisure activities, and relating to aging parents.
- Late adulthood (65 years and older): Developmental tasks are adjusting to decreased physical strength and loss of health, adjusting to retirement and reduced income, coping with the death of one's partner, developing new friends and relationships, and preparing for one's own death.

CRITICAL THINKING IN PRACTICE

You are caring for a 2-year-old boy. You take the child to another room to weigh him. The child's mother stays in his room with her infant. You ask the child to stand on the scale. He says: "No." You reach for him to place him on the scale. He cries and runs from you. Is this response normal? What could have been done to avoid this?

REVIEW QUESTIONS

Answers to these questions are at the bottom of page 319.

Circle the BEST answer.

1. Changes in psychological and social functioning are called:
   A. Growth
   B. Development
   C. Reflexes
   D. A stage
2. Which is true about growth and development?
   A. They occur from the complex to the simple.
   B. They do not occur in an orderly pattern.
   C. They occur at specific rates.
   D. It is common for people to skip stages.
3. The stage of infancy is the first:
   A. 4 weeks of life
   B. 3 months of life
   C. 6 months of life
   D. 1 year of life
4. Which reflexes in the infant are needed for feeding?
   A. The Moro and startle reflexes
   B. The rooting and sucking reflexes
   C. The grasping and Moro reflexes
   D. The rooting and grasping reflexes
5. Solid foods are usually given to an infant during the:
   A. Fifth month to the seventh month
   B. Eighth month
   C. Ninth or tenth month
   D. Eleventh or twelfth month
6. The toddler can:
   A. Use a spoon and cup
   B. Ride a bike
   C. Help set the table
   D. Name parts of the body
7. Playing with other children begins during:
   A. Infancy
   B. The toddler years
   C. The preschool years
   D. Middle childhood
8. Peer-group activities become more important at the age of:
   A. 4 to 6 years
   B. 7 to 9 years
   C. 10 to 12 years
   D. 13 to 15 years
9. Reproductive organs begin to function and secondary sex characteristics appear during:
   A. Late childhood
   B. Preadolescence
   C. Puberty
   D. Early adulthood
10. Which of the following is true?
    A. Boys reach puberty earlier than girls do.
    B. Most girls reach puberty between the ages of 10 and 14 years.
    C. Menopause marks the onset of puberty in girls.
    D. A growth spurt occurs during the toddler stage.
11. Dating usually begins:
    A. During late childhood
    B. With "crowd" dating
    C. With "pairing off"
    D. During late adolescence
12. Adolescence is usually a time when parents and children:
    A. Talk openly about sex
    B. Express love and affection
    C. Disagree
    D. Do things as a family

13. Which of the following is a developmental task of young adulthood?
- A. Adjusting to changes in the body and in physical appearance
- B. Becoming independent
- C. Choosing an occupation
- D. Relating to aging parents

14. Middle adulthood occurs at about:
- A. 25 to 35 years
- B. 30 to 40 years
- C. 40 to 50 years
- D. 40 to 65 years

15. Middle adulthood is usually a time when:
- A. Families are started
- B. Physical energy and free time are gained
- C. Children have grown up and left home
- D. People need to prepare for death

Answers: 1.B, 2.B, 3.D, 4.B, 5.A, 6.A, 7.C, 8.C, 9.C, 10.B, 11.B, 12.C, 13.C, 14.D, 15.C

Chapter opener image: Suzanne Tucker/Shutterstock.com

CHAPTER 19

Caring for Mothers and Infants

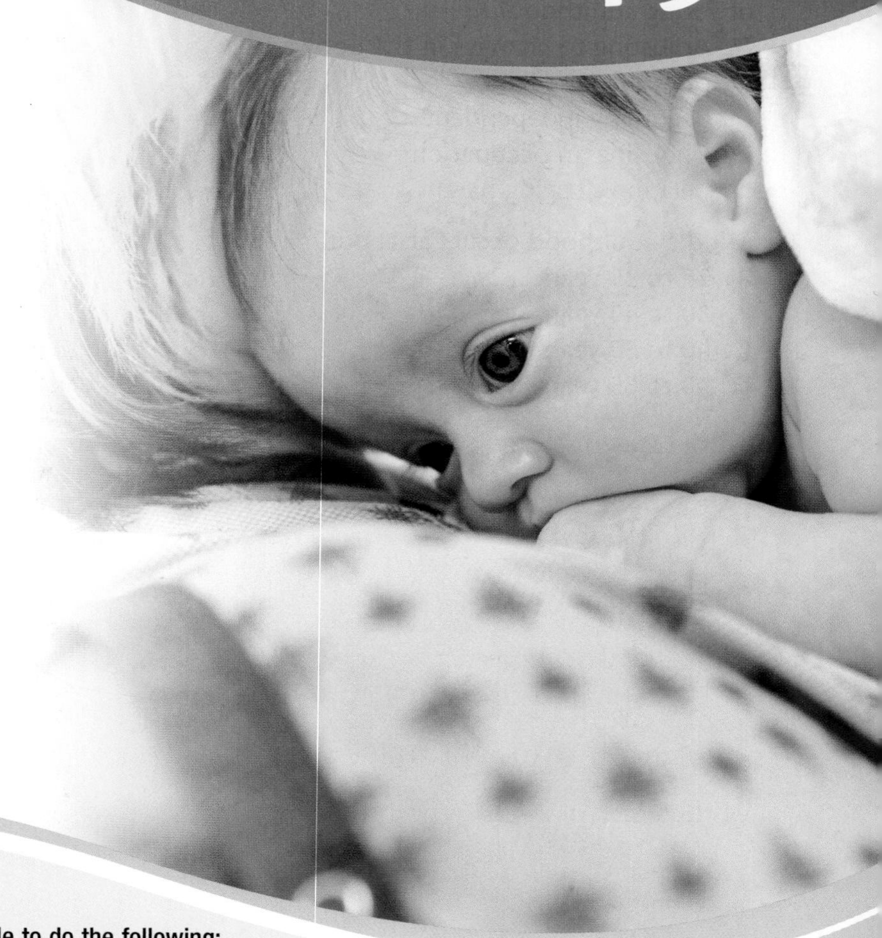

OBJECTIVES

After reading this chapter, the learner should be able to do the following:

- List physical and emotional changes a new mother may experience.
- Identify the signs and symptoms of postpartum complications.
- Identify some common disorders in infants.
- Identify the signs and symptoms of serious illness in infants.
- Describe how to hold and comfort infants.
- List precautions that reduce the risk of sudden infant death syndrome (SIDS).
- Describe how to help mothers with breastfeeding and bottle-feeding.
- Describe how to burp and diaper an infant.
- Describe how to provide cord care and circumcision care.
- Describe how to bathe infants.
- State why infants are weighed.
- Describe your role in providing child care.
- Apply the procedures described in this chapter to your clinical practice properly.

KEY TERMS

Caesarean section A surgical incision into the abdominal and uterine walls; the baby is delivered through the incision. *p. 324*
cervical mucus A viscous discharge secreted by the glands in the cervix. *p. 323*
circumcision The surgical removal of foreskin from the penis. *p. 340*
congenital Present at birth. *p. 330*
cradle cap (seborrheic dermatitis) A skin condition in which yellowish, scaly, or crusty patches, made up largely of oil and dead skin cells, appear on the scalp. *p. 328*
engorged breasts Breasts that are overfilled with milk, which makes them swollen, hard, and painful. *p. 324*
episiotomy An incision made in the perineum to increase the size of the vaginal opening for the delivery of the baby. *p. 323*
jaundice A yellowing of the skin and the white part (sclera) of the eyes. *p. 331*
lactation The process of producing and secreting milk from the breast. *p. 324*
leukocytes White blood cells that are part of the blood; the cells are part of the immune system that fight infection. *p. 323*
lochia Postpartum vaginal discharge that begins as a bloody discharge and then changes in colour and decreases in amount after 4 to 6 weeks. *p. 322*
mastitis An infection (*itis*) of the breast (*mast*). *p. 325*
postpartum After (*post*) childbirth (*partum*). *p. 322*
postpartum blues Feelings of sadness or mild depression in the mother during the first 2 weeks after childbirth; *baby blues*. *p. 325*
postpartum depression Major depression in the mother at any point during the first year after childbirth. *p. 326*
postpartum psychosis The most severe form of postpartum depression; the mother may experience delusions, hallucinations, and suicidal thoughts. *p. 326*
sudden infant death syndrome (SIDS) The sudden, unexplained death of an apparently healthy infant under 1 year of age. *p. 329*
thrush A common yeast infection that resembles cottage cheese or milk curds and is found on the sides, roof, and sometimes the tongue of a baby's mouth. *p. 330*
toxic shock syndrome (TSS) A rare, often life-threatening, illness that develops suddenly after an infection. *p. 323*
umbilical cord The structure that carries blood, oxygen, and nutrients from the mother to the fetus. *p. 339*

Support workers are sometimes required to care for new mothers and infants and must report any concerns about the infant's or mother's health to either the nurse in charge (if in a hospital or acute-care setting) or to the supervisor or public health nurse (if working in a home care or community setting). Caring for an infant provides a valuable service to the mother because it enables her to have more time and energy for herself and her family. It is important that you, as the support worker, respect the family's routines, schedules, and ways of doing things. Remember to follow the mother's standards and preferences whenever possible. As with all of the duties that you perform, it is your responsibility to follow your clients' care plan, know the limits of your scope of practice, and know whom to turn to if you have any questions about the client (see the *Supporting Leslie and Milton: Knowing Whom to Turn to for Answers* box).

CARING FOR NEW MOTHERS

Support workers employed in acute-care settings, such as hospitals, may be assigned to units where babies and new mothers are admitted.

In community settings, a new mother may require home care services in the following situations:

- She experienced complications before or after the birth.
- She needs help caring for her other young children at home.

Supporting Leslie and Milton: Knowing Whom to Turn to for Answers

Leslie, 17, mother of 2-week-old Milton, is a single mother who is new to your community. Milton's father left Leslie during her pregnancy while they were both in drug rehab, and she does not have any contact with her family. You are the support worker assigned to Leslie after a public health nurse reported that Leslie had troubles bathing and feeding Milton and adjusting to her new role as a mother. You are to report any concerns to your supervisor. Leslie is currently breastfeeding Milton. Milton weighed 3.6 kg (8 lb.) at birth and, according to his pediatrician, has grown and gained weight well. On the two last visits, Leslie seemed to have no trouble changing him, bathing him, or knowing when to bring him to his doctor for weekly visits.

On your visit today, Leslie greets you at the door, carrying Milton in one arm and holding a cigarette in her other hand. She looks as if she has been crying. Milton is crying, wet, and obviously needs a diaper change. Leslie says that she thinks that her decision to keep Milton was a wrong one and that she wants to spend more time with her friends. While you watch Leslie change Milton's diaper, you notice her hands are shaking. Leslie then says that she has been feeling very lonely and sad lately and asks if smoking a "joint" (i.e., marijuana cigarette) to help her relax will be harmful to Milton.

You are unsure how to answer Leslie's question. What should you do? What can you say to her? Who can she turn to for help in your community?

- She had a multiple birth (twins, triplets, or more).
- She has an infant with special needs who requires extra time and attention.
- She has a physical or mental disability.
- She has difficulty adjusting to her new responsibilities.

When assisting a new mother, you usually do one or more of the following:

- Provide physical care for the mother
- Provide care for the newborn
- Help with child care when other young children are in the home
- Help with home management tasks such as meal preparation and housekeeping

The **postpartum**—after (*post*) childbirth (*partum*)—period starts with the birth of the baby and ends 6 weeks later. During this time, the mother begins to adjust physically and emotionally to the effects of childbirth, and her uterus and the rest of her body begin to return to their normal (prepregnant) state. Because of the many changes experienced during the postpartum period, the mother needs to rest and recover. Encourage her to rest or nap when the baby is sleeping and to take time for herself and her partner. During this time, she also has important nutritional needs (see Chapter 28).

Lochia

In the first few weeks to months after giving birth, the mother's hormone levels will change dramatically, and her uterus will begin to contract to its prepregnant size. Blood and other substances will be expelled from the uterus; this vaginal discharge, called **lochia** (from the Greek word *lochos*, which means "childbirth"), is made up of blood, mucus, and placental tissue.

Lochia will typically increase with breastfeeding (*nursing*) and activity, but the amount of flow should return to normal after the mother rests. The mother wears clean sanitary pads to absorb the discharge, which eventually decreases in amount.

Lochia generally has an odour similar to that of normal menstrual discharge. Any offensive odour indicates a possible infection and should be reported to a health care provider. The mother should shower daily, change her sanitary pad frequently (at least every 4 hours, or after each time she urinates), practise hand hygiene before and after changing her

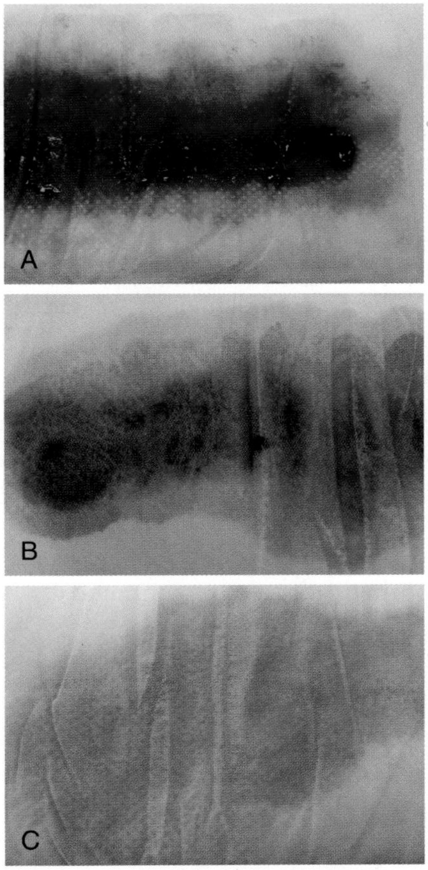

FIGURE 19–1 **A,** Lochia rubra; **B,** Lochia serosa; **C,** Lochia alba. (**Source:** Dr. Ursula Osteneck. Copyright: Saskatchewan Polytechnic.)

sanitary pad (see Chapter 23), and check her lochia for signs of infection (such as an offensive odour and greenish colour). You should check for fever and pelvic pain, which are also signs of infection.

Lochia typically continues for 4 to 6 weeks after childbirth and progresses through three stages. These stages (see **FIGURE 19–1**) describe the changes in the colour of the postpartum flow:

1. ***Lochia rubra (or "red" lochia)***—the first discharge, red because of the large amount of blood it contains. It typically lasts no longer than 3 to 5 days after childbirth.
2. ***Lochia serosa (or "watery" lochia)***—thinned discharge that has turned brownish or pink. It contains blood, water, red blood cells, white blood cells, and **cervical mucus**. This stage continues until around the tenth day after delivery.

BOX 19–1 Signs and Symptoms of Postpartum Complications

- Fever of 38°C (100.4°F) or higher
- Chills, poor appetite, fatigue, nausea, or vomiting
- Lochia that soaks a sanitary pad within 1 hour of application
- Foul-smelling lochia
- Large number of clots in the lochia
- Painful, burning, or difficult urination
- Severe abdominal or perineal pain
- Bleeding, redness, swelling, or drainage from a Caesarean-section incision (see next page)
- Leg pain, tenderness, or swelling
- Breast pain, tenderness, or swelling (see **BOX 19–2**)
- Feelings of depression (see **BOX 19–3**, on p. 326, and Chapter 35)

3. ***Lochia alba (or "white" lochia)***—discharge that has turned whitish or yellowish-white. It typically lasts from the second through the third to sixth week after delivery. It contains fewer red blood cells and is made up mainly of **leukocytes**, epithelial cells, cholesterol, fat, and mucus.

It is important to note that the mother should not use tampons during the postpartum period, as the risk of **toxic shock syndrome (TSS)** is very great, especially if the mother had an episiotomy or vaginal tear. TSS is a rare, often life-threatening, illness that develops suddenly after an infection. It can quickly affect several different organ systems, including the liver, lungs, and kidneys.

It is important that you observe these changes, as postpartum hemorrhage, infection of the uterine lining, and other complications are possible. Tell your supervisor immediately if you notice any of the signs or symptoms listed in **BOX 19–1**.

Perineal Care and Episiotomies

An **episiotomy** is an incision (*otomy*) in the perineum performed to increase the size of the vaginal opening for delivery of the baby or to decrease the risk of perineal tearing. The physician or midwife performs this procedure, and the incision is sutured after the delivery. After the episiotomy, the perineal area may become swollen, sore, and tender. The episiotomy prevents perineal tearing, which will cause severe pain, swelling, or more severe problems in the mother's perineal area. Unfortunately, in spite of every precaution, perineal tearing does occur during childbirth in some women, and repair and suturing are then needed. As a result, women who have had perineal tearing and subsequent repair may be quite bruised and sore and may require a longer healing time.

Some women do not require an episiotomy, especially if (1) the woman has had previous vaginal deliveries; (2) the woman experiences a very long labour, allowing her perineum to have an opportunity to stretch sufficiently; or (c) the woman's doctor or birthing midwife thinks it is unnecessary.

Complications can develop after an episiotomy or vaginal tearing and suturing, so it is very important that the mother practises strict perineal care and proper hand hygiene (see Chapter 23) while she has lochia. She should be instructed to clean her perineum by using a squirt bottle filled with warm water, and then wiping away all remaining drainage with a clean, wet cloth (a baby wipe will be useful), change her sanitary pad, and practise hand hygiene each time she urinates. Complications of an episiotomy include infection and wound separation (*dehiscence*). Tell your supervisor if the client complains of pain in the perineum.

The physician may order pain relief medications and cold packs to the perineum for the client's comfort. Physicians may also order *sitz baths* to promote comfort and hygiene (see Chapter 44). A warm bath also may relieve perineal pain and soreness. Make sure the tub is disinfected before each use, and have clean washcloths and towels available for the client.

The client will be advised by her doctor, nurse practitioner, or midwife about the safe time to resume sexual activity, which is usually 6 weeks after delivery.

Care of Caesarean-Section Incisions

Some clients may have had a Caesarean section. A **Caesarean section** (C-section) is a surgical incision into the abdomen and uterine wall through which the baby is delivered. A C-section is done in the following situations:

- The baby must be delivered quickly to save the baby's or the mother's life.
- The baby is too large to pass through the birth canal or is in a position that would make vaginal delivery difficult or dangerous to either the baby or the mother.
- The mother has a vaginal infection that could be transmitted to the baby.
- A vaginal delivery is expected to cause difficulties for the baby or the mother. In consultation between the mother and her doctor, a C-section delivery may been deemed the best course of action.
- The mother's doctor recommends a C-section because of a previous C-section.

The mother requires recovery time because not only has she just given birth, she has also had a major surgery (C-section). In the first few weeks after surgery, she may feel weak and tired. The physician may order her to avoid any lifting or housework during at least the first week. You may be required to help with housekeeping tasks and child care, or you may bring the baby to her for feedings.

The C-section incision also needs to heal (see Chapter 24). Tell your supervisor or nurse in charge if the client complains of pain around the incision site. Also, tell your supervisor or nurse in charge if you observe bleeding, redness, swelling, or drainage from the incision.

Breast Care

Lactation—the process of producing and secreting milk from the breasts—usually begins around the third day after childbirth. Occasionally, the new mother's breasts may become overfilled with milk. **Engorged breasts** are swollen, hard, and painful, but once breastfeeding is established or the milk dries up (if the mother chooses not to breastfeed), engorgement decreases within 1 or 2 days. Cold packs applied to the breasts or warm showers promote comfort. A well-fitting nursing bra worn day and night supports the breasts and increases comfort during engorgement. Follow the care plan to promote the client's comfort.

Although uncommon, some women are unable to breastfeed for a variety of reasons. New mothers experiencing this difficulty may be very upset by it and will need to be supported.

Sometimes, clients feel a tender lump in a breast, which usually is a symptom of a *plugged duct*. Milk drains into ducts that open onto the nipple (see **FIGURE 17-30**, on p. 298). When the milk does not drain properly through the duct, it builds up within the breast. An untreated plugged duct can cause a breast infection. Tell your supervisor if you suspect the mother has a plugged duct. Treatment usually involves:

- Encouraging frequent nursing
- Keeping pressure off the clogged duct by ensuring that the clothes and the bra are not too tight
- Applying warm washcloths to the affected area or having warm showers to promote drainage

Mastitis is an infection (*itis*) of the breast (*mast*). The following are risk factors for mastitis while breastfeeding:[1]

- Previous mastitis
- Delaying or skipping breastfeeding or pumping sessions, causing engorgement and possible blockage of milk ducts
- Cracked or irritated nipples, often caused by poor positioning or poor latching on, through which bacteria can enter
- Anemia, which can lower resistance to infection

One way the client can help prevent mastitis is to practise proper hand hygiene each time she touches her nipples.

Mastitis is usually very painful, so early treatment is essential. Tell your supervisor as soon as signs or symptoms appear (**BOX 19–2**). Medications and rest may be ordered by the client's doctor or nurse practitioner.

Breastfeeding during treatment for mastitis is usually encouraged because it keeps the milk flowing and speeds recovery. The client should breastfeed as much as possible from the affected breast, even if it is painful at first.[2]

BOX 19–2 Signs and Symptoms of Mastitis

- Pain, heat, tenderness, red streaks, or swelling in a breast
- Tender lump or hardened area in the breast
- Fever: 38°C (100.4°F) or higher
- Chills
- Fatigue
- General body ache
- Cracked nipples or cracked skin around the nipples

Postpartum Blues, Depression, and Psychosis

The postpartum period is also a time of emotional changes. Lack of sleep, more responsibilities, and her new role may affect the new mother's moods. These and other issues such as isolation, disappointment, anxiety, poor body image, and lack of support from a partner or spouse, as well as the changes in hormone levels, may contribute to **postpartum blues** ("baby blues"), which are feelings of sadness or mild depression during the first 2 weeks after childbirth.

Common symptoms of postpartum blues include:

- Insomnia
- Mood changes
- Weepiness
- Fatigue
- Headaches
- Poor concentration
- Feelings of sadness, anger, or anxiety
- Agitation or irritability
- Changes in appetite
- Feeling withdrawn or unconnected
- Lack of pleasure or interest in most or all activities
- Loss of concentration

Health Canada estimates that up to 80% of Canadian women who give birth experience postpartum blues.[3] Symptoms usually begin in the first days after delivery and disappear, even without treatment, after 1 to 2 weeks. Your encouragement and emotional support during this time may be very helpful to the mother.

A smaller but still significant number of Canadian women suffer postpartum depression—about 10% to 15%.[4] **Postpartum depression** is major depression that begins any time within the first year after childbirth (see Chapter 35 for a discussion of major depression). Usually, it begins within 2 weeks to 6 months after childbirth. Professional care is needed as soon as possible, as postpartum depression can worsen over time.

Postpartum psychosis is a severe form of postpartum depression. It is relatively rare, affecting about 1 woman per 1 000.[5] The mother with postpartum psychosis loses touch with reality and has delusions, hallucinations, or suicidal thoughts (see Chapter 35). She could harm or neglect her child, so she must not be left alone with the infant or other children. ***Tell your supervisor or the nurse in charge immediately if the mother shows any of the signs or symptoms listed in*** BOX 19–3.

A client diagnosed with postpartum depression may be ordered medications and may need help with home management or child care so that she has time to rest. Your understanding and emotional support are essential at this time.

CARING FOR INFANTS

Since infants are helpless and cannot care for or protect themselves and must depend on others for their basic needs, as a support worker, you must ensure their safety (see Chapter 22) as well as meet their physical and emotional needs while they are in your care. Because infants have a delicate immune system, it is important for everyone to remember to practise proper hand hygiene (see Chapter 23) each time infants are touched or picked up.

Newborns and infants change and grow quickly, and their physical and emotional needs will also change as they grow. Review the normal growth and development patterns of newborns and infants (see Chapter 18). Follow the care plan to meet the infant's needs.

BOX 19–3 Signs and Symptoms of Postpartum Depression

- Crying
- Feelings of sadness, hopelessness, or guilt
- Difficulties sleeping
- Inability to cope with everyday problems
- Avoiding visiting with others
- Feelings of anger toward the baby
- Fatigue
- Extreme anxiety
- Delusions or hallucinations
- Thoughts of harming the baby or self

Holding the Infant

Pay particular attention to hygienic measures when handling infants. You should always practise proper hand hygiene before and after handling the infant. You should wear a clean top (or gown) for each baby that you hold. If you are caring for a client and her baby in a home care setting, you should, if feasible, change into your clean uniform when you arrive at the client's house. If changing is not feasible, you should protect your clean uniform by wearing a covering garment over it until you are in the client's home and are about to pick up the infant.

Most infants are comforted when they are held and cuddled, and it helps them feel loved and secure. Always handle a baby with gentle, smooth movements; avoid sudden or jerking movements, as these may startle or upset the baby.

Use both hands to lift a newborn. Always support the entire body, especially the head and the neck (because a baby's neck is very weak for about the first 3 months) when lifting and holding the infant. Do not let the baby's arms or legs dangle. Hold the baby securely and close to your body. FIGURE 19–2 shows how to hold a baby. Do not forget to practise proper hand hygiene before touching the infant.

Swaddling the Infant

Swaddling an infant, a technique that is practised throughout the world in many cultures, provides warmth, comfort, and security to an infant by *securely* wrapping the baby (but not too tightly). Many parents also report that their infants sleep better

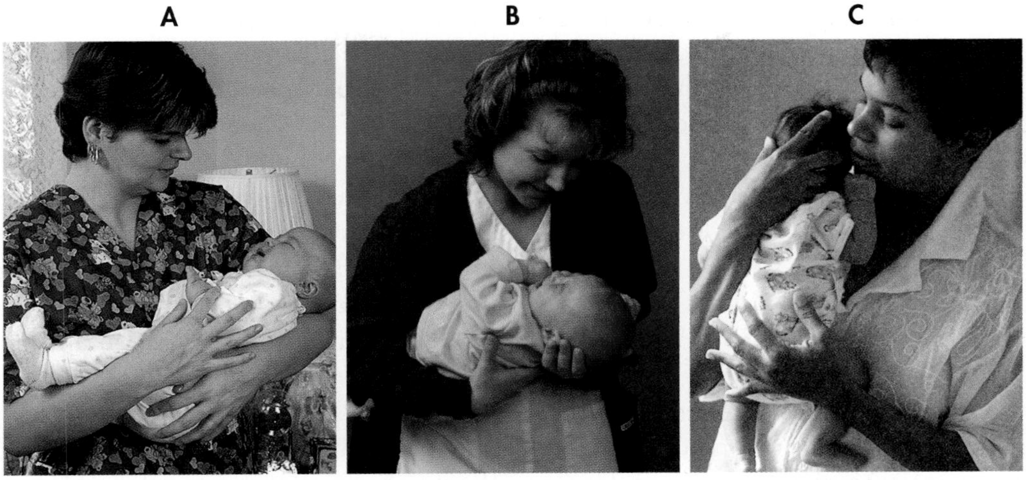

FIGURE 19–2 Support the head and neck with one hand and the legs and back with the other. Hold the baby close to your body. **A,** The cradle hold. **B,** The football hold. **C,** The shoulder hold. Note how each support worker is looking at the baby she is holding.

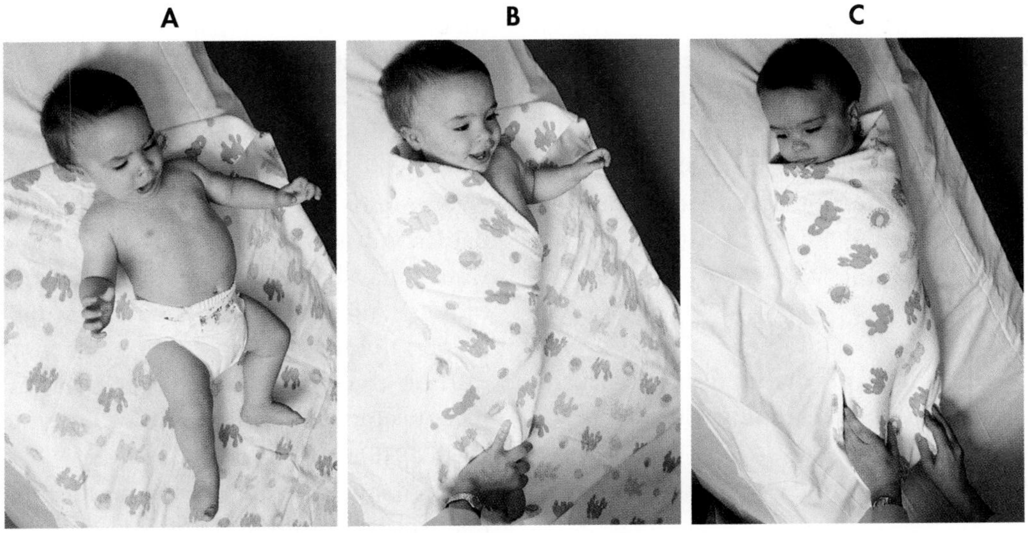

FIGURE 19–3 Swaddling an infant. Lay out the receiving blanket in a diamond shape, and bring the top corner of the blanket down. **A,** Place the baby's shoulders in line with the top edge of the blanket. **B,** Take the left side of the blanket and bring it over the baby's chest. Tuck the baby's right arm inside. Tuck the blanket under the baby. **C,** Take the bottom of the blanket and fold it up on top of the baby's body. Bring the right side of the blanket around the baby, making sure the arm is at the baby's side. Tuck the end of the blanket under the baby. (**Source:** Hockenberry, M.J., Wilson, D., Winkelstein, M.L., et al. (2003). *Wong's nursing care of infants and children* (7th ed., p. 1139). St. Louis, MO: Elsevier/Mosby.)

when they are swaddled. Swaddling holds infants securely so that they do not flail their limbs and startle themselves. Many infants sleep better on their backs (the proper way for babies to sleep) while they are swaddled. Some babies like being swaddled, but some dislike it, so you should always check with the parents before swaddling. To promote the baby's safety, it is important to check frequently to ensure the baby is not overheating. Loosened blankets in the crib could increase the risk for suffocation. When swaddled, the baby should be able to easily move and bend her hips to prevent hip problems.

To swaddle an infant, begin by performing hand hygiene; when your hands are completely dry, lay a receiving blanket on a flat surface, and fold a top corner down. Place the baby supine with the head on the folded corner and the baby's shoulders in line with the top edge of the blanket (FIGURE 19–3, *A*). Bring the left side of the blanket over the baby's chest. Tuck the right arm inside. Tuck the blanket under the baby. (**FIGURE 19–3, *B***). Pull the bottom corner up over the baby's body and to the chest. Bring the right side of the blanket over the baby's left arm and across the chest, and tuck it under the back on the baby's right side (**FIGURE 19–3, *C***). The blanket should be wrapped loosely but securely enough so that the baby's arms and legs do not come out of the blanket.

Comforting the Crying Infant

Infants cry to communicate a number of things, including that they are wet, hungry, hot, cold, tired, uncomfortable, in pain, overstimulated, or lonely. You should respond to the baby's crying immediately to help the baby feel safe and secure. ***An infant cannot be spoiled with too much attention and comfort.***

Some babies cry a lot, and the parents have to figure out what comforts them. Ask the mother how she soothes her baby. You may have to try different things to find a method that works (**BOX 19–4**). Tell your supervisor if you are not able to comfort the baby.

BOX 19–4 Guidelines for Soothing a Crying Infant

- Ensure all physical needs are met. Determine if the baby needs a diaper change or is hungry, hot, cold, tired, or in pain.
- Use gentle motions, such as rocking, swinging, or walking back and forth with the baby.
- Hold the baby close to your chest so that the baby can hear your heartbeat.
- Rub the baby's back or stomach.
- Swaddle the baby.

Cradle Cap, Diaper Rash, and Thrush

Many babies get "cradle cap," diaper rash, or thrush. None of these issues is life-threatening, but each may cause discomfort to the baby.

Cradle Cap

Cradle cap (seborrheic dermatitis) is a skin condition in which yellowish, scaly, or crusty patches, made up largely of oil and dead skin cells, appear on the scalp. The condition is most common in infants, but it may be seen occasionally in children up to the age of 5 years. These patches appear most often on the scalp and may even extend onto the forehead. They may also appear in the skin fold behind the baby's ears, on the ears, or in the diaper area. The most typical location is over the soft spot (anterior fontanelle) on the top of the baby's head.

Cradle cap is quite common and not difficult to treat. Mild cases usually clear up when the baby is shampooed daily with regular baby soap applied on a wet, rough facecloth wrapped around your hand. Remember to always rinse the soap completely from the baby's skin. Check the baby's care plan or check with your supervisor for details on how to provide care for cradle cap on an infant. One common treatment is to soften the crusts first by massaging a small amount of baby oil into the baby's scalp and letting it remain there overnight.

Diaper Rash

Diaper rash is a very common condition that most babies will develop at one time or another. Diaper rashes may be caused by medications (such as antibiotics), moisture, urine, or irritating chemicals in diapers (cloth or disposable). When you observe a rash on the baby you are caring for, make a note of its appearance, location, and other typical symptoms (**BOX 19–5**).

There are different types of rashes that have different causes. Always remember to practise proper hand hygiene before and after changing the baby. If it is stated in the baby's care plan, you may have to wear gloves for changing the baby's diaper. ***Always report a rash that is new, a rash that seems to be spreading in spite of treatment, or one that is present for longer than a day.*** Common types of rashes include the following:

- ***Simple diaper rash.*** Simple diaper rashes are red, slightly rough, and scaly and may appear over the whole area touched by the diaper. The skin may be irritated by chemicals used in laundering cloth diapers—detergent, bleach, whitener, water softener, or soap. Plastic or rubber pants worn over cloth diapers sometimes affect the skin. The skin may also react to the chemicals used in the

Think About Safety

Laying the Infant Down to Sleep

When laying the baby down to sleep, safety precautions must be taken to prevent **sudden infant death syndrome (SIDS)**—the sudden, unexplained death, usually during sleep, of an apparently healthy infant under 1 year of age.

When laying the baby down to sleep, remember the following:

- ***Always lay babies on their backs for sleep.*** Babies who sleep on their stomachs or sides have an increased risk of SIDS. However, some babies have medical conditions that *require* them to sleep on their stomachs, so it is important to check with your supervisor and the care plan. Babies can lie on their stomachs *when they are awake and being supervised.*
- ***Do not lay the baby on soft bedding products.*** These include fluffy, plush products such as sheepskin pillows, quilts, comforters, memory foam mattresses or mattress pads, or soft toys. Remove these items from the crib. Soft products might cause large amounts of carbon dioxide to pool around the baby's head, which may result in SIDS. The soft bedding also can cover the baby's nose and mouth and cause suffocation.
- ***Make sure the baby is warm but never hot.*** Overheating is thought to increase the risk of SIDS. Do not overdress the baby at bedtime. If the room temperature feels comfortable for you, it is also right for the baby. Use a lightweight blanket that you can add or remove, depending on the room temperature. To check if the baby is too hot, place your hand on the back of the baby's neck. If the neck is sweaty, the baby is too warm.

BOX 19–5 Treating Simple Diaper Rash or Ammonia Rash

- Always practise proper hand hygiene (see Chapter 23).
- Keep the baby as dry as possible; change diapers frequently, even if they are only slightly wet; and avoid any airtight coverings.
- If using cloth diapers, use double diapers during the daytime and triple diapers at night.
- Wash the diaper area with plain water each time you change the baby. Be sure to remove any old creams that might remain on the baby's skin. Dry the baby's skin thoroughly, taking care to dry the baby's skin folds well. If instructed in the baby's care plan, apply a protective cream or ointment (such as zinc oxide, petroleum jelly, or an ointment combining zinc oxide, cod liver oil, petrolatum, and lanolin). Use only one type of ointment at a time unless the client's care plan has instructed you to use more than one.
- Do not dust the baby's skin with cornstarch, a practice that was once commonly recommended; it has been found to encourage the growth of fungi.
- Try a different brand of laundry soap on cloth diapers. Do not use fabric softener with every wash because the baby may be sensitive to a buildup of it.
- Give cloth diapers a try if you have been using disposables, or switch brands. Try disposables if you have been using cloth diapers.
- Cut down on the use of commercial baby wipes, powders, and oils for the baby, and ensure that whatever products you use are mild and nonallergenic.
- To further promote healing, place a pad under the baby and let the baby lie undiapered, whenever possible, to expose the baby's skin to air.

Source: Baby Center. (2014). *Diaper rash 101*. Retrieved from http://www.babycenter.ca/a81/diaper-rash-101.

manufacture of disposable diapers as well as in commercial baby wipes.

- ***Ammonia rash.*** Ammonia rash is a form of diaper rash caused by urine. The skin is literally burned by the ammonia that is formed when urine is decomposed by normal bacteria on the skin. Not surprisingly, ammonia rash is worse after the baby has been asleep for a long period without a diaper change. You can identify it by the noticeable ammonia smell when you change the diaper. The baby's skin should be washed with mild soap and warm water and then dried thoroughly. Be sure to dry in between the baby's skin folds.
- ***Other types.*** Besides these two basic types of diaper rashes, a variety of other rashes may appear in the diaper area, including those caused by an allergy to a food or a drug, a skin infection, or a contagious disease such as chicken pox or measles.

Thrush

Thrush is a common yeast infection that resembles cottage cheese or milk curds and is found on the sides, roof, and sometimes the tongue of a baby's mouth (**FIGURE 19–4**). Unlike milk residue, which leaves a white coating on the baby's tongue that easily comes off, the white patches associated with thrush do not come off easily. If one of these patches is accidentally scraped away, you will find underneath, a raw, red area that may bleed. Thrush is not life-threatening, but it can be very sore and would prevent the baby from feeding, which would lead to dehydration.

You may first suspect thrush if the baby starts crying while breastfeeding or sucking on a pacifier or a bottle. It is most common in babies 2 months and younger but can appear in older babies, too. ***If the baby develops a fever, your supervisor should be notified immediately, as the baby may have another type of infection.***

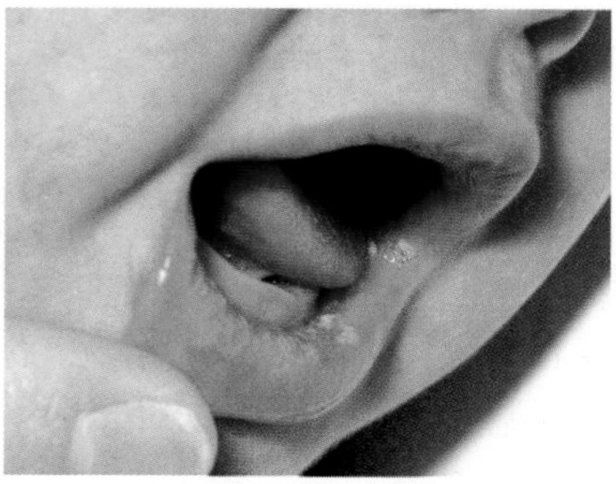

FIGURE 19–4 Thrush. (**Source:** Alamy Stock Photo)

Cause

Yeast is present in the human body as the normal flora of the digestive system, but when the balance is disturbed, an infection sets in. Sometimes, hormonal changes or the use of antibiotics (in the mother or the baby) during the period of breastfeeding can cause this imbalance.

Some babies, such as low-birth-weight babies, premature babies, babies born to mothers with diabetes, or babies with some type of **congenital** (present at birth) disorder are more susceptible to infections than others are. Some babies are infected by their mothers during delivery through the birth canal.

Treatment

If you suspect the baby has thrush, you should immediately report it to your supervisor. Some doctors may prescribe medicated drops that the mother must place in her baby's mouth before feeding. If she is breastfeeding the baby, she may be prescribed an antifungal cream to be applied on her nipples so that she and her baby will not re-infect each other. It may take a week for the thrush to clear up after medication has been started. It is important that everyone who has contact with the baby practise proper hand hygiene. Soothers may trap the yeast particles and re-infect the baby, so they should be replaced with either new soothers or ones that have been properly sterilized.

Signs and Symptoms of Potentially Serious Illness

Infants can become ill quickly. Signs and symptoms may be sudden, so you must be very alert to note them. Your observations are important for the infant's safety and well-being. Tell your supervisor when the sign or symptom began. If the infant has any of the signs or symptoms listed in **BOX 19–6**, tell your supervisor immediately. Your supervisor will tell you which care method to use.

You may need to take an infant's or child's temperature and count respirations (see Chapter 15). Axillary (between skin folds in the armpit) temperatures are taken on infants, and tympanic (external

BOX 19–6 Signs and Symptoms of Possible Serious Illness in Infants

- **Jaundice**—a yellowish colour to the skin and whites of the eyes
- Redness or drainage around the cord stump or circumcision (see p. 339)
- High temperature (over 38°C)
- Limpness; slow response
- Screaming or crying for a long time
- Flushed or pale skin
- Heavy perspiration
- Rash
- Noisy, rapid, difficult, or slow respirations
- Coughing or sneezing
- Reddened or irritated eyes
- Turning the head to one side or putting a hand to one ear (signs of an ear infection)
- Not feeding
- Vomiting most of the feeding or vomiting between feedings
- Hard, formed stools
- Frequent watery, green, mucous, or foul-smelling stools
- Signs of dehydration:
  - Fewer than six wet diapers a day
  - Dark yellow urine
  - Decreased saliva and tears
  - Dry lips
  - Dry, wrinkled skin
  - Sunken eyes and top of head
- Stiff neck; head not pulling forward toward the chest

ear canal) or axillary temperatures are taken on children younger than 5 years. Apical (over the apex of the heart) pulses are taken on both infants and young children.

Helping Mothers Breastfeed

Mothers who breastfeed are aware of the health benefits to the baby associated with breastfeeding. Usually, both mothers and babies learn the process in a very short time. However, some mothers and babies can have difficulties in the first few weeks, which may be a stressful time for the mother. Provide a calm, reassuring, supportive, and positive atmosphere. Tell your supervisor if the mother is having difficulties with breastfeeding, as she may require additional support. Whether the baby is being bottle-fed or breastfed, without sufficient feeding, the baby can become dehydrated. Signs and symptoms of dehydration that you should be aware of are in **BOX 19–6**.

Breastfed newborns usually nurse every 2 to 3 hours throughout the day and night. Babies are fed on-demand—that is, they are fed whenever they are hungry, not on a schedule. When babies want to eat, they often become restless, suck on their fists, and cry.

At first, babies breastfeed for a short time—maybe only 5 minutes at each breast. Eventually, total nursing time may take between 20 and 30 minutes. Mothers might need help getting ready to breastfeed. Assist the mother, as needed. The mother may require assistance to position herself and her baby until she is comfortable doing so on her own. Refer to **FIGURE 19–5** on page 332 to see various breastfeeding positions. If you leave the room while the mother is breastfeeding, stay within hearing distance in case she needs help. Some mothers want privacy while breastfeeding, and some others may want you to stay with them. Ask the mother what her preference is. **BOX 19–7** describes how you can help with breastfeeding.

Helping Mothers Bottle-Feed

Formula milk is given to infants who are not breastfed. It provides the essential nutrients the infant needs. Formula comes in three forms: The *ready-to-feed* formula is poured directly from the can into the baby bottle (**FIGURE 19–6**); water is added to *powdered* and *concentrated* formulas. The formula container has directions about the amount of formula and amount of water to be added.

Infants under 4 months of age are especially at risk for a severe, even life-threatening diarrheal infection if the bottles and other items have not been sterilized. It is important that all items that come into contact

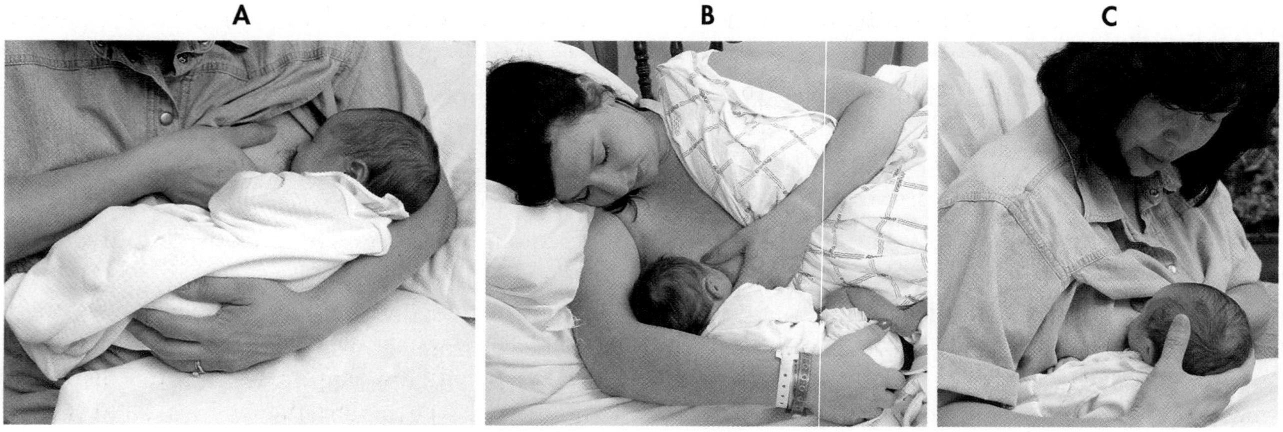

FIGURE 19–5 Breastfeeding positions: **A,** regular position; **B,** side-lying position; and **C,** football hold. Positions B and C are often used after a Caesarean section so that the baby is not resting on the mother's abdomen. Position C can be used to breastfeed twins at the same time by placing one baby at each breast. (**Source:** James, S.R., & Ashwill, J.W. (2007). *Nursing care of children: Principles and practices* (3rd ed.). St. Louis, MO: Saunders.)

BOX 19–7 Guidelines for Helping With Breastfeeding

- Perform proper hand hygiene, and remind the mother to do so also, as it is necessary before she handles her breasts.
- Help the mother into a comfortable position. She may want to breastfeed sitting up in bed or in a chair, or she may prefer the side-lying position (**FIGURE 19-5, *B***). If the mother is recovering from a Caesarean section or has a sore perineum after an episiotomy, she may prefer the side-lying position.
- Change the baby's diaper if necessary. Bring the baby to the mother.
- Mothers often appreciate help getting ready for breastfeeding. Assist her, as needed. For example, bring supportive pillows and make her comfortable; provide a drink (many women get thirsty while breastfeeding), a quiet room, or a comfortable chair.
- Offer the mother a blanket to cover the baby and her breast to promote privacy during the feeding. Some women may find that using a blanket makes nursing difficult. Follow the mother's preferences.
- Help the mother burp the baby if necessary. The baby is burped after nursing at each breast.
- Change the baby's diaper after the feeding if necessary.
- Place the baby in the crib if the baby has fallen asleep. ***Remember, place the baby on the back. Do not place the baby on the stomach or side unless the care plan instructs you to do so.***
- Record what time the baby was nursed and how long on each side. Report any problems or concerns.

with the infant's formula be sterilized. Preboiled, cooled tap water should be mixed with the formula. All mixing containers, spoons, funnels, forceps, nipples, and bottles that are used in formula preparation or feeding must be sterilized (see Chapter 23, p. 442, for tips on how to sterilize baby bottles and equipment). Boil the tap water that is to be mixed with the concentrated formula or formula powder for at least 2 minutes to destroy microbes. Use tap water from the cold tap. Check with the supervisor before using hot tap water, well water, bottled water, or water that has been filtered or treated. Follow the care plan, and contact your supervisor if you have any questions.

Bottles are prepared one at a time or in batches for the whole day. Bottles not needed immediately are capped (FIGURE 19–7) and stored in the refrigerator. The prepared bottles should be used within 24 hours. After 24 hours, the formula must be discarded.

Cleaning the Equipment

Baby bottles, caps, and nipples must be thoroughly cleaned. Reusable bottle-feeding equipment is carefully washed in hot, soapy water or in a dishwasher. Complete rinsing is needed to remove all of the soap. Some mothers use plastic nursers, which require plastic liners that are used once and then discarded.

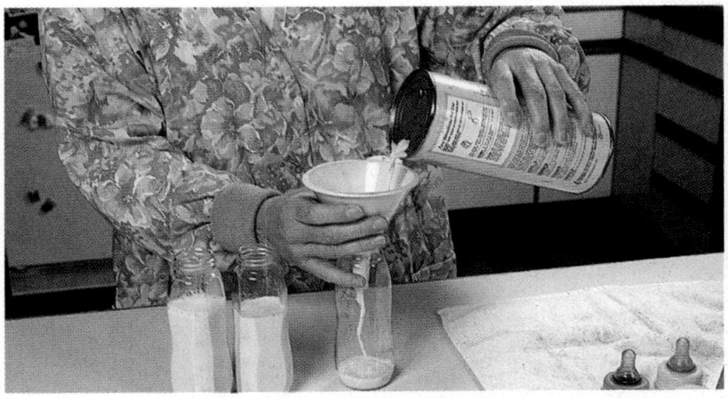

FIGURE 19–6 Ready-to-feed formula is poured from the can into the bottle. Use a clean funnel to avoid spilling.

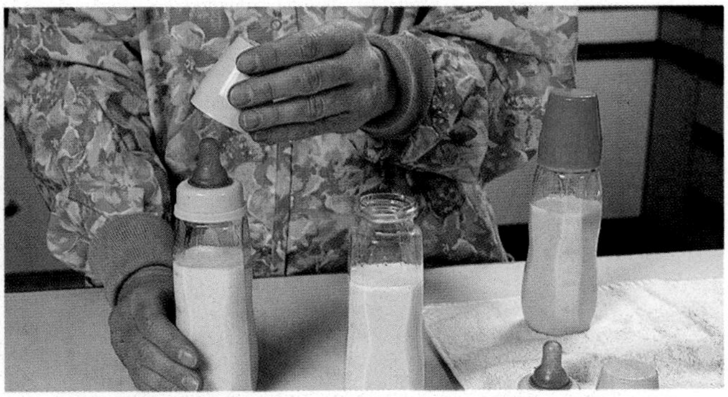

FIGURE 19–7 Bottles are capped for storage in the refrigerator.

Cleaning Bottle-Feeding Equipment 123

Advocate on behalf of the client's quality of life by promoting:

Dignity • Independence • Preferences • Privacy • Safety *(see BOX 1-4, on p. 17)*

PRE-PROCEDURE

1 Practise proper hand hygiene
2 Collect the following supplies:
- ☐ **Bottles, nipples, and caps**
- ☐ **Funnel**
- ☐ **Can opener**
- ☐ **Bottle brush**
- ☐ **Dishwashing soap**
- ☐ **Other items needed to prepare formula**
- ☐ **Clean dishtowel**

It is important to plan thoroughly before starting any procedure. By collecting all the necessary equipment beforehand, you will not have to leave your client's side and can eliminate wasting time and energy in obtaining the forgotten equipment.

Continued

Cleaning Bottle-Feeding Equipment—cont'd

PROCEDURE

3 Wash the bottles, nipples, caps, funnel, and can opener in hot, soapy water. Wash other items used to prepare the formula.
Babies can develop severe diarrhea from contaminated feeding utensils.

4 Clean the inside of the baby bottle with a bottle brush. (**FIGURE 19–8**).
Dried formula can stick to the curves inside the bottle, unless removed by a bottle brush.

5 Squeeze hot, soapy water through the nipple (**FIGURE 19–9**).
This helps remove all traces of the formula from it.

6 Rinse all items thoroughly in hot water.
Soap residue can cause diarrhea in babies.

7 ***If the infant is 4 months of age or under:***
  a All items must be sterilized after being thoroughly washed and rinsed. Boil items at least 15 minutes and allow to cool.
  b After cooling, remove items from the water with sterile forceps. Do not touch the parts that will be in contact with the baby's mouth.
Infants under 4 months of age are at risk of developing severe life-threatening diarrhea from contaminated feeding items.
When the baby is older than 4 months of age or older:
  a Place a clean towel on the countertop.
  b Stand the bottles upside down to drain. Place the nipples, caps, and other items on the towel.

8 Allow the items to dry completely.

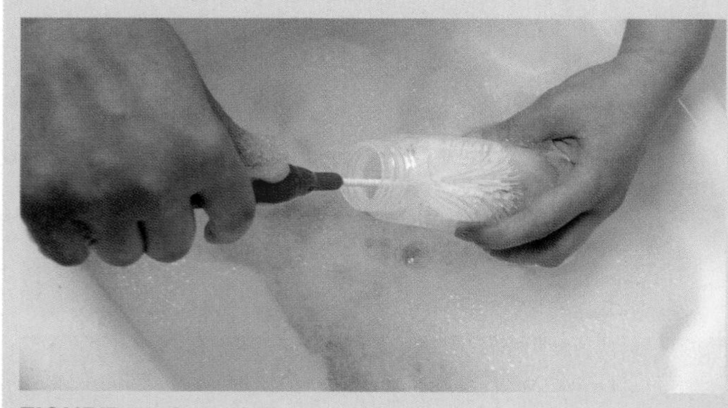

FIGURE 19–8 A bottle brush is used to clean the inside of the bottle.

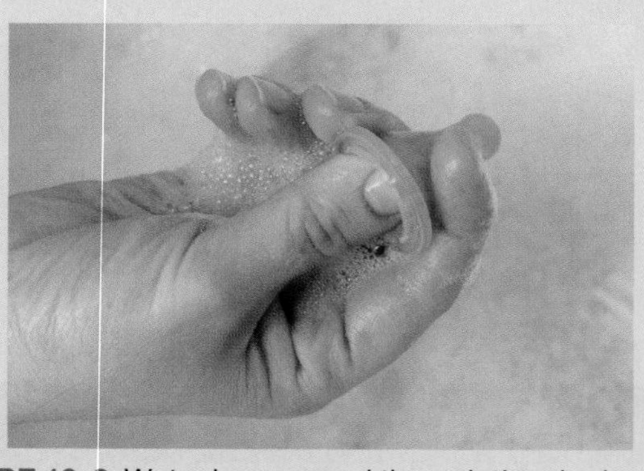

FIGURE 19–9 Water is squeezed through the nipple during cleaning.

Bottle-Feeding the Infant

Bottle-fed babies usually want to be fed every 3 to 4 hours. The care plan or the mother tells you how much formula a baby needs at each feeding. Babies usually take as much formula as they need; however, a newborn should not take in more than 60–90 mL with each feeding because of the small size of the baby's stomach. When full, the baby stops sucking and turns away from the bottle.

Babies should not be given cold formula out of the refrigerator. The bottle must be warmed in a bowl of warm water before the feeding. The formula should feel warm to the touch. Test the temperature by sprinkling a few drops on the inside of your wrist (**FIGURE 19–10**). When feeding the baby, the bottle should be tilted so the formula fills the bottle neck and nipple (**FIGURE 19–11**). The baby should be held throughout the entire feeding. Never place a baby in

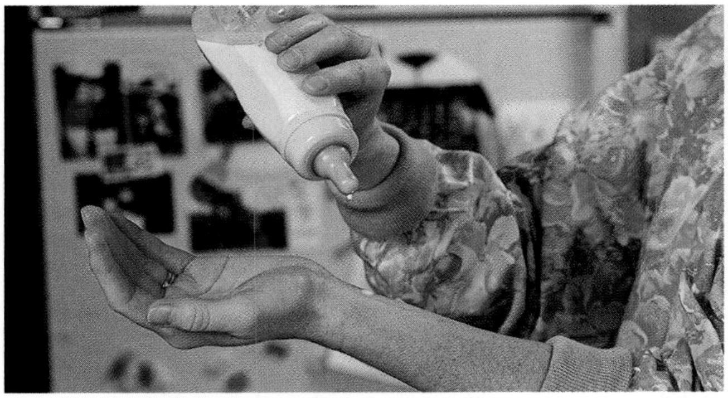

FIGURE 19–10 The formula should feel warm on the wrist.

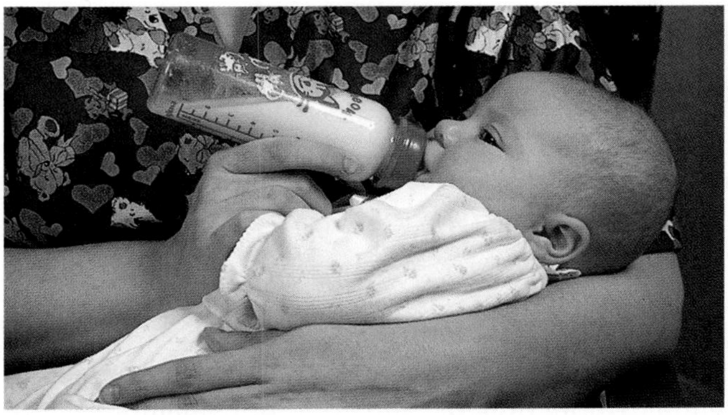

FIGURE 19–11 Tilt the bottle so that the formula fills the bottle neck and nipple.

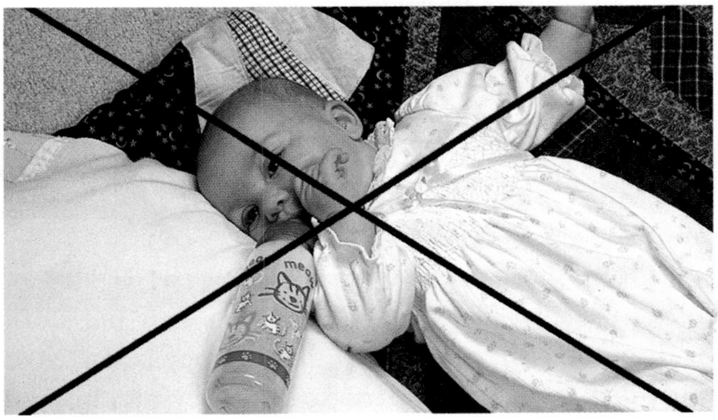

FIGURE 19–12 Do not prop the bottle to feed the baby.

BOX 19–8 Guidelines for Bottle-Feeding Infants

- Practise proper hand hygiene.
- Place the bottle in a bowl of warm water until the formula feels warm on your wrist.
- Tilt the bottle to check the flow of formula dripping out of the nipple. Two or three drops should drip out per second. Too few drops indicates that the hole in the nipple is too small, and too many drops indicates that the hole is too large. Change the nipple if the hole is not right, and test again.
- Assume a comfortable position for the feeding.
- Hold the baby close to you. Relax, and snuggle the baby.
- Tilt the bottle so that the neck of the bottle and the nipple are always filled (see **FIGURE 19–11**). Otherwise, some air might remain in the neck or nipple. Swallowing air may later cause the baby discomfort and cramping.
- ***Do not lay the baby down and prop the bottle for the feeding*** (**FIGURE 19–12**). This positioning puts the baby at risk for choking.
- Burp the baby after about half the formula has been taken and at the end of the feeding.
- Do not expect the baby to always finish all of the formula. The feeding is over when the baby stops sucking and turns the head away from the bottle. Your supervisor, the care plan, or the doctor will indicate the amount of formula the baby should be taking at each feeding.
- Discard the remaining formula.
- Wash the bottle, cap, and nipple after the feeding (see the procedure box *Cleaning Bottle-Feeding Equipment* on p. 333).

bed with the bottle propped up (**FIGURE 19–12**). This positioning can cause the baby to aspirate on formula.

Do not leave the bottle out for the formula to reach room temperature. Not only does this method take too long; it allows the growth of microbes. Also, do not heat formula in a microwave oven. It can heat unevenly and burn the baby's mouth. Some warming devices for the home or the car are popular. However, caution should be taken NEVER to leave the baby bottle in the device for long periods because the milk or formula can curdle. At all times, carefully follow the manufacturer's instructions for these devices.

The guidelines in **BOX 19–8** will help you bottle-feed babies.

Burping the Infant

Babies swallow some air during feeding, whether they are breastfed or bottle-fed. However, bottle-fed babies swallow more air. Air in the stomach and intestines

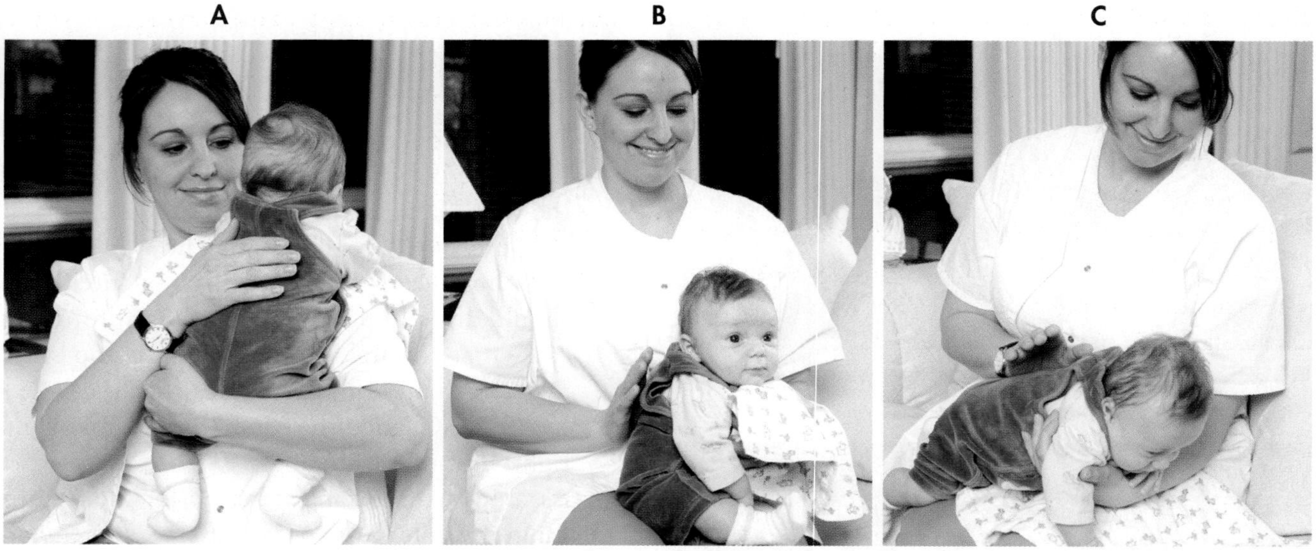

FIGURE 19–13 Burping a baby. **A,** The baby is held over the shoulder for burping. **B,** The baby is supported in the sitting position for burping. **C,** The baby is placed on the stomach for burping.

will cause the baby discomfort and cramping, which can lead to fussiness and vomiting. Burping helps get rid of the swallowed air. Most babies need to be burped after they have finished half the formula, after which they may want to continue feeding. They should be burped again at the end of the feeding.

There are three ways to position the baby for burping (**FIGURE 19–13**). One way is to hold the baby over your shoulder. Place a clean diaper or towel over your shoulder to protect your clothing in case the baby "spits up." The second way is to support the baby in a sitting position on your lap. If the baby is younger than 3 months, support the head and neck by cupping your hand under the baby's chin. Hold a towel or diaper in front of the baby. Gently pat the baby's back or rub it in circular motions until the baby burps, which may take up to 5 minutes. The third way is to sit, then lay the baby on the stomach across your knees and pat the back.

Diapering

Babies usually urinate several times a day. A baby who is only breastfed usually has stools that are bright yellow, are sweet smelling, and have the consistency of scrambled eggs. Breastfed babies usually have bowel movements after feedings. If you introduce anything other than breast milk into a baby's diet—for example, formula or solids—then the stools will change, usually to become more like an adult's (more brown, solid, and foul-smelling). Until they are fed solid foods, babies usually have stools that are soft and unformed. Bottle-fed babies may have three bowel movements a day.

Hard, formed stools indicate that the baby has constipation, and watery stools indicate diarrhea, which is very serious in babies, as their fluid balance can be upset quickly (see Chapter 28). Inform your supervisor immediately if you suspect a baby has constipation or diarrhea.

Diapers should be changed when they get wet or soiled, usually after a feeding. Parents may use cloth or disposable diapers. Cloth diapers may be fastened with diaper pins or Velcro strips. They are covered with plastic pants to protect against leaks. When changing a soiled cloth diaper, empty the stool into the toilet if possible. Place used diapers and plastic pants in the diaper pail to be laundered later. They should be washed in hot water with a laundry detergent made especially for baby clothes. Putting them through the wash cycle a second time without detergent helps remove all soap. They should be dried thoroughly and folded for reuse.

Disposable diapers help keep the baby dry because they absorb moisture. However, they still need to be changed whenever they become wet or soiled. When changing a soiled disposable diaper, empty the stool into the toilet if possible. Place the diaper in the garbage. Do not flush disposable diapers or wipes down the toilet.

Changing diapers whenever they become wet helps prevent diaper rash. Moisture, stool, and urine irritate the baby's skin. If a diaper rash develops, tell your supervisor and the mother immediately. Make sure the baby is clean and dry before you apply a clean diaper. Health Canada advises that gloves are not necessary for routine diaper changes if you can avoid touching the stool or urine with your hands.[6] Check your employer's policy for the use of gloves when diapering. Always wash your hands before and after changing diapers.

To prevent falls, never turn your back on the baby when changing diapers. Gather all supplies before starting the procedure. Arrange them in an easy-to-reach place. If the baby is on a change table, keep one hand on the baby at all times.

Diapering the Baby

123

Advocate on behalf of the client's quality of life by promoting:

Dignity • Independence • Preferences • Privacy • Safety

(see BOX 1-4, on p. 17)

PRE-PROCEDURE

1 Practise proper hand hygiene.
2 Collect the following supplies:
- ☐ **Clean diaper**
- ☐ **Waterproof changing pad**
- ☐ **Disposable or flushable wipes, or small facecloth**
- ☐ **Basin of warm water**
- ☐ **Baby soap**
- ☐ **Baby lotion or cream if necessary**

By collecting all the necessary equipment beforehand, you will not have to leave the baby's side and can eliminate wasting time and energy in obtaining the forgotten equipment. ***For safety reasons, babies should never be left unattended while on a diaper table or in a tub, even for a second!***

PROCEDURE

3 Unfasten the dirty diaper. Place diaper pins out of reach of the baby or other children.
Diaper pins can be a safety hazard to the baby or older siblings.

4 Wipe the genital area with the front of the diaper if the diaper is dry enough (FIGURE 19–14). Wipe from the front to the back.
Wiping from front to back ensures that fecal pathogens are not deposited in the baby's skin folds.

5 Fold the diaper so that urine and stool are well inside. Set the diaper aside.
Folding helps contain diaper contents and their smells.

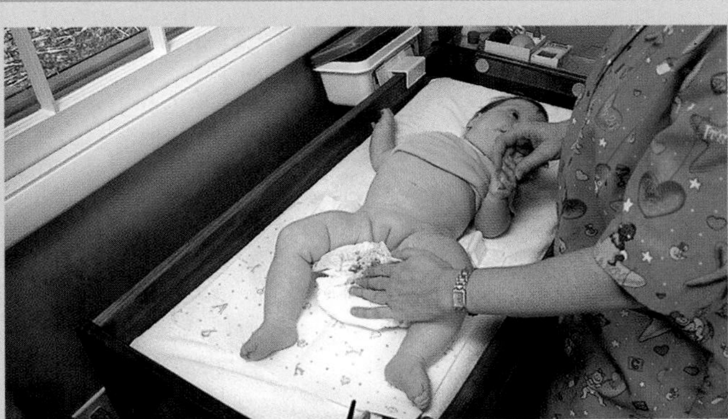

FIGURE 19–14 Clean the genital area with the front of the diaper.

Continued

Diapering the Baby—cont'd

6 Clean the genital area from the front to back using a wet washcloth, disposable or flushable wipes, or small facecloth.
Wiping with a wet cloth softens the stool on the skin and makes it easier to clean the skin.

7 Paying particular attention to the baby's skin folds, wash with mild soap and warm (not hot) water if there is a lot of stool or if the baby has a rash.
Traces of urine and stool can collect in the baby's skin folds, which can cause skin irritation and infections. Rinse thoroughly, and pat the area dry.

8 Give cord care (p. 339) and circumcision care (p. 340).

9 Apply cream or lotion to the genital area and buttocks if specified in the care plan. Do not use too much.
Caking can occur if too much cream or lotion is used. Caking is wasteful and actually decreases the effectiveness of the cream or lotion.

10 Raise the baby's legs. Slide a clean diaper under the buttocks.

11 For boys, fold a cloth diaper so that the extra thickness is in the front (**FIGURE 19–15, *A***).
The extra thickness allows better absorption over the baby's urethral area.
For girls, fold the diaper so that the extra thickness is in the back (**FIGURE 19–15, *B***).

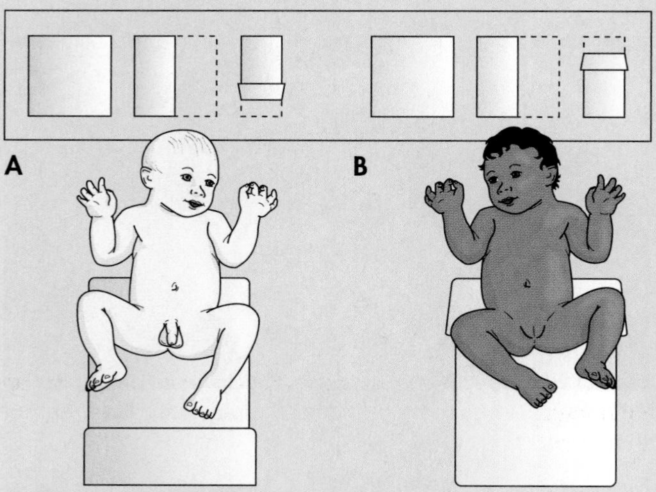

FIGURE 19–15 **A,** Fold a cloth diaper in the front for boys. **B,** Fold the diaper in the back for girls.

12 Bring the diaper between the baby's legs.

13 Make sure the diaper is snug around the hips and abdomen. It should be loose near the penis if the circumcision has not healed.
Applying the diaper snugly ensures that stool or urine will not leak out the sides of the diaper.
The diaper should be below the cord stump.
Keeping the top of the diaper below the cord stump helps prevent the diaper irritating it and prevents the cord stump from being contaminated by urine.

14 Secure the diaper in place.
  a Use the tabs on disposable diapers (**FIGURE 19–16, *A***), making sure the tabs stick in place.
  b Use diaper pins or Velcro strips for cloth diapers. Pins should point away from the abdomen (**FIGURE 19–16, *B***).
This helps ensure that the pin cannot stab the baby's abdomen accidentally.

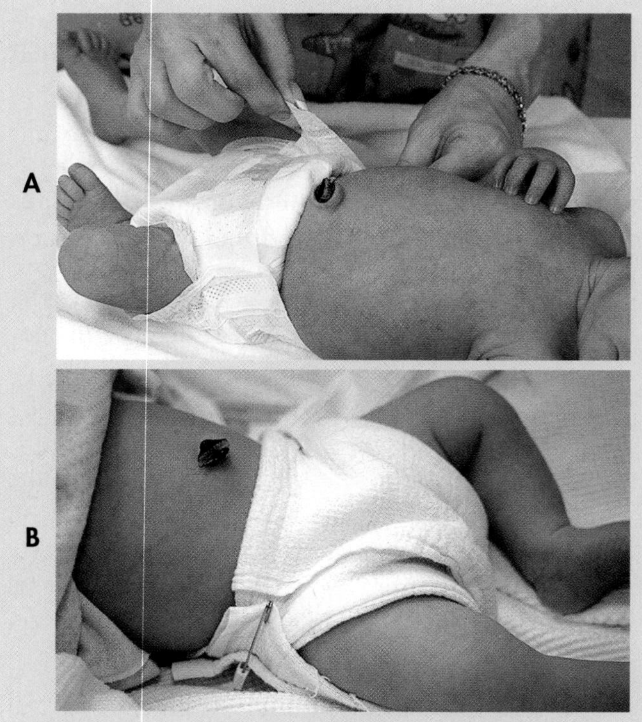

FIGURE 19–16 Securing a diaper. **A,** Secure the disposable diaper in place with tabs. **B,** Diaper pins are sometimes used to secure cloth diapers. Point pins away from the baby's abdomen.

Continued

Diapering the Baby—cont'd

15 Apply plastic pants if cloth diapers are used. Do not use plastic pants with disposable diapers.
Disposable diapers already have waterproof protection. Wearing plastic pants on top would make the baby very warm and uncomfortable.

16 Put the baby in the crib, infant seat, or other safe location.
This helps ensure the baby's safety.

POST-PROCEDURE

17 Rinse the stool from the cloth diaper in the toilet. Empty the stool from the disposable diaper into the toilet if possible.
Rinsing the stool in the toilet softens and disposes of the stool in the most appropriate manner.

18 Store used cloth diapers in a covered pail or plastic bag. Roll the disposable diaper into a ball, and secure it with its tabs. Put the disposable diaper in the garbage.
Rolling the soiled diaper in a ball keeps the spoiled contents and smell contained.

19 Clean the changing area.
Cleaning the area makes it ready to use the next time it is needed.

20 Practise proper hand hygiene.

Report and Record your actions and observations, according to employer policy.
This is for legal reasons and to keep the rest of the health care team informed.

Care of the Umbilical Cord[7]

The **umbilical cord** connects the mother and the fetus (unborn baby) and carries blood, oxygen, and nutrients from the mother to the fetus (**FIGURE 19–17**). The umbilical cord is not needed after birth, so shortly after delivery, the physician or midwife clamps and cuts the cord. The stump of cord that is left on the baby dries up and falls off in 7 to 14 days. Slight bleeding may occur when the cord comes off. Do not pull the cord off—even if it looks ready to fall off.

The cord stump provides an area for the growth of microbes, so you need to ensure that it is clean and dry at all times. Cord care is done with each sponge bath and is continued for 1 to 2 days after the cord comes off. The care plan and your supervisor will advise you on cord care, which usually consists of the following:

- Keep the cord dry.
- Wash your hands before and after contact with the umbilical area.
- Keep the cord clean using a mild soap and water. Gently wipe around the base of the cord with a clean, small facecloth or a gauze square moistened

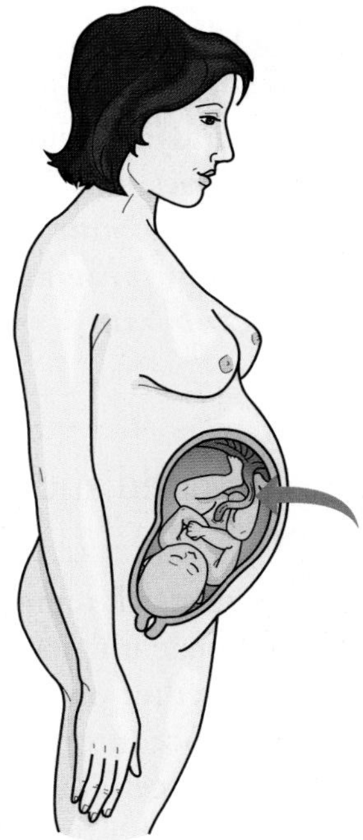

FIGURE 19–17 The umbilical cord connects the mother and the fetus.

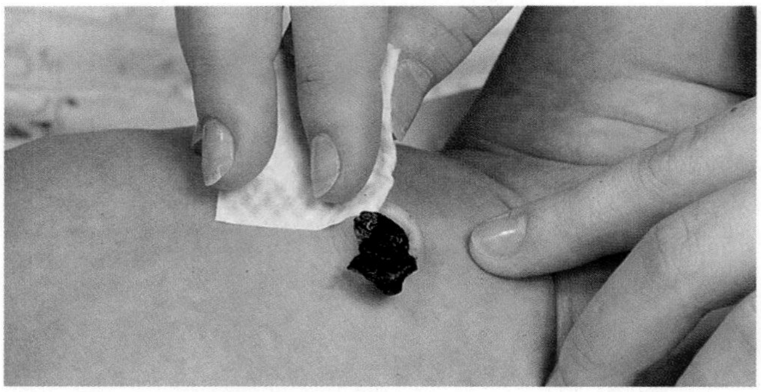

FIGURE 19–18 Wipe the cord stump at the base with a clean, small facecloth moistened with warm water.

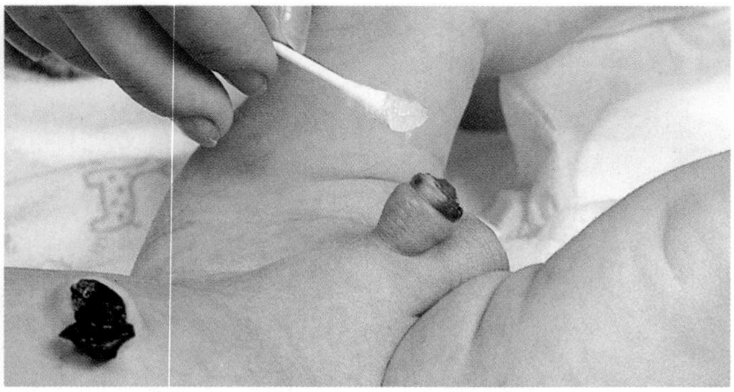

FIGURE 19–19 Use a cotton swab to carefully apply petroleum jelly to the circumcised penis.

with warm water (**FIGURE 19–18**). (Note: Alcohol swabs are not recommended.)

- Keep the top of the diaper below the cord to prevent the diaper from irritating the cord and to prevent the cord from being contaminated by urine.
- Repeat cord care daily and any time the cord gets wet or soiled.
- Report any signs of infection such as redness, odour, or drainage from the cord.
- Give sponge baths to the baby until the cord falls off, after which the baby can be given a tub bath. In some provinces, it is now acceptable practice to immerse newborns into a shallow tub of water, providing the cord does not get soaked. ***It is important to check with your supervisor what the practice is for your province and whether giving a newborn a tub bath is included in your scope of practice.***

Caring for Uncircumcised and Circumcised Babies[8]

Circumcision is the surgical removal of foreskin from the penis. Not all male infants are circumcised, as the parents decide whether or not they want the procedure done. The procedure promotes hygiene and is thought to prevent certain cancers. Circumcision is usually done in the hospital before the baby goes home. In the Jewish faith, the procedure is mandatory and is conducted as a religious ceremony by a *mohel* (one who performs circumcision on a Jewish male as a religious rite).

The uncircumcised penis can easily be kept clean by gently washing the genital area while bathing. Do not apply antiseptics of any kind. In uncircumcised baby boys, the foreskin ***usually does not retract for several years and should never be forced.*** Whether circumcised or not, the penis should be thoroughly cleaned at each diaper change, especially after the baby has a bowel movement. Use mild soap and water or commercial wipes.

After circumcision, a gauze square covered in petroleum jelly may be applied on the baby's penis. In some provinces, it is common practice to wait until this gauze falls off, whereas in other provinces, the gauze square is removed (it may need to be soaked off) and replaced at each diaper change. It is important to check with your supervisor or the baby's care plan as to what is appropriate for the baby. The penis will look red, swollen, and sore for the first couple of days after the surgery, but the circumcision does not interfere with urination. The area should be completely healed in 10 to 14 days. Report observations of bleeding, odour, or drainage.

If the baby has been circumcised, apply the diaper loosely to prevent the diaper from irritating the penis. Some physicians recommend carefully applying a teaspoonful of petroleum jelly to the penis to protect it from urine and stool. It also prevents the penis from sticking to the diaper. Use a cotton swab to carefully apply the petroleum jelly (**FIGURE 19–19**). Your supervisor will tell you if other measures are needed.

Bathing the Infant

Baths are very important not only to maintain cleanliness and hygiene but also to comfort and relax

Think About Safety

Bathing the Infant

The following safety measures are very important:

- Never leave the baby alone on a table or in the bathtub.
- Hold the baby securely throughout the bath. Babies are very slippery when they are wet. A wet, squirming baby can be hard to hold, so pay close attention to what you are doing.
- Room temperature for the bath should be 24°C to 27°C (75°F to 80°F). Turn up the thermostat, and close windows and doors for about 20 minutes before the bath, even if the room temperature is uncomfortably warm for you. You may need to remove your sweater or roll up your sleeves before starting the baby's bath.
- Pay special attention to water temperature. Babies have delicate skin that is easily burned. Bathwater temperature should be 37.8°C to 40.6°C (100°F to 105°F). Bathwater temperature is measured with a bath thermometer. If one is not available, test the water temperature with the inside of your wrist (**FIGURE 19–20**). The water should feel warm and comfortable on your wrist.
- Although the baby's bath should not be rushed, it is important that you are well prepared to bathe the baby to avoid wasting time since babies can get chilled very easily during bathing.

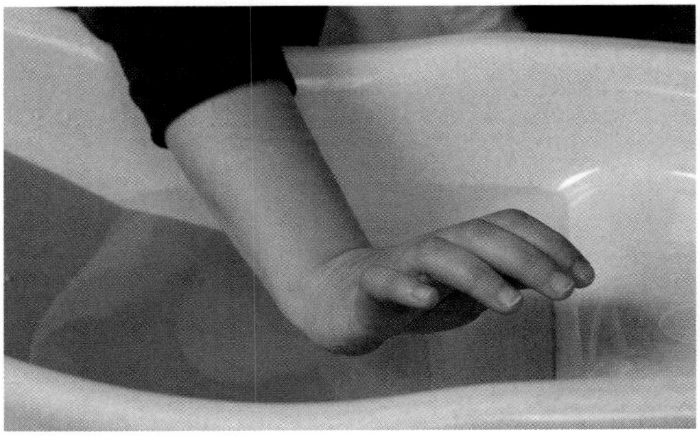

FIGURE 19–20 Use the inside of your wrist to test the temperature of the bathwater.

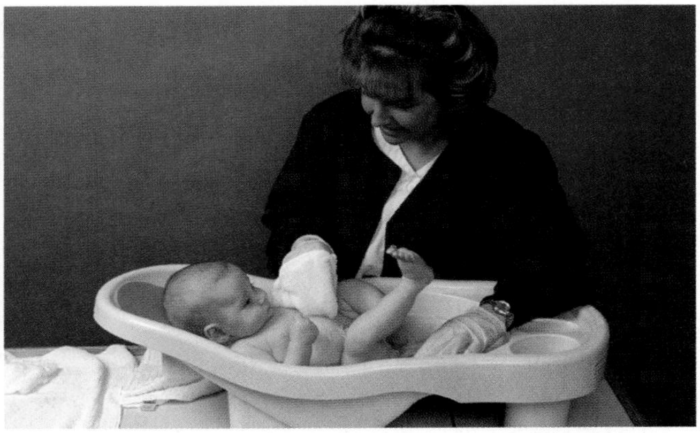

FIGURE 19–21 The baby is given a tub bath.

babies. Bath time provides a wonderful opportunity to hold, touch, and communicate with the baby. It should be part of the baby's daily routine. Some mothers like to bathe their babies in the morning, and some in the evening. Follow the family's routine.

Planning and preparation are an important part of the bath routine. You cannot leave the baby alone because you forgot something and have to go and get it. Gather all necessary equipment, supplies, and the baby's clothes *before* you start the bath, and place everything you need within your reach.

When bathing the baby, you should pay particular attention to the folds in the baby's skin, such as in the neck area and on the arms and legs. These folds can trap moisture, sweat, and lint from fabrics. The neck folds can also trap breast milk or formula. When skin is not cleaned thoroughly and dried, it can become excoriated (red and irritated).

In some provinces, two bath procedures are used for babies: (1) Sponge baths are given until the baby is about 2 weeks old or until the cord stump has fallen off and the cord site and circumcision have healed. (2) Tub baths (**FIGURE 19–21**) are given after the cord site and circumcision have healed. As mentioned, some provinces allow all babies to be bathed in a shallow tub of water, although usually only nurses are assigned to bathe a newborn. ***It is important to check what procedures are done in your province and if bathing the baby is within your scope of practice.***

Giving the Baby a Sponge Bath

123

Advocate on behalf of the client's quality of life by promoting:

Dignity • Independence • Preferences • Privacy • Safety

(see BOX 1-4, on p. 17)

PRE-PROCEDURE

1 Practise proper hand hygiene.
2 Collect the following supplies:
- ☐ **Bath basin**
- ☐ **Bath thermometer**
- ☐ **Bath towel**
- ☐ **Two hand towels**
- ☐ **Receiving blanket**
- ☐ **Washcloth**
- ☐ **Clean diaper**
- ☐ **Clean baby clothing**
- ☐ **Baby soap**
- ☐ **Baby shampoo**
- ☐ **Baby lotion**

It is important to plan thoroughly before starting any procedure. You should never leave the baby's side at any time while the baby is on a change table or in the bath.

3 Fill the bath basin with warm water. Water temperature should be 37.8°C to 40.6°C (100°F to 105°F). Check the water temperature with the bath thermometer, or use the inside of your wrist. The water should feel warm and comfortable on your wrist.
Babies' skin is delicate, and if the water is too hot, the baby can easily suffer from skin burns.

PROCEDURE

4 Undress the baby. Leave the baby's undershirt and diaper on.
Leaving the baby partially covered ensures warmth and privacy for the baby.

5 Wash the baby's eyelids (**FIGURE 19–22**):
- a Dip a clean, small facecloth into the water.
- b Squeeze out excess water.
- c Wash one eyelid from the inner part to the outer part.
- d Dry gently with a towel.
- e Repeat this step for the other eye with a fresh corner of the facecloth.

The eyes are regarded to be the cleanest area on the body, so this is the first step taken for bathing babies.

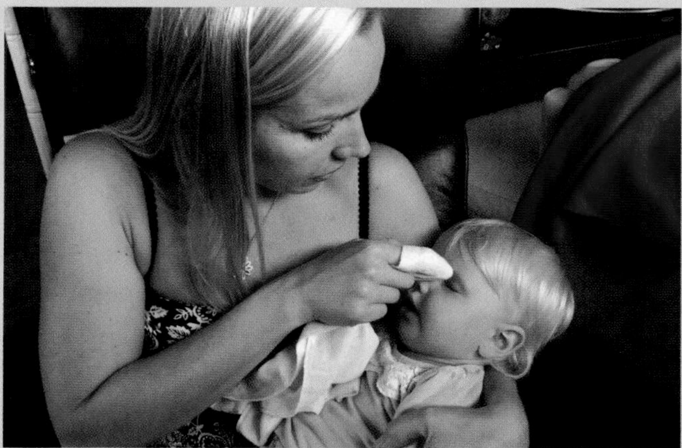

FIGURE 19–22 Wash the baby's eyelids. (Courtesy of the Kruusmann family, photo by Isabel Paul.)

6 Moisten the washcloth. Clean the outside of the ear and then behind the ear, paying attention to all skin folds. Dry with the towel. Repeat this step for the other ear. Be gentle.
The ear region can trap dried skin and soap, particularly behind the ears, leading to skin irritation.

7 Rinse and squeeze the washcloth. Make a mitt with the washcloth (**FIGURE 19–23**).
A mitt keeps bathwater contained and retains heat more than an open cloth can.

8 Wash the baby's face (see **FIGURE 19–23**). Wipe around the mouth and nose and then the cheeks and forehead. ***Do not use cotton swabs to clean inside the ears or nostrils.*** Pat the face dry.
Cotton swabs can damage or perforate the delicate mucous membranes of a baby.

Continued

Giving the Baby a Sponge Bath—cont'd

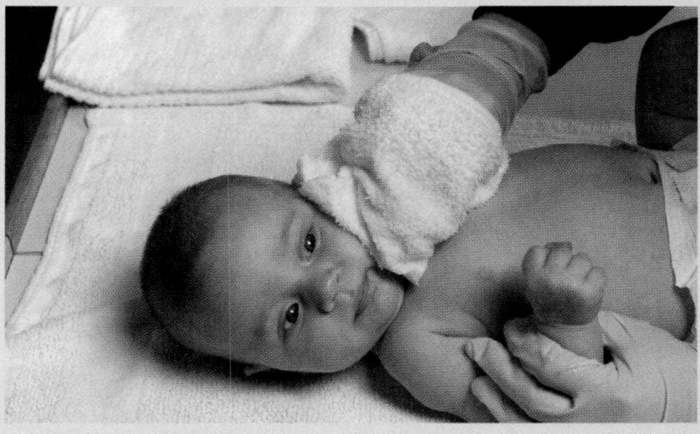

FIGURE 19–23 Wash the baby's face with a mitted washcloth.

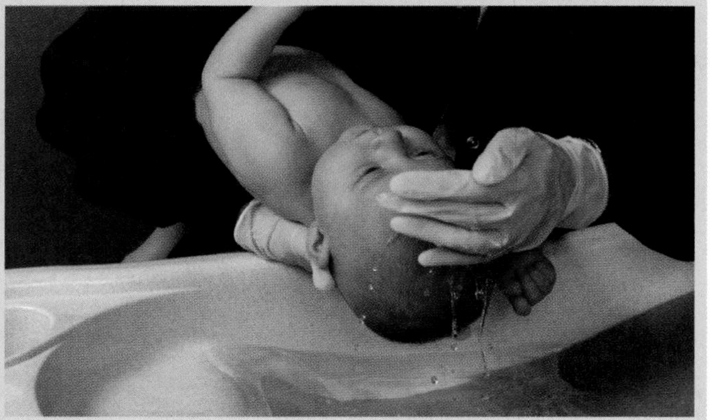

FIGURE 19–24 Wash the baby's head over the basin.

9 Wipe under the baby's chin and in the neck creases. Dry well.
The baby has a lot of creases in the neck area that can trap leaked food and become irritated. The skin in the creases can get even more irritated if wet.

10 Pick up the baby. Hold the baby over the bath basin using the football hold. Support the baby's head and neck with one wrist and hand, while using the washcloth in your opposite hand to wash the baby.
This positioning helps you hold the baby securely and avoid dropping the baby or causing head or neck injury to the baby.

11 Wash the baby's head (**FIGURE 19–24**):
- **a** Squeeze a small amount of water from the washcloth onto the baby's head.
- **b** Apply a small amount of baby shampoo to the head.
- **c** Wash the head using circular motions.
- **d** Rinse the head by squeezing water from a washcloth over the baby's head. Be sure to rinse thoroughly. Avoid getting soap in the baby's eyes.
- **e** Use a small hand towel to dry the head.

Washing the baby's head while the baby is still in the shirt and diaper and then drying the head carefully prevents the baby from getting chilled.

12 Lay the baby on the table.
Putting the baby down makes it easier to handle the baby safely.

13 Remove the undershirt and the diaper.

14 Wash the front of the body. Use a soapy washcloth. You may also apply soap to your hands and wash the baby with your hands. Do not get the cord wet, according to the care plan. Rinse thoroughly. Pat the skin dry, being sure to wash and dry all creases and skin folds.
Thorough rinsing is important since soap residue dries the baby's skin.

15 Wash and dry baby's hands, feet, and between the fingers and toes.
These areas collect lint and soap and need to be cleaned and dried carefully.

16 Place the baby in the prone position. Wash the back and buttocks using a soapy washcloth or your hands. Rinse thoroughly. Pat dry.

17 Give cord care (p. 339) and circumcision care (p. 340).

18 Apply baby lotion to the baby's body, as directed by the care plan.
Lotion keeps the skin moist and soft.

19 Put a clean diaper and clean clothes on the baby.

20 Wrap the baby in the receiving blanket. Put the baby in the crib or other safe location.
The blanket ensures warmth, and placing the baby in the crib ensures safety for the baby.

Continued

Giving the Baby a Sponge Bath—cont'd

POST-PROCEDURE

21 Clean and return equipment and supplies to their proper places. Do this step when the baby is settled.
Returning them makes them easier to find the next time they are needed.

22 Practise proper hand hygiene.

Report and Record your actions and observations, according to employer policy.
This is for legal reasons and to keep the rest of the health care team informed.

Giving the Baby a Tub Bath

123

Advocate on behalf of the client's quality of life by promoting:

Dignity • Independence • Preferences • Privacy • Safety *(see BOX 1-4, on p. 17)*

PROCEDURE

1 Follow steps 1 through 13 in the Procedure box *Giving the Baby a Sponge Bath* on page 342.

2 Hold the baby as in **FIGURE 19–25**:
   a Place your right hand* under the baby's shoulders. Your thumb should be over the baby's right shoulder. Your fingers should be under the right arm.
   b Use your left hand to support the baby's buttocks. Slide your left hand under the thighs. Hold the right thigh with your left hand.

It is important to have a good grasp on the baby, especially since the baby will be wet and slippery.

3 Lower the baby into the water, feet first.
Putting the baby in the water feet first is least traumatic.

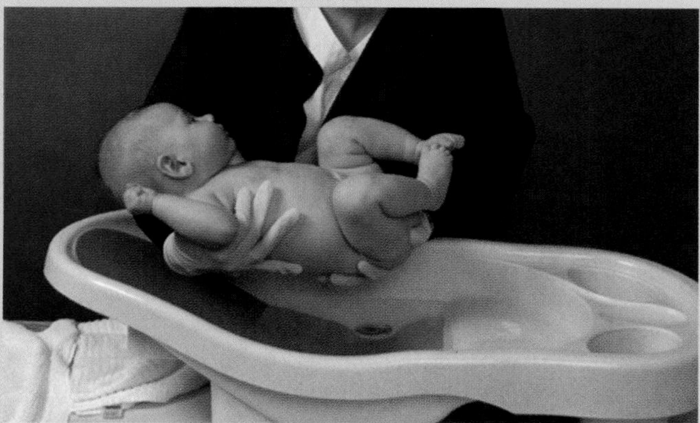

FIGURE 19–25 The baby is held for a tub bath.

4 Wash the front of the baby's body. Be sure to wash all skin folds and creases. Rinse thoroughly.
The baby has a lot of skin creases that can become soiled and irritated. The skin in the creases can get even more irritated if food traces or soap residue is left behind.

5 Reverse your hold. Use your left hand to hold the baby.

6 Wash the baby's back. Rinse thoroughly.
Thorough rinsing is important since soap residue dries the baby's skin.

7 Reverse your hold again. Use your right hand to hold the baby.

8 Wash the genital area.

9 Lift the baby out of the water and onto a towel.

10 Wrap the baby in the towel, taking care to cover the baby's head.
Wrapping the baby ensures warmth and comfort.

11 Pat the baby dry. Be sure to dry all skin folds and creases.
Patting the skin is less harsh than rubbing it.

12 Follow steps 18 to 22 in the Procedure box *Giving the Baby a Sponge Bath*.

Report and Record your actions and observations, according to employer policy.
This is for legal reasons and to keep the rest of the health care team informed.

*This procedure was written for right-handed people. Reverse the hand positions if you are left-handed.

Nail Care

The baby's fingernails and toenails should be kept short; otherwise, the baby could scratch himself and others. However, if the care plan or supervisor instructs you to cut the nails, extreme care should be taken not to cut them too short since the nail tips are highly vascular and could bleed a lot if accidentally cut. Some doctors suggest gently tearing or ripping the nails to keep them short. In some cultures, mothers are taught to bite off their baby's nails to shorten them. If you do choose to cut them, nails are best cut when the baby is sleeping so that the baby does not squirm or fuss during the procedure. Use nail clippers or file nails with an emery board. If using nail clippers, clip nails straight across as for an adult (see **FIGURE 31-9** on page 667).

Weighing Infants

Infants are weighed at birth since the birth weight is the baseline for measuring the infant's growth. Your supervisor will tell you when to weigh the baby. While you are weighing the baby, you must meet the baby's safety needs. Protect the baby from chills by keeping the room warm and free of drafts. Also, protect the baby from falling by always keeping a hand over the baby when measuring the weight, especially if you need to look away.

Weighing the Baby 123

Advocate on behalf of the client's quality of life by promoting:

Dignity • Independence • Preferences • Privacy • Safety *(see BOX 1-4, on p. 17)*

PRE-PROCEDURE

1 Practise proper hand hygiene.
2 Collect the following supplies:
- ☐ **Baby scale**
- ☐ **Paper for the scale**
- ☐ **Items for diaper changing** (see the Procedure box *Diapering the Baby* on p. 337)

It is important to plan thoroughly before starting any procedure. You should never leave a baby unattended while the baby is on a scale or on a surface where the baby can roll off.

PROCEDURE

3 Place the paper on the scale.
4 Adjust the scale to zero (0).
This ensures accuracy in measurement.
5 Undress the baby, and remove the diaper. Clean the genital area.
Urine or stool should never be left on a baby's delicate skin.
6 Lay the baby on the scale. Keep one hand over the baby without touching the baby.
A hand nearby helps prevent the baby from falling without adding to the baby's measured weight.
7 Read the digital display (**FIGURE 19–26**), or move the pointer until the scale is balanced.

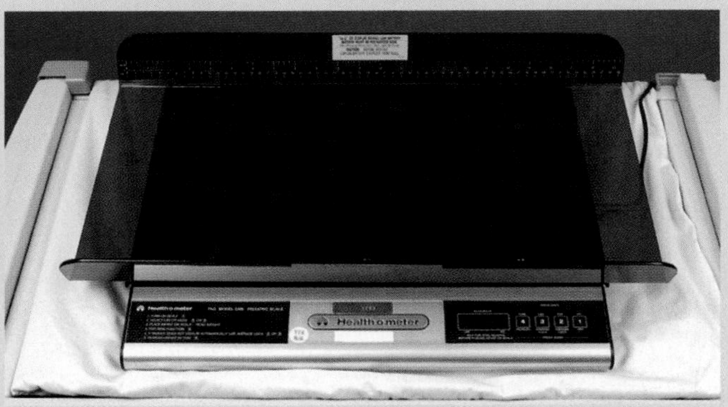

FIGURE 19–26 Digital infant scale.

8 Diaper and dress the baby. Lay the baby in the crib.
The baby should be kept warm and safe at all times.

Continued

Weighing the Baby—cont'd

POST-PROCEDURE

9 Return the scale to its proper place.
This makes it easier to find the next time it is needed.

10 Practise proper hand hygiene.

Report and Record the weight and your observations according to employer policy.
This is for legal reasons and to keep the rest of the health care team informed.

CHAPTER REVIEW

KEY POINTS

- Support workers sometimes give care to new mothers and infants, usually in a home care setting. Providing this service leaves the mother more time and energy for herself and her family.
- Respect the family's routines, schedules, and ways of doing things. As much as possible, follow the mother's standards and preferences. As with all of the duties that you perform, follow your clients' care plan and know the limits of your scope of practice.
- The postpartum period starts with the birth of the baby and ends 6 weeks later.
- As a support worker, you need to know how to care for a new mother and baby in the following areas: (1) lochia, (2) perineal care, (3) abdominal incision care, (4) breast care, (5) holding the infant, (6) comforting the infant, (7) assisting a new mother with breastfeeding, (8) preparing infant formula, (9) feeding the baby, (10) diapering the baby, (11) caring for the umbilical cord, (12) caring for a circumcised or uncircumcised baby's penis, (13) bathing the baby, and (14) weighing the baby.
- The support worker must be able to identify abnormal findings during the care of mothers and infants and should know who to report these findings to.

CRITICAL THINKING IN PRACTICE

You have been assigned to care for Sue Smith, a new mother who is trying to breastfeed her baby after a Caesarean section. You have never breastfed a baby, so you are uncertain about how to position the baby so she can breastfeed comfortably. You also cannot answer her questions about whether or not the baby is getting enough nourishment. What should you do? What resources can you check and recommend to Sue?

REVIEW QUESTIONS

Answers to these questions are at the bottom of page 348.

Circle the BEST answer.

1. A new mother has a red discharge evident on her pad the first few days after childbirth. This is:
   A. Lochia
   B. Menstrual flow
   C. Discharge from her rectum
   D. A very rare occurrence

2. A Caesarean delivery involves:
   A. A vaginal incision
   B. A perineal incision
   C. An abdominal incision
   D. A normal delivery through the vagina

3. A symptom of mastitis is:
   A. Engorgement
   B. Postpartum blues
   C. Thirst while breastfeeding
   D. Pain and redness in a breast

4. Zach is a newborn. Which of the following should be reported?
   A. Zach looks flushed and is perspiring.
   B. Zach has a soft spot on the top of his head.
   C. Zach spits up a small amount when burped.
   D. Zach has soft, unformed stools several times a day.

5. When holding Zach, you should:
   A. Support his head
   B. Tell him to stop crying
   C. Let his arms and legs dangle
   D. Bounce him up and down vigorously

6. When laying down Mehreen, who is an infant, for her sleep, you should:
   A. Place her on her back
   B. Place pillows under her head
   C. Place her on her stomach with her head turned to the side
   D. Place stuffed animals in her bed to give her something to look at

7. A breastfed baby is burped:
- A. Every 5 minutes
- B. After the feeding
- C. After the baby has been fed from both breasts
- D. After the baby has been fed from one breast and then again after having been fed from the other

8. You are required to warm a baby bottle. Which of the following is true?
- A. The formula should feel warm on your wrist.
- B. The bottle should be left out for the formula to get to room temperature.
- C. The bottle is warmed for 3 minutes in the microwave.
- D. The formula is warmed on the stovetop for 5 minutes.

9. When bottle-feeding, you should:
- A. Burp the baby every 5 minutes
- B. Save remaining formula for the next feeding
- C. Lay the baby down with the bottle propped on a pillow
- D. Tilt the bottle so that formula fills the neck of the bottle and the nipple

10. When the umbilical cord stump has not yet healed, the diaper should be:
- A. Disposable
- B. Below the stump
- C. Snug over the stump
- D. Loose over the stump

11. Cord and circumcision care are given:
- A. Once a day
- B. Three times a day
- C. At every diaper change
- D. Whenever the baby has had a bowel movement

12. When bathing babies, you should:
- A. Keep the room temperature slightly cool
- B. Gather supplies before beginning the bath
- C. Not use soap until the cord and circumcision have healed
- D. Have the water temperature between 38.9°C and 43.3°C (102°F to 110°F).

Answers: 1.A, 2.C, 3.D, 4.A, 5.A, 6.A, 7.D, 8.A, 9.D, 10.B, 11.C, 12.B

Chapter opener image: Tyler Olson/Shutterstock.com

CHAPTER 20

Caring for the Young

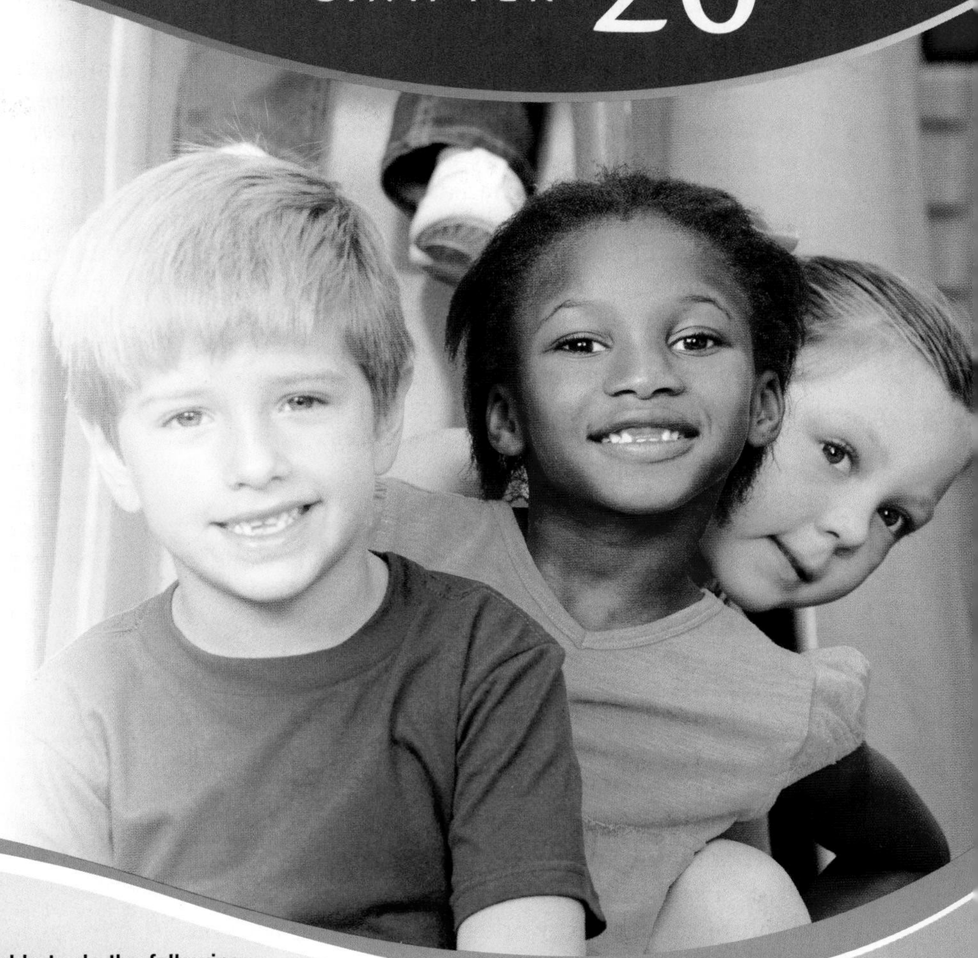

OBJECTIVES

After reading this chapter, the learner should be able to do the following:

- Identify the role of the support worker when caring for the young.
- List ways to assist an infant or child to meet nutritional needs.
- Identify the principles for dealing with a challenging child.
- Identify causes of early childhood deaths from injury.
- List ways to prevent falls in children.
- List ways to prevent choking in children.
- List ways to prevent burns in infants and children.
- List ways to prevent accidental poisoning in children.
- Explain how the developmental stage a child is in can influence the risk for injury.
- Describe ways to prevent or minimize childhood infections.
- List the most common reasons for children missing school.
- Apply the information in this chapter to clinical practice.

KEY TERMS

conjunctivitis An inflammation of the clear membrane that covers the white part of the eye and lines the inner surface of the eyelids. The nonmedical term is **pink eye**. *p. 362*
ear infection See **otitis media**. *p. 364*
eustachian tube The tiny drainage pipe in the middle ear. *p. 364*
gastroenteritis More commonly known as "stomach flu," this illness causes vomiting and diarrhea and can lead to dehydration, particularly in very young children and frail older adults. *p. 364*
negative reinforcement Encouraging a behaviour by penalizing the person when that behaviour is not demonstrated. *p. 363*
obesity Excess fat accumulation that puts a person's health at risk. *p. 352*
otitis media Infection (*itis*) of the middle (*media*) ear (*ot*), caused by either a virus or bacteria. Also known as **ear infection**. *p. 364*
pink eye See **conjunctivitis**. *p. 362*
positive reinforcement Encouraging a behaviour by rewarding the desired behaviour after it is demonstrated. *p. 363*
Reye's syndrome A rare but potentially fatal disease causing inflammation of the brain, which can occur during the recovery stage of flu or chicken pox. It has been seen in children who take Aspirin. *p. 358*
strep throat A throat that is infected with **streptococci**. *p. 362*
streptococci (singular, *streptococcus*) A type of bacteria that cause **strep throat** and other medical issues. *p. 364*
upper respiratory infections (URIs) The medical term for colds and other viral illnesses that affect the throat, nose, and sinuses. *p. 363*

This chapter presents a discussion of the need to provide a safe environment for the young, discusses the role of the support worker when dealing with the family, and explores some of the difficulties support workers may experience when working with children. It also offers a list of ways to deal with challenging children. In addition, this chapter includes the common causes for children missing school.

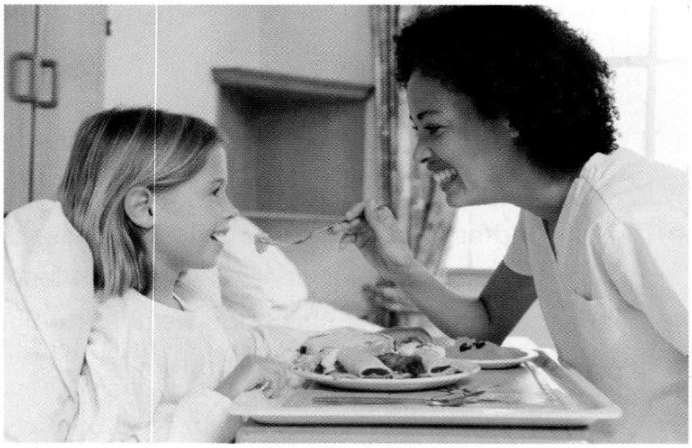

FIGURE 20–1 The support worker provides care to a sick child. (**Source:** © Monkey Business Images/Dreamstime.com.)

SUPPORTING THE INFANT, CHILD, OR TEEN

As a support worker, you will be expected to provide care and support to people of all ages, including the young. The young person that you are assigned to support may be a family member of your primary client (see the *Supporting Jane Smith: Families as Clients* box on p. 360) or may be your assigned client (see the *Supporting Jamie: Offering Respite to Family* box on p. 361). Always consult your supervisor if you have questions or concerns when working with children (**FIGURE 20–1**).

When providing support to the young, you must always remember that they have rights, too. Promote the priorities of support work when working with children. When dealing with both the young and their families, you must remember to follow the principles of DIPPS (dignity, independence, privacy, preferences, and safety) just as you would for any other client (see the *Providing Compassionate Care: Working With Children* box).

Your Role

As a support worker, your goal is to provide a stable, secure, and safe atmosphere for the family. Such an environment is very important for children who have illnesses and for those who are experiencing stress when a family member is ill.

Your responsibilities will vary in each family situation. However, the following are usually included:

- Developing positive relationships with all family members. A positive relationship is one that is friendly, respectful, and trusting.
- Maintaining the existing rules of behaviour.
- Maintaining daily routines, as much as possible.
- Being alert to situations that may create stress or cause harm to the family. Report these situations to your supervisor (see the *Think About Safety: Family Situations That Must Be Reported* box on page 361).

Follow the guidelines in **BOX 20–1** when interacting with children. Check with your supervisor and refer to the care plan for instructions for each child.

ASSISTING INFANTS AND CHILDREN TO MEET NUTRITIONAL NEEDS

Infants and children require proper, nutritional food to grow and develop each body system to its maximum potential. The nutritional requirements for children are discussed in Chapter 28. However, getting children to eat properly is often an ongoing challenge for parents and caregivers. As a support worker, you should be aware that a number of children in Canada face nutritional challenges.

Understanding the Challenges That Children and Families Face

Working with children and their families can be stressful for support workers. Some of the children that you care for may have physical or developmental challenges that you may be unfamiliar with, so it is very important that you understand your duties before you start working with children. In some cases, the child's family situation may create a stressful working environment for you.

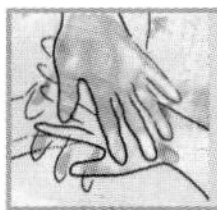

Providing Compassionate Care
Working With Children

- ***Dignity.*** Children have the right to be treated with respect and in a manner that promotes their dignity. Never tease or laugh at children, as their feelings are easily hurt. Remember to include children in conversations when appropriate. Do not talk about the child in front of him. Also, remember to say "please" and "thank you" to children. Treat each child as an individual of worth.
- ***Independence.*** Even very young children should be allowed and encouraged to do what they can for themselves.
- ***Preferences.*** It is usually not difficult to find out a child's preferences. However, often, the child cannot have what she wants, possibly because the child's wishes may be unsafe or unhealthy. Whenever possible, offer limited choices that are equally acceptable. For example, instead of saying, "What do you want for a snack?" say, "Would you like an apple or an orange for your snack?" This way, you are able to accept the child's preference.
- ***Privacy.*** Privacy is especially important to middle school–aged children and adolescents. Unless the care plan directs otherwise, let them have privacy when using the bathroom, bathing, and using the phone. Do not pry into their affairs, and respect their belongings.
- ***Safety.*** Ensuring the child's safety is essential. Children are at high risk for accidental injuries. Young children are curious about everything around them, and most are very active, but they do not usually understand danger. Provide constant supervision for babies, toddlers, and young children. When you are responsible for them, do not let them out of your sight. Review the safety measures in Chapter 22.

BOX 20–1 Guidelines for Caring for Children in the Home

Communication

- Use active listening skills. Maintain eye contact, and concentrate on what is being said.
- Watch for nonverbal communication cues from the child, such as frowning, lack of eye contact, and lack of smiling.
- Provide nonverbal communication by way of comforting the child with a touch on the shoulder or arm or a hug (according to acceptable custom and culture).
- Speak to children in a manner that is appropriate for their developmental level or age. If the child (or teen) has a developmental delay, speak using clear instructions, being careful about your body language and nonverbal cues. Ask the child's family for suggestions on how to best communicate with the child.
- Answer the child's questions simply, honestly, and clearly. Difficult questions about a family member's illness or death should be handled carefully. Ask your supervisor for guidance in advance.
- Offer praise for something well done.
- Give encouragement when the child attempts to improve behaviour, even when there is only slight progress.
- Use positive suggestions rather than negative words. Avoid using "Don't" and "No."

Rest, Sleep, Play, and Exercise

- Maintain the child's bedtime and naptime routines. Routines and rituals provide comfort and, therefore, are usually very important to children. Going to sleep at the right time is also very important for most children because they will become overtired, overactive, or cranky without enough sleep.
- Supervise playtime. Encourage active exercise, if allowed.
- Avoid taking sides when a disagreement occurs among children.
- Do not give extra attention to one child and ignore others.
- Ignore tattling if it is used to get attention.
- Distract the child if he begins to misbehave. If possible, play with the child or provide a different toy or activity.

Mealtime

- Prepare foods that the child will eat. Follow the care plan. Check whether the child has any food allergies or sensitivities (see Chapter 28).
- Do not force a child to eat. When the child feels full, the meal is over.
- Serve meals and snacks on time. Many children become cranky if they do not eat on time.

Here are a few of the many challenges that children and their families face and that a support worker may find stressful:

- More than 1.2 million Canadian children live in poverty, including one in five under the age of 7 years. Children from economically poor families are more likely to have chronic health problems and difficulties at school and are less likely to feel good about themselves.
- One fifth of school-aged children spend some time alone at home and tend to make decisions by themselves about what and when to eat. Almost 30% of these "latch-key" kids are between 6 and 9 years of age.
- Obesity appears to be increasingly prevalent among Canadian children, mainly because of their limited physical activity and high-calorie food choices. **Obesity** is excessive fat accumulation that puts a person's health at risk.
- Most young people, especially girls, are concerned about their appearance and weight and may feel a need to diet. Some have low self-esteem, which increases their risk for eating disorders. By Grade 9, only 26% of girls report having high self-esteem compared with 40% of boys.
- About 13% of Canadians speak a language other than English or French at home and come from different backgrounds; their cultural diversity is reflected in their eating patterns.

Helping a Child Eat Well

Setting the Stage for Pleasant Mealtimes

- The family should eat together as often as possible. A regular mealtime gives family members a chance to talk and relax together and helps them develop healthy attitudes about food.
- The meal table should be viewed as a positive, conflict-free zone. Problem solving and difficult discussions should be saved for a different time and place.
- Avoid distractions such as reading, playing with toys, watching television, or answering the phone. The family should relax, eat, and talk together instead.
- Adults must teach and model good table manners and respectful behaviour.

Avoiding Power Struggles and Learning to Trust the Child's Food Choices

- Most children self-correct their undereating, overeating, and weight issues when the power struggle is taken out of their mealtimes. Parents and caregivers should avoid using comments such as "Eat at least one bite of the vegetable," "That's a lot of bread you're eating," "Clean your plate," and "No seconds." Children have an internal hunger gauge that controls how much they eat. By overriding the child's signals, you will prevent the child from easily tuning in to that internal hunger gauge.
- If the child skips certain foods, eats lightly, or eats more than you would like him to, do the following:
  - As the support worker, check the family's diet, and ask: Are there any foods that the family eats that are not good for them? Is the child watching the behaviours of adults? If so, you can politely make suggestions to the family to improve the situation.
  - Let the child decide when she is full. You can remind her of the next scheduled meal or snack time: "Just make sure that you've eaten enough to hold you till snack time, which is after we get back from your swim class." This reminder can help the child make a wise decision about what and how much to eat now.
- Although it can be tempting to give in to the child's demands, if you give consistent messages to him about eating and mealtimes, the child will eventually become more comfortable with the division of responsibility.
- Gradually, the child's eating habits will balance out. You will notice that as long as you provide nutritious choices, the child will eat a healthy variety and amount of food each week. Try to relax through this change in roles, and you will see that the child relaxes, too.

Adjusting Your Approach According to the Child's Age

- ***Feeding an infant***. From birth, infants follow their internal hunger and fullness cues. They eat when they are hungry, and they stop eating when they are full. Experts recommend that newborns be fed on demand and not on a schedule.
- ***Feeding a child***. As you introduce new foods to a young child's diet, you are encouraging a love of variety, texture, and taste in foods. The more adventurous a child feels about foods, the more balanced and nutritious her weekly intake will be. Remember that it is normal to need to present a new or different food as many as 15 times or more before a child will be comfortable trying it. The key is to offer the new food in a relaxed manner without pressuring the child.

Getting Help for a Child's Eating Habits

As the support worker providing care to a child, if you are worried about the child's eating habits, you can call your supervisor, who may suggest that you ask the family doctor for help. Calling your supervisor is especially important if the child has a major change in appetite or weight—for example, eating too much or too little, or gaining or losing weight. Other concerns might include the following:[1]

- Eating issues have turned the family's mealtimes into a battleground.
- The child may have an eating disorder (see Chapter 35), such as anorexia nervosa (eating too little) or bulimia nervosa (eating too much and then vomiting the food and possibly abusing laxatives or enemas to reduce the likelihood of absorbing food to avoid weight gain).

Your supervisor (or the child's doctor) can advise you on the actions you can take or direct you to seek out assistance from someone with specific expertise, such as:

- ***Registered dietitians***, who teach people about nutrition, develop diets to promote health, and specialize in counselling to help treat food-related problems, including eating disorders
- ***Pediatricians***, who may have special training and experience in caring for children with eating issues
- ***Therapists or counsellors***, who can help the family cope with power struggles over eating
- ***Psychiatrists***, who can provide counselling and medication
- ***Pediatric gastroenterologists***, who can rule out or treat conditions of the digestive system that could be causing the eating disorder
- ***Pediatric endocrinologists***, who can rule out or treat hormone-related conditions that can lead to weight issues

PROTECTING CHILDREN FROM INJURY

As a support worker, it is your responsibility to ensure that children (regardless of age) are protected from harm. Injuries (from accidents, falls, choking, burns, abuse, poisonings, and other causes) are the leading cause of death in children over 1 year and are responsible for more deaths and disabilities in children than all causes of disease combined.[2] The developmental stage of the child (see Chapter 18) can help predict the injuries that a child may be prone to.

Despite various safety efforts, one of the leading causes of death among children over the age of 1 year in Canada is accidents, including motor vehicle collisions, falls, poisoning, drowning, suffocation, fire, and being struck with an object (such as a puck).[3] **BOX 20–2** gives an overview of consumer product–related injuries, and **BOX 20–3** lists risk factors for childhood injuries. You should also refer to Chapter 22 for further discussion of potential hazards in the home.

BOX 20–2 Consumer Product–Related Injuries

Canadian Hospitals Injury Reporting and Prevention Program (CHIRPP) data were analyzed to look at consumer product–related injuries in children and youth. Details on the circumstances surrounding injuries included the following:

Bunk Beds

- Bunk beds can result in injuries such as falls and strangulations.
- Between 1990 and 2007, there were 5 403 reported cases of injuries associated with bunk beds.
- People who sustained injuries involving a top bunk were almost twice as likely to be admitted to the hospital.

Magnets

- Magnet-related injuries have increased sharply in recent years.
- Between 1993 and 2007, there were 328 reported cases of children aged 13 years or younger who had injuries from magnets.
- Just over half of these incidents involved ingestion of a magnet.
- About 60% of the magnets were associated with a toy and about 25% involved jewellery.

Baby Walkers

- In April 2004, Health Canada acted to ban the sale, advertisement, and importation of baby walkers in Canada.
- Between 1990 and 2007 there were 2 192 reported injuries from baby walkers among children aged 5 months to 14 months.
- Of the children in baby walkers who fell down stairs or fell from a height, 88.8% sustained head injuries and 8.2% required admission to hospital.

Other Household Products

- Numerous products in and around the home present an injury risk to children and youth.
- Trampoline-related injuries have become increasingly common in recent years. Falls from the trampoline involving impact with the ground are the most severe, generating almost two-thirds of all fractures and one in five patients admitted to hospital.

Continued

BOX 20–2 Consumer Product–Related Injuries—cont'd

- Drownings and near-drownings can occur in association with bath seats, in particular when a child is left unattended.
- Children playing around dangling blind or curtain cords are exposed to a strangulation hazard.
- Furniture, televisions, and large appliances are frequently associated with injuries. Between 1990 and 2007, these items resulted in an average of about 9 000 injury cases per year, 71% of which involved children less than 5 years of age.

Source: *Child and Youth Injury in Review, 2009 Edition – Spotlight on consumer product safety*. Public Health Agency of Canada, 2012. Adapted and reproduced with permission from the Minister of Health, 2016.

BOX 20–3 Risk Factors for Childhood Injuries

- ***Gender:*** The majority of children injured are males mainly because of the prevalence of behavioural characteristics such as aggression.
- ***Temperament:*** Highly active children are at greater risk for injury.
- ***Stress:*** Stress predisposes the child to increased risk-taking and self-destructive behaviours, usually combined with a general lack of self-protection.
- ***Alcohol and drug use:*** This factor is associated with a higher incidence of motor vehicle injuries, drownings, homicides, and suicides.
- ***History of previous injury:*** A history of injury is associated with an increased likelihood of future injuries, especially if the initial injury required hospitalization.
- ***Developmental characteristics:***
  - Mismatch between the child's developmental level and skill required for the activity (such as driving all-terrain vehicles)
  - Natural curiosity to explore the environment
  - Desire to assert self and challenge rules
  - In the older child, desire for peer approval and peer acceptance
- ***Cognitive characteristics*** (age-specific):
  - ***Infant***—this age group explores the environment through taste and touch, which may lead to accidental poisonings or burns.
  - ***Young child***—this age group:
    - Tends to actively search for attractive objects
    - Is unaware of "cause and effect" (consequential) dangers
    - May fail to learn from experiences (e.g., falling from a step is not perceived as the same type of danger as climbing a tree)
    - Cannot comprehend dangers to themselves or others (e.g., children may accidentally poison themselves)
  - ***School-age child***—this age group is generally unable to fully comprehend "cause and effect," so they may attempt dangerous acts without thinking of the consequences (e.g., too few children wear safety helmets when riding bicycles).
  - ***Adolescent***—adolescents' preoccupation with abstract thinking may cause them to feel invulnerable (e.g., drowning, diving in shallow water).
- ***Anatomical characteristics*** (especially in young children):
  - ***Large head***—predisposes to cranial injury
  - ***Large spleen and liver***—predisposes to trauma in these areas
  - ***Small and light body***—may be thrown easily, especially out of a moving vehicle
  - ***Left-handedness***—environmental biases (things built for people who are right-handed) may predispose left-handed people to injury
- ***Other factors:***
  - Poverty (and living in substandard housing), family stress (such as maternal illness or recent environmental change), substandard (below-average) alternative child care, young maternal age, low maternal education, and multiple siblings may also increase a child's risk for injury.

Source: Hockenbury, M., Wilson, D., Winkelstein, M., et al. (2013). *Wong's nursing care of infants and children* (9th ed., p. 7). St. Louis, MO: Mosby.

Preventing Falls

Falls are the leading cause of injuries in children, and accidental injuries are the leading cause of death among Canadian children.[3] Infants can easily roll off a change table or bed. Falls out of highchairs and infant seats and falls down the stairs are also common accidents among babies and children. Older children often fall when running or playing. When children are tired, they may not pay close attention to the potential dangers around them and may also have a delay in reaction time, which contributes to risk for an injury.

Children are at an increased risk for being accidentally hurt during times of stress or changes in the family's routine, because the caregiver's attention is divided and supervision may not be as careful as usual. For example, when a family member is ill, the caregiver may be focused on the person with the illness rather than on the child. Support workers can provide care and support to clients and their families at such times of stress and at times of change.

As a support worker, when you are working with or around children, you must always be aware of possible dangers to them. It is your responsibility to always practise safety measures to prevent falls, burns,

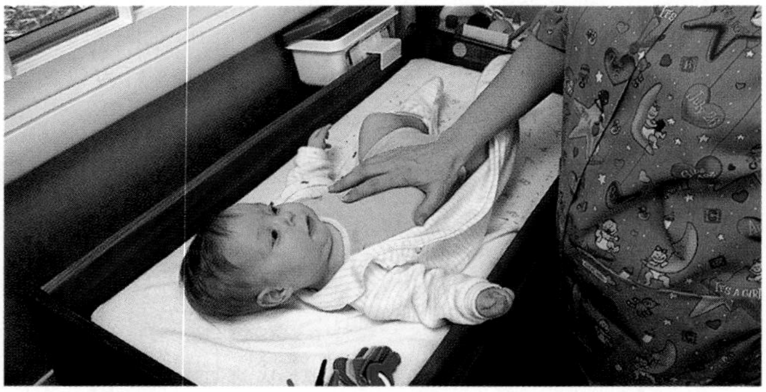

FIGURE 20–2 Keep one hand on a child on a change table.

Think About Safety

Safety Measures to Prevent Falls Among Infants and Children

- Do not leave infants and young children unsupervised. Never leave them unattended in highchairs or on a table, couch, bed, or other high surface.
- Secure the child in a highchair or infant seat. Use both the waist and crotch straps. Lock the highchair tray after securing the child in the chair. Keep highchairs away from stoves, tables, and counters. The child could push off against these and fall backwards.
- Do not use baby walkers; they have caused many serious falls and injuries.
- Use safety gates at the top and bottom of stairs. Make sure the child cannot get caught in the slats.
- Keep one hand on a child lying on a scale, bed, change table, or other furniture (FIGURE 20–2).
- Keep one hand on the baby when changing diapers. Gather supplies before changing diapers or bathing an infant. Place supplies within easy reach.
- Keep crib rails up and in the locked position. Frequently check children in cribs.
- Make sure there is nothing in the crib that the baby can stand on (like large stuffed toys or firm bumper pads). Standing on something in the crib could cause the baby to fall over the top of the railing.
- Do not let children under 6 years of age sleep or play on the top bed of a bunk bed.
- Keep children away from windows. Do not let them sit on windowsills or lean on windows. Window screens are not strong enough to prevent a child from falling out. Do not put furniture underneath or near windows. Children could climb on it to reach the window.
- Do not let children run with objects in their hands or mouths (like baby bottles, soothers, or sticks). The object could cause injury if the child falls.
- Take measures to prevent furniture such as TVs, bookcases, dressers, and tables from falling on children. Injuries and deaths can occur when children climb, pull on, sit on, lean on, or try to move furniture. Heavy furniture should be anchored to the wall.

Think About Safety

Ways to Prevent Choking in Children

- Always supervise children when they are eating. Grate, mash, blend, or chop food into very small pieces before giving it to a baby. Do not give infants and young children hot dogs, raw carrots, peanuts, popcorn, whole grapes, raisins, hard candy, or gum.
- Do not prop bottles on a rolled towel or blanket. Hold the baby and the bottle during feedings.
- Check for small objects such as coins, buttons, marbles, pins, and paper clips lying on the floor, and remove them. Children can choke on them.
- Do not allow children to blow balloons or put one in their mouths. Immediately dispose of any broken balloon pieces.
- Keep all plastic bags and wrappings away from children.
- Do not let children wear necklaces, strings, cords, or other items around their necks. These can become tightly twisted or get caught on furniture. Remove bibs before placing infants in cribs.
- Remove or tie up cords or drawstrings on all articles of children's clothing, including drawstrings in the hood, at the neckline, and at the waist.
- Keep cords for blinds, curtains, and drapes out of children's reach. Tie up cords, or use a cord shortener. Make sure cribs and playpens are placed far away from blinds, shades, or drapes. Items with strings, cords, or elastic should not be hung around cribs or playpens.
- Position infants on their backs for sleep.
- Make sure crib mattresses fit snugly and are very firm. The space between crib rail slats must be no more than 6.3 cm (2½ in.). Never let infants sleep on a waterbed. They should sleep only on firm, flat surfaces.
- Do not use pillows to position infants or prevent them from falling off beds or furniture.
- Remove pillows, comforters, quilts, sheepskin, stuffed toys, and other soft items from the crib when the baby is sleeping.
- Always supervise children who are in or near water, including tubs, toilets, sinks, buckets and containers, wading pools, and swimming pools.
- Keep bathroom doors closed to prevent children from entering the bathroom without supervision and drowning in toilets or bathtubs. Keep toilet seats down, and use toilet safety locks.
- Keep sinks, tubs, basins, and buckets empty when not in use.
- Keep diaper pails locked.
- Do not leave children unattended in a vehicle. They can suffocate very quickly in high temperatures in the summer or suffer from extreme cold temperatures in the winter inside the vehicle.

poisoning, and suffocation. Use common sense and follow the safety rules of your agency and the client's care plan at all times. Refer to the *Think About Safety: Safety Measures to Prevent Falls Among Infants and Children* box and the *Think About Safety: Ways to Prevent Choking in Children* box for ways to help ensure a child's safety.

Protecting Children From Burns

Burns are common in children and can cause significant morbidity (illness) and mortality (deaths). They constitute one of the leading causes of accidental death in children.[4] Degrees of burns are determined by the extent of tissue damage. Children and older adults are both at great risk for burns.

Hot liquids such as coffee or tap water are often responsible for childhood burns. For example, a child may get in the way when an adult is carrying a hot drink, and the adult may trip over the child and spill the hot liquid on the child (see the *Think About Safety: Protecting Children From Burns* box).

Preventing Accidental Poisoning

All children, especially when they are very young, put things in their mouths as part of learning and exploring their world. This natural instinct is one reason

Think About Safety

Protecting Children From Burns

- Do not drink or carry hot liquids near infants and children. Make sure children are not in your way when you are carrying anything hot, including drinks, clothes irons, or dishes from the oven.
- Do not heat a baby bottle or baby food in a microwave oven. Always shake the bottle or stir the food and test the temperature before giving it to the baby.
- Keep hot foods and liquids away from counter and table edges where children can reach them.
- Avoid using tablecloths or placemats that can be pulled down by a child.
- Always test the temperature of the bathwater before bathing a child. Position the child facing away from water faucets, and do not let children touch faucet handles.
- Never leave a "live" extension cord lying around (that is, one end is plugged in, and the other end is free). A child could pick it up and put it in the mouth, which would result in severe burns to the child's mouth.
- Put safety plugs in all unused electrical outlets (FIGURE 20–3).
- Keep pot handles pointed toward the back of the stove. Use the back burners on the stove rather than the front, whenever possible, when children are around. Turn off the stove and the burners when they are not in use.
- Do not let very young children help you cook on the stove.
- Do not let electrical cords from irons, coffee pots, toasters, and so on hang down where children could pull on them.
- Do not let children play near hot stoves, space heaters, fireplaces, and other heat sources.

hundreds of children every year are victims of accidental poisonings.[3] Parents, guardians, and caregivers can prevent many of these accidents by identifying and locking away toxic materials.

Accidental poisoning is most common in children between the ages of 1 and 4 years, when they are crawling or walking and exploring their environments. Eating substances such as Aspirin, cigarette butts, or vitamin pills is a common cause of childhood poisoning. Poisoning also occurs when certain poisonous substances—for example, oven cleaner or pesticide—spill on the skin and are absorbed into the body.[3] (See the *Think About Safety: Ways to Prevent Accidental Poisoning* box.)

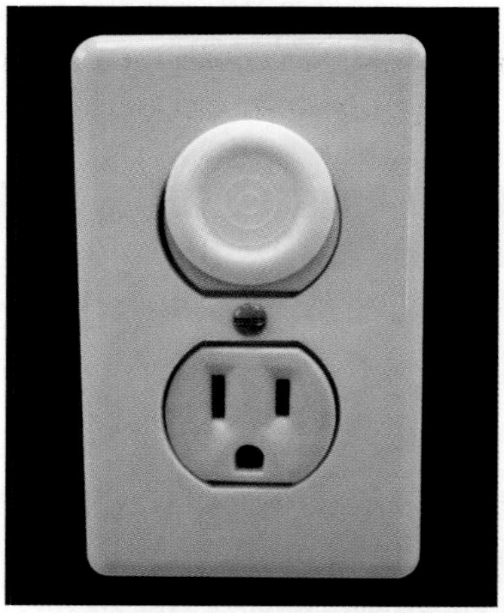

FIGURE 20–3 Safety plug in an outlet. (**Source:** © Can Stock Photo Inc./thesupe87.)

Reye's Syndrome

In cooperation with the Canadian Paediatric Society, Health Canada issued a warning about ASA (acetylsalicylic acid, commonly referred to as *Aspirin*) and products containing ASA, advising that it not be used for treating symptoms of the flu or chicken pox in those younger than 20 years of age.[5] In addition, manufacturers of products containing ASA are now putting warnings on their labels saying that a doctor should be consulted before giving ASA to children or teenagers who have the flu or chicken pox.

These warnings are based on research that has linked the use of ASA to treat the flu or chicken pox and the development of a condition called **Reye's syndrome**, which involves inflammation of the brain. Reye's syndrome is a rare but often fatal

Think About Safety

Ways to Prevent Accidental Poisoning

- ***Read the labels on all household products before buying them, and try to use the least toxic ones.*** Among the household products generally considered less hazardous are nonchlorine bleaches, vinegar, borax, beeswax, mineral oil, and compressed air drain openers (rather than corrosive liquids).
- ***Lock up all medicines and harmful substances.*** Secure all cupboards that contain poisonous substances, even those you might assume to be out of reach. Poison experts have come across numerous cases of toddlers dragging a chair over to a kitchen counter, climbing onto the counter or even the refrigerator, and opening a cupboard that is then at eye level.
- ***Do not rely on childproof container lids.*** These are not always childproof. No bottle top can be made so fail-safe that a child cannot find a way to get it off. It is not unusual for a 2-year-old, left alone for 30 minutes, to break into even the "safest" devices of a manufacturer.
- ***Keep medicines, pesticides, and even detergents in their original containers.*** Rewrite any labels that get smudged so that you know exactly what is in each bottle. Never put poisonous or toxic products in containers that were once used for food. Emergency medical staff have heard far too many horror stories of toxic liquid put into an unmarked container and having been mistaken for juice.
- ***Never refer to any kind of medicine as "sweets."*** Even if you are trying to get a reluctant toddler to take his cough syrup, do not present it as something good to eat. Children learn by imitation, so when you are taking your own medications, make sure that they are not watching.
- ***Never let children play with chipped or flaking paint.*** Old paint contains lead, which is a toxic substance known to cause neurological problems in children. Remove all chipped paint, and consult your local poison control centre or a reputable paint store for ways to remove the lead paint from your walls and woodwork.

Examples of Materials Found in the Home That Are Toxic to Children

- ***Household cleaning products.*** Assume that they are all dangerous. The safest thing to do is to keep them all out of the reach of children, including drain cleaner, oven cleaner, toilet cleaner, dishwasher detergent, and rust remover. Even if children do not ingest them, they may spray themselves with them, burning their eyes or skin.
- ***Pills and medicines.*** Always assume that any medicine your child takes, whether prescribed for you or for him, can be dangerous. Even vitamin supplements can be fatal in large doses, so keep them locked in a cupboard. Prescription drugs, especially antidepressants and time-release drugs, have a cumulative effect. Travel medicines, too, can be dangerous; keep them all inside a locked medicine cupboard.
- ***Cosmetics.*** Lock cosmetics in the medicine cabinet. Even an everyday product such as hair remover can be dangerous if swallowed.
- ***Household plants.*** Many garden plants are poisonous, especially philodendron, rue, privet, laurel berries, yew berries, and laburnum seeds. Make sure that you and all of the child's caregivers know the names of all the plants and trees inside and outside the home, just in case. It is a good idea for caregivers to leave the tags on all items that are brought home from a plant nursery. An expert from a plant nursery can help identify the plant and also provide tags to place near the plants.
- ***Paint thinner and paint remover, gasoline, paraffin, and metal polishes.*** Keep these items locked out of children's reach in the garage, and do not let children into the workshop unsupervised.
- ***Pesticides.*** Lock them away, even the "friendly" replacements for pesticides since they can also make pets and children ill.

condition that can occur during the recovery stage of the flu or chicken pox.[6] A health care professional will advise when it is appropriate to treat the child's fever and suggest ways to do so. The symptoms of Reye's syndrome are as follows:[6]

- A viral illness (such as the flu or chicken pox) that seems to last longer than in others who have the same illness
- Frequent or persistent nausea and vomiting
- A change in personality, confusion, agitation, or combativeness (being eager to fight)
- Coma
- Seizures

If these symptoms occur in a child or teenager who has been given ASA for the flu or chicken pox, you should seek medical attention immediately.

Discipline

When supervising or caring for children, you need to reinforce the rules of acceptable behaviour in the home. The system of rules that governs how we act is called *discipline*. Discipline is a *positive* way of teaching responsible behaviour. It sets limits and provides guidelines so that children can learn how to behave in an appropriate way. A support worker should never use physical force, such as spanking or pinching, at any time.

Discipline should be consistent. Each time a rule is broken, the consequence should be the same. For example, Noah (age 4 years) forgets to remove his boots and gets the floor dirty. He must get a cloth and help clean the floor, and he is not allowed to play until he does so. Noah knows the rules and what will happen if a rule is broken. The child feels secure when he or she knows the caregiver's expectations.

Recognize the child's efforts when he tries to follow the rules of the household. Praising these efforts encourages acceptable behaviour. Being positive with children is always more effective than being negative. For example, if Noah gets the floor dirty, it is better to say, "Let's clean up the mess" than "Shame on you for making that big mess." After he cleans up the mess, you could say, "Thank you for doing such a fine job." This show of appreciation would help to make Noah feel good about his accomplishment. Praise and acknowledgement also promote a child's dignity and show respect for the child.

Supporting Jane Smith: Families as Clients

Jane Smith is a 29-year-old woman who has terminal cancer. She is the mother of four young children, aged 6 months to 4 years. Her husband is a truck driver and is often away from home during the week but takes care of Jane and the children on weekends. During the week, Jane's mother (who is herself not in good health) takes the three older children to and from day care and assists with the family's shopping and laundry.

Jane was diagnosed with ovarian cancer during her pregnancy but waited until after her baby was born to start cancer treatments. Last month, Jane tripped over one of her children's toys, fell, and broke her ankle. While her ankle was being X-rayed, it was discovered that Jane's cancer had spread (metastasized) to her bones. Further tests revealed that it had also spread to her liver and brain. The doctors gave Jane only months to live.

Jane has a support worker in her home for 4 hours a day to assist with morning care for her and her baby. Jane's baby is a happy, active infant who is beginning to crawl. The support worker's responsibilities also include caring for the baby while Jane sleeps (she takes frequent naps throughout the day), light housekeeping (which includes ensuring that toys are not left on the floor), and preparing the family's dinner. Because Jane's husband's insurance covers the cost of a support worker for only up to 20 hours per week, Jane is worried about what will happen to her family when her condition declines further. Jane has often told the support worker just how grateful she is to have this assistance.

Supporting Jamie: Offering Respite to Family

Jamie is a happy, fun-loving boy who has just celebrated his twelfth birthday. Like many preteens his age, he likes to watch television and listen to music. Jamie is in Grade 8 and is looking forward to attending high school next year. He does well in school, but he is not sure yet about the career he wants to pursue. Jamie is just beginning his growth spurt. His family has noticed that he has grown taller and his voice is getting deeper. He has three younger brothers, and his mother and stepfather care for Jamie when he is home from school.

Jamie has cerebral palsy and is wheelchair dependent. He is often incontinent of urine, so he must wear incontinence products. Because of his ever-increasing size, his mother (who has always been his primary caregiver) has rented a mechanical lift and is able to use it to toilet, bathe, and move Jamie from the bed to his chair. Jamie also requires assistance with eating. He communicates by way of a computer, which sounds out the words that he types using the keyboard.

After putting off surgery on her knee for several years, Jamie's mother is now going to have a total knee replacement and will therefore not be able to care for Jamie for several weeks. You are one of the support workers who will be caring for Jamie in his home during this time. Your duties are to assist with his activities of daily living (ADLs) and occasionally arrange for his wheelchair taxi to drive him to school. You will get to know all of Jamie's family, as they will be home during the afternoon and evening hours when you are there.

Think About Safety

Family Situations That Must Be Reported

- Violent behaviour of a family member (see Chapter 16)
- Frequent visits by "strangers," who seem to make the members of the household fearful or uneasy
- Suspected drug abuse—for example, the presence of instruments or equipment for drug use
- Excessive drinking, as evidenced by the presence of liquor bottles hidden throughout the house or the child's parent or caregiver being inebriated
- Electricity, heat, or water turned off
- Severe shortage of food or clothing—for example, no food in the cupboards or refrigerator, or the child being dressed inappropriately for the weather (such as no coat in winter)
- Illness of a child that has been unreported to you
- Sudden departure of caregiver
- Unexpected return of a family member

Your role in disciplining the child is to:

- Know the rules of acceptable behaviour in each family situation
- Ask an appropriate family member to clarify the rules if you are unsure
- Reinforce existing rules
- Be consistent when using discipline
- Praise the child's efforts at following the rules

Some parents may have very few rules of discipline, or the existing rules may seem too harsh or too loose. In such a case, you should contact your supervisor. New rules may need to be set, but you should not set discipline rules without the guidance of your supervisor.

Punishment

Punishment is a harsh response that occurs when a discipline rule is broken. ***Punishing a child for failing to follow the rules of the household is not your responsibility.*** If a family member asks you to do so, explain that it is against your agency's policy to carry out punishment. Ask the family member to contact your supervisor if she has further questions. Record this information, and tell your supervisor about the situation.

SUPPORTING THE CHALLENGING CHILD

Children raised in troubled environments may become troubled themselves. These challenging children may be verbally aggressive, resistant to rules and regulations, or have difficulty forming bonds with others.

Why Do Some Children "Act Out"?

Children of all ages sometimes express their feelings of anger, frustration, fear, guilt, or shame through their behaviour because it is the only way they know how to convey what they feel. Some children display emotional or behavioural outbursts, whereas others will demonstrate that they feel overwhelmed, tired, or physically unwell. Children may behave this way if there are too many changes in their lives; if they have recently experienced painful losses; or if they have problems at school, such as difficulty learning, too much peer pressure, or bullying.

Some children may have suffered or witnessed physical abuse, emotional abuse, or sexual abuse, or they may be using drugs or alcohol. In cases in which children have been hospitalized for much of their lives, they may have difficulty accepting limits, especially if their parents tend to overindulge them, as parents are tempted to do if they think the child may die or if they feel a need to reduce their own feelings of guilt regarding the child's illness.

It is the support worker's responsibility to provide care in a nonjudgemental and supportive manner no matter the reason a child is "acting out." Some ways to successfully manage a challenging child are discussed in **BOX 20–4**.

PREVENTING INFECTIONS

When children start child care or school, it may seem as if they get sick all the time. This pattern is normal, as all children's immune systems are developing, and their resistance to infection develops only after exposure to a multitude of germs. Young children in large groups are breeding grounds for organisms that cause illnesses. Little hands rub drippy noses and then transfer infectious agents to other children or to shared toys.

Children who have physical or developmental delays may be even more prone to infectious illnesses, as they may have a fragile immune system. As a support worker, you have a responsibility to ensure that you always practise hand hygiene (see Chapter 23) to prevent spreading infections from yourself to these children. By simply following proper hygiene practices, you may reduce the likelihood that a contagious infection will keep the child home from school or child care. The guidelines for hand hygiene should also be followed in your own household to reduce transmission of germs and infectious illnesses from your client's home to you or your own family.

Prevention of Childhood Infections

When a child sneezes or coughs, he sprays germs into the air, which land on other children, who are then infected. A child's hands can become vehicles for carrying viruses and bacteria from toys and other frequently handled objects to other children's eyes, noses, or mouths, which are the usual points of entry for germs that cause illness.

The single most important thing anyone can do to prevent illness is to wash his hands thoroughly and frequently. The Centers for Disease Control and Prevention recommend that people wash their hands with soap and warm water for 15 seconds—about as long as it takes to sing the "Happy Birthday" song twice. Alcohol-based hand sanitizers come in disposable wipes or in gel form, require no water, and help keep hands clean (see Chapter 23).

How Long Should Sick Children Stay Home?

Each facility generally has its own rules, but most will not let children attend school or child care if they have a fever of more than 38°C (100.4°F), are vomiting, or have diarrhea. In addition, some facilities require that children with **strep throat** or bacterial **conjunctivitis** (**pink eye**) be on antibiotic therapy for 24 hours before returning.

BOX 20–4 Twelve Principles for Supporting a Challenging Child

1. Be specific about your expectations, and stick to them!
2. Put first things first. Keep your focus on important issues, and choose your battles wisely. This reaction will teach the child to make *good decisions*, not to win power struggles.
3. Praise, praise, and praise some more! **Positive reinforcement** (encouraging a behaviour by rewarding the desired behaviour after it is demonstrated) is much more effective than **negative reinforcement.**
4. Be knowledgeable about the child's specific problem(s) and difficulties. The child's parents, siblings, or caregivers may be able to assist you with finding solutions.
5. Follow the client's care plan for the amount of time and activity you should provide for the child. If you can, spend some one-on-one time focusing only on positives.
6. Be specific about positive and negative consequences ("rewards and punishments"), and follow through with them *consistently*. You should also consistently ensure your words and actions are straightforward and clear so that the child cannot misinterpret you.
7. Act quickly, and speak calmly. Never yell, scream, or swear, as these behaviours will only aggravate the situation.
8. Give bonuses, and focus on the positive. For example, if a child puts his clothes away, reward him by placing a gold star on his "Activities" sheet. Display the sheet where others can see it.
9. Seek out the middle ground. Know when to negotiate and when to stand firm. For example, if a child wants to watch television for more time than usual and her request is reasonable, and if the parent permits it, negotiate with her the length of time she can have.
10. Practise forgiveness and patience. Children need to know that they are still valued and cared for in spite of their naughty behaviour.
11. Use others for support, and seek assistance when appropriate. Consult your supervisor if the child's behaviour worsens or if you are unsure about what you should do.
12. Remember to take care of yourself. You have needs, too! Pay attention to your own cues that you may be losing patience. It is better to silently count to ten than to lose your cool!

Adapted from David P. Fago, Ph.D., The Maryland Institute, Twelve Principles for Dealing with a Difficult Child. Retrieved from http://dpfago.wix.com/david-fago#!difficult-children. Reprinted with permission.

Generally, however, children can return to school when the following are true:

- They have no fever.
- They can eat and drink normally.
- They are rested and alert enough to pay attention in class.
- They have completed any period of medically recommended isolation.

Resistance Comes With Time

Despite the best efforts, most children will get sick, especially during the first few years of contact with larger groups of children. Most children's immunity does improve with time, with school-age children gradually becoming less prone to common illnesses and recovering more quickly from the illnesses they do catch. If you have any questions about the child that you are supporting and his immunity, you should ask your supervisor.

The Top Five Reasons Children Miss School or Child Care

1. ***Colds.*** The most common childhood illnesses are **upper respiratory infections (URIs),** the medical term for colds and other viral ailments that affect the throat, nose, and sinuses. Whereas adults, on average, experience 2 to 4 colds a year, children typically experience 6 to 10. Children also tend

to have more severe and longer-lasting symptoms than adults do.

Studies have shown that there is no benefit in treating children's colds with antihistamines, decongestants, or cough suppressants. If a child you are looking after is ill, you should discuss the appropriate medication to reduce fever. Children should never be given Aspirin because it may trigger Reye's syndrome, a rare but potentially fatal disease (see p. 358).

2. ***The stomach flu (gastroenteritis).*** The second most common childhood illness is **gastroenteritis**, more commonly known as the "stomach flu." This childhood illness causes vomiting and diarrhea and can lead to dehydration, particularly in very young children. Signs and symptoms of dehydration include the following:
   - Excessive thirst
   - Dry mouth
   - Little or no urine, or dark yellow urine
   - Decreased tears
   - Severe weakness or lethargy

   Your client may be required to drink an oral rehydration solution (e.g., special frozen treats or Pedialyte), which can help replace lost fluids, minerals, and salts. ***(These items would be on the client's care plan and should not be given unless specified there.)*** When food is re-introduced, easy-to-digest items such as broth, toast, bananas, and rice should be given first. Avoid dairy products, which can be hard to digest.

   Often, parents assume that any kind of stomach upset in a child is the result of an infection, when the real culprit could be simple indigestion or constipation. Some children get stomach aches when they are worried about things either at home or at school. The dread of facing a bully or taking a test, for example, can make a child's stomach hurt. It is important for a doctor to determine the cause of a child's symptoms before prescribing treatment.
3. **Ear infection (otitis media).** Ear infections most often occur in children under the age of 2 years, but they can also be common between the ages of 5 and 6 years, triggered by the respiratory illnesses picked up in kindergarten or Grade 1. Colds or allergies cause congestion, which may squeeze shut the child's **eustachian tube**, the tiny drainage pipe for the middle ear. Fluid trapped in the middle ear can become a breeding ground for viruses or bacteria.

   It can be difficult to distinguish between ear infections caused by bacteria and those caused by viruses. The distinction is important, however, because antibiotics will cure bacterial—but not viral—infections. And using antibiotics when they are not necessary has serious consequences, most notably the emergence of bacterial strains with built-in resistance to drugs that fight infection. For that reason, doctors today often wait to see if an ear infection will clear up on its own before prescribing antibiotics.
4. ***Pink eye (conjunctivitis).*** Pink eye (conjunctivitis) is an inflammation of the clear membrane that covers the white part of the eye and lines the inner surface of eyelids. When caused by viruses or bacteria, conjunctivitis is highly contagious. It is typically treated with antibiotic eye drops or ointment. Warm or cool compresses may ease the child's discomfort.
5. ***Sore throat.*** Most sore throats are caused by viruses and are usually associated with other respiratory signs and symptoms such as a runny nose and cough. But about 15% of children's sore throats are caused by **streptococci**, bacteria that cause strep throat.

   Fevers above 38°C (100.4°F) are common with strep throat, and swallowing can be so painful that the child may have difficulty eating. Antibiotics are required to combat strep throat. Left untreated, the bacteria can eventually trigger an abnormal immune response, which can lead to rheumatic fever. Complications of rheumatic fever include damaged heart valves and stiff, swollen joints.[7]

Vaccinations to Prevent Serious Infectious Illnesses

Canadian babies and children require routine administration of vaccinations to be able to fend off contagious infections and illnesses such as measles, mumps, pertussis (whooping cough), diphtheria, tetanus, certain types of meningitis, and polio.[5] Vaccines are so effective that most of the diseases that they help prevent have now become rare in Canada.

Updated immunization schedules are available from family doctors, local health units, or the Public Health Agency of Canada website at http://www.phac-aspc.gc.ca/publicat/cig-gci/p01-12-eng.php#tab1. This website will ask for your province or territory and the child's date of birth.

What Would Happen if We Stopped Vaccinating?

In the past several years, vaccination has become a subject of controversy. However, in countries where fewer people were immunized, the diseases quickly returned. For example:

- In 2000, the number of measles cases in Ireland increased from 148 to more than 1 200 in just 1 year because vaccination had been reduced to 76%, and several children died as a result.
- In 1999, there was a large outbreak of rubella (German measles) in Nebraska. All 83 adults who were affected had not been vaccinated; most of them came from countries where rubella vaccine is not routinely administered. Rubella is extremely dangerous in pregnant women, and can cause the unborn infant either to die or to become severely handicapped.[8]
- In 2014, there were confirmed outbreaks of measles in British Columbia, Alberta, Saskatchewan, and Ontario.[9] Measles is highly contagious and can lead to serious complications or death for children under the age of five.

Why Do People Choose Not to Immunize Their Children?

There are parents who do not immunize their children due to medical, religious, or ideological reasons. In 1998, *The Lancet* (a medical journal that is highly regarded throughout the world) published a study based on fraudulent (falsified) data linking the measles, mumps, and rubella (MMR) vaccine to autism. Although this finding has been disproven, many people have lost confidence in the MMR vaccine as a result of this article.

In Canada, only Ontario, Manitoba, and New Brunswick have legislation that mandates children be vaccinated in order to attend school.[9] For a child to attend school without immunizations in those provinces, a notarized statement of the reasons for opting out of vaccinations must be provided to the school by the child's physician or nurse practitioner. In the case of an outbreak, children who are not vaccinated may be excluded from child care facilities or schools at the discretion of the Medical Office of Health.

Do the Benefits of Vaccination Outweigh the Possible Adverse Effects?

The short answer is yes. If there were no vaccines, there would be more cases of disease, more serious adverse (harmful) effects from disease, and more deaths. ***The diseases that vaccines help prevent lead to pneumonia, deafness, brain damage, heart problems, blindness, and paralysis in children who are not vaccinated.*** Canadian children are very fortunate to have vaccines that prevent diseases that still kill and disable children in some other parts of the world every day. The risks of not being vaccinated are much greater than any risk from vaccination itself.

CHAPTER REVIEW

KEY POINTS

- Support workers provide care and support to people of all ages, including the young. A young person that you are assigned to support may be your assigned client and have physical or developmental challenges or he or she may be a family member of your primary client.
- As a support worker, you need to adjust your approach according to the child's age.
- Your responsibilities will vary in each family situation but usually will include (1) developing positive relationships with all family members, (2) maintaining the existing rules of behaviour, (3) maintaining daily routines as much as possible, (4) being alert to situations that may create stress or cause harm to the family, and (5) reporting any issues to your supervisor.
- In regard to children, support workers are responsible for helping the child to (1) eat well, (2) prevent injuries, (3) prevent falls, (4) prevent burns, (5) prevent accidental poisoning, and (6) prevent infections.
- As a support worker, you should be aware of the general guidelines for caring for children in the home regarding (1) communication; (2) rest, sleep, play, and exercise; (3) mealtime; and (4) discipline.
- Your role, as a support worker, in disciplining the child is to (1) know the rules of acceptable behaviour in each family situation, (2) ask an appropriate family member to clarify the rules if you are unsure, (3) reinforce existing rules, (4) be consistent when using discipline, and (5) praise the child's efforts at following the rules.
- Generally, children with signs or symptoms of illness can return to school when they (1) have no fever, (2) can eat and drink normally, (3) are rested and alert enough to pay attention in class, and (4) have completed any period of medically recommended isolation.
- The top five reasons children miss school or child care are (1) colds, (2) stomach flu (gastroenteritis), (3) ear infection (otitis media), (4) pink eye (conjunctivitis), and (5) sore throats.
- Support workers should be aware of the reasons some children "act out."

CRITICAL THINKING IN PRACTICE

While his mother is in the hospital recuperating from abdominal surgery, you are caring for a 5-year-old boy who is usually home-schooled. At lunchtime, you warm up his meal, place it on the table and ask him to wash his hands. The boy refuses to do so and then begins throwing his toy building blocks at you, runs into his room, and hides. You do not know what to do and debate whether or not you should go after him in his room. You also do not know how much firmness to use when insisting that he eat. How much discipline should you use? Does this incident warrant a call to your supervisor? What can you do in this instance? Can you identify reasons for this child's behaviour?

REVIEW QUESTIONS

Answers to these questions are at the bottom of page 367.

Circle the BEST answer.

1. Your role when providing child care includes:
   A. Maintaining your rules of behaviour
   B. Providing punishment, when necessary
   C. Maintaining the family's daily routines
   D. Ignoring situations that may add stress or cause harm to the family
2. The leading cause of death in children over the age of 1 year is:
   A. Cancer
   B. Starvation
   C. Injuries
   D. Pneumonia

3. Why is it important to understand the relationship between a child's developmental level and his risk factors for injuries?
- A. You can more easily anticipate which injuries the child may get.
- B. The older the child, the less likely it is that he will get injured.
- C. Older children are more likely to get injured than toddlers are.
- D. There is no relationship between a child's developmental level and the risk for injuries.

4. Why are boys more likely to become injured than girls are?
- A. Girls have smaller heads.
- B. Girls play more computer games.
- C. Boys are usually more physically aggressive.
- D. Boys are usually poorer eaters than girls and are, therefore, more likely to get injured.

5. A teen who is under stress is more at risk for injury because she:
- A. Is less active
- B. Engages in riskier behaviours
- C. Eats more fast food
- D. Has more friends than happy teens do

6. How can an infant most likely be injured in his own crib or playpen?
- A. He can burn himself on a nearby space heater.
- B. He can get head and neck injuries by crawling around.
- C. He can get injured trying to climb out of his crib.
- D. He might choke on his toys.

7. Young children are at risk for injuries because they:
- A. Do not know that some things may be poisonous
- B. Usually engage in risk-taking behaviours
- C. Are prone to depression and suicidal behaviours
- D. Want peer acceptance and approval

8. You are caring for an infant and some young children. Which of the following measures is safe?
- A. Using a safety strap when putting a child in a highchair
- B. Ironing the clothes while the children play near your feet
- C. Placing stuffed animals and toys in the crib at naptime
- D. Allowing a child to play with empty pill bottles

9. One of the main illnesses that cause children to miss school or child care is:
- A. Stomach flu
- B. Headaches
- C. Chicken pox
- D. Head lice

10. Children can usually return to school after a contagious illness when:
- A. They have a fever of just below 38°C
- B. Their parents must go to work
- C. They can eat and drink normally
- D. They miss a day of school

11. In time, most school-age children become less prone to common infectious diseases because:
- A. Older children eat more vegetables
- B. They eventually learn how to avoid getting sick
- C. Their immune system matures, making them more resistant to illnesses
- D. They are given decongestants and antihistamines by their parents

Answers: 1.C, 2.C, 3.A, 4.C, 5.B, 6.D, 7.A, 8.A, 9.A, 10.C, 11.C

Chapter opener image: Robert Kneschke/Shutterstock.com

CHAPTER 21

Caring for Older Adults

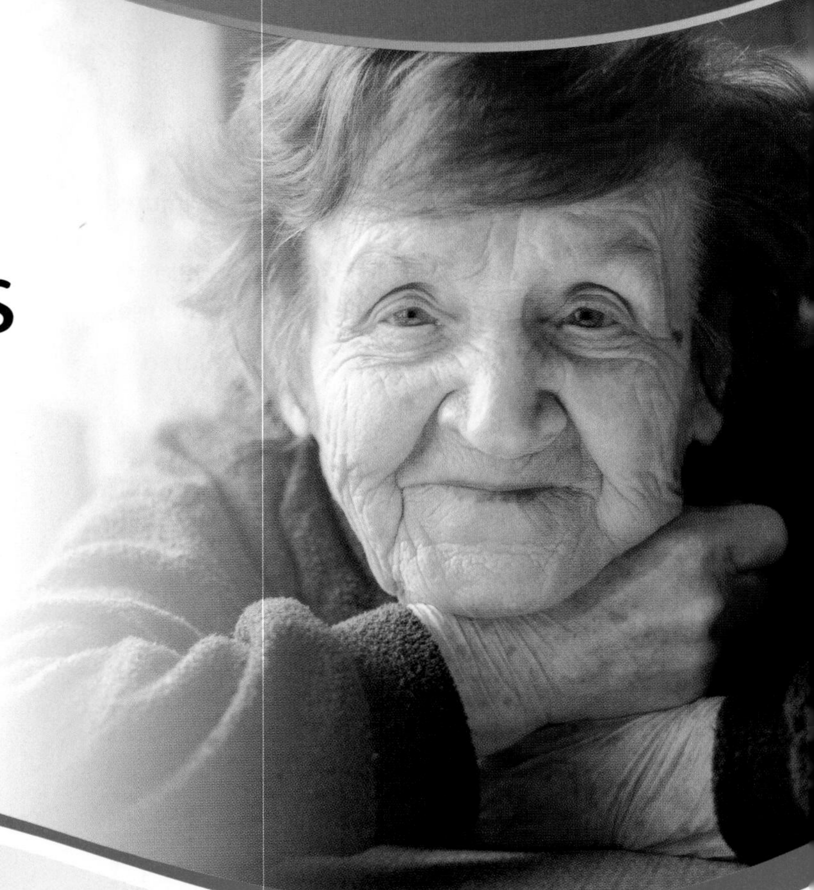

OBJECTIVES

After reading this chapter, the learner should be able to do the following:

- Describe the effects of retirement.
- Identify the social changes common in older adulthood.
- Describe how a partner's death affects the survivor.
- Describe the changes that occur in the body's systems during aging and the care required.
- Explain how aging affects sexuality in older adults.
- Describe how the health care team promotes the client's sexuality.
- Explain the effect of ageism on older adults.

KEY TERMS

atrophy A decrease in size or wasting away of tissue. *p. 376*

dysphagia Difficulty (*dys*) swallowing (*phagia*). *p. 377*

dyspnea Difficult, laboured, or painful breathing. *p. 377*

geriatrics The branch of medicine that provides care for older adults. *p. 369*

gerontology The study of the aging process. *p. 369*

The number of older adults is increasing every day in Canada. People are living longer and are healthier and more active than ever before, so most people can expect to live into their seventies, or even into their eighties or nineties (see **FIGURE 21–1**). There are more 100-year-olds now than ever before. After a lifetime of working, raising children, and making a difference in their communities, older adults have the knowledge, wisdom, and experience that we can all benefit from.

As *baby boomers* (people born during the post–World War II years, from 1946 to mid-1960s) age, Canada is increasing its efforts to better understand the implications of the aging population on health and long-term care needs and costs.[1] For example, "active aging" is becoming the norm, meaning that older adults are increasingly contributing to society through unpaid activities and paid employment. Older adults contribute to society as workers, volunteers, grandparents, and caregivers to family members and friends who need care. As the workforce ages and labour-force growth slows, older workers are increasingly important to the Canadian economy.

The older adults of the future are likely to have higher levels of education, better health, and longer life expectancy. They will be more ethnoculturally diverse. They are likely to remain active during retirement, whether through continuing their employment, perhaps in a new career; returning to school; caring for grandchildren; volunteering; or travelling. They are more likely to have smaller and more diverse families and few or no children. Those who are married may be in a second or subsequent marriage.

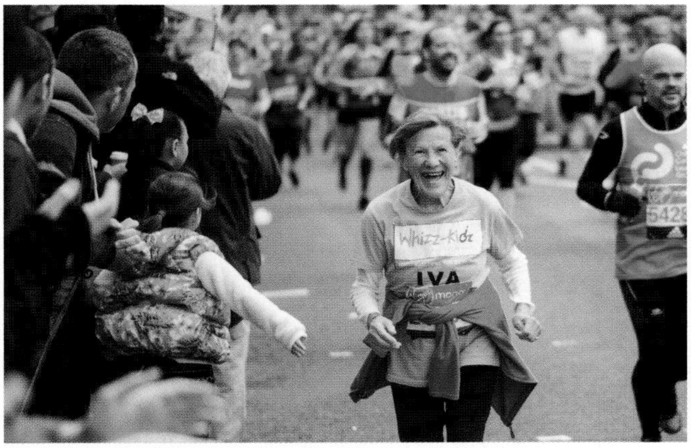

FIGURE 21–1 Many seniors live healthy and active lives. (**Source:** Roomanald/Shutterstock.com)

Moreover, baby boomers, particularly women, will retire with different work histories and pension coverage than people of previous generations did, a situation that will greatly impact their retirement income.

Gerontology is the study of the aging process. **Geriatrics** is the branch of medicine that provides care for older adults. Aging, or growing old, is a normal process during which normal changes in body structure and function occur, increasing the risk for illness, injury, persistent illness, and disability. These changes, however, are usually gradual. Emotional and social changes also occur, and most older adults adjust to these changes well and live healthy and happy lives. Older adults may continue to live in their own homes by themselves or with their partners or live with their adult children or other family members. Some move into assisted-living facilities, and those who require 24-hour care move into long-term care facilities.

As stated in Chapter 18, the developmental tasks of late adulthood are as follows:

- Adjusting to decreased physical strength and loss of health
- Adjusting to retirement and reduced income
- Coping with the death of a partner
- Developing new friends and relationships
- Preparing for one's own death

CARING FOR OLDER CLIENTS

Mainstream North American culture tends to over-value youth, as reflected in media messages that stress the importance of looking and acting young. There are ads for hair dyes that cover grey hair and lotions that reduce wrinkles so that people can look younger than they are. Media images often also stereotype older adults. Many greeting cards and cartoons portray older adults as grouchy, unproductive, simple (not very intelligent), and slow. Remember, older adults are not all alike. Every person—young, middle-aged, or old—is unique, and every person develops and ages in his or her own way. Treating older people as if they are boring, useless, or child-like is ageism.

Older adults can think and make decisions for themselves. Failure to recognize this fact can result in your making a person feel that he is being treated like a child. How would you feel if a younger person made your decisions for you? Would you feel insulted or angry? Would you feel useless? Treating older adults disrespectfully threatens their dignity and sends the message that they are no longer useful, productive members of society.

Older people are often coping with the loss of loved ones, friends, and health. The loss of dignity and self-esteem in addition to all that can be too much for them to bear, and they face the risks of withdrawal from social contact and depression. As a support worker, by treating older clients with respect, you help them maintain emotional and social health.

To care for older clients effectively, you need to understand the emotional, social, and physical changes that occur with aging and also be aware of each client's health status and needs. Always follow the individual care plan for each older client (see the *Providing Compassionate Care: Supporting Older Clients* box).

EMOTIONAL AND SOCIAL CHANGES

Greying hair, wrinkles, and slowing movements are physical reminders that one is growing old, and retirement and the deaths of partners, family members, and friends are social reminders. Physical and social changes have emotional effects on older adults and also have an impact on their basic needs of love and belonging and self-esteem.

Retirement

Most people look forward to their retirement. People usually retire at the age of 65 years, but some may choose to retire earlier or work after they turn 65. Retirement is a reward for a lifetime of work. The person has earned the right not to work any longer and can now relax and enjoy life. Travel, leisure, spending time with family, and doing only what one wants to do are retirement "benefits." Nowadays, more and more retired people are interested in furthering their education.

Most people enjoy their retirement, but some are not so fortunate. Some are forced to retire because of persistent illness or disability, and poor health can make retirement very difficult. Retirement is often a person's first real experience with aging.

Work has social and emotional effects. It helps meet the basic needs of love and belonging and self-esteem and brings fulfillment and a feeling of usefulness. Many people enjoy a sense of pride, identity, and status associated with their occupation or title. They take pride in a day's work or a job well done. Friendships form; co-workers share daily events; and leisure time, recreation, and companionship often involve co-workers. Some people thus need work for emotional and social fulfillment, and for such people, retirement can be hard. Some retired people, therefore, take on part-time jobs or volunteer work (**FIGURE 21–2**) because such activities promote a sense of purpose, usefulness, and well-being.

Retirement allows many people the opportunity to pursue hobbies and activities that they have always

Providing Compassionate Care
Supporting Older Clients

- ***Dignity.*** Show respect for your older clients. Avoid using terms, gestures, or a tone of voice that could be considered patronizing (see Chapters 5 and 10). For example, never use the term "girl" when addressing an older female client. Some older clients find it disrespectful to be addressed by their first names, especially by younger people. Ask your clients how they would like to be addressed. Never assume you can use a client's first name, even if you have heard your co-workers use it. Do not talk about the client with others. Do not exchange glances with co-workers when reacting to something an older client has said or done.
- ***Independence.*** Help clients only when necessary. Respect their routines. Do things the way clients are used to doing them. Allow time for rest, and avoid rushing them.
- ***Preferences.*** Older clients have the right to make choices, so you must have their consent for all procedures. They can make decisions regarding their care and also choose when to get up and when to go to bed, what to wear, what activities to participate in, and what to eat. Always ask about and accommodate a client's preferences.
- ***Privacy.*** Provide for privacy, and keep information about the client confidential. All clients should be given privacy when they are visiting with others or using the telephone. Use draping and screening to avoid exposing the client's body during procedures. Provide for privacy during elimination.
- ***Safety.*** Be alert to safety hazards in the client's environment. Practise the safety measures discussed in Chapter 22 to prevent falls, burns, poisoning, and suffocation. Apply restraints only if ordered by a physician and only once the task has been properly delegated to you.

Note that older clients may not show the usual signs of infection such as fever, pain, inflammation, and swelling (see Chapter 23). The only signs may be changes in behaviour, so observe for any such changes, including sudden confusion; urinary incontinence; a fall; or a change in mood, energy levels, or eating habits. Immediately report all changes in your client's behaviour and health to your supervisor.

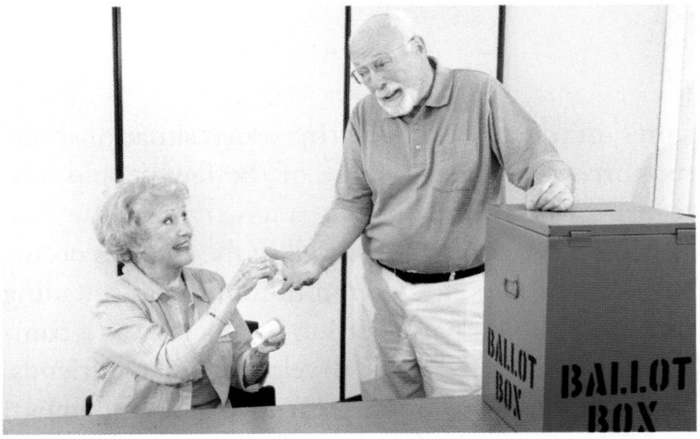

FIGURE 21–2 These retired people volunteer. (**Source:** © Can Stock Photo Inc./lisafx)

enjoyed or the time to take up new ones. However, for people who have never cultivated interests or hobbies outside of their job, retirement can cause a very abrupt and upsetting change of lifestyle that they have difficulties adjusting to.

It is important to record and report any signs of depression that you observe in your client or that your client expresses after retirement. Your client may feel lonely and isolated from former co-workers and friends.

Reduced Income

Retirement income is often less than half of a person's full income during her work years. For some retired people, the Canada Pension Plan (CPP) may be the only source of income, but, unfortunately, CPP has not kept pace with the rising cost of living. More people qualify for the Old Age Security pension (OAS) than CPP. OAS is a monthly payment available to most people 65 years of age and older who meet the Canadian legal status and residency requirements. Employment history is not a factor in determining eligibility for OAS. You can receive OAS pension even if you have never worked or are still working.[2]

Being an older adult and being retired do not mean one has fewer expenses. Older adults still need to make rent or mortgage payments, buy food and clothing, spend on transportation and utilities, and pay taxes. They must also pay for medications that are not covered under government drug plans.

Reduced income during retirement may force lifestyle changes such as limiting social and leisure activities and finding cheaper housing or moving in with children or other relatives. Some older adults must rely on family for money or needed items; others live in poverty if they do not have an adequate pension income or assets. While the cost of living is rising in Canada, the old-age pension is not increasing at the same rate, so the gap between income and need is widening each year.

Some older adults do not face a reduction in their income because when they were working, they were able to provide for their retirement through their savings, investments, retirement plans, and insurance. For these older adults, the retirement years are financially comfortable.

Social Relationships

Social relationships change throughout life (see the *Respecting Diversity: Older Adults From Different Cultures* box). Children grow up, leave home, and have their own families. Some of them live far away from their parents. Older friends and family move away, die, or become disabled. Some older people have regular contact with children, grandchildren, brothers and sisters, nieces and nephews, and other relatives and friends. But some others may feel isolated and lonely because of separation or distance from their children, their peers' dying, and an overall lack of companionship.

Some older adults develop mobility issues, which may interfere with their pursuing interests that they previously enjoyed, independently or in groups, such as gardening or boating or bicycling. Others may begin to feel isolated if they are no longer able to drive and must learn how to get around using public transportation. Some older people live in remote areas of the country and may not have easy access to stores or doctors' offices. In some situations, the support worker may be one of the few people who regularly visits with them.

Most older adults adjust well to the changes occurring in their lives. Many find fulfillment in spending time on hobbies, participating in religious and community activities, and developing new friends. Grandchildren can bring great love and enjoyment, and taking part in family activities not only gives companionship but also helps the older person to feel useful and wanted.

Some home care plans include a "friendly visitor" program for older adults living alone. Older adults who move into retirement homes and long-term care facilities often make new friends and take part in social activities offered in the facilities (**FIGURE 21–3**).

Respecting Diversity

Older Adults From Different Cultures

Some older adults who have moved to Canada from another country may not speak English or French. In Canada, they may have lived and worked in a community of people from their home country. When family and friends move away or die, these people may be left with no one to talk to. If the health care workers also do not speak their language or understand their culture, these older adults feel lonely and isolated.

Some older adults born into Indigenous communities may experience this isolation, too. They may have grown up, been educated, worked, and socialized within this same Indigenous community, and reached older age with the same peer group. They will have depended on the support of their family and community in a way that people outside their community may not understand.

As a support worker, you need to realize the possible effects on your clients of being removed from their support system in their community and placed in a long-term care facility. They could feel very isolated. You need to be sensitive to clients in this situation.

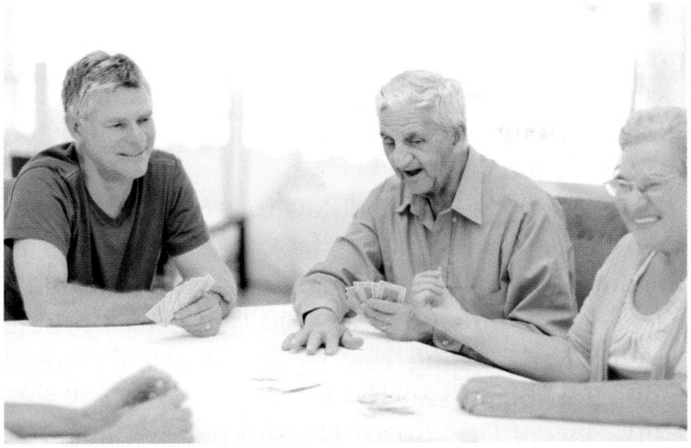

FIGURE 21–3 Older adults enjoy companionship with people their own age. (**Source:** © Can Stock Photo Inc./4774344sean.)

Children as Caregivers

Sometimes, parents and children exchange roles, and the adult child cares for the aging parent. This role exchange and dependency on their children can make some older adults feel more secure but make others feel unwanted, in the way, and useless. Some may feel that they have lost their dignity and self-respect, so tensions may develop among the child, parent, and other household members.

From the other perspective, being a caregiver to a parent can be very stressful. The caregiver often has to meet the needs of the parent as well as those of her own children. If the parent has a medical condition, the caregiver has even more responsibilities; she may need to quit work to care for the parent, and the resulting loss of income may cause financial difficulties. Lack of privacy is also a common problem for both the caregiver and the parent.

Death of a Partner, Significant Other, or Pet

As a couple grows older, the chances that one partner will die increase. Women usually live longer than men do, and most women will, therefore, become widows.

Even when a person tries to be emotionally prepared for a partner's death, when death occurs, the loss is devastating. No amount of preparation is ever enough to cope with the emptiness that results. With that one death, the surviving partner loses a friend, lover, companion, and confidant, so the grief is great and can lead to serious physical and mental health problems. The grieving partner may lose the will to live or may even attempt suicide. Support from family, friends, and religious, social, or recreational groups is very important at this time to help the surviving partner cope.

Some older adults can also be devastated by the loss of a close friend or a pet that has been a constant companion for many years. As with the death of a partner, many older adults experience profound feelings of sadness and loss in these events.

DEPRESSION IN OLDER ADULTS[3,4]

Depression is ***not*** an inevitable part of aging, but because of life changes that older adults face—losses of loved ones, retirement, persistent health problems, loss of independence, and increased isolation—many older adults experience depression. Signs and symptoms of depression are listed in Chapter 35. While people can experience depression at any age, depression in older adults may go unrecognized because many of the signs and symptoms occur gradually or may be mistaken for normal signs of aging. Many older adults do not readily admit to feelings of depression because of the stigma associated with any mental health disorder (see Chapter 35). However, depression can increase the risk of death in older adults by two or three times.[4] See **BOX 21–1** for some common signs and symptoms of depression in the older adult.

If your client exhibits any signs or symptoms of depression, it is important that you report them to your supervisor. Once depression is recognized, the treatment for it in the older adult involves mainly psychological therapy, instead of medication. The client's physician may also prescribe antidepressant medications, but the client must be closely monitored to observe for adverse effects. Some common therapies used include the following:[4]

- Cognitive behavioural therapy, which helps the client learn ways to identify and correct negative ways of thinking
- Interpersonal therapy, which helps the client deal with stresses and challenges
- Problem-solving therapy, which helps the client manage difficulties through problem-solving
- Reminiscence therapy, which helps the client revisit past good memories and feelings of self-worth

BOX 21–1 Common Signs and Symptoms of Depression in Older Adults

- Sadness
- Loss of energy and feeling of tiredness
- Memory problems
- Irritability
- Neglecting personal care
- Loss of interest in hobbies or interests
- Reluctance to be with friends or engage in activities
- Difficulty falling asleep or staying asleep
- Oversleeping
- Feelings of being burdensome or worthless
- Increased use of alcohol or medications
- Fixation on death or suicidal thoughts
- Increase in physical complaints, such as of arthritis or headaches

PHYSICAL CHANGES

Certain physical changes are a normal part of aging and occur in everyone (**BOX 21–2**). Some changes are a result of lifestyle choices. Physical processes slow down, and energy level and body efficiency decline. The rate and degree of change vary with each person. Influencing factors include diet, general health, exercise, stress, environment, and heredity. Most of these normal changes are gradual and, therefore, not immediately noticed. Some older adults also experience physical changes caused by disease, illness, or injury (see Chapter 37).

Normal aging does not mean loss of health, so quality of life does not have to change with aging. The older person can adjust to the normal changes that occur with age, but some do have at least one persistent illness.

The Integumentary System

In older adulthood, the skin loses its elasticity, strength, and fatty-tissue layer. As a result, the skin thins and sags, and folds, lines, and wrinkles appear. Dry skin develops because of decreased secretions from oil and sweat glands, so the skin becomes fragile and is easily injured. Skin breakdown, skin tears, and pressure ulcers are some of the risks older adults face (see Chapter 24). Brown spots, often called "age spots" or "liver spots," appear on the skin, usually on the wrists and hands.

As a person ages, blood flow to the skin decreases, resulting in fewer or less effective nerve endings in the skin. The loss of nerve endings interferes with the client's ability to sense heat, cold, and pain. Bruising and delayed healing can result from a decreased number of blood vessels.

The loss of fatty tissues beneath the skin increases sensitivity to cold, so the client needs to be protected from drafts and extreme cold. Sweaters, lap blankets, socks, and higher thermostat settings are often needed.

Nails become thick and tough, and feet usually have poor circulation. A nick or cut can lead to a serious infection (see Chapter 31 for a description of nail and foot care).

Dry skin is easily damaged and causes itching, so older adults with dry skin should avoid having daily showers or tub baths. A complete bath once a week and partial baths on the other days should be enough to maintain hygiene. Wash the client's face with water only, as soap can dry the skin too much. Use mild soaps when washing the other parts of the body. Lotions, oils, and creams are often recommended to prevent drying and itching. Deodorants usually are not needed because sweat gland secretion decreases (see Chapter 30 for a discussion on hygiene). Be sure to follow the care plan for these clients.

Older clients may complain of cold feet. For warmth, provide socks that are not too tight to avoid cutting off circulation to the toes. Do not use hot-water bottles and heating pads on the client because of the risk for burns. Fragile skin, poor circulation, and decreased sensitivity to heat contribute to the increased risk for burns. A doctor's order is necessary for applying heat or cold to your client. When applying either, you must check the area every 15 minutes (see Chapter 44). If the area where heat is applied turns red, report it immediately to your supervisor. If the area where you are applying cold appears blue, report it immediately to your supervisor. Report to your supervisor immediately if your client complains of any discomfort.

BOX 21–2 Physical Changes That May Occur During the Aging Process

Integumentary System

Skin becomes less elastic
Skin loses its strength
Brown spots ("age spots" or "liver spots") appear on the wrists and hands
Nerve endings decrease in number
Blood vessels decrease in number
Fatty tissue layer is lost
Skin thins and sags
Skin becomes fragile and is easily injured
Folds, lines, and wrinkles appear
Secretion from oil and sweat glands decreases
Skin becomes dry
Skin becomes itchy
Sensitivity to extreme heat and to cold environments decreases
Sensitivity to pain decreases
Nails become thick and tough
Hair whitens or greys
Hair thins
Facial hair appears in some women
Hair becomes dry

Musculo-Skeletal System

Muscles atrophy
Strength decreases
Bones become brittle; can break easily
Joints become stiff and painful
Height gradually decreases
Mobility decreases

Nervous System

Vision and hearing decrease
Senses of taste, smell, and touch decrease
Sensitivity to pain is reduced
Blood flow to the brain is reduced
Cells shrink
Memory becomes shorter (forgetfulness)
Ability to respond slows
Sleep patterns change
Dizziness occurs

Circulatory System

Heart pumps with less force
Arteries narrow and are less elastic
Less blood flows through narrowed arteries
Weakened heart has to work harder to pump blood through narrowed vessels

Respiratory System

Respiratory muscles weaken
Lung tissue becomes less elastic
Breathing becomes difficult
Strength for coughing decreases

Digestive System

Saliva production decreases
Swallowing becomes difficult
Appetite decreases
Secretion of digestive juices decreases
Digesting fried and fatty foods becomes difficult
Indigestion occurs
Teeth fall out
Peristalsis decreases, causing flatulence and constipation

Urinary System

Blood supply to kidneys is reduced
Kidneys atrophy
Kidney function decreases
Urine becomes concentrated
Urinary frequency, urgency, and incontinence may occur
Nighttime urination may occur

Female Reproductive System

Menstruation stops
Estrogen production decreases
Ovaries and uterus decrease in size
Vaginal walls become thinner, drier, and less elastic
Fat and elastic tissue in external genitalia decrease
Breasts become less firm

Male Reproductive System

Testosterone production decreases
Force of ejaculation decreases
Sperm count is reduced
Testes become smaller
Prostate gland enlarges
Erections develop more slowly

Most older adults have grey or white hair, and some of them may choose to colour their hair. Hair loss and thinning occur in both men and women as they age. Thinning occurs on the head, in the pubic area, and under the arms. Facial hair grows above the lips and on the chin of some older women. Decreased scalp oils lead to dry hair in older adults. Brushing helps stimulate circulation and oil production. The frequency of shampooing is a matter of personal choice and should be done as often as necessary for the client's hygiene and comfort. Follow the care plan for the client. Note that some Indigenous people believe their hair should not be put in garbage receptacles but that it should be collected from hairbrushes, sinks, drains, and so on and burned in a sacred fire or in a ceremony.

Signs of age are often visible on a person's skin. Older adults themselves as well as others can see their grey hair, bald patches, brown spots, wrinkles, and sagging skin, and these reminders of old age can affect an older adult's self-esteem and body image.

The Musculo-Skeletal System

Muscles **atrophy** (shrink) and decrease in strength. Bones lose strength, become brittle, and break easily, so sometimes just turning in bed can cause fractures (broken bones). Vertebrae shorten, joints become stiff and painful, and hip and knee joints flex (bend) only slightly. These changes result in a gradual loss of height, loss of strength, and decreased mobility.

Activity and an appropriate diet can help slow the rate of these changes, so older adults need to be as active as possible. A regular exercise program, including range-of-motion (ROM) exercises, is helpful; bathing, dressing, grooming, and other activities of daily living (ADLs) are forms of physical activity that are also helpful (see Chapter 26). In addition, an older adult's diet should be high in protein, calcium, and vitamins.

Remember, the bones of older adults can break easily, so protect these clients from injury and take measures to prevent falls (see Chapter 22). Turn and move your client gently and carefully. Some older clients need help and support for getting out of bed or walking.

The Nervous System

Aging affects the senses—hearing and vision losses may occur (see Chapter 37 for more details). The senses of taste and smell may become dull; touch, sensitivity to pain and pressure, and the ability to feel heat and cold are reduced. These changes increase the risk for injury, as the older adult may not feel pain when ill or injured, or pain may be perceived as only minor. Protect older clients from injury (see Chapter 22), provide skin care, check for signs of skin breakdown, and prevent pressure ulcers (see Chapters 24 and 30).

Aging affects brain cells, causing them to shrink; also, blood flow to the brain is reduced. These changes affect response time, energy levels, and memory, so reflexes become slower. The client may tire more easily. Forgetfulness may occur but is not a normal part of aging. The reduction in blood flow to the brain may also cause dizziness, which increases the risk for falls. As a support worker, take measures to prevent falls (see Chapter 22). Remind your older clients to rise slowly from their beds or chairs to help prevent dizziness.

Sleep patterns may change with age. Some older adults have difficulty falling asleep or wake often during the night, so they may rest or nap during the day to prevent fatigue.

The Circulatory System

The heart muscle weakens with age, so the heart pumps blood through the body with less force. This decreased blood force may not cause problems during rest, but when activity, exercise, excitement, or illness increases the body's needs for oxygen and nutrients, a weaker heart may not be able to meet them.

In the older adult, arteries narrow and become less elastic, so less blood is able to flow through them, causing poor circulation in many body parts. A weak heart must work harder to pump blood through narrowed vessels. Clients with severe circulatory problems need rest periods throughout the day. They should not engage in activities that cause overexertion—for example, walking long distances, climbing many stairs, or carrying heavy things. Personal care items, television controls, and other needed items should be kept close at hand.

Moderate daily exercise, however, stimulates circulatory, respiratory, digestive, and musculo-skeletal functions and helps prevent blood clots (thrombi) in the leg veins. Some older adults are able to engage in activities such as walking, biking, golf, tennis, swimming, and other forms of exercise. Active or passive ROM exercises are necessary for clients on bed rest (see Chapter 26). Follow the care plan for exercise and activity levels.

The Respiratory System

Respiratory muscles weaken with age, and lung tissue becomes less elastic. These changes may not be noticed at rest, but difficult, laboured, or painful breathing (**dyspnea**; *dys* means difficult, and *pnea* means breathing) may occur with activity. Older clients may lack the strength to cough and clear the airway of secretions, which puts them at risk for respiratory infections (such as pneumonia) and other diseases that can be life threatening.

The following help to promote normal breathing in older clients:

- Avoiding use of heavy bed linens over the client's chest, which can prevent normal chest expansion
- Encouraging the client to turn, reposition, and breathe deeply to help prevent respiratory complications that can arise from continuous bed rest
- Resting in the semi-Fowler's position (see Chapter 25)
- Encouraging the client to be as active as possible

The Digestive System

Changes in the digestive system caused by aging include the following: (1) Salivary glands produce less saliva, causing difficulty swallowing (**dysphagia**); (2) secretion of digestive juices decreases, resulting in difficulty digesting fried and fatty foods; and (3) peristalsis (the involuntary contractions of intestinal muscles) decreases, so the stomach and colon empty at a slower rate, leading to flatulence and constipation. Other physical changes such as dulled senses of taste and smell affect appetite and enjoyment of food. Some older adults may have lost teeth from illness or lifestyle choices. This loss of teeth and the presence of ill-fitting dentures make chewing difficult (see Chapter 28 for a discussion on diet changes that help older adults address eating and digestive issues).

The Urinary System

Kidney function declines with age. Blood flow to the kidneys is reduced, and the kidneys atrophy. As a result, the removal of body wastes is less efficient, and urine is more concentrated. Not drinking enough fluids can also cause urine to become more concentrated.

Since bladder muscles weaken and the size of the bladder decreases, it is able to hold very little urine, resulting in urinary frequency or urgency. Some older adults experience *nocturia*, which is the need to urinate several times during the night. In some others, urinary incontinence (the inability to control passing urine) may occur, but it is not a normal part of aging (see Chapter 32).

In older men, the prostate gland enlarges, which causes pressure on the urethra. As a result, difficulty urinating and frequent urination are common problems.

Older adults, especially women, are at risk for urinary tract infections. To avoid them, clients should drink adequate fluids, including water, fruit juices, and milk. As a support worker, you should allow clients personal choice in beverages. Most fluids should be ingested before 1700 hours (5:00 p.m.) to help reduce the need to urinate during the night. Bladder control training programs may be necessary for those with urinary incontinence. However, fluids should never be restricted just to reduce the need to urinate at night (see Chapter 32 for a discussion on urinary elimination).

The Reproductive System

In older men, the hormone testosterone decreases. Since the decrease in this hormone affects physical strength, sperm production, and reproductive tissues, it has a negative impact on sexual activity. It takes longer for erection and orgasm to occur, and orgasm is weaker than in younger years. The erection is lost quickly after orgasm, and the time between erections lengthens. Older men may need to have the penis stimulated for sexual arousal. These changes result in decreased frequency of sexual activity.

During perineal care, your male client may develop an erection, which is a normal physical reaction to the wiping of sensitive perineal nerve endings. Bringing attention to the client's physical reaction may cause embarrassment. Simply provide privacy by covering his penis with a towel and continue wiping in another area as needed. When his erection is over, you may resume cleansing his perineal area.

Mental and physical fatigue, overeating, and excessive drinking can also affect the ability to have erections. Some men fear performance problems and may therefore avoid sexual activity.

In women, menopause occurs around 50 years of age. At menopause, a woman stops menstruating, and her reproductive years come to an end, as ova cease to be produced. Female hormones (estrogen and progesterone) decrease, and this reduction affects reproductive tissues. The uterus, the vagina, and the external genitalia all begin to atrophy, and breasts become less firm. Intercourse may be uncomfortable or painful because of thinning vaginal walls and vaginal dryness. Older women also experience changes in sexual excitement. Arousal takes longer, and the time between arousal and orgasm is longer. Orgasm is less intense, and the pre-excitement state returns more quickly.

Frequency of sexual activity decreases for many older intimate couples because of weakness, mental and physical fatigue, pain, persistent illness, and reduced mobility.

THE OLDER ADULT AND SEXUALITY

Love, affection, and intimacy are needed throughout life, as sexuality is part of the whole person. These needs do not disappear (**FIGURE 21–4**); older adults have the right—and it is normal—to be sexual and to form sexual relationships.

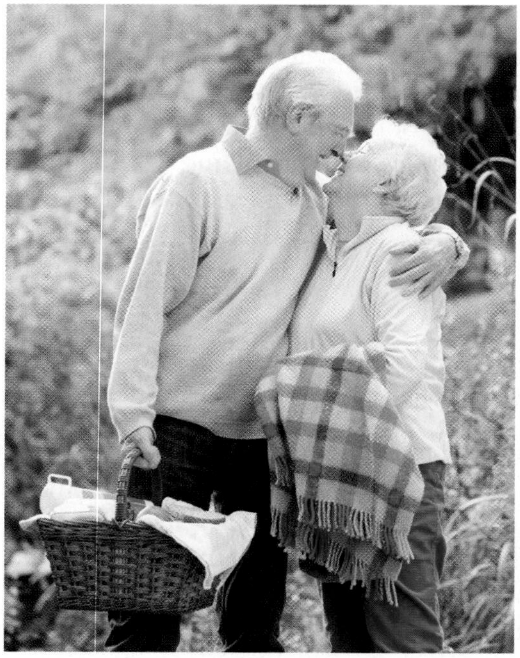

FIGURE 21–4 Love and affection are important to older adults. (**Source:** © Can Stock Photo Inc./monkeybusiness.)

Some older people are not able to have sexual intercourse, but this inability does not mean that they have lost their sexual needs or desires. They can express their feelings in other ways—for example, hand holding, touching, caressing, and embracing—that can bring closeness and intimacy.

Members of the health care team must respect their clients' sexuality and allow and promote ways for clients to meet their sexual needs (see **BOX 21–3** and the *Focus on Long-Term Care: Residents' Sexual Rights* box).

BOX 21-3 Respecting and Promoting the Client's Sexuality

- ***Respect your client's clothing and grooming routines.*** Appearance is often an important part of sexual identity and expression. The client may want to spend extra time on grooming. Assist as needed.
- ***Accept the client's sexual relationships.*** Your client may not share your sexual attitudes, values, practices, or standards. The older person may have a marital, premarital (before marriage), extramarital (outside marriage), or same sex relationship. Do not judge or gossip about relationships.
- ***Allow privacy.*** Privacy is key to sexual expression. Knock before entering the client's room to show respect for privacy. Knocking also saves you and the client possible embarrassment. Privacy is sometimes hard to find, especially in a facility. Remember the following if you work in a facility:
  - You can usually tell when two people want to be alone. If the client has a private room, close the door for privacy. It is ideal for facilities to have *Do Not Disturb* signs for doors. Let the client and partner know how much time they will have alone. For example, remind them about mealtimes or medication rounds. Tell other staff members to avoid disturbing the couple.
  - Consider the client's roommate. Privacy curtains provide little privacy. Arrange for privacy when the roommate is out of the room. Sometimes, roommates offer to leave the room for a while. If the roommate cannot leave, the nurse should find another private area for the client.
  - Allow privacy for masturbation. It is a normal form of sexual expression and release. Close the privacy curtain and the door. Sometimes, people who are confused masturbate in public areas. Lead the person to a private area, or distract him or her with an activity.

FOCUS ON LONG-TERM CARE

Residents' Sexual Rights

Couples within an intimate union in long-term care facilities are allowed to share the same room if one is available. Long-term care legislation in some provinces even requires it (see Chapter 9). A couple who have lived together for many years have the right to stay together in a facility when possible and can share the same bed if their conditions permit. Sometimes family members are embarrassed by the sexual expression of their parents and may not see the need to provide privacy for their parents' need for sexual expression.

It is important to demonstrate respect for the couple by always knocking before you enter their room. If you do happen to find clients engaging in intimate activity, show respect by politely excusing yourself from the room, closing the door and allowing the couple some uninterrupted time together. Do the same for any client you find masturbating. Politely excuse yourself, provide privacy, and allow the client some uninterrupted time alone. It would be disrespectful and unprofessional to bring up this sexual activity to the client(s) or your co-workers in a joking manner.

In some cases, couples may have lived apart and may not want to share a room. As a support worker, you must respect their decision. After losing a sexual partner through death or divorce, a resident may develop a relationship with another resident. This couple, too, have the right to spend time together.

As a support worker, you must keep in mind that clients who are cognitively impaired could become victims of sexual abuse. They could mistake someone else for their spouse. If you find an inappropriate person in your client's room, ensure that you record and report the finding to your supervisor.

CHAPTER REVIEW

KEY POINTS

- Retirement affects older adults in many ways. Some clients may be happy to retire and look forward to more leisure time, whereas others may have been forced into retirement because of a persistent illness or a disability. As a support worker, be sensitive to your client's reactions and their effect on the family.
- Financial concerns can cause stress to your client and her family. In most cases, income will be reduced after retirement, and in some cases, expenses may go up because of lack of insurance coverage for medications. Older clients still need to deal with the expenses of living.
- Social interactions change as a client ages. Children grow up and may move away. In some cases, they become the caregivers for their parents. A client who has been living in her home and then needs to move to supportive housing may lose contact with friends.
- Depression is not a normal part of aging. You should look for the signs and symptoms of depression and report any to your supervisor. Psychological therapy is the main treatment for depression in the older adult.
- Keep in mind that numerous changes occur in an older person's body systems. Your supervisor will direct your care for your client. Changes occur in the (1) integumentary, (2) musculo-skeletal, (3) nervous, (4) circulatory, (5) respiratory, (6) digestive, (7) urinary, and (8) reproductive systems of older adults.
- Love, affection, and intimacy are needed throughout life, as sexuality is part of the whole person. There are ways you, as a support worker, can respect and promote your client's sexuality.

CRITICAL THINKING IN PRACTICE

You assist a client onto the commode. The person is unsteady, and the care plan states the person is not to be left alone. The person says, "I'm not a baby! I can't go with you standing here." What do you do? How will you provide privacy and safe care?

REVIEW QUESTIONS

Answers to these questions are at the bottom of page 381.

Circle the BEST answer.

1. Which of the following is a developmental task of late adulthood?
   A. Adjusting to increased physical strength
   B. Adjusting to physical changes
   C. Seeking employment
   D. Selecting a partner
2. Retirement usually results in:
   A. A lower income
   B. Physical changes caused by aging
   C. Less free time
   D. Financial security
3. Skin changes occur with aging. Care should include the following:
   A. Daily baths
   B. Not applying lotion
   C. Using soap daily
   D. Providing good skin care
4. An older adult has cold feet. You should:
   A. Provide socks
   B. Apply a hot-water bottle
   C. Soak the client's feet in hot water
   D. Apply a heating pad
5. Changes occur in the musculo-skeletal system with aging. Which of the following is true?
   A. Bones do not become brittle.
   B. Older adults should avoid exercise.
   C. Joints become less stiff.
   D. Range-of-motion exercises help slow the rate of musculo-skeletal changes.
6. In older adults, arteries lose their elasticity and become narrow. These changes result in:
   A. A slower heart rate
   B. Lower blood pressure
   C. Poor circulation to many body parts
   D. Less blood in the body

7. Mr. Steinberg, 88, has severe circulatory problems. You should do the following:
   A. Ignore his complaints of discomfort
   B. Follow the care plan
   C. Plan physically demanding activities
   D. Allow him to carry heavy bags
8. Respiratory changes occur with aging. Which of the following is true?
   A. Heavy bed linens prevent normal chest expansion.
   B. The person should not be turned and repositioned frequently.
   C. The side-lying position is best for breathing.
   D. The person should not be physically active.
9. Older adults should avoid fried and fatty foods because of:
   A. Decrease in saliva secretion
   B. Ill-fitting dentures or loss of teeth
   C. Decreased amount of digestive juices
   D. A decreased sense of taste
10. A physician orders increased fluid intake for an older client. You should:
    A. Give most of the fluid before 1700 hours (5:00 p.m.)
    B. Provide mostly water
    C. Start a bladder training program
    D. Insert an indwelling urinary catheter
11. The health care team in a long-term care facility should:
    A. Discourage older clients from sexual expression and activity
    B. Allow and promote sexual expression and activity in older adults
    C. Expect every client to have the same attitudes toward sex
    D. Not allow clients to masturbate, even in private

Answers: 1.B, 2.A, 3.D, 4.A, 5.D, 6.C, 7.B, 8.A, 9.C, 10.A, 11.B

Chapter opener image: De Visu/Shutterstock.com

CHAPTER 22

Safety

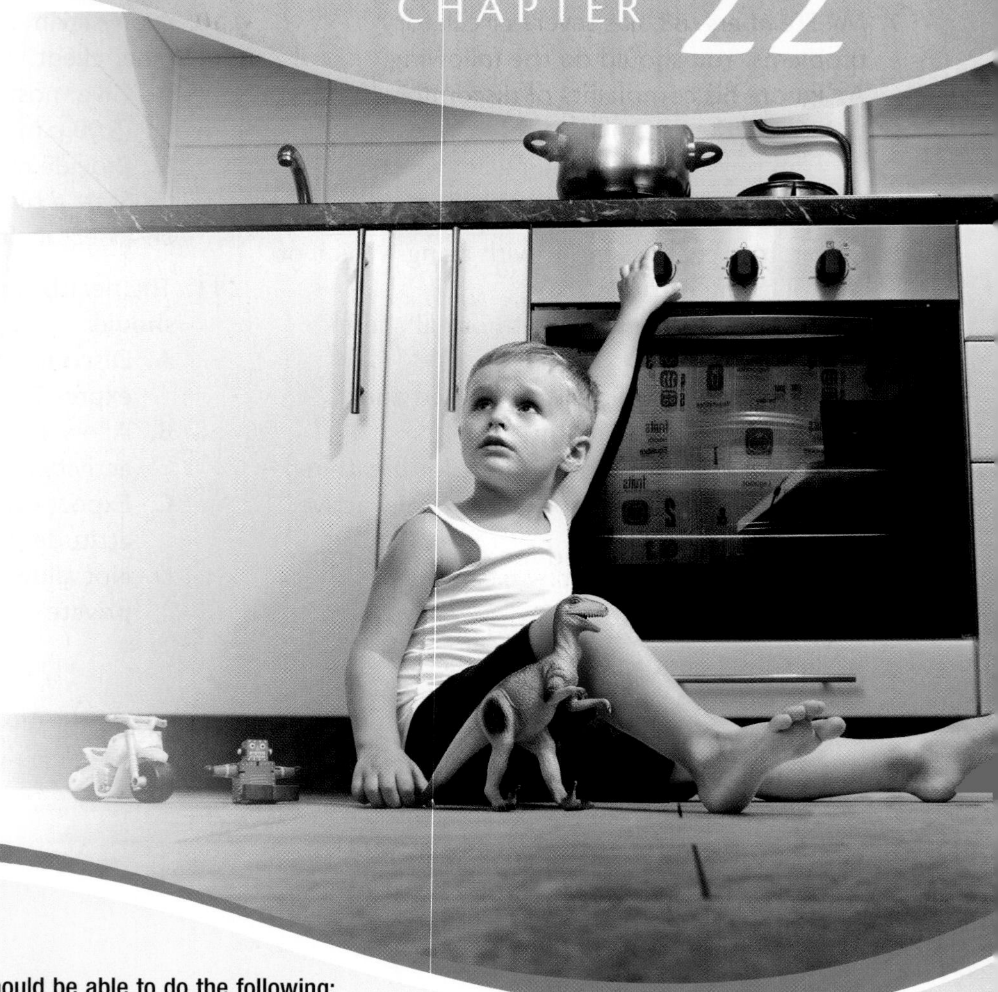

OBJECTIVES

After reading this chapter, the learner should be able to do the following:

- List the risk factors for accidents.
- Describe how identifying the client, providing call bells, and correctly using bed rails promote client safety.
- Identify the safety measures to prevent falls.
- Describe how restraints can cause injury to clients and why they should be avoided.
- Identify how a client's quality of life can suffer as a result of being restrained.
- Identify the safety measures to prevent poisoning, suffocation, and burns.
- Identify fire prevention measures.
- Describe what to do during a fire.
- Describe the causes of and emergency care for burns.
- Describe how to prevent equipment accidents.
- List the steps to reporting a workplace injury, as identified by the Workplace Safety and Insurance Board.
- Apply the information provided in this chapter to protect yourself in the workplace.

KEY TERMS

bed rails The metal or plastic sides of a hospital bed that are used to prevent a client from falling out of bed. *p. 397*

call bell A safety device for clients in facilities that enables them to notify staff that they need assistance. *p. 407*

chemical restraints Medication that is ordered by a doctor and given to a client to control unsafe, undesirable, or bizarre behaviour or movement. *p. 396*

environmental restraints Barriers, furniture, or devices that prevent a client from having free movement. *p. 396*

hazardous material Any substance that presents a physical hazard or a health hazard in the workplace. *p. 411*

incident report A report submitted whenever an accident, error, or unexpected problem arises in the workplace. Also known as an **occurrence report**. *p. 411*

mobility The ability to move around. *p. 384*

occurrence report See **incident report**. *p. 411*

OH&S (occupational health and safety) legislation Federal and provincial laws designed to protect employees from injuries and accidents in the workplace; these laws outline the rights and responsibilities of employers, supervisors, and workers. *p. 410*

physical restraints Garments or devices used to restrict movement of the whole body or parts of the body. *p. 396*

restraint Any device, garment, barrier, furniture, or medication that limits or restricts freedom of movement or access to one's own body. *p. 388*

suffocation A lack of oxygen that causes breathing to stop. *p. 402*

Workplace Hazardous Materials Information System (WHMIS) A national system that provides safety information about hazardous materials; includes labelling, material safety data sheets (MSDSs), and employee education. *p. 411*

workplace violence Any physical assault or threatening behaviour that occurs in a work setting that is directed toward clients, members of the health care team, or both. *p. 413*

Safety is a basic need and a right. People need to both be safe and feel safe, in all circumstances, even electronically. You, as the support worker, your clients, and your co-workers have the right to safety, whether in a client's home or in a facility where you are employed. Promoting client safety is one of the priorities of support work. Because of age or a physical or mental health condition, many clients are at great risk for accidents and injuries, so facilities and community care agencies try to create and maintain a safe environment for their clients.

In a safe environment, clients face little risk of accidents or injuries, and they feel safe and secure, physically and emotionally. You and your employer share the responsibility of ensuring client and worker safety. Your employer must ensure that workplace safety rules are followed and provide training to staff to update their knowledge about lifts, WHMIS (see p. 411), fire safety, smoking, and other safety-related topics. It is your responsibility to know and practise the basic safety measures that you have learned to protect your clients, yourself, and others.

Past measures for protecting clients from harm included the use of restraints. In many cases, however, clients were harmed *because* of their restraint. This chapter discusses safety, including reasons for *not* using restraints and alternatives to restraint use.

ACCIDENT RISK FACTORS

Anyone can be accidentally injured, but children, older adults, and people living with illnesses or disabilities are especially vulnerable to accidents. Factors that increase their risk for accidental injury are given below.

The Client With Awareness Challenges

To protect themselves from injury, people need to be aware of their surroundings. Those who are unconscious are unaware of their surroundings and are unable to react or respond to danger. An unconscious person, therefore, relies on others for protection.

As well, people who have intellectual disabilities or who are confused or disoriented might not be able to recognize and avoid danger and could, therefore, harm themselves. For example, a confused client may wander outside in the middle of winter without a coat, gloves, or boots.

People (including health care workers!) who are preoccupied with things other than the task they are doing are more likely to have accidents because of a decreased awareness regarding their surroundings. Some may just be tired; according to newspaper reports, fatigue is a factor in many motor vehicle accidents along Canada's highways.

Some prescribed medications can cause drowsiness and thus reduced awareness of surroundings. People should always follow the instructions provided by their health care providers and heed the warnings on prescription containers.

The influence of drugs or alcohol (or both) can compromise a person's reflexes, vision, balance, or coordination. Some overconfident people have what can be called "a sense of invincibility." They simply do not believe that they would ever have an accident or be injured. These are the people who tend to speed or text while driving, do not wear their seatbelts, ignore health warning signs, do not get medical checkups, and engage in unsafe habits such as smoking or unprotected sex. These people learn about safety the hard way!

The Client With Vision Challenges

Poor vision can lead to falls. People may not be able to see the obstacles in their path (such as toys, small rugs, furniture, or electrical cords), or they may not be able to judge distances or depth correctly. They may also have problems reading labels on medicines, cleaners, and other containers, which can result in poisonings.

Some people who have decreased eyesight might require eyeglasses but refuse to wear them. Others might wear their eyeglasses all the time but not see clearly because they have not kept their prescriptions up to date. As a support worker, you should always ensure that your client's glasses are properly cleaned (see Chapter 40).

The Client With Hearing Challenges

People with impaired hearing have problems hearing explanations and instructions or may not hear warning signals or fire alarms. Since they are not alerted to danger, they do not know that they must move to safety. Chapter 40 deals with ways to communicate with people with hearing problems.

The Client With Taste, Smell, and Touch Challenges

Diminished senses of taste and smell may cause someone to eat spoiled food or not be aware of a gas leak. A diminished sense of touch may make a person unable to feel heat and cold, as well as pain and discomfort. For example, Mrs. Gagnon has poor circulation to her legs and feet, and so she does not feel the presence of blisters on her feet caused by her new shoes. There is a risk for the blister becoming a serious wound.

The Client With Mobility Challenges

Mobility means the ability to move around. Aging, disease, and injury can affect mobility, so some people cannot walk or use wheelchairs. Being unable to move oneself out of danger is a serious safety risk, and even minor changes in mobility increase accident risks. For example, someone with a sore knee may not be able to recover her balance from a stumble and end up falling.

Medications

Some medications have adverse effects such as loss of balance, drowsiness, lack of coordination, reduced awareness, confusion, and disorientation, among others. Certain medications can even make people fearful and uncooperative. These effects increase the risk for accidents, so they must be reported to your supervisor.

Think About Safety

Risk Factors for Accidents and Falls in Older Adults

One estimate suggests that approximately half of all continuing care clients fall in any 1-year period. Ninety percent of hip fractures are caused by falls, and even non-injurious falls can result in post-fall anxieties that inhibit day-to-day activities.[1] Any injury may be serious for older adults because their bodies take longer to heal and recover. In fact, an injury that may be minor to a younger person (such as a broken bone) may be life threatening to an older adult.

It is true that proper nutrition and lifestyle choices will enable older adults to live longer and healthier lives than ever before. However, a number of them will still experience age-related changes, which will increase their risk for falls and other accidents (see Chapter 21). These changes include the following:

- Weaker muscles
- Slower, less steady movements
- Slowed reaction time
- Balance problems
- Reduced sensitivity to heat
- Decreased vision
- Hearing problems
- Dulled senses of smell, taste, and touch
- Memory problems
- Joint pain and stiffness
- Low blood pressure

In addition to the above, most common physical changes, other factors that can predict the likelihood of an older adult falling include the following:

- A history of falls
- Foot problems
- Ill-fitting shoes
- Elimination problems—incontinence or frequent urination
- Dizziness and light-headedness, especially on standing
- Depression
- Poor judgement or dementia
- Unfamiliar surroundings
- Treatment equipment (intravenous [IV] poles, drainage tubes and bags, and others)
- Improper use of wheelchairs, walkers, canes, and crutches

Age

Children and older adults are at risk for injuries (see Chapters 20 and 21 and the *Think About Safety: Risk Factors for Accidents and Falls in Older Adults* box).

IDENTIFYING THE CLIENT

As a support worker, you will be required to care for many people, each having different treatments, therapies, and activity limits. Before performing a procedure, make sure you are giving the right care to the right person. Follow employer policies and procedures for identifying clients. Life and health are threatened if you give wrong care to a client.

In home care settings, identifying the client is easy, as there is usually only one client per home. Make sure you bring the right assignment sheet for the right home. In other community settings, such as group homes and assisted-living facilities, you might have more than one client in the home. Read the name on the care plan for each client carefully and confirm the person's identity.

In continuing care facilities, you will often care for the same people over an extended period. You will get to know these clients very well and will easily recognize them. Nevertheless, be certain to give each client the right care. Check the client's name and room number on the assignment sheet carefully. Do not confuse one client's care plan with another's. Some continuing care facilities use a photograph identification system. The client's picture is taken on admission and the photo placed in the person's medical record. Other facilities post identifying information in the client's room. Learn about your employer's policies and procedures for identifying clients.

In hospitals, clients usually are admitted and discharged within a short period, and it may not be easy

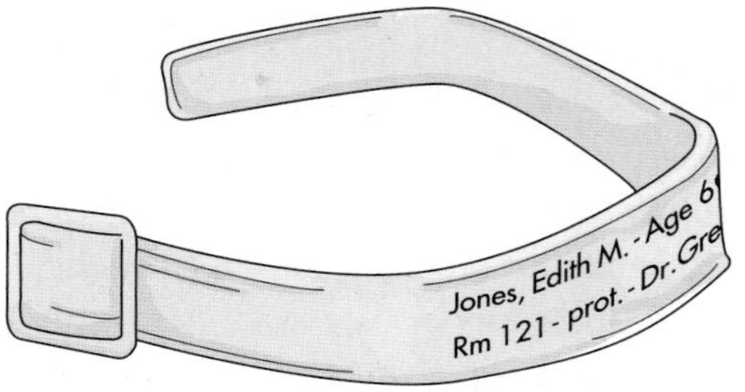

FIGURE 22–1 ID bracelet.

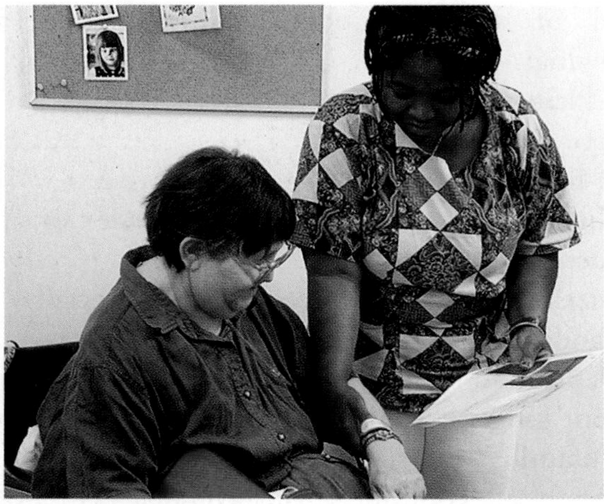

FIGURE 22–2 In hospitals, compare the ID bracelet against the assignment sheet to accurately identify the client.

to identify every client on sight. Therefore, hospitals usually assign identification (ID) bracelets to clients (**FIGURE 22–1**) containing information that includes the client's name, room number and bed number, age, gender, and physician.

Read the ID bracelet to identify the client before giving care. Treatment cards or assignment sheets specify the care to be given. To identify a client in a hospital, do as follows:

- Compare identifying information on the treatment card or assignment sheet with that on the ID bracelet (**FIGURE 22–2**). Carefully check the client's full name. Some people share the same first and last names—for example, common names such as John Smith.
- Call the client by name when you check the ID bracelet. Using the client's name is both a courtesy that you extend as you touch the client and before giving care and also a way of confirming the client's identification. However, just calling a client by name may not be enough to identify the person accurately: clients who are confused, disoriented, drowsy, hearing-impaired, or distracted may answer to any name.

SAFETY MEASURES AT HOME AND IN THE WORKPLACE

Safety is something we take for granted until someone we know or love is injured. We need to be aware of safety hazards in our homes as well as in our workplaces, wherever that may be. As a support worker, you have the responsibility of ensuring your clients' and co-workers' safety as well as your own. Doing so begins with the recognition of common safety hazards (see the *Supporting Mrs. Gerhlbardt: Creating a Safer Environment* box) and reporting any lapses in safety measures immediately to the proper authority, usually your supervisor.

Most accidents can be prevented by using simple safety measures and common sense. The safety measures discussed in this chapter apply to both facility and community settings. Whatever the setting, your employer will have safety policies to protect clients and staff. In the community, case managers, for example, check the client's home for safety hazards during the assessment phase. Any safety hazards identified are then corrected by the case manager, other professionals, or the client's family. In continuing care facilities, there are policies and procedures aimed at protecting the safety of clients and staff. Finally, all community and facility settings have individualized client care plans, which list the safety measures needed by each client.

It is important to follow all safety policies and care plans. Despite careful planning and policies, avoidable accidents can still happen when employees fail to follow the care plan and safety policies.

Preventing Falls and Injuries

Falls are the most common cause of accidental injuries in all settings, and children (see Chapter 20) and older adults are at greatest risk. ***While you should always supervise all of your clients, you should pay particular attention to children, clients in wheelchairs, clients with a history of injury, sedated clients, older clients, and cognitively impaired***

Supporting Mrs. Gerhlbardt: Creating a Safer Environment

Maria Gerhlbardt is an 80-year-old widow who lives alone in her own home, a small, clean, comfortable two-storey house. Her bedroom is on the main floor, but the house's only bathroom is on the second floor. Mrs. Gerhlbardt and her husband bought this home 50 years ago when they first came to Canada from Europe. Mrs. Gerhlbardt is proud of her house, and it is easy to see that she is a very tidy person.

Mrs. Gerhlbardt is able to care for herself in most ways, although she does need some assistance in the winter to go out for banking, shopping, and doctor's appointments. As her support worker, you have arranged to visit her for 45 minutes a day, 5 days a week, to assist her with dressing and cooking. She hired you privately after you answered her personal ad for a support worker in the newspaper and is paying you directly.

Mrs. Gerhlbardt is a very friendly, mentally alert woman. However, she has such severe osteoarthritis and osteoporosis that she is bent over whenever she stands up. To avoid going up and down the stairs to use the bathroom, Mrs. Gerhlbardt has placed an old china bowl on a chair next to her bed to use as a bedside commode. She also has such severe arthritis in her hands and feet that she often has difficulty getting dressed. Her kitchen is very clean and always smells of cooking, but you have noticed that the light bulbs in her kitchen are either burned out or very dim, leaving it very dark. Mrs. Gerhlbardt, however, seems to know where everything is in her kitchen.

You have also noticed that Mrs. Gerhlbardt has many throw rugs, which cover her gleaming floors. She has told you that they were the last purchase she and her husband made together before he died of a heart attack 20 years ago and that she will "never get rid of them." She is particularly fond of the rug at the top of her stairs.

How would you go about providing safe support care for Mrs. Gerhlbardt? Identify the potential safety hazards in Mrs. Gerhlbardt's home.

clients, as they are at greatest risk for injuries related to falls.

The risk for falls increases with age and illness (see the *Think About Safety: Risk Factors for Accidents and Falls in Older Adults* box on page 385). Falls may result in death, serious injuries, or changes in the older person's quality of life. For example, after a fall, an older adult may avoid leaving the house for fear of falling, and staying in the house may lead to feelings of isolation, anxiety, and depression. It may also lead to increased dependency on others.

Clients in long-term care facilities are at greater risk for falls than are older adults living at home.[1] Clients in facilities tend to be older, use more medications, and require more assistance with their activities of daily living (ADLs). Some have impairments that affect their abilities to think, remember, communicate, or concentrate—for example, brain injuries, mental health disorders, dementia, and other conditions that cause confusion and disorientation—which increase clients' risk for falls.

Many facilities have fall prevention programs, which incorporate a variety of strategies to prevent falls. Some of these strategies include the following:

- Clients in facilities are assessed to determine their risk for falls, and those who are at high risk are provided extra supervision and assistance.
- Staff who work with clients receive up-to-date information and training on how to move and care for clients at risk for falls. This education for staff includes training on how to use equipment properly and how to avoid getting injured themselves.
- Methods used to identify clients at risk include a colour-coded bracelet worn by the client and a sign, sticker, or tag placed on the client's chart, at the nurses' station, or, in a few agencies, above the client's bed to indicate that the client is at greater risk of falling. Wherever these signs are used, they should be placed in such a way as to be respectful of the client's right to privacy.

- Since most falls occur in bedrooms, bathrooms, and on stairs, particular attention is paid to making these areas as safe as possible.
- Since falls sometimes occur when clients rush to get to the bathroom or commode without help, they are repeatedly reminded to ask for assistance.
- Most falls in facilities occur in the evening, between 1800 hours (6:00 p.m.) and 2100 hours (9:00 p.m.), when the hallways may be darker than they were during the day. For this reason, keep hallways well lit and free of obstacles or clutter.
- Falls also are more likely during shift changes, when most of the staff are trying to listen to the shift report. To remedy this risk, many agencies use overlapping shifts so that staff remains available to check on clients while the shift report is taking place.
- The safety measures listed in the *Think About Safety: Measures to Prevent Falls Among Older Adults and Others at Risk* box help prevent falls in home and facility settings. Most of these measures are included in fall prevention programs and care plans. Always follow the client's care plan for specific safety measures. Students and staff alike could benefit from participating in any fall prevention workshops offered by the facility.

RESTRAINTS AND HOW TO AVOID THEM

A **restraint** is any device, garment, barrier, furniture, or medication that limits or restricts freedom of movement or access to one's own body. Restraints are rarely used now; only a small number of the types of restraints that were allowed in the past are still allowed in Canada today. Only restraints currently in use will be discussed in this textbook.

It is important to know that every effort is made to protect clients without resorting to the use of restraints. In the past, people have been severely injured (or even died) as the result of restraint application, so laws that prohibit their general use have since been enacted. ***Restraints can cause emotional harm and serious physical injury*** (see the *Providing Compassionate Care: Understanding the Effects of Restraints on Clients* box on page 391). ***Restraints require a physician's order, after consultation with the client's family.***

In most provinces, the client or substitute decision maker (power of attorney; see Chapter 9) must sign a consent form that allows restraints to be used. ***Support workers never decide if restraints are to be used.*** Under our Canadian Charter of Rights and Freedoms, threatening a client with applying a restraint is considered an assault, and using a restraint on a client without a doctor's order is considered false imprisonment (see Chapter 9).

Guidelines Regarding the Use of Restraints

All support workers need to keep in mind the guidelines discussed in this book regarding restraints. Remember that:

- Unnecessary restraint is false imprisonment (see Chapter 9). There must be a written consent in the client's chart for using the restraint, and it must be indicated in the client's care plan.
- Restraints are never used to discipline a client. *Discipline* is any action that punishes or penalizes.
- Restraints are never used for staff convenience. They should not be used to make the staff's jobs easier. If a restraint must be used, the least restrictive method is chosen ***by the physician***. If clients are in danger of harming themselves or others, physicians usually advise them to enter a facility, where safe care can be provided.
- Always try to determine the cause of the client's agitation or behaviour (see the section "Managing Challenging or Responsive Behaviours" in Chapter 36). If the cause is known and addressed, the need for restraints can usually be prevented. When determining the causes of harmful behaviour, health care providers consider some of the following questions:
  - Is the client injured or in pain? Clients who feel uncomfortable may react in an agitated and even aggressive manner.
  - Is the client afraid?
  - Is the client seeing, hearing, or feeling things that are not real?
  - Is the client confused or disoriented?
  - Are medications causing the behaviour? ***A recent change in the client's medications can***

Think About Safety

Measures to Prevent Falls Among Older Adults and Others at Risk

- Report throw rugs and small mats that are not secure. They can be secured with carpet tape or nonskid backing. Make sure throw rugs and small mats are not in high-traffic areas or at the tops of stairways.
- Report loose floorboards and tiles. Report frayed, torn, or bumpy rugs and carpets.
- Keep traffic areas free of telephone and electrical cords. Cords and wires can be taped to the wall so the client will not trip over them.
- Keep the floors and stairways free of clutter. Never leave items on the stairs.
- Use only nonglare and nonslip floor wax.
- Clean up water and other spills immediately.
- Ensure proper lighting, especially near stairways and bathrooms. Offer to replace burned-out light bulbs.
- Turn on night lights in the halls, especially near the bathroom, in case the client has to get up in the middle of the night.
- Keep a clear path from the bedroom to the bathroom.
- Do not rearrange the client's furniture.
- Use nonslip rubber bath mats or nonslip strips in bathtubs and showers.
- Make sure the client's footwear and clothing fit properly. Shoes and slippers must have nonskid soles. Long shoelaces should be avoided. Clothing should not be loose or drag on the floor. Belts must be tied or secured in place.
- Ensure crutches, canes, and walkers have nonskid tips. Make sure the client uses these devices correctly.
- Remember that clients have *the right to live at risk of injuring themselves*. For example, even if they understand that their scatter rugs are a potential hazard, they may choose to keep them.
- Check wheelchair brakes. Make sure they can be locked and unlocked. Remind the client to keep the brakes locked when not moving the wheelchair, as the brakes prevent the chair from moving when the client transfers to or from the chair. Lock both brakes before you transfer the client to or from the wheelchair. Do not let the client stand on the footrests. Make sure front wheels point forward to keep the wheelchair balanced and stable. Remove the armrests and footrests (if removable) when the client transfers to or from the wheelchair (see Chapters 25 and 26).
- Encourage clients to wear their glasses or hearing aids, as needed. Reading glasses should not be worn when the client is walking.
- Position the client in bed, in a chair, or in a wheelchair properly. Use pillows, wedge pads, or seats, as directed by the care plan.
- Check the client often. Careful and frequent observation is important, especially for those with risk factors.
- Electronic warning devices may be used for some clients. Weight-sensitive alarms placed on beds or wheelchairs detect movement or absence of weight and sound an alarm (**FIGURE 22–3**).
- Respond to all alarms at once.
- Clients at risk for falls can wear hip or coccyx protectors to minimize the risk for injury if a fall occurs. ***But these devices do NOT replace frequent monitoring!***
- Place the call bell within the client's reach. Ask the client to call for assistance when getting out of bed or a chair or when walking. Answer calls as soon as possible, before the client tries to get up without help.
- Offer assistance often to clients who need help with elimination. Help them to the bathroom as soon as requested, or offer a bedpan, urinal, or commode regularly.
- Keep the bedpan or urinal within easy reach of clients able to use them without help.
- Keep beds in the lowest position, except when giving bedside care.
- Never leave the client alone when the bed is raised.
- Use bed rails strictly according to the care plan. If a client tends to get up without calling for assistance, the care plan may state that bed rails be left down. For other clients, the care plan may call for raised bed rails. Know your employer's rules for using bed rails. Bed rails can be unsafe

Continued

Think About Safety—cont'd

if used incorrectly. Follow the care plan for more safety rules regarding bed rails.

- Floor cushions (**FIGURE 22–4**) provide a soft landing spot if the client does fall out of bed. The bed should always be left at its lowest level.
- Roll guards can prevent a client from rolling out of bed (**FIGURE 22–5**).
- Encourage clients to use handrails and grab bars. Facilities provide them in hallways, bathrooms, and on both sides of stairways to provide support for those who are unsteady when walking (**FIGURE 22–6**).
- Use barriers to prevent wandering (**FIGURE 22–7**).
- Lock the wheels on bed legs when giving bedside care and transferring the client.
- In facilities, be careful when turning corners, entering corridor intersections, and going through doors. A person coming from another direction could be injured in a collision.
- In both facilities and homes, perform a safety check of the room after visitors leave. They may have lowered a bed rail, removed the call bell, or moved a walker out of reach. They also may have brought an item that could harm the client.
- In facilities, family and friends are usually allowed to visit during busy times or during the evening and night shifts. A warm drink, soft lights, or a back massage may be used to calm the client who is agitated after visits. Companions are provided to sit with the client who is agitated or restless.

A

B

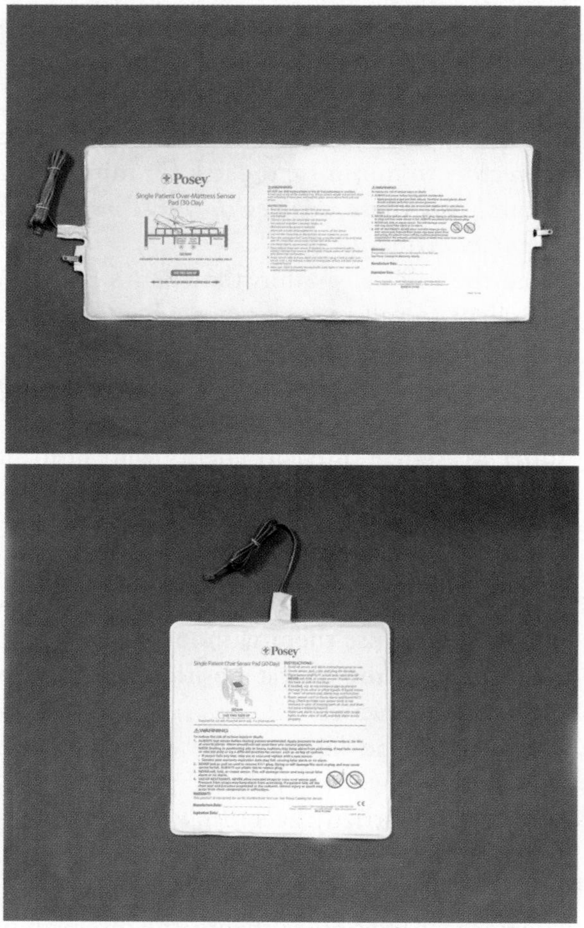

FIGURE 22–3 Many facilities are now using weight-sensitive mats, which trigger an alarm at the central desk to notify staff when the client is climbing out of bed. Weight-sensitive alarms may be used on beds **(A)** or on chairs and wheelchairs **(B)**. (Courtesy J.T. Posey Co., Arcadia, CA.)

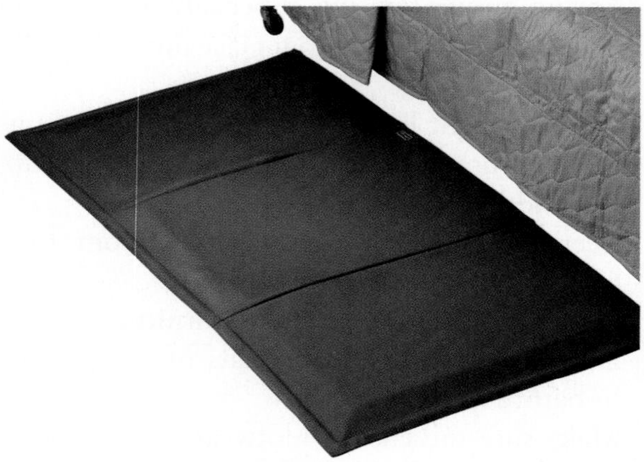

FIGURE 22–4 Floor cushion. (Courtesy J.T. Posey Co., Arcadia, CA.)

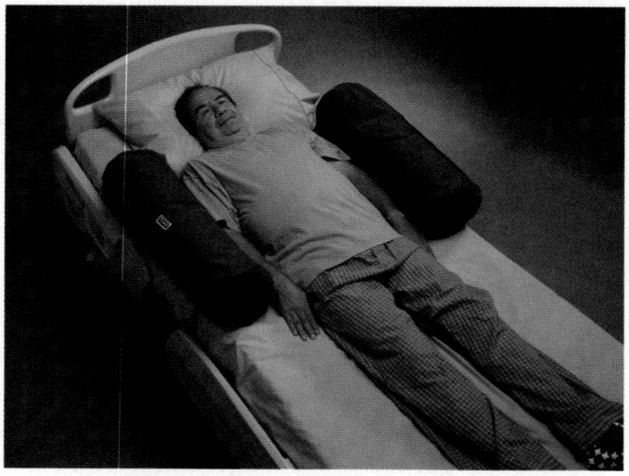

FIGURE 22–5 Roll guard. (Courtesy J.T. Posey Co., Arcadia, CA.)

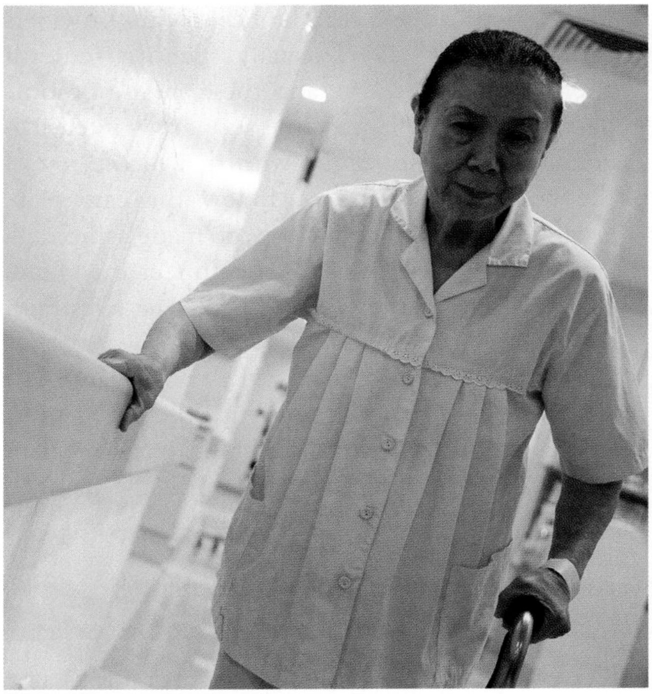

FIGURE 22–6 Handrails provide support to clients when walking. (**Source:** © Corbis RF/Alamy.)

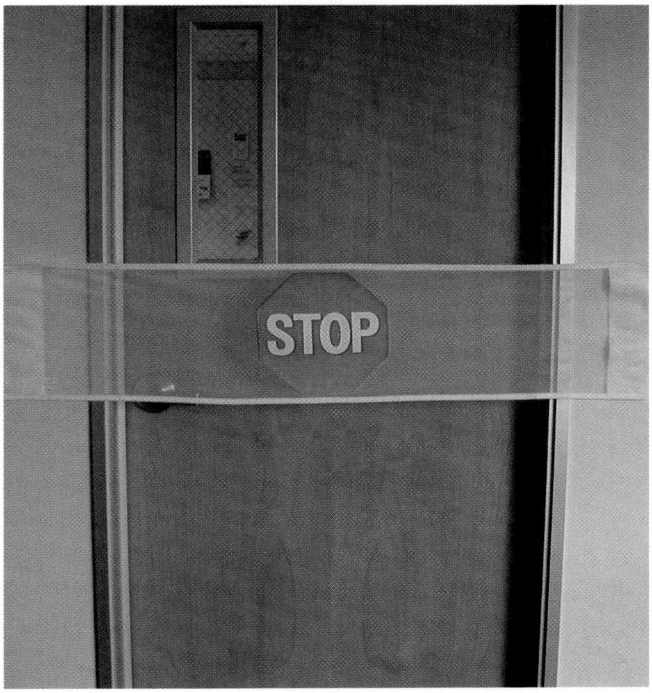

FIGURE 22–7 Barriers safely prevent clients from wandering. Some agencies use wordless, brightly coloured strips of fabric across doorways to signify an entry barrier. Most entry barriers are held in place with hook-and-loop strips on either side of the doorway. (Courtesy J.T. Posey Co., Arcadia, CA.)

Providing Compassionate Care
Understanding the Effects of Restraints on Clients

A common misunderstanding is that restraints will decrease agitated behaviour and the likelihood of one falling. In fact, restraints often make people more agitated, confused, or combative. Clients are also more likely to sustain injury when restrained. People who are restrained may not understand what is happening to them and may try to get out of the restraint. They may beg anyone who passes by to free them.

Try to put yourself in the client's situation to better understand how the client might be feeling. Imagine what it would be like to have your hands and arms restrained:

- Your nose itches, but you cannot scratch it.
- You need to use the bathroom, but you cannot get up, so you soil yourself.
- You are thirsty, but you cannot reach for your glass of water.
- You are not wearing your eyeglasses, so you cannot identify people coming into and out of your room.
- You are lying in an uncomfortable position, but you cannot turn or move in bed.
- You hear the fire alarm, but you cannot get up and move to a safe place. You must wait until someone rescues you.

What would you do? Would you calmly lie or sit there? Would you try to get free from the restraint? Would you cry out for help? What would the staff think? Would they think that you are agitated and uncooperative or just uncomfortable?

Treat a restrained client as you would want to be treated in a similar situation—with kindness, caring, respect, and dignity. Meet the client's food, fluid, and elimination needs, and make sure the client is as comfortable as possible. Restrained clients need repeated explanations and reassurance. Visit with the client often, and be a good listener. Spending time with the client may have a calming effect.

cause a change in behaviour. This reaction should be reported immediately to the supervisor.
- Is the behaviour occurring because the client has not taken the medication?
- Does the client need to urinate or defecate?
- Is clothing or a dressing tight or causing other discomfort?
- Is the client's position uncomfortable?
- Is the client too hot, too cold, hungry, or thirsty?
- Are body fluids, secretions, or excretions causing skin irritation?

- Restraint use should always be avoided. Most agencies have a "No Restraint" policy that staff must strictly adhere to. The health care providers caring for the client usually identify restraint alternatives (**BOX 22–1**), and these should become part of the care plan. As the support worker, it is your responsibility, along with that of the rest of the health care team, to follow the care plan. Changes to the care plan may be made as needed. If restraint alternatives do not protect the client, the physician may, as a last resort, order a restraint to be applied.
- Informed consent is required. Restraints cannot be used without informed consent. The client must understand the reason for the restraint. The client is told how the restraint will help in the planned

BOX 22–1 Alternatives to Restraints

- The client living at home may be moved into a facility.
- Diversion, such as TV, videos, music, games, books, relaxation tapes, back massages, exercise programs, outdoor time, and the assignment of simple tasks can calm or distract the client.
- Lifelong habits and routines—for example, showers before breakfast, walks before lunch, TV after lunch—provide comfort.
- Activities that occupy the client's time and energies (such as gardening or birdwatching) may be suggested, according to the client's care plan, needs, and abilities. Sometimes, a client who has dementia may try to do something that she "used to do" and will become agitated if confined or not allowed to do it (see the *Supporting Mr. Lee: Finding a Safe Alternative to Restraints* box for an example of a solution).
- Support workers, family, friends, and volunteers visiting with the client provide attention and companionship. Visits and observations made frequently can help keep the client calm.
- A calm, quiet setting and reduced noise levels are beneficial.
- Care should be consistent, and procedures and care measures, explained.
- The client should be encouraged to spend time in supervised areas—for example, in the lounge or near the nurses' station.
- The client can be allowed to walk around in safe areas, though the entire staff should be informed.
- Confused clients should be helped to orient themselves to people, time, and place. Place calendars and clocks so that they are easily seen by clients.
- The call bell must be within reach of the client.
- Food, fluid, and elimination needs must be met; ensure the bedpan, urinal, or commode is within reach.
- Clients who need to be toileted may demonstrate agitated behaviours. Toileting them at regular intervals will be helpful.
- Lighting should meet the client's needs and preferences.
- The client should be uninterrupted while sleeping.
- Rooms and furniture must meet safety and comfort needs (e.g., lower bed, reclining chair, cushioned walls and furniture). Use warning devices on beds, chairs, and doors, and use knob guards on doors.
- Pillows, wedge cushions, and posture and positioning aids can prevent clients from falling out of bed.

Supporting Mr. Lee: Finding a Safe Alternative to Restraints

Won Lee, a 76-year-old man, is a client in a continuing care facility. He has dementia and did not remember his wife or daughters at their last visit. Lately, he has also seemed unable to speak or understand English.

The staff members at the facility where Mr. Lee resides have noticed that he becomes very agitated in the early mornings. He has fallen several times trying to get out of bed, and more recently, before his bath, he tries to pull the towels away from the staff. He has scratched several of the support workers who have tried to remove the linens from his hands.

Support workers have tried toileting him more frequently, but nothing they have tried seems to decrease Mr. Lee's agitation. Mr. Lee has become so agitated that the staff members are afraid that he will hurt himself or others, so they suggest holding a client conference to discuss ways to safely care for Mr. Lee.

Mr. Lee's family members, his doctor, the occupational therapist, and some of the nurses and support workers who care for him attend the family conference. Mr. Lee's family members are very concerned after hearing of his increasing agitation and wish to discuss the routines he kept when he was younger. Mrs. Lee tells the staff that waking up very early to get to work had been part of her husband's routine his entire adult life. She also informs them that they used to own a large laundry company, where he had worked for over 50 years.

Mrs. Lee says that when her husband was stressed at work, he would always do something physical, such as folding linens or ironing shirts. At Mrs. Lee's suggestion, it is agreed that when he wakes up the next morning, the night staff will help Mr. Lee to get out of bed and sit by the nursing station, where he will be allowed to fold linens. It is hoped that this will "settle" him.

The next morning, when Mr. Lee begins to become agitated in his bed, the staff quickly toilet him and assist him to a chair by the nursing station, where a large laundry basket of freshly laundered towels and facecloths has been placed. Mr. Lee sits quietly and folds the linens. He is neither agitated nor aggressive, and he smiles while he is "working." Before lunchtime, he is given the opportunity to fold clients' clothing protectors and linen napkins in the dining room. The staff members are surprised at Mr. Lee's change in disposition and decide that they will maintain this new routine the next day as well to see if it continues to reduce Mr. Lee's agitation.

treatment and what the risks of restraint use are. The client has the choice to give or withhold consent. If the client is not capable of giving informed consent, a family member or substitute decision maker is given the information, and this person must decide whether or not to give consent. Only the physician or nurse can provide the necessary information and obtain informed consent.

- ***Restraints are used only in extreme cases and when necessary to prevent harm.*** Restraints can hurt a person's dignity, so they are used only after other measures fail to protect the client or others. Some clients with physical, emotional, or behavioural problems may act in ways that are harmful to themselves or others. The following are examples of harmful behaviour:
  - Mr. Gorsky, 22, suffers from a severe mental health disorder. He tries to strangle a staff member, putting her life in danger.
  - Nicole Black, 3, tries to rip out the stitches in her chest. The wound could become infected, putting her life in danger.
  - Mr. Najjar has dementia. He constantly scratches his thighs. Unfortunately, his doctors have never been able to determine why he does this, and no medication seems to help. In the past, Mr. Najjar had scratched himself so hard that he had deep, bleeding wounds on his thighs, which caused a severe skin infection requiring hospitalization.
- ***Restraints require a physician's order.*** Restraints cannot be used without consent and a physician's

order. The physician explains to the staff as well as to the client and family why the restraint is needed, which one to use, and how long to use it. This information is recorded on the care plan and on your assignment sheet.

- ***The least restrictive method is used.*** For example, most environmental restraints are less restrictive than physical restraints.
- ***The manufacturer's instructions on restraints must be followed.*** The manufacturer of a restraining device provides instructions on applying and securing it, and failure to follow these instructions could harm the client. You could be found negligent if you improperly apply or secure a restraint. ***You are never allowed to use items, such as bedsheets, that are not standard restraints to restrain a client.***
- ***Restraints are applied only by knowledgeable workers. You must receive proper training and instruction before applying restraints.*** Some facilities require you to obtain certification to apply restraints. Make sure you know what is required of you.
- ***The client's basic needs are met.*** The restraint must be snug and firm but not tight. Tight restraints affect circulation and breathing. The client must be comfortable and able to move the restrained part to a limited and safe extent. Food, fluid, comfort, exercise, and elimination needs must be met. Ensure that the client has adequate support even while staff members are taking breaks.
- ***More than one staff member may be needed to safely apply the restraint.*** Clients in immediate danger of harming themselves or others are restrained quickly. Combative and agitated clients can hurt themselves and the health care worker when restraints are being applied. Two or more workers may be needed to complete the task safely and quickly.
- ***The client's quality of life is protected.*** Restraints are used for as short a time as possible. The care plan must show how to reduce restraint use. The goal is always to meet the client's needs with as little restraint as possible. Visit with the client, and offer reassurance.
- ***The client is observed at least every 15 minutes or more often, as required by the care plan.*** Restraints can be dangerous, and injuries and deaths can occur from improper use and poor observation. Frequent observation alerts the staff to complications such as breathing and circulation problems. Practise the safety measures listed in the *Think About Safety: Safety Measures for Using Restraints* box.

Think About Safety

Safety Measures for Using Restraints

- Use the restraint specified in the care plan. The least restrictive device is used.
- Follow employer policies and procedures.
- Use only restraints that have manufacturer instructions and warning labels.
- Follow the manufacturer's instructions for snug fitting and for specific use. Some restraints are safe for use with beds, chairs, and wheelchairs, whereas some others are used only with certain equipment.
- Do not use sheets, towels, tape, rope, straps, bandages, or other items to restrain a client.
- Use only intact restraints. Check for tears, cuts, or frayed fabric or straps.
- Do not use restraints to position a client on the toilet.
- Do not use restraints to position a client on furniture that does not allow for correct application. Follow the manufacturer's instructions.
- Position the client in good body alignment before applying the restraint (see Chapter 25).
- If mitt restraints are applied, you should be able to slide one or two fingers under the restraint (**FIGURE 22-8**). Check the client's circulation every 15 minutes. You should feel a pulse at a

Continued

Think About Safety—cont'd

pulse site below the restraint. Fingers or toes should be warm and pink. Tell the nurse at once if any of the following situations arises:
   - You cannot feel a pulse.
   - The client's fingers are cold, pale, or blue.
   - The client complains of pain, numbness, or tingling in the restrained hand.
   - The client's skin is red or damaged.
- Use a belt restraint with chairs or wheelchairs. Position the client in the chair so that the hips are well to the back of the chair. Apply the belt restraint at a 45-degree angle over the hips (**FIGURE 22–9**). If a belt restraint is used, check the client at least every 15 minutes. The client should be able to breathe easily.
- Bed rails are one type of environmental restraint. Use them only if indicated in the care plan. Check with your supervisor and the care plan for instructions on when to raise or lower bed rails. According to your supervisor's instructions, use bed rail covers or gap protectors, which prevent the client from getting trapped between the rails or the bed rail bars.
- Check the client at least every 15 minutes for safety and comfort. For example, clients can easily slip down in Geri chairs and become injured.
- Remove the restraint and reposition the client every 2 hours. Meet the client's basic needs during this time, and whenever necessary do the following:
   - Meet elimination needs.
   - Give skin care.
   - Perform range-of-motion exercises or help the client ambulate (see Chapter 26). Follow the care plan.
   - Offer food and fluids.
   - Record what was done, the care given, your observations, and the time and details of what you reported to the nurse. Follow your employer policy for recording.
- Keep the call bell within the client's reach.
- Report to the nurse every time you checked the client and released the restraint. Report your observations and the care given. Follow your employer policy for reporting.

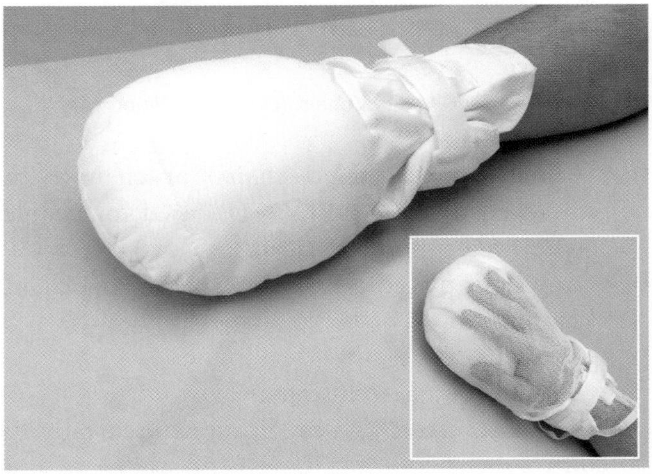

FIGURE 22–8 Mitt restraint. (Courtesy J.T. Posey Co., Arcadia, CA.)

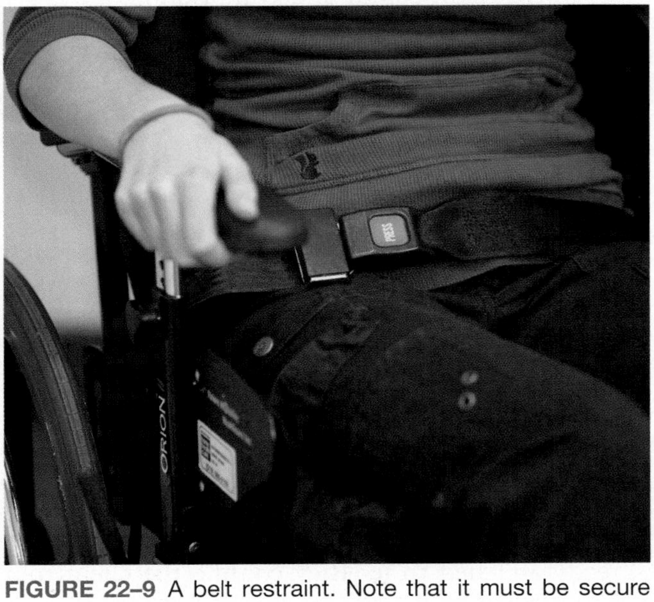

FIGURE 22–9 A belt restraint. Note that it must be secure enough to prevent sliding, but never applied too tightly. (**Source:** Brian Hillier.)

- ***The restraint is removed, the client is repositioned, and basic needs are met at least every 2 hours.*** These needs include food, fluid, elimination, skin care, and range-of-motion exercises. The client is helped to ambulate (walk) according to the care plan.
- ***Information about restraints must be recorded in the client's chart.*** When caring for restrained clients, give verbal reports to your supervisor. The following information should be charted *when the restraint is applied (or removed)*:
  - The type of restraint applied
  - The reason for the application
  - Safety measures taken, as listed in the care plan (e.g., bed rails padded and up)
  - The time you applied the restraint
  - The time you removed the restraint
  - The care given when the restraint was removed
  - Client's skin colour and condition
  - The pulse rate in the restrained part
  - Complaints of a tight restraint; difficulty breathing; and pain, numbness, or tingling in the restrained part (report these complaints to your supervisor at once)

If you are allowed to chart, include this information *when supporting a client who is restrained*:

- Safety measures taken, as listed in the care plan (e.g., bed rails padded and up)
- Client's skin colour and condition
- The pulse rate in the restrained part

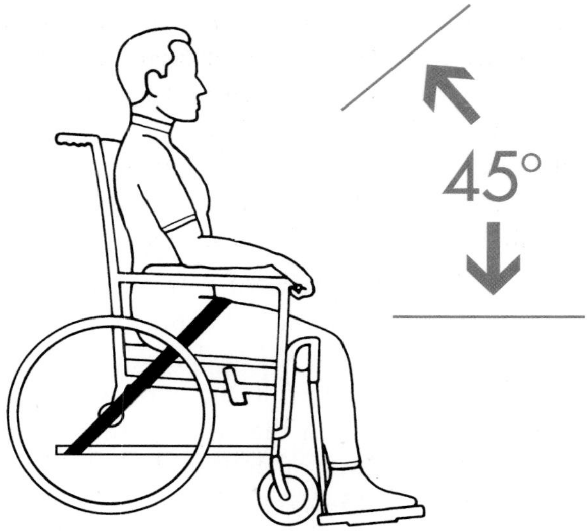

FIGURE 22–10 The safety belt is at a 45-degree angle over the hips. (Courtesy J.T. Posey Co., Arcadia, CA.)

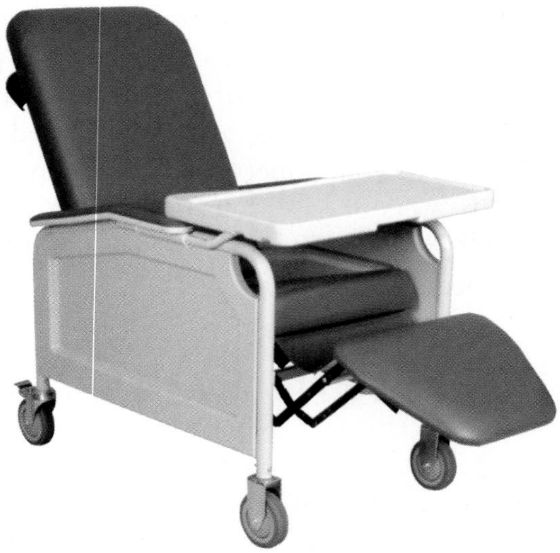

FIGURE 22–11 A Geri chair. (Courtesy Winco Mfg.)

Types of Restraints

There are three types of restraints:

1. **Physical restraints**—garments or devices used to restrict movement of the whole body or parts of the body. They are attached to a body part (e.g., a mitt restraint) or go around the client's waist and wheelchair (e.g., a belt restraint) (**FIGURE 22–10**).
2. **Environmental restraints**—barriers, furniture, or devices that prevent free movement. Environmental restraints are near the body, but not directly attached to it. They confine the client to a specific place such as a bed, chair, or room. Examples of environmental restraints include the following:
   - Geriatric chairs (Geri chairs) or chairs with attached trays (**FIGURE 22–11**), used for people who need support to sit up
   - Any chair placed close to a wall so that a client cannot move
   - Bed rails
   - Locked rooms, seclusion areas
3. **Chemical restraints**—medications used only to control behaviour or movement; they are not otherwise required for the client's medical condition. Sometimes confused and disoriented clients become anxious, agitated, or aggressive, and the physician may order medications to control these behaviours without making the client sleepy or impairing function. Like all restraints, chemical

restraints *must not be used for discipline or staff convenience.* They must not be used if they impair physical or mental function and should be used only for as long as indicated. Administering chemical restraints is out of your scope of practice, as support workers are never permitted to administer medications. Only a physician or nurse can administer chemical restraints.

Using Bed Rails

An important part of safe client care is using the **bed rails** on hospital beds correctly. Bed rails are raised and lowered according to the care plan. Bed rails are half, three-quarters, or the full length of the bed and lock in place with levers, latches, or buttons. When half-length rails are used, each side may have two rails—one for the upper part of the bed and the other for the lower part.

When to Use Bed Rails

Your supervisor and the care plan will tell you when to raise the bed rails. For example, clients who are unconscious or sedated, as well as those who are confused or disoriented, need the bed rails raised. Some clients just feel safer with the bed rails up, and some others use them to change positions in bed. If the care plan calls for raised bed rails, keep them up at all times, except when giving bedside care. Beds should also be lowered to their lowest setting, except when bedside care is given.

In the past, health care providers were taught that bed rails on a bed should always be placed up. However, having the bed rails up all the time can cause some clients to become restless. Check the client's care plan, and report any observations of increased restlessness to your supervisor.

Hazards Associated With Bed Rail Use

Bed rails present certain hazards (**FIGURE 22–12**). The client can fall while trying to climb over them, or a client can get caught, trapped, or entangled in the following gaps:

- Between the bars of the bed rail
- Between two half-length rails
- Between the bed rail and the headboard or footboard
- Between the bed rail and mattress

Injury or death can occur if the client's head, neck, chest, arm, or leg becomes trapped in these gaps.

Who Is at Greatest Risk for Injury With Bed Rails?

Clients at greatest risk are as follows:

- Clients who are confused or disoriented
- Clients who are restrained
- Small clients
- Clients who have poor muscle control or tend to have seizures

For an adult client's safety, all bed rail gaps should be no more than 10 cm (4 in.). Sometimes, padding is placed over the bed rails to cover the gaps in the rails (**FIGURE 22–13**). Gap protectors may also be used for split bed rails (**FIGURE 22–14**). Follow the manufacturer's instructions and employer policy for the use of gap protectors or padded bed rails.

Because bed rails prevent the client from getting out of bed, they are considered environmental restraints. They cannot be used unless they are needed to treat the client's medical symptoms. The client or the substitute decision maker must give consent for the use of raised bed rails. The need for bed rails must be carefully noted in the client's chart and care plan.

Check clients often when raised bed rails are used. Always adjust the bed height to its lowest position whenever bed rails are in use and whenever the client is not directly supervised by the staff. In some instances, instead of using bed rails, a client's mattress could be placed on a lower bed frame or placed directly on the floor during the night to ensure that the client will not fall out of bed, thus reducing the risk for injury. The mattress that is placed on the floor during the night would be returned to the bed in the morning to preserve the client's dignity and privacy.

How to Use Bed Rails

A number of procedures described in this book include using bed rails, so doing these procedures will help you learn how to use them correctly. However, remember that not all beds have bed rails and not all clients who have beds equipped with bed rails use them. Your supervisor, the care plan, and your assignment sheet will tell you which clients will need the use of bed rails. To give care when bed rails are used, lower the rail that is near you, and leave the

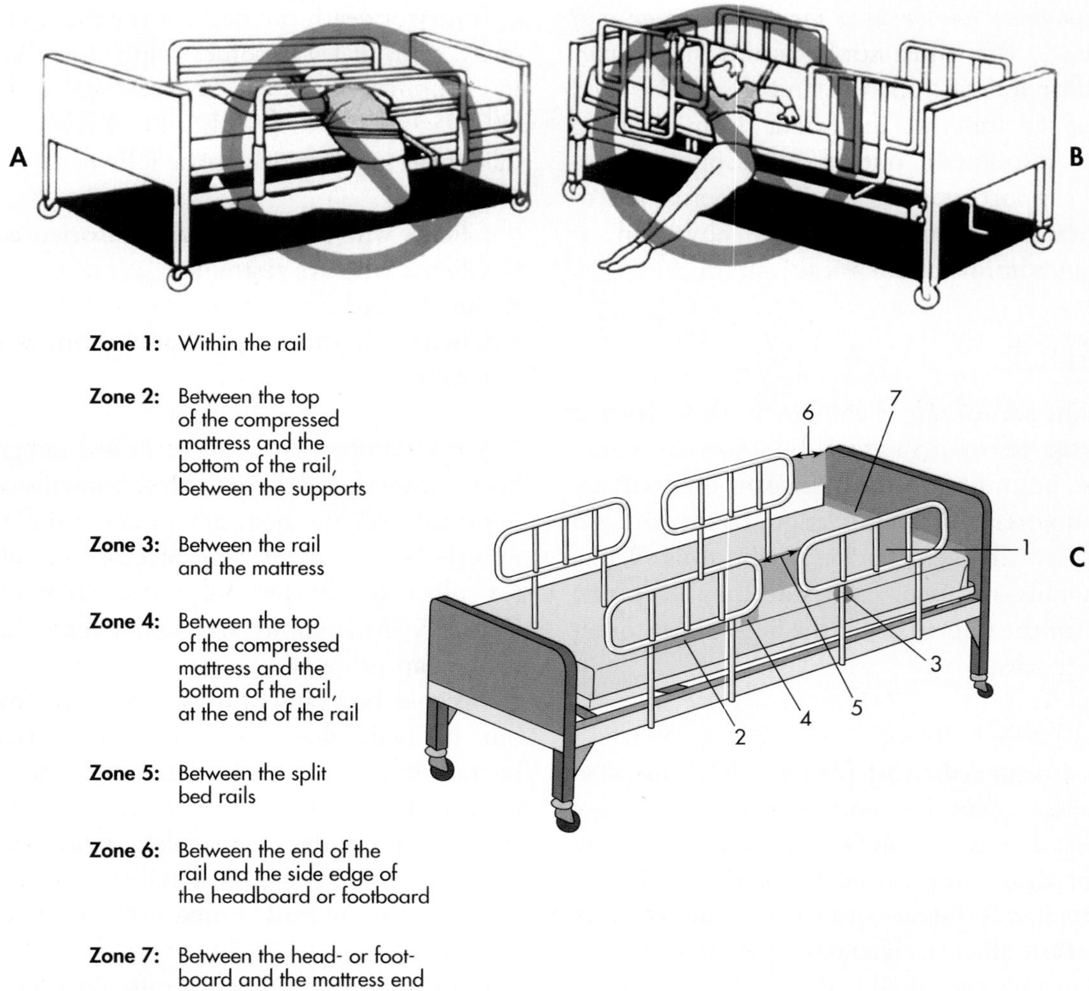

FIGURE 22–12 Bed rail hazards. **A,** The client is trapped between the bed rail bars. **B,** The client is trapped between two half-length rails. **C,** Bed rail hazard zones. (**Sources:** (for *A* and *B*) Images provided courtesy Posey Company, Arcadia, CA; (for *C*) Redrawn from Food and Drug Administration. (2006). *Guidance for industry and FDA staff: Hospital bed system dimensional and assessment guidance to reduce entrapment.*)

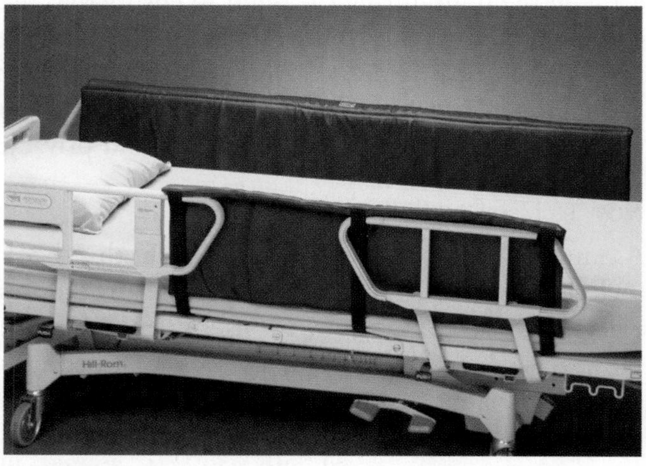

FIGURE 22–13 Padded bed rails. (Courtesy J.T. Posey Co., Arcadia, CA.)

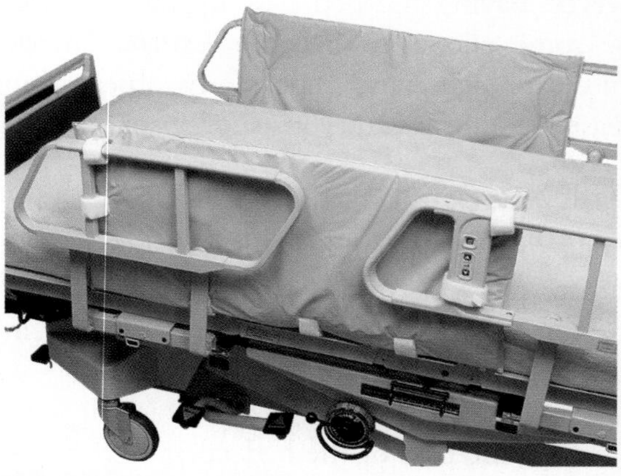

FIGURE 22–14 Gap protectors. (Courtesy J.T. Posey Co., Arcadia, CA.)

bed rail raised on the opposite side. Keep both bed rails raised if you need to leave the bedside for any reason. Remember to raise the rail again after completing the procedure.

PREVENTING POISONING

The most common ways adults are poisoned are by eating or drinking contaminated food and water and by overdosing on medications. Carelessness, confusion, and difficulty reading medication labels can lead to accidental overdose. For example, confused or disoriented adults may eat poisonous substances. Sometimes, poisoning occurs as a suicide attempt. The safety measures for children listed in Chapter 20 should be followed for adults as well (**FIGURE 22–15**). Common harmful substances include the following:

- Medications and vitamins
- Household cleaners, such as bleach; drain cleaner; floor wax; furniture polish; soaps; detergents; and toilet, window, and oven cleaners
- Personal care products, such as aftershave, rubbing alcohol, nail polish and remover, shampoo and conditioner, bath oil, bubble bath, cosmetics, perfumes, deodorant, mouthwash, diaper wipes, and baby oils and powders
- Houseplants
- Insecticides, fertilizers, and insect sprays
- Alcohol and tobacco products, including nicotine gum, patches, and sprays

What to Do if You Suspect Poisoning

In community settings, the phone number for the local poison control centre should always be posted near the telephone, programmed into your cellphone, or carried in your bag. You might suspect poisoning if you find empty pill bottles or hazardous products lying around. You might also suspect poisoning if the client suddenly collapses, vomits, or has difficulty breathing. If you suspect poisoning, follow these steps:

1. Contact the emergency medical services (EMS) for your area by dialing 9-1-1 on the telephone. The EMS operator will give you clear instructions.
2. Gather any empty pill bottles or other evidence of poisoning to determine what has been ingested and how much.
3. Stay with your client. Be sure to remain calm.

PREVENTING BURNS

Often, burns to older adults occur in the kitchen—for example, while cooking, the person may be wearing clothes with loose-fitting sleeves, which could dangle over the burner and catch fire. Bathwater and heating pads that are too hot can cause burns. Careless smoking or unattended cigarette butts in ashtrays are also common causes of burns (see the *Think About Safety: Measures to Prevent Burns* box).

A

B

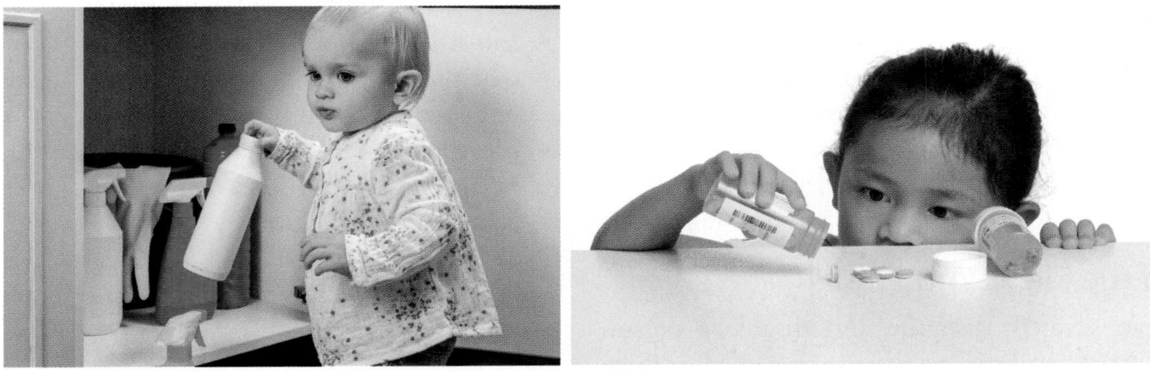

FIGURE 22–15 Harmful substances must be kept in locked areas, out of the reach of children and confused adults. **A,** Household cleaners are within reach when placed in low cabinets. **B,** The bathroom medicine chest holds many hazardous substances. (**Sources:** (for *A*) Red pepper/Shutterstock.com; (for *B*) Thomas M Perkins/Shutterstock.com.)

Think About Safety

Measures to Prevent Burns

To protect older adults and others at risk from burns, do the following:

- Educate clients about the dangers of wearing clothes with loose-fitting sleeves while cooking.
- In facilities, ensure that clients smoke only in designated smoking areas, if at all. Most facilities no longer allow smoking on their premises. Clients who smoke must be a designated distance away from the doors of the facility.
- Supervise clients who smoke and who cannot protect themselves. Some facilities insist that some or all of the clients who smoke wear "smoking jackets," which are made of nonflammable material, to prevent burns in the case of a dropped cigarette.
- Do not allow clients to smoke in bed. The client could fall asleep and drop the cigarette onto the bedsheets or on clothing and start a fire.
- Follow safety guidelines when applying heat and cold (see Chapter 44).
- Before feeding clients who cannot feed themselves, test the temperature of the food by dipping a clean spoon into the food and touching the inner aspect of your lower arm with the spoon. Remember to then place the spoon into the used cutlery container, and use a clean spoon to feed the client.
- Always test the temperature of the water in the tub, shower, or basin, with either a water thermometer or your wrist or elbow, before bathing an adult client or helping the client bathe. Check for "hot spots" in the water, and mix the water well by moving your hand back and forth in the water.
- Test the water temperature in a tub even if the tub has an electronic temperature sensor, in case it is not working properly.
- Assist clients with eating and drinking, as needed. Spilled hot foods and fluids can cause burns, which can be minor or severe.

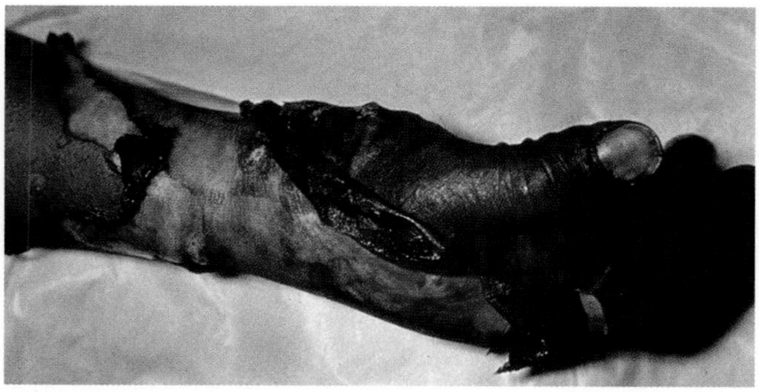

FIGURE 22–16 An example of a severe burn. (**Source:** Ignatavicius, D.D., & Workman, M.L. (2010). *Medical-surgical nursing: Critical thinking and collaborative care* (6th ed., p. 524). Philadelphia, PA: Saunders.)

Care of the Client With Burns

Burns can severely disfigure and disable a person (**FIGURE 22–16**) and can even cause death. Most burn injuries occur in the home. Infants and children as well as older adults are at highest risk. Burns are described as being *first degree* (red, painful skin that is not blistered); *second degree*, which affects the epidermis and dermis layers (resulting in pain, redness, blistering, and swelling of the skin); and *third degree*, which extends below the dermis to underlying layers and nerves (resulting in blackened, charred skin, which may be numb).

Causes of burns include the following:

- Dry heat—fire, stoves, space heaters
- Moist heat—hot liquids, steam
- Chemicals—oven cleaner, drain cleaner, rust remover, and so on
- Electricity—faulty electrical equipment, live wires, or lightning (**FIGURE 22–17**)
- Radiation—sunlight

Burns are more severe and require emergency help in the following circumstances:

- They are located on the head, face, neck, hands, feet, or genitals.
- They are spread over a large area of the body.

A

B

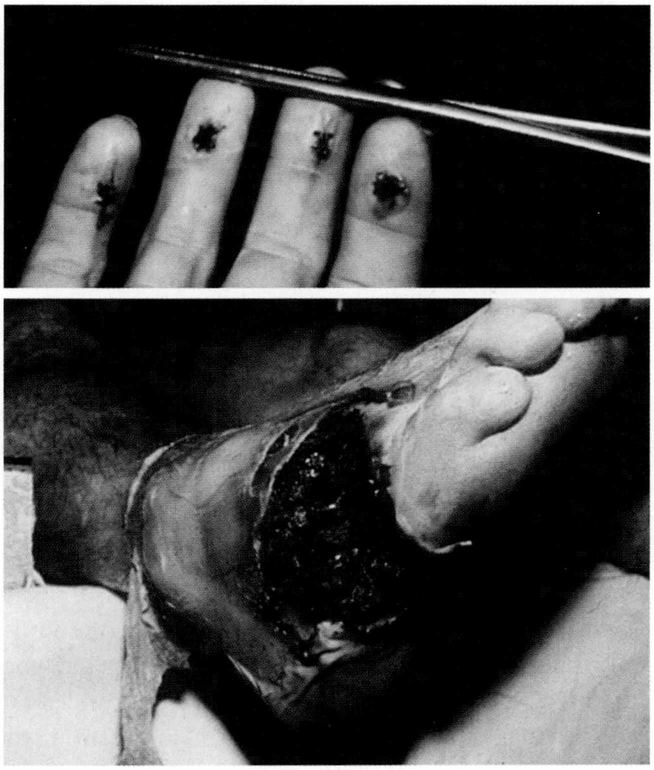

FIGURE 22–17 An electrical burn. **A,** The electrical current enters through the hand. **B,** The electrical current exits through the foot. (**Source:** Sanders, M. (1994). *Mosby's paramedic textbook.* St. Louis, MO: Mosby.)

- The burned person is under 2 or over 50 years of age or has a pre-existing medical condition (such as diabetes or hypertension).

The size and depth of the burn also affect its severity.

First Aid for Minor Burns

For minor burns that are limited to a small area, do the following:

- Immediately cool the injured area to reduce pain, swelling, blistering, and tissue damage. Immerse the area of the burn in a sink of cool water, run cool water over it, or cover it with a clean, wet, cool cloth.
- Once pain is reduced, gently pat the skin dry and cover it with a dry, lint-free, clean cloth or gauze. Secure the dressing with tape, being careful not to touch the burn with the tape.
- Do not apply oil, butter, salve, or ointments on a burn.
- Report the burn to your supervisor. Seek medical attention, if necessary.

What to Do if the Burn Appears Serious

Emergency care of severe burns includes the following:

- Activate the EMS system for your area, usually by dialing 9-1-1 by telephone.
- For *chemical burns*, carefully and quickly brush off any loose chemical powder with a cloth. Flush the area with large amounts of cool water (such as in a shower) for 15 to 20 minutes. Carefully remove contaminated clothing while flushing the area.
- For *electrical burns*, secure your safety first. Do not touch the person if he or she is still in contact with the electrical source. Have the power source turned off, or remove the electrical source first. Use an object that does not conduct electricity (rope or wood) to remove the electrical source. Do not apply water on the burn, as water may increase the risk of shock.
- For *heat source burns*, stop the burning process. Protect yourself from the source of the burn. Extinguish flames with water, or roll the person in a blanket, coat, sheet, or towel.
- Remove burned clothing that is not sticking to the skin. Do not pull at clothing if it is sticking to the burn. Remove any jewellery, tight clothing, or belts before the injured area swells.
- Administer rescue breathing and cardiopulmonary resuscitation (CPR), as needed.
- Cool the burned skin with cool water, not ice. Do not use cold water on large, third-degree burns. Do not immerse the burn in ice water. Cover the burn with a clean, cool, moist compress. (Use a towel, a sheet, or any other clean cloth.) Reapply the cool compress for up to 20 minutes (for burns on the hands, feet, or face) or up to 1 hour (for second-degree burns). Pat the area dry.
- Loosely cover the burn wounds with a clean, dry covering. Thick, sterile gauze is preferable, but you can use towels, sheets, or any other clean cloth. Tape the covering in place, being careful not to touch the burn with the tape.
- Do not put oil, butter, salve, or ointments on the burn.

- Do not break the blisters.
- Cover the client with a blanket or coat to prevent heat loss.
- Watch for signs of shock:
  - Lack of alertness
  - Loss of consciousness
  - Rapid heartbeat, weak pulse, and rapid breathing
  - Sweating, paleness
  - Rapid breathing
  - Decreased or no urine output
- Stay with the client until help arrives.

PREVENTING SUFFOCATION

Suffocation occurs when breathing stops due to lack of oxygen. Brain damage or death may occur, depending on how long the person has been deprived of oxygen, sometimes within 3 to 4 minutes. Common causes of suffocation include choking, drowning, inhaling gas or smoke, strangulation, and electrical shock. Children under 1 year, clients who have difficulties chewing and swallowing, and clients with serious mobility disorder or intellectual disability are at risk for suffocation (see the *Think About Safety: Measures to Prevent Suffocation in Adults* box).

Carbon Monoxide Poisoning

Carbon monoxide (CO), also sometimes known as the "silent killer," is a colourless, odourless, tasteless gas, produced by the burning of material containing carbon, such as in common household appliances or fireplaces. CO is also present in car exhaust fumes, so vehicles running in confined spaces can cause CO poisoning. When automobiles, appliances, or fireplaces are not properly ventilated, carbon monoxide can build up in the air and enter the bloodstream of the unsuspecting people or animals that inhale the air. They have no idea what is happening to them—that this gas, instead of oxygen, is quickly binding to the hemoglobin in their red blood cells, which can be fatal (see Chapter 41).

Early symptoms of carbon monoxide poisoning—such as headaches, nausea, and fatigue—are often mistaken for flu symptoms because this deadly gas goes undetected in a home. Prolonged exposure can lead to brain damage and even death. As in suffocation, the person dies from a lack of oxygen to the brain.

Carbon Monoxide Detectors

Carbon monoxide detectors are strongly recommended for all homes, especially in areas of the home

Think About Safety

Measures to Prevent Suffocation in Adults

- When feeding adult clients, do not rush them. Cut food into small, bite-sized pieces for those who cannot do so themselves.
- Observe and report any indication that the client is having difficulty swallowing, such as drooling, pocketing food, or coughing (see Chapter 28).
- If the client has had any of the above signs of swallowing difficulties, choose foods that he can easily swallow. Note that foods such as canned peaches might easily become lodged in the client's throat during eating.
- Make sure the client's dentures fit properly and are in place. Report any loose teeth or dentures.
- Before serving any food or fluids, check the care plan about dealing with clients' swallowing problems. Clients may ask for something that they cannot swallow.
- Tell your supervisor at once if the client has problems swallowing.
- Do not give food or fluids orally to clients with feeding tubes, unless it is stated in their care plan. Remember that all clients who are NPO (not by mouth) for any reason must not receive foods or fluids orally.
- Open doors and windows if you notice gas odours. Immediately report gas odours to your supervisor, or dial 9-1-1 if the odour is strong. Assist your client to move out of the area.
- Position the client in bed properly (see Chapter 25).
- Use bed rails properly (see pp. 397–399).

where the family members gather and spend the most time, such as kitchens and bedrooms. It is important that the manufacturer's instructions are followed and that the devices are checked periodically to ensure that they work properly. Some CO detectors are connected to household electricity (they may be hard-wired or plugged in), and some work on batteries. Batteries must be replaced routinely, according to manufacturer's instructions. Carbon monoxide detectors are inexpensive, but they can save lives!

PREVENTING ACCIDENTS WITH EQUIPMENT

As a support worker, you will be required to use equipment such as household appliances, mechanical lifting devices, wheelchairs, and walkers in clients' homes as well as in facilities. All equipment is unsafe if broken, not used correctly, or not working properly.

When using any type of equipment, you must know what you are doing. You also must make sure that the equipment is in safe working order (see the *Think About Safety: Measures to Prevent Equipment Accidents* box).

PREVENTING FIRES

Fires are a constant danger in homes and facilities. Unsafe smoking, cooking accidents, faulty electrical equipment and wiring, and heating equipment are major causes. The entire health care team must be vigilant to prevent fires (see the *Think About Safety: Fire Prevention Measures* and the *Focus on Home Care: Fire Safety* boxes).

Think About Safety

Measures to Prevent Equipment Accidents

- Follow your employer's policies and procedures.
- Follow the manufacturer's instructions.
- Read all cautions and warning labels.
- Do not use unfamiliar equipment. Ask for needed training. Ask for supervision the first time you use the item.
- Use equipment only for its intended purpose.
- Inspect all equipment before use. Check for broken or damaged parts. Check for cracks, chips, rough or sharp edges, or loose bolts and screws. These defects can cause cuts, stabs, or scratches. Do not use or give damaged items to clients.
- Notify your supervisor immediately about the broken equipment. Follow your employer's policies for reporting equipment in need of repair or equipment-related accidents.
- Do not try to repair broken equipment yourself.
- Make sure electrical cords are not frayed or damaged in any way (**FIGURE 22–18**). Make sure that not too many cords are plugged into one electrical outlet (**FIGURE 22–19**). Frayed cords and overloaded electrical outlets can cause electric shocks.
- Inspect electrical equipment to ensure that the plug's grounding prong was not removed. Three-pronged plugs (**FIGURE 22–20**) are designed to allow two of the prongs to carry the electrical current, while the third prong grounds the current and carries leaking electricity to the earth and away from the item, preventing electric shocks.
- Stop using any electrical equipment and ***immediately report it*** to your supervisor in the following cases:
  - It gives you a shock.
  - It produces sparks, buzzing sounds, or a burning odour.
  - Lights dim or flicker.
  - The power shuts down.
- Immediately report any shock received while using a piece of equipment.
- Keep electrical equipment away from water (water conducts electricity).
- Hold on to the plug (not the cord) when removing it from an outlet.
- Turn off equipment when you are finished using it.

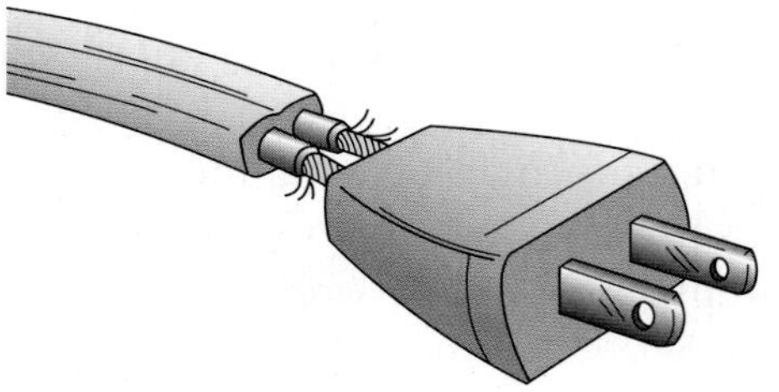

FIGURE 22–18 A frayed electrical cord.

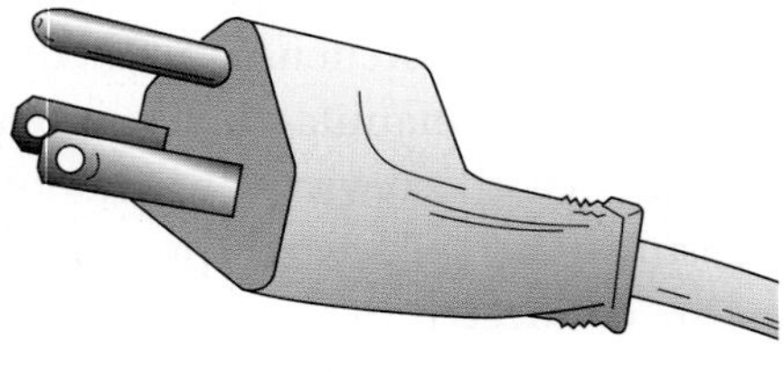

FIGURE 22–20 A three-pronged plug.

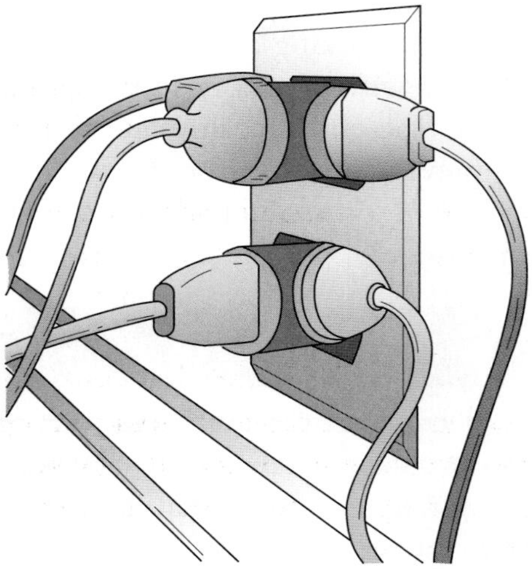

FIGURE 22–19 An overloaded electrical outlet.

FOCUS ON HOME CARE

Fire Safety

It is essential to have working smoke detectors on every floor of the home and ideally outside each sleeping area. Always identify all smoke detectors in clients' homes, and make sure they are working. Notify your supervisor and the family if you find a smoke detector that is not working.

Think About Safety

Fire Prevention Measures

- Smoke only in areas where smoking is allowed. Do not smoke in the client's home.
- Supervise clients who smoke. Supervision is very important for clients who are confused, disoriented, or sedated.
- Provide ashtrays for clients who are allowed to smoke.
- Check smoking areas, especially furniture, for dropped cigarettes and ashes.
- Be sure all ashes, cigars, and cigarettes are put out before emptying ashtrays.
- Empty ashtrays into a metal container partially filled with sand or water. Do not empty them into plastic containers or wastebaskets lined with paper or plastic bags.
- Do not allow clients to smoke in bed or while lying down; they could fall asleep and drop a lit cigarette onto the sheets or cushion, starting a fire.
- Do not light matches or lighters or smoke around flammable liquids or materials.
- Keep matches and lighters out of the reach of children.
- Avoid deep-frying in oil, since oil is highly flammable. If you must deep-fry, use a deep-fryer rather than a shallow pan.
- Do not drape tea towels or other material over the oven door.
- Use potholders to remove hot items from the oven. Do not use tea towels.
- Follow the manufacturer's instructions when using space heaters. Keep them at least 1 m

Continued

Think About Safety—cont'd

(3 ft.) away from curtains, drapes, and furniture, and do not leave them unattended.
- Keep flammable liquids and materials away from fireplaces, radiators, heat registers, and other sources of heat or flame.
- Store flammable liquids in their original containers.
- Do not run electrical cords under carpets.
- Use extension cords only as a temporary measure.
- Prevent equipment accidents. Follow the guidelines in the *Think About Safety: Measures to Prevent Equipment Accidents* box.
- Follow the safety measures for oxygen use (see the *Think About Safety: Safety Guidelines for Oxygen Therapy* box in Chapter 41).

Fires and the Use of Oxygen

Some clients have difficulty breathing or do not receive enough oxygen from the air, so oxygen therapy is prescribed by physicians. Oxygen therapy provides additional oxygen through a nasal tube or face mask. The oxygen is supplied through portable oxygen tanks, wall outlets, or oxygen concentrators (see Chapter 41).

Oxygen systems are widely used in facilities and in home care. However, oxygen is a serious fire hazard, as it supports combustion (see the *Think About Safety: Using Oxygen Equipment Properly* box on page 406). Therefore, you should ensure that combustible items (such as petroleum jelly on the client's lips, or clothing, towels, and sheets that are static charged) are kept away from the source of the oxygen to reduce the risk of a fire. Special safety measures are needed where oxygen is used and stored (see the *Think About Safety: Fire Prevention Measures* box).

What to Do During a Fire

The health care team must act quickly and responsibly during a fire. The key to surviving a fire is to be prepared before one starts. Know your employer's policies and procedures for fire emergencies. Know where to find fire alarms, fire extinguishers, and emergency exits. Facilities conduct fire drills to practise emergency fire procedures (see the *Focus on Home Care: Being Prepared for a Fire* box).

The acronym *RACE* will help you remember what to do if you discover a fire in a home or a facility:

R—for **R**escue. Rescue people in immediate danger. Move them to a safe place.

A—for **A**larm. Sound the nearest fire alarm. Notify the switchboard operator. Or call 9-1-1 if in a client's home.

C—for **C**onfine. Close doors and windows to confine the fire. Turn off oxygen or electrical equipment in use in the general area of the fire.

E—for **E**xtinguish or **E**vacuate. Use a fire extinguisher on a small fire that has not spread to a larger area. If the fire cannot be easily extinguished, evacuation will be necessary. Always keep equipment away from all exits so exits remain passable.

Using a Fire Extinguisher

In some facilities, only supervisory or registered staff are allowed to use a fire extinguisher, whereas in others, all employees are required to demonstrate use of a fire extinguisher. It is your responsibility to know the rules of your agency and to receive the proper training regarding the use of a fire extinguisher. Fire extinguishers are readily available in facilities; however, home care clients should also have them available. If the client has a fire extinguisher in the home, identify it and make sure that (1) the pin is intact, (2) the plastic seal is secured to the body of the extinguisher, and (3) the pressure dial reads "full." Notify your supervisor and the family if the fire extinguisher does not have any of these components.

Never attempt to fight a large or spreading fire with an extinguisher. Fire extinguishers are useful only against small fires that have not spread from where they started—for example, a wastebasket or a cushion. Do not use a fire extinguisher on a fire that is fed by gas or flammable liquid.

Think About Safety

Using Oxygen Equipment Properly

- Never smoke around oxygen equipment. Remove all items related to smoking (such as ashtrays and lighters) from the room.
- "No Smoking" and "Oxygen in Use" signs should be placed on the front door of the client's home, apartment, or room and near the area where the oxygen is being directly used. Some people ignore such rules; however, be sure to remind the client, family, and visitors never to smoke around oxygen equipment.
- Keep oxygen tanks away from open flames (such as pilot lights, candles, and incense) and heat sources (such as stoves, heating ducts, radiators, and space heaters).
- Remove from the room materials that can ignite easily—for example, alcohol, nail polish remover, oils, and greases.
- Make sure the client does not use toiletry items that are flammable, such as perfume, petroleum jelly, hairspray, and aftershave lotion, when receiving oxygen.
- Turn off electrical items before unplugging them. Sparks can occur when electrical items are unplugged while still on.
- Use electrical equipment, including shavers, hair dryers, radios, and stereo equipment, only if the prongs are intact and the equipment is in good working order.
- The oxygen source should be shut off and removed from the client prior to shaving the client with an electric shaver, drying a client's hair with a blow dryer, or using a curling iron on the client's hair because of the risk of sparks from such equipment.
- Remove all wool and synthetic fabrics from the room because they could create static electricity. Wear cotton uniforms, and use cotton blankets and clothing for the client.
- Have the phone numbers of the oxygen supply company readily available in the event of an emergency.

FOCUS ON HOME CARE

Being Prepared for a Fire

Plan what to do in each client's home before a fire occurs. The first time you enter a client's home, plan two fire escape routes from every room. If the client lives in an apartment building, identify the fire alarms in the hallways in case you ever need to use them.

Types of Fire Extinguishers

Different extinguishers are used for different kinds of fires. Use the ABCs to remember the types of extinguishers:

- Class A: **A**sh. Materials that burn and leave ash, such as paper and wood.
- Class B: **B**urn/**B**oil. Materials that can burn or boil, such as oil and grease.
- Class C: **C**urrent. Materials that have an electric current, causing electrical fires.

Using the wrong extinguisher on a fire makes the fire worse. A number of extinguishers are multipurpose ones, designed to fight all types of fires. Learn how to use a fire extinguisher *before* an emergency, and when you must use a fire extinguisher, remember the acronym *PASS* (**FIGURES 22–21 and 22–22**).

P—Pull the pin out.
A—Aim at the base of the fire.
S—Squeeze the handle.
S—Sweep from side to side, spraying the contents of the extinguisher.

Evacuating

When evacuating a facility or a home, several safety measures apply (**BOX 22–2**). Facilities have evacuation policies and procedures. If evacuation is necessary,

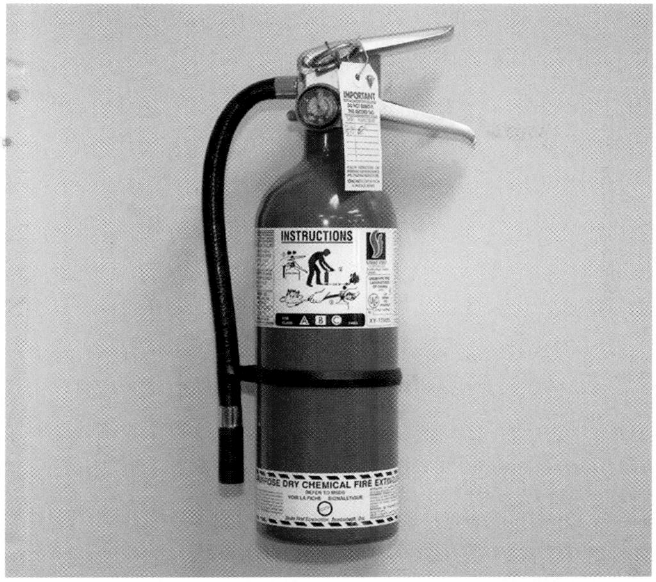

FIGURE 22–21 A typical fire extinguisher. (**Source:** Brian Hillier.)

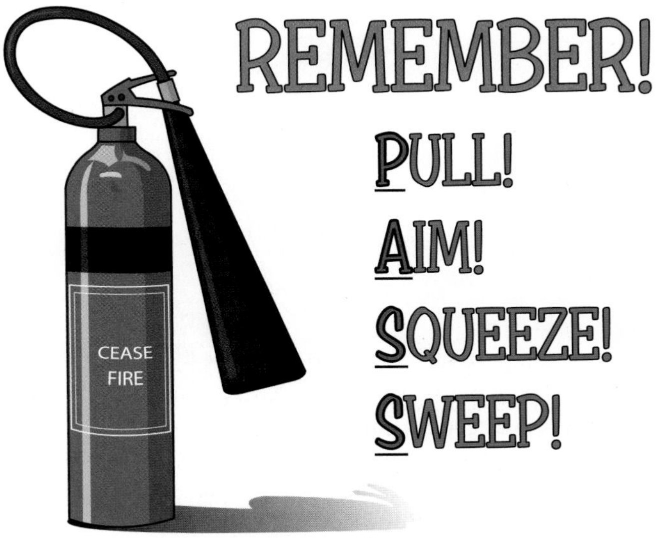

FIGURE 22–22 P.A.S.S.

clients closest to the danger are taken out first. Those who can walk are given blankets to wrap around themselves and escorted by a staff member to a safe place. FIGURE 22–23 and FIGURE 22–24 show how to rescue people who cannot walk. ***Remember that these procedures are for emergency evacuation only and are not intended to be used routinely to move a client.*** Once firefighters arrive, they direct the rescue efforts.

BOX 22–2 Important Information About Evacuating in the Event of a Fire

- Never use elevators when there is a fire in the building. Elevators can quickly fill with smoke and may stop working if there is a power outage.
- Touch doors before opening them. Do not open a hot door. Use another way out. If the door is cool, open it carefully. If heat and smoke rush in, shut the door again.
- If smoke is present, look for another escape route that is smoke-free. If you must exit through smoke, cover your nose and mouth with a damp cloth. Do the same for the client and family. Have everyone crawl to the nearest exit to stay below the smoke.
- If your clothes catch on fire, do not run. Drop to the ground, cover your face, and roll to smother the flames. If possible, wrap a rug or blanket around yourself. If a client's clothing is on fire, get the client to roll on the floor until the fire is out. Alternatively, cover the person with a blanket or coat; start by protecting the client's head and neck, and then lay out the blanket or coat over the burning area. Pat the burning area until the fire goes out.
- Once you and your client get out of the burning building, do not go back in.
- If you get trapped by fire or smoke in a room, shut the door and block any gaps, such as under a door, with blankets or other thick material that will keep smoke from entering the room. If possible, call 9-1-1 or the fire department and tell them exactly where you are in the building. Go to the window and shout for help, and hang a large piece of material such as a towel, sheet, or clothing from the window to attract the firefighters' attention.

USING THE CALL BELL

Call bells are important safety devices for clients in facilities such as hospitals and long-term care residences. A **call bell** enables a client to call for assistance. Different facilities use different call systems. The term *call bell* is used in this book when

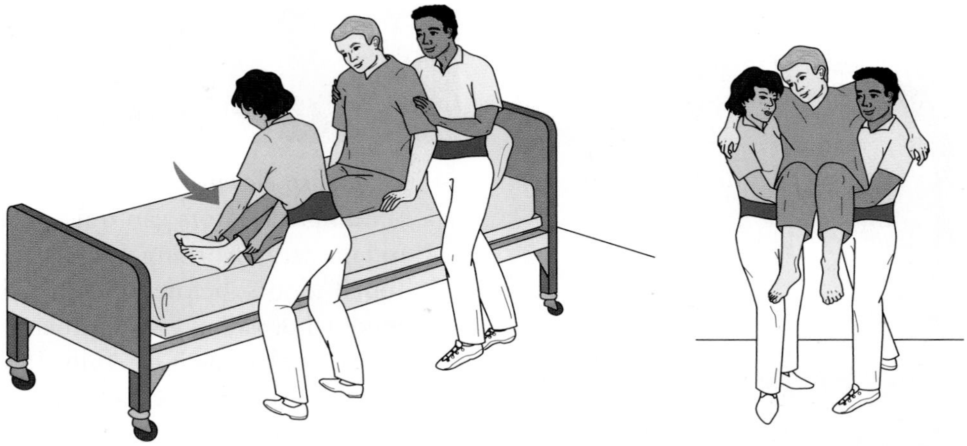

FIGURE 22–23 Swing carry technique. **A,** Assist the client to a sitting position. As a co-worker grasps the client's ankles, you work together to turn the client so that he sits on the side of the bed. **B,** Pull the client's arm over your shoulder. With one arm, reach across the client's back to your co-worker's shoulder. Reach under the client's knees and grasp your co-worker's arm. Your co-worker does the same.

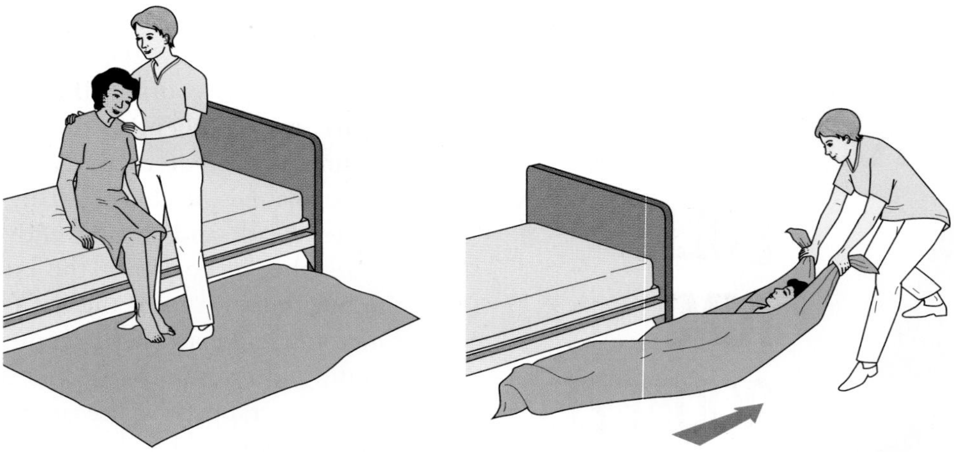

FIGURE 22–24 One-rescuer carry. **A,** Spread a blanket on the floor. Make sure the blanket will extend beyond the client's head. Help the client sit on the side of the bed. Place one of your knees on the bed near the client's side. From behind the client's back, grasp the client under the arms with both of your arms, and cross your hands over her chest. Lower the client to the floor by sliding her down one of your legs. **B,** Wrap the blanket around the client. Grasp the blanket over the head area. Pull the client to a safe area.

referring to any one of a number of call systems that a facility may use. Most systems consist of a cord that is attached to the bed or a chair. A button is at the end of the cord (FIGURE 22–25). To get help, the client presses the button, which causes a signal to ring at the nurses' station. Or pressing the button may turn on a light above the client's door and at the nurses' station (FIGURE 22–26, *A*). These signals alert the health care team that the client needs assistance.

Some call bells are also connected to an intercom at the nurses' station (see FIGURE 22–26, *B*). Using the intercom, a support worker or a nurse can talk with the client who has called for help. In newer facilities, the call bell system may be directly connected to cordless phones carried by the staff. As a support worker in the facility, you would respond directly to the client by phone, and the client can tell you what is needed. However, be careful when using an intercom or a cellphone, as people nearby can hear

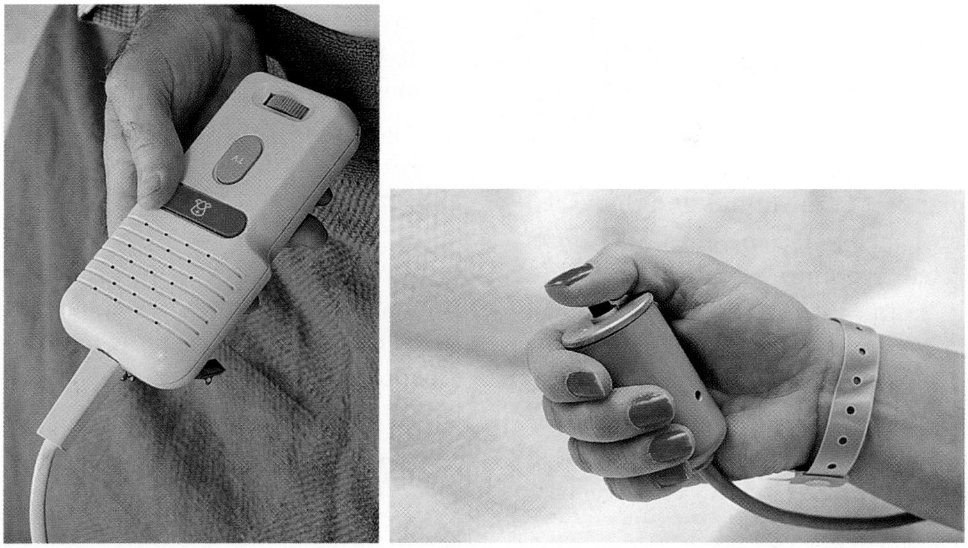

FIGURE 22–25 Clients press the call bell button when needing assistance.

A

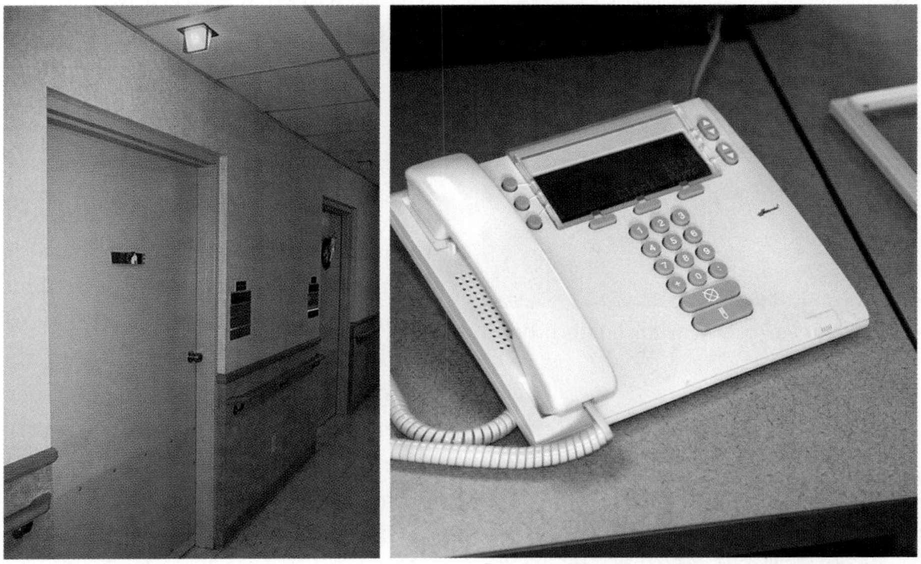

B

FIGURE 22–26 **A,** The light above the door of the client's room. **B,** Light panel of intercom system at the nurses' station. In newer facilities, the call bell may be directly connected to a cordless phone carried by the staff. The support worker would then respond to the client by phone. (**Source** (for *B*)**:** Brian Hillier.)

what you say; keep in mind the client's right to confidentiality.

Clients with limited hand mobility may need a special call bell that is turned on by tapping it with a hand or fist (**FIGURE 22–27**).

Clients are taught how to use the call bell when admitted to a facility. Some clients, however—for example, clients who are confused or in a coma—cannot use call bells. Check the care plan carefully for special communication methods for these clients. Check on them often, and make sure that their needs are met (see the *Focus on Home Care: Call Bells* box).

Whenever you finish a procedure and leave the client's room, make sure the call bell is within the client's reach. You must do the following:

- Keep the call bell within the client's reach in the room, bathroom, and shower or tub room. Even if the client cannot use the call bell, keep it within

FOCUS ON HOME CARE

Call Bells

Some home care clients are unable to move out of bed or a particular part of the home, and they need a way to call for help. Tap bells, dinner bells (**FIGURE 22–28**), baby monitors, and other devices are all useful in home care settings. Or you can give the client a small can with a few coins inside that can be rattled to get your attention. Children's toys with bells, horns, and whistles may also be useful. Whatever the client decides to use, keep the calling device within the client's easy reach.

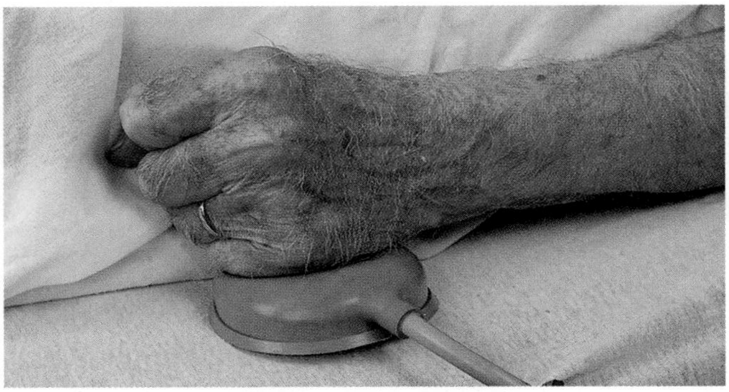

FIGURE 22–27 Call bell for a client with limited hand mobility.

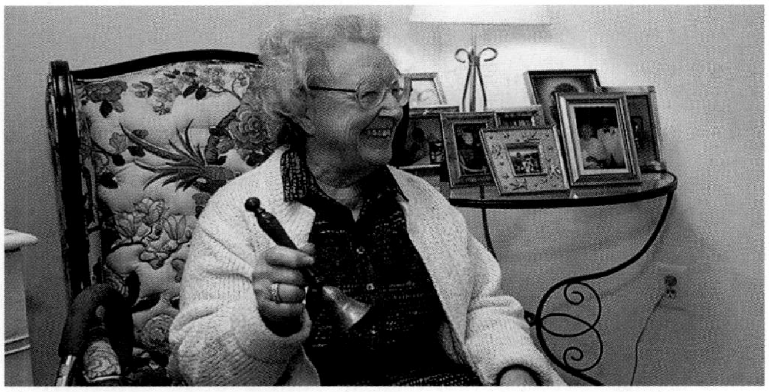

FIGURE 22–28 This woman rings a dinner bell when she needs assistance at home.

reach of visitors and staff, as they may need to call for help.

- Place the call bell on the client's strong (unaffected) side.
- Remind the client to use the call bell when help is needed.
- Answer call bells promptly. The client may have an urgent need to use the bathroom. You can prevent the client's embarrassment by promptly helping her to the bathroom. A prompt response also helps prevent infection, skin breakdown, pressure ulcers, and falls.

Leaving a client without a call bell can be considered by the client to be negligence or punishment. It is certainly regarded as emotional abuse (see Chapter 16).

PROMOTING YOUR PERSONAL SAFETY

As a support worker, you are sometimes exposed to safety hazards on the job. You could have an accident if your workplace environment is not safe. You could be injured when working with hazardous materials. You might also be at risk for workplace violence.

Creating a Safe Workplace

In Canada, each province and territory has occupational health and safety (OH&S) legislation. **OH&S legislation** is designed to protect employees from injuries and accidents in the workplace. The name of this legislation varies across the country but, in most places, is called the *Occupational Health and Safety Act* (http://www.canoshweb.org/en/legislation.html). It is revised regularly to reflect changes in policies.

The details of the legislation also vary from one place to another, but the basic elements are similar. In general, the legislation assumes that all people in the workplace—employers, supervisors, and workers—are responsible for their own health and safety and also have certain rights and duties.

Employers' and Supervisors' Responsibilities

According to OH&S legislation, your employer and supervisor must take every reasonable precaution to protect your health and safety (see the *Focus on Home Care: OH&S Legislation* box).

Your employer is responsible for the following:

- Having written policies that promote safety
- Training and educating you about these policies

> **FOCUS ON HOME CARE**
>
> **OH&S Legislation**
>
> When you are providing services to a home care client, the client's home is considered a workplace, and the home care agency is considered your employer. Therefore, agencies have the same obligations to provide for the safety of their employees as facilities do.

- Creating a health and safety committee to identify hazards in the workplace and investigate accidents
- Responding to reports of workplace hazards
- Warning you about safety hazards and correcting these hazards, whenever possible
- Reporting all accidents promptly to the government department responsible for occupational health and safety
- Making sure that all necessary equipment (including personal protective equipment such as gloves and masks) is available and is kept in good working order

Employees' Responsibilities

You are responsible for the following:

- Following all safety policies and procedures
- Using all recommended protective equipment and clothing
- Reporting all safety hazards and concerns immediately to your supervisor or a representative of your health and safety committee
- Completing an **incident report** (also known as an **occurrence report**). This report is submitted to an employer whenever an accident, error, or unexpected problem arises in the workplace. **FIGURE 22–29** shows an example of a generic incident report. Your agency's incident reports may differ slightly.

According to the OH&S legislation, you have the right to refuse to do unsafe work. This right applies whether you are working in a facility or in a community setting. However, you cannot refuse to work if (1) the danger is a normal part of the job and (2) your refusal would endanger the client. For example, you could not refuse to provide care to a client with a communicable disease because you are afraid of getting the disease. However, you could refuse to provide care to a client with a communicable disease if protective gloves, masks, and gowns are not available.

Handling Hazardous Materials

A **hazardous material** is any substance that presents a physical hazard or a health hazard in the workplace. *Physical hazards* can cause fires or explosions. *Health hazards* are chemicals that can cause acute or chronic health problems—for example, kidney or lung damage, cancer, or burns. Support workers may work with or around hazardous materials in some settings—for example, the following:

- Drugs used in cancer therapy (chemotherapy, anticancer drugs)
- Gases used to sterilize equipment
- Oxygen used in oxygen therapy
- Certain disinfectants and cleaning solutions

OH&S legislation requires that health care employees understand the risk of hazardous materials and know how to handle them safely. To provide this information, the Canadian government created the **Workplace Hazardous Materials Information System (WHMIS)** and has aligned with the Globally Harmonized System of Classification and Labelling for chemicals (GHS). WHMIS is a comprehensive system for providing health and safety information on the safe use of hazardous products used in Canadian workplaces. It includes hazard identification and product classification, cautionary labelling of containers, the provision of material safety data sheets (MSDSs), and worker education and training programs. The key duties of suppliers, employers, and workers in regard to WHMIS are listed below. For more details about WHMIS and GHS, visit the Canadian Centre for Occupational Health and Safety website.

Suppliers' Duties Under WHMIS[2]

Suppliers, the organizations that sell or import hazardous products, must ensure the appropriate

Find information about hazardous material in the MSDS binder.
Check MSDS for directions on how to clean up a hazardous
Spill

REPORT OF INCIDENT AND INJURY

PLEASE PRINT IN INK To be completed by Employee

Employer ______________________ Location ______________________

Name of Client ______________________ Identification No. ______________________

Birth Date ______________ Sex ☐ Male ☐ Female Telephone (   ) ______________

Name of employee (if incident included them) ______________________ Shift ______________

Occupation ______________________ Department ______________________

If you did see incident occur:

Date of incident ______________ Time of incident ______________ ☐ am ☐ pm

Describe what caused the injury/symptoms, what you were doing just before the incident, and what you did after the incident (if you need more space, write on the back of this form). Be specific – name any objects or substances involved:

____

____

____

Describe what you saw:

____

____

____

Did anyone else see the incident? ☐ Yes ☐ No If yes, who? ______________________

Did you report this incident to anyone? ☐ Yes ☐ No If not, why not? ______________________

If yes, to whom did you report it? ______________ Title/Position ______________ When? ________

What part(s) of the body was/were affected? (BE SPECIFIC: for example, right elbow, left knee, right index finger)

____

What type of injury resulted? (BE SPECIFIC: for example, bruise, scrape, laceration, pull)

____

Was any first aid provided at the scene? ☐ Yes ☐ No If yes, describe: ______________________

Was other medical treatment sought? ☐ Yes ☐ No If yes, when? ______________________

Where? ______________________ If treatment was not sought immediately, explain why:

____

If this injury happened to you: Is this an aggravation of a previous injury/symptom? ☐ Yes ☐ No If yes, when were you last treated for the previous injury? ______________ By whom or where? ______________

Have you ever had a similar injury? ☐ Yes ☐ No If yes, describe other injury: ______________________

____

FIGURE 22–29 A sample incident report. (Courtesy St. Joseph's at Fleming, Peterborough, ON.)

classification of hazardous products. When a product is considered to be a "hazardous product," the supplier must label the product or container and must provide a safety data sheet (SDS) to its customers. The purpose of the label is to clearly identify the hazardous product, the supplier, the hazards, and precautionary measures. The SDS provides more information about that product.

Employers' Duties Under WHMIS[2]

- Educate and train workers on the hazards and safe use of products
- Ensure that hazardous products are properly labelled
- Prepare workplace labels, as needed
- Prepare SDSs, as necessary (e.g., if an employer manufactures a hazardous product that is used on-site)
- Provide access to up-to-date SDSs to workers
- Ensure appropriate control measures are in place to protect the health and safety of workers

Workers' Duties Under WHMIS[2]

- Participate in WHMIS education and training programs
- Take necessary steps to protect themselves and their co-workers
- Participate in identifying and controlling hazards

Consumer Products' Use in the Workplace

Consumer products are those products that can be purchased in a store and are generally intended for use in the home. They include cleaning products, adhesives, or lubricants. These products are labelled according to other legislation, not covered by WHMIS.

A comprehensive chemical safety program would include both hazardous products as regulated by WHMIS and any other products that a worker may be exposed to (including consumer products). Workers should receive education and training for safe use of all these products.

Components of the WHMIS Labels

WHMIS labels provide the essential information needed to handle a controlled product safely (**FIGURE 22–30**), including hazard pictograms representing the kind of danger the product presents (**FIGURE 22–31**).

Read and follow all warning labels. A container must have a label, and this label must not be removed

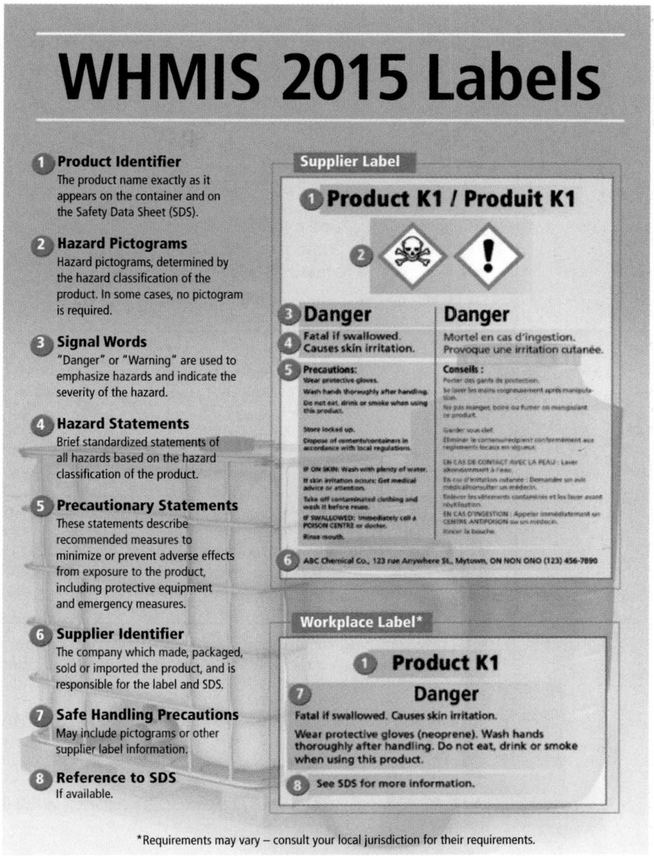

FIGURE 22–30 Sample WHMIS 2015 labels. (**Source:** Canadian Centre for Occupational Health and Safety. (2015) Retrieved October 12, 2015 from http://www.ccohs.ca/products/posters/pdfs/labelElements.pdf. Canadian Centre for Occupational Health and Safety (CCOHS), 2015. Reproduced with the permission of CCOHS, 2016.)

or damaged in any way. If a warning label is removed or damaged, do not use the product. Take the container to your supervisor and explain the problem. Do not leave the container unattended.

The supplier label contains the product identifier, hazard pictograms, signal words, hazard statements, and precautionary statements. Workplace labels provide the product identifier, safe handling precautions, and a reference to the SDS.

Reducing Personal Security Risks

Workplace violence is any physical assault or threatening behaviour that occurs in a work setting. It includes the following:

- Psychological trauma—threat, obscene phone call, and harassment of any nature (e.g., being followed, sworn at, or shouted at)

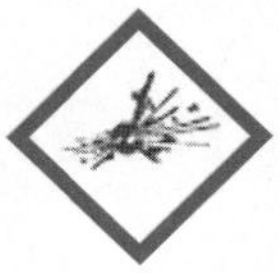	**Exploding bomb** (for explosion or reactivity hazards)		**Flame** (for fire hazards)		**Flame over circle** (for oxidizing hazards)
	**Gas cylinder** (for gases under pressure)	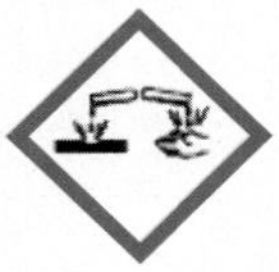	**Corrosion** (for corrosive damage to metals, as well as skin, eyes)		**Skull and Crossbones** (can cause death or toxicity with short exposure to small amounts)
	**Health hazard** (may cause or suspected of causing serious health effects)		**Exclamation mark** (may cause less serious health effects or damage the ozone layer*)	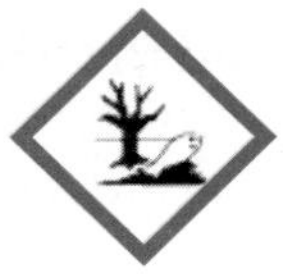	**Environment*** (may cause damage to the aquatic environment)
	**Biohazardous Infectious Materials** (for organisms or toxins that can cause diseases in people or animals)				

*The GHS system also defines an Environmental hazards group. This group (and its classes) was not adopted in WHMIS 2015. However, you may see the environmental classes listed on labels and Safety Data Sheets (SDSs). Including information about environmental hazards is allowed by WHMIS 2015.

FIGURE 22–31 WHMIS 2015 pictograms. (**Source:** Canadian Centre for Occupational Health and Safety. (2015) Retrieved October 12, 2015 from www.ccohs.ca/oshanswers/chemicals/whmis_ghs/pictograms.html. Canadian Centre for Occupational Health and Safety (CCOHS), 2015. Reproduced with the permission of CCOHS, 2016.)

- Robbery
- Rape
- Kidnapping
- Beating, stabbing, or shooting
- Murder

Workplace violence can occur in any environment where an employee is carrying out a work-related task, including buildings, parking lots, field locations, homes, and means of travel to and from work assignments.

Home care workers, especially, have personal security risks. They work alone in an unknown, uncontrolled environment and often work early or late hours. Clients, family members, or any person in the home could act violently toward them.

You can expect your employer to make your workplace as safe as possible. However, you must also protect yourself from harm (see the *Think About Safety: Personal Safety Measures* box). Follow the personal safety measures all the time. Most of the rules presented apply to support workers working in facilities and in the community.

Think About Safety

Personal Safety Measures

When Considering Your Own Safety, Be Sure to Also Take Steps Toward Your Electronic Safety:

- Do not provide personal information about yourself that can give strangers access to you on any electronic website, chat room, or social networking site.
- Take electronic threats directed toward you as seriously as you would any threat received in person. Report it to your local police department. If the threat has come from a co-worker or client, notify your supervisor.
- Do not respond to any electronic threat, as responding may only make the situation worse.

Continued

Think About Safety—cont'd

If possible, print off a hard copy of the threat or save it electronically to provide proof of receiving the threat.

When Driving to and From Work, Take the Following Precautions:

- Familiarize yourself with the area where you will be driving. Plan your route in advance, keeping to well-travelled streets and routes that you know. Note the locations of nearby police stations, gas stations, and other public buildings that may be of help in an emergency.
- Let your supervisor and a member of your family know the route you will take.
- Keep with you the phone number of a reliable tow truck company.
- Keep maps or a global positioning system (GPS) in the car.
- Maintain your car in good working order at all times.
- Always use a seat belt.
- Be prepared for winter driving conditions. Keep a survival kit in the car—booster cables, shovel, extra clothing, a blanket, sand, and road flares.
- Keep cash with you for gas or to make a phone call.
- Have a cellphone for emergencies on the road, and program emergency numbers into the phone. Do not use the phone while driving. Pull off the road if you need to make a call.
- Pull over to a safe spot away from traffic if you have car trouble. Put on your hazard lights, and call for help if you have a cellphone. Keep your doors locked and windows rolled up until help arrives. Never leave the car and walk off alone for help.
- Check for places to park. Choose a well-lit, busy area. If using a parking garage, park near entrances or exits and on a lower level. Try to stay close to the parking attendant if possible. Be aware of passengers sitting in parked cars, and avoid parking by these cars if possible. Lock your car doors as you leave.
- Ask for an escort to walk you back to your car after work. Some facilities provide this service. In a home setting, ask a family member to escort you.
- Have your car key ready so you can get into the car quickly. Do not fumble for keys on the way to or at the car. If necessary, you can use your house or car keys as a weapon. Carry them in your strong hand. Have one key extended (**FIGURE 22–32**). If you are attacked, slash at the attacker's face with the key.
- Check for a possible intruder in the front and back seats before getting into your car.
- If you think someone is following you, cross the street or change directions. Head toward a public building or a lighted house. If you are scared, yell for help.
- Lock the car doors when you get in the car. Keep the windows rolled up.
- Keep purses, backpacks, and other valuables under the seat or near your side. Do not leave them on the seat. They are easy targets for robberies.
- Do not carry valuables. Do not bring your purse or valuables into clients' homes. Leave them at home or in the car trunk. If an attacker demands something you have, give it. The only thing of value is you. Report the crime to the police.
- Carry a whistle or a "shriek alarm." Carry a travel size can of aerosol hairspray. Aim for the attacker's face. If someone tries to force you into a vehicle, do whatever you can to resist being pulled in. Fight back even if you see a weapon (yell, kick, push your thumbs into the attacker's eyes). You are at much greater risk if you are forced into the vehicle.

When Visiting a Client, Take the Following Precautions:

- Call your supervisor when you arrive at and leave a client's home.
- Be cautious in hallways, elevators, and stairwells in apartment buildings. Do not get on an elevator with a stranger who makes you nervous.
- Stay in the centre of the hallways and avoid hidden corners in apartment buildings. If someone threatens you, knock on as many doors

Continued

Think About Safety—cont'd

as possible and yell to get attention. If you are attacked, pull the fire alarm.

- Pause for a few seconds when entering someone's home. Assess the environment. Check any threats to your safety, including used syringes, strange odours, clutter, unfamiliar people, or household items that could be used as weapons. Note the location of the phone. Note any obstacles blocking exits.
- Keep your shoes on. In an emergency, you may need to leave in a hurry. In the winter, bring a pair of shoes for indoor use.
- Leave if a client or anyone else is abusive or makes sexual comments or suggestions.
- If you feel uncomfortable or threatened in any way, go to a safe place and immediately call your supervisor.
- Let the client lead the way down corridors, up staircases, and so on.
- Leave an exit route, or place yourself between the exit and the client. Never allow yourself to be cornered. Decide whether you should leave a door open or unlocked. Tell the client not to shut or lock a door if the action makes you uncomfortable.
- Sit in a hard-backed chair. You can get up faster from a firm chair than from a soft chair or sofa.
- Sit with your strong leg back and your other leg forward. This position lets you get out of your seat quickly without using your hands.
- Ask that pets be restrained or kept out of the room if you are nervous about them.
- If a client or family member becomes angry and begins to scream, stay calm. (Refer to the *Think About Safety: The ABCDs of Managing Responsive or Challenging Behaviours* box in Chapter 36).
- Report any unusual incidents to your supervisor as soon as possible.

Source: Health Care Health and Safety Association of Ontario (HCHSA) & Workplace Safety and Insurance Board (WSIB) of Ontario. (2003). *Health and safety in the home care environment* (pp. 14–26, 40–47). Toronto, ON: HCHSA.

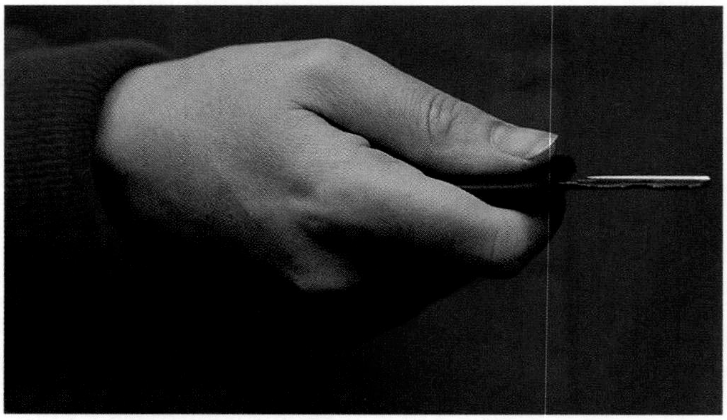

FIGURE 22–32 Car or house keys can be used as a weapon.

CHAPTER REVIEW

KEY POINTS

- Because of age or physical or emotional health condition, clients may be at great risk for accidents and injuries. It is up to facilities and community care agencies to try to create and maintain a safe environment for their employees and their clients.
- Older adults, children, and people living with illnesses or disabilities are especially vulnerable to accidents. Some of their accident risk factors include (1) impaired awareness of surroundings, (2) impaired vision, (3) impaired hearing, (4) impaired taste, smell, or touch, (5) impaired mobility, (6) medication effects, and (7) age.
- Health care workers must implement safety measures aimed at preventing falls among older adults and other clients at risk.
- Although you should always supervise all of your clients, you should pay particular attention to children, clients in wheelchairs, clients with a history of injury, sedated clients, older adults, and clients who are cognitively impaired, as they are at greatest risk for injuries related to falls.
- A restraint is any device, garment, barrier, furniture, or medication that limits or restricts freedom of movement or access to one's own body. Restraints can cause emotional harm and serious injury.
- The use of restraints requires a physician's order after consultation with the client's family.
- Support workers should be aware of the many alternatives to using restraints.
- Restraints can be classified as (1) physical restraints, (2) environmental restraints, and (3) chemical restraints.
- All health care workers should be aware of (1) common poisonous substances and what to do if a poisoning is suspected, (2) ways to prevent burns in older adults and others at risk, (3) ways to prevent suffocation in adults, (4) ways to prevent equipment accidents, and (5) safety measures for preventing fires, including how to use oxygen safely and how to assist in the evacuation of a building in the case of a fire.
- Occupational health and safety laws require health care employees to understand what hazardous materials are and how to safely handle the ones that they may be in contact with. This educational system is called WHMIS, or the Workplace Hazardous Materials Information System.
- Health care workers should be aware of the measures to prevent personal injury both at work and outside of work and be prepared to use them if necessary.

CRITICAL THINKING IN PRACTICE

You are assisting Mr. Park with feeding. He begins to cough loudly. He can speak a few words. You hear wheezing between breaths. What do you do? Mr. Park is suddenly unable to cough, speak, or breathe. What do you do?

REVIEW QUESTIONS

Answers to these questions are at the bottom of *page 419.*

Circle T if the answer is true, and circle F if the answer is false.

1. T F Older adults are at risk for accidents because of changes in the body.
2. T F The use of medications may increase a client's risk for accidents.
3. T F Restraints can be used for staff convenience.
4. T F A device is a restraint only if it is attached to the person's body.
5. T F Bed rails are restraints.
6. T F Restraints can be used to protect the client from harming others.
7. T F Unnecessary restraint is false imprisonment.
8. T F Informed consent is needed for restraint use.
9. T F You can apply restraints when you think they are needed.

10. T F You should remove restraints every 2 hours to reposition the client and give skin care.
11. T F Some medications are restraints.
12. T F Children are not at increased risk for accidents during times of stress or change.
13. T F Middle-aged women have the greatest risk of falling.
14. T F Falls in facilities are more likely to occur during the evening.
15. T F Rushing to get to a bathroom or commode is a major cause of falls.
16. T F Socks and bedroom slippers help prevent falls.
17. T F Childproof caps should be kept on medications and harmful products.
18. T F Medicines and harmful products can be stored in food containers out of the reach of children.
19. T F Do not carry or drink hot liquids while holding a child.
20. T F You are not responsible for reporting if any equipment is broken or damaged.
21. T F To correctly identify a hospital client, call the person by name.
22. T F Smoking is allowed where oxygen is used.
23. T F Hazardous materials must have warning labels.

Circle the BEST answer.

24. What is the most common accident in all settings?
    A. Burns
    B. Suffocation
    C. Falls
    D. Poisoning
25. Signs of shock include which of the following?
    A. Rapid pulse and breathing
    B. Flushed face
    C. Increased blood pressure
    D. Heightened awareness of surroundings
26. Mr. Higgins is 86 years old. Which of the following are *unsafe* for him?
    A. Nonglare, waxed floors
    B. Electrical cords and other items on the floor in high-traffic areas
    C. Safety rails and grab bars in the bathroom
    D. Nonskid shoes
27. To prevent falls, you should do the following:
    A. Wipe up spills right away
    B. Avoid night lights, as they can cause eye strain
    C. Discourage the use of handrails and grab bars
    D. Keep the bed in the highest position
28. Which of the following actions *best* prevents falls?
    A. Assisting the client to the washroom once each shift
    B. Answering calls for assistance promptly
    C. Keeping the bed in the highest position
    D. Always using bed rails for clients in continuing care facilities
29. Mrs. Carrera often tries to get up without help. You should do the following:
    A. Remind her to call for assistance
    B. Check on her twice per shift
    C. Allow her to go to the washroom on her own
    D. Decide on your own to keep the bed rails up
30. Which of the following is a common cause of burns?
    A. Hot bathwater and heating pads
    B. Spilling of cold liquids
    C. Using a microwave oven
    D. Suffocation
31. In the home, a working smoke detector should be present:
    A. In every room
    B. Near the front door
    C. On every floor
    D. In every bathroom

32. To prevent equipment accidents, you should do the following:
- A. Fix broken or cracked equipment using duct tape
- B. Fix broken items yourself
- C. Stop using electrical equipment if it produces a burning odour
- D. Remove the third prong on plugs if you have only two-prong outlets

33. You are using certain equipment. Which of the following is *unsafe*?
- A. Following the manufacturer's instructions
- B. Keeping electrical items away from water and spills
- C. Pulling on the cord to remove a plug from an outlet
- D. Turning off electrical items after using them

34. A fire alarm sounds. Which of the following is *unsafe*?
- A. Turning off oxygen
- B. Moving clients to a safe place
- C. Using elevators for a quick exit
- D. Closing doors and windows

35. Your clothing is on fire. Which is the *best* first thing you should do?
- A. Pour the first liquid you can grab on your burning clothes
- B. Run outside
- C. Dial 9-1-1 and wait for help
- D. Roll on the ground to smother the flames

36. Bed rails are raised when:
- A. The client tries to get up without assistance
- B. Your supervisor and the care plan tell you to raise them
- C. The client has a seizure
- D. You decide they should be raised

37. Which of the following is a common hazard of bed rails?
- A. Burns
- B. Strangulation
- C. Infections
- D. Pressure sores

38. According to the occupational health and safety legislation, employers are responsible for:
- A. Expecting employees will educate themselves about safety policies
- B. Doing the unsafe work themselves
- C. Warning employees of any potential and existing safety hazards
- D. Forcing employees to do unsafe work

39. You gave Mr. Ford the wrong treatment. What should you do?
- A. Report the error at the end of the shift
- B. Take action only if Mr. Ford was harmed
- C. Ask Mr. Ford what to do
- D. Complete an incident report as soon as you realize the error

40. You are working with a WHMIS-controlled product. You should:
- A. Use a liquid even though the label is damaged and unreadable
- B. Wear any needed personal protective equipment
- C. Remove the label after using the product
- D. Review instructions on the material safety data sheet after using the material

41. You work the night shift. Which of the following is *unsafe*?
- A. Parking in a well-lit area
- B. Locking your car
- C. Looking for your keys while at the car
- D. Checking the back seat before entering your car

Answers: 1.T, 2.T, 3.F, 4.F, 5.T, 6.T, 7.T, 8.T, 9.F, 10.T, 11.T, 12.F, 13.F, 14.T, 15.T, 16.F, 17.T, 18.F, 19.T, 20.F, 21.F, 22.F, 23.T, 24.C, 25.A, 26.B, 27.A, 28.B, 29.A, 30.A, 31.C, 32.C, 33.C, 34.C, 35.D, 36.B, 37.B, 38.C, 39.D, 40.B, 41.C

Chapter opener image: Oleksandr Khmelevskyi/Shutterstock.com

CHAPTER 23

Preventing Infection

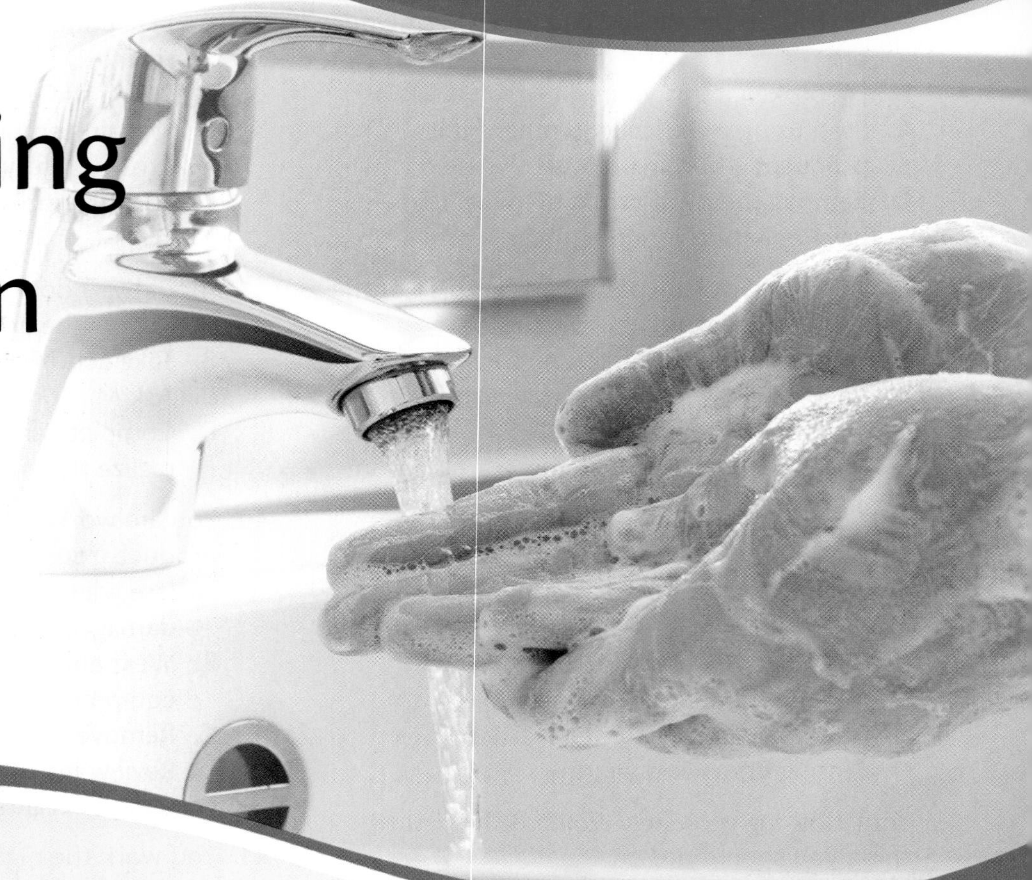

OBJECTIVES

After reading this chapter, the learner should be able to do the following:

- Distinguish between pathogens and nonpathogens.
- Summarize what microbes require to live and grow.
- Differentiate between bacteria, viruses, fungi, and parasites.
- List the signs and symptoms of infection.
- Describe the chain of infection.
- List ways in which microbes are transmitted.
- Define what a multidrug-resistant organism (MRO) is and state why it can be difficult to treat.
- List risk factors for infection.
- Describe common aseptic practices.
- Explain why handwashing is important.
- Describe when to wash your hands and general guidelines for handwashing.
- Describe cleaning, disinfection, and sterilization methods.
- Compare and contrast the principles and practices of Standard Practices and Transmission-Based Practices.
- Summarize how to use personal protective equipment (PPE).
- Describe the principles and practices of surgical asepsis.
- Apply the procedures described in this chapter to your clinical practice properly.

KEY TERMS

asepsis The practice of reducing or eliminating potential pathogens (bacteria, viruses, fungi, and parasites). There are two levels of asepsis: (1) **medical asepsis** and (2) **surgical asepsis**. *p. 432*

bacteria Single-celled microbes that naturally occur on living, dead, or inanimate objects. *p. 423*

biohazardous waste Items that may be harmful to others because they are contaminated with blood, body fluids, secretions, or excretions; *bio* means life and *hazardous* means dangerous or harmful. *p. 453*

carriers Persons who are able to transfer a pathogen to others without getting an active infection themselves. *p. 427*

clean technique See **medical asepsis**. *p. 432*

Clostridium difficile (C. difficile) A bacterium that causes diarrhea and colitis. It is the most common cause of infectious diarrhea in hospitalized people in the industrialized world and one of the most common infections in hospitals and long-term care facilities. *p. 425*

colonize To establish a habitat; for example, bacteria grow on or in specific regions of the body and survive as part of that person's **normal flora**. *p. 425*

communicable disease A disease caused by microbes (disease-causing organisms) that spreads easily. Also known as **contagious disease**. *p. 426*

communicable phase The period when a person is infectious and can spread pathogens to others. *p. 427*

contagious disease See **communicable disease**. *p. 426*

contamination The process of being exposed to microorganisms, including pathogens. *p. 435*

disinfection The process of destroying pathogens. *p. 441*

droplet A drop of liquid. *p. 431*

endospore The protective shell that surrounds dormant bacteria and viruses, which protects them from external harm. *p. 423*

febrile respiratory illness (FRI) A term used to describe a wide range of respiratory infections, such as colds, influenza, influenza-like illness (ILI), and pneumonia, spread through droplets. *p. 431*

fomite Any nonliving object that is capable of carrying infectious organisms and that may serve as a mode of transmission. *p. 430*

fungi Microbes that live only on organic matter such as plants and animals. *p. 423*

hand hygiene The process of cleaning hands. *p. 435*

handwashing The process of removing soil, dead skin cells, and excess microbes from the hands, using soap, friction, and running water. It is one form of **hand hygiene**. *p. 435*

health care–associated infection (HAI) An infection acquired while a person is a patient, client, or resident in a health care facility or while receiving care from a health care provider. This term has replaced the term **nosocomial infection**. *p. 427*

incubation period The time between exposure to a pathogenic organism and the appearance of signs and symptoms. *p. 427*

infection A disease state resulting from the invasion and growth of pathogens in the body. *p. 426*

infection control Policies and procedures to prevent the spread of infection within health care settings. *p. 422*

influenza ("the flu") A highly contagious infection of the respiratory tract by the causative (disease-causing) virus in airborne droplets. Symptoms include sore throat, cough, fever, muscular pains, and weakness. *p. 429*

isolation precautions Guidelines for preventing the spread of pathogens; include **Standard Practices** and **Transmission-Based Practices**. *p. 442*

medical asepsis Practices that reduce the number of pathogens and prevent their spread. Also known as **clean technique**. *p. 432*

methicillin-resistant *Staphylococcus aureus* (MRSA) A type of multidrug-resistant organism that is resistant to the antibiotic methicillin. *p. 425*

microbe See **microorganism**. *p. 422*

microorganism A form of life (*organism*) that is so small (*micro*) it can be seen only with a microscope. Also known as a **microbe**. *p. 422*

multidrug-resistant organism (MRO) A strain of bacteria that is very difficult to treat with common antibiotics. *p. 424*

nonpathogen A microbe that does not usually cause infection or disease and is not harmful to humans. *p. 423*

normal flora The microorganisms (primarily bacteria and yeast) that are usually found on the surface of skin, mucous membranes, and in the gastro-intestinal tract. *p. 423*

nosocomial infection See **health care–associated infection (HAI)**. *p. 427*

organism Any single-celled or multicellular living thing. *p. 422*

pandemic An epidemic that spreads quickly over a large region or even worldwide. *p. 429*

parasites Organisms that derive nourishment and protection from other living organisms, known as *hosts*. *p. 423*
pathogen A microbe that can cause harm, such as an infection or a disease. *p. 423*
personal protective equipment (PPE) Special clothing and equipment that act as a barrier between microbes and a person's hands, eyes, nose, mouth, and clothes; includes gloves, gowns, masks, and eye protection. *p. 441*
reservoir The environment in which microbes live and grow; host. *p. 423*
Routine Practices See **Standard Practices.** *p. 444*
sharps Equipment or items that may pierce the skin; include needles, razor blades, and broken glass. *p. 446*
Standard Practices Guidelines to prevent the spread of infection from blood, body fluids, secretions, excretions, non-intact skin, and mucous membranes. Also known as **Routine Practices or Standard Precautions**. *p. 444*
Standard Precautions See **Standard Practices**. *p. 444*
sterile Free of all microbes, both pathogens and nonpathogens, as well as their spores. *p. 435*
sterile field A work area free of all microbes, both pathogens and nonpathogens. *p. 455*
sterile technique See **surgical asepsis**. *p. 435*
sterilization The process of destroying *all* microbes. *p. 435*
surgical asepsis Practices that keep equipment and supplies free of *all* microbes. Also known as sterile technique. *p. 435*
Transmission-Based Practices Guidelines to contain pathogens within a certain area, usually the client's room. *p. 445*
tuberculosis (TB) A persistent bacterial infection generally transmitted by the inhalation or ingestion of infected droplets and usually affecting the lungs, although infection of multiple organ systems occurs. *p. 432*
vaccine A suspension containing a live (attenuated) or killed bacterium or virus that is administered for the purpose of inducing active immunity to a specific infectious disease. Vaccines are available in either oral or injectable suspensions. *p. 423*
vancomycin-resistant *Enterococcus* (VRE) A type of multidrug-resistant organism made up of bacterium. *p. 425*
vector An organism that spreads infection by transmitting pathogens from one host to another but is not the cause of the infection. *p. 430*
viruses Infectious particles that are much smaller than bacteria and infect living cells to grow and multiply. *p. 423*
waterless, alcohol-based hand rubs Hand hygiene products that are rubbed into the hands and then allowed to dry completely, thereby killing most microbes on the skin's surface in seconds. Also called *waterless antiseptic handwash. p. 436*

Infection can be a serious safety and health hazard. Some infections cause only minor symptoms, whereas others are much more serious. They may delay a person's recovery, create long-term health problems, or even cause death in some situations. Older adults, people with health challenges, and people with disabilities are at increased risk of developing infections. Infections can easily spread from worker to client, from client to client, or from client to worker.

All members of the health care team must take every precaution to protect clients and themselves from infection. As a support worker, in order to prevent infection, you must understand how infections spread and also must follow your employer's infection-control policies. **Infection control** refers to policies and procedures to prevent the spread of infection within health care settings. ***Proper hand hygiene—the easiest way to reduce the risk for infection spread to yourself and others—should always accompany any other infection-control efforts.***[1]

MICROORGANISMS

A **microorganism** (**microbe**), sometimes called a "germ" or "bug," is a form of life (**organism**) that is so small (*micro*) it can be seen only with a microscope. Microbes live and grow everywhere—in and on water, air, food, soil, plants, animals, and inanimate (nonliving) objects such as clothing, furniture, medical equipment, and personal care items. Microbes also live and grow on and in people—on the skin and in the mouth, nose, respiratory tract, stomach, and intestines.

Most microbes usually do not cause infection or disease; these are called **nonpathogens**. Microbes that are harmful and can cause infection or disease are called **pathogens**.

Types of Microorganisms

Within health care settings, the four types of microbes that cause the greatest risk for infection are bacteria, viruses, fungi, and parasites.

1. **Bacteria**—single-celled microbes that naturally occur on living, dead, or inanimate objects. They can multiply rapidly or, if necessary for survival, can remain dormant (nonactive), surrounded by a protective shell called an **endospore**. Several types of bacteria can form endospores (primarily *Bacillus* and *Clostridium* [botulism] species), which protect them from harsh environmental conditions, making them difficult to kill. In the right conditions, bacteria can become active again and resume multiplying rapidly. They can be nonpathogenic, or they can cause serious infections in any body system. Infections caused by bacteria are usually treated with antibiotics. Examples of bacteria include: *Salmonella enteritidis*, *Helicobacter pylori*, *Staphylococcus epidermidis*, and *Staphylococcus aureus*.
2. **Viruses**—infectious particles that are much smaller than bacteria and infect living cells to grow and multiply. They take over the cells' machinery to produce new virus particles. Viruses can kill their host cells while producing new virus particles (lytic cycle), or they can incorporate into a host cell's DNA (deoxyribonucleic acid) and remain dormant for a certain period (lysogenic cycle). Acquired immune deficiency syndrome (AIDS), hepatitis, influenza, herpes, and the common cold are examples of infections caused by viruses. Antibiotics are not effective against viruses, but a few antiviral medications that can kill specific viruses are available. Some viral diseases (such as measles, mumps, rubella, polio, and influenza) can be prevented by vaccination. A **vaccine** is a suspension containing a live or killed bacterium or virus that is administered for the purpose of inducing active immunity to a specific infectious disease. Examples of viruses include chicken pox (varicella zoster); hepatitis A, B, and C; herpes simplex ("cold sore virus"); and influenza.
3. **Fungi**—microbes that live only on organic matter such as plants and animals. Certain types of yeasts and moulds are common fungi that can be pathogenic. In humans, fungi can infect the mouth, vagina, skin, feet, and other body areas. Most fungal infections, such as athlete's foot, are mild, but fungi can also cause life-threatening infections, especially in susceptible people. Examples of common fungal infections include athlete's foot (tinea pedis), ringworm (tinea corporis), scalp fungus (tinea capitis), and *Candida* (found in the mouth [thrush], intestines, or vagina).
4. **Parasites**—organisms that derive nourishment and protection from other living organisms, known as *hosts*. Parasites may be transmitted from animals to humans, from humans to humans, or from humans to animals. They may be transmitted from host to host through consumption of contaminated food and water—for example, by putting something that has touched the feces of an infected animal or human into the mouth. The illnesses they can cause range from mild discomfort to severe illness and possibly death. Parasites range in size and shape from tiny, single-celled, microscopic organisms to worms that can be seen without a microscope.[2] Parasites are more common in developing countries. Common parasites in Canada include lice, mites, pinworms, *Giardia*, and *Trichomonas* (a sexually transmitted parasitic infection).

All four types of microbes require certain conditions to live and grow. The **reservoir** (host) is the environment where the microbe lives and grows. Microbes grow in reservoirs that are *warm* and *dark*, and they need *water* and *nourishment*. Most microbes also need *oxygen*, although some can thrive without it. Microbes that infect humans have evolved to grow best at body temperature but are destroyed by heat and light.

Normal Flora

Normal flora are made up of the microbes that naturally live and grow in certain locations on or in the human body. Certain microbes, for example, are found on the skin and in the respiratory tract, digestive system, eyes, ears, and vagina. These microbes are harmless (nonpathogens) and are beneficial to the body ("good bacteria"). The normal flora contain organisms (bacteria) that play a number of essential roles in the health of humans: They aid digestion, produce some vitamins, and help fight off infections of pathogenic organisms. If a bacterium in the normal flora is transferred to another site in the body, it can cause serious disease. For example, *Escherichia coli* (*E. coli*) is a bacterium normally found in the colon that assists with food metabolism, but if *E. coli* enters the bloodstream or the urinary tract, it can cause a serious infection.

The numbers of microbes that make up the normal flora of a body surface are constantly affected by certain factors, including infection by pathogenic organisms. Maintenance of healthy normal flora, therefore, is a delicate number balance of all types of beneficial bacteria that share the same body area. When a person is ill or on medications (such as antibiotics), some of the normal flora can be killed, disrupting this balance. The person can then develop a potentially harmful infection. Probiotic foods such as yogourt, cheeses, pickled foods, and so on can be very beneficial in maintaining the normal flora, especially while a person is on antibiotic medication.

Antibacterial soaps—intended for handwashing or for washing contaminated substances from skin—have been blamed for certain illnesses because their *overuse* (using them for bathing, for example) can destroy the delicate balance of a person's normal flora. It is important to recognize that the normal flora play a critical role in helping our immune system protect us from infection, and overuse of antimicrobial soaps and alcohol-based sanitizers can damage our beneficial bacterial organisms.

Multidrug-Resistant Organisms

Bacteria reproduce rapidly, and their large numbers can quickly make a person ill if there are not enough "good bacteria," or normal flora, to stop them from multiplying. Misuse and overprescribing of antibiotics in the past have led certain strains of bacteria to mutate (change) to become more resistant to most antibiotics. Many bacteria now have DNA that allow them to make membrane proteins that eliminate antibiotic medications, which then have no effect on the bacteria. Some bacteria have developed resistance by producing proteins that neutralize or deactivate antibiotic medications. In addition, many bacteria have the ability to undergo "conjugation," which allows them to transfer antibiotic-resistant genes between different species of bacteria, meaning that some people will get infections that are resistant to most antibiotics.

Bacteria that are resistant to more than one antibiotic are known as **multidrug-resistant organisms (MROs)**, sometimes called "superbugs." Infections with MROs are becoming increasingly common and are easily spread among people at risk for infection (such as babies, older adults, and people with serious medical conditions or a weakened immune system). Since MROs are difficult to treat, they can be fatal if the infection is severe. As a result, MROs pose a serious threat to clients in health care facilities.

The most common MROs in Canada are methicillin-resistant *Staphylococcus aureus* (MRSA), vancomycin-resistant *Enterococcus* (VRE), and *Clostridium difficile* (*C. difficile*, which causes diarrhea infection common in hospitalized clients on antibiotic treatment), although new strains of MROs are continually being reported throughout the world by health care officials. One MRO that is increasingly associated with urinary tract infections, wound infections, pneumonia, and bloodstream infections is extended-spectrum beta-lactamase (ESBL). It is treated in a similar manner as MRSA or VRE (see **BOX 23–1**).

As a support worker, you will be trained to take special precautions when you are in contact with clients who are infected, or suspected of being infected, with MROs, and you should be aware of the precautions you must take for any new MRO that you may come into contact with. Many healthy health care workers can become carriers for these infections and spread them to susceptible clients without having symptoms themselves. It cannot be emphasized enough that hand hygiene (especially handwashing and wearing gloves when moving from working with one infectious client to another) is a necessary component in the fight against the spread of MROs.

BOX 23–1 Multidrug-Resistant Organisms: *C. difficile*, MRSA, and VRE

C. difficile

Clostridium difficile (C. difficile) is a bacterium that causes mild to severe diarrhea and intestinal conditions like pseudomembranous colitis (inflammation of the colon). *C. difficile* is the most frequent cause of infectious diarrhea in hospitals and long-term care facilities in Canada, as well as in other industrialized countries. Symptoms include watery diarrhea, fever, loss of appetite, nausea, and abdominal pain/tenderness.

Most cases of *C. difficile* occur in patients who are taking certain antibiotics in high doses or over a prolonged period of time. Some antibiotics can destroy a person's normal bacteria found in the gut, causing *C. difficile* bacteria to grow. When this occurs, the *C. difficile* bacteria produce toxins, which can damage the bowel and cause diarrhea. However, some people can have *C. difficile* bacteria present in their bowel and not show symptoms.

As with any infectious disease, frequent hand hygiene is the most effective way of preventing the transmission of health care–associated infections. Handwashing with soap and water is important during *C. difficile* outbreaks and is one of the best defences against further spread of the bacteria. If you do not have access to soap and water, frequent use of alcohol-based hand rubs is encouraged. Most health care facilities provide alcohol-based hand rubs at entrances. Be sure to use them, but be aware that they are less effective than washing with soap and water as they do not destroy *C. difficile* spores.

For people with mild symptoms, no treatment may be required. For more severe cases, medication and sometimes surgery may be necessary. There are also new treatments, such as fecal transplantation, currently being studied for treating persistent *C. difficile* infection.

MRSA

Methicillin-resistant *Staphylococcus aureus* (MRSA) is a type of common bacterium that is not killed by most antibiotics. The symptoms of MRSA depend on which body system is infected. MRSA can cause pneumonia, sepsis, toxic shock syndrome, and necrotizing fasciitis (flesh-eating disease). Most people with MRSA do not have signs or symptoms of an infection but carry the bacteria on the skin, in the nose, or in the gastro-intestinal tract. These people are known as *carriers*. A person who is a carrier of MRSA bacteria may not carry these bacteria forever, as they can be treated with certain powerful antibiotics, or the problem may resolve itself. *S. aureus* is a normal flora bacterium that normally **colonizes**, or grows in, the nostrils and the respiratory tract.

Hospital inpatients who have incisions, wounds, or tubes, which make it possible for the germs to enter their bodies, are prone to MRSA infections, which are most likely spread in hospitals or long-term care settings through person-to-person contact, through contact with infected wound discharge or urine, or through health care workers who fail to practise hand hygiene or fail to wear proper gloves.

A test can be done to confirm the presence of the MRSA germ. If the test proves positive for MRSA, multiple powerful IV antibiotics are prescribed.

VRE

Enterococci are bacteria that are normally found in the digestive tract and are not dangerous in healthy people with strong immune systems, as the balance of healthy flora in their digestive tracts helps keep the bacteria from getting out of control. Because of overuse of antibiotics, however, a strain of *Enterococcus*, called **vancomycin-resistant *Enterococcus* (VRE)**, has become resistant to all antibiotics, including vancomycin. It is most commonly spread from the hands of health care workers who acquired VRE after contact with clients colonized or infected by the bacteria or from handling contaminated material or equipment.

VRE is dangerous because it cannot be controlled with antibiotics, and it causes life-threatening infections in people with compromised immune systems—clients who are very young, very old, and very ill. Also, it can easily pass on the resistance gene to other, more dangerous bacteria such as *Staphylococcus* and *Streptococcus*.

There are other ways that VRE can be spread—for example, from contact with contaminated

Continued

BOX 23–1 Multidrug-Resistant Organisms: C. *difficile*, MRSA, and VRE—cont'd

surfaces such as call bells, bed rails, blood pressure cuffs, and other equipment. Contamination of the environment with VRE is more likely when a client has diarrhea.

Both MRSA and VRE can cause serious infections. The best way to stop the spread of both the MRSA and VRE bacteria is by careful handwashing with an antibacterial soap; when gloves are necessary, health care workers should always change them between clients. As well, the number of people visiting a very sick person should be limited to one, and visitors should be sure to wash their hands well. Residents of long-term care facilities who have recently been admitted to a large hospital are usually tested for MROs before they are transferred back to their facilities. If they are found to have drug-resistant bacteria, they are then isolated from other residents.

Sources: © All rights reserved. *Fact Sheet – Clostridium difficile (C.difficile)*. Public Health Agency of Canada, 2014. Adapted and reproduced with permission from the Minister of Health, 2016. Government of Ontario, Ministry of Health and Long-Term Care, Provincial Infectious Diseases Advisory Committee. (2007, March). *Best practices for infection prevention and control of resistant Staphylococcus aureus and Enterococci*. Toronto, ON; Falcao, R. (n.d.). *Vancomycin-resistant Enterococcus*. Mountain View, CA. Retrieved from http://www.gentlebirth.org/vre/vremain.html#What.

THE SPREAD OF PATHOGENS

An **infection** is an illness or disease state resulting from the invasion and growth of pathogens in the body. These pathogens may have been introduced into the body from an inanimate object (such as a soiled sheet) or from another person who has a **communicable disease** (**contagious disease**). A communicable disease—for example, the common cold, influenza, chicken pox, hepatitis, pneumonia, and tuberculosis—is caused by pathogens that spread easily.

A *local infection* is an infection that occurs in one body part, such as an infected cut on the arm. A *systemic infection* involves the whole body, and the affected person would have *generalized* (entire body) signs and symptoms of infection. Some or all of the signs and symptoms of infection are listed in **BOX 23–2** (also see the *Focus on Older Adults: Signs and Symptoms of Infection* box).

BOX 23–2 Signs and Symptoms of Infection

- Fever and chills
- Increased pulse and respiratory rates
- Aches, pain, or tenderness
- Fatigue and loss of energy
- Loss of appetite
- Nausea
- Vomiting
- Diarrhea
- Rash
- Sores on mucous membranes
- Redness and swelling of a body part
- Discharge or drainage from the infected area that may have a foul odour
- New or increased cough, sore throat, or runny or stuffy nose
- Burning pain when urinating or the need to urinate more often or with increased urgency
- Behavioural changes in older adults

Being exposed to pathogens *does not always* result in an infection, as the body can protect itself from infection. There are three possible outcomes of exposure to a pathogen:

1. ***The immune system destroys the pathogen.*** The pathogen does not live and grow within the body, so an infection does not occur (see Chapter 17 to review the discussion of the immune system). If the person has been infected by that pathogen previously, his body may have "immunological memory," thereby fighting the infection without causing symptoms.
2. ***The immune system does not destroy the pathogen, and yet an infection does not develop.*** Some people remain healthy because of a strong immune

FOCUS ON OLDER ADULTS

Signs and Symptoms of Infection

Older adults are especially at risk for infections because of the normal age-related changes occurring in their bodies. If they had a serious health concern before they were infected, they are also more likely than younger adults to become seriously ill or to die from an infection; for example, pneumonia and influenza are often life-threatening illnesses in older adults because their immune systems are not as capable of mounting a strong reaction to new infections as the immune systems of younger, healthier people.

Older adults often do not show the usual signs of infection. Fever, pain, and swelling, for instance, are usually absent in older adults, who tend to have lower body temperatures and decreased pain sensation, because these symptoms are caused by the immune response, which can be greatly decreased in older people.

Sometimes, the only sign of infection in older adults is a change in behaviour. If an older client displays any of the following, report it to your supervisor:

- New or increased confusion or delirium
- New or increased incontinence
- Loss of appetite
- Decreased ability to perform activities of daily living (ADLs)
- Falls
- Changes in mood—for example, a client who is usually talkative, cheerful, and cooperative becomes unusually quiet, moody, and uncooperative

response. They are healthy and have no other illnesses or infections to deal with, but the pathogen can still be present within the body and can be transmitted to others; these persons would be considered **carriers**. The pathogens are not harmful to these persons but might be harmful to others who have a weakened immune system for certain reasons such as fatigue, stress, malnourishment, or other illnesses.

3. ***An infection develops sometime after exposure to the pathogen.*** The period between exposure to the pathogen and the onset (beginning) of illness is called the **incubation period**, which may be relatively short (hours to days) or may last for years. During the incubation period, the person can transfer the pathogen to others. The time during which a person is at risk of transferring pathogens to others (putting people at risk of "catching" the illness) is known as the **communicable phase**. The incubation period and length of time of the communicable phase vary from pathogen to pathogen.

Infections in Health Care Settings

A **health care–associated infection (HAI)** is an infection acquired after admission to a health care facility or acquired from any type of health care provider. In the past, HAIs were called ***nosocomial infections***, so you might hear this term used where you work. Infections can also be acquired in home care and other community settings. Health care workers can heal from the infections they are frequently exposed to and can develop "memory cells," which make them less likely to develop *symptoms* from the infection. But these memory cells may make them more likely to carry pathogens to unhealthy clients or to vulnerable people around them. The health care workers themselves might also have some or all of the risk factors for infection listed in **BOX 23–3**.

Microbes can enter the body through equipment used in treatments, therapies, and tests, so it is important that all equipment be kept free of pathogens. Workers can transfer microbes from client to client and from themselves to clients. **BOX 23–4** lists ways the support worker can reduce the risk of spreading infections to others or even to themselves and their families.

The most common infections that occur within health care settings include respiratory tract infections (colds, pneumonia, bronchitis, and influenza), urinary tract infections, gastro-intestinal tract infections (causing nausea or diarrhea), and skin infections (such as wound or intravenous [IV] site infections).

Sick, frail, and older clients have a hard time fighting infections, so it is up to the health care team to

BOX 23–3 Factors That Increase the Risk for Infection

- Extremes of age (the very young and the very old are most at risk)
- Poor nutrition
- Stress
- Lack of sleep
- The presence of disease or illness, which themselves or the treatments for them weaken the immune system—for example, AIDS, cancer (especially if the person is receiving chemotherapy or radiation therapy), organ transplantations, and kidney failure
- Certain medications
- Invasive procedures—for example, intubations and surgeries
- Invasive devices—for example, intravenous lines (IVs) and urinary catheters
- Open wounds
- Living in close contact with people who have communicable diseases
- Having contact with multiple caregivers

BOX 23–4 Ways the Support Worker Can Break the Chain of Infection

1. Take care of yourself to keep your immune system strong. Get enough rest, and eat nutritious food. Do not smoke. Get immunized. Stay physically active. **BOX 23–3** lists other factors that increase the risk for infection.
2. Bathe frequently, and ensure that your hair, teeth, and nails are clean and pathogen-free. You should never wear artificial nails when providing care! Wear a clean uniform and clean socks and underwear daily.
3. Practise proper hand hygiene between contacts with clients (follow the steps listed in this box and in **BOXES 23–5, 23–6, AND 23–7**).
4. Practise proper hand hygiene after removing used gloves and before putting clean gloves on.
5. Don gloves just prior to completing a care task that requires gloves and remove gloves immediately following the procedure. Perform hand hygiene immediately after removing gloves.
6. Never take "shortcuts" when it comes to hand hygiene, such as using waterless hand sanitizer on your gloved hands to avoid changing gloves. This is poor technique!
7. Avoid touching your face, hair, or clothing after completing hand hygiene.
8. Keep common surfaces (such as doorknobs, light switches, telephones, and keyboards) clean and disinfected to prevent the spread of pathogens. Practise this both at home and at work.
9. If you must cough or sneeze, do so into your arm, not your hand. If you use a tissue, dispose of it as soon as possible, and wash your hands immediately.
10. Keep all of your immunizations up to date.
11. Avoid going to work if you have a fever. Some agencies provide masks to wear if either you or someone you are caring for has a cough or runny nose (see **FIGURE 23–1** for an illustration of how a sneeze can spread infection).
12. Never place linens—clean or soiled—on the floor. This is a sure way to infect others!
13. If you are in a client's home, practise the points outlined in the "Focus on Home Care" boxes in this chapter.
14. Always use PPE properly. Refer to **BOXES 23–10** and **23–11** on page 449.

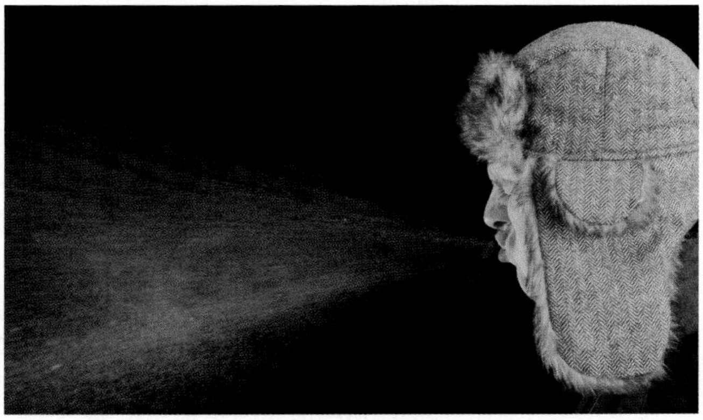

FIGURE 23–1 Droplets propelled into the air by a sneeze. During a common cold, most of the droplets contain virus particles. (**Source:** riopatuca/Shutterstock.com)

prevent the spread of infection. In health care settings, the three practices that help prevent infections are as follows:

1. Medical asepsis (especially hand hygiene) (see p. 432)
2. Isolation precautions (see p. 442)
3. Surgical asepsis (see p. 455)

A pandemic occurs when a communicable illness or infection spreads quickly throughout the population of a country or even throughout the world. The Canadian government, for example, is preparing for an influenza ("the flu") pandemic. Normally, people are exposed to different strains of the influenza virus frequently during their lives, so even though the virus may change (or mutate), previous exposures to influenza may offer some protection against infection. This protection results from viruses mutating only some of the proteins on their surface each year. We usually have memory cells that will recognize at least some of the proteins, allowing us to recover quickly. However, for unknown reasons, three to four times in a century, a radical change takes place in the influenza A virus, causing a new strain to emerge.[3] Then, we have no memory cells for any antigen, which can lead our immune systems to overreact, causing death, as occurred in the SARS (severe acute respiratory syndrome) epidemic in 2002 and 2003. In such cases, even young, healthy people can die from influenza, as they did during the flu pandemic of 1918. In the past, radical mutation in pathogens has resulted in widespread illness and deaths, especially among the young, the ill, and the very old. Across Canada, public health care departments are involved in attempts to prevent such a disaster from happening through widespread health teaching and influenza vaccinations.

H1N1 Virus and New Strains

In past years, the Canadian government took precautions against a new strain of influenza, the H1N1 virus, which has affected primarily young people. The H1N1 virus emerged in the spring of 2009 in people in North America. Because humans had little to no natural immunity to this new virus, it caused serious and widespread illness. The H1N1 flu virus (and all subsequent viruses that have since emerged from that strain) is contagious and is spread the same way as regular seasonal influenza: an infected person coughing or sneezing and germs from them entering the nose, eyes, or throat of another person. These germs can also rest on hard surfaces such as counters and doorknobs and can be transferred to hands and transmitted to the respiratory system when someone touches the mouth, nose, or both. Although the illness was originally called "swine flu," it is not possible to catch by eating pork or pork products or through blood transfusions.

The main symptoms of H1N1 infection are fever and cough. If you suspect that you have H1N1 infection, you should be seen by a health care provider. According to the Canadian government, more investigation is needed on how long a person can be infectious (able to spread the virus to others), but it is believed that this period is 24 hours before the onset of symptoms and continues for approximately 7 days after symptoms have started.[4]

The Chain of Infection

A number of factors work together for an infection to develop. The spread of infection involves a process known as the *chain of infection* (FIGURE 23–2).

The links in the chain are as follows:

- ***Pathogen***—a microbe capable of causing disease.
- ***Reservoir***—the environment where the pathogen lives before it infects a person. Remember, a pathogen can live on or in a person or animal (a host), food, water, soil, or inanimate objects.

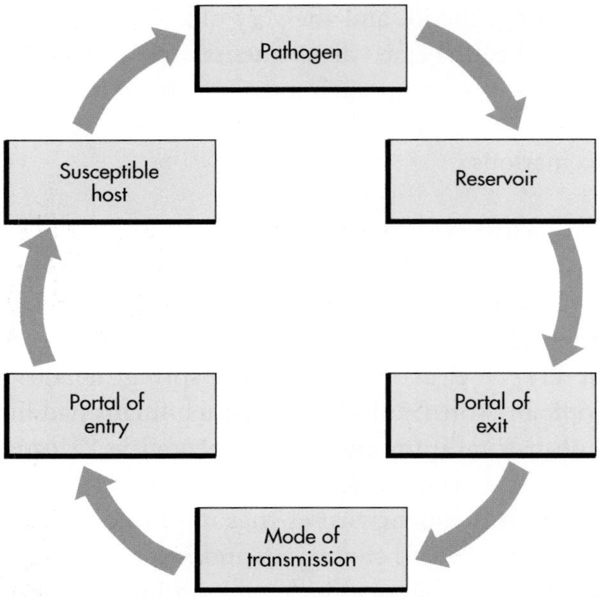

FIGURE 23–2 The chain of infection. (**Source:** Redrawn from Potter, P.A., & Perry, A.G. (2009). *Fundamentals of nursing* (rev. 7th ed., p. 642). St. Louis, MO: Mosby.)

- ***Portal of exit***—the path by which the pathogen leaves the reservoir. Portals of exit in the human body are the body openings (mouth; nose; and rectal, vaginal, and urethral openings), breaks in the skin (a scrape, cut, or other wound), and breaks in the mucous membranes (in the mouth, eyes, nose, vagina, and rectum). Pathogens are carried through the portals of exit by blood, body fluids, excretions, or secretions. These include urine, stool, vomitus, saliva, mucus, pus, vaginal discharge, semen, wound drainage, and sputum (respiratory secretions).
- ***Mode of transmission***—how the pathogen travels from the portal of exit to the next reservoir or host. Microbes can be transmitted by physical contact (direct and indirect); droplets in the air; air currents; an infected vehicle, or **vector** (such as a mosquito); or a **fomite** (any nonliving material, such as bed linen). The mode of transmission depends on the type of microbe. Some microbes are transmitted in more than one way (TABLE 23–1).

TABLE 23–1 Modes of Transmission of Microorganisms

Mode of Transmission and Examples of Infectious Diseases	Description
1. Contact Transmission Multidrug-resistant organisms Gastro-intestinal (GI, enteric) organisms Skin infections Wound infections	Occurs by transfer of microbes through physical touch. Contact transmission is by direct or indirect contact.[1] 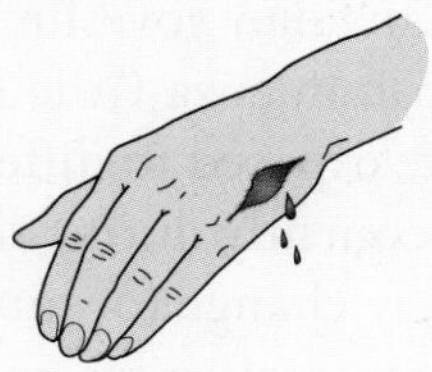
Direct Contact Transmission	Occurs by touching an infected or colonized person. Many personal care activities require direct (skin-to-skin) contact, such as bathing or turning a client in bed. Even shaking hands transmits microbes. 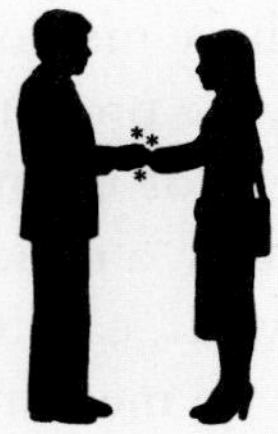
Indirect Contact Transmission	Occurs by touching a contaminated object, such as soiled linen, a tissue, eating and drinking utensils, dressings, equipment, and surfaces in the client's room. 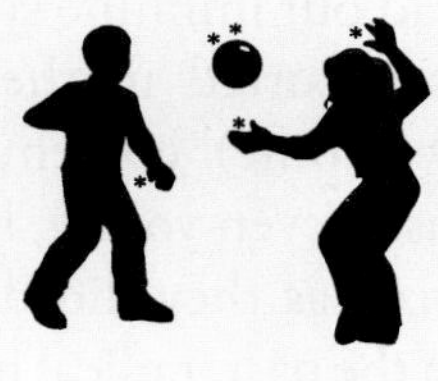

Continued

TABLE 23–1 Modes of Transmission of Microorganisms—cont'd

Mode of Transmission and Examples of Infectious Diseases	Description
2. Droplet Transmission Meningitis Pneumonia Influenza (including H1N1 virus) Mumps	Occurs when microbes are spread across short distances (less than 1 m) in the air by **droplets**. Coughing, sneezing, and talking propel droplets that carry microbes from the respiratory system through the air (**FIGURE 23–1**); the droplets settle on another person or object in the environment. 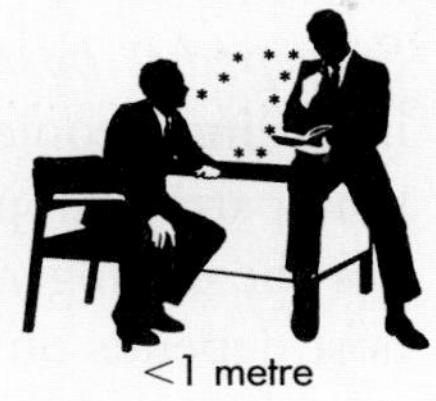
3. Airborne Transmission Measles Chicken pox Tuberculosis (TB) SARS **Febrile respiratory illness (FRI)**	Occurs when microbes are transmitted across long distances (farther than 1 m) by air currents. These microbes are contained in dust particles (acting as fomites) or evaporated droplets in the air. Microbes carried in this manner can travel across a room or even farther. People may then inhale the microbes or have contact with them if they are deposited on the skin. 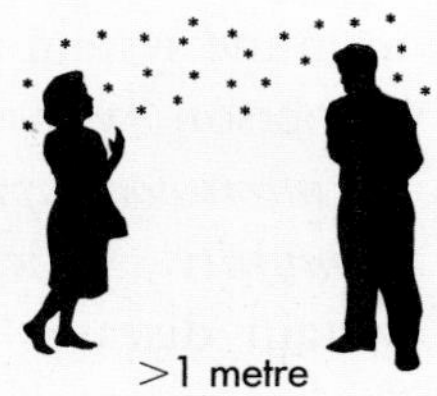
4. Vehicle Transmission Hepatitis A, B, and C Human immunodeficiency virus/ Acquired immune deficiency syndrome (HIV/AIDS)	Occurs when microbes are transmitted by a contaminated source (vehicle). Common vehicles of transmission include food, water, medication, and invasive medical equipment, as well as body fluids. One vehicle can transmit microbes to many people, resulting in an outbreak. 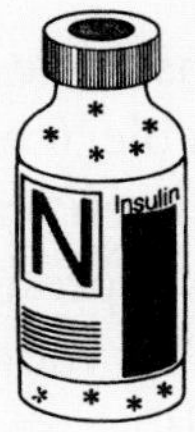
5. Vectorborne Transmission West Nile virus Lyme disease	Occurs when insects (fleas, ticks, mites, mosquitoes) or pests (mice) transmit microbes to humans. These other species are known as vectors. This type of transmission is rare in health care settings. 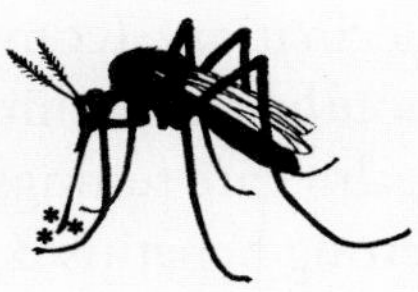

Source: © All rights reserved. *Routine Practices and Additional Precautions for Preventing the Transmission of Infection in Health Care* (Vol 25S4). Public Health Agency of Canada, 1999. Adapted and reproduced with permission from the Minister of Health, 2016.

- ***Portal of entry***—where the pathogen enters the new host's body. Portals of entry are the same as the portals of exit (in the human body)—body openings and breaks in the skin or mucous membranes.
- ***Susceptible host***—a person at risk for infection, including people who have not been exposed to that particular pathogen previously. Whether or not the pathogen grows and multiplies in the new host depends on the state of the person's immune system and the presence of memory cells from a previous exposure. For example, people who have had chicken pox usually do not have symptoms again if they are re-exposed. Remember, the immune system protects the body from infection. A person whose immune system is weakened is *immunocompromised*. (*Immuno* comes from *immunity*, which means protection against a certain disease. *Compromised* means weakened.) Such a person is more likely to get the infection.

There are numerous factors that increase the risk of infection (see **BOX 23–3** on page 428).

Vaccinations

Vaccinations have been proven to prevent serious communicable (contagious) illnesses in the people who have been vaccinated against those illnesses. TABLE 23–2 presents a chart listing the routine vaccinations and the recommended ages for receiving them. Health care agencies require workers to have their routine vaccinations up to date before they start work.

In addition to these vaccinations, the hepatitis B vaccination (comprising three injections over 6 months) is recommended for all those working in health care settings. This vaccination protects against getting hepatitis B from clients (see Chapter 37). The antibody levels can be checked periodically after vaccination to ensure immunity to hepatitis B. Some health care facilities suggest that their employees be vaccinated for hepatitis A (usually given along with hepatitis B vaccine), especially if the workers handle food. Check with your local health unit (or employer) for more information about this vaccine.

A yearly influenza vaccination is also highly recommended (and sometimes required) for anyone working in the health care field. This vaccine is very important to protect both health care workers and clients from influenza, which can be very dangerous to older adults and people with weakened immune systems.

Tuberculosis (TB) is a highly infectious bacterial disease, to which some of the older adults now living in long-term care facilities might have been exposed in their youth, when TB was much more common. TB is still a global health concern—more common among people with immune problems (such as those with HIV or AIDS), in places where people live in crowded situations (such as group homes, prisons, and long-term care facilities), and in developing countries that lack adequate health care. New staff and residents of long-term care facilities are required to have a two-step TB skin test (or a chest X-ray, if the doctor thinks it is necessary) so that they do not risk spreading or contracting TB. As a support worker, it is very important that you inform your doctor if you think you may have been exposed to a client or family member suspected of having TB.

MEDICAL ASEPSIS

Asepsis is the practice of reducing or eliminating potential pathogens (bacteria, viruses, fungi, and parasites). There are two levels of asepsis: (1) medical asepsis, for which the goal is to exclude *all pathogenic microorganisms* through medical aseptic technique, and (2) surgical asepsis, which aims to exclude *all microorganisms* and their spores through surgical aseptic technique.[6]

Medical asepsis (or **clean technique**) refers to the practices that:

- Reduce the number of pathogens
- Prevent the spread of pathogens from person to person or place to place

Medical asepsis is the most common technique, and it should be practised by *all* health care workers, who have an important role in preventing the spread of infection to others. Hand hygiene is the most important part of medical asepsis that health care workers can practise to prevent the spread of illnesses caused by pathogens.

In most health care units, the term *clean* is used to refer to anything that has no visible contaminants.

TABLE 23–2 Communicable Illnesses and Diseases: Care and Immunization

Illness	How Contracted	Signs and Symptoms; Incubation Period	Care	Immunization
Chicken pox (shingles) *Virus [Varicella zoster]*	Airborne	Fever, painful vesicles (fluid-filled sacs)—with shingles, the vesicles are usually along a nerve root on one section of the body; 14–21 days	Rest; do not scratch or irritate the vesicles. In the case of shingles, see the doctor for medication or treatment; isolate from people who have not had chicken pox	Chicken pox immunization may be given as long as the person does not have symptoms
Clostridium difficile (C. difficile) (see **BOX 23–1**) *Bacteria*	Direct contact	Severe diarrhea and abdominal cramping; 1–10 days	Rest, fluids, treating the symptoms. The person should be under a doctor's care. Handwashing (over and above the use of hand rubs) is very important because hand rubs do not kill these bacteria. Isolate from others, as very easily spread	None
Febrile respiratory illness (FRI) *Virus [Influenza A]*	Droplet-spread respiratory infections, such as colds, influenza-like illness (ILI), and pneumonia	Fever greater than 38°C (100.4°F) and new shortness of breath. *Note:* Some older people or those with immune problems may not have a high fever[4]; within days after exposure[5]	Rest, fluids, treating the symptoms. The person should be under a doctor's care. Airborne isolation precautions	Influenza vaccine (for certain viral strains)
Measles *Virus [Paramyxovirus family]*	Airborne; direct droplet transmission of virus	Fever and rash, often mild and passes unnoticed; 6–19 days	Rest, isolation, cool sponge baths	Immunization given with that for mumps and rubella (MMR)

Continued

TABLE 23–2 Communicable Illnesses and Diseases: Care and Immunization—cont'd

Illness	How Contracted	Signs and Symptoms; Incubation Period	Care	Immunization
Rubella *Virus [Rubivirus]*	Droplet, airborne	Begins with symptoms of upper respiratory infection and fine, raised rash; 14–23 days	Rest; isolate from people who have not had vaccine	Vaccine (MMR); Never give vaccine to women who are pregnant or trying to get pregnant
Hepatitis (A, B, and C) *Virus*	Hepatitis A is spread through direct contact with fecal-contaminated water or food. Hepatitis B and C are spread by direct contact with contaminated blood or body fluids	Jaundice, swollen liver, loss of appetite, changes in urine or stool colours; hepatitis A: 2–6 weeks; hepatitis B: 4–20 weeks; hepatitis C: 2–26 weeks	Must consult a doctor for medical treatment; if hepatitis B and C, avoid contact with blood or body fluids	Vaccine available for hepatitis A and B, but not for hepatitis C
Human immunodeficiency virus (HIV) and acquired immune deficiency syndrome (AIDS) *Virus*	Spread by direct contact with contaminated blood or body fluids	Chills, fever, cough, tiredness, confusion, stiff neck, oral lesions, nausea, vomiting, etc.; 3–8 weeks	Must consult a doctor for medical treatment; avoid contact with blood or body fluids	No vaccine currently available
Human papilloma virus (HPV) *Virus*	More than 100 types of HPV; 30–40 types are most commonly spread through sexual contact and may cause cervical cancer in women	May have visible warts on hands and feet or oral, anal, and genital cavities; 1 month to 2 years	Must consult a doctor for medical treatment; avoid contact with infected areas, blood, or body fluids; avoid sexual contact	There are two vaccines currently available that can prevent infection from types 16 and 18 (which cause 70% of cervical cancer). Prior to receiving it, the client should discuss its suitability

Continued

TABLE 23–2 Communicable Illnesses and Diseases: Care and Immunization—cont'd

Illness	How Contracted	Signs and Symptoms; Incubation Period	Care	Immunization
Multidrug-resistant *Staphylococcus aureus* (MRSA) *Bacteria* (see **BOX 23–1**)	Direct contact with people who have MRSA or direct contact with a contaminated object	Same symptoms as any other skin infection; MRSA can also cause pneumonia and necrotizing fasciitis (flesh-eating disease); 2–3 days	Avoid contact with infected items or people; infections require medical care	No vaccine currently available
Vancomycin-resistant *Enterococcus* (VRE) *Bacteria* (see **BOX 23–1**)	Direct contact with people who have VRE or direct contact with a contaminated object	Same symptoms as any other skin or diarrheal infection; 1–8 weeks	Avoid contact with infected items or people; infections require medical care	No vaccine currently available

For example, after we have washed our hands or our clothes, we refer to them as being "clean." We use clean gloves (not sterile surgical gloves), and we change them between clients. We use the word *contaminated* (unclean) to describe anything that has been exposed to pathogens, whether or not the contamination is visible (such as soiled bed linen). **Contamination** is the process of exposure to pathogens.

A *clean* environment is different from a *sterile* environment. **Sterile** means free from *all* microbes, including pathogens, nonpathogens, and their spores. Because infection is a risk, microbes cannot be present during surgery or invasive procedures, so operating rooms and instruments inserted into the body must be sterile. **Surgical asepsis** (also called **sterile technique**) refers to the practices that keep equipment and supplies free of *all* microbes and their spores. **Sterilization** is the process of destroying *all* microbes, both pathogens and nonpathogens, and their spores.

HAND HYGIENE

Handwashing ***with soap and running water, using friction, or applying waterless, alcohol-based hand rubs is the easiest and most important way to prevent the spread of infection.*** You use your hands in almost every task you perform as a support worker. Your hands can easily pick up microbes from any client, place, or thing, and then transmit the microbes to other clients, places, or things. If you touch your eyes, nose, or mouth with your contaminated hands, you can also transfer microbes into your own body. **Hand hygiene** should therefore be practised before and after client contact of any kind. Because hands are contaminated very easily, you need to practise hand hygiene often and properly. Although hand hygiene is a simple procedure, many health care workers do it incorrectly. You should remember that gloves never take the place of hand hygiene. Your skin will breed microbes in the dark, warm, moist environment of your gloved hands. You should always wash or sanitize your hands after removing your gloves and before putting new ones on. BOX 23–5 lists guidelines for proper hand hygiene.

Waterless, alcohol-based hand rubs clean hands effectively and are convenient to use. Some manufacturers of these hand rubs recommend that you wash your hands with water and soap after a maximum of 10 applications of their product to remove accumulated dead skin and bacteria on your hands. Always wash your hands when they become visibly soiled. Your hands must be dry before you apply a hand rub because moisture dilutes the alcohol in the rub and makes it less effective. The hand rub is also not effective if your hands are visibly soiled.

BOX 23–5 When to Practise Hand Hygiene

- ***Immediately before and after giving care***—even though it may seem you just cleaned your hands after giving care, wash them again immediately before you care for the next client
- Whenever your hands are visibly soiled
- After contact with your own or another person's blood, body fluids, secretions, or excretions
- After touching objects that are contaminated, such as soiled linens, tissues, toilet paper, garbage bags, bedpans, diapers, or adult incontinence products
- Before and after preparing, handling, and eating food
- Before and after feeding a client
- Before putting on disposable gloves and after removing them
- After personal body functions, such as urinating or defecating; changing tampons or sanitary pads; and sneezing, coughing, or blowing your nose

Note: If you have touched any object that has been contaminated with pathogens (such as feces), or you can see visible contamination on your hands, you should thoroughly wash your hands with soap and running water instead of using waterless hand sanitizer to clean your hands.[7]

Handwashing

123

Advocate on behalf of the client's quality of life by promoting:

Dignity • Independence • Preferences • Privacy • Safety *(see BOX 1–4, on p. 17)*

1 Ensure the following supplies are available:
- ☐ **Soap**
- ☐ **Paper towels**
- ☐ **A wastebasket**

Being organized reduces wasting time and avoids missing important steps.

2 Push your watch and sleeves up well over your wrists. Remove rings.

Pathogens multiply in warm, dark, and moist environments such as under rings and jewellery.

3 Stand away from the sink. Do not let your hands, body, or uniform touch the sink. Stand such that the soap and faucet are easy to reach.

The sink is considered to be contaminated. Touching it would increase your risk for pathogen contamination. (FIGURE 23–3).

Continued

Handwashing—cont'd

4 Turn on and adjust the water until it feels warm. Always wash your hands under warm running water.
Warm water opens your skin pores, allowing more pathogens to exit the skin. It is also more comfortable to wash in warm (not hot) water than in cold water.

5 Wet your wrists and hands thoroughly under running water. Keep your hands at a level lower than your elbows (**FIGURE 23–3**).
Soap can irritate dry skin, so it is important to first wet the areas that you plan on washing! If you hold your hands and forearms up, dirty water runs from hands to elbows, and those areas become contaminated as well.

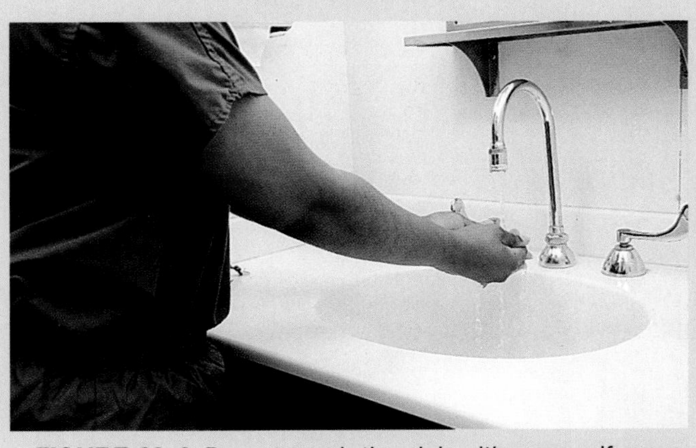

FIGURE 23–3 Do not touch the sink with your uniform.

6 a Apply about 5 mL (1 teaspoon) of liquid soap to your hands. If using bar soap, do not touch the soap dish when you pick up the soap. Rinse the bar soap well before you use it.
Rinsing the bar of soap helps to wash away any loose dead skin cells that may be present on the bar.

b Do not touch the soap dish as you put the soap back. Do not use too much soap.
Too much soap may be hard to rinse off and will dry the skin, causing irritation.

7 Rub your palms together, and interlace your fingers to work up a good lather (**FIGURE 23–4**).
This rubbing action helps loosen and remove microbes and dirt.
Microbes and pathogens can hide in skin folds.

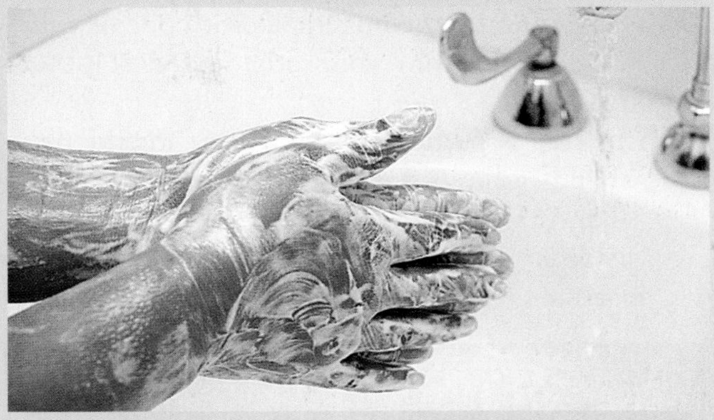

FIGURE 23–4 Rub your palms together to work up a good lather. This step should last at least 15 seconds. Pay attention to areas often missed during handwashing: thumbs, knuckles, sides of the hands, little fingers, and under the nails.

8 Wash each hand and wrist thoroughly. Clean well between the fingers.
Washing thoroughly reduces the chance of leaving pathogens on the skin.

9 a Clean the fingernails by rubbing the fingertips of one hand against the palm of the other hand (**FIGURE 23–5**).

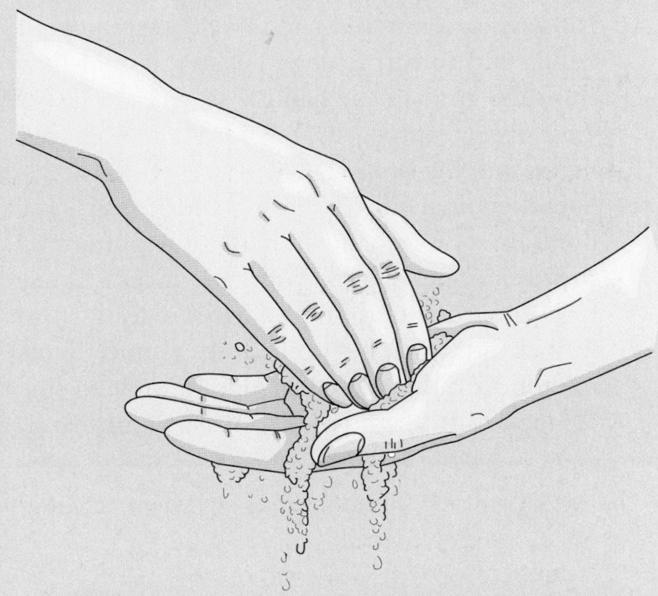

FIGURE 23–5 Rub your fingertips against your palm to clean the fingernails.

Continued

Handwashing—cont'd

b Clean under the fingernails with one of your fingernails from your other hand (**FIGURE 23–6**).

This step is particularly important for the first handwashing of the day and any time your hands are highly soiled.

Microbes and pathogens easily grow under fingernails.

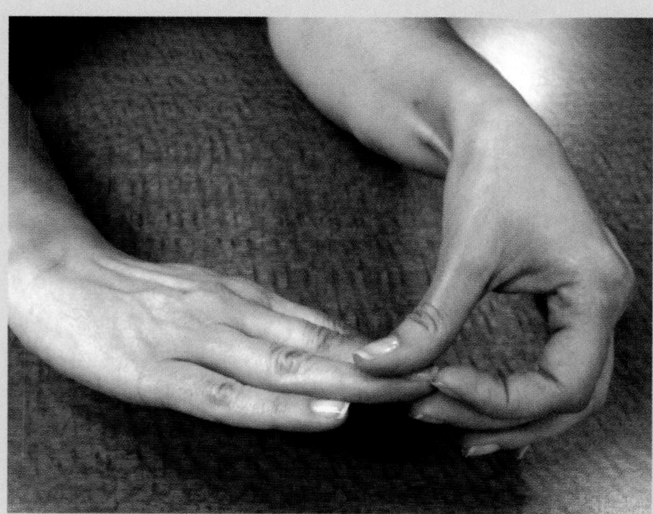

FIGURE 23–6 Use a fingernail to clean under your other fingernails. (**Source:** © Kristiina Paul)

10 Rinse your wrists and hands well, keeping your hands and forearms down. Water should flow from the arms to the hands.

This allows pathogens to naturally exit your hands into the sink.

11 Spend enough time lathering and rinsing. The duration of the handwash is as important as the technique. Check your employer's policy regarding the duration required. At least 15 to 20 seconds will be needed to remove most microbes on the skin (the length of time to sing "Happy Birthday" twice!). Wash your hands longer if they are dirty or soiled with blood, body fluids, secretions, or excretions.

The longer you scrub, the more likely you are to remove harmful pathogens from your skin.

12 Repeat steps 6 through 11, if needed.

13 Pat dry by starting with your forearms and working down to your fingertips.

The forearms are cleaner than the fingertips. Drying this way will dry the cleanest area first.

Dry hands thoroughly.

Microbes and pathogens flourish in a moist environment.

14 Turn off the faucet using a clean paper towel (**FIGURE 23–7**).

The faucets are contaminated, and using paper towels prevents clean hands from becoming contaminated again.

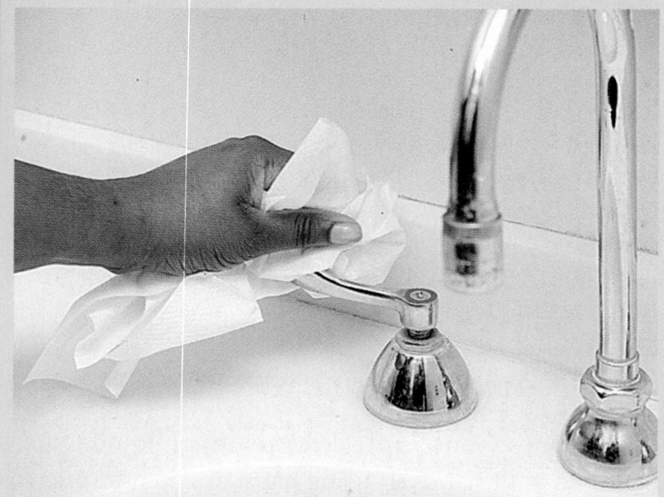

FIGURE 23–7 Use a paper towel to turn off the faucet.

15 Apply hand lotion or cream after washing your hands.

This prevents skin from chapping and drying. Skin breaks can occur in chapped and dry skin. Remember, skin breaks are portals of entry for microbes.

Using Waterless, Alcohol-Based Hand Rubs

123

Advocate on behalf of the client's quality of life by promoting:

Dignity • Independence • Preferences • Privacy • Safety *(see BOX 1–4, on p. 17)*

1 Pour about 3 to 5 mL (½ to 1 teaspoon) of waterless, alcohol-based hand rub onto both hands.
This amount of hand rub is adequate to kill the pathogens that may be present on your hands.

2 Rub hands together. Make sure that all areas of the hands are covered, including between the fingers. Rub hands together for about 15 seconds.
Rubbing this long will properly spread the waterless, alcohol-based hand rub.

3 Clean under the fingernails by rubbing fingertips on the wet palms.
Pathogens thrive under fingernails and between skin folds.

4 Rub hands until they are dry, between 30 seconds and 1 minute.
This allows the alcohol-based rub to evaporate and dry properly.

5 Never try to dry hands using a towel or paper napkin.
Drying your hands with these will defeat the pathogen-killing effectiveness of the waterless, alcohol-based hand rub.

Wearing Gloves

Disposable gloves provide a protective barrier between your hands and the client's blood, body fluids, secretions, excretions, non-intact skin, and mucous membranes. Gloves protect you from acquiring microbes from the client and protect the client from acquiring microbes that are on your hands. However, gloves are used as additional protection and not as a substitute for handwashing.

Gloves are not required for most routine support care activities during which contact is limited to a client's intact skin. Do not wear gloves when they are not needed. Your hands will sweat and then become dry, and the skin will eventually crack if gloves are worn continuously. Remember, cracked skin is a portal of entry for microbes.

Gloves are often made of latex (a rubber product), and some people are allergic to latex. This allergy can cause skin rashes as well as more serious problems such as asthma and shock. If you experience skin rashes or difficulty breathing, report it to your supervisor right away. If you have a latex allergy, you need to wear latex-free gloves. If your clients are allergic to latex, you cannot wear latex gloves when caring for them. Check their care plan for this information.

No special technique is required to put on disposable gloves. Be careful not to tear them when putting them on as pathogens can enter through the tear. Carelessness, long fingernails, and rings can tear the gloves. Remember the following about wearing gloves:

- Wear gloves if you have cuts or abrasions on your hands or bitten fingernails.
- Wash and dry your hands before putting on gloves.
- Use a new pair of gloves for every client.
- Remove and discard torn, cut, or punctured gloves right away. Wash your hands. Then put on a new pair.
- Practise hand hygiene each time you remove your gloves.
- Wear gloves only once. Discard them after use.
- Do not use waterless hand rubs on gloves. These rubs can weaken the gloves, increasing the risk for tearing.
- Put on clean gloves before touching mucous membranes or broken (non-intact) skin.
- Wear gloves when contact with surfaces or items contaminated by blood, body fluids, secretions, or excretions is likely (for example, when handling bedpans, cleaning a bathroom floor, or removing soiled linens).
- Put on new gloves as soon as gloves become contaminated with blood, body fluids, secretions, or excretions. You may need more than one pair of gloves for a single task to prevent cross-contamination of different body sites.
- Replace gloves if you touch an unclean surface.

Removing Gloves

123

Advocate on behalf of the client's quality of life by promoting:

Dignity • Independence • Preferences • Privacy • Safety (see BOX 1–4, on p. 17)

1 Make sure that gloves touch only gloves. Do not let gloves touch the skin on your wrists or arms.
Skin is regarded as contaminated. Touching skin with gloves would defeat the purpose of wearing gloves.

2 Grasp a glove just below the cuff with the gloved fingers of your opposite hand. Grasp it on the outside. (**FIGURE 23–8, *A***).
Grasping the glove by the outside ensures that your gloved fingers do not touch the skin of the wrist.

3 Pull the glove down over your hand so it is turned inside out. (**FIGURE 23–8, *B***).
This traps the pathogens, reducing the chance of their spreading.

4 Hold the removed glove with your gloved hand.
Remember that the contaminated side should never be touched by skin.

5 Insert two fingers of your bare hand inside the cuff of the remaining glove. (**FIGURE 23–8, *C***).
Inserting fingers into the glove keeps them away from the outside (or contaminated) side of the glove.

6 Pull the glove down (inside out) over your hand and the already removed glove (**FIGURE 23–8, *D***).
This traps the two contaminated gloves together and eliminates the chance of spreading the pathogens that exist on the outsides of the gloves.

7 Drop both gloves together into the appropriate container. Follow employer policy.
It is important to dispose of soiled gloves appropriately to avoid spreading pathogens to others.

8 Practise hand hygiene.
Pathogens and microbes multiply in warm, dark, moist environments, which is exactly the environment under your gloves! Hand hygiene kills any new pathogens that would have multiplied on your hands while you were wearing your gloves.

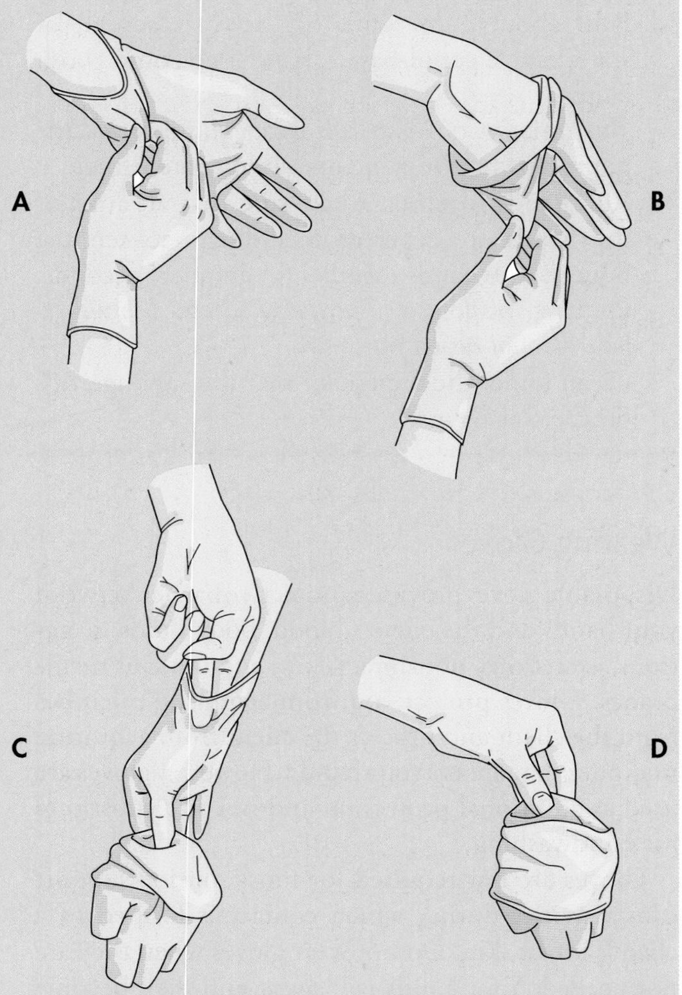

FIGURE 23–8 Removing gloves. **A,** Grasp the glove below the cuff. **B,** Pull the glove down over the hand. The glove is inside out. **C,** Insert the fingers of your ungloved hand inside the other glove. **D,** Pull the glove down over your hand and the other glove. The glove is inside out.

FOCUS ON HOME CARE

Hand Hygiene

A client's home might not have everything you need for proper handwashing, such as soap or paper towels. Do not use the client's cloth towels for drying your hands, but use paper towels instead. Check with your supervisor before visiting the client. Most agencies provide workers with needed basic supplies to take with them on visits. Bring paper towels with you for home visits. You should always carry waterless, alcohol-based hand rub when you go on home visits in case the home lacks available hand hygiene supplies.

Care of Supplies and Equipment

Remember, microbes live on people and on objects. Contaminated equipment and supplies can easily become a source of infection.

Most items used in facilities and home care are disposable, which means they are used only once and then discarded. In these cases, cleaning them is not an issue. Some items, however, are reused—for example, bedpans, urinals, washbasins, water pitchers, and drinking cups. In facilities where reusable items are used, they are labelled with the client's name, room, and bed number. They are never used or "borrowed" for another client.

Reusable items must be decontaminated. There are three levels of decontamination: *cleaning, disinfection*, and *sterilization*.

Cleaning

Cleaning reduces the number of microbes present on an item. It also removes any visible organic material such as dirt, blood, body fluids, secretions, and excretions. For some equipment, periodic cleaning is all that is required. For example, items such as crutches and blood pressure cuffs need to be cleaned only when visibly soiled and between uses on different clients. Follow employer policy about when and how to clean items. The following guidelines apply when cleaning equipment:

- Wear personal protective equipment when cleaning items that may be contaminated with blood, body fluids, secretions, or excretions. **Personal protective equipment (PPE)** consists of special clothing and equipment that act as a barrier between microbes and your hands, eyes, nose, mouth, and clothes such as gloves, gowns, masks, and eye protection (goggles or face shields) (see p. 445). Follow your employer's policies for the use of PPE when cleaning equipment.
- Rinse the item first in cold water to remove any organic material. Warm or hot water makes the protein in organic material thick, sticky, and hard to remove, similar to the way the protein in an egg will permanently change texture when it is heated.
- Wash the item with soap and hot water.
- Scrub the item thoroughly. Use a brush, if necessary.
- Rinse the item in warm water.
- Dry the item.
- Disinfect or sterilize the item.
- Disinfect equipment and the sink used in the cleaning procedure.
- Discard gloves and other PPE.
- Practise hand hygiene.

Disinfection

Disinfection is the process of destroying all pathogens except their spores. Spores can be destroyed only by the sterilization process. An item must be thoroughly cleaned before it is disinfected.

Reusable items are disinfected with chemicals such as alcohols or chlorines (*chemical disinfectants*). Such items include:

- Metal bedpans
- Commodes
- Countertops
- Tubs
- Room furniture

Follow your employer's policies regarding when and how to disinfect equipment and supplies (see the *Focus on Home Care: Disinfectants* box).

Chemical disinfectants can burn and irritate the skin. Wear utility gloves or rubber household gloves that are waterproof to prevent skin irritation. Do not wear disposable gloves when using disinfectants, as the chemicals in the disinfectants will degrade (break down) the gloves. Some chemical disinfectants have

FOCUS ON HOME CARE

Disinfectants

Detergent and hot water are common disinfectants for utensils, linens, and clothes. Many commercial products are available for household surfaces, including sinks, countertops, floors, toilets, tubs, and showers. In home care settings, use the products preferred by the client's family or as instructed by your supervisor.

Vinegar is an effective and cheap disinfectant. You can use it to clean bedpans, urinals, commodes, and toilets. To make a vinegar solution, mix 250 mL (1 cup) of white vinegar and 750 mL (3 cups) of water. Make sure you label the container properly as "vinegar solution." Also, put the date and your name on the container.

special measures for use and storage. Check the material safety data sheet (MSDS) before handling a disinfectant (see Chapter 22). Follow your employer's policies.

Sterilization

Sterilization destroys all nonpathogens and pathogens, including spores. Very high temperatures are used because most microbes can be destroyed only by heat.

Boiling water, radiation, liquid or gas chemicals, dry heat, and steam under pressure are sterilization methods. Items that enter the body or are used during surgery—for example, IV catheters, urinary catheters, and needles—have to be sterilized. In facilities, specially trained workers are responsible for carrying out the sterilization process. Therefore, support workers are *not* responsible for sterilizing equipment. However, you may be required to clean the items in preparation for sterilization (see the *Focus on Home Care: Sterilization* box).

See **BOX 23-6** for guidelines on how to follow medical asepsis measures.

FOCUS ON HOME CARE

Sterilization

In home care, almost all medical items that must be sterile are commercially prepared and are disposable. However, you may be required to sterilize noninvasive items such as cloth diapers or glass baby bottles.

Cloth diapers and other colour-fast linens can be sterilized by soaking them in a solution of 1 part household bleach and 10 parts water. One cup of bleach can be added to the wash when laundering items soiled with blood and body fluids. Always check with your client and your supervisor for direction before using bleach. Some linens cannot be bleached, so check the labels on clothes before using bleach to wash them (see Chapter 42).

Glass baby bottles and other such items can be sterilized in boiling water. Place the items in a large pot filled with cold water. Cover the pot and bring the water to a full boil. Boil the items for at least 15 minutes; then turn off the heat and allow the water and the items to cool. Use tongs to remove the items, and let them air dry on a clean towel. Although boiling water is a convenient and inexpensive method of sterilization in the home, it does not always kill all the spores and viruses. Therefore, facilities do not use boiling water for sterilizing items.

ISOLATION PRECAUTIONS

Along with medical asepsis, infection-control policies use isolation precautions to reduce the risk for infection. **Isolation precautions** are guidelines for preventing the spread of pathogens. The most recent isolation precautions were developed in 1996 in the United States by the Centers for Disease Control and Prevention (CDC). These precautions have been accepted by Health Canada and are currently used in most Canadian health care facilities and community care agencies.

There are two types of isolation precautions: Standard Practices (also known as Routine Practices) and Transmission-Based Practices. Both types of precautions provide guidelines on how to contain microbes. Standard Practices are practised at all times, whereas Transmission-Based Practices are

BOX 23–6 Medical Asepsis Measures You Should Follow

Controlling Reservoirs

- Maintain your personal hygiene. Bathe, shampoo your hair, brush your teeth, and change clothes daily.
- Never wear artificial nails when providing care. They trap many microorganisms (including pathogens), can scratch your client, and can tear your gloves if they are worn. Jewellery such as rings, bracelets, or watches can also cause these problems.
- Make sure your vaccinations are up to date (see TABLE 23–2 on page 433).
- Dispose of or store soiled tissues, linens, and other materials in leak-proof plastic bags.
- Empty garbage at least once a day.
- Keep tables, countertops, wheelchair trays, and other surfaces clean and dry.
- Wash contaminated areas with soap and water. Stool, urine, and blood contain microbes, as do other body fluids, secretions, and excretions.
- Clean work surfaces after completing a task, when they are dirty, and after blood or other potentially infectious material is spilled. Follow employer policies.
- Provide for the client's hygiene (see Chapter 30).
- Keep drainage containers below the drainage site (see Chapter 32).
- Cook meats and poultry adequately. Wash fruits and raw vegetables before eating or serving them. Handle and store all foods safely (see Chapter 28).
- Wash all cooking and eating utensils with soap and water after use.

Controlling Portals of Exit

- Cover your nose and mouth when coughing or sneezing. Wash your hands immediately.
- Give tissues to clients to use when coughing or sneezing.
- Wear personal protective equipment, as needed.
- Check your hands frequently for cuts, scrapes, or other breaks in the skin. Report any to your supervisor.

Controlling Transmission

- Wash your hands properly and at appropriate times (see **BOXES 23–4** on page 428 and **23–5** on page 436).
- Assist clients with hand hygiene:
  - Before and after handling or eating food
  - After elimination
  - After coughing, sneezing, or blowing the nose
  - After changing tampons, sanitary pads, incontinence products, or other personal hygiene products
  - After contact with blood, body fluids, secretions, or excretions
  - Any time their hands are soiled
- Make sure all clients have their own care equipment, including wash basins, bedpans, urinals, commodes, and glass thermometers. Make sure all clients have their own toothbrush, drinking glass, towels, washcloths, eating and drinking utensils, and other personal care items. Make sure that these items are not shared among clients or among the client's family members.
- Do not take equipment and supplies from one client's room to use for another client—even if the item is unused.
- Hold equipment and linens (clean or contaminated) away from your uniform to prevent the transfer of microbes from the equipment to your uniform and from your uniform to the equipment (**FIGURE 23–9**).
- Prevent dust movement, as dust carries microbes. Do not shake linens. Use a damp cloth for dusting.
- Remove soiled linens by folding them so that the dirtiest areas are in the centre.
- Clean from the cleanest area to the dirtiest to prevent soiling a clean area.
- Clean away from your body. Do not dust, brush, or wipe toward yourself. Otherwise, you transmit microbes to your skin, hair, and clothing.
- Flush urine and stool down the toilet. Avoid splatters and splashes by pouring carefully and closing the toilet lid prior to flushing. Cover

Continued

BOX 23–6 Medical Asepsis Measures You Should Follow—cont'd

bedpans and commodes with a lid when transporting them in order to contain microbes as well as odours.
- Pour contaminated liquids directly into sinks or toilets. Avoid splashing them onto other areas. Clean and disinfect the sink and contaminated areas immediately.
- Avoid sitting on a client's bed. You will pick up microbes and transfer them to the next surface that you sit on, possibly another client's bed.
- Do not use items that have touched the floor, as the floor is contaminated. Do not let linens (clean or soiled) touch the floor.
- Disinfect tubs, showers, shower chairs, bedpans, urinals, and commodes after each use. Follow your employer's disinfection procedures.
- Report pests in the room—ants, spiders, mice, and so on.

Controlling Portals of Entry
- Provide good skin care and oral hygiene according to the care plan (see Chapter 30). Good hygiene and skin care promote intact skin and mucous membranes. Damaged skin and mucous membranes provide portals of entry.
- To protect the client's skin from injury, do not let the client lie on tubes or other items.
- Make sure linens are dry and wrinkle-free so as to protect the client's skin from injury (see Chapters 24 and 34).
- Turn and reposition the client, as directed in the care plan, to protect the client's skin from injury (see Chapters 24 and 25).
- Assist with or clean the client's genital area after elimination, called *perineal care,* as needed (see Chapter 30). Wipe and clean from the urethra (the cleanest area) to the rectum (the dirtiest area). This method helps prevent urinary tract infections.
- Make sure drainage tubes are properly connected. Otherwise, microbes can enter the drainage system.

Protecting the Susceptible Host
- Follow the care plan to meet hygiene needs and thereby protect the skin and mucous membranes of the client.
- Follow the care plan to meet nutrition and fluid needs to keep the immune system strong and prevent infection.
- Assist with coughing and deep-breathing exercises, as directed, to help prevent respiratory infections.

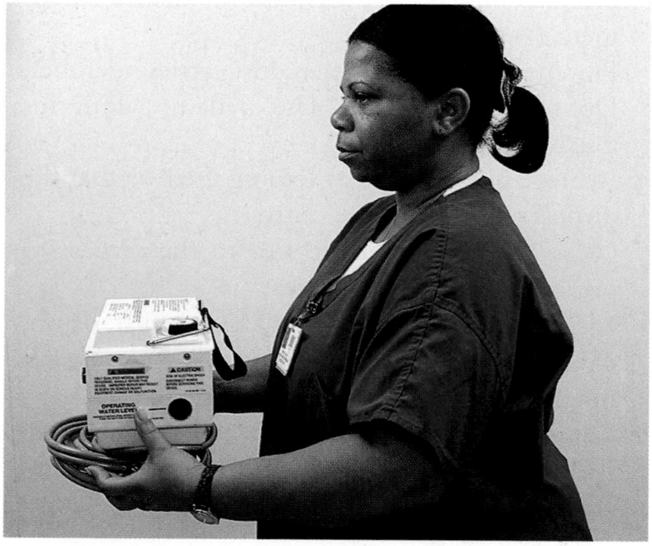

FIGURE 23–9 Hold equipment away from your uniform.

practised when caring for clients with certain communicable diseases.

Standard Practices

Standard Practices (sometimes called **Routine Practices** *or* **Standard Precautions**, depending on the province you live in) are guidelines to prevent the spread of infection from the following:

- Blood
- All body fluids, secretions, and excretions (except sweat), whether or not blood is visible
- Non-intact skin (skin with open sores, wounds, cuts, scrapes, or other breaks)
- Mucous membranes (including the membranes in the nose, eyes, mouth, vagina, and rectum)

BOX 23–7 summarizes the Standard Practices. Because you cannot tell by looking at people whether or not they carry pathogens, everyone must be considered a potential source of infection. Therefore, ***Standard Practices should be used when caring for all clients in all settings.***

Transmission-Based Practices

Some clients have (or are suspected of having) communicable diseases, which are highly contagious. In certain cases, additional isolation precautions are required to protect staff, visitors, and other clients from the infection. **Transmission-Based Practices** are guidelines to contain pathogens within one area, usually the client's room. Only clients infected or colonized with certain pathogens are placed under Transmission-Based Practices. These precautions are followed in addition to Standard Practices. You will be told when Transmission-Based Practices are ordered for a client.

There are three types of Transmission-Based Practices: (1) airborne precautions, (2) droplet precautions, and (3) contact precautions (BOX 23–8).

BOX 23–7 Standard Practices

Hand Hygiene

- Wash your hands after touching blood, body fluids, secretions, excretions, non-intact skin, mucous membranes, and contaminated items. Wash your hands even if you wore gloves.
- Practise hand hygiene immediately before putting on gloves and immediately after removing gloves.
- Practise hand hygiene between client contacts.
- Practise hand hygiene, whenever necessary, to avoid transferring microbes to other people or areas.
- Practise hand hygiene between tasks and procedures on the same client to prevent cross-contamination of different body sites.
- Use plain soap for routine handwashing. Your supervisor will tell you when other types of soap or agents are needed.

Gloves

- Wear gloves when touching blood, body fluids, secretions, excretions, non-intact skin, mucous membranes, and contaminated items. Clean, disposable, nonsterile gloves are adequate.
- Change gloves between tasks and procedures on the same client.
- Change gloves after contact with material that may be highly contaminated.
- Remove gloves promptly after use.
- Remove gloves before touching uncontaminated items and surfaces.
- Remove gloves before going to another client.
- Practise hand hygiene immediately after removing gloves to prevent the transfer of microbes to other clients or areas.

Masks and Eye Protection

- Wear a mask and eye protection (goggles or a face shield) during procedures and tasks that are likely to cause splashes or sprays of blood, body fluids, secretions, or excretions to protect your eyes, nose, and mouth from contact with splashes or sprays (see FIGURE 23–11 on p. 450).

Gowns

- Wear a gown during procedures and tasks that are likely to cause splashes or sprays of blood, body fluids, secretions, or excretions. The gown protects the skin and also prevents contamination of clothing. A clean, nonsterile gown is adequate.
- Remove a used gown as soon as possible.
- Practise hand hygiene after removing the gown to prevent transfer of microbes to other clients or areas.

Care of Equipment

- Handle used care equipment carefully. Equipment may be contaminated with blood, body fluids, secretions, or excretions. Do not let the equipment touch your skin, mucous membranes, or clothing. Also, prevent the transfer of microbes to other clients or areas.

Continued

BOX 23–7 Standard Practices—cont'd

- Do not use one client's reusable items for another client. The item must be cleaned and disinfected or sterilized before it is used again.
- Discard disposable (single-use) items properly.

Environmental Control

- Follow employer procedures for the routine care, cleaning, and disinfection of surfaces, including environmental surfaces, bed rails, bedside equipment, and other frequently touched surfaces.

Linen

- Follow employer policy for linen that is soiled with blood, body fluids, secretions, or excretions. The policy describes how to handle, transport, and process soiled linen.
- Do not touch soiled linen to your skin, mucous membranes, or clothing.
- Do not shake linens so as to prevent the transfer of microbes to other clients and the surrounding area.

Occupational Health and Blood-Borne Pathogens

- Use extreme care when handling **sharps** (equipment or items that may pierce the skin, such as needles, scalpels, razor blades, lancets, and broken glass).
- Use extreme care when handling sharp instruments after procedures.
- Use extreme care when cleaning used instruments.
- Use extreme care when disposing of used needles.
- Never recap used needles. Do not handle them with both hands. Never direct the needle point toward any body part. Use a one-handed "scoop" technique or a mechanical device that holds the needle sheath.
- Do not remove used needles from disposable syringes by hand.
- Do not bend, break, or otherwise handle used needles by hand.
- Place used disposable syringes and needles, scalpel blades, and other sharp items in puncture-resistant containers.
- Place reusable syringes and needles in a puncture-resistant container for transport to the reprocessing area.
- Use barrier devices for rescue breathing in emergencies.

Client Placement

- A private room is used if the client:
  - Contaminates the area
  - Does not or cannot assist in maintaining hygiene or environmental control
- Follow your supervisor's instructions if a private room is not available.

BOX 23–8 Types of Transmission-Based Practices

Airborne Precautions

For known or suspected infections caused by microbes transmitted by airborne droplets.

Examples: Measles, chicken pox, TB, FRI, and SARS.

Practices:

- Follow Standard Practices.
- Assign client to a private room.
- Keep the room door closed and the client in the room.
- Wear respiratory protection (such as an N-95 respirator) when entering the room of a client with known or suspected TB or SARS (see **BOX 23–11**). A disposable surgical mask does not provide enough protection. Follow employer policy for care of clients with TB.
- Do not enter the room of a client with known or suspected measles or chicken pox if you are susceptible to the disease. If you are susceptible but must enter the room, wear respiratory

Continued

BOX 23–8 Types of Transmission-Based Practices—cont'd

protection (not needed if you are immune). A disposable surgical mask does not provide enough protection.

- Limit moving and transporting the client from the room. The client must be made to wear a mask when being moved or transported from the room for any reason.
- For home care clients, revise these precautions as necessary. For example, wear respiratory protection (if not immune) when in the client's home. Check with your supervisor and the care plan before entering the home.

Droplet Precautions

For known or suspected infections caused by microbes transmitted by droplets produced by coughing, sneezing, or talking.

Examples: Meningitis, pneumonia, influenza, and mumps.

Practices:

- Follow Standard Practices.
- Assign a private room if possible.
- Keep the room door closed unless the bed is more than 1 m (3 ft.) from the door
- Wear a disposable surgical mask when working within 1 m (3 ft.) of the client. (Wear a mask on entering the room if required by employer policy.)
- Limit moving and transporting the client from the room. The client should wear a mask when she has to be moved or transported from the room for any reason.
- For home care clients, revise these precautions as necessary. Household members should avoid sharing common articles or eating utensils. Check with your supervisor and the care plan before entering the home.

Contact Precautions

For known or suspected infections caused by microbes transmitted by (1) direct contact with the client (skin-to-skin contact that occurs during care) or (2) indirect contact (contact with surfaces or care items in the client's room).

Examples: MROs and gastro-intestinal, respiratory, skin, or wound infections.

Practices:

- Follow Standard Practices.
- Assign a private room if possible.
- Leave the room door open as per client's preference.
- Wear gloves when entering the room.
- Wear a gown when entering the room if the client is incontinent or has diarrhea, an ileostomy, a colostomy, or wound drainage not contained by a dressing.
- Make sure gloves cover your wrists and the cuff of your sleeve or gown (see **FIGURE 23-13** on page 452).
- Change gloves after touching anything that might have high concentrations of microbes (for example, fecal material or wound discharge).
- Remove gloves, ensuring they are turned inside out, before leaving the client's room (see the procedure *Removing Gloves* on p. 440).
- Discard gloves in a container for contaminated waste (see p. 453). Follow employer policy.
- Practise hand hygiene immediately after removing gloves. Your supervisor will tell you what agent to use (usually an antimicrobial agent or a waterless, alcohol-based hand sanitizer).
- Do not touch potentially contaminated surfaces or items after removing gloves and washing hands.
- When opening the door, use a paper towel to touch the doorknob. Discard the paper towel in the garbage pail inside the room as you leave.
- Remove the gown before leaving the client's room. Make sure your clothing does not touch potentially contaminated surfaces in the client's room.
- Limit moving or transporting the client from the room. Maintain precautions if moving or transporting the client is necessary.
- For home care clients, revise these precautions as necessary. Check with your supervisor and the care plan before entering the home.

The choice of precautions depends on how a particular pathogen is spread.

When clients in a facility are under Transmission-Based Practices, they are usually placed in private or semi-private rooms in order to isolate their germs from infecting others. The isolation room must have handwashing and toilet facilities. It also must have wastebaskets and laundry and garbage containers lined with plastic bags. An isolation sign that states that precautions are in place is usually displayed on the outside of the room door.

Sometimes, Transmission-Based Practices are necessary for home care clients to protect other household members and home care workers. For example, if a client is infected with an MRO, Transmission-Based Practices might be required. As a member of the home care team, you will be told of the need for these precautions. An isolation sign is not needed in the home.

The rules in **BOX 23–9** are a guide for giving safe care when Transmission-Based Practices are used. Your employer may follow these or other guidelines. Know your employer's policies about isolation precautions.

Protective Measures

Standard Practices and Transmission-Based Practices involve wearing personal protective equipment, also known as PPE (gloves, mask, gown, and eye protection). Your supervisor and employer policy will guide you about when to use PPE. **BOX 23–10** lists the proper order for putting on and taking off a full set of PPE. Standard Practices also involve careful handling of sharps. Transmission-Based Practices involve extra measures when removing linens, garbage, and equipment from the room. Special measures are also needed when transporting clients.

Wearing Masks and Respiratory Protection

Masks (also called *surgical masks*), which are disposable, prevent pathogens from entering your mouth and nose; protect you from splashes or sprays of blood, body fluids, secretions, or excretions; and prevent the spread of microbes from your respiratory tract. Breathing can cause masks to become wet or moist. A wet or moist mask is considered to be contaminated, so you must apply a new mask if yours becomes damp (see the procedure *Wearing a Mask*).

BOX 23–9 General Rules for Transmission-Based Practices

- Wear personal protective equipment, as required.
- Collect all needed equipment before entering the room. Limit the number of trips in and out of the room.
- Prevent contamination of equipment and supplies. If you drop anything on the floor, consider the item contaminated, and do not use it.
- Use mops wetted with a disinfectant solution to clean floors. Floor dust is contaminated.
- Prevent drafts. Pathogens are carried in the air by drafts.
- Use paper towels to handle contaminated items.
- Remove items from the room in sturdy, leak-proof plastic bags.
- Double-bag items if the outer part of the bag is or can be contaminated (see p. 453).
- Follow employer policy for removing and transporting disposable and reusable items.
- Return reusable dishes, eating utensils, and trays to the food service department or kitchen. Discard disposable dishes, eating utensils, and trays in the waste container in the client's room.
- Do not touch your hair, nose, mouth, eyes, or other body parts when providing care.
- Do not touch any clean area or object if your hands are contaminated.
- Place clean items or objects that you bring into the room on paper towels.
- Do not shake linen.
- Use paper towels to turn faucets on and off.
- Tell your supervisor if you have fever, cuts, open skin areas, vomiting, diarrhea, a sore throat, or a cough.

BOX 23–10 Order for Putting on and Taking off a Full Set of Personal Protective Equipment

Put on PPE in the following order (wash hands first):

- Mask
- Goggles or face shield
- Gown
- Gloves

Take off PPE in the following order:

- Gloves
- Gown
  (Perform hand hygiene.)
- Goggles or face shield
- Mask
  (Perform hand hygiene.)

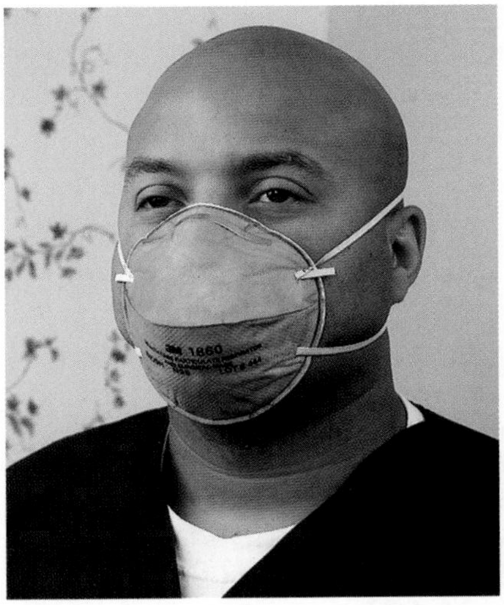

FIGURE 23–10 The N-95 respirator. Respiratory protection is used when caring for clients with TB and other infections requiring airborne precautions.

There are different types of masks for different situations. If you are required to wear *respiratory protection*, you must wear a special face mask that filters the air—for example, the N-95 respirator used for clients under airborne isolation precautions (**FIGURE 23–10**). **BOX 23–11** discusses different types of masks. It is *your responsibility* to be fitted for the correct type of mask and to wear it properly, following employer policy. When airborne and droplet precautions are in place, everyone—staff, clients, and visitors—needs to wear these masks.

BOX 23–11 Particulate Respirator Masks

Special masks (such as the N-95 mask in **FIGURE 23–10**) are designed to provide respiratory protection against certain airborne infections such as TB and SARS. The N-95 mask is the most common size of mask—that is, it fits most people—but it is not intended to be used by people who have beards.

If the N-95 mask does not fit, you need to be "fit-tested" with other available mask sizes. It may be your employer's responsibility to make sure that you have been fit-tested. Under specific conditions, a trained fit-tester will spray a special solution of either a very sweet or a bitter substance toward you to find out if you can taste it through your mask.

If you *do* taste the sweet or bitter solution through your mask, the mask does not have the proper seal around your nose and mouth. Without a good seal, you may be at risk for exposure to an airborne pathogen since you will not be able to prevent the pathogen from entering your body.

Wearing Personal Protective Equipment

Gowns, plastic aprons, shoe covers, boots, and leg coverings prevent the spread of microbes by protecting your clothes, wrists, and arms from contact with blood, body fluid, secretions, and excretions. They also protect against splashes and sprays.

Gowns must completely cover your clothing. The sleeves are long with tight cuffs. The gown opens at the back and is tied at the neck and waist. The inside and neck are *clean*, and the outside and waist strings are *contaminated*. Gloves should be worn so that they cover the cuffs of the gown (see **FIGURE 23–13** on p. 452). Gowns are used only once. A wet gown is contaminated and must be replaced with a dry one. Disposable gowns are made of paper and should be discarded after one use. Reusable gowns are made of cloth and must be laundered before reuse.

Wearing a Mask

123

Advocate on behalf of the client's quality of life by promoting:

Dignity • Independence • Preferences • Privacy • Safety

(see BOX 1–4, on p. 17)

1 Practise hand hygiene.

2 Pick up the mask by its upper ties. Do not touch the part that will cover your face.
This will reduce the chances of contaminating the part of the mask that you must breathe through.

3 Place the mask over your nose and mouth (**FIGURE 23–11, *A***).

4 Place the upper strings over your ears. Tie the strings in the back toward the top of your head. (**FIGURE 23–11, *B***).
Tying above and below the ears ensures a more secure fit.

5 Tie the lower strings at the back of your neck (**FIGURE 23–11, *C***). The lower part is under your chin.

6 Pinch the metal band around your nose. The top of the mask must be snug over your nose. If you wear glasses or protective eyewear, the top of the mask must be snug over your nose and under the bottom edge of the eyewear.
This ensures that air breathed through the mask is filtered by the mask, reducing your risk for harm.

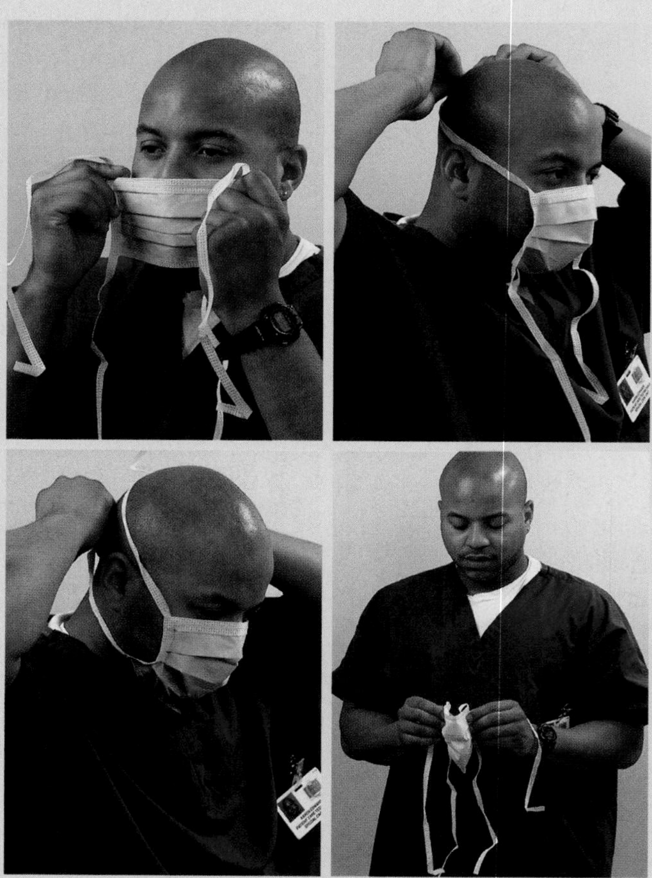

FIGURE 23–11 Donning a mask. **A,** Cover your nose and mouth with the mask. **B,** Tie upper strings at the back of your head. **C,** Tie lower strings at the back of your neck. **D,** Fold the inside of the mask together after removing it.

Continued

Wearing a Mask—cont'd

7 Practise hand hygiene.

8 Put on gloves, if needed.

9 Provide care to the client. Avoid coughing, sneezing, and unnecessary talking.
Coughing, sneezing, and unnecessary talking increase the risk for spreading airborne microbes and pathogens.

10 Change the mask if it becomes moist or contaminated.
Microbes thrive and multiply in a moist environment.

11 When the task has been finished, remove and discard the gloves. Wash your hands.

12 Remove the mask:
- a Untie the lower strings.
- b Untie the top strings.
- c Hold the top strings. Remove the mask.
- d Bring the strings together. The inside of the mask folds together (see **FIGURE 23–11, *D***). Do not touch the inside of the mask.

The ties are the least contaminated parts of the mask, and the face part is the most contaminated part (especially if it is damp). Avoiding the most contaminated areas will reduce the risk of spreading pathogens.

13 Discard the mask. Follow employer policy.
Masks trap moisture, which attracts airborne pathogens. Masks should be discarded after each use to reduce the spread of pathogens.

14 Practise hand hygiene.
The mask that you just discarded is full of microbes and pathogens. Practising hand hygiene will reduce your risk of being contaminated by them.

Donning and Removing a Gown

123

Advocate on behalf of the client's quality of life by promoting:

Dignity • Independence • Preferences • Privacy • Safety *(see BOX 1–4, on p. 17)*

1 Remove your watch and all jewellery.
These items may harbour microbes and pathogens. Removing them reduces the risk of contaminating your gown or work surface.

2 Roll up uniform sleeves.

3 Practise proper hand hygiene.
Hand hygiene reduces dead skin cells and microbes present on the skin.

4 Pick up a clean gown. Hold it out in front of you, and let it unfold. Do not shake the gown.
Shaking the gown can scatter microbes and pathogens and contaminate your work surface.

5 Put your hands and arms through the sleeves (**FIGURE 23–12, *A***).

6 Make sure the gown covers the front of your uniform and is snug at the neck.
By covering the front of your uniform, you are reducing the risk of contaminating yourself.

7 Tie the strings at the back of the neck (**FIGURE 23–12, *B***).

8 Overlap the back of the gown. Make sure the gown covers your uniform. The gown should be snug, not loose. (**FIGURE 23–12, *C***).
Uncovered uniform sections will most likely become contaminated.

9 Tie the waist strings at the back.
Tying the strings ensures the gown will stay in place.

Continued

Donning and Removing a Gown—cont'd

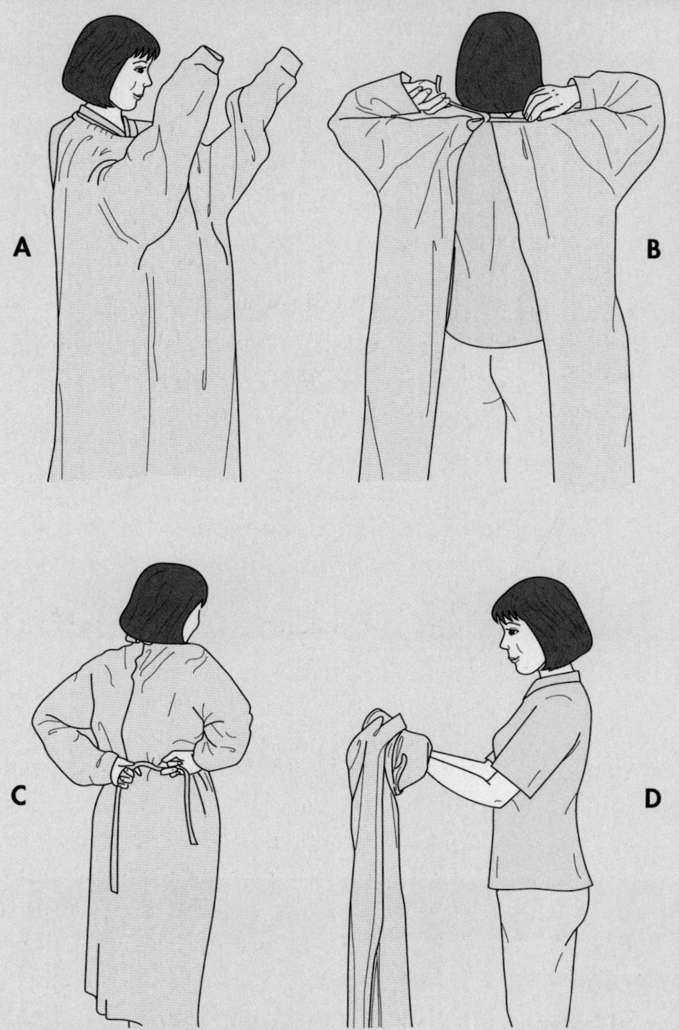

FIGURE 23–12 Gowning technique. **A,** Put your arms and hands through the sleeves. **B,** Tie the strings at the back of your neck. **C,** Overlap the gown in the back to cover your entire uniform. **D,** Turn the gown inside out as you remove it.

10 Put on gloves. Ensure they cover the cuffs of the gown (**FIGURE 23–13**).
This prevents contaminating your wrists.

11 Provide care to the client.

12 Remove and discard the gloves. Practise hand hygiene.

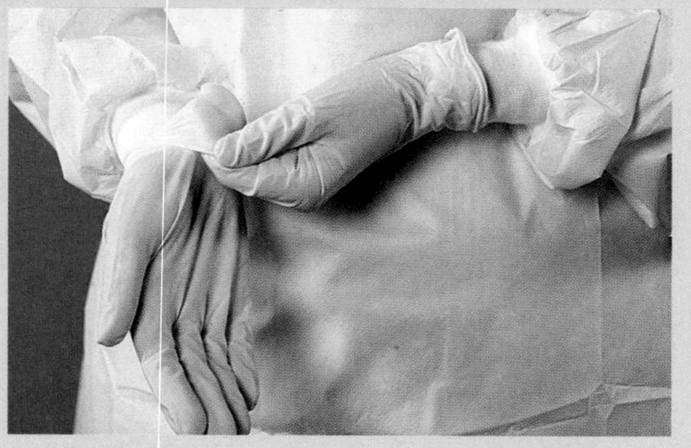

FIGURE 23–13 The gloves cover the cuffs of the gown.

The gloves are considered the most contaminated items, so they should be removed and discarded first.

13 Remove the gown:
- a Untie the waist strings.
- b Practise proper hand hygiene.
- c Untie the neck strings. Do not touch the outside of the gown.
- d Peel the gown away from the neck and shoulders. Pull the gown down from the shoulders.
- e Turn the outside toward the inside.
- f Hold the gown at the inside shoulder seams and bring your hands together (**FIGURE 23–12,** *D*).

14 Roll up the gown away from you. Keep it inside out.
Turning the gown inside out keeps the contamination contained and away from your uniform and skin.

15 Discard the gown. Follow employer policy.
Discarding the gown immediately prevents accidental cross-contamination.

16 Practise hand hygiene.
Hand hygiene reduces dead skin cells and microbes present on the skin.

Wearing Eye Protection and Face Shields

Goggles and face shields protect your eyes, mouth, and nose from the splashing or spraying of blood, body fluids, secretions, or excretions. You may need such protection when giving care to clients, cleaning instruments, or disposing of contaminated fluids.

Discard disposable eye protection after use. Reusable eye protection should be cleaned with soap and water and then disinfected before reuse.

Disposing of Sharps

Although, as a support worker, you do not administer injections, you may come across needles that are improperly disposed of. Improper disposal is especially common in home care. For example, while changing sheets for a client who has diabetes, you may find a forgotten needle in the bed. Or while emptying the garbage can, you could find an IV device that was mistakenly tossed into it. You must always watch out for stray sharps, especially if you know the client frequently uses needles.

Standard Practices say that used needles must not be bent or broken. Place them and other sharps into a container that is tightly capped, puncture-resistant, and leak-proof. This container, usually provided by an employer, may be made of steel or heavy plastic. The container should be labelled. Other containers can be used as long as they follow the criteria (see the *Focus on Home Care: Sharps Containers* box).

If your skin is pierced by a needle stick or another sharp, you must report the incident at once (see Chapter 22). Such an incident puts you at risk for infections, including HIV, hepatitis B, and hepatitis C. Assume that all clients are potential carriers of these viruses. ***Never ignore a sharps injury.***

Immediately after being poked by a sharp, encourage bleeding from the site of your injury and flush the area with large amounts of water for about 5 minutes. You should then seek prompt medical attention, according to employer policy. Your client may be asked to consent to testing for the above-mentioned viruses to help with managing your exposure. As always, confidentiality is important through this process. You will be told of evaluation results and also of any medical conditions that may need treatment.

FOCUS ON HOME CARE

Sharps Containers

Home care agencies often use sharps containers that are different from those used in facilities. Safe sharps containers used in home care include empty bleach bottles, coffee cans with the plastic lids taped closed, and plastic milk bottles. Glass or clear plastic containers should not be used. The home care agency is responsible for collecting the containers and disposing of them according to agency policy and local laws.

Bagging and Disposing of Waste Items

Items contaminated with blood, body fluids, secretions, or excretions are called **biohazardous waste** and may be harmful to others. (*Bio* means life, and *hazardous* means dangerous or harmful.) These items are considered infectious and must be disposed of in specially marked containers, according to employer policy. Biohazardous waste includes used gloves, dressings, incontinence products, and soiled linen. Containers for these items are lined with sturdy, leak-proof plastic bags that may be colour-coded. The containers are labelled with the universal *BIOHAZARD* symbol (**FIGURE 23–14**).

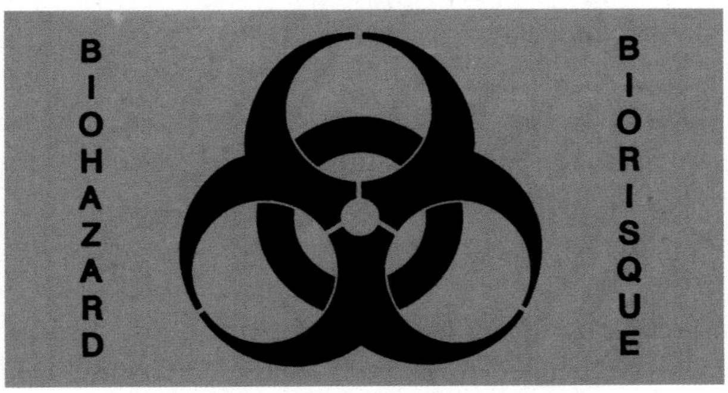

FIGURE 23–14 *BIOHAZARD* symbol.

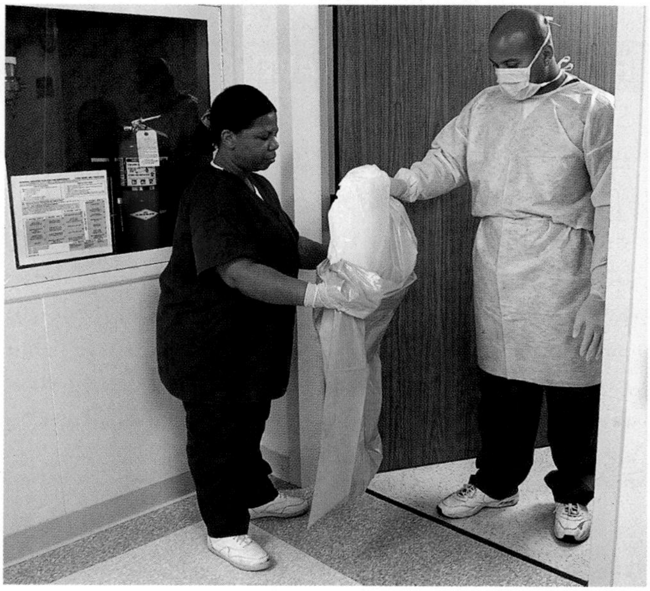

FIGURE 23–15 Double-bagging. One worker is in the room inside the doorway; the other is outside the room. The contaminated bag is placed inside the clean bag.

Follow employer policy for bagging and transporting biohazardous waste. One bag is usually adequate. Double-bagging (see **FIGURE 23–15**) is not needed unless the contaminated waste touches the outside of the first bag or the bag contains linens that are wet or soiled. Two staff members are needed for double-bagging in isolation rooms:

- The worker in the room places contaminated items into a bag and then seals the bag.
- The worker outside the room holds open another bag. This bag is clean. A wide cuff is made on the clean bag to protect hands from contamination.
- The contaminated bag is placed in the clean bag at the doorway.

Handle soiled linen as little as possible, and bag it in a linen bag with the *BIOHAZARD* symbol immediately ***in the room where it was used***. Do not sort it or rinse it in client care areas. Do not overfill the bag because it is important to be able to tie the bag securely. Linen that is very wet or soiled should be double-bagged to prevent leakage. Place the linen bag in a laundry hamper lined with a biohazard plastic bag.

Transporting Clients on Transmission-Based Practices

Clients on Transmission-Based Practices usually do not leave their rooms. However, they may have to go to another area of the facility for special treatments or tests.

Transporting procedures vary among facilities. Some require transport by bed, which prevents contaminating wheelchairs and stretchers. Other facilities use wheelchairs and stretchers.

A safe transport protects other residents or patients, staff, and visitors from infection. Follow employer policies and the following guidelines to safely transport clients:

- Ensure the client is wearing a clean gown or pyjamas and an isolation gown.
- Put a mask on a client on airborne or droplet precautions.
- Cover any draining wounds.
- Give the client tissues and a leak-proof bag in which to place used tissues.
- Wear a gown, mask, and gloves, as required by the isolation precaution.
- Place an extra layer of sheets and absorbent pads on the stretcher or wheelchair to protect against draining fluids.
- Do not allow anyone else into the elevator so as to reduce exposure to the infection.
- Alert staff in the receiving area about the isolation precautions. They should wear gowns, masks, protective eyewear, and gloves, as needed.
- Disinfect the stretcher or wheelchair after use.

Basic Needs and Transmission-Based Practices

All clients have love, belonging, and self-esteem needs, but often care is not taken to meet them when Transmission-Based Practices are used. Visitors and staff tend to avoid the client, as the extra effort required to put on PPE may discourage them from visiting. Some visitors may be afraid of getting the disease and feel anxious during the visit and unsure about what they can touch safely. Without intending to, visitors and staff can make the client feel ashamed and guilty about having a contagious disease. As a result, the client can feel lonely, unloved, and rejected. Self-esteem is easily damaged, and depression is a risk.

It is important to understand the reasons for using Transmission-Based Practices. Do not be afraid of the client. Remember, the precautions enable you to interact safely with the client and help meet the client's need for belonging and self-esteem. The following actions are helpful:

- Remember that it is the pathogen that is undesirable, not the client.
- Treat the client with respect, kindness, and dignity.
- Allow the client to make choices and decisions whenever possible.
- Provide newspapers, magazines, and other reading material to the client.
- Provide hobby materials, if possible.
- Place a clock or radio in the client's room.
- Encourage the client to telephone family and friends.
- Provide a current television schedule.
- Organize your work so that you can stay to visit with the client.
- Say hello from the doorway often if the door can be left open.

Young children and clients with dementia do not understand the need for isolation precautions. PPE may frighten children. It also may increase confusion and cause fear and agitation in adults with dementia. The following measures can help in such situations:

- Let the client see your face before putting on a mask or protective eyewear.
- Tell the client who you are and what you are going to do.
- Use a calm, soothing voice.
- Do not hurry the client.
- Follow the care plan and your supervisor's instructions for individual approaches.
- Report signs of increased confusion or changes in behaviour to your supervisor.

SURGICAL ASEPSIS

As was previously mentioned in this chapter, there are two levels of asepsis: (1) medical asepsis, discussed on pages 432–442, and (2) surgical asepsis. Surgical asepsis (sterile technique) refers to practices that keep equipment and supplies free of *all* microbes—pathogens and nonpathogens. Surgical asepsis is required any time the skin or sterile tissues are penetrated.

Procedures that require surgical asepsis include catheterizations, IV administrations, suctioning, sterile dressing changes, and blood collection. Support workers are not normally authorized to do these procedures. However, you could be delegated to do them, or you might assist with these procedures. You should, therefore, understand the principles of surgical asepsis.

Principles of Surgical Asepsis

To prevent introducing microbes into the client, sterile procedures require the use of sterile gloves and sterile equipment. If an item is contaminated, the client is at risk for infection, so maintaining a sterile field is very important. A **sterile field** is a work area free of pathogens and nonpathogens (including spores). Remember that *clean* is different from *sterile*! All items in contact with the client must be kept sterile. **BOX 23–12** lists the principles and practices of surgical asepsis. Follow them to maintain a sterile field when assisting with a sterile procedure.

You must also wear PPE to prevent contact with blood, body fluids, secretions, and excretions.

BOX 23–12 Principles and Practices of Surgical Asepsis

- A sterile item can touch only another sterile item.
- If a sterile item touches a clean item, the sterile item is contaminated.
- A sterile package that is open, torn, punctured, wet, or moist is contaminated.
- A sterile package is contaminated after the expiration date on the package.
- Place only sterile items on a sterile field.
- Apply sterile gloves (**FIGURE 23–16**) or use sterile forceps to handle other sterile items.
- Consider any item to be contaminated if you are unsure of its sterility.
- Do not use contaminated items. They must be discarded or resterilized.
- A sterile field or sterile items are always kept within your vision and above the level of your waist. If an item is below the level of your waist, the item is contaminated.
- Keep sterile gloved hands above the level of your waist and within your sight.
- Do not leave a sterile field unattended or turn your back on a sterile item or a sterile field. If you cannot see an item, the item is contaminated.
- Airborne microbes can contaminate sterile items or a sterile field.
- Prevent drafts. Close the door and avoid extra movements.
- Ask other staff in the room to avoid extra movements.
- Avoid coughing, sneezing, talking, or laughing over a sterile field. Turn your head away from the sterile field if you must talk.
- Wear a mask if you need to talk during the procedure.
- Do not assist with sterile procedures if you have a respiratory infection.
- Do not reach over a sterile field.
- Fluids flow downward because of gravity; therefore, hold wet items down. For example, if you have wet hands and hold them up, water will run down your arms.
- The sterile field is kept dry to avoid contamination; if the sterile field gets wet, it is then contaminated.
- Avoid spilling and splashing when pouring sterile fluids into sterile containers.
- The edges of a sterile field are contaminated.
- A 2.5-cm (1-in.) margin around the sterile field is contaminated (**FIGURE 23–17**).
- Place all sterile items inside the 2.5-cm margin of the sterile field.
- Items outside the 2.5-cm margin are contaminated.
- Honesty is essential to sterile technique. You know when you have contaminated an item or sterile field. Be honest with yourself even if no other staff members are present. Remove the contaminated item and correct the situation. If necessary, start over with sterile supplies. Report the contamination to your supervisor.

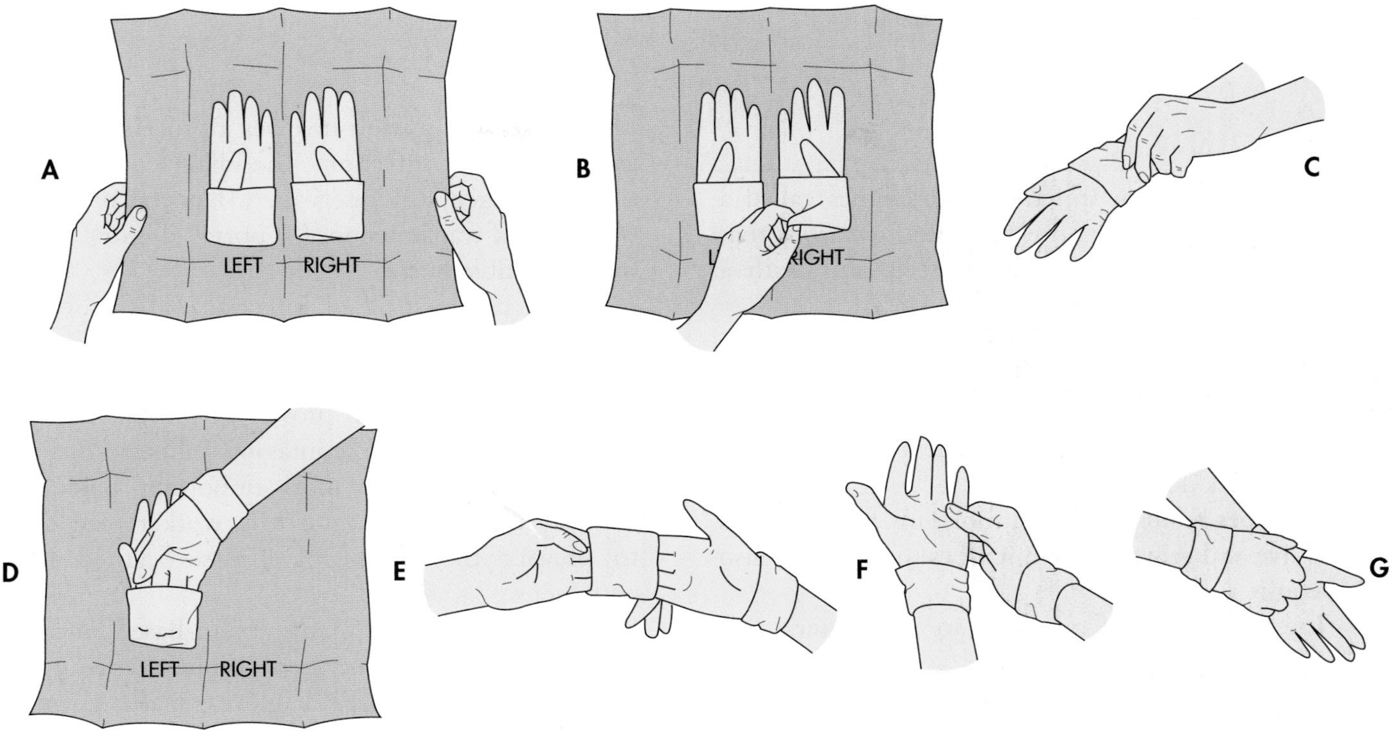

FIGURE 23–16 Donning sterile gloves. **A,** Open the inner wrapper to expose the gloves. **B,** Pick up the glove at the cuff with your thumb and index finger. **C,** Slide your fingers and hand into the glove. **D,** Reach under the cuff of the other glove with your fingers. **E,** Pull on the glove. **F,** Adjust each glove for comfort. **G,** Slide your fingers under the cuffs to pull them up.

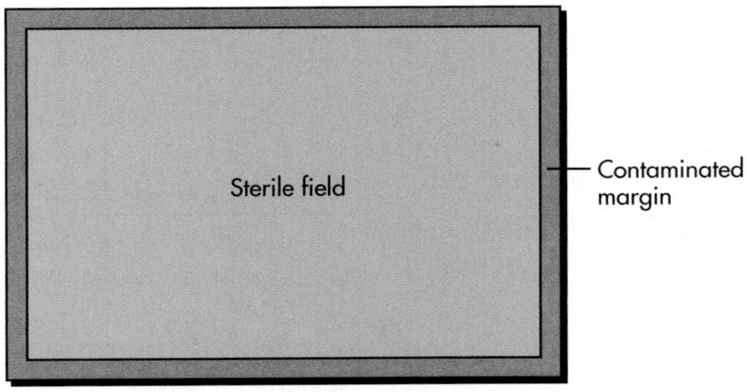

FIGURE 23–17 The 2.5-cm (1-in.) margin around a sterile field is considered contaminated.

CHAPTER REVIEW

KEY POINTS

- A microorganism (microbe), sometimes called a "germ" or "bug," is a form of life (*organism*) that is so small (*micro*) it can be seen only with a microscope.
- Normal flora contain microbes that naturally live and grow in certain locations on or in the human body.
- Nonpathogens do not cause illness or disease, but pathogens do.
- Microbes require warmth, moisture, and darkness to live and grow. Many microbes (but not all) also require oxygen.
- The three types of microbes are (1) bacteria, (2) viruses, and (3) fungi.
- Microbes are transmitted through (1) contact, (2) droplet, (3) airborne, (4) vehicle, and (5) vector modes of transmission.
- Signs and symptoms of infection include (1) fever and chills; (2) increased pulse and respiratory rates; (3) aches, pain, or tenderness; (4) fatigue and loss of energy; (5) loss of appetite; (6) nausea; (7) vomiting and diarrhea; (8) rash; (9) sores on mucous membranes; (10) redness and swelling of a body part; (11) discharge or drainage from the infected area that may have a foul odour; (12) new or increased cough, sore throat, or runny or stuffy nose; and (13) burning pain when urinating, or the need to urinate more often or with increased urgency.
- Older adults' signs and symptoms of infection may differ in part because older adults tend to have lower body temperatures, decreased pain sensation, and less immune response to infection. Sometimes, the only sign of infection is a change in behaviour.
- A *local* infection is an infection that occurs in one body part, such as an infected cut on the arm. A *systemic* infection involves the whole body, and the affected person would have generalized (entire body) signs and symptoms of infection.
- A multidrug-resistant organism (MRO) is a pathogen that has developed resistance to most (or all) available antibiotics.
- The spread of infection involves a process known as the chain of infection. The chain consists of a (1) pathogen, (2) reservoir, (3) portal of exit, (4) mode of transmission, (5) portal of entry, and (6) susceptible host.
- A health care–associated infection (HAI) is an infection acquired from a health care provider or in a health care facility.
- Vaccinations have been proven to prevent many serious communicable (contagious) illnesses.
- Hand hygiene is the most important part of medical asepsis that health care workers can do to prevent the spread of illnesses caused by pathogens.
- Standard Practices and Transmission-Based Practices involve wearing personal protective equipment, also known as PPE (gloves, mask, gown, and eye protection).

CRITICAL THINKING IN PRACTICE

A nurse enters the room of a person who requires contact precautions. The nurse is not wearing PPE. What do you do? What PPE is needed? What precautions are needed upon entering and leaving the room and while in the room?

REVIEW QUESTIONS

Answers to these questions are at the bottom of page 459.

Circle T if the answer is true, and circle F if the answer is false.

1. T F A pathogen can cause an infection.
2. T F Multidrug-resistant organisms are easily treated with antibiotics and, because of that, are not a risk in facilities.
3. T F Older adults often do not show the usual signs of infection.
4. T F A person who is colonized by a pathogen cannot transfer the pathogen to others.
5. T F The presence of illness and the use of invasive devices increase the risk of infection.

6. T F Wash your hands before *or* after giving care.
7. T F You should hold your hands and forearms up during the handwashing procedure.
8. T F The duration of the handwash is not important.
9. T F Disinfecting items usually involves chemicals.
10. T F Unused items in a client's room can be used for another client.
11. T F Isolation precautions include Standard Practices *and* Transmission-Based Practices.
12. T F Standard Practices are used only when the client has a specific contagious disease.
13. T F Transmission-Based Practices are guidelines that help keep pathogens within one area, usually the client's room.
14. T F Gloves are worn at all times.
15. T F A mask is contaminated when moist.
16. T F Goggles, masks, and gowns are worn when there is a risk of splashing blood or body fluids.
17. T F You do not need to report a sharps injury if the bleeding is not severe.
18. T F Double-bagging always requires two people.
19. T F An item is sterile if nonpathogens are present.
20. T F A sterile item can touch only another sterile item.
21. T F The 2.5-cm edge around a sterile field is considered contaminated.

Circle the BEST answer.

22. Most pathogens are destroyed by:
    A. Water
    B. High heat
    C. Oxygen
    D. Nourishment

23. Aseptic practices:
    A. Destroy spores
    B. Reduce the number of microbes
    C. Are a link in the chain of infection
    D. Destroy all microbes—pathogens and nonpathogens

24. Standard Practices:
    A. Are used for all clients
    B. Involve surgical asepsis
    C. Prevent the spread of airborne pathogens
    D. Are not necessary for children or older clients

25. Gloves are always worn in the following situations:
    A. When washing a person's face
    B. When the client has a cold
    C. While washing spilled juice from the floor
    D. If you bite your fingernails

26. Proper use of personal protective equipment involves the following:
    A. Reusing your face mask after your break
    B. Using waterless hand sanitizer on disposable gloves for reuse
    C. Removing personal protective equipment after leaving the work area
    D. Wearing gloves when touching contaminated items or surfaces

27. Circle the words that indicate signs of infection: fever, vomiting, pain, tenderness, constipation, hunger, redness, fatigue, bluish skin around the mouth, a change in behaviour, bleeding, swelling, loss of appetite.

Answers: 1.T, 2.F, 3.T, 4.F, 5.T, 6.F, 7.F, 8.F, 9.T, 10.F, 11.T, 12.F, 13.T, 14.F, 15.T, 16.T, 17.F, 18.F, 19.F, 20.T, 21.T, 22.B, 23.B, 24.A, 25.D, 26.D, 27. Fever, vomiting, pain, tenderness, redness, fatigue, a change in behaviour, swelling, loss of appetite

CHAPTER 24

Skin Care and Prevention of Wounds

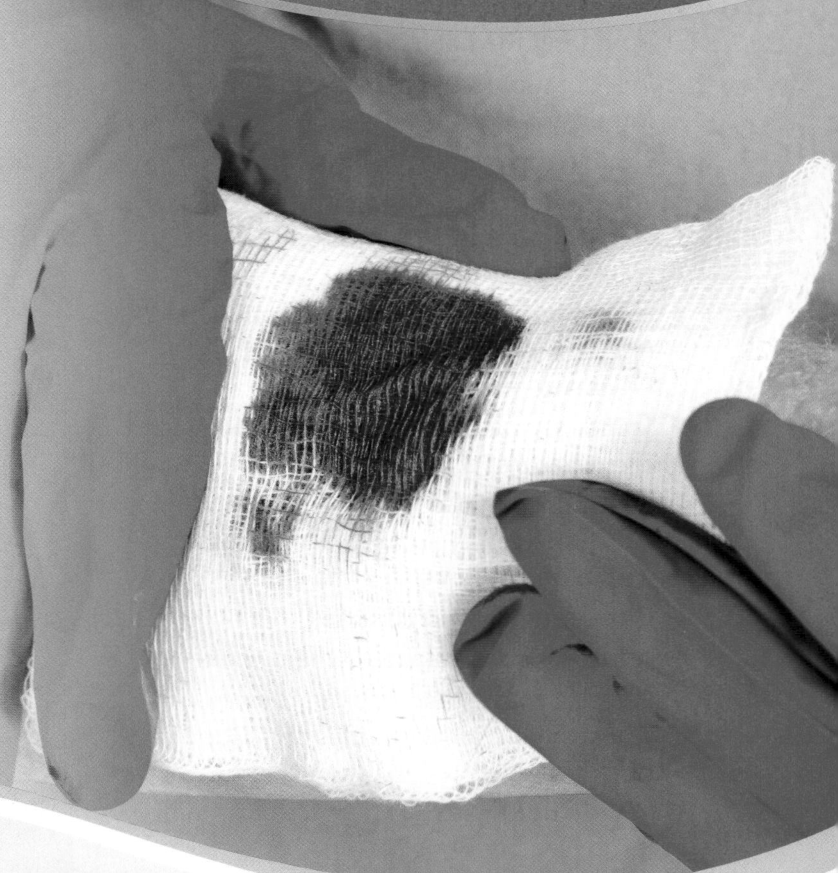

OBJECTIVES

After reading this chapter, the learner should be able to do the following:

- List clients at risk for skin tears and pressure ulcers.
- Describe the causes of skin tears and how to prevent them.
- Describe the signs, symptoms, and causes of pressure ulcers and ways to prevent them.
- Identify the pressure points in the basic bed positions and sitting positions.
- Describe the causes of leg and foot ulcers and ways to prevent them.
- Describe the process, types, and complications of wound healing.
- Describe what to observe about wounds and wound drainage.
- Explain how to secure dressings.
- Explain the guidelines for applying dressings.
- Describe how to meet the basic needs of clients who have wounds.
- Apply in your practice the procedures described in this chapter.

KEY TERMS

abrasion A partial-thickness wound caused by the scraping away or rubbing of skin. *p. 463*

arterial ulcer An open wound on the lower legs and feet caused by poor arterial blood flow. *p. 475*

bedsore See **pressure ulcer**. *p. 465*

bony prominence An area on the body where the underlying bone seems to "stick out." *p. 465*

Braden Scale A scale used to predict the likelihood of a client developing a pressure ulcer. *p. 467*

bruise See **contusion**. *p. 463*

chronic wound A wound that does not heal easily in a timely manner. *p. 463*

circulatory ulcer An open wound on the lower legs and feet caused by decreased blood flow through arteries or veins. Also known as **vascular ulcer**. *p. 473*

clean-contaminated wound A wound occurring from the surgical portal of entry into the urinary, reproductive, or digestive system. *p. 463*

clean wound A wound that is not infected; microbes have not entered the wound. *p. 463*

closed wound A wound in which tissues are injured but skin is not broken. *p. 463*

contaminated wound A wound with a high risk for infection; microbes have entered the wound. *p. 463*

contusion A closed wound caused by a blow to the body. Also known as a **bruise**. *p. 463*

decubitus ulcer See **pressure ulcer**. *p. 465*

dehiscence The separation of wound layers along a surgical suture line. *p. 476*

dirty wound See **infected wound**. *p. 463*

edema Swelling in tissues caused by an accumulation of fluid. *p. 473*

evisceration Separation of the wound accompanied by protrusion of abdominal organs. *p. 476*

friction Resistance that skin encounters when it rubs against another surface such as clothing, bedding, or another fold of skin. *p. 463*

full-thickness wound A wound in which the dermis, epidermis, and subcutaneous tissue are penetrated; muscle and bone may be involved. *p. 463*

gangrene A condition in which tissue dies and then decays. *p. 473*

hematoma The collection of blood under skin and tissues. *p. 476*

hemorrhage The excessive loss of blood within a short period. *p. 476*

incision An open wound with clean, straight edges; usually intentionally created with a sharp instrument. *p. 463*

infected wound A wound containing a large amount of bacteria and showing signs of infection. Also known as **dirty wound**. *p. 463*

intentional wound A wound created for treatment. *p. 463*

laceration An open wound with torn tissue and jagged edges. *p. 463*

necrotic tissue Localized tissue death as a result of disease or injury. *p. 482*

open wound A wound in which skin or the mucous membrane is broken. *p. 463*

partial-thickness wound A wound in which the dermis and epidermis of skin are broken. *p. 463*

penetrating wound An open wound in which skin and underlying tissues are pierced. *p. 463*

peri-wash A type of gentle soap for skin. It is used primarily as a cleanser and deodorizer of the perineal area soiled by urine and feces. *p. 480*

picture-frame dressing A type of dressing in which tape is applied to all four edges to reduce the likelihood of the dressing wrinkling or falling off. *p. 484*

pitting edema A type of edema that is evident by an impression left in the skin upon compressing the fingers into the swollen tissues and then removing the fingers. *p. 473*

pressure points Bony prominences that bear the weight of the body in certain positions and may lead to **pressure ulcers**. *p. 465*

pressure sore See **pressure ulcer**. *p. 465*

pressure ulcer Any injury caused by unrelieved pressure. Also known as **decubitus ulcer**, **bedsore**, or **pressure sore**. *p. 465*

puncture wound An open wound made by a sharp object; entry into skin and underlying tissues may be intentional or unintentional. *p. 463*

purulent drainage Thick drainage from a wound or body orifice, which may have a foul odour; purulent drainage is yellow, green, or brown and may indicate an infection. *p. 478*

sanguineous drainage Bloody drainage. *p. 478*

serosanguineous drainage Thin, watery drainage that is blood-tinged (*sanguineous*). *p. 478*

serous drainage Drainage that is clear and watery fluid. *p. 478*

shearing Tearing of skin tissue caused when the skin sticks to a surface (usually the bed or chair) and deeper tissues move downward, exerting pressure on the skin. *p. 464*

shock The condition that results when there is not enough blood supply to organs and tissues. *p. 476*

skin tear A break or rip in skin; the epidermis separates from the underlying tissue. *p. 463*

stasis ulcer See **venous ulcer**. *p. 473*

Steri-Strip A proprietary type of adhesive bandage; thin strips are applied across a skin tear to bring the skin edges together and hold them together while the wound heals. *p. 464*

trauma An accident or violent act that injures skin, mucous membranes, bones, or internal organs (*physical trauma*) or causes an emotionally painful, distressful, or shocking result (*emotional trauma*), which often leads to lasting mental and physical effects (*psychological trauma*). *p. 462*

unintentional wound A wound resulting from trauma. *p. 463*

vascular ulcer See **circulatory ulcer**. *p. 473*

venous ulcer Open wounds on the lower legs and feet caused by poor blood return through the veins. Also known as **stasis ulcer**. *p. 473*

wound A break in the skin or mucous membrane. *p. 462*

Skin is the body's first line of defence. It protects the body from microbes that cause infection and disease. As a support worker, you have to consider providing good skin care to your clients one of your most important tasks. Infants, older adults, and clients who have disabilities are at greatest risk for skin breakdown because their skin can be easily injured due to limited mobility and certain health conditions that make their skin more susceptible to injury. It should be noted that the skin of infants and the skin of older adults are quite different from one another. Support workers should also be aware that clients who are diabetic or have circulation challenges (see Chapter 37) are prone to delayed healing times and wound and skin infections. Support workers should look for signs of skin problems and report them immediately to either the nurse or their supervisor, depending on their workplace. **BOX 24–1** lists the common causes of skin breakdown.

A **wound** is a break in the skin or the mucous membrane, which becomes a portal of entry for microbes. Wounds have many causes. A surgical incision leaves a wound, for example, and wounds often result from **trauma**—an accident (such as a fall or vehicular accident) or violent act (such as a gunshot or stabbing) that injures skin, mucous membranes, bones, or internal organs. Other wounds may result from immobility or poor blood circulation.

The support worker's role in wound care depends on provincial or territorial laws, job description, and the client's condition. Whatever your role, you need to know the types of wounds, how wounds heal, and how to promote wound healing. You must prevent skin injury and give good skin care. When injury *does* occur, infection is a major threat, so wound care is important for preventing infection and further injury to the wound and nearby tissues.

BOX 24–1 Common Causes of Skin Breakdown

- Age-related changes in the skin
- Skin dryness
- Fragile and weak capillaries
- General thinning of the skin
- Loss of fatty layer under the skin
- Decreased sensation to touch, heat, and cold
- Decreased mobility
- Sitting in a chair or lying in bed most or all of the day
- Persistent diseases (e.g., diabetes, high blood pressure)
- Diseases that decrease circulation
- Poor nutrition
- Poor hydration
- Incontinence
- Moisture in the dark areas of the body (skin folds, under breasts, between toes, and perineal areas)
- Pressure on bony parts (see **FIGURE 24–1** on page 466)
- Poor care of fingernails or toenails
- Friction and shearing

BOX 24–2 Types of Wounds

Intentional Wound and Unintentional Wound

- **Intentional wound**—created for treatment; for example, surgical incisions, as well as sterile venipunctures (vein punctures) for starting intravenous (IV) therapy or for collecting blood specimens
- **Unintentional wound**—results from trauma—for example, falls, vehicle accidents, gunshots, stabbings

Open Wound and Closed Wound

- **Open wound**—a break in the skin or mucous membrane; intentional and most unintentional wounds are open
- **Closed wound**—injury to tissues without breaking the skin; for example, bruises, twists, and sprains

Clean Wound and Contaminated Wound

- **Clean wound**—not infected, meaning microbes have not entered the wound; closed wounds and intentional wounds created under surgically aseptic conditions are usually clean; because the urinary, respiratory, and digestive systems are not entered, there is a reduced risk of infection
- **Clean-contaminated wound**—result of the surgical entry (sterile technique used) of the urinary, reproductive, or digestive system; because these systems are not sterile and contain normal flora, the risk for infection is greater than with a clean wound
- **Contaminated wound**—unintentional wound (such as from a stabbing) that is not created under sterile conditions and is generally contaminated and has a high risk for infection; wound contamination can also occur from a break in surgical asepsis and from the spillage of intestinal contents; tissues may show signs of inflammation
- **Infected wound (dirty wound)**—wound containing a large amount of bacteria and showing signs of infection; for example, old wounds, surgical incisions into infected areas (such as a ruptured appendix), and traumatic injuries that rupture the bowel
- **Chronic wound**—one that does not heal easily in a timely manner, such as a pressure ulcer or circulatory ulcer (see pp. 465–475); any wound that is continually exposed to friction, pressure, or moisture can become chronic

Partial- and Full-Thickness Wounds (Described by Wound Depth)

- **Partial-thickness wound**—the dermis and epidermis of the skin are broken
- **Full-thickness wound**—the dermis, epidermis, and subcutaneous tissue are penetrated; muscle and bone may be involved

TYPES OF WOUNDS

Wounds are described in many ways (**BOX 24–2**), including the following:

- **Abrasion**—a partial-thickness wound caused by the scraping away or rubbing of skin
- **Contusion**—a closed wound caused by a blow to the body (a **bruise**)
- **Incision**—an open wound with clean, straight edges; usually intentionally created with a sharp instrument
- **Laceration**—an open wound with torn tissues and jagged edges
- **Penetrating wound**—an open wound in which skin and underlying tissues are pierced
- **Puncture wound**—an open wound made by a sharp object; entry into skin and underlying tissues may be intentional or unintentional

SKIN TEARS

A **skin tear** is a break or rip in the skin. The epidermis (top skin layer) separates from the underlying tissue. The hands, arms, and lower legs are common sites for skin tears. Many older adults have very thin and fragile skin, and even slight pressure or friction can cause a skin tear. **Friction** is the resistance that skin encounters when it rubs against another surface such as clothing, bedding, or another fold of skin. Clients who are most likely to have skin tears are those with very dry and paper-thin skin.

Causes of Skin Tears

Skin tears occur due to friction, shearing, pulling, or direct pressure on skin. **Shearing** is the tearing of skin tissues as a result of skin sticking to a surface (usually the bed or chair) and deeper tissues moving downward, exerting pressure on the skin (see Chapter 25). Blood vessels and tissues become damaged, reducing blood flow to the area and increasing the risk for a pressure ulcer. Shearing occurs when the client slides down in the bed or chair. Skin tears are commonly caused by the following:

- Bumping a hand, arm, or leg on any hard surface such as a bed, bed rail, chair, wheelchair footrest, or table
- Holding on to a client's arm or leg too tightly
- Repositioning, moving, or transferring a client without a transfer sheet or other nonfriction surface, the absence of which can cause the client's skin to rub against the surface and even tear
- Bathing, dressing, and other tasks
- Pulling buttons or zippers across fragile skin

It is always your responsibility to be careful when moving, repositioning, or transferring clients. Skin tears are painful, and they can become portals of entry for pathogens. Tell your supervisor at once if you cause or find a skin tear, bruise, bump, or scrape (see the *Supporting Mrs. Nippeskaya: Preventing Further Skin Injuries in a Frail Client* box).

Supporting Mrs. Nippeskaya: Preventing Further Skin Injuries in a Frail Client

You are the support worker assigned to care for Mrs. Nippeskaya, 56, a widow with ovarian cancer currently living at the long-term care facility where you are employed. Her daughter is trying to make arrangements to move her mother to the town where she lives. Because of Mrs. Nippeskaya's illness and her treatments, she has lost approximately 50 kg (110 pounds) over the past year.

Mrs. Nippeskaya has been very weak and dizzy for several months now, and while at home, she was frequently falling or bumping into the corner of her bed or dresser. Since being admitted to your facility, she has been advised to ask for assistance to go to the washroom. Yesterday, however, she did *not* ask for assistance, and when she stood up on her own, she lost her balance and fell to the floor, hitting the side of her bed.

The nursing staff heard Mrs. Nippeskaya fall and came to her side immediately. Upon examination, they observed a 3.75-cm (1.5-in.) tear on her right buttock and a 2.5-cm (1-in.) tear on her right forearm around her elbow. She also had several bruises and scrapes on her right arm and had difficulty moving her leg. Mrs. Nippeskaya was taken by ambulance to the local hospital, where she was examined, her leg was X-rayed, and her skin tears were covered with **Steri-Strip** bandages (which hold the skin edges together during healing). Back at the facility, she agreed to be lifted with a mechanical lift (see Chapter 25) for toileting.

Today, you and your co-worker apply the mechanical lift sling carefully and properly under Mrs. Nippeskaya's hips, according to your agency's policy. However, while raising her up, you notice that there is blood on her pants over her buttock area. You carefully lower her and remove her pants to find the source of the blood.

You discover that her buttock skin tear has reopened due to the friction of the mechanical lift sling on her skin. While your co-worker stays with Mrs. Nippeskaya, you summon assistance from the nurse. You are instructed to document everything you have observed and to switch to another mechanical device that does not require placing a sling around the client's buttocks. The nurse then applies clean Steri-Strips to Mrs. Nippeskaya's skin tear and fills out an incident report (see Chapter 22).

Clients at Risk for Skin Tears

Clients at risk for skin tears include the following:

- Those who require moderate to complete help in moving
- Those who have poor nutrition or are very thin
- Those who are poorly hydrated
- Those with altered mental awareness; for example, clients with dementia may resist care and move quickly and without warning, which can cause skin tears
- Those who are older

Prevention and Treatment of Skin Tears

Giving careful and safe care helps prevent skin tears and further injury. Follow the guidelines in **BOX 24–3**.

The physician and the nurse direct skin care treatment and may order dressings. Elastic wraps protect the skin from injury and help the healing process. Follow the care plan and your supervisor's instructions.

BOX 24–3 Guidelines for Preventing Skin Tears

- Follow the care plan for moving, lifting, repositioning, transferring, dressing, and bathing the client.
- Keep the skin moisturized, as per the care plan.
- Offer fluids, as per the care plan.
- Dress and undress the client carefully.
- Dress the client in soft clothing with long sleeves and long pants. Allow the client to make choices.
- Keep your fingernails short and filed smooth.
- Keep the client's fingernails short and filed smooth. Report to your supervisor if the client's toenails are long and rough.
- Do not wear rings with large or raised stones or edges that could snag on anything.
- Follow safety guidelines when transferring or lifting the client to and from a bed or wheelchair (see Chapter 25).
- Prevent friction and shearing during lifting, moving, transferring, and repositioning.
- Use a turning sheet to move and turn the client in bed.
- Use pillows to support arms and legs, as per the care plan.
- Be patient and calm when the client is confused or agitated or resists care.
- Ensure that bed rails and wheelchair arms, footrests, and leg supports are padded. Follow the care plan.
- Ensure that body parts are not pressing on each other by placing padding such as pillows, soft blankets, or towels between them.
- Provide good lighting to prevent the client from bumping into furniture, walls, and equipment.

PRESSURE ULCERS

A **pressure ulcer** (also called a **decubitus ulcer**, **bedsore**, or **pressure sore**) is any injury caused by unrelieved pressure. It usually occurs over a **bony prominence**—an area where the bone seems to "stick out" and is compressed under the client or between the client's skin folds. The shoulder blades, elbows, hip bones, sacrum (the bone in the lower part of the spine), knees, ankle bones, heels, and toes are all bony prominences.

These bony prominences are called **pressure points** because they bear the weight of the body in certain positions (**FIGURE 24–1**). Pressure from body weight can reduce blood supply to the area, which results in a pressure ulcer. Pressure points that are moist with perspiration or body excretions are especially prone to developing a pressure ulcer, as well as bacterial infections that are very difficult to treat once they set in.

Causes of Pressure Ulcers

Pressure, friction, and shearing are common causes of skin breakdown and pressure ulcers. Other factors include breaks in skin; poor circulation to an area; moisture (such as perspiration or urine); dry, flaky skin; and irritation from urine and stool. Pressure occurs when the skin over a bony prominence is squeezed between hard surfaces (the bone itself and another surface, such as a chair seat or mattress). In obese people, pressure ulcers can develop in areas where friction is caused by skin-to-skin contact.

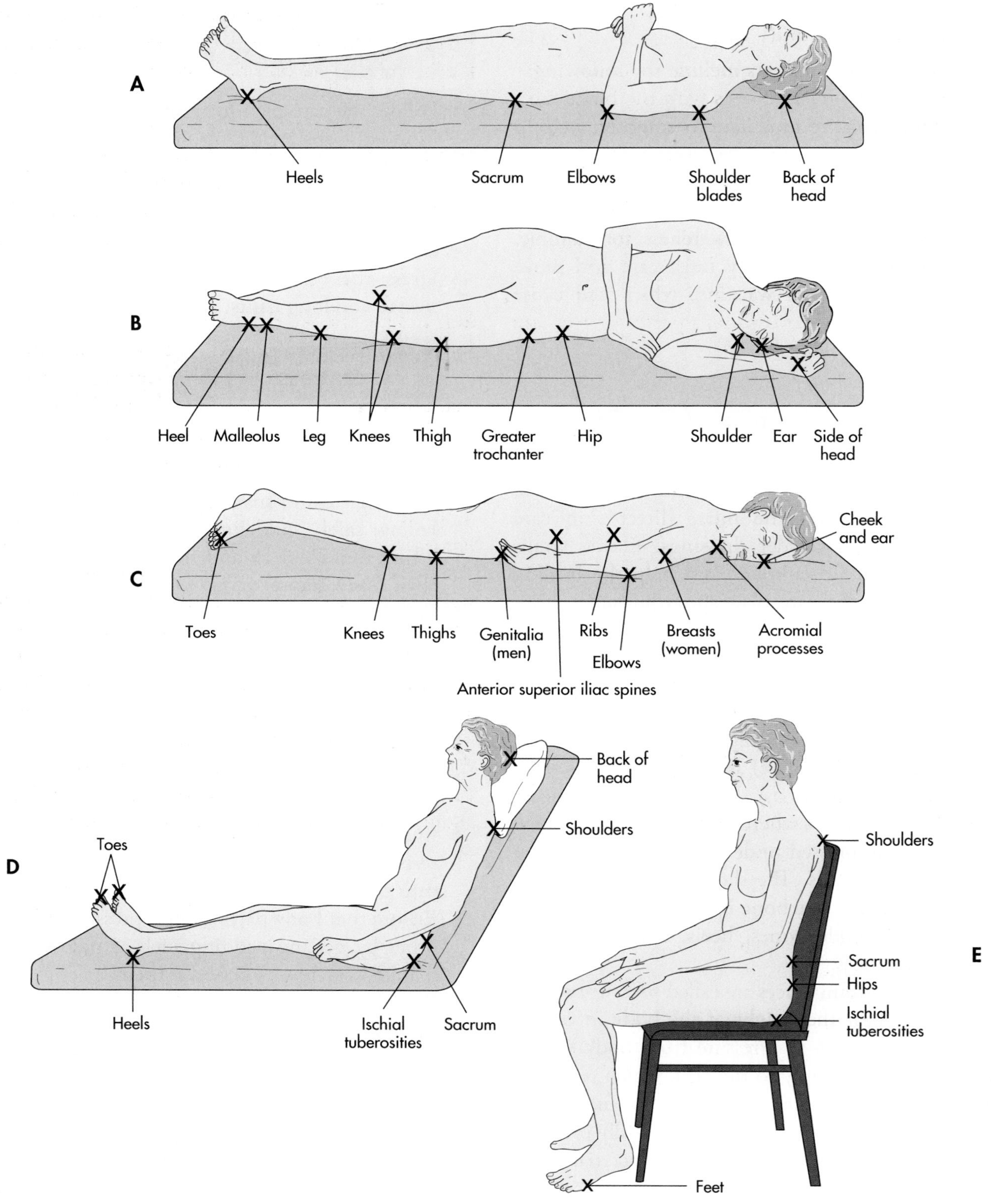

FIGURE 24–1 Pressure points: common pressure ulcer sites. **A,** The supine position. **B,** The lateral position. **C,** The prone position. **D,** Fowler's position. **E,** The sitting position.

Pressure ulcers can also occur in thin people when two bony areas are in direct contact with each other (such as knees or ankles rubbing together). This squeezing or pressure interferes with the blood flow to the skin and underlying tissues, preventing oxygen and nutrients from reaching cells (see the *Supporting Mr. Hansen: How Pressure Can Result in Skin Blistering* box) and causing the death of the skin and tissues in the area (**FIGURES 24–2 AND 24–3**). In many settings in both the U.S. and Canada, health care providers use the **Braden Scale**, which is used to predict the likelihood of a client developing a pressure ulcer (see **FIGURE 24–4**). It takes into account the client's sensory function, skin moisture, activity level, nutrition, and likelihood of friction and shear when the client is moved.

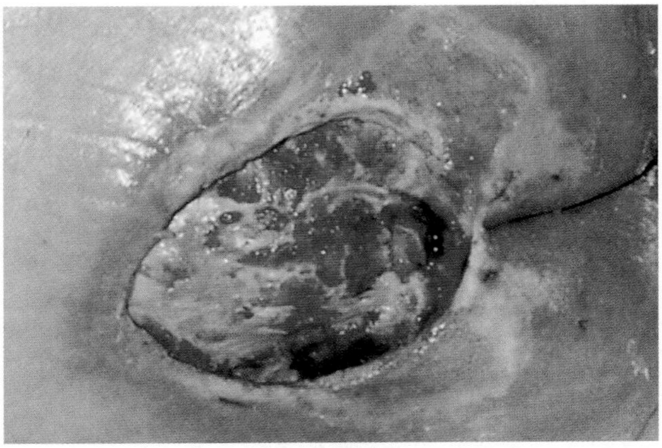

FIGURE 24–2 A pressure ulcer. (**Source:** HMP Communications. (2005, February). Proceedings from the November National V.A.C.(R). *Ostomy Wound Management, 51*(2A, Suppl.): 7S. Used with permission.)

Friction scrapes skin, and the resulting wound creates a portal of entry for microbes. For the scraped area to heal, a good blood supply to the area and prevention of infection are necessary. A poor blood supply or an infection can lead to a pressure ulcer.

Other High Risk Areas

Skin fold areas—under breasts, between abdominal folds, on legs and buttocks, and between toes—are also at risk for infection (which can lead to the formation of pressure sores). These areas, often missed during a bed bath, are frequently warm and moist because of perspiration and infrequent exposure to air. In addition, some clients use body lotions that tend to add moisture to the skin in these areas, increasing the risk for infection. It is your responsibility, as a support worker, to wash these body areas well, ensure they are dried thoroughly, and report any signs of redness or skin irritation to your supervisor. A small piece of cloth or gauze inserted under a large breast can help prevent moisture and friction—and thus skin redness and breakdown—whenever a bra is not worn. Some nurses apply barrier cream to the washed and dried skin fold areas. The client is then dressed. Consult with your supervisor (or the client) before trying this cream on a client.

A

B

C

D

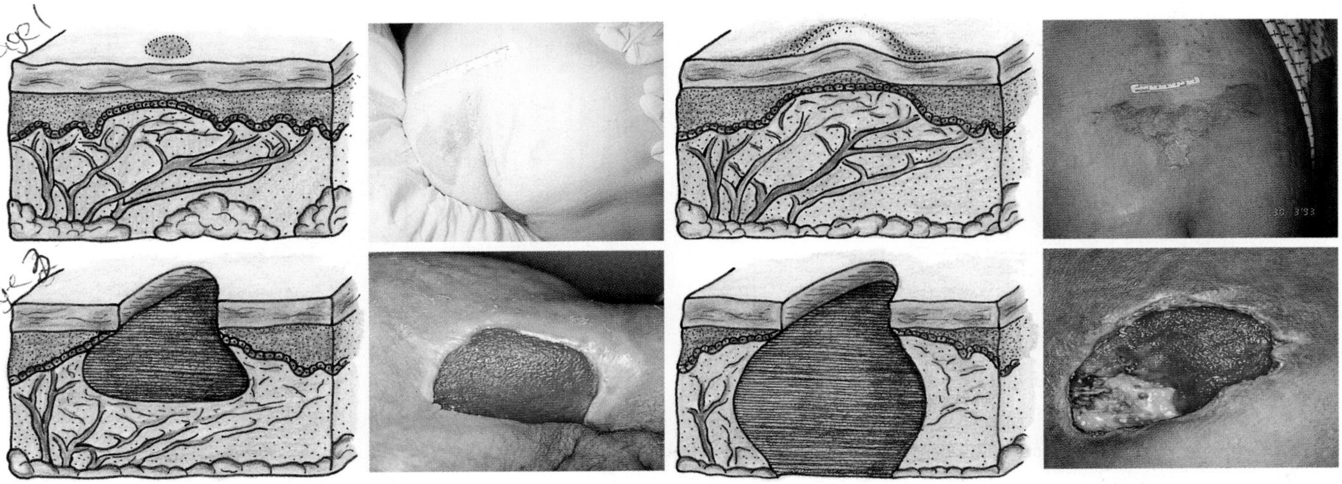

FIGURE 24–3 Stages of pressure ulcers. **A,** Stage 1. **B,** Stage 2. **C,** Stage 3. **D,** Stage 4. (Photos courtesy of Laurel Wiersema-Bryant, RN, MSN, Clinical Nurse Specialist, Barnes-Jewish Hospital, St. Louis, MO.)

Veterans Affairs Canada   Anciens Combattants Canada

Protected when completed.

Braden Scale for Predicting Pressure Sore Risk

Client's name	File No.	Date of assessment

Sensory Perception Ability to respond meaningfully to pressure-related discomfort.	**1. Completely Limited** Unresponsive (does not moan, flinch or grasp) to painful stimuli, due to diminished level of consciousness or sedation OR limited ability to feel pain over most of body.	**2. Very Limited** Reponds only to painful stimuli. Cannot communicate discomfort except by moaning or restlessness OR has a sensory impairment which limits the ability to feel pain or discomfort over ½ of body.	**3. Slightly Limited** Responds to verbal commands, but cannot always communicate discomfort or the need to be turned OR has some sensory impairment which limits ability to feel pain or discomfort in 1 or 2 extremities.	**4. No Impairment** Responds to verbal commands. Has no sensory deficit which would limit ability to feel or voice pain or discomfort.	**Sensory Perception Score**
Moisture Degree to which skin is exposed to moisture.	**1. Constantly Moist** Skin is kept moist almost constantly by perspiration, urine, etc. Dampness is detected every time patient is moved or turned.	**2. Very Moist** Skin is often, but not always moist. Linen must be changed at least once a shift.	**3. Occasionally Moist** Skin is occasionally moist, requiring an extra linen change approximately once a day.	**4. Rarely Moist** Skin is usually dry, linen only requires changing at routine intervals.	**Moisture Score**
Activity Degree of physical activity.	**1. Bedfast** Confined to bed.	**2. Chairfast** Ability to walk severely limited or non-existent. Cannot bear own weight and/or must be assisted into chair or wheelchair.	**3. Walks Occasionally** Walks occasionally during day, but for very short distances, with or without assistance. Spends majority of each shift in bed or chair.	**4. Walks Frequently** Walks outside room at least twice a day and inside room at least once every two hours during waking hours.	**Activity Score**
Mobility Ability to change and control body position.	**1. Completely Immobile** Does not make even slight changes in body or extremity position without assistance.	**2. Very Limited** Makes occasional slight changes in body or extremity position but unable to make frequent or significant changes independently.	**3. Slightly Limited** Makes frequent, though slight, changes in body or extremity position independently.	**4. No Limitation** Makes major and frequent changes in position without assistance.	**Mobility Score**
Nutrition Usual food intake pattern.	**1. Very Poor** Never eats a complete meal. Rarely eats more than 1/3 of any food offered. Eats 2 servings or less of protein (meat or dairy products) per day. Takes fluids poorly. Does not take a liquid dietary supplement OR is NPO and/or maintained on clear liquids or IV's for more than 5 days.	**2. Probably Inadequate** Rarely eats a complete meal and generally eats only about ½ of any food offered. Protein intake includes only 3 servings of meat or dairy products per day. Occasionally will take a dietary supplement OR receives less than optimum amount of liquid diet or tube feeding.	**3. Adequate** Eats over half of most meals. Eats a total of 4 servings of protein (meat, dairy products) per day. Occasionally will refuse a meal, but will usually take a supplement when offered OR is on a tube feeding or TPN regiment which probably meets most of nutritional needs.	**4. Excellent** Eats most of every meal. Never refuses a meal. Usually eats a total of 4 or more servings of meat and dairy products. Occasionally eats between meals. Does not require supplementation.	**Nutrition Score**
Friction and Shear	**1. Problem** Requires moderate to maximum assistance in moving. Complete lifting without sliding against sheets is impossible. Frequently slides down in bed or chair, requiring frequent repositioning with maximum assistance. S pasticity, contractures or agitation leads to almost constant friction.	**2. Potential Problem** Moves feebly or requires minimum assistance. During a move skin probably sllides to some extent against sheets, chair, restraints or other devices. Maintains relatively good position in chair or bed most of the time but occasionally slides down.	**3. No Apparent Problem** Moves in bed and in chair independently and has sufficient muscle strength to lift up completely during move. Maintains good position in bed or chair.		**Friction and Shear Score**

Signature	Designate	Date

Total Score

VAC 656e (2007-05)

Ce formulaire est disponible en français.

FIGURE 24–4 The Braden Scale. © Copyright Barbara Braden and Nancy Bergstrom, 1988. All rights reserved.

Supporting Mr. Hansen: How Pressure Can Result in Skin Blistering

Mr. Hansen, a 75-year-old man, has been cared for by his wife (a retired nurse) at home since his stroke 5 years ago. He has limited use of his left side; however, being right-handed, he is able to assist his wife with his care in a number of ways. His wife was admitted recently to the hospital for pneumonia, so your agency has been hired to provide respite personal care and support to Mr. Hansen while she is recovering.

Today, while you are washing Mr. Hansen's feet, you notice a large doughnut-shaped blister on his left heel. When you ask him about the blister, Mr. Hansen tells you that when a pressure ulcer developed on his heel, his wife made something to prevent his heel from getting any worse. When he shows it to you, you see that it is a doughnut-shaped object made by wrapping a gauze strip around a circular object. The blistered area seems to be the same size and shape as the "doughnut dressing."

Uncertain about what to do about the blister, you call your supervisor, who says that Mr. Hansen should discard the "doughnut dressing." She explains that although it might prevent the heel from getting a blister, that circular surface will suffer from increased pressure and decreased blood flow when Mr. Hansen is lying in bed with his heel resting flat on the bed, causing a pressure ulcer to develop on the skin under the doughnut dressing. You convey to Mr. Hansen what your supervisor has said. After thinking about it, he asks you how he can prevent getting blisters (or pressure sores) on his heel in the future. What will you advise him?

Clients at Risk for Pressure Ulcers

Clients at risk for pressure ulcers are the following:

- Those who must stay in bed or in a chair
- Those who require moderate to complete help in moving
- Those with loss of bowel or bladder control
- Those with poor nutrition
- Those with altered mental awareness
- Those with problems sensing pain or pressure
- Those with circulatory problems
- Those who are older
- Those who are obese or very thin

Signs of Pressure Ulcers

The first sign of a pressure ulcer is pale or greyed skin or a warm, reddened area. Colour changes in skin may be hard to notice in dark-skinned clients, so if the client is complaining of pain, burning, itching, or tingling in the area (common signs and symptoms of poor blood flow to the area), you should report the complaint to your supervisor. However, some clients may not feel anything unusual, so it is important that you observe your client and look for other signs of poor blood flow to the area. BOX 24–4 describes pressure ulcer development. It is your responsibility to check your client's skin every time you provide personal care. You should also immediately notify your supervisor if you observe any signs of a pressure ulcer.

BOX 24–4 Stages of Pressure Ulcers

Stage 1	The skin is redder than surrounding skin and does not return to its natural colour when relieved of pressure (see FIGURE 24–3, *A*). This finding must be reported to the nurse or supervisor promptly.
Stage 2	The skin cracks, blisters, or peels (see FIGURE 24–3, *B*). There may be a shallow crater.
Stage 3	The skin is gone, and the underlying tissues are exposed and damaged (see FIGURE 24–3, *C*). There may be drainage from the area.
Stage 4	Muscle and bone are exposed and damaged (see FIGURE 24–3, *D*). Drainage is likely.

Prevention and Treatment of Pressure Ulcers

Pressure ulcers develop over time. The longer pressure is exerted on skin, the greater the risk is that a pressure ulcer will develop.

Preventing pressure ulcers is much easier than healing them. Good support care (which includes frequent position changes and ensuring a proper diet with lots of fluid), cleanliness, and skin care are essential. The *Think About Safety: Guidelines for Preventing Pressure Ulcers* box lists guidelines for preventing skin breakdown and pressure ulcers. As always, it is important that you also follow your client's care plan and adhere to the preventive measures described on it.

Clients at risk for pressure ulcers are placed on a surface that reduces or relieves pressure—for example, foam, air, alternating air, gel, or water mattresses. The health care team decides on the best surface for the client.

A physician orders specific pressure ulcer treatment—wound care products, medications, treatments, and special equipment—for each client. Your supervisor and the care plan tell you what to do. Special beds and other protective devices, described below, are often ordered to prevent and treat pressure ulcers and other types of skin breakdown.

Think About Safety

Guidelines for Preventing Pressure Ulcers

- Follow the repositioning schedule in the care plan. Some clients have to be repositioned at least every 2 hours and some every 15 minutes. Each client's care plan should have specific instructions in regard to that client.
- Position the client as specified in the care plan. Use pillows for support, as instructed by your supervisor. The 30-degree lateral position is recommended (**FIGURE 24–5**).
- Use proper lifting, positioning, and transferring procedures to prevent friction and shearing (see Chapter 25).
- To reduce the likelihood of shearing, do not raise the head of the bed to more than 30 degrees. Always follow your client's care plan.
- Provide good skin care. The skin must be clean and dry after bathing and kept free of moisture from urine, stool, perspiration, and wound drainage.
- Minimize exposure of skin to moisture. Check incontinent clients (those with loss of bowel or bladder control) frequently. Also check clients who perspire heavily and those with wound drainage, paying particular attention when drying between the client's toes and between skin folds. Change linens and clothing as needed. Give good skin care.
- Check with your supervisor before using soap on a client. Soap can dry and irritate the skin.
- Apply a moisturizer on dry areas—hands, elbows, legs, ankles, and heels—but ***not on the areas under the breasts, between skin folds, and between toes***. Your supervisor will tell you what to use and where to apply it. As a very wise nurse once stated, "***Never grease a crease!***"
- Give a back massage after repositioning the client. Do not massage bony areas or pressure points. ***Never rub or massage reddened areas, but massage the skin around the reddened area. Be careful to never scratch or irritate the skin.***
- Keep linens clean, dry, and wrinkle-free.
- Do not irritate the skin. Avoid scrubbing or rubbing when bathing or drying the client.
- Use pillows and blankets to prevent skin-to-skin contact and to reduce moisture and friction.
- Keep the client's heels off the bed. Use pillows or other devices as directed. Place the pillows or devices under the lower legs from mid-calf to ankle.

Continued

Think About Safety—cont'd

- Use protective devices as instructed by your supervisor and the care plan.
- Remind clients sitting in chairs to shift their positions every 15 minutes to decrease pressure on bony points. Assist if requested.
- Report any signs of skin breakdown or pressure ulcers at once. Record your observations, according to employer policy.
- Remember that areas that had pressure ulcers in the past (but are now healed) are always at risk of redeveloping the ulcers. Pay particular attention to these areas, and follow the above guidelines.

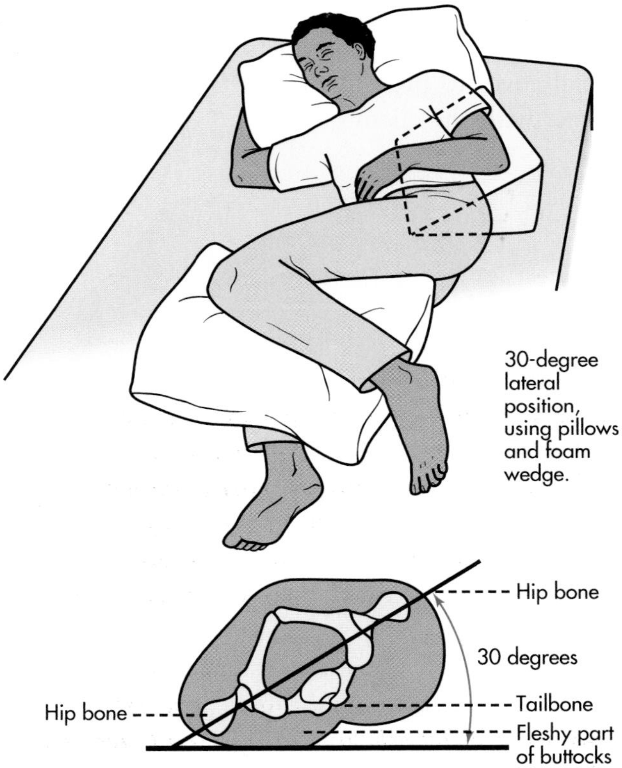

FIGURE 24–5 The 30-degree lateral position. Pillows are placed under the head, shoulder, and leg. This position inclines (lifts up) the hip to avoid pressure on the hip. The client does not lie on the hip as in the side-lying position.

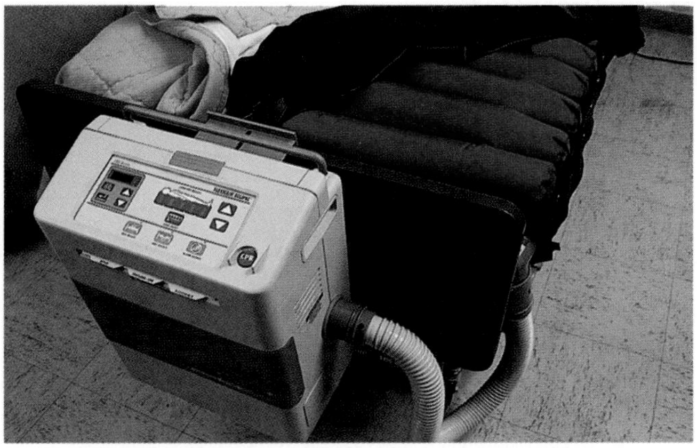

FIGURE 24–6 Air flotation bed.

Special Beds

Some beds may have air flowing through the mattress (**FIGURE 24–6**), may be made out of a gel-like substance, or may be made out of a special foam material that conforms to the body. On these mattresses, the client seems to float, which allows body weight to be evenly distributed and reduces pressure on bony parts.

Another type of bed allows you to reposition clients without having to move them. Depending on the bed, the client is turned to the prone or supine position (see Chapter 25), or the angle of the bed is tilted so the entire bed is angled side to side. Body alignment does not change, but pressure points change as the position changes, and friction is reduced. Some beds continually rotate from side to side and are useful for clients with spinal cord injuries.

If you are caring for a client in this type of special bed, it is your responsibility to inquire about the type of bedding that is required when making the bed. Some mattresses require that incontinence or transfer pads (see Chapter 34) *not* be placed under the client, as this additional padding reduces the effectiveness of the special mattress. For other mattresses, it is recommended that the bottom sheet not be tucked under it.

Bed Cradle

A bed cradle (Anderson frame) is a metal frame placed on the bed and over the client. Top sheets are brought over the cradle to prevent pressure exerted by these sheets on legs and feet (**FIGURE 24–7**). Top sheets either are folded back to expose the feet, if the client is too warm, or tucked in at the bottom of the mattress and mitred, if the client prefers it. They are also tucked under both sides of the mattress to protect the client from air drafts and chilling (see the *Focus on Home Care: Bed Cradles* box.)

Elbow Protectors

Elbow protectors, made of foam rubber or sheepskin, prevent friction between the bed and the elbow. They fit the shape of the elbow (**FIGURE 24–9**); some have straps to secure them in place.

Heel Elevators

Pillows or special cushions raise the heels off the bed (**FIGURE 24–10**). Special braces and splints also keep pressure off the heels.

Flotation Pads

Flotation pads or cushions (**FIGURE 24–11**) are like waterbeds, but they are made of a gel-like substance with an outer case of heavy plastic. The pads can be placed in chairs and wheelchairs, allowing the client to sit comfortably without the risk of developing pressure ulcers. The pad is placed in a pillowcase or special cover to prevent the plastic from coming in contact with the client's skin.

FOCUS ON HOME CARE

Bed Cradles

A sturdy cardboard box can be used as a bed cradle (**FIGURE 24–8**). Your supervisor would tell you how to line the box to prevent pressure on the heels.

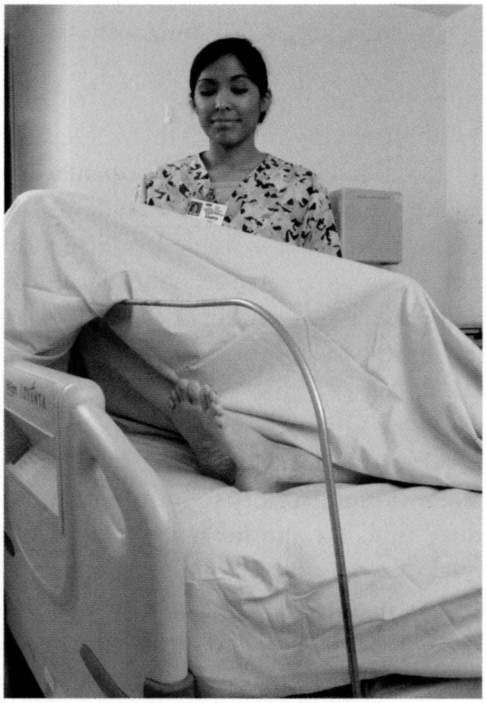

FIGURE 24–7 A bed cradle is placed on top of the bed. Linens are brought over the top of the cradle.

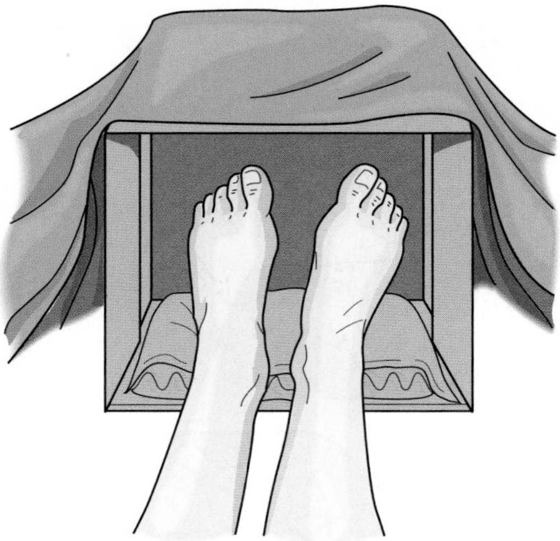

FIGURE 24–8 A cardboard box serves as a bed cradle. It keeps top linens off the client's feet.

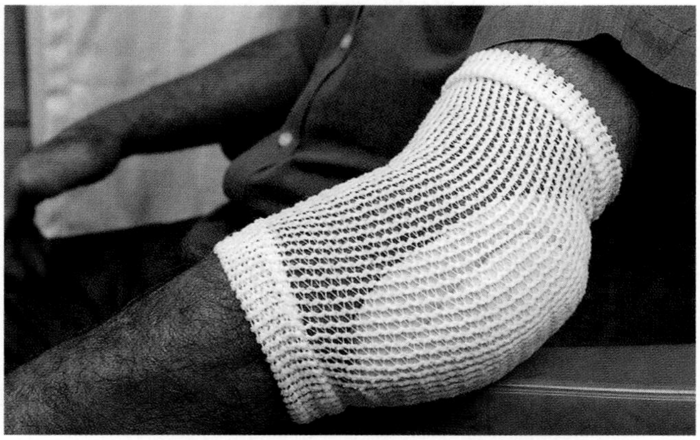

FIGURE 24–9 Elbow protector.

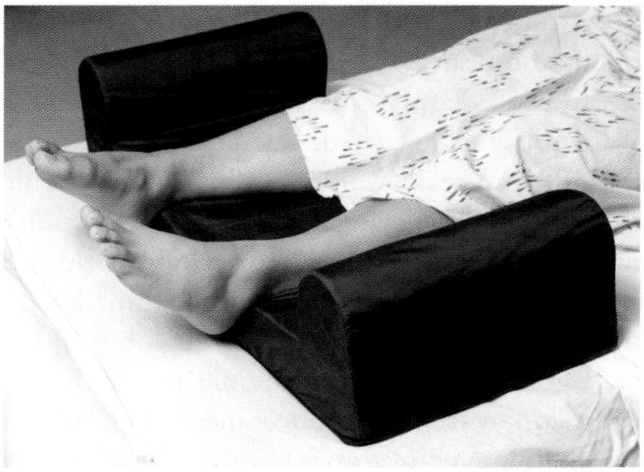

FIGURE 24–10 Heel elevator. Image provided courtesy Posey Company, Arcadia, CA.

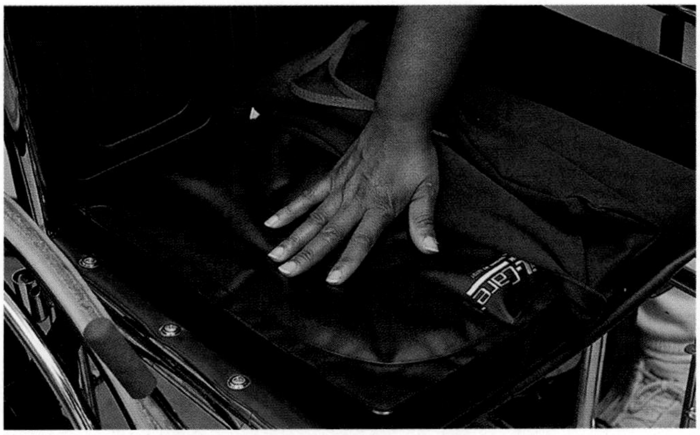

FIGURE 24–11 Flotation pad.

Egg Crate–Like Mattress

The egg crate–like mattress is a foam pad that looks like an egg carton with peaks that distribute the client's weight more evenly. This mattress is placed on top of the regular mattress and encased in a special cover that protects it against moisture and soiling. Only a bottom sheet covers the mattress. ***Many agencies do not use this type of mattress because it can aggravate pressure points and may be a fire hazard since it is made of flammable material.*** They are, however, inexpensive and commercially available, and some family physicians still recommend them to their clients for home use. Although clients should never smoke in bed, it is important to warn them of the particular dangers of doing so when using this or any other type of flammable mattress pad.

Other Equipment

Trochanter rolls and footboards are also used to prevent pressure ulcers (see Chapter 26).

LEG AND FOOT ULCERS

Some diseases may affect blood flow to and from the legs and feet, which can cause pain, open wounds, and **edema** (swelling caused by fluid collecting in tissues). Infection and gangrene can result from the open wound and poor circulation. **Gangrene** is a condition in which tissue dies and then decays. Gangrenous tissue may be black and have a foul smell (see Chapter 37).

Clients with leg and foot ulcers need special skin care, as directed by a physician. The nurse uses the care-planning process to prevent skin breakdown on legs and feet.

Circulatory Ulcers

Circulatory ulcers (**vascular ulcers**) are open wounds on the lower legs and feet caused by decreased blood flow through arteries or veins. People with diseases affecting blood vessels are at risk for these ulcers on legs and feet, which can be painful and hard to heal. Depending on where they originate, they are classified as *venous ulcers* or *arterial ulcers.*

Venous Ulcers

Venous ulcers (**stasis ulcers**) are open wounds on the lower legs and feet caused by poor blood return through veins (**FIGURE 24–12**, *A*). Blood travelling from the feet to the heart must defy gravity. In people who are active, the use of leg muscles assists the valves in their leg veins to pump the blood upward.

Unfortunately, in some clients who are not active, who are extremely obese, or who have circulatory problems, blood will pool in the leg veins, or the valves will not close well. As a result, blood will not be pumped back to the heart normally, and blood and fluid will collect in their legs and feet, resulting in edema in their legs and feet. If you compress your fingers into the swollen, edematous tissue and then take away your fingers, you will notice that your fingers have left a skin impression, which is called **pitting edema.**

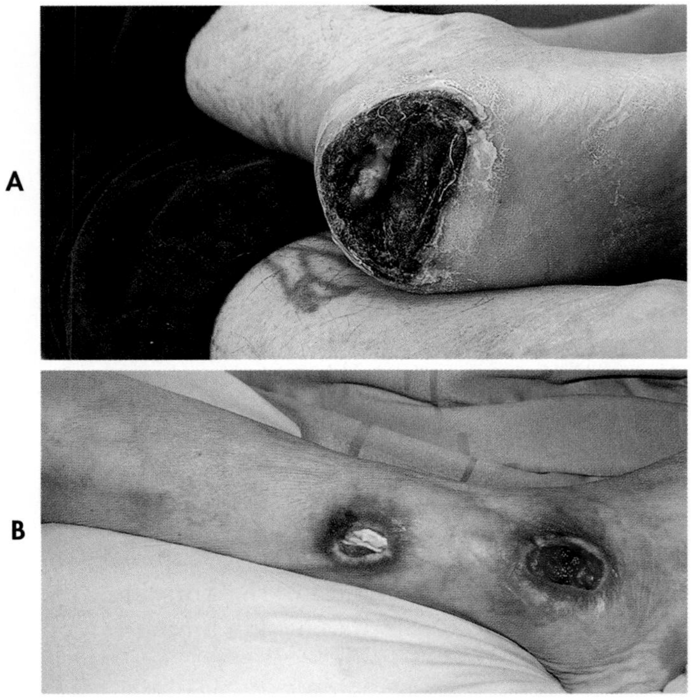

FIGURE 24–12 **A,** Venous ulcer. **B,** Arterial ulcer. Compare their appearances and how they differ from each other. (Source (for *B*): Black, J.M., & Hawks, J.H. (2005). *Medical-surgical nursing: Clinical management for positive outcomes* (7th ed.). St. Louis, MO: W.B. Saunders.)

Appearance

Edema in tissues will give them a swollen appearance. If the edema is fairly recent, skin can also appear shiny and stretched. Edema and venous ulcers are painful and make walking difficult. Venous ulcers may "weep" fluid. Healing is slow, and infection is a great risk. If the edema lasts for a long period, skin will change in appearance and texture. Small veins in skin can rupture, allowing the hemoglobin in blood (which gives blood its red colour) to enter tissues, causing skin to darken and become dry, leathery, and hard. Itching is common.

Causes

Heels and the inner sides of ankles are common sites for venous ulcers because these areas can be easily injured. Scratching is also a common cause of venous ulcers. Some ulcers occur spontaneously, without any specific cause.

Prevention

It is important to prevent skin breakdown caused by poor circulation because skin breakdown leads to venous ulcers, which are hard to heal. The *Think About Safety: Guidelines for Preventing Venous Ulcers* lists guidelines that may be part of the client's care plan.

Think About Safety

Guidelines for Preventing Venous Ulcers

- Apply elastic stockings or elastic wraps according to the care plan if it is within your scope of practice to do so (see Chapter 31).
- Remind the client not to sit with legs crossed.
- Do not use elastic garters to hold socks or hose in place. Ensure that the tops of stockings are not so tight as to be restrictive. Provide good skin care daily. Clean and dry between the toes.
- Avoid injury to the client's legs and feet.
- Keep linens clean, dry, and wrinkle-free.
- Follow the care plan for walking and exercise, as movement increases venous blood flow.
- Reposition the client at least every 2 hours. Follow the care plan.
- When positioning the client in bed, ensure that there is adequate padding between the client's body parts, through the use of pillows, soft blankets, or towels.
- Elevate the client's legs according to the care plan.
- Have the client wear comfortable socks and shoes.
- Do not do anything that may irritate the skin. Avoid scrubbing or rubbing when bathing or drying the client.
- Avoid massaging over pressure points. ***Never rub or massage reddened areas.***
- Keep the heels off the bed. Use pillows or other devices, as instructed by your supervisor. Place the pillows or devices under the lower legs from mid-calf to ankle.
- Use protective devices, as directed by your supervisor and the care plan.
- Report signs of skin breakdown, venous ulcers, or pressure ulcers at once.

The physician may order elastic stockings or elastic bandages (see Chapter 31), which promote comfort and circulation by providing support and pressure to the veins. Foot care by a professional with specialized training in foot care, as well as medications or wound care products, may be ordered by the client's physician or nurse practitioner.

Arterial Ulcers

Arterial ulcers are open wounds on the lower legs and feet caused by poor arterial blood flow.

Appearance

The affected leg and foot may feel cold and look grey or blue or shiny (**FIGURE 24–12**, *B*). The ulcer is often painful during rest and is usually worse at night. Arterial ulcers are found between toes, on the tops of toes, and on the outer sides of ankles. Heels are common sites for arterial ulcers in people on bed rest. Arterial ulcers can also occur in pressure sites from shoes that fit poorly.

Causes

These ulcers are caused by diseases or injuries that decrease arterial blood flow to the legs and feet—such as high blood pressure, diabetes, and narrowing of arteries due to aging. Smoking is a significant risk factor for vascular disease, such as atherosclerosis, arteriosclerosis, venous ulcers, or arterial ulcers.

Treatment and Prevention

The physician directs the client's care by treating the disease that caused the ulcer and ordering medications, wound care, and a walking program. ***You should never provide foot care to a client with an arterial ulcer unless it is specified in the client's care plan to prevent further injury.*** See the *Think About Safety: Guidelines for Preventing Arterial Ulcers* box.

> **Think About Safety**
>
> **Guidelines for Preventing Arterial Ulcers**
>
> - Urge a client who smokes to quit smoking.
> - Remind clients not to sit with legs crossed.
> - Avoid exposing the client to cold.
> - Do not use elastic garters to hold socks and hose in place. Ensure that the tops of stockings are not so tight as to be restrictive.
> - Make sure the client's shoes fit well.
> - Keep feet clean and dry.
> - Keep pressure off heels and other bony points.
> - Avoid pressure under the knees.
> - Check the client's legs and feet daily. Report changes in skin colour or breaks in the skin to your supervisor.
> - Avoid massaging over pressure points. ***Never rub or massage reddened or newly discoloured areas.***
> - Use protective devices, as directed by your supervisor and the care plan.

WOUND HEALING

The healing process has three phases:

- ***Inflammatory phase*** (3 days). Bleeding stops, and a scab forms over the wound, which prevents microbes from entering the wound. Blood supply to the wound increases, and the blood brings nutrients and healing substances. Because blood supply increases, signs and symptoms of inflammation—redness, swelling, heat or warmth, and pain—may appear, and there may be some loss of function.
- ***Proliferative phase*** (day 3 to day 21). *Proliferate* means multiply rapidly. Tissue cells multiply to repair the wound.
- ***Maturation phase*** (day 21 to 1 or 2 years). The scar tissue gains strength and appears red and raised but eventually becomes thin and paler than surrounding skin.

Types of Wound Healing

The healing process occurs through primary intention, secondary intention, or tertiary intention. With *primary intention* (also called *first intention* or *primary closure*), the wound is closed with sutures (stitches), staples, clips, or adhesive strips to hold the wound edges together.

Secondary intention (also called *second intention*) is used in contaminated and infected wounds. Wounds are cleaned and dead tissue removed. Wound edges are not brought together—the wound is left gaping. Healing occurs naturally but takes longer, and a larger scar is formed. These wounds have a high risk of infection.

Tertiary intention (also called *third intention* or *delayed intention*) involves leaving a wound open for a time before then closing it. Thus, tertiary intention combines secondary and primary intentions. Infection and poor circulation are common reasons for choosing tertiary intention.

Complications of Wounds

Many factors affect healing and could increase the risk for complications—for example, the client's age, general health, nutritional status and lifestyle, and the type and location of the wound. Clients with diabetes are at increased risk for infection. The client might be very old, might have a medical condition (such as circulatory disease or diabetes), or may have a lifestyle risk factor (such as smoking or poor diet) that might slow down the healing process. Other clients may be on certain medications (such as warfarin or heparin) that will prolong bleeding and possibly delay healing.

Wound healing is dependent on good blood circulation to the wound as well as good nutrition for the client, with a diet rich in fluids (needed for tissue hydration), protein, and vitamin C (needed for tissue growth and repair). The wound must be protected from infection. Sometimes, the client's doctor may prescribe antibiotics to prevent the development of an infection.

Hemorrhage

Hemorrhage is excessive loss of blood within a short period. If bleeding is not stopped, death results. Hemorrhage may be internal or external. Internal hemorrhage, when bleeding occurs into tissues and body cavities, cannot be seen. It leads to a **hematoma**, which is a collection of blood under skin and tissues. The area appears swollen and has a reddish-blue or grey colour. Shock, vomiting blood, coughing up blood, and loss of consciousness are signs of internal hemorrhage. External bleeding is visible as bloody drainage or through dressings soaked with blood. As with internal hemorrhage, shock can occur.

Shock is a result of there not being enough blood supply to organs and tissues. Signs and symptoms of shock include low or falling blood pressure; rapid and weak pulse; rapid respirations; and cold, moist, and pale or greyish skin. A client experiencing shock is restless and may complain of thirst. Confusion and loss of consciousness eventually occur.

Hemorrhage and shock are emergencies, so notify your supervisor immediately, and assist as requested. Remember to follow Standard Practices when in contact with blood. Gloves should always be worn, and gowns, masks, and eye protection are necessary when blood splashes and splatters are likely.

Infection

Wound contamination can occur at any time during or after an injury or surgery. Trauma often results in contaminated wounds, and surgical wounds can be contaminated during or after surgery. An infected wound has drainage and is painful and tender to the touch (**BOX 24–5**). A client with an infected wound may have a fever.

Dehiscence

Dehiscence is the rupture or sudden separation of the wound layers along a surgical suture line (**FIGURE 24–13**). Separation may occur just at the skin layer or affect underlying tissues, as usually seen in abdominal wounds. Coughing, vomiting, and abdominal distension place stress on the wound. The client often describes a sensation of the wound popping open.

Evisceration

Evisceration is the separation of the wound, which is accompanied by protrusion of abdominal organs

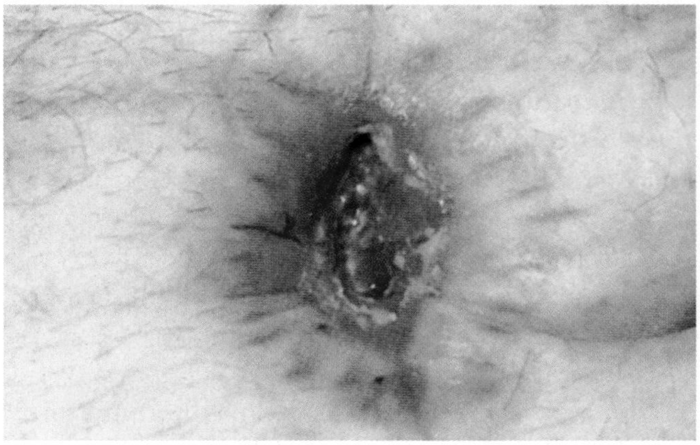

FIGURE 24–13 Wound dehiscence. (**Source:** Morison, M. (1992). *A colour guide to the nursing management of wounds.* London, U.K.: Wolfe Medical Publishers.)

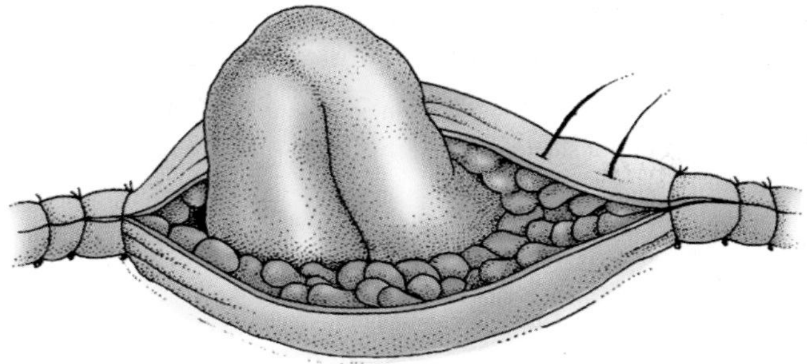

FIGURE 24–14 Wound evisceration. (**Source:** Ignatavicius, D.D., & Workman, M.L. (2002). *Medical-surgical nursing: Critical thinking for collaborative care* (4th ed.). Philadelphia, PA: Saunders.)

(**FIGURE 24–14**). Causes are the same as those of dehiscence.

Dehiscence and evisceration are surgical emergencies. Tell your supervisor at once if you see them. A nurse will cover the wound with a large sterile dressing saturated with sterile saline, and the client will need emergency medical care.

Wound Appearance

During the healing process, physicians and nurses routinely observe the wound and its drainage for healing and complications. As a support worker, you also need to make certain observations when assisting with wound care. You should report your observations to your supervisor, and record them, according to employer policy. **BOX 24–5** lists questions to consider when observing wounds.

Wounds Under Casts and Dressings

If you work in an acute-care setting, you may be responsible for caring for a client who has a wound that you cannot see, such as one inside a cast or under a large, bulky dressing. It is your responsibility to observe the wound area and to report your observations. For example, if you discover that the client has blood seeping through a freshly applied cast or dressing, you must report the discovery to the nurse. You may be instructed to mark the outline of blood seepage through the cast or dressing and report any further drainage. In this case, the client will also be monitored for signs of blood loss, such as low blood pressure and a high pulse rate.

BOX 24–5 Wound Observations

Wound Location

- Where is the wound located on the body? Is there more than one wound? (Multiple wounds may exist from surgery or trauma.)

Wound Appearance

- Is the wound red and swollen?
- Is the area around the wound warm to the touch?
- Are sutures, staples, or clips intact or broken?
- Are wound edges closed or separated? Did the wound break open?

Drainage

- Is there drainage?
- What is the amount of drainage?
- Is the drainage:
  - Clear?
  - Bloody?
  - Watery and blood-tinged?
  - Thick and green, yellow, or brown?

Odour

- Does the wound or drainage have an odour?

Surrounding Skin and Tissues

- Is surrounding skin intact?
- What is the colour of the surrounding skin?
- Are the surrounding tissues swollen?

Wound Drainage

During injury and during the inflammatory phase of wound healing, fluid and cells escape from tissues. The amount of drainage may be small or large, depending on wound size and location and the presence of bleeding or infection. Although the nurse is responsible for changing dressings, you need to observe and report to the nurse any type of wound drainage. You may also be shown how to measure the amount of drainage and to document the amount of drainage, depending on your employing agency and your scope of practice in your province.

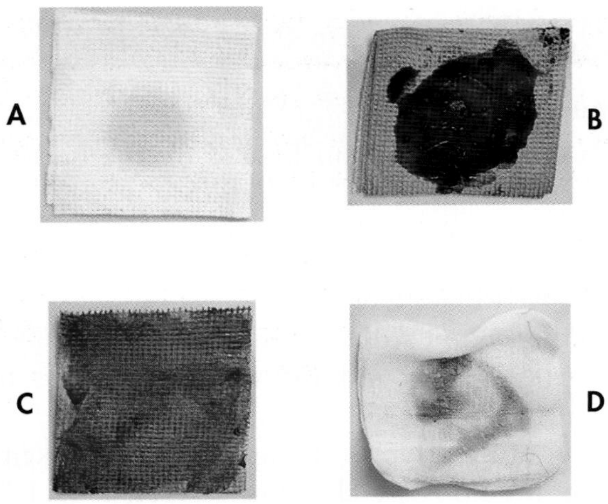

FIGURE 24–15 Wound drainage. **A,** Serous drainage. **B,** Sanguineous drainage. **C,** Serosanguineous drainage. **D,** Purulent drainage. (**Source:** Potter, P.A., & Perry, A.G. (2009). *Fundamentals of nursing* (rev. 7th ed., p. 1287). St. Louis, MO: Mosby.)

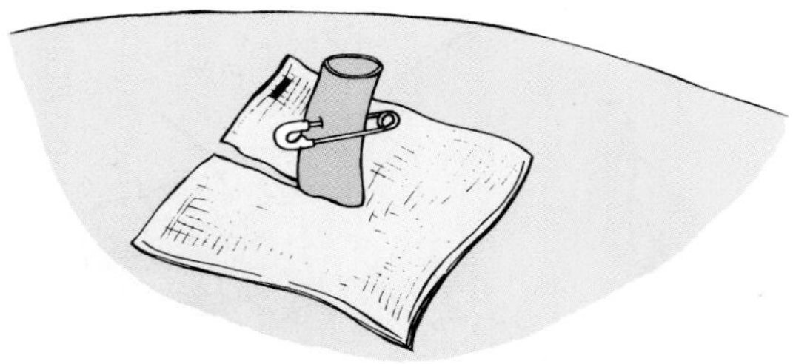

FIGURE 24–16 A Penrose drain. The safety pin prevents the drain from slipping into the wound. (**Source:** Potter, P.A., & Perry, A.G. (2009). *Fundamentals of nursing* (rev. 7th ed., p. 1297). St. Louis, MO: Mosby.)

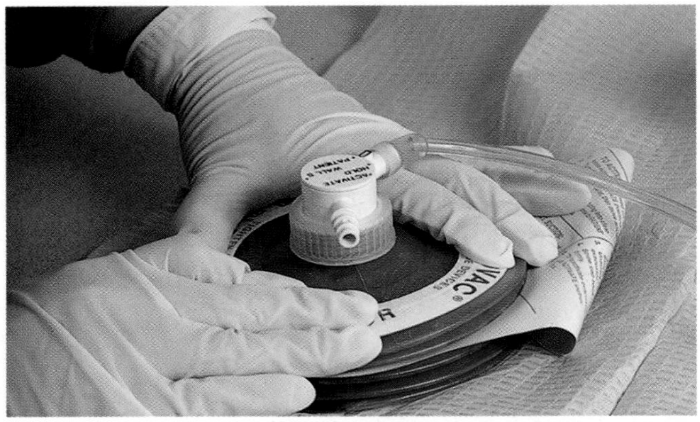

FIGURE 24–17 Hemovac. Drains are sutured to the wound and connected to the reservoir. (**Source:** Potter, P.A., & Perry, A.G. (2009). *Fundamentals of nursing* (rev. 7th ed., p. 1329). St. Louis, MO: Mosby.)

Major types of wound drainage are as follows:

- **Serous drainage**—clear, watery fluid (**FIGURE 24–15**, *A*). The fluid in a blister is serous (from the Latin word *serum*, meaning clear, thin, fluid portion of blood). Serum does not contain blood cells or platelets.
- **Sanguineous drainage**—bloody drainage (**FIGURE 24–15**, *B*). The amount and colour of sanguineous (from the Latin word *sanguis*, which means blood) drainage are important. Hemorrhage is suspected when large amounts are present. Bright red drainage means fresh bleeding, whereas older bleeding is darker.
- **Serosanguineous drainage**—thin, watery drainage (*sero*) that is blood-tinged (*sanguineous*) (**FIGURE 24–15**, *C*).
- **Purulent drainage**—thick drainage that is green, yellow, or brown and may have a foul odour (**FIGURE 24–15**, *D*).

Drainage must leave the wound for healing to occur. If drainage is trapped inside the wound, underlying tissues swell. The wound may heal at the skin level, but underlying tissues do not close, and infection and other complications can occur. When large amounts of drainage are expected, the physician will insert a drain. A Penrose drain is a rubber tube that drains onto a dressing (**FIGURE 24–16**). Because it is an open drain, it can act as a portal of entry for microbes.

Closed drainage systems prevent microbes from entering the wound. A drain is placed in the wound and attached to suction—for example, the Hemovac (**FIGURE 24–17**) and Jackson-Pratt (**FIGURE 24–18**) systems. Depending on the wound type, size, and location, other systems may be used.

A nurse measures drainage in two ways:

- ***Noting the number and size of dressings with drainage***—the amount and kind of drainage are described. Are dressings saturated? Is the drainage on just part of the dressing? If so, which part? Is the drainage occurring through some or all layers?
- ***Measuring the amount of drainage in the collecting receptacle***—if closed drainage is used.

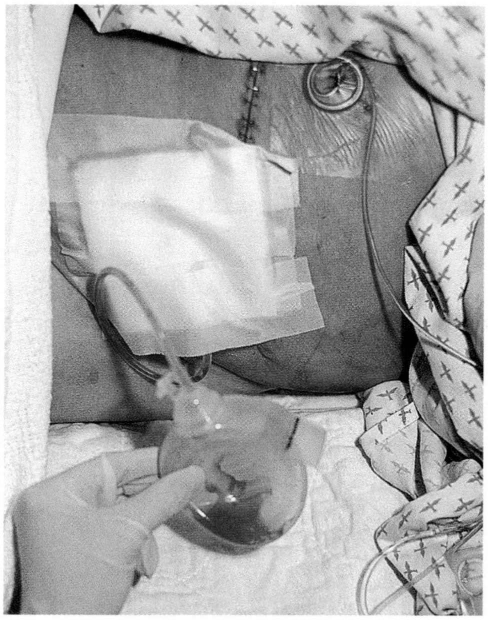

FIGURE 24–18 Jackson-Pratt drainage system. (**Source:** Potter, P.A., & Perry, A.G. (2009). *Fundamentals of nursing* (rev. 7th ed., p. 1298). St. Louis, MO: Mosby.)

DRESSINGS

Wound dressings have many functions:

- They protect wounds from injury and microbes.
- They absorb drainage.
- They remove dead tissue.
- They promote comfort.
- They cover unsightly (ugly) wounds.
- They provide a moist environment for wound healing.
- When bleeding is a problem, pressure dressings help control bleeding.

Sterile Dressings

The type and size of dressing used depend on many factors—(1) the type of wound, (2) its size and location, (3) the amount of drainage, (4) the presence or absence of infection, (5) the dressing's function, and (6) the frequency of dressing changes. The physician and nurse choose the best type of dressing for each wound. In many agencies, wound care is assessed by a nurse who specializes in skin care of wounds and around ostomies (see Chapters 32 and 33). You may be asked to assist in the application of a sterile dressing (see Chapter 23). ***Because there is such a wide range of sterile dressing types and indications for the use of each, and because it is beyond your scope of practice to decide on the type of dressing, this chapter focuses on the support worker's responsibilities in regard to a client's dressing.***

Although you are not responsible for sterile dressing changes or for skin assessment (these tasks are the responsibility of the nurse), you should function as the "eyes and ears" of the client, reporting important details about the dressings to the nurse (**BOX 24–6**).

Types of Dressings

Dressings are described by the material used and application method. Many products are available for dressing wounds. Dressings may be dry, moist, or hydrocolloid (a substance that forms a gel in the presence of water). The following are common dressings:

- ***Gauze***—comes in squares, rectangles, pads, and rolls (**FIGURE 24–19**). Gauze dressings absorb moisture.
- ***Non-adherent gauze***—a gauze dressing with a nonstick surface. It does not stick to the wound and is removed easily without injuring the tissue.
- ***Vapour-permeable transparent adhesive film***—air can reach the wound but fluid and microbes cannot. The wound is kept moist. Drainage is not absorbed. The transparent film allows wound observation.

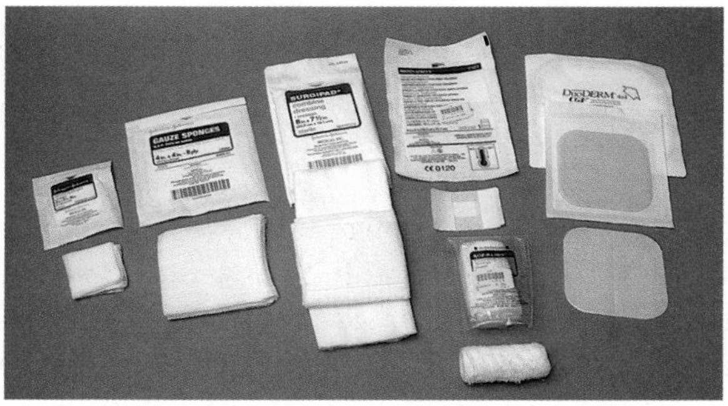

FIGURE 24–19 Different types of gauze dressings. (**Source:** DeWit, S.C. (2000). *Fundamental concepts and skills for nursing* (3rd ed.). St. Louis, MO: Saunders.)

BOX 24–6 The Support Worker's Responsibilities to Clients With Wounds

Specific Areas	Your Responsibilities
1. *Overall*	• Follow the client's care plan. • Document all wound care or observations that you have made. • Participate in the interprofessional efforts by all team members (Chapter 6) for wound care. • Use proper hand hygiene and follow the rules of asepsis at all times. • Report and document any observations you have made about your client in any of the areas noted below.
2. *Prevention of Pressure Sores* It is important that you observe your client's skin, especially over the bony prominences, and report any reddened areas. Remember that irritated areas can quickly become pressure sores!	• Remove any restrictive clothing such as socks that are too tight, which can prevent blood circulation, leading to skin breakdown. • Ensure the client is repositioned at least every 2 hours (***or more frequently if specified by the client's care plan!***). • Inspect bony prominences that have been compressed by any type of surface. • Ensure that the client is correctly using the gel pad seat cushion (used to reduce pressure on areas prone to pressure ulcers). • Keep bony prominences and skin folds clean and dry. Wash skin after each soiling, and then rinse and pat dry. • Pad between body parts to reduce likelihood of creating pressure sores or skin irritation. • Avoid oily soaps that trap bacteria, or drying, antiperspirant soaps that can cause the skin to dry and crack. If possible, use **peri-wash** (a gentle pH-balanced soap), which does not leave a residue on the client's skin. • Massage only *around* reddened areas, never directly on the area, so as not to remove more skin cells. • ***Never*** perform nail care if the client has diabetes or if the client's care plan states to avoid it. Nail care for some clients should be done only by a professional with specialized training in foot care. Always report reddened areas or ingrown toenails so that these can be treated as soon as possible. • Report and record your findings, according to your agency's policies.

Continued

BOX 24–6 The Support Worker's Responsibilities to Clients With Wounds—cont'd

Specific Areas	Your Responsibilities
3. *Pain and Comfort* A client in pain will probably not eat or participate in care. Pain may affect your client's breathing and moving, turning, repositioning, and walking. In addition, pain is exhausting and can make the client depressed or irritable. It is important that the client be made as comfortable as possible.	• Observe to find out if the client is in pain (look for grimacing, holding a body part for a long period, or tensing up during repositioning). If you find the client to be in pain, determine where, the amount, the intensity, aggravating factors, and the cause so that you can report and record this information appropriately. • Handle the client gently. • Report the client's pain and details to the appropriate nurse, who can give the client pain medication if it is ordered and appropriate. • Allow pain medications to take effect before giving care (at least 1 hour). • Assist the client into a comfortable position, and frequently turn the client (according to the care plan) to avoid placing pressure on compromised areas. • If specified in the client's care plan, massage around the client's bony prominences. Assist the client into a proper body alignment, and position the client with pillows. • Ensure that the client who is in bed is lying on a wrinkle-free foundation.
4. *Movement and Ambulation* Movement is important for everyone because it encourages deeper respirations and better blood circulation, reduces the risk of pressure ulcers developing, increases the body's metabolism, promotes peristalsis, and improves digestion. Clients with painful wounds are often reluctant to move or to ambulate, and those with wounds that are foul smelling may be self-conscious about leaving their rooms, even if they can.	• Encourage the client to move in bed, take deep breaths, and turn independently as much as possible. • Following the client's care plan, assist the client into a chair (or wheelchair) or to ambulate as often as stated. If the person is unable to ambulate, turn the client frequently, as indicated in the care plan. • Schedule activities around the time the client receives pain medication (at least 1 hour after) so that the client is as comfortable as possible before attempting to ambulate. • Have another worker on hand to help, in case the client feels light-headed or faint. • Encourage the client to rise slowly and to take a few deep breaths before standing up to help eliminate any potential feeling of light-headedness.
5. *Dressings* Depending on the type of dressing that is ordered for your client, the appearance, care, and maintenance of the dressing may vary. Regardless of type, all dressings should be kept clean.	• Depending on where you live in Canada, dressing application may be a delegated task from a nurse. • Observe if the client's dressing is clean and free from bodily fluids (such as urine or feces). Report pertinent information. • If required, assist the nurse with the client's dressing change. If the wound is particularly unsightly, be careful to control your facial expressions so as not to alarm the client.

Continued

BOX 24–6 The Support Worker's Responsibilities to Clients With Wounds—cont'd

Specific Areas	Your Responsibilities
6. *Nutrition and Hydration* The client's wound cannot heal with a diet that is poor in protein or vitamin C. In addition, the client must have adequate fluid to replace any lost in wound drainage. The client who is anemic will not have enough hemoglobin to bind with oxygen, so the client must also eat an iron-rich diet.	• Take the client's care plan, dietary needs, and preferences into account, and prepare tasty treats that are high in protein, vitamin C, and iron. • If the client has diabetes, ensure that caloric restrictions are not exceeded. • Offer liquids frequently throughout the day to ensure the client is adequately hydrated. Observe and report if the client's urine output is low or dark in colour (see Chapter 32).
7. *Oxygenation* Oxygen is a requirement for healing. On a cellular level, oxygen must bind itself to hemoglobin (part of a red blood cell) and be transported throughout the body.	• Help the client to maintain positions that will maximize lung expansion. • Gently remind the client to take several deep breaths at least every hour.
8. *Odour* Some wounds, especially those with **necrotic tissue** (dead tissue), may be very foul smelling, which can embarrass the client and ruin the appetite.	• Keep drainage containers out of the client's sight. • Open windows, whenever possible, to allow fresh air to enter the client's room. • Ensure that dressing materials are removed promptly and placed in a plastic bag that is tied to contain the odour (see Chapter 23). • Discreetly use room air fresheners to mask any odour. • If possible, move the client into another room for meals.
9. *Temperature* Fever is the body's way of fighting infection by increasing white blood cells and blood flow to the area. ***Not all clients who have an infection will have a fever when you take the temperature.*** Some clients (such as older adults or clients with immune challenges) may not have a fever in the presence of an infection.	• Take the client's temperature, according to the care plan (see Chapter 15), and if there is a fever, report it. Often, fever is a sign of infection. • Report any abnormal findings at once. It is common for older adults to have a normally low body temperature, so they may not seem to have a fever even if there is an infection. ***Observe for other signs that indicate an infection*** (such as redness or swelling around the wound, tenderness, and warmth to the touch).
10. *Skin Care* Clean, dry skin is less likely to harbour pathogens than moist, soiled skin. Pathogens can cause skin infections, which, in turn, can lead to skin ulceration and breakdown.	• Keep the client's skin clean and dry. Avoid the use of powders, which may dry out the skin too much and may irritate the client's airway. • After washing the client's skin, rinse it thoroughly and pat it dry. Do not towel-dry roughly, as this action can actually tear the skin of some frail clients. • Report and record any observations of edema, bruising, swelling, or any other abnormal feature.

Continued

BOX 24–6 The Support Worker's Responsibilities to Clients With Wounds—cont'd

Specific Areas	Your Responsibilities
11. *Maintaining Skin Integrity* Intact skin is the body's first line of defence against pathogens. It is important that skin is kept intact, as it is easier to prevent a skin infection than it is to cure one.	• Transfer or position the client gently. Use equipment properly. Use friction-reducing equipment, such as sliding boards (see Chapter 25). • Never apply straps or boards directly on the skin, as this contact can increase the client's risk of getting scratched or bruised. • Ensure that the client's skin remains clean and dry at all times. Follow all of the above steps to ensure the client's skin is not damaged at any time. • Avoid tight, restrictive clothing.

12. *Complications and Concerns*
Delayed healing is a risk for clients who are older or obese or who have poor nutrition. Poor circulation and diabetes also affect healing.
Survivors of violence have many other concerns. Fear of future attacks, concerns about the attacker being found and convicted, and fear for family members are common.
The wound may be disfiguring. Whatever the wound's location or size, the client's body image and self-esteem are often affected.
Amputation of a finger, hand, arm, toes, foot, or leg can affect the client's function, daily activities, and job.
The wound may be large or small. It may be visible to others—on the face, arms, or legs—or hidden by clothing. If the client had surgery, anaesthesia and pain medication can affect eating and elimination.
	• Be aware of the following:
	  • These conditions are risk factors for infection.
	  • Survivors of abuse often hide the true source of their injuries.
	  • The wound may affect the client's sexual performance or the client's sense of being sexually attractive.
	  • Eye injuries can affect vision.
	  • Many clients with serious and disfiguring wounds have an increased need for love and acceptance.
	  • The client may have fears about scarring, disfigurement, delayed healing, and infection or may have fears about the wound "popping open."
	• Be empathetic to the client's feelings. The client may be sad and tearful or angry and hostile. Adjustments may be hard and rehabilitation necessary. Be gentle and kind, give compassionate care, and practise good communication.
	• Work in cooperation with other health care team members—social workers, psychiatrists, therapists, and spiritual advisors—who may be involved in the client's care.

Some dressings contain special agents to promote wound healing. If it is considered within your scope of practice, and you are to assist with a dressing change, your supervisor will explain the use of the dressing to you. Dressing application methods involve a number of dressing types, depending on the client's particular type of wound. Your supervisor or the nurse will direct you in regard to the particulars of dressing change and care for each client.

Securing Dressings

Dressings must be secure over wounds to avoid microbes entering the wound and drainage escaping

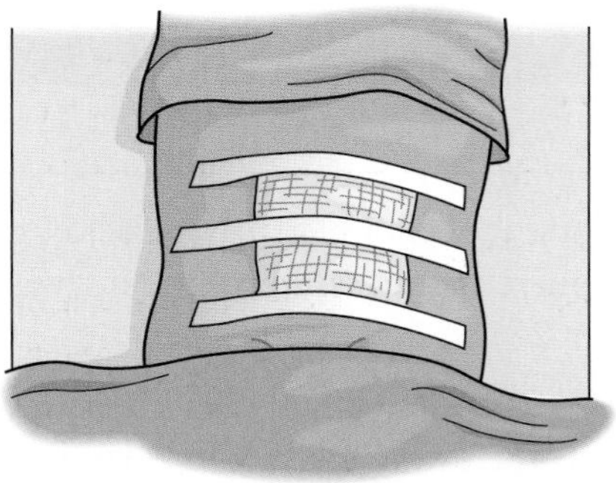

FIGURE 24–20 Tape is applied at the top, middle, and bottom of the dressing. Note that the tape extends several centimetres beyond both sides of the dressing.

(see the *Focus on Children: Dressings* box on this page and *Focus on Older Adults: Dressings* box on p. 485).

Tape

Adhesive, paper, plastic, and elastic tapes are common. Adhesive tape sticks well to the skin, but removing the remaining adhesive can be difficult, and the adhesive can irritate the skin. Some skin may come off with the tape, causing an abrasion. For clients who are allergic to adhesive tape, paper and plastic tapes are used since they do not usually cause allergic reactions. Elastic tape allows easier movement of the body part.

Tape is applied to secure the top, middle, and bottom of the dressing (**FIGURE 24–20**). The tape extends several centimetres beyond each side of the dressing. ***The tape must not encircle the entire body part. If swelling were to occur, circulation to the part would be impaired.***

If the client can tolerate it, a **picture-frame dressing**—where the tape is applied to all four edges—can be used. This method of wound dressing is less likely to wrinkle or fall off. Many simple bandages already have adhesive tapes on all four edges or are transparent and allow for vapour and oxygen exchange through it (**FIGURE 24–21**).

Applying Dressings

Your supervisor may ask you to assist with dressing changes. Some employers allow support workers to apply simple, dry, nonsterile dressings to simple wounds. **BOX 24–7** lists guidelines for applying nonsterile dressings (see the *Focus on Home Care: Changing Dressings* box).

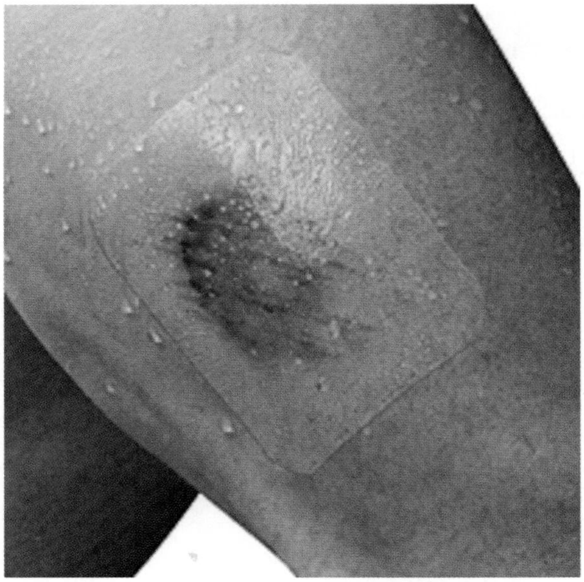

FIGURE 24–21 This type of dressing (shown here is Nexcare™ Tegaderm™ Transparent Waterproof Dressing) is clear and allows the wound to be observed while protecting it. For wounds that may drain, there are bandages with a small gauze square surrounded by the adhesive. These bandages promote healing by allowing vapour and oxygen to penetrate the clear membrane. (**Photo source:** Copyright ©3M IPC 2016. All rights reserved. This material is reproduced by courtesy of 3M. No further reproduction is permitted without 3M's prior written consent.)

FOCUS ON CHILDREN

Dressings

Children are often afraid of dressing changes. Tape removal is often painful for them, and the wound's appearance can be frightening. It is important to ensure that the child is calm and cooperative, or the sterile field could become contaminated. A parent or caregiver should hold the child so that the wound can be reached with ease. Holding or playing with a favourite toy is often comforting to the child. To help decrease the child's fear and apprehension about dressings, you can suggest that the child apply a dressing to a doll (and remove it).

HEAT AND COLD APPLICATIONS

Physicians and nurses often order heat and cold applications for wound care (see Chapter 44) to promote healing and comfort and to reduce tissue swelling.

FOCUS ON OLDER ADULTS

Dressings

As we age, skin becomes thinner and more fragile, so skin tears are more common in older adults. Extreme care is, therefore, necessary when removing tape. One method that many nurses suggest using is to "peel" the tape off by folding the edge of the tape over and dragging it back. This technique avoids lifting the skin, which can be uncomfortable to the client and can injure the client's skin.

FOCUS ON HOME CARE

Changing Dressings

Your supervisor may ask you to telephone after removing the client's old dressing. During this telephone call, you should report your observations, and your supervisor will give you instructions on how to proceed further. Follow your employer policy for disposing of dressings. Usually, employers require you to do the following:

- Place the used dressing in a plastic bag
- Fasten the bag securely
- Dispose of the bag in the household garbage

BOX 24–7 Guidelines for Applying Nonsterile Dressings

- Make sure your province or territory allows you to perform the procedure.
- Make sure the procedure is in your job description.
- Apply dressings only under a nurse's direction and supervision.
- Review the procedure with the nurse.
- Allow time for pain medications to take effect, as the client may experience discomfort during the dressing change. The nurse will give the medication and tell you how long to wait.
- Provide for the client's fluid and elimination needs before starting the procedure.
- Collect needed equipment and supplies before you begin.
- Be aware of your nonverbal communication. Wound odours, appearance, and drainage may be unpleasant, but take care not to communicate your thoughts and reactions to the client.
- Follow Standard Practices. Wear personal protective equipment, as necessary. Never touch a wound with ungloved hands.
- Remove dressings in a way that prevents the client from seeing the soiled side. The drainage and its odour may upset the client.
- Do not force the client to look at the wound, as the appearance of the wound can affect body image and self-esteem. The nurse will address the client's concerns about the wound.
- Remove the tape by pulling it toward the wound. You can ensure that the tape does not stick to the skin by, again, folding it back on itself.
- Remove the dressing gently. If the dressing sticks to the wound and surrounding skin, ask your supervisor if the wound can be dampened (for example, by applying sterile normal saline) to loosen the dressing from the wound.
- Observe the wound, and report and record your observations, according to employer policy (see **BOX 24–5** on p. 477).

Applying a Dry Nonsterile Dressing

123

Advocate on behalf of the client's quality of life by promoting:

Dignity • Independence • Preferences • Privacy • Safety

(see BOX 1–4, on p. 17)

PRE-PROCEDURE

1 Review the procedure with your supervisor.
Being familiar with the procedure before beginning will reduce your anxiety and, in turn, the client's.

2 Identify the client, according to employer policy.
This eliminates the possibility of mistaking one client for another.

3 Explain the procedure to the client.

4 Allow time for pain medication to take effect (injectable medication may begin to work within minutes, but oral pain medication may take at least 1 hour).
This will make the procedure more comfortable for the client.

5 Provide for the client's fluid and elimination needs.
This will make the client more comfortable during the procedure.

6 Practise proper hand hygiene.

7 Collect the following supplies:
- ☐ **Gloves**
- ☐ **Personal protective equipment**, as needed
- ☐ **Tape**
- ☐ **Dressing**, as directed by the care plan
- ☐ **Dressing tray**, as directed by the care plan
- ☐ **Clean, small gauze squares** to wipe wound area, as directed by the care plan
- ☐ **Normal saline** to clean the wound, as directed by the care plan
- ☐ **Adhesive remover**
- ☐ **Scissors**
- ☐ **Leak-proof plastic bag**
- ☐ **Bath blanket or clean sheet**

By collecting all the necessary equipment beforehand, you will not have to needlessly leave your client's side and can eliminate wasting time and energy in obtaining the forgotten equipment. You will also avoid tiring the client needlessly.

8 Provide for privacy.

9 Arrange items on your work area.

10 Raise the bed to a comfortable working height. Follow the care plan for bed rail use.*
Raising the bed will reduce your risk for back strain. Lowering the head of the bed will make it easier to slide the client up to a better position.

PROCEDURE

11 Lower the bed rail near you if it is up.

12 Help the client to a comfortable position.

13 Cover the client with a bath blanket or clean sheet. Fan-fold the client's top linen to the foot of the bed.
A fan-folded sheet is easier for the client to grasp when it is time to cover up.

14 Expose the affected body part, leaving the rest of the client as covered as possible.
This respects the client's need for privacy and prevents the client from being needlessly chilled.

15 Make a cuff on the plastic bag. Place it within reach and in a place that avoids crossing over the wound with soiled wipes.

16 Wear a gown and mask if necessary as directed by the care plan.
These measures decrease the risk for pathogen spread.

17 Put on gloves.

18 Remove tape by holding the skin down and gently pulling the tape toward the wound.
Pulling the tape toward the wound is more comfortable for the client than pulling away from it. It can also reduce the chance of reopening the wound if it has not yet healed.

19 Remove adhesive from the skin. Wet a 10 × 10 cm (4 × 4 in.) gauze dressing with the adhesive remover. Clean *away* from the wound.

Continued

Applying a Dry Nonsterile Dressing—cont'd

Adhesive left behind irritates the skin, so it should always be removed. Cleaning away from the wound decreases the chance of introducing pathogens or adhesive into the wound.

20 Remove the gauze dressing. Start with the top dressing. Keep the soiled side of the dressing out of the client's sight.
Keeping the soiled dressing out of sight reduces the client's anxiety.

21 Place the dressing in the leak-proof bag. It must not touch the outside of the bag.
The outside of the bag must remain clean and uncontaminated to reduce the risk for pathogen spread.

22 Remove the dressing directly over the wound very gently.
The old dressing may stick to the wound. By being rough, you can reopen a wound that hasn't yet healed.

23 Observe the wound and drainage (see BOX 24–5, on p. 477). Avoid showing the drainage to the client.
Seeing the drainage may be upsetting to the client.

24 Remove gloves. Put them in the bag. Practise proper hand hygiene. (If used, raise the bed rail before leaving the bedside. Lower it when you return.)

25 Open the dressing tray. Unfold the clean or sterile wrapper and ensure it stay opens.
The new dressing tray is opened after *the soiled dressing is removed to reduce the risk of contaminating it.*

26 Pour the normal saline into the dressing tray, being careful not to splash it on the wrapper.
Splashing will contaminate the wrapper.

27 Open the small gauze square package and, using the forceps supplied in the dressing tray, place five or six onto the dressing tray or on the clean wrapper, staying as close to the centre of the wrapper and the tray as possible.
The small gauze squares will be used to cleanse the wound. Old drainage and dried blood left behind on a wound can be a source of infection and should be removed.
The outer 2.5 cm of the wrapper is regarded as contaminated.

28 Cut the length of tape needed.

29 Put on clean gloves.

30 Using either the forceps supplied in the dressing tray or your clean, gloved hand, pick up a small gauze square. Dip it into the normal saline solution.

31 Wipe the wound in one long stroke down the middle of the wound from top to bottom. Discard the gauze square into the leak-proof bag. If you are using a cleaning cloth, use a fresh corner for each stroke you use. Do not touch the wound again with a soiled gauze square or cleaning cloth.
The wound is wiped in long strokes, and the gauze wipe is discarded after each wipe to prevent pathogen spread.

32 Wipe down the middle of the wound again and then on either side of the wound.
Wiping is always done from the centre of the wound to the outside to prevent contaminating the wound.

33 Apply dressing, as directed by the care plan.

34 Secure the dressing in place using tape.
Tape prevents the dressing from falling off.

35 Remove your gloves. Put them in the bag. Practise proper hand hygiene.
These steps decrease the risk for pathogen spread.

Continued

Applying a Dry Nonsterile Dressing—cont'd

POST-PROCEDURE

36 Provide for safety and comfort.
37 Cover the client and remove the bath blanket or clean sheet.
38 Place the call bell within reach.*
This provides an easy, safe way for the client to contact the staff if necessary.
39 Return the bed to its lowest position. Follow the care plan for bed rail use.*
40 Remove privacy measures.
41 Discard supplies into the leak-proof bag. Tie the bag closed. Dispose of the bag, according to employer policy.
42 Clean your work surface, according to employer policy.
This reduces the risk for pathogen contamination of anything placed on that surface after the dressing change.
43 Practise proper hand hygiene.

Report and Record your actions and observations, according to employer policy.
This is done for legal reasons and to keep the rest of the health care team informed.

*Steps marked with an asterisk may not apply in community settings.

* Sitz bath (See page 1020).

CHAPTER REVIEW

KEY POINTS

- Skin is the body's first line of defence, protecting the body from invading pathogens.
- A wound is a break in skin or mucous membranes and becomes a portal of entry for microbes and pathogens.
- The support worker's role in wound care depends on provincial or territorial laws, job description, and the client's condition.
- Types of wounds include (1) intentional, (2) unintentional, (3) open, (4) closed, (5) clean, and (6) contaminated. Wounds can also be described according to their depth, such as (1) partial-thickness or (2) full-thickness.
- Skin tears occur due to friction, shearing, pulling, or direct pressure. They should always be reported to the supervisor.
- Pressure ulcers are caused by unrelieved pressure over a bony prominence. All support workers should know who is at risk for pressure ulcers and should observe for them and report any found immediately to the supervisor.
- Support workers should know ways to prevent pressure ulcers.
- Circulatory ulcers include (1) venous ulcers and (2) arterial ulcers. Their causes, appearances, and treatment differ from each other.
- Complications of wounds include (1) hemorrhage, (2) infection, (3) dehiscence, and (4) evisceration.
- Wound drainage types include (1) serous, (2) sanguineous, (3) serosanguineous, and (4) purulent.
- Support workers should be familiar with the responsibilities of caring for clients with wounds.

CRITICAL THINKING IN PRACTICE

You are dressing an older resident with thin, fragile skin. You notice a new skin tear on the person's arm. What do you do? How can you prevent skin tears?

REVIEW QUESTIONS

Answers to these questions are at the bottom of page 490.

Circle T if the answer is true, and circle F if the answer is false.

1. T F Good nutrition and hydration can help prevent skin breakdown.
2. T F White, greyish, or reddened skin is the first sign of a pressure ulcer.
3. T F Pressure ulcers do not usually occur over a bony area.
4. T F Pressure ulcers can develop from failing to reposition the client often enough.
5. T F Shearing and friction can cause pressure ulcers.

Circle the BEST answer.

6. A child fell off her bike. She has a laceration on her right leg. She has a(n):
   A. Closed wound
   B. Infected wound
   C. Contaminated wound
   D. Intentional wound
7. Mrs. Katz had rectal surgery. What type of wound does she have?
   A. A clean wound
   B. A dirty wound
   C. A clean-contaminated wound
   D. A contaminated wound
8. The piercing of skin and underlying tissues is called a(n):
   A. Penetrating wound
   B. Hematoma
   C. Contusion
   D. Abrasion

9. Which of the following can cause skin tears?
- A. Keeping your nails trimmed and filed smooth
- B. Dressing clients in clothing with long sleeves and long pants
- C. Hurrying when lifting and transferring clients
- D. Padding wheelchair footrests

10. Which of the following causes pressure ulcers?
- A. Repositioning the client every 2 hours
- B. Scrubbing and rubbing the skin
- C. Applying lotion to dry areas
- D. Keeping linens clean, dry, and wrinkle-free

11. Which of the following are used to treat or prevent pressure ulcers?
- A. Hospital beds
- B. Waterbeds and flotation pads
- C. Plastic drawsheets and waterproof pads
- D. Heel "doughnut dressings"

12. You can help prevent stasis ulcers by:
- A. Using elastic garters to hold socks in place
- B. Keeping the client in bed as much as possible
- C. Encouraging the client to sit with legs crossed
- D. Avoiding injury to the legs and feet when giving care

13. Which of the following areas is a common site for arterial ulcers?
- A. On the scalp
- B. On top of the nose
- C. On the outer side of the ankle
- D. Behind the knee

14. A wound appears red and swollen. The area around it is warm to the touch. These signs occur during:
- A. The inflammatory phase of wound healing
- B. The proliferative phase of wound healing
- C. Healing by primary intention
- D. Healing by secondary intention

15. A wound is healing by primary intention. While assisting with a dressing change, you note that the wound is separating. This is called:
- A. Dehiscence
- B. Tertiary intention
- C. Evisceration
- D. Hematoma

16. You see clear, watery drainage from a wound. This drainage is called:
- A. Purulent drainage
- B. Serous drainage
- C. Seropurulent drainage
- D. Serosanguineous drainage

17. Which of the following does a dressing do?
- A. Protects the wound from injury
- B. Reduces swelling
- C. Prevents healing too fast
- D. Prevents oxygen from entering the wound

18. You are securing a dressing with tape. Tape is applied:
- A. Around the entire body part
- B. To the top and bottom of the dressing
- C. To the top, middle, and bottom of the dressing
- D. As the client prefers

Answers: 1.T, 2.T, 3.F, 4.T, 5.T, 6.C, 7.C, 8.A, 9.C, 10.B, 11.B, 12.D, 13.C, 14.A, 15.A, 16.B, 17.A, 18.C

Chapter opener image: Joe Belanger/Shutterstock.com

CHAPTER 25

Body Mechanics: Moving, Positioning, Transferring, and Lifting the Client

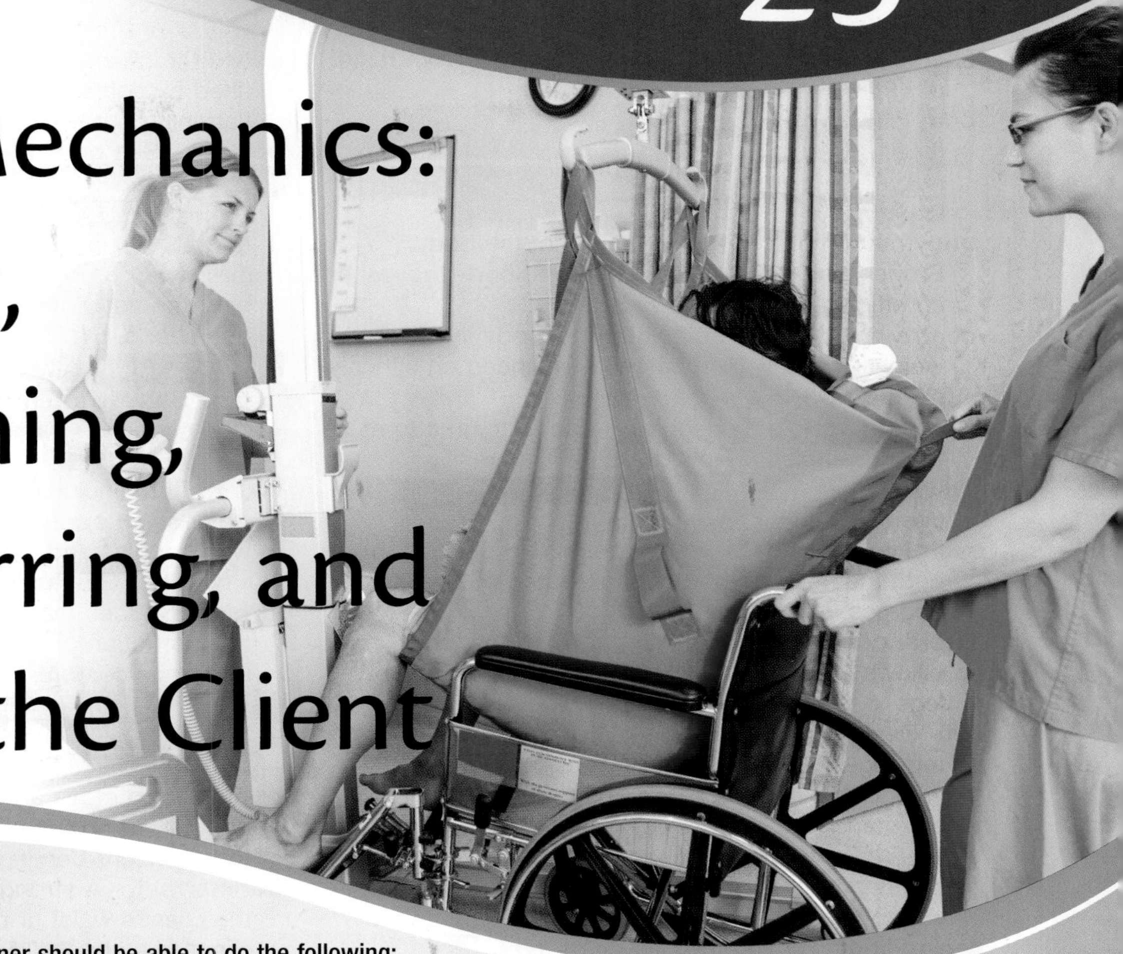

OBJECTIVES

After reading this chapter, the learner should be able to do the following:

- List the purpose and rules of using good body mechanics.
- Describe why good body alignment and position changes are important for the client.
- Identify the comfort and safety measures for positioning clients in bed.
- Describe how to position a client in the basic bed positions and in a chair.
- Describe comfort and safety measures for moving, turning, and lifting clients in bed.
- Differentiate between a transfer and a lift.
- Identify safety measures used when transferring clients.
- Identify the purpose of a transfer belt and a transfer board.
- Demonstrate how to move a client in bed.
- Apply the information provided in this chapter by performing the procedures described.

KEY TERMS

base of support The area on which an object rests. *p. 494*

body alignment The way in which body parts (head, trunk, arms, and legs) are positioned in relation to one another, whether lying, sitting, or standing. Also known as **posture**. *p. 493*

body mechanics The movement of the body. Proper body mechanics ensure the body moves in an efficient and careful way. *p. 493*

centre of gravity The point in the body in which weight is evenly distributed or balanced on either side. *p. 493*

fan-fold To fold a sheet back and forth, in a form that resembles a fan. *p. 499*

Fowler's position A semi-sitting to upright sitting position in bed. *p. 510*

high Fowler's position A semi-sitting position in bed; the head of the bed is elevated 45 to 90 degrees. *p. 510*

lateral position A side-lying position that uses pillows to support the back and separate the lower legs. *p. 511*

lift Device used to move—or the action of moving—a client from one place to another, without the client's weight-bearing or assistance. *p. 524*

line of gravity An imaginary vertical line that extends from the centre of gravity to the base of support. *p. 493*

log-rolling Turning the person as a unit, in alignment, with one motion. *p. 498.*

low Fowler's position A semi-sitting position in bed; the head of the bed is elevated 15 to 30 degrees. *p. 510*

lunge (or stride) stance A position whereby you place one foot in front of the other foot, keeping both feet about a shoulder-width apart. *p. 494*

manual lift Physically picking up a client who cannot weight-bear, without the assistance of a mechanical lift. *p. 524*

mechanical lift A device that can elevate and move the person while in a special body sling. *p. 515*

no-lift policy Agency regulations that prohibit workers from manually lifting clients and instruct them to use a mechanical lifting device instead. *p. 494*

pelvic tilt A standing position whereby the pelvis is tilted by tightening the stomach muscles and flattening out the small of the back. *p. 494*

posture See **body alignment**. *p. 493*

prone position A front-lying position on the abdomen, with the head turned to one side. *p. 512*

semi-Fowler's position A semi-sitting position in bed; the head of the bed is elevated 30 to 45 degrees. *p. 510*

Sims' position A left-side-lying position; the right leg is sharply flexed so that it is not on the left leg, and the left arm is positioned along the client's back. *p. 512*

slider Item (including *slider sheet*, *slider board*, and *slider sheet system*) made of low-friction material with handles and used to move clients. *p. 498*

sliding pad See **turning pad**. *p. 497*

stroke Sudden loss of brain function because of the disruption of blood supply to the brain. Also known as *cerebral vascular accident (CVA). p. 515*

supine position A back-lying position; the legs are together. Also called *dorsal recumbent position* or *horizontal position. p. 511*

transfer To move a person from one place to another, using the client's assistance with partial to full weight-bearing. *p. 514*

transfer belt A strong strap that is secured around the client's waist or hips to help and support the client to stand, sit, and walk. It is removed after the activity is completed. *p. 516*

transfer board A smooth board placed between two surfaces (e.g., a chair and a wheelchair) that allows the client to slide over more easily. *p. 518*

turning pad A small pad or folded sheet placed on top of the bottom sheet and extending from the client's head to above the knees. Also known as a **sliding pad**, *turning sheet*, *transfer sheet*, or *lift pad*. A turning pad is sometimes (inaccurately) referred to as a *drawsheet*. *p. 497*

weight-bear To shift body weight onto feet while attempting to stand. *p. 514*

As a support worker, you will find that your daily activities often include lifting, moving, and carrying items—for example, lifting grocery bags, pushing wheelchairs, moving the client's bed, or carrying garbage and laundry bags. You also move, turn, and reposition clients in their beds. You will assist clients from the bed to another supporting surface such as a chair or wheelchair and back again. In some settings, you may be required to lift a client while providing care. Note that some agencies have a no-lift policy. In such an agency, you will be responsible for following agency policies when lifting clients mechanically.

You must always protect yourself and the client during moving, positioning, and transferring activities. Knowing and using proper body mechanics and lifting techniques will help you prevent injuries. Exercise regularly to maintain strong abdominal and quadriceps muscles, the main muscles used in lifting. Back injuries and muscle and joint strains are serious and common injuries among health care workers and support workers. Use your body correctly. If you experience an injury, report it immediately. Seeking medical attention promptly may reduce the long-term complications of injuries, including back injuries.

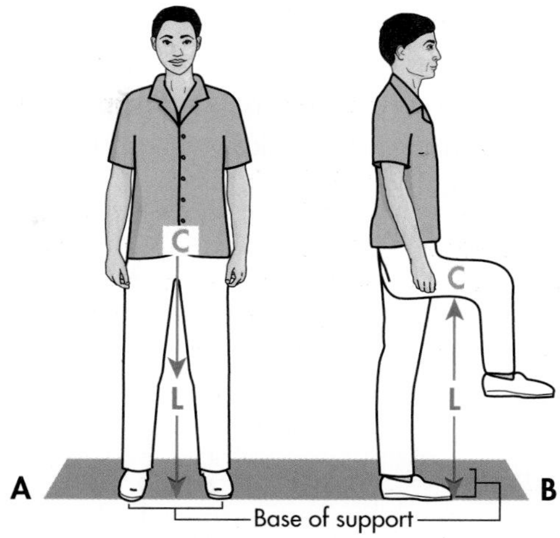

FIGURE 25–1 Proper body alignment when standing. Note how feet are placed apart for a wide base of support. Note where the line of gravity (L) and centre of gravity (C) are. In image *B*, the centre and line of gravity have moved to accommodate the person's change of position.

BODY MECHANICS

The term **body mechanics** refers to the movement of the body. Proper body mechanics include moving in an efficient and careful way and having good posture and balance, as well as using the strongest and largest muscles for work. (Review the structure and function of the musculo-skeletal system in Chapter 17.) Good body mechanics reduce the risk for injury. Fatigue, muscle strain, and injury can result from the improper use and positioning of the body during activity or rest, so you must be aware of both your client's and your own body mechanics.

Body alignment (or **posture**) is the way the body parts (head, trunk, arms, and legs) are positioned in relation to one another. Good body alignment enables the body to move and function with strength and efficiency, reduces strain on the muscles and joints, and prevents injury. For people with limited mobility, correct body alignment helps prevent disabling complications such as muscle atrophy and contractures (see Chapter 26).

A client who is placed in poor body alignment may develop serious effects on all body systems. For example, a client who is poorly positioned in a stooped-over position will probably not be able to breathe deeply and bring oxygen into the lungs. Or if positioned flat on the back with no pillows under the knees, a client may experience severe pain in the lumbar spine region. As a support worker, you must constantly watch to see that clients are positioned (or repositioned) properly.

FIGURE 25–1 shows a person standing with good body alignment. Notice that both sides of the body are in line with each other—in the centre is the **line of gravity**. Body balance is achieved when a relatively low **centre of gravity** (the point in the body at which weight is evenly distributed on either side) is balanced over a wide, stable base. Imagine a vertical line falling from the centre of gravity and through the centre of the base of support.

Good posture in a standing position has the following traits:

- The head and neck are erect and straight.
- Shoulders and hips are parallel to each other.
- Shoulders are back.
- The chest is out.
- The spine maintains a natural lumbar curve.

- The abdomen is tucked in and the pelvis tilted in (also known as a **pelvic tilt**). This positioning helps improve the posture, strengthen the lower spine, and reduce the risk for back injury.
- Knees are slightly flexed.
- Arms are hanging comfortably at the sides.
- Feet are about shoulder-width apart.
- Toes are pointing forward; one foot is slightly forward.

Lying down and sitting also require good alignment.

The position of the feet is especially important for good body mechanics because feet provide the base of support. A **base of support** is the area on which an object rests. A wide base of support provides more stability and balance than a narrow base of support. You should stand with your feet and legs apart for a wide base of support, especially when moving, lifting, or transferring weight. A **lunge (or stride) stance** has one foot in front of the other, with the two about shoulder-width apart. This stance will enable you to keep your balance while performing the various tasks described in this chapter.

The strongest and largest muscles are in the shoulders, upper arms, hips, and thighs. These muscles should be used for lifting and moving. Using smaller and weaker muscles, such as those in the lower back, will strain your back and lead to back fatigue and injury. Follow the guidelines in the *Think About Safety: Guidelines for Good Body Mechanics* box to move clients and objects safely and efficiently.

MOVING CLIENTS IN BED

Some clients can move and turn in bed themselves, whereas others may need some help. Although many may not be able to move independently, they can often work with you as you move them. Some clients, such as those who are unconscious, paralyzed, or very weak, are unable to move at all or even help when others move them. In some cases, assistive devices may be necessary—for example, a turning pad (see p. 497) or a mechanical lift (see pp. 524–525). Occasionally, two or three workers may be needed to move or turn a client in bed.

Check with the care plan, your supervisor, and the client to find out if the client can help with moving. ***Do not attempt to move a client by yourself if you think you may not be able to do it safely. If your agency has a no-lift policy, you should never attempt moving or lifting the client without using the proper equipment, having the correct number of qualified assistants, and checking first with your supervisor.*** You must consider the client's safety and your own safety (see the *Focus on Home Care: Getting Help With Moving and Repositioning a Client* box).

Think About Safety

Guidelines for Good Body Mechanics

- Assess the situation before you begin any attempt to move the client. Get help if you think the client's weight is more than you can safely turn or transfer. Many employers have a **no-lift policy**, in which case, workers are not allowed to lift or move clients without mechanical aid and qualified assistance. ***Always check the care plan and know employer policy before moving a client.***
- Face your work area to prevent unnecessary twisting. Remember to stand with a wide base of support.
- Bend at your knees and hips and squat when lifting or setting down objects below your waist. Do not bend forward from your waist, or you will strain your small back muscles (**FIGURE 25–2**).
- Tighten your stomach muscles and tuck in your pelvis as you lift. Keep your back straight. Use your leg and thigh muscles as you lift an item to waist level. Your legs should be bearing the weight, not your back.
- Hold objects *close* to your body when lifting, moving, or carrying them, activities that involve the upper arm and shoulder muscles (see **FIGURE 25–2**). Holding objects away from your body

Continued

Think About Safety—cont'd

places a strain on the small muscles in your lower arms. Do not lift objects higher than chest level. Use both hands and arms to lift, move, or carry heavy objects.

- Avoid unnecessary bending and reaching. If your client is on a hospital bed, raise the bed so that it is close to the height of your waist. Adjust the overbed table so that it is at your waist level. Arrange all equipment and supplies in a convenient, easy-to-reach location before you begin a task. If necessary, move a chair next to the bedside and arrange your supplies on it. If an object is higher than chest level, use a stepstool to reach it.
- Turn your whole body as one unit when changing the direction of your movement. Do not twist your body. Move your feet in the direction of the turn. Work with smooth and even movements. Avoid sudden or jerky motions. Take your time.
- Push, slide, or pull heavy objects whenever you can, rather than lifting them. Pushing with your body weight is easier than pulling. Widen your base of support when pushing or pulling: Move your front leg forward when pushing; move your rear leg back when pulling (**FIGURE 25–3**).

FOCUS ON HOME CARE

Getting Help With Moving and Repositioning a Client

Some clients you care for may have mechanical lifting devices in their homes. However, although assistance with lift devices is always available in facilities, usually you will not have a co-worker to help you move home care clients. In that case, plan your duties ahead of time with your supervisor.

In home care settings, it is common for a client's family members, the primary caregiver, or another person in the home to want to assist you in moving their loved one. ***Remember, whereas a helper in a facility is a co-worker, a helper in a home care setting is usually a trained family member or primary caregiver.*** A nurse or physiotherapist is responsible for teaching the client's family or primary caregiver about body mechanics and moving, positioning, and transferring the client. It is your responsibility to make sure that anyone who helps you has received training.

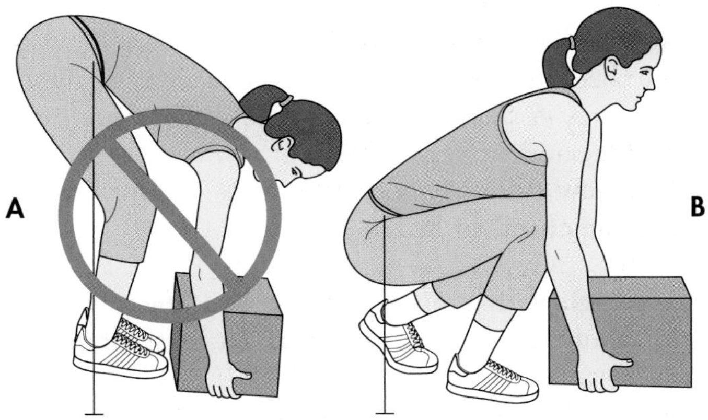

FIGURE 25–2 Picking up a box using incorrect ***(A)*** and good ***(B)*** body mechanics. (**Source:** Potter, P.A., & Perry, A.G. (2009). *Fundamentals of nursing* (rev. 7th ed., p. 1246). St. Louis, MO: Mosby.)

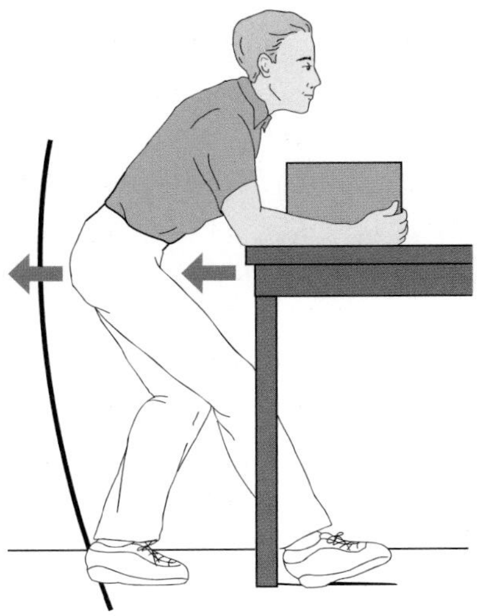

FIGURE 25–3 Move your rear leg back when pulling an item.

Comfort and Safety Measures

The client's skin must be protected when you are moving and repositioning the client. Otherwise, friction and shearing can injure the skin and cause infection and pressure ulcers (see Chapter 24). As defined in Chapter 24, *friction* is the resistance the skin encounters when it rubs against another surface, such as clothing, bedding, or another fold of skin. *Shearing* is the tearing of skin tissues caused when the skin sticks to a surface (usually the bed or chair) and deeper tissues move downward, exerting pressure on the skin (**FIGURE 25–4**). Shearing can happen when a client slides down in bed or is moved in bed. Shearing can be very painful and can lead to serious skin and health problems.

Reduce friction and shearing by rolling or lifting the client. A quilted turning pad (see p. 497) is used by some employers to reduce friction while moving the client in bed (see the *Focus on Older Adults: Shearing* box). A slider is used to slide a client from one bed to another (see p. 498).

Follow these comfort and safety measures when moving clients in bed:

- Check with your supervisor and the care plan about limits or restrictions in positioning or moving the client (see Chapter 26). For example, clients with severe arthritis and osteoporosis may experience pain or injury when being moved. Your supervisor will tell you what measures to take when moving these clients.
- Decide how to move the client and how much help you need *before* attempting the move. Then ask for help *before* starting the move.
- Communicate directions to your helper. Count 1-2-3 and then move together. ***Decide BEFORE you attempt this whether you both should move at the count of three or immediately after.***
- Move the client in small steps. Several small movements may be easier than one large movement.
- Cover and screen the client to protect privacy rights.
- Protect tubes or drainage containers connected to the client. Make sure that the tubing is not pulled, tangled, or pinched during the move.
- Position clients in good body alignment after lifting or moving them.
- After moving the client, make sure all linens under any of the client's body surfaces (such as under the client's back or head) are wrinkle-free. Straighten the linens, as needed.

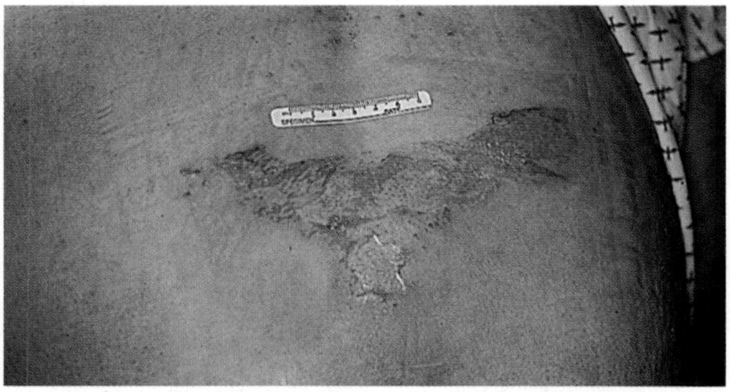

FIGURE 25–4 Shearing often occurs over the coccyx bone, just above the buttocks. When the head of the bed is raised for the sitting position, the skin on the client's buttocks stays in place, but internal structures move forward as the client slides down in bed. Skin that is pinched between the mattress and the hip bones can become scraped or even torn. To prevent shearing when moving a client up in bed, always use turning pads. (**Source:** Potter, P.A., & Perry, A.G. (2005). *Fundamentals of nursing* (6th ed., p. 1486). St. Louis, MO: Mosby.)

Moving the Client up in Bed

When sitting up in bed, the client can easily slide down toward the middle or the foot of the bed (**FIGURE 25–5**). The client then needs to be moved up in the bed to maintain good body alignment and

FOCUS ON OLDER ADULTS

Shearing

Older adults are at great risk for shearing. Their skin is fragile and easily torn. ***Always*** use a turning pad when lifting and moving older adults. Remember that older clients usually have less body fat, which means that their bony areas are more pronounced. The skin over bony areas is more likely to shear (tear and scrape) than that over other parts of the body.

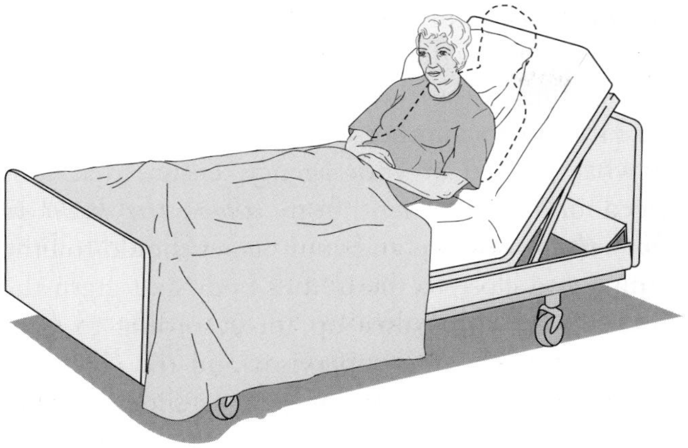

FIGURE 25–5 A client in poor alignment after sliding down in bed—shoulders are slouched, head and neck are forward, and the spine is curved.

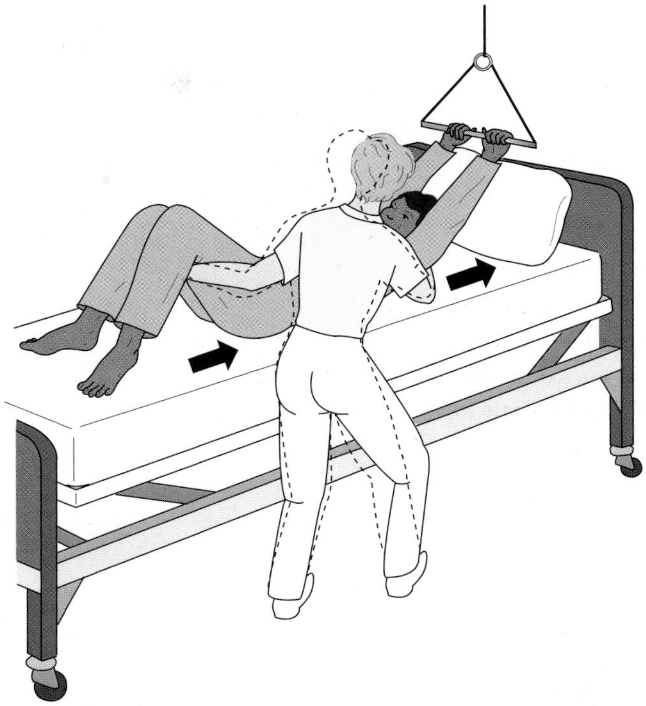

FIGURE 25–6 The client grasps a trapeze and flexes the knees. Shift your body weight from the rear leg to the front leg as you assist the client to move herself up in bed. Make sure the client does not shear the buttocks when moving this way.

comfort. Moving the client up in bed is also usually done before providing bedside care.

Check for agency or provincial guidelines that may indicate acceptable size or weight limits governing what you can do to assist a client by yourself. In some agencies, you might be allowed to move children and lightweight adults up in bed by yourself if the clients are able to help. The client helps by pushing with hands or feet to move up in bed. Or the client may have a trapeze (FIGURE 25–6) to aid with moving. A trapeze is a device that attaches to the bed or to a frame over the bed; the client grasps the bar of the trapeze and pulls.

Clients who are very heavy or weak need two people to move them and, usually, must be moved using a mechanical lift. ***You should be aware of your agency's caregiver lifting programs and familiarize yourself with your agency's safety policies and procedures. These are in place both to ensure client safety and to reduce workplace injuries.*** Remember to check with your supervisor or the client's care plan before attempting to move a client. Having someone help you protects you and the client from injury.

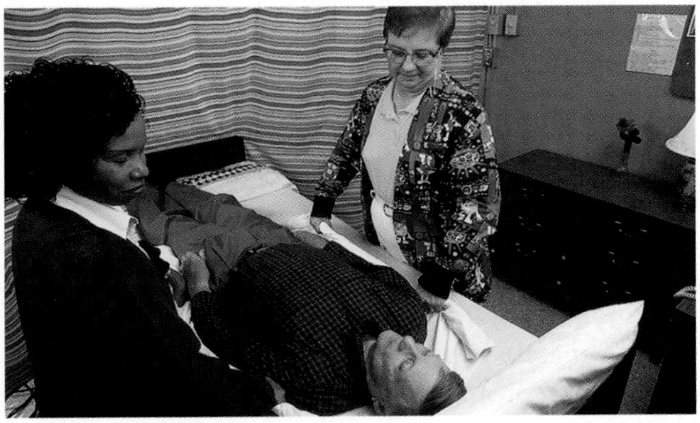

FIGURE 25–7 A turning pad is used in some agencies to move the client up in bed. Hold it close to the client near the client's shoulders and buttocks. Follow your agency's policies regarding whether to place your palms inward or outward while grasping the turning pad, as policies may differ from one agency to another.

Turning Pads and Sliders

A **turning pad** (also known as **sliding pad**, *turning sheet, transfer sheet, lift pad,* and, inaccurately, *drawsheet*) is a small pad or folded sheet placed on top of the bottom sheet and extending from the client's head to above the knees; it helps keep the mattress and bottom linens clean and dry (FIGURE 25–7). The turning pad can be made from a waterproof material or even a folded sheet (see Chapter 34). Some agencies use reusable waterproof incontinence pads as turning pads.

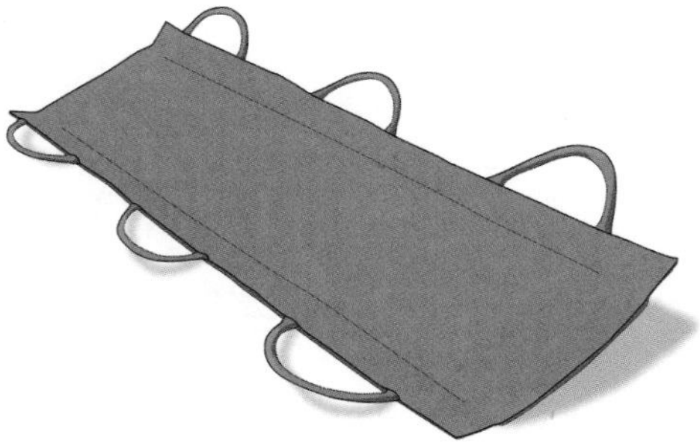

FIGURE 25–8 Slider sheets have replaced turning pads in many agencies. Notice the placement of the handles, which makes grasping the sheet easy for workers. (**Source:** Monica Schroeder/Science Source)

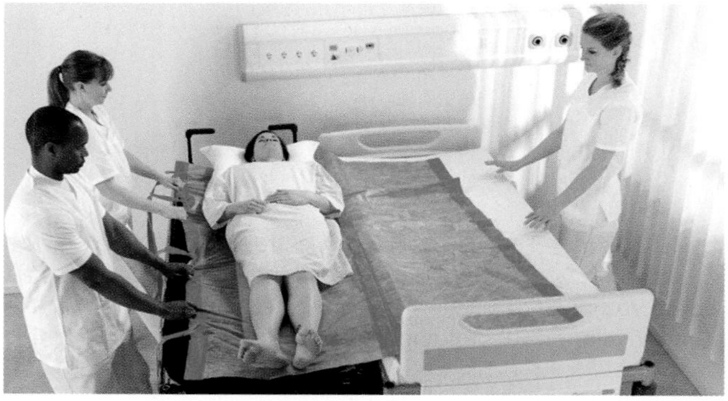

FIGURE 25–9 Using a slider sheet to transfer a client to a stretcher. The stretcher is placed against the bed, which is raised to stretcher height, and both are held firmly in place. Note how both workers' legs are placed to increase their centre of gravity and reduce strain on the back. In this photo, the client, on one slider sheet, was carefully dragged over the second slider sheet on the bed. (**Source:** Courtesy Arjo-Huntleigh Inc.)

Sliders are used to move clients. Made of a low-friction material with handles, the slider (*slider sheet, slider board,* or *slider sheet system*) is placed under the client, grasped by the handles, and then slid. Their use decreases the likelihood of client or worker injury. Sliders have replaced turning pads in many facilities (**FIGURE 25–8**). Some facilities use slider sheet systems, which are two slider sheets used together to reduce friction between the client and the bed surface. ***It is important to always use the equipment that your employer recommends.***

The slider or turning pad is used to reposition clients such as older adults, large clients, clients with mobility challenges (e.g., arthritis, spinal cord injuries, paralysis), and clients who are unconscious. They prevent pain, skin damage, and bone and joint damage by protecting the client's skin from friction and shearing as the client is slid or transferred from one location to another (**FIGURE 25–9**). Depending on what is used at your agency, ensure that it is placed under the client from ***above the head to above the knees.*** You and your helper should roll the turning pad close to the client's body and grasp the sheet firmly, with palms up (or according to your agency's policy). Your supervisor and the care plan will note whether a turning pad or slider sheet is required for each client.

When moving a client in bed, it is very important that you pay close attention to your own body alignment and posture. First, you can reduce your risk for injury if you do a few simple stretching exercises before beginning. Then, to reduce your risk for back injury, you should either raise the level of the client's bed or, if the bed cannot be raised, place your knee (the one closest to the client's head) on the bed. By placing your knee on the bed, you will not have to bend as far and will be less likely to hurt your back. While moving your client, avoid twisting or bending your back. Last, remember that it is safer for both you and your client to use the turning pad or slider instead of grasping the client.

Rolling Versus Log-Rolling a Client

Clients who have suffered a severe injury to their spinal cord or hip or who are recovering from neck, back, or spinal surgery often need to keep their spinal column in straight alignment to prevent further injuries. The client will need to be rolled as one unit, with care taken to prevent any twisting of the spinal column, from the neck to the tailbone. This special type of turn is called **log-rolling.**

Clients who are *not* severely injured or recovering from neck, back, or spinal surgery—if stated in the client's care plan—may be turned (or "rolled") in bed. For these clients, it can be easiest to bend the client's knee to assist you with the turn. Bend the knee opposite to the direction of the turn. For example, to turn the client onto her right side, bend her left knee and roll the client to the right, avoiding any twisting of the spine.

Moving the Client Up in Bed

123

Advocate on behalf of the client's quality of life by promoting:

Dignity • Independence • Preferences • Privacy • Safety (see BOX 1–4, on p. 17)

PRE-PROCEDURE

1 a Identify the client according to employer policy.
This eliminates the possibility of mistaking one client for another.
b Check the care plan for a description of the client's abilities or limitations.
Care must be taken in order to prevent injuring yourself or others.

2 Obtain slider sheet (FIGURE 25–8) or turning pad (FIGURE 25–7), as determined by your agency.
These decrease the friction created when moving a client in bed and help to prevent injuries to the client and to workers.

3 Ask someone to help you.
Two caregivers' working together makes moving the client easier, reduces time, and decreases the risk for skin shearing.

4 Perform hand hygiene.

5 Explain the procedure to the client.

6 Provide for privacy.

7 Raise bed to a comfortable working height for this procedure. Make sure bed wheels are locked. Follow the care plan for bed rail use. Lower the head of the bed to a level appropriate for the client. It should be as flat as possible.*
Raising the bed will reduce the risk for back strain. Lowering the head of the bed will make it easier to slide the client up to a better position.

PROCEDURE

8 You and your helper should stand on either side of the bed. Lower one of the bed rails. You and your helper should communicate directions throughout the procedure.
By working as a team, you will reduce the risk for client or worker injury.

9 Roll the client to one side (see the procedure *Log-Rolling the Client*) so that the client is facing the bed rail that is up.
Rolling ensures that the client's spine is not twisted, which could cause discomfort or injury.

10 The worker on the side facing the client should hold and support the client. Ensure that the client is in proper body alignment and safely positioned. Some clients feel better if they can hold on to the bed rail; if this is the case, keep the bed rail up.

11 The other support worker should **fan-fold** a slider sheet or turning pad and place it behind the client from the back of the head to below the thighs. The fan-folded slider sheet or turning pad should be tucked as close to the client's body as possible. Ensure the client's skin is protected at all times.
A fan-folded turning pad or slider sheet will be easier to grasp and to straighten out than one that is rolled up, reducing the time that the client has to lie on one side.

12 Inform the client that he will be rolling over a "bump" in the bed. Assist the client to log-roll over to the opposite side. Place the bed rail facing the client in the "up" position to allow the client to grasp it.
Informing the client of the "bump" may decrease anxiety and feelings of helplessness.

13 Lower the bed rail on the opposite side, grasp the turning pad or slider sheet and straighten it out.
It is important to straighten out the pad or sheet, as wrinkles may cause pressure sores.

Continued

Moving the Client Up in Bed—cont'd

14 Assist the client to log-roll onto the back. Lower the raised bed rail.

15 Grasp the handles of the slider sheet or roll the sides of the turning pad up close to the client.
Grasping the handles of the slider sheet on either side of the client will ensure easier client moving (see **FIGURE 25–8** *and* **FIGURE 25–9**)*. Rolling the sides of the turning pad will provide a good "handle" for staff to grasp.*
Note: If it is more comfortable for both you and the client, place your knee closest to the client's head on the bed.

16 Ensure that the client's head is supported.
When clients do not have the strength to hold their heads up for this procedure, supporting the head will reduce the risk for injury.

17 Place the client's pillow against the headboard if the client can do without the pillow.
The pillow acts as padding and prevents head injury.

18 Move the client up in bed on the count of three. The workers should shift their weight from the rear leg to the front leg.
Working together in synchronous actions makes this procedure easier for the workers and for the client.

19 Unroll the turning pad.
The rolled edge could cause pressure sores if the client were to lie on it.

20 Provide for safety and comfort. Position the client in good body alignment according to the care plan. Straighten linens.

21 If the client is lying in a hospital bed, the easiest and safest method to raise the client's head and shoulders is to raise the head of the bed. Use the electronic control to raise the head of the bed.

POST-PROCEDURE

22 Put the pillow under the client's head and shoulders. Tidy up the bed linens. Place the call bell within reach.*
These steps allow the client to feel respected, comfortable, safe, and secure.

23 Provide for safety and comfort. Check again that the client is positioned in good body alignment.
The client can slide down in bed after being repositioned.

24 Return the bed to the lowest height position if it was moved. Follow the care plan for bed rail use.*

25 Remove privacy measures.

26 Perform hand hygiene.

Report and Record your actions and observations, according to employer policy.
This is done for legal reasons and to keep the rest of the health care team informed.

*Steps marked with an asterisk may not apply in community settings.

Log-Rolling the Client (Note: This Procedure Requires Three Team Members.) 123

Advocate on behalf of the client's quality of life by promoting:

Dignity • Independence • Preferences • Privacy • Safety *(see BOX 1–4, on p. 17)*

PRE-PROCEDURE

1 a Identify the client according to employer policy.
This eliminates the possibility of mistaking one client for another.
b Check the care plan for a description of the client's abilities or limitations.
Care must be taken in order to prevent injuring yourself or others.

2 Ask two other team members to assist you to log-roll the client.
Three caregivers working together makes moving the client easier and reduces the risk for client and worker injury.

3 Perform hand hygiene.

4 Explain the procedure to the client.

5 Provide for privacy.

6 Raise the bed to a comfortable working height. Make sure the bed wheels are locked. Follow the care plan for bed rail use. Lower the head of the bed to a level appropriate for the client. It should be as flat as possible.*
Raising the bed will reduce the risk for back strain. Lowering the head of the bed will make it easier to slide the client up to a better position.

PROCEDURE

7 Place a pillow between the client's knees.
This prevents tension on the client's spinal column and adduction of the hip.

8 Cross the client's arms across the chest.
This prevents injury to the client's arms.

9 Two team members stand on the side of the bed opposite to the third team member. Each should communicate directions throughout the procedure (**FIGURE 25–10, *A***).
This will make log-rolling the client easier while using less energy. By working as a team, you will reduce the risk for client or worker injury.

10 Lower the bed rails on either side of the client.

11 a On the count of three, using the slider sheet or turning pad, move the client as a unit in a smooth, continuous motion to the side of the bed (**FIGURE 25–10, *B***).
This will ensure proper body alignment of the neck and spinal column by moving all body parts at the same time.

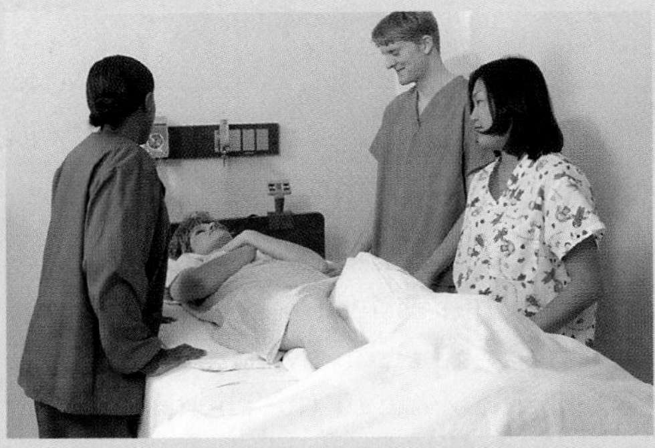

FIGURE 25–10 A Position the team members on either side of the client. (**Source:** Potter, P.A., & Perry, A.G. (2005). *Fundamentals of nursing* (5th Canadian ed., p. 1229). Toronto, ON: Elsevier.)

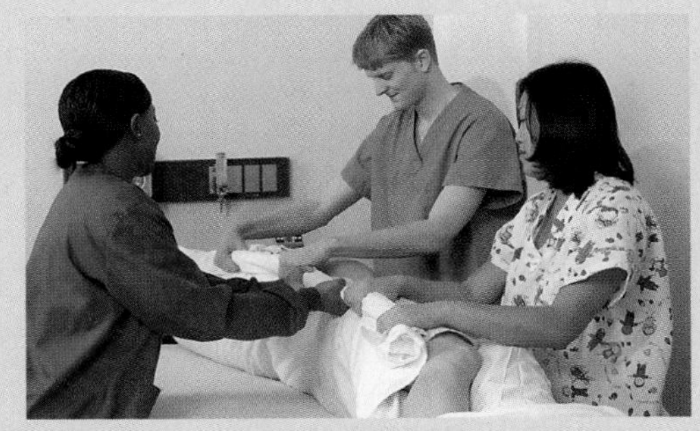

FIGURE 25–10 B Maintain the client's correct body alignment by moving all body parts at the same time. (**Source:** Potter, P.A., & Perry, A.G. (2005). *Fundamentals of nursing* (5th Canadian ed., p. 1229). Toronto, ON: Elsevier.)

Continued

Log-Rolling the Client (*Note: This Procedure Requires Three Team Members.*)—cont'd

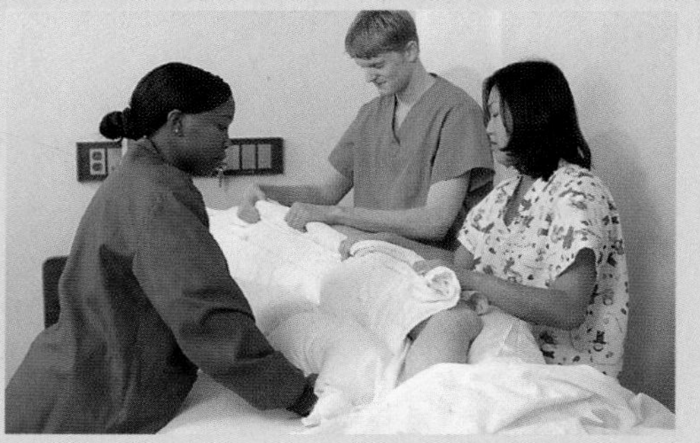

FIGURE 25–10 C Place pillows along the client's body for support. (**Source:** Potter, P.A., & Perry, A.G. (2005). *Fundamentals of nursing* (5th Canadian ed., p. 1229). Toronto, ON: Elsevier.)

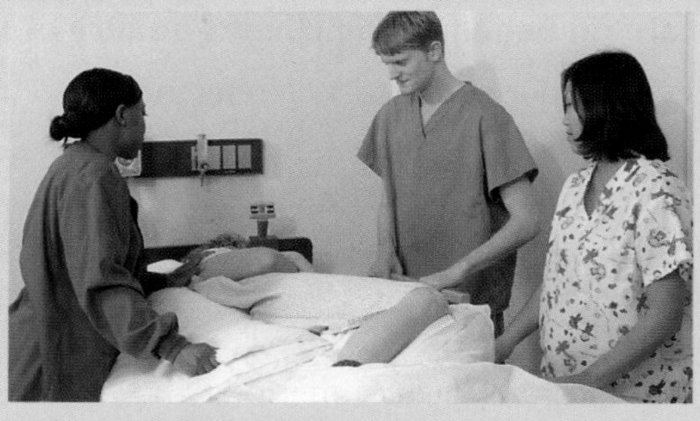

FIGURE 25–10 D Gently lean the client back toward the pillows. (**Source:** Potter, P.A., & Perry, A.G. (2005). *Fundamentals of nursing* (5th Canadian ed., p. 1229). Toronto, ON: Elsevier.)

b The solo team member on the opposite side of the bed places pillows along the length of the client (**FIGURE 25–10, *C***).

c Ensure the pillow surface next to the client is wrinkle-free.

Positioning a client with pillows decreases muscle fatigue and increases comfort.

d Tuck the pillow in toward the client.

12 Gently lean the client as a unit back toward the pillows for support (**FIGURE 25–10, *D***).

13 a Carefully adjust the pillow under the client's head, ensuring the head is in proper alignment.

b Adjust the shoulder. The client should not lie on an arm.

c Bend the upper arm toward the client's head. Place a small pillow under the upper hand and arm to keep the client in proper alignment.

POST-PROCEDURE

14 Provide for safety and comfort.

15 Place the call bell within reach.*

16 Return the bed to its lowest position. Raise or lower the bed rails according to the care plan.*

17 Remove privacy measures.

18 Perform hand hygiene.

Report and Record your actions and observations, according to employer policy.
This is done for legal reasons and to keep the rest of the health care team informed.

*Steps marked with an asterisk may not apply in community settings.

Turning the Client

Turning clients onto their sides helps prevent complications from bed rest. Certain care procedures require the side-lying position so that clients are turned toward you or away from you. The direction depends on the client's condition and on the situation. If you are going to turn clients over in bed, it is usually safer and easier to try to roll them. *Rolling* is the turning of a person over from the back or side to the other side. One of the client's knees (the one opposite the side the client is being turned onto) may be bent, if necessary (and if stated in the client's care plan), ***but you must always make sure the client is in good body alignment. You must always turn the***

client's neck and spine in one step, making sure they are never twisted.

Many clients have conditions such as arthritis in the spine or knees that make turning painful for them. When turning these clients, it is best to roll them using a turning pad. Remember to check with your supervisor and the care plan to determine the correct procedure to use for each client.

Some clients will need a minimum of two people to roll them, and if a client is tall or heavy, even three people may be needed. Clients who will need three people to roll them include the following:

- Clients with arthritic spines or knees (common in older adults)
- Clients recovering from hip fractures
- Clients with spinal cord injuries (the spine must be kept straight at all times following spinal cord injury)
- Clients recovering from spinal surgery (the spine must be kept straight at all times following spinal cord surgery)

Moving the Client From a Bed to a Stretcher

Stretchers are sometimes used to transport clients to other areas in a facility. In particular, they are used for the following:

- Clients who cannot sit up
- Clients who must stay in a lying position
- Clients who are seriously ill
- Clients who are waiting for or returning from surgery

The stretcher is covered with a folded flat sheet. A pillow and extra blankets are kept at hand. With your supervisor's permission, raise the head of the stretcher to the semi-Fowler's position (see "Positioning the Client," pp. 509–514). This position is more comfortable for most clients.

A slider board is used to assist in moving the client. Placed between the bed and the sheet the client is lying on, the slider board allows the staff to move the client with less friction. Its handles on either side allow for easy grasping. At least three staff members are needed to safely move a client from a bed to a stretcher. Remember, keep the client in good body alignment, and use good body mechanics.

After the client has been moved to the stretcher, fasten the safety straps across the client's chest. The stretcher's side rails are kept up during transport of the client. Clients should be moved feet first in the stretcher so that they can observe where they are going. As you push the stretcher, you should observe the client's breathing and colour during the transport. Never leave a client unattended on a stretcher.

Moving the Client From a Bed to a Stretcher 123

Advocate on behalf of the client's quality of life by promoting:

Dignity • Independence • Preferences • Privacy • Safety *(see BOX 1–4, on p. 17)*

PRE-PROCEDURE

1 a Identify the client according to employer policy.
This eliminates the possibility of mistaking one client for another.
b Check the care plan for a description of the client's abilities or limitations.
Care must be taken in order to prevent injuring yourself or others.

2 Ask two co-workers to help you.
Three caregivers working together makes moving the client easier, reduces time, and decreases the risk for skin shearing.

3 Explain the procedure to the client.

4 Collect the following supplies:
- ☐ **Stretcher covered with a sheet**
- ☐ **Sheet**

Continued

Moving the Client From a Bed to a Stretcher—cont'd

- ☐ **Slider board**
- ☐ **Pillow(s), if needed**

By collecting all the necessary equipment beforehand, you will not have to leave your client's side and can eliminate wasting time and energy in obtaining the forgotten equipment.

5 Perform hand hygiene.

6 Provide for privacy.

PROCEDURE

7 Raise the bed to a height equal to the height of the stretcher.
This reduces the risk for back strain.

8 You and your co-workers should position yourselves properly. Two workers stand on the side of the bed where the stretcher will be. The third worker stands on the other side of the bed. You and your helpers should communicate directions throughout the procedure.

9 Cover the client with a sheet.
This keeps the client warm and covered for privacy.

10 Fan-fold top linens to the foot of the bed.
A fan-folded sheet is easier to grasp and to straighten out than a rolled-up sheet would be.

11 Lower the head of the bed so that it is as flat as possible.
This ensures client safety and comfort by keeping the two surfaces as level as possible.

12 Lower bed rails, if used.

13 Being careful to secure the client's safety, log-roll the client onto one side. Place the slider board underneath the client, from the head to the legs, between the bed and the bottom sheet. Do not place the slider board directly next to the client's skin.
Log-rolling ensures that the client has better body alignment while inserting the slider board.

14 Log-roll the client onto the back. Position the client in good body alignment. Place the pillow under the client's head, and ensure that the client is comfortable. The top sheet may remain on the client, if the client so desires.
Leave the client in proper body alignment and in a comfortable position to decrease discomfort and muscle fatigue.

15 Ask your co-workers to help move the client to the side of the bed by grasping the handles of the slider board.

16 Protect the client from falling, and have your co-workers position the stretcher next to the bed. They should stand behind the stretcher.
By keeping the bed and stretcher together, you reduce the risk of the client falling between the two mattresses.

17 Lock the bed and stretcher wheels.
Locking the wheels reduces the chance of the bed moving.

18 Roll up and grasp the slider board as shown in FIGURE 25–11. (*Note:* To prevent back injuries to themselves, staff may have to kneel on the bed.)
This supports the entire length of the client's body.

19 Transfer the client to the stretcher on the count of three by lifting and pulling the client. Make sure the client is centred on the stretcher.
The slider board is safer to use when the client is properly centred on it.

20 Place a pillow or pillows under the client's head and shoulders, if allowed.
Pillows help to decrease discomfort and muscle fatigue in the client.

21 Provide for safety and comfort.

22 Fasten the safety straps. Raise the stretcher side rails.
Safety straps help secure the client, and side rails will prevent the client from rolling off the bed.

23 Unlock the stretcher's wheels. Transport the client.

Continued

Moving the Client From a Bed to a Stretcher—cont'd

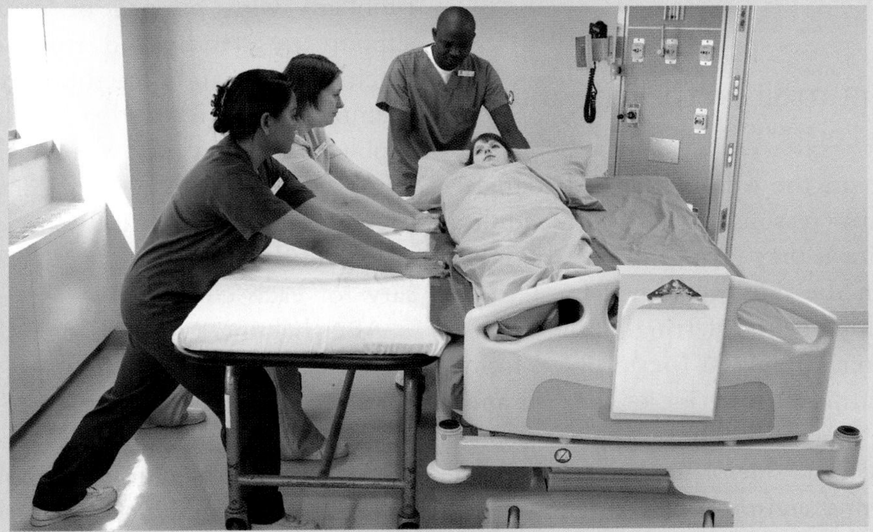

FIGURE 25–11 Moving the client to a stretcher. At this agency, a slider board is used to smoothly move the client from the bed to the stretcher. Regardless of what is used to assist the client to transfer, it is always important to make sure that the stretcher is against the bed with the brakes locked. (**Source:** Brian Hillier.)

POST-PROCEDURE

24 Perform hand hygiene.

25 Reverse the procedure to return the client to bed.

Report and Record your actions and observations, according to employer policy. Include the following:

☐ The time of the transport
☐ Where the person was transported
☐ Who went with the client
☐ How the transfer was tolerated

This is done for legal reasons and to keep the rest of the health care team informed.

Moving the Client to the Side of the Bed

Many care procedures—for example, a bed bath—require moving the client to the side of the bed. By moving the client to the side of the bed, you do not have to reach or stretch too much when doing the procedure. Also, you usually move clients to the side of the bed before repositioning or turning (log-rolling) them.

One method for moving a client involves moving the client in segments. You can usually do this method by yourself. However, as mentioned, some clients, such as older adults, people with arthritis, and people with spinal cord injuries, cannot be moved in segments. For these clients, using a turning pad helps prevent pain and skin damage, as well as injury to the bones, joints, and spinal cord. When using a turning pad to move a client to the side of the bed, it is best to have some help. Check with your supervisor for the correct procedure to use with each client.

Helping the Client to Sit on the Side of the Bed (Dangle the Legs)

Clients need to sit on the side of the bed (dangle their legs) for many reasons. Many older adults become dizzy or faint if they get out of bed too fast. They need to sit on the side of the bed for 1 to 5 minutes before walking or transferring. Some clients need to increase activity in stages. They progress from resting in bed to sitting on the side of the bed and then to sitting in a chair. Walking is the next step.

Some clients sit on the side of the bed when they need to perform their exercises. While dangling their legs, they cough and deep breathe. They also move their legs back and forth and in circles to stimulate circulation. The procedure is also part of preparing clients to walk or transferring them to a chair or wheelchair.

You might need a helper when assisting a client to sit on the side of the bed. If the client has problems with balance or coordination, provide support by standing in front of the client and placing your hands on the client's shoulders. For example, people recovering from a stroke often have problems with balance when sitting up. They must always be supported when dangling their legs to prevent falls and injuries. Check with your supervisor and the care plan for safety precautions necessary for each client.

After helping a client dangle the legs, report and record the following:

- Pulse and respirations (if instructed to measure)
- Pale, greyish, or bluish skin colour (cyanosis)
- Complaints of dizziness, light-headedness, or difficulty breathing
- How well the activity was tolerated
- The length of time the client dangled the legs
- The amount of help needed
- Other observations or complaints

Moving the Client to the Side of the Bed

123

Advocate on behalf of the client's quality of life by promoting:

Dignity • **I**ndependence • **P**references • **P**rivacy • **S**afety

(see BOX 1–4, on p. 17)

PRE-PROCEDURE

1 a Identify the client according to employer policy.
This eliminates the possibility of mistaking one client for another.
b Check the care plan for a description of the client's abilities or limitations.
Care must be taken in order to prevent injuring yourself or others.

2 Ask someone to help you if you need assistance.
Two caregivers working together makes moving the client easier, reduces time, and decreases the risk for skin shearing.

3 Perform hand hygiene.

4 Explain the procedure to the client.

5 Provide for privacy.

6 Raise the bed to a comfortable working height. Make sure the bed wheels are locked. Follow the care plan for bed rail use. Lower the head of the bed to a level appropriate for the client. It should be as flat as possible. You and your helper should communicate directions throughout the procedure.
These steps help ensure safety. By working as a team, you reduce the risk for client or worker injury.

Continued

PROCEDURE

7 Stand on the side of the bed to which you will move the client.
It is easier to move a client toward you rather than away from you.

8 Lower the bed rail near you if it is up.
It is awkward to work over a raised bed rail.

9 Stand with your feet about 30 cm (12 in.) apart and one foot in front of the other. Flex your knees.
This provides a good base of support.

10 Cross the client's arms over the chest.
This prevents the risk of injuring the client during the procedure.

11 ***Method 1: Moving the client without a helper (in segments)***

a Place your arm under the client's neck and shoulders.

b Place your other arm under the middle of the client's back.

c Rock backward and shift your weight to your rear leg.
Rocking slightly reduces the amount of energy that you would need to perform the procedure.
This moves the upper part of the client's body toward the edge of the bed (**FIGURE 25–12, *A***).

d Place one arm under the client's waist and one under the thighs.

e Rock backward, moving the middle part of the client to the edge of the bed (**FIGURE 25–12, *B***).

f Place one arm under the client's thighs and one under the calves.

g Rock backward, moving the client's legs to the edge of the bed (**FIGURE 25–12, *C***).

h Repeat steps *a* through *g*, as necessary.

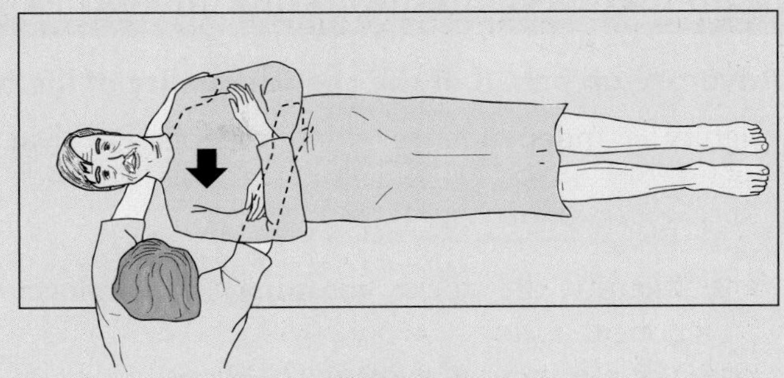

FIGURE 25–12 A

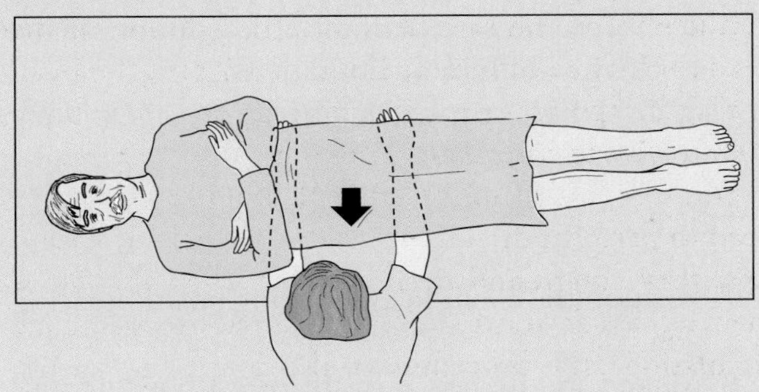

FIGURE 25–12 B

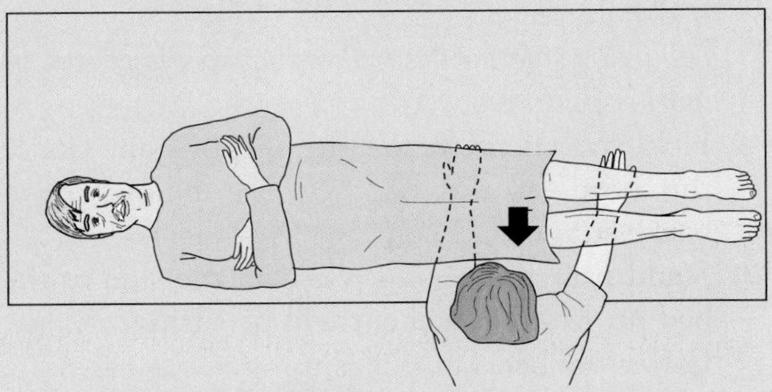

FIGURE 25–12 C

12 ***Method 2: Moving the client with a turning pad***

a Roll the turning pad up close to the client. Your helper does the same.

b Grasp the rolled-up turning pad near the client's shoulders and buttocks. Your helper does the same. Make sure you support the client's head.

c Rock backward on the count of three, moving the client toward you. Your helper rocks backward slightly and then forward toward you while keeping the arms straight. Repeat, if necessary.

d Unroll the turning pad.

13 Reposition the pillow under the client's head and shoulders.

POST-PROCEDURE

14 Follow steps 14 through 18 in the procedure *Log-Rolling the Client* on page 502.

Report and Record your actions and observations, according to employer policy.
This is done for legal reasons and to keep the rest of the health care team informed.

Helping the Client Sit on the Side of the Bed (Dangle the Legs) 123

Advocate on behalf of the client's quality of life by promoting:

Dignity • Independence • Preferences • Privacy • Safety *(see BOX 1–4, on p. 17)*

PRE-PROCEDURE

1 a Identify the client according to employer policy.
This eliminates the possibility of mistaking one client for another.

b Check the care plan for a description of the client's abilities or limitations.
Care must be taken in order to prevent injuring yourself or others.

2 Explain the procedure to the client.

3 Perform hand hygiene.

4 Decide which side of the bed to use.
It is important to plan thoroughly before starting any procedure.

5 Move furniture away from the work area.
This provides space to move.

6 Provide for privacy.

PROCEDURE

7 Position the client in a side-lying position facing you.

8 Make sure the bed is in its lowest position and bed wheels are locked. Follow the care plan for bed rail use.*
Following safety rules will reduce risk for client or worker injuries.

9 Help the client to the sitting position. (Raise the head of the bed, or use pillows or a backrest.)

10 Stand near the client's waist on the side of the bed on which the client will be sitting.

11 Lower the bed rail if it is up.

12 Turn so that you face the client. Stand with a broad base of support.
A broad base of support will prevent you from losing your balance while performing this procedure.

13 Slide one arm under the client's neck and shoulders. Grasp the far shoulder. Place your other arm over the client's thighs near the knees. Grasp under the thighs (**FIGURE 25–13,** ***A***).

14 Pivot back toward the head of the bed while pulling the client's feet, and lower the client's legs over the edge of the bed.
This keeps the client's body in the best alignment possible.

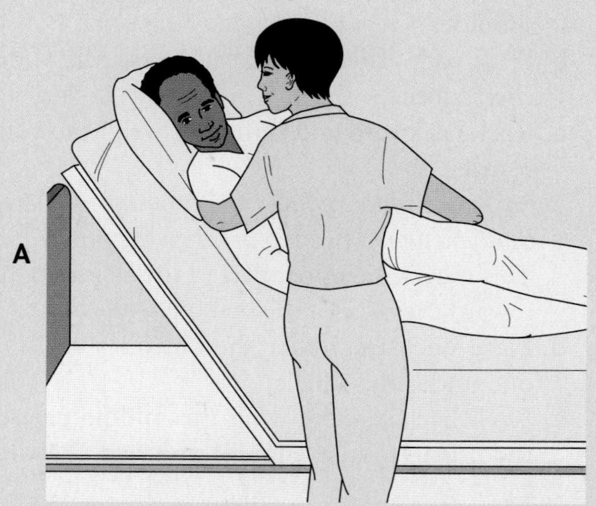

FIGURE 25–13 A Assist the client to a sitting position by placing one arm under the client's shoulders and the other behind the client's knees.

15 Help the client sit upright. Do not pull the client too close to the edge of the bed. Only the client's knees should be at the edge, not the thighs or buttocks (**FIGURE 25–13,** ***B***).
If the client is too close to the edge of the bed , falling or injury can result.

16 Ask the client to hold on to the edge of the mattress. Allow the client to have the feet touch the floor.
This supports the client in the sitting position.

Continued

Helping the Client Sit on the Side of the Bed (Dangle the Legs)—cont'd

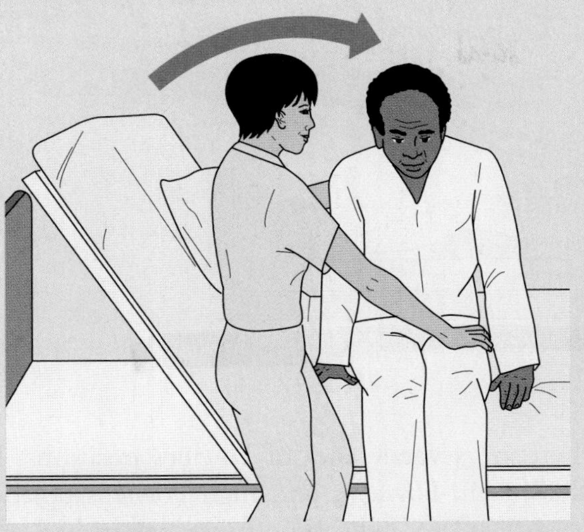

FIGURE 25–13 B Assist the client to a sitting position by bringing the client's legs and feet over the edge of the bed. Do this in one step, and hold on to the client for safety.

17 Do not leave the client alone. Remain in front of the client. Place both hands on the client's shoulders to provide support if necessary.
This prevents the client from falling back onto the bed.

18 Check the client's condition:
- **a** Ask how the client feels. Also, ask if the client feels dizzy or light-headed.
- **b** Check pulse and respirations.
- **c** Check for difficulty breathing, pale skin, or *cyanosis* (greyish or bluish skin colour).
- **d** Ensure the client is well enough to sit unassisted before you leave the client's side.

19 If the client feels dizzy or weak, help the client lie back down.
Assisting the client reduces the risk for injury.

20 Reverse the procedure to return the client to bed.

POST-PROCEDURE

21 Provide for safety and comfort. Help the client move to the centre of the bed. Position the client in good body alignment, according to the care plan.

22 Place the call bell within reach.*
This provides an easy, safe way for the client to contact staff, if necessary.

23 Follow the care plan for bed rail use.*

24 Return furniture to its proper location.
This reduces risk of losing equipment and makes it easier to find the next time it is required.

25 Remove privacy measures.

26 Perform hand hygiene.

Report and Record your actions and observations, according to employer policy.
This is done for legal reasons and to keep the rest of the health care team informed.

*Steps marked with an asterisk may not apply in community settings.

POSITIONING THE CLIENT

The client must be properly positioned at all times. Regular position changes and good body alignment promote comfort and well-being, make breathing easier, and promote circulation. Proper positioning also helps prevent many complications such as pressure ulcers (see Chapter 24) and contractures (see Chapter 26).

Most clients can move and reposition themselves. Some need reminding to adjust their position, while others need help or depend entirely on the health care team for position changes.

Comfort and Safety Measures

Whether in a bed or a chair, clients are repositioned at least every 2 hours, and some more often. Follow your supervisor's instructions and the care plan.

The physician may order certain positions or position limits. Every time you position a client, check

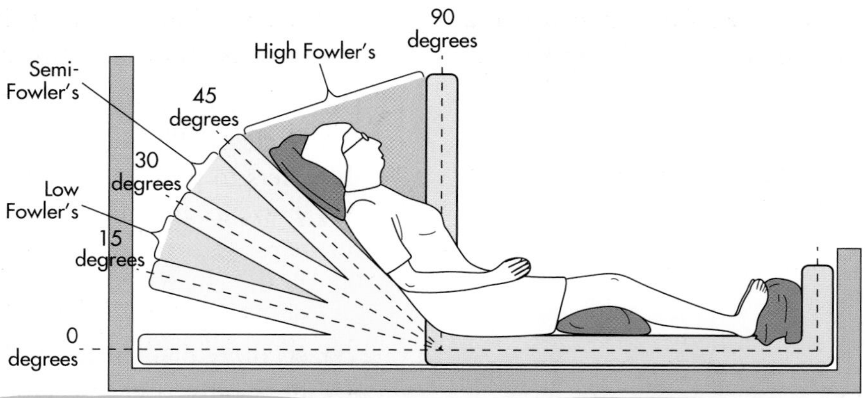

FIGURE 25–14 Head of bed positioning for low-Fowlers, semi-Fowler's, and high Fowler's positions.

the skin for signs of redness, paleness, or discoloration. Report any of these observations immediately.

To safely position a client, follow these guidelines:

- Check with your supervisor and the care plan for the best positions for each client.
- Follow the scheduled times for repositioning the client.
- Use good body mechanics.
- If necessary, ask for help *before* beginning.
- Explain the procedure to the client.
- Be gentle when moving the client.
- Provide for privacy.
- Leave the client in good body alignment; use pillows as directed in the care plan for comfort and support.
- Make sure linens are wrinkle-free; change or straighten them, as needed.
- Place the call bell (in facilities) within the client's reach.

Fowler's Positions

Fowler's position is a semi-sitting to upright sitting position in bed. It is used to relax tense abdominal muscles, allowing for improved breathing in clients. It is also used for women in the postpartum period after delivery to improve uterine drainage. Most clients find that it is more comfortable to have their legs slightly bent and their arms supported on pillows while in this position. Supporting the client's arms on pillows may also prevent the client from slipping to one side of the bed.

There are several types of Fowler's positions: low Fowler's, semi-Fowler's, and high Fowler's positions (**FIGURE 25–14**). Clients who must stay in bed often use one of these positions when eating, having visitors, taking medications, reading, and watching TV.

To place a client in the **low Fowler's position**, raise the head of the bed to an angle of 15 to 30 degrees. The client's head and shoulders can alternatively be raised with extra pillows.

For the **semi-Fowler's position**, raise the head of the bed to an angle of 30 to 45 degrees and reposition the client's shoulders and head on the pillow. The foot of the bed may be raised at the knee so that the client does not slide down in the bed. However, raising the knee portion can interfere with leg circulation, so some care plans suggest placing a small pillow under the client's knees instead of raising the knee portion of the bed.

To place a client in the **high Fowler's position**, raise the head of the bed 45 to 90 degrees and reposition the client's shoulders and head on the pillow. (Clients are usually not positioned above a 60-degree sitting position, as they are too uncomfortable at that angle.) This position is the best position for clients who must use a bedpan in bed. Some clients who must eat or drink while in bed may need to be placed in an almost 90-degree sitting position, especially if they have difficulty swallowing. The support worker should consult the client's care plan or supervisor's directions on proper positioning during meals.

People with heart and respiratory disorders also usually breathe better in the high Fowler's position. However, many clients find it difficult to sit in a 90-degree sitting position. ***Frail clients should never***

be left unattended while sitting upright in a 90-degree position because they could tip forward, fall to one side of the bed, or even fall out of bed.

The following are important points about positioning a client in Fowler's positions:

- Follow the client's care plan for positioning the client.
- If the client is in a hospital bed and the care plan allows it, raise the client's knees slightly using the knee gatch control on the bed.
- If the client's bed is not adjustable or the client's care plan specifies it, place a small pillow under the client's lower calves to keep the knees flexed. Raising the client's knees slightly can reduce back strain, prevent the client from sliding down toward the foot of the bed, and minimize shearing on the client's coccyx area.
- You can use a backrest, a foam wedge pillow, or sofa pillows to support the client in this position. If using pillows for support, make sure the headboard is sturdy or the head of the bed is against the wall (see Chapter 34).
- Make sure the client is positioned in good alignment. The spine should be straight and the hips should be directly against the bend in the bed or the pillows.
- Place a small pillow behind the head and neck.
- Place small pillows under the arms and hands.
- Place small pillows under the lower back, thighs, and ankles if your supervisor tells you to do so.
- Use the angle indicator built into the supporting frame of most hospital beds to measure the angle of the head of the bed, instead of using personal judgement only.

Supine Position

The **supine position** is the back-lying position (**FIGURE 25–15**) that is used for sleeping and resting.

To place a client in the supine position, do the following:

1. Make sure the bed is flat. Lower the head of the bed if necessary.
2. Place a small pillow under the head and shoulders.
3. Place the person's arms along the person's sides, palms facing down.
4. Place a small pillow under the arms and hands.
5. Place a small pillow under the client's knees to keep them flexed. This can reduce back strain.
6. Place small pillows or rolled towels under the lower back, thighs, and ankles if your supervisor tells you to do so.

Lateral Position

The **lateral position** is the side-lying position (**FIGURE 25–16**). Most clients can lie on one side or the other. Check the client's care plan for any positioning restrictions, such as a pressure sore on the hip area. Check often to make sure that the client is not

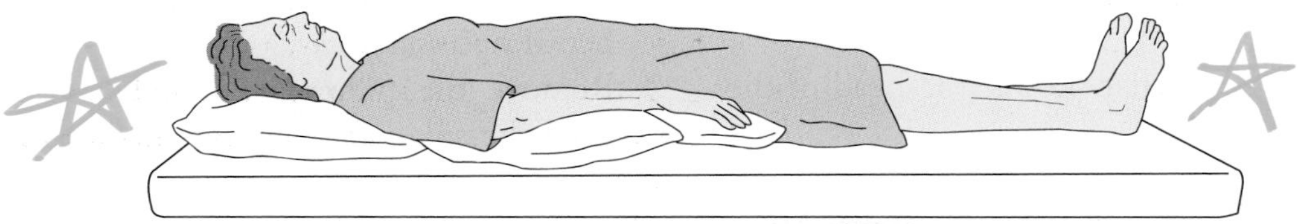

FIGURE 25–15 Supine position.

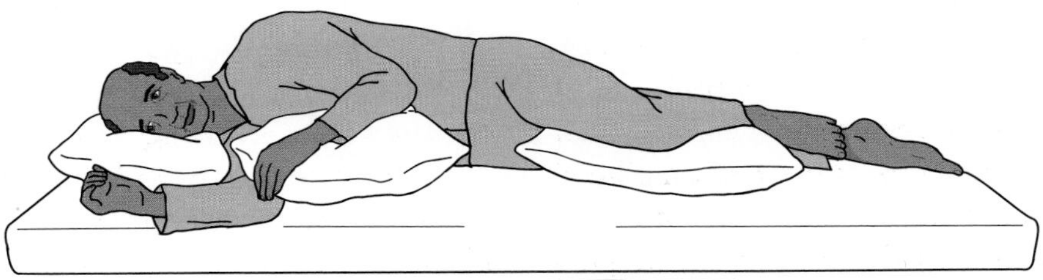

FIGURE 25–16 Lateral position.

experiencing pain, numbness, or discomfort in this position.

To place a client in the lateral position, do the following:

1. Make sure the bed is flat. Lower the head of the bed if necessary.
2. Position the client onto the side (see the procedure *Log-Rolling the Client*, on pp. 501–502).
3. Bend the upper leg at the knee. Position the upper leg in front of the lower leg.
4. Place a small pillow under the head and neck.
5. Place small pillows under the upper leg and thigh.
6. Place small pillows under the upper hand and arm.
7. Position a small pillow against the client's back.

Sims' Position

Sims' position is the left-side-lying position in which the right leg is sharply flexed so that it is not resting on the left leg. The left arm is positioned along the client's back. This position, in which the client is lying partly on the abdomen (**FIGURE 25–17**), is used for administering enemas and other procedures. It can also be used for resting if the client is comfortable in this position. It is, however, usually *not comfortable* for older adults, so if you must put them in this position, position them well with plenty of pillows. Check with your supervisor before positioning an older adult in Sims' position. Check the client frequently for comfort and circulation in the lower arm and hand.

To place a client in Sims' position, do the following:

1. Make sure the bed is flat. Lower the head of the bed if necessary.
2. Position the client onto the left side (see the procedure *Log-Rolling the Client*, on pp. 501–502).
3. Bend the upper (right) leg, and position it such that it does not lie on the lower (left) leg.
4. Bend the upper (right) arm, and position the hand, palm down, near the head.
5. Place the lower (left) arm behind the client, palm facing up. If the client cannot tolerate this position, move this arm to a more comfortable position.
6. Place a small pillow under the head and neck. Ensure that the pillow is not covering the client's face and that the client can breathe freely.
7. Place small pillows under the upper arm and hand and under the upper leg.

Prone Position

The **prone position** is the front-lying position on the abdomen, with the head turned to one side (**FIGURE 25–18**). Most clients, especially clients with limited range of motion in their necks, cannot tolerate the prone position. It is usually used, if at all, for only a short period at a time. The prone position is used mainly to prevent shortening (contractures) of the thigh muscle in clients who have had leg amputations and sit in a wheelchair for long periods. The prone position will help keep the thigh muscles in the amputated leg stretched. Use the prone position only if it is called for in the care plan.

To place a client in the prone position, do the following:

1. Make sure the bed is flat. Lower the head of the bed if necessary.
2. Remove the pillows. Carefully turn the client onto the side and then onto the abdomen.

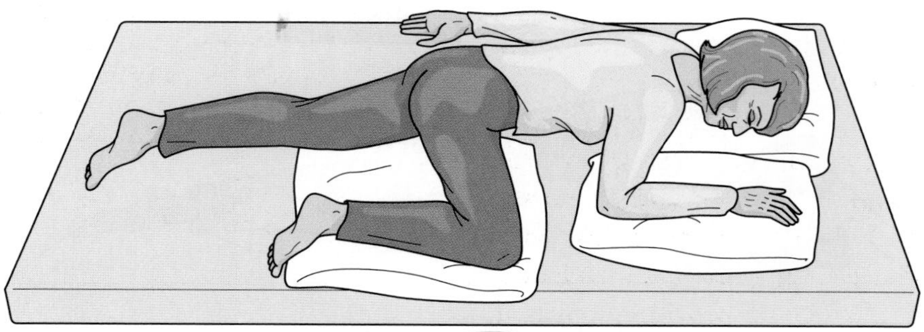

FIGURE 25–17 Sims' position.

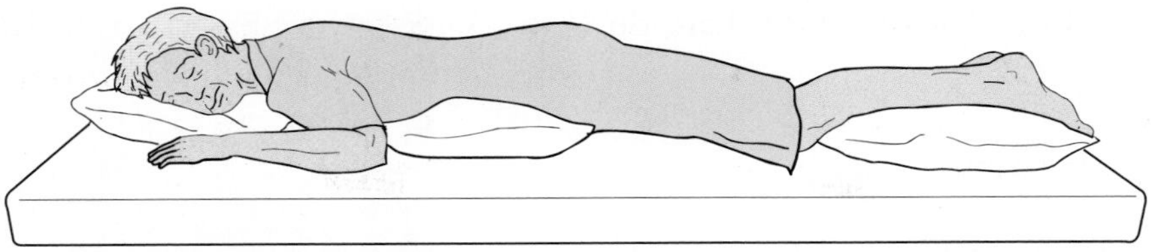

FIGURE 25–18 Prone position. If the client is tall, you may choose to dangle the feet over the end of the mattress.

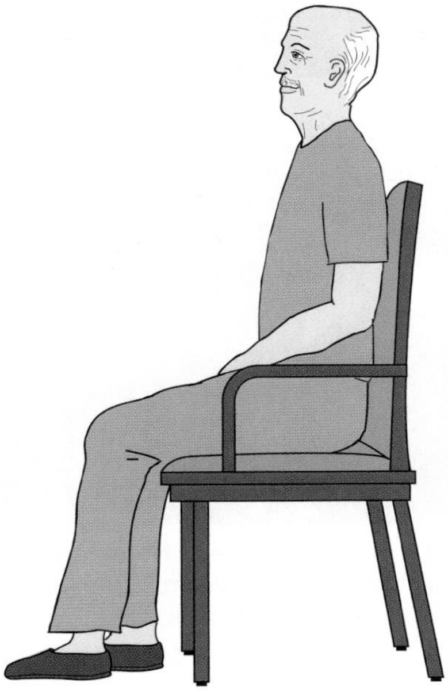

FIGURE 25–19 Client positioned in a chair. The client's feet are flat on the floor; the calves do not touch the chair; and the back is straight and against the back of the chair.

3. Turn the client's head to one side.
4. Bend the arms at the elbows, and place the hands near the head.
5. Place small pillows under the client's head, abdomen, and lower legs (see **FIGURE 25–18**). If the client is positioned with the feet hanging over the end of the mattress, do not place a pillow under the lower legs.

Sitting Position

Clients in chairs or wheelchairs must hold the upper body and head erect to avoid poor alignment (**FIGURE 25–19**). Clients who cannot keep the upper body erect require postural supports (**FIGURE 25–20**), which help maintain good alignment. The health care team selects the best product for the client's needs, with consideration for the client's dignity, independence, preferences, and safety. Assist with providing postural supports, as needed.

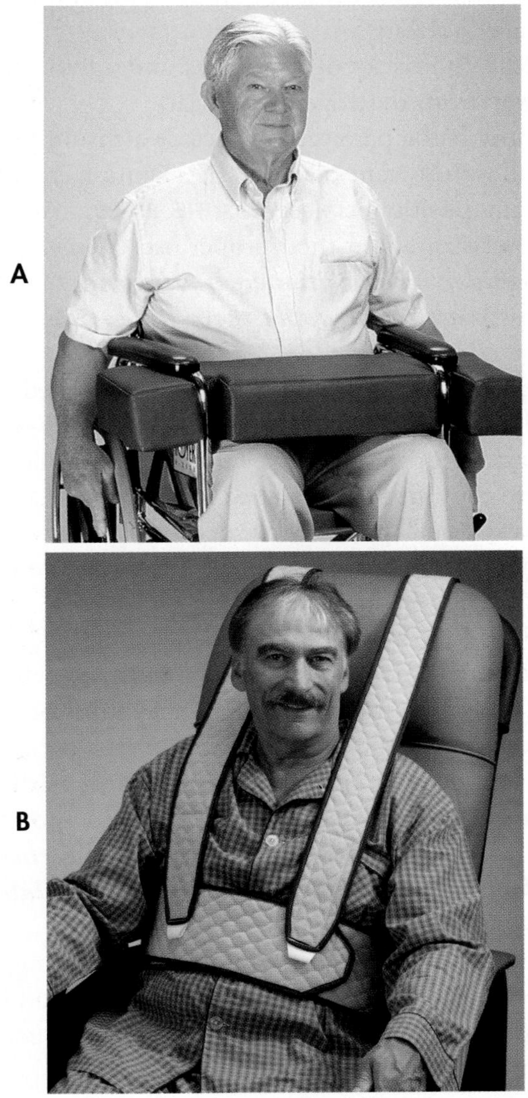

FIGURE 25–20 Postural supports. **A,** Pelvic holder. **B,** Torso support. These supports must be ordered by the client's doctor. It is your responsibility to check the client's skin under the supports every hour to watch for friction and irritation. (Images provided courtesy Posey Company, Arcadia, CA.)

To position a client in a chair or wheelchair, do the following:

1. Position the client's back and buttocks against the back of the chair.
2. Make sure the back is straight. The client should not be leaning to the side.
3. Place the client's feet flat on the floor or on wheelchair footrests.
4. Place the backs of the knees and calves slightly away from the edge of the seat.
5. Support the paralyzed (affected) arms on pillows. Follow the care plan. Some clients have special foam positioners (see **FIGURE 25–20**). Ask your supervisor about their proper use. ***Some agencies consider such positioners a restraint. Therefore, you must never apply them unless they are in the client's care plan.***
6. Position the client's wrists at a slightly flexed angle. Elevated wheelchair armrests (**FIGURE 25–21**) are suitable for some clients who have the tendency to lean toward their paralyzed (affected) side.
7. Place a small pillow between the client's lower back and the chair if your supervisor tells you to do so.

Repositioning the Client in a Chair or Wheelchair

Clients can sometimes slide down in their chairs. For good body alignment and safety, they must be repositioned so that their backs and buttocks are against the backs of their chairs. Although transfer belts are recommended to facilitate repositioning the client, some agencies do not carry them. ***Always check to see if this type of safety equipment is available at your agency.***

Some clients can help with repositioning, but some others cannot. Use the following method if the client is alert, is cooperative, can follow instructions, and has the strength to help:

1. Lock the wheelchair wheels.
2. Stand in front of the client. Block the client's knees and feet with your knees and feet.
3. Place your knees in front of the client's knees.
4. Apply a transfer belt (see pp. 516–517), if they are used in your agency.
5. Position the client's feet flat on the floor. If wheelchair foot pedals are in place, swing them out of the way.

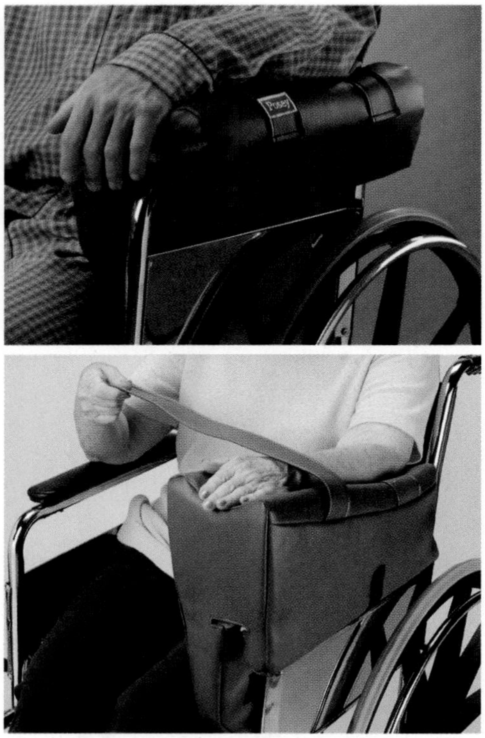

FIGURE 25–21 Elevated armrest. Note how the client's arm would be positioned with the Velcro strap. (Images provided courtesy Posey Company, Arcadia, CA.)

6. Position the client's arms on the armrests.
7. Grasp the transfer belt on each side behind the client's armpits while the client leans forward. Or if a transfer belt is not available, put your arms under the client's arms and place your hands around the client's shoulder blades.
8. Ask the client to push with the feet and arms on the count of three.
9. Lift the client back into the chair on the count of three. ***Ensure that your back maintains its natural curve; otherwise, this activity can cause back injury.***
10. As the client pushes with the feet and arms (**FIGURE 25–22**), push the client's knees with your knees. The client will naturally be repositioned back into the wheelchair.

TRANSFERRING THE CLIENT

The term **transfer** means helping a client move from one place to another. See the box *Think About Safety: The Difference Between a Lift and a Transfer* for the difference between a lift and a transfer. For a transfer, the client must be able to **weight-bear** (have the

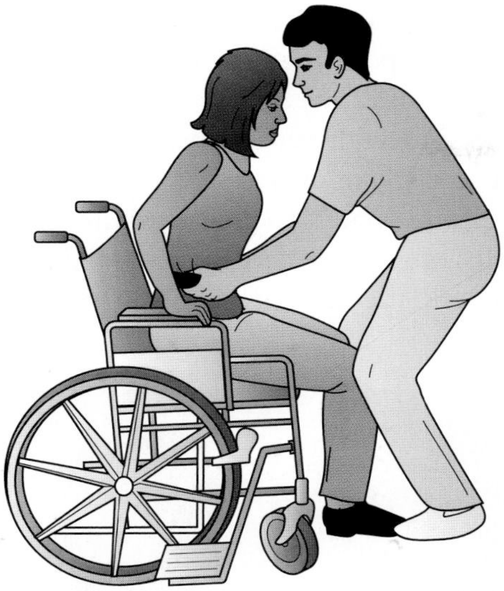

FIGURE 25–22 Repositioning the client in a wheelchair. Use a transfer belt to lift the client to the back of the chair.

ability to shift body weight) to any degree. Clients are often moved from their beds to chairs, wheelchairs, commodes, toilets, or stretchers. Some clients need only minimal help with transferring, but others need two (or occasionally three) people to help them. Your supervisor and the care plan will tell you how much help a client needs. Place the chair or wheelchair with its back aligned with the head of the bed. Lock the bed and wheelchair wheels, and raise the footrests.

Know the Client

Never attempt a transfer without assistance if the client cannot help. Always make sure that you have enough room for a safe transfer. Clear the area of potential hazards. You may have to move furniture to make room for a chair, wheelchair, or stretcher. Before transferring a client, check the care plan or ask your supervisor if the client has a weaker side (or *affected side*), which is the side affected by disease or disability. The strong side (or *unaffected side*) is the side not affected by disease or disability, and it pulls the weak side along.

Transfers from the weak side are awkward and unsafe and may also frighten the client. The client may have limited vision on the affected side, and the weak arm and leg may not be able to bear any of the client's weight. For example, if a client's left side is weak from a stroke, the right side is the stronger side; plan to move the client so that the right side moves first.

Think About Safety

The Difference Between a Lift and a Transfer

It is important that you know the difference between a *transfer* and a *lift*. A transfer is the method used to move a client who is able to weight-bear to any degree. If the client cannot assist you by weight-bearing, or if the client is too unsteady to safely transfer, a lift is used. In most settings, clients who require lifting must be lifted with the use of a mechanical lift, especially if they are large, heavy, or restless. Because of the serious risk for back injury to workers, most (if not all) long-term care agencies have a strict no-lift policy, preventing staff from manually lifting clients. ***In addition, most agencies have a two-person lift policy, meaning that there must be two people present who are trained to use mechanical lifts whenever a mechanical lift is used.*** It is your responsibility to know if your agency has a no-lift policy and what it entails *before* providing care to your clients.

Follow Principles of Safety and Good Body Mechanics

The number of people needed for a transfer depends on the client's physical capabilities, condition, and size. You should always check the care plan to see what equipment and how many people are required to transfer that client. Many long-term care facilities require the use of transfer belts when residents are transferred to or from chairs or wheelchairs.

The rules of good body mechanics apply to transfers also. They will help you reduce the risk for injury to yourself and to the client. Follow the same comfort and safety measures listed for lifting and moving clients.

After transferring a client, report and record the following:

- Pulse rate (if it is to be measured, as directed) before and after the transfer
- Complaints of light-headedness, pain, discomfort, difficulty breathing, weakness, or fatigue
- The amount of help needed to transfer the client
- How the client helped with the transfer

Applying Transfer Belts

A **transfer belt** (**FIGURE 25–23, *A***) is used in some agencies to transfer unsteady clients and those with disabilities. It helps prevent falls and other injuries. In many agencies, the belt goes around the client's waist, although some agencies require you to place the transfer belt around the client's hips. You should be aware of your agency's policies for placement before using a transfer belt. Grasp the belt, with your folded fingers pointing up, to support the client during the transfer.

A wider belt with vertical handles (**FIGURE 25–23, *B***), called a *walking* or *gait belt*, is used for walking with a client. Many facilities require staff to use these belts when transferring or walking a client. Always check the client's care plan before using a transfer belt.

A 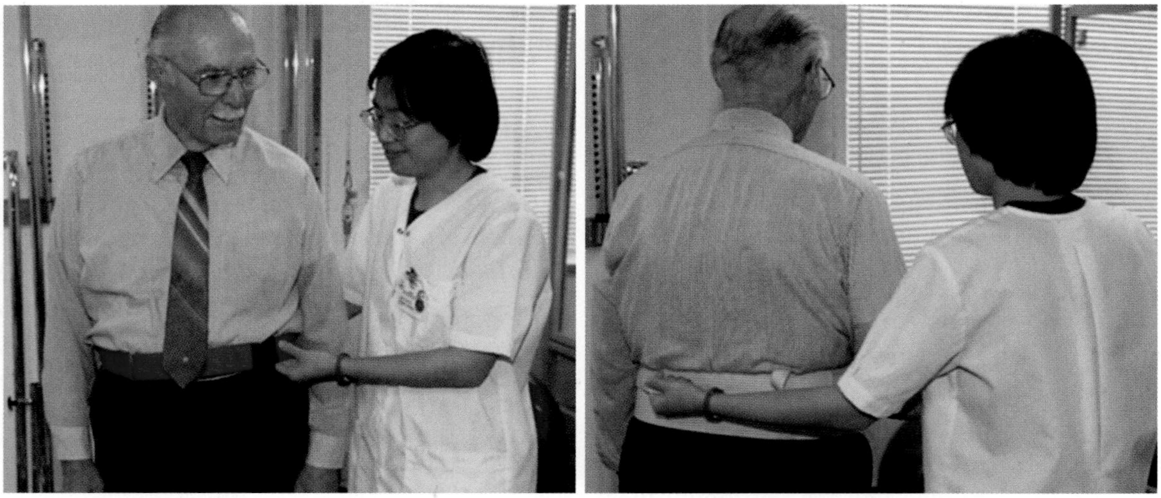 B

FIGURE 25–23 Note the different types of transfer belts. **A,** Position the belt buckle off centre in the front. Grasp under the belt, with your fingers pointing up. **B,** Walking or gait belt. The belt buckle has padding under it and remains in front of the client. This wider belt has vertical and horizontal handles for the support worker to hold on to while assisting the client to walk.

Applying a Transfer Belt

123

Advocate on behalf of the client's quality of life by promoting:

Dignity • Independence • Preferences • Privacy • Safety *(see BOX 1–4, on p. 17)*

PROCEDURE

1 a Identify the client according to employer policy.
This eliminates the possibility of mistaking one client for another.
b Check the care plan for a description of the client's abilities or limitations.
Care must be taken in order to prevent injuring yourself or others.
2 Explain the procedure to the client.
3 Perform hand hygiene.
4 Provide for privacy.
5 Assist the client to the sitting position.
6 Apply the belt around the client's waist over clothing. Do not apply it over bare skin. (*Note:* Some agencies require you to place the transfer belt around the client's hips.)
Having equipment next to a client's skin may tear the skin and increases the risk for pathogen transfer from one person to another.
7 Tighten the belt so that it is snug. It should not cause discomfort or impair breathing. You should be able to slide your fingers under the belt.
A snug-fitting belt reduces the risk of its slipping off while it is being used.

Continued

Applying a Transfer Belt—cont'd

8 Make sure that a woman's breasts are not caught under the belt.
This promotes comfort and safety.
9 Place the buckle off centre in the front or in the back for the client's comfort (see **FIGURE 25–23**, *A*). The buckle should not be over the spine.
10 Grasp the transfer belt from underneath when using it to transfer a client.
11 Return the transfer belt to its correct storage place.
12 Practice hand hygiene.

FOCUS ON LONG-TERM CARE

Transferring and Lifting Safety Precautions

In long-term care facilities, it is important to identify the amount of assistance each resident requires to move each individual safely, as well as what equipment is required.

Most agencies have a system that classifies the type of assistance each resident requires and will post this information somewhere, usually on the client's care plan, along with details necessary to ensure the safety of that client. Regardless of where it is posted, it should respect the client's right to confidentiality and privacy. Examples of transferring and lifting safety-precaution levels that you may find in long-term care include the following:

- Independent with no assistance (or "No assistance")
- Standby (or "Observe and supervise")
- Transfer board required (e.g., some clients with paraplegia may have enough upper body strength to transfer themselves using a transfer board)
- One-person transfer
- Two-person transfer
- One-person lift*
- Two or more people to lift*
- Mechanical lift (see **FIGURE 25–30**, pp. 526–527) (or "MediLift/Argo**/Ground-based lift")
- Ceiling lift (**FIGURE 25–24**)
- Standing lift (or "Sit-to-stand") (see **FIGURE 25–31**, p. 528)

*Not used in agencies that have a no-lift policy.
**This is an example of a specific name brand. Your agency may use another name.

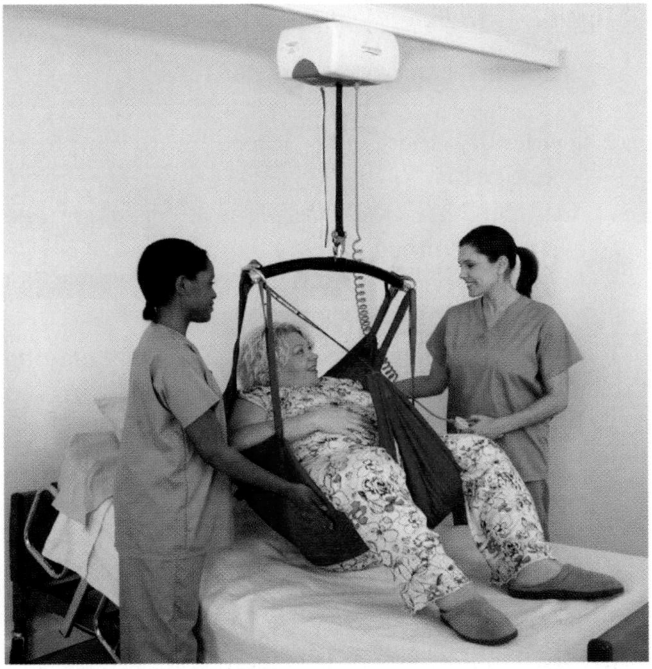

FIGURE 25–24 Ceiling lift. This type of ceiling lift is very useful in a home or residential setting. Note the handheld controls, which operate the client's movements up, down, or sideways along a ceiling track. (**Source:** Courtesy of Prism Medical)

Transferring a Client From the Bed to a Chair or Wheelchair

It is important to ensure safety during chair and wheelchair transfers. You must prevent falls in clients and protect your back from injury. Always hold the client securely during the procedure. Make sure the client wears nonskid footwear to prevent sliding or slipping. The chair or wheelchair must be able to support the client's weight. See the *Focus on Long-Term Care: Transferring and Lifting Safety Precautions* box.

Some agencies use **transfer boards** to assist certain clients to slide from their bed or chair to a wheelchair. Transfer boards are mostly used when the client is able to assist the staff. The client must have adequate padding on the buttocks, and the staff must ensure that shearing does not occur while sliding the client. Most bedside chairs and wheelchairs have vinyl seats and backs, and because vinyl holds in body heat and can stick to the client, you should cover the back and seat with a folded blanket to promote comfort. Place small pillows or cushions behind the client's back, as instructed by your supervisor. As a support worker, you must take necessary steps to promote comfort, prevent pressure ulcers, and maintain proper posture in the client.

Transferring the Client to a Chair or Wheelchair 123

Advocate on behalf of the client's quality of life by promoting:

Dignity • Independence • Preferences • Privacy • Safety *(see BOX 1–4, on p. 17)*

PRE-PROCEDURE

1 a Identify the client according to employer policy.
This eliminates the possibility of mistaking one client for another.
b Check the care plan for a description of the client's abilities or limitations.
Care must be taken in order to prevent injuring yourself or others.
2 Explain the procedure to the client.
3 Ensure the client is fully dressed or robed and is wearing nonskid footwear.
4 Familiarize yourself with the client's care plan.
The client's care plan will contain details pertinent to the client, necessary for safely transferring the client.
5 Collect the following supplies:
☐ **Wheelchair or armchair**
☐ **One or two sheets**
☐ **Transfer belt, if required by your agency**
☐ **Transfer board (if your agency uses them)**
☐ **Seat cushion, if used by the client**
By collecting all the necessary equipment beforehand, you will not have to leave your client's side and can eliminate wasting time and energy in obtaining the forgotten equipment.
6 Perform hand hygiene.
7 Provide for privacy.
8 a Decide which side of the bed to use. Move furniture away to provide space to move.
It is important for the client's safety to try to plan thoroughly before starting any procedure.
b You and your helper must communicate directions throughout the procedure.
By working as a team, you will reduce the risk for client or worker injury.

PROCEDURE

9 Place the back of the chair so that it is aligned with the headboard.
This reduces the distance the client has to move.
10 Place the client's gel-seat pad or cushion on the seat, if stated in the care plan.
This pads the seat and reduces pressure on the buttocks' bony prominences, reducing the risk for pressure ulcers. Padding the seat of a wheelchair also makes sitting in a wheelchair for an extended length of time more comfortable for the client.
11 Lock the wheelchair wheels. Raise the footrests, or swing them out of the way.
12 Lower the bed to its lowest position or as specified in the client's care plan. Lock the bed wheels. Lower the bed rail near you if it is up.
This ensures safety by reducing the risk of falling.
13 Fan-fold top linens to the foot of the bed.
A fan-folded sheet is easier to grasp and to straighten out than a rolled-up sheet would be.

Continued

Transferring the Client to a Chair or Wheelchair—cont'd

14 Help the client dangle the legs (see the procedure *Helping the Client Sit on the Side of the Bed* on pp. 508–509). Make sure the client's feet touch the floor.

Touching the floor with the feet is very reassuring to the client. The client will be less likely to be tense and will be more willing to proceed with this procedure.

15 Apply the transfer belt if it will be used.

16 ***Method 1: Using a transfer belt***

a A transfer belt is used to help stabilize the client while eliminating the need to grasp the client's clothing or easily damaged skin.

b Stand in front of the client. Stand with your feet apart. Flex your hips and knees. Align your knees with the client's knees.

c Have the client hold on to the mattress or place the fists on the bed by the thighs.

d Make sure the client's feet are flat on the floor.

e Have the client lean forward.

f Grasp the transfer belt at each side.

g Brace your knees against the client's knees. Block the client's feet with your feet (**FIGURE 25–25, A**).

h Tell the client to push down on the mattress and to stand on the count of three. Pull the client into a standing position as you straighten your hips and legs. Keep your knees slightly flexed (see **FIGURE 25–25, B**).

17 ***Method 2: Without using a transfer belt***

a Follow steps 16 a–c.

b Place your hands under the client's arms and around the client's shoulder blades.

c Have the client lean forward.

d Brace your knees against the client's knees. Block the client's feet with your feet.

This helps to stabilize the client and reduces the chance of the client slipping.

e Tell the client to push down on the mattress and to stand on the count of three. Pull the client up into a standing position as you straighten your hips and legs. Keep your knees slightly flexed.

This uses proper body mechanics when assisting the client, reducing the risk of either the client or worker losing balance.

18 Support the client in the standing position. Hold the transfer belt, or keep your hands around the person's shoulder blades. Continue

A

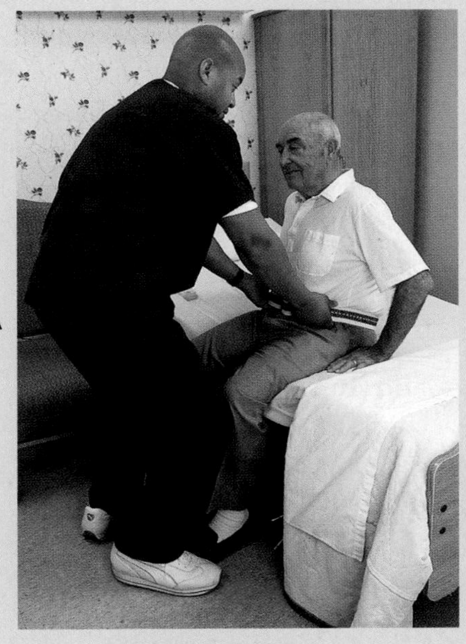

FIGURE 25–25 A

B

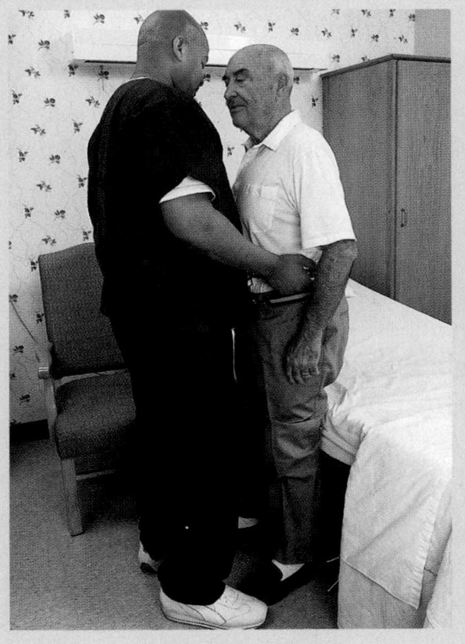

FIGURE 25–25 B

Continued

Transferring the Client to a Chair or Wheelchair—cont'd

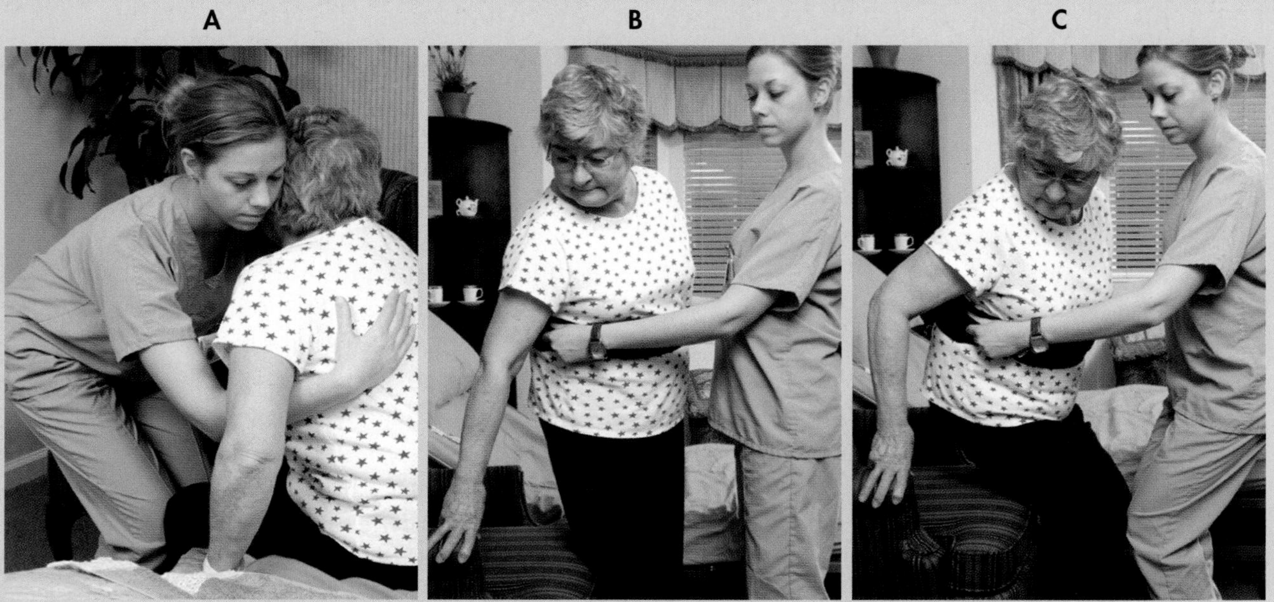

FIGURE 25–26 When the client is getting ready to sit, provide support as the client grasps the far arm of the chair. The client's legs are against the chair. Lower the client into the chair while the client holds on to the armrests, leans forward, and bends the elbows and knees.

to block the client's feet and knees with your feet and knees.

19 Pivot on your foot and turn the client so that the client can grasp the far arm of the chair. The client's legs will touch the edge of the chair.

20 Continue to turn the client until the client grasps the other armrest.

21 Lower the client into the chair as you bend your hips and knees. Keep your back straight, with your lumbar area curved. The client assists by leaning forward and bending the elbows and knees (see **FIGURE 25–26**).

22 Make sure the client's buttocks are to the back of the seat. Position the client in good alignment.

23 Position the client's feet on the wheelchair footrests.

24 Cover the client's lap and legs with a sheet or blanket, keeping it off the floor and the wheels.

25 Remove the transfer belt if it was used.

26 Position the chair as the client prefers. Lock the wheelchair wheels.
Locking prevents the wheelchair from accidentally slipping and injuring the client.

POST-PROCEDURE

27 Provide for safety and comfort.

28 Place the call bell within reach.*
This enables the client to notify the staff if necessary.

29 Remove privacy measures.

30 Perform hand hygiene.

31 Reverse the procedure to return the client to bed.

Report and Record your actions and observations, according to employer policy.
This is done for legal reasons and to keep the rest of the health care team informed.

*Steps marked with an asterisk may not apply in community settings.

Other Transfers

The basic transfer from a bed to a chair, commode chair, or wheelchair can be modified for other situations. You can transfer a client from a wheelchair to a commode chair, shower chair, or bath chair (**FIGURE 25–27** and **FIGURE 25–28**). You can also transfer a client to and from a toilet. Carefully consider how to proceed. It is your responsibility to check first with your supervisor and the care plan to determine the client's physical abilities and limitations. Also, consider the client's environment. How much space do you have available to move about? Are there assistive devices, such as grab bars or slider boards? Use good body mechanics, and apply the general safety and comfort rules.

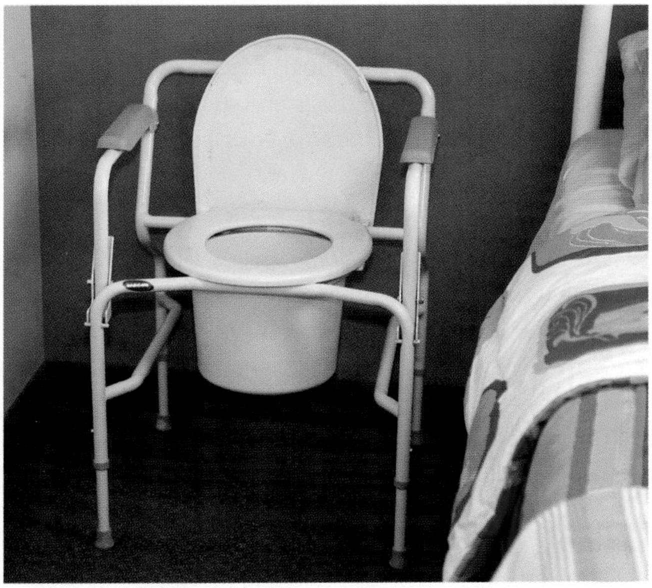

FIGURE 25–27 The bedside commode has a toilet seat with a container beneath it. The container slides out from under the toilet seat for emptying. Many clients prefer to use this type of chair instead of a regular toilet because it offers supportive arms on either side, which can help them remain balanced. This commode is extra-wide to accommodate large clients. (**Source:** Brian Hillier.)

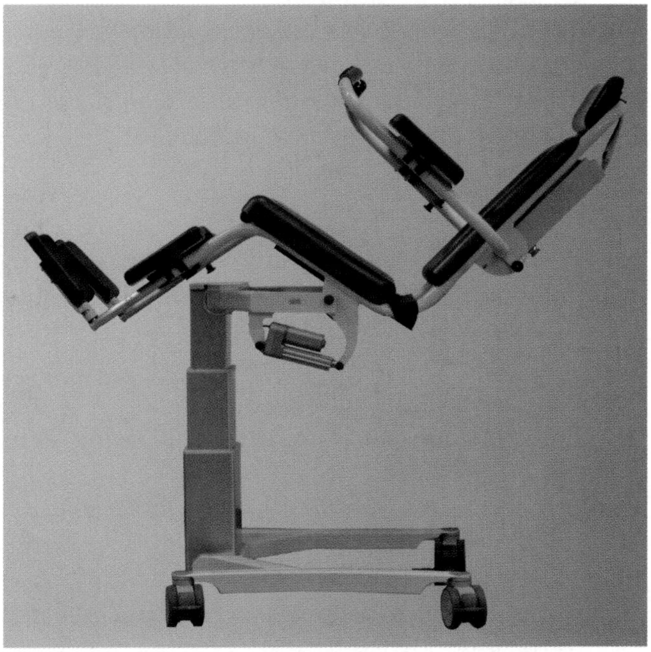

FIGURE 25–28 Tilt shower chair. Note the back of the chair can be lowered, making shampooing easier for the client. (Courtesy of Tollos)

Transferring the Client From a Wheelchair to a Shower, Commode, or Bath Chair 123

Advocate on behalf of the client's quality of life by promoting:

Dignity • Independence • Preferences • Privacy • Safety *(see BOX 1–4, on p. 17)*

PRE-PROCEDURE

1 a Identify the client according to employer policy.

This eliminates the possibility of mistaking one client for another.

b Check the care plan for a description of the client's abilities or limitations.

Care must be taken in order to prevent injuring yourself or others.

Continued

Transferring the Client From a Wheelchair to a Shower, Commode, or Bath Chair—cont'd

2 Explain the procedure to the client.
3 Collect the necessary equipment, such as:
- ☐ **Shower, commode, or bath chair**
- ☐ **Sheet**
- ☐ **Towel**
- ☐ **Transfer belt, if used**

By collecting all the necessary equipment beforehand, you will not have to leave your client's side and can eliminate wasting time and energy in obtaining the forgotten equipment.

4 Perform hand hygiene.
5 Provide for privacy.
6 Check that the shower chair is securely positioned and locked in place. Do not transfer the client if the shower chair is not secure.
Thorough checking reduces the risk for client injury.
7 Check the grab bars near the shower. Do not transfer the client if the grab bars are not secure. Report loose grab bars to your supervisor.

PROCEDURE

8 Position the wheelchair at a 90-degree angle to the shower chair. The client's strong side should be near the shower chair.
This reduces the risk for client injury.
9 Lock the wheelchair wheels.
10 Raise the footrests. Remove them or swing them out of the way.
This reduces the risk for client or worker injury.
11 Prepare the water. Test it to confirm it is the correct temperature.
This ensures the water is not too hot or too cold before immersing the client in it.
12 Apply the transfer belt if used.
13 Help the client stand and turn to the shower chair (see the procedure *Transferring the Client to a Chair or Wheelchair*, steps 16 and 17 on page 519). The client uses the grab bars or shower chair armrests for support.
14 Provide support, as necessary, while the client undresses. Hold the transfer belt, or keep your hands around the client's shoulder blades. Continue to block the client's feet and knees with your feet and knees. Instruct the client to hold on to the grab bars or armrests for support.
This ensures client safety while assisting the client to undress.
15 Lower the client onto the shower chair.
16 Remove the transfer belt if it was used.

POST-PROCEDURE

17 Help the client dry off after the shower. Cover the client with a sheet.
This reduces the risk for client injury or chilling.
18 Reverse the procedure to transfer the client from the shower chair to the wheelchair.
19 Help the client put on clean clothing while maintaining warmth and privacy for the client.
20 Perform hand hygiene.

Report and Record your actions and observations, according to employer policy.
This is done for legal reasons and to keep the rest of the health care team informed.

Transferring the Client to and From the Toilet Seat 123

Advocate on behalf of the client's quality of life by promoting:

Dignity • Independence • Preferences • Privacy • Safety *(see BOX 1–4, on p. 17)*

PRE-PROCEDURE

1 a Identify the client according to employer policy.
This eliminates the possibility of mistaking one client for another.
b Check the care plan for a description of the client's abilities or limitations.
Care must be taken in order to prevent injuring yourself or others.

2 Perform hand hygiene.

3 Provide for privacy.

4 Make sure the client has an elevated toilet seat so that the toilet seat and wheelchair are at the same level.
This reduces the risk for injury to the client when sitting.

5 Check the grab bars near the toilet. If they are loose, tell your supervisor. Do not transfer the client to the toilet if the grab bars are not secure.
Equipment that is not safe can lead to client or worker injury.

PROCEDURE

6 Have the client wear nonskid footwear.
This reduces the risk for client injury.

7 Position the wheelchair next to the toilet if there is enough room. If not, position the wheelchair at a right angle to the toilet (**FIGURE 25–29**). It is best if the client's strong side is near the toilet.

8 Lock the wheelchair wheels.
These safety steps will reduce the risk for client or worker injury.

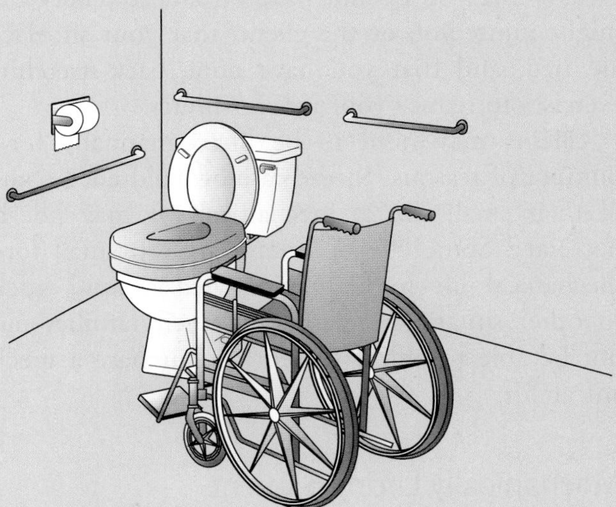

FIGURE 25–29 Position the wheelchair at a right angle to the toilet.

9 Raise the footrests. Remove them or swing them out of the way.

10 Apply the transfer belt if used.

11 Help the client unfasten clothing.

12 Help the client stand and turn toward the toilet, using the grab bars (see the procedure *Transferring the Client to a Chair or Wheelchair*, steps 16 and 17 on page 519).

13 Provide support while the client lowers clothing. Hold the transfer belt, or keep your hands around the client's shoulder blades. Continue to block the client's feet and knees with your feet and knees. Have the client hold on to the grab bars for support.
This reduces the risk of the client's slipping and falling during this step. Lower the client's pants and undergarments.

14 Lower the client onto the toilet seat.

15 Remove the transfer belt if used.

16 Tell the client that you will stay close by and to use the call bell (in facilities) or to call for you when help is needed. ***(Because of their increased risk of falling, some clients must have someone stay right by their side while they are toileting. Check with your supervisor if you are unsure!)***
This allows clients to be assisted while ensuring their rights to privacy and dignity.

Continued

Transferring the Client to and From the Toilet Seat—cont'd

17 Close the bathroom door to provide privacy.
18 Stay near the bathroom. In the meanwhile, you may complete other tasks in the client's room.
19 Knock on the bathroom door when the client calls for you.
20 Help with wiping, perineal care, flushing, and handwashing, as needed. Wear gloves for this step.
21 Apply the transfer belt if used.
22 Help the client stand, and support the client in the standing position. Hold the transfer belt, or keep your hands around the client's shoulder blades. Continue to block the client's feet and knees with your feet and knees.
23 Help the client pull up and secure clothing.
This preserves the client's dignity.
24 Transfer the client to the wheelchair (see the procedure *Transferring the Client to a Chair or Wheelchair*, steps 18 through 26 on pages 519 and 520).

POST-PROCEDURE

25 Provide for safety and comfort.
26 Place the call bell within reach.*
This provides a way for the client to contact the staff.
27 Perform hand hygiene.

Report and Record your actions and observations, according to employer policy.
This is done for legal reasons and to keep the rest of the health care team informed.

*Steps marked with an asterisk may not apply in community settings.

LIFTING A CLIENT

Some clients need to be lifted when they cannot help with a transfer by weight-bearing. **Lifts** are used to physically move clients from one place to another—for example into chairs, stretchers, tubs, shower chairs, toilets, whirlpools, and vehicles. Because of the serious risk for back injury, most long-term care agencies no longer allow staff members to manually lift clients, enforcing a strict no-lift policy.

Manual Lifts

When working in the home care sector, you might be responsible for **manual lifts** (physically picking up a client who cannot weight-bear), done with the assistance of a family member. You must know your agency's policies regarding lifts *before* going into a client's home. Before assisting with a manual lift, be certain that you do not have on any jewellery that might injure you or the client, that your shoelaces are tied, and that you have done back-stretching exercises to reduce your risk for injury.

Clients may need to be lifted manually for a number of reasons. In the case of children, because of their small size, a mechanical lift may not be necessary. Some clients' homes are too small for a mechanical lift to be manoeuvred around safely. In other situations, clients and their families may not be able to afford to rent or purchase a mechanical lift.

Mechanically Lifting a Client

There are different kinds of lifts—mechanical and electric (**FIGURE 25–30** on page 526 and **FIGURE 25–31** on page 528). Knowing how to use one type of lift does not mean that you know how to use others. Always follow the manufacturer's instructions. Employers usually provide special training for the use of mechanical lifts. You may also be required to take yearly refresher courses to keep your skills current. If you have questions, ask your supervisor (see *Supporting Mrs. Quouong: Understanding the No-Lift Policy*). ***If you have not used a certain type of lift before, it is your responsibility to ask your supervisor to show you how to use it safely.***

Before using a lift:

- Make sure you are trained in its use.
- Make sure the lift works.
- Compare the client's weight and the lift's weight limit. Do not use the lift if a client's weight exceeds the lift's capacity.
- At least two people are usually needed to work a mechanical lift. Get a co-worker or a trained member of the client's family to help you.

Supporting Mrs. Quouong: Understanding the No-Lift Policy

You have recently been hired as a support worker, and today is your first full day working alongside the staff. You have learned in your orientation that there are signs posted inside each client's bedside locker, stating the type of lift or transfer that they require. This facility has a strict no-lift policy of anybody or anything over 23 kg (50.7 lb.). During your morning care rounds, you and Rosie, the support worker you are working with, enter the room of Mrs. Lua Quouong.

Mrs. Quouong, a 90-year-old client, is very small, weighing only 36 kg (80 lb.), and has very swollen ankles. In her care plan is a sign that indicates that she must be moved by using a mechanical lift. Rosie closes the door to Mrs. Quouong's room and tells you to help her manually lift Mrs. Quouong. Rosie explains that it is easier and faster to manually move Mrs. Quouong than it is to move her mechanically. Besides, she explains, Mrs. Quouong is so small that if the two of you lifted her together, each of you would be lifting only 18 kg. Rosie tells you that for these reasons, all the staff members usually manually lift Mrs. Quouong. You are unsure about what you should do.

Using a Mechanical Lift to Move a Client

123

The following procedure is a general guideline based only on principles of moving and body mechanics. The mechanical lift that your employer uses may be different and may require different actions. Check with your employer to see what your responsibilities are.

Advocate on behalf of the client's quality of life by promoting:

Dignity • Independence • Preferences • Privacy • Safety *(see BOX 1–4, on p. 17)*

PRE-PROCEDURE

1 a Identify the client according to employer policy.
This eliminates the possibility of mistaking one client for another.

b Check the care plan for a description of the client's abilities or limitations.
Care must be taken in order to prevent injuring yourself or others.

Continued

Using a Mechanical Lift to Move a Client—cont'd

2 Ask someone who is properly trained to use this type of lift to help you.
It is the policy of most agencies to have two workers assist with mechanical lifts to reduce the risk for client or worker injury.
3 Explain the procedure to the client.
4 Collect the following supplies:
- ☐ **Mechanical lift**
- ☐ **Armchair or wheelchair**
- ☐ **Client footwear**
- ☐ **Cushion or towel**
- ☐ **Blanket to cover the client with afterward.**

By collecting all the necessary equipment beforehand, you will not have to leave your client's side and can eliminate wasting time and energy in obtaining the forgotten equipment.
5 Perform hand hygiene.
6 Provide for privacy.

PROCEDURE

7 a Put the footwear on the client. *Footwear prevents foot injury.*
b Centre the sling under the client (FIGURE 25–30, *A*).
c Turn the client from side to side—as if making an occupied bed (see Chapter 34)—to position the sling. Position the sling according to the manufacturer's instructions.
d You and your helper must communicate directions throughout the procedure.
By working as a team, you will reduce the risk for client or worker injury.
8 Place the chair at the head of the bed. It should be aligned with the headboard and about 30 cm (1 ft.) away from the bed. Place a folded towel or cushion in the chair if needed for hygiene or privacy.
The towel or cushion will be used to maintain privacy for the client by covering exposed body parts.
9 Lock the bed wheels, and lower the bed to its lowest position.*
This prevents the bed from slipping during this procedure.
10 Raise the lift so that it can be positioned over the client.
11 Position the lift over the client (FIGURE 25–30, *B*).
12 Lock the lift wheels in position.
13 Attach the sling to the swivel bar (FIGURE 25–30, *C*).
14 Assist the client to the sitting position. Raise the head of the bed or use pillows for support.

A
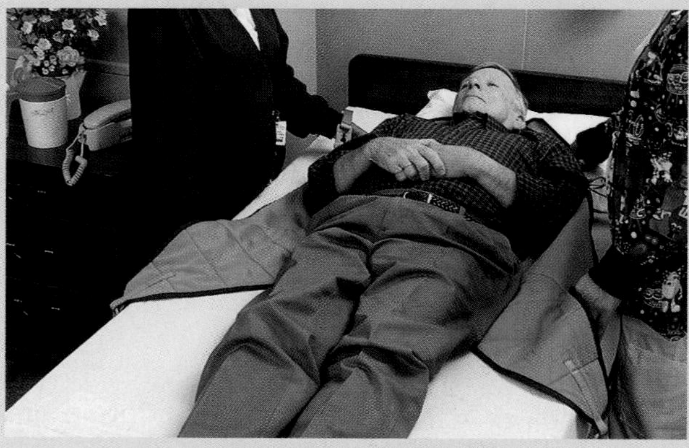
FIGURE 25–30 A

B
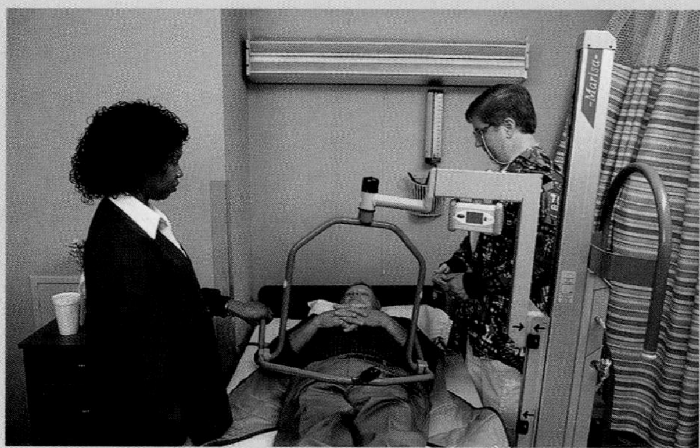
FIGURE 25–30 B

Continued

Using a Mechanical Lift to Move a Client—cont'd

C

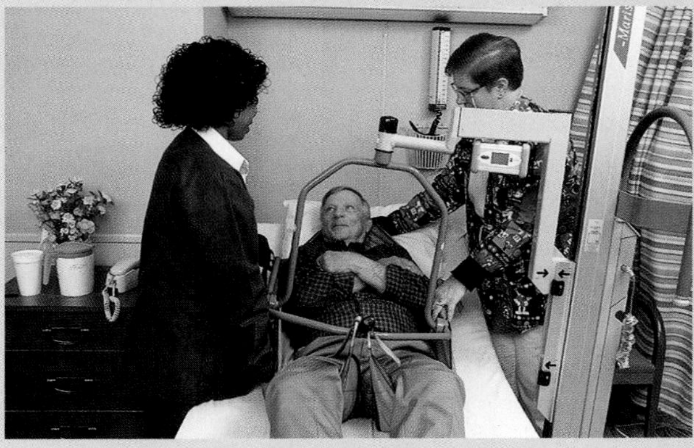

FIGURE 25–30 C

D

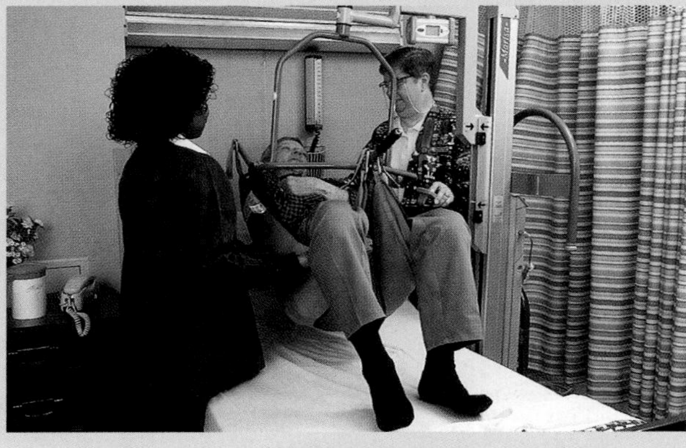

FIGURE 25–30 D

E

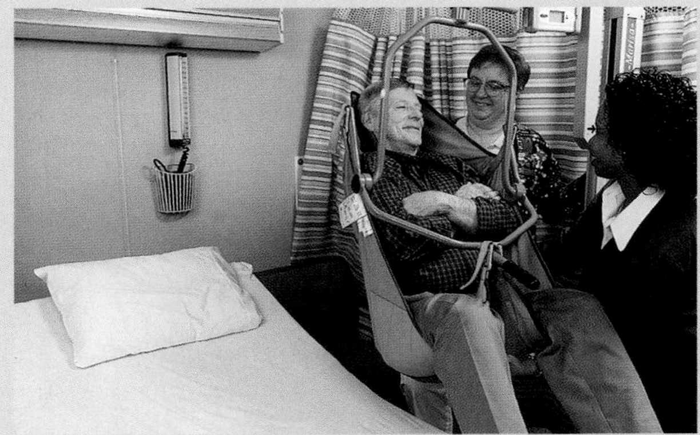

FIGURE 25–30 E

F

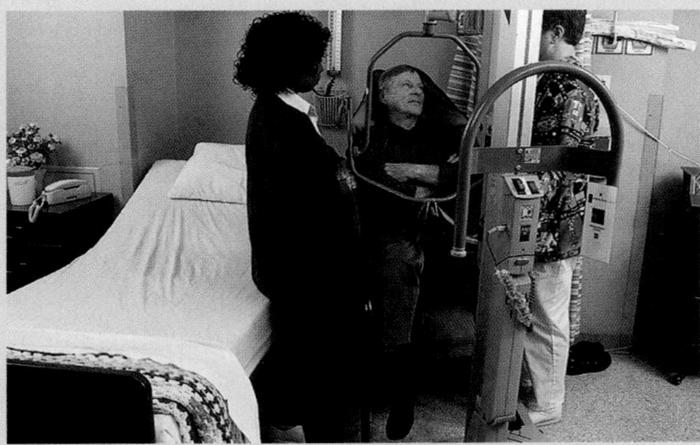

FIGURE 25–30 F

15 Cross the client's arms over the chest. Let the client hold on to the straps or chains, but not to the swivel bar.
This prevents client injury.

16 Raise the lift high enough that the client and the sling are free of the bed (**FIGURE 25–30, *D***).
By elevating the client above the bed, workers can check to see if the client is in a safe position before moving the client.

17 Ask your helper to support the client's legs as you move the lift and client away from the bed (**FIGURE 25–30, *E***).
This prevents client injury and reassures the client.

18 Position the lift so that the client's back is toward the chair.

19 Position the chair so that you can lower the client into it safely.
Judging the appropriate position of the chair is often difficult until the sling is right above it.

20 Lower the client into the chair, following the lift manufacturer's instructions. Guide the client into the chair (**FIGURE 25–30, *F***).

21 Lower the swivel bar to unhook the sling. Remove the sling from under the client, unless instructed otherwise.

22 Position the client's feet on the wheelchair footrests.
This reduces the risk for foot injury.

23 Cover the client's lap and legs with a blanket. Keep the blanket off the floor and wheels.
If the blanket is allowed to drag on the floor, it can become caught in the wheels.

24 Position the chair as the client prefers. Lock the wheelchair wheels.
This reduces the risk for client injury.

Continued

Using a Mechanical Lift to Move a Client—cont'd

POST-PROCEDURE

25 Provide for safety and comfort.
26 Place the call bell within reach.*
This provides an easy, safe way for the client to contact staff if necessary.
27 Perform hand hygiene.
28 Reverse the procedure to return the client to bed.

Report and Record your actions and observations, according to employer policy.
This is done for legal reasons and to keep the rest of the health care team informed.

*Steps marked with an asterisk may not apply in community settings.

The Sit-to-Stand Mechanical Lift

The sit-to-stand mechanical lift is commonly used in long-term care agencies and in private homes. The sit-to-stand lift is a mobile lift that allows for client transfers from one seated position to another. This lift is used for bed-to-chair transfers and for toileting, performing perineal care, or changing incontinence briefs.[1]

The sit-to-stand lift (**FIGURE 25–31**) differs from the sling-type mechanical lift in that it is suitable only for clients who are cognitively aware enough to cooperate with instructions. In addition, clients must possess some muscle tone in at least one leg and have some upper body muscle tone to be suitable to be safely lifted in this type of lift.

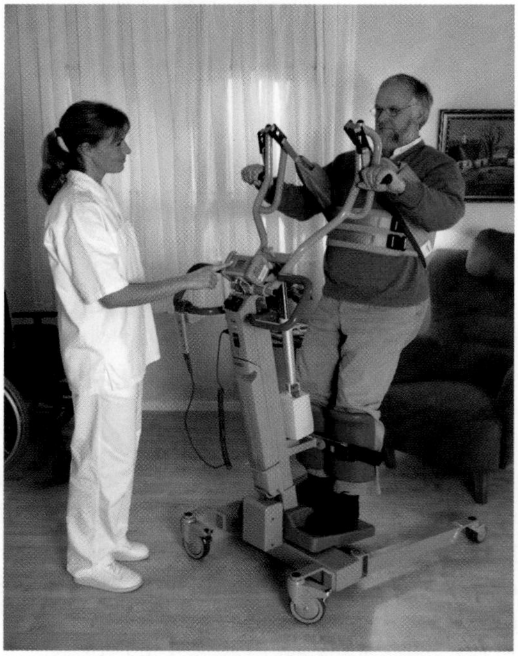

FIGURE 25–31 Sit-to-stand lift. This type of lift is useful for moving seated clients from chair to toilet or the reverse. Because there are no straps around the client's buttocks, that entire area can be thoroughly washed and inspected. The lift is operated with a handheld device. ***(Note: There should always be two workers operating this mechanical device. Check your agency's policy.)*** (Courtesy ArjoHuntleigh Inc.)

Using a Sit-to-Stand Mechanical Lift to Move a Client From a Chair to a Commode

123

The following procedure is a general guideline only. *The mechanical lift that your employer uses may be different and may require different actions.* Check with your employer to find out what your responsibilities are.

Advocate on behalf of the client's quality of life by promoting:

Dignity • Independence • Preferences • Privacy • Safety *(see BOX 1–4, on p. 17)*

PRE-PROCEDURE

1 a Identify the client according to employer policy.
This eliminates the possibility of mistaking one client for another.
b Check the care plan for a description of the client's abilities or limitations.
Care must be taken in order to prevent injuring yourself or others.

2 Ask someone who is properly trained to use this type of lift to help you.
It is the policy of most agencies to have two workers assist with mechanical lifts to reduce the risk for client or worker injury.

3 Explain the procedure to the client.

4 Collect the following supplies:
- ☐ **Mechanical sit-to-stand lift**
- ☐ **Commode chair**
- ☐ **Cleaning supplies required to perform perineal care after the client has used the commode chair** (see "Perineal Care" in Chapter 30).

By collecting all the necessary equipment beforehand, you will not have to leave your client's side and can eliminate wasting time and energy in obtaining the forgotten equipment.

5 Perform hand hygiene.

6 Provide for privacy.

PROCEDURE

7 Since the client is already in a chair, the person should already be wearing supportive footwear. However, if this is not the case, put footwear on the client.
Proper footwear prevents foot injury.

8 You and your helper must communicate directions throughout the procedure.
By working as a team, you will reduce the risk for client or worker injury.

9 Ensure the chair the client is sitting in will not slide. If the client is in a wheelchair, lock the wheelchair wheels.
This prevents the chair from slipping during this procedure.

10 a Position the harness properly around the client's trunk, underneath the armpits, extending down around the client's lower back region.
This reduces the risk of the client slipping down through the harness.
b Tighten the inner belts so they fit snugly to the client.
c Apply leg straps if applicable.

11 Position the sit-to-stand mechanical lift with the base of the lift open so that it is facing the client.

12 Lock the lift wheels in position.

13 Instruct the client to place feet in the footplate of the lift.
This reduces the risk for foot injury.

14 Attach the strap of the harness to the lift without lifting or tugging.
Lifting or tugging can increase the risk for client injury.

15 Instruct or assist the client to grasp the handles of the lift. The client's arms should be on the *outside* of the harness.
Having the arms on the outside of the harness prevents the client from sliding through the harness.

Continued

Using a Sit-to-Stand Mechanical Lift to Move a Client From a Chair to a Commode—cont'd

16 Close the leg base of the lift. Do not move the lift with the lift leg base open.
This prevents client injury.

17 **a** Verbally prepare the client for moving.
This reassures the client.
b Instruct client to lean back into the back harness.

18 Slowly lift the client minimally from the floor.
This prevents client injury while workers check to ensure the client is in a safe position before moving any further.

19 **a** Bring the lift-supported client to the commode.
b Undo the client's pants and lower them enough to allow the client to be toileted.

20 Position the commode under the client.
The commode should be in a position to allow the client to be safely lowered onto it.
a Lower the client into the commode chair, following lift manufacturer's instructions. Guide the client onto the commode.
b Once the client is on the commode, open the lift base legs.
Opening the lift's legs provides a wider base of support, preventing the risk of tipping.

21 Allow the client to toilet, providing privacy as instructed in the client's care plan.

22 **a** After the client has finished toileting, elevate the lift and move the client so you have access to the perineal area. Perform perineal care while the client is supported by the sit–stand harness (see the procedure *Giving Perineal Care to a Female Client*, p. 643, or *Giving Perineal Care to a Male Client*, p. 646).
b Assist the client with hand hygiene.

23 Re-dress the client, making sure the clothing is not twisted or bunched.
This ensures client privacy, dignity, warmth, and security.

24 Reverse the procedure to return the client to the chair.

POST-PROCEDURE

25 Provide for safety and comfort.
26 Place the call bell within reach.*
27 Perform hand hygiene.

Report and Record your actions and observations, according to employer policy.
This is done for legal reasons and to keep the rest of the health care team informed.

*Steps marked with an asterisk may not apply in community settings.

CHAPTER REVIEW

KEY POINTS

- Using good body mechanics will help you protect yourself and your client from injury during moving, positioning, transferring, and lifting activities.
- Remember to use good hand hygiene practices before and after any moving, positioning, transferring, or lifting activity.
- *Body mechanics* refers to the movement of the body in an efficient and careful way, the use of good posture and balance, and the use of the longest and largest muscles of the body.
- *Body alignment* is the way the body parts are positioned in relation to one another. Good body alignment allows the body to move with strength and efficiency, reduces strain on muscles and joints, and prevents injury.
- When positioning clients, ensure that they are left in a safe, wrinkle-free, and comfortable position. Ensure that pillows, padding, or stabilizers are used correctly.
- Regular position changes and good body alignment promote comfort and well-being, make breathing easier, and promote circulation.
- Always check the client's care plan, and know employer policy before moving a client.
- The client's skin must be protected from friction and shearing when the client is being moved.
- Know what turning pads are and how to use them properly. They must be positioned from the head to the mid-thigh, keeping the client's neck in a stable position.
- All movements with another worker or helper should be done in a synchronous manner (at the same time) to prevent injury.
- A transfer is the method used for moving a client who can weight-bear to any degree. If a client cannot assist by weight-bearing, a lift is used.
- Most agencies have a no-lift policy because of the serious risk for back injury to the workers.
- The DIPPS principles should always be observed whenever a client is moved, positioned, transferred, or lifted at any time.

CRITICAL THINKING IN PRACTICE

A resident needs to go to the bathroom right away. She uses a mechanical lift to transfer safely. You do not see another staff member nearby to help. What will you do?

REVIEW QUESTIONS

Answers to these questions are at the bottom of page 532.

Circle T if the answer is true, and circle F if the answer is false.

1. T F *Body mechanics* refers to the way in which body parts are positioned in relation to one another.
2. T F Good body mechanics help you protect yourself and the client from injury.
3. T F Body mechanics involve the use of small muscles.
4. T F Base of support is the area on which an object rests.
5. T F You should keep objects far away from the body when lifting, moving, or carrying them.
6. T F You should face the direction you are working in to prevent unnecessary twisting.
7. T F You should push, slide, or pull heavy objects rather than lift them.
8. T F Sliding the client reduces friction and shearing.
9. T F You should ask your supervisor about limits or restrictions in positioning or moving a client.
10. T F The right to privacy should be protected when you are moving, lifting, or transferring clients.
11. T F A turning pad should extend from below the client's shoulders to above the knees.

12. T F A client should be moved to the side of the bed before being turned to the side-lying position.
13. T F Log-rolling is rolling the client in segments.
14. T F Clients with spinal cord injuries are log-rolled.
15. T F Repositioning prevents prolonged pressure on body parts.
16. T F The head of the bed is elevated 45 to 60 degrees for the supine position.
17. T F Sims' position is the left-side-lying position.
18. T F A transfer belt is part of a mechanical lift.
19. T F A client is being transferred from the bed to a chair. He needs nonskid footwear.
20. T F You are going to transfer a client from the bed to a chair. You should move the person from the direction of the weak side of the body.

Circle the BEST answer.

21. Good body alignment means:
    A. The area on which an object rests
    B. Having the head, trunk, arms, and legs aligned with one another
    C. Using muscles, tendons, ligaments, joints, and cartilage correctly
    D. The back-lying or supine position
22. Support workers are at great risk for:
    A. Friction and shearing
    B. Arm and hand injuries
    C. Back injuries
    D. Falls
23. A client's skin rubs against the sheet. This is called:
    A. Shearing
    B. Friction
    C. Transferring
    D. Posture
24. Clients who are immobile must be repositioned at least every:
    A. 30 minutes
    B. 1 hour
    C. 2 hours
    D. 3 hours
25. The back-lying position is called:
    A. Fowler's position
    B. The supine position
    C. The prone position
    D. Sims' position
26. A client is positioned in a chair. The feet:
    A. Must be flat on the floor
    B. Are crossed
    C. Dangle
    D. Must be positioned on pillows
27. When transferring a client to bed, a chair, or the toilet:
    A. The client's strong side is moved first
    B. The weak side is moved first
    C. Pillows are used for support
    D. The transfer belt cannot be used
28. These statements are about transfers to and from a toilet. Which is false?
    A. The client wears nonskid footwear.
    B. Wheelchair brakes must be locked.
    C. The wheelchair is positioned so that the client's strong side is near the toilet.
    D. The client uses the towel bars for support.

Answers: 1.F, 2.T, 3.F, 4.T, 5.F, 6.T, 7.T, 8.F, 9.T, 10.T, 11.F
12.T, 13.F, 14.T, 15.T, 16.F, 17.T, 18.F, 19.T, 20.F, 21.B, 22.C,
23.B, 24.C, 25.B, 26.A, 27.A, 28.D

CHAPTER 26

Exercise and Activity

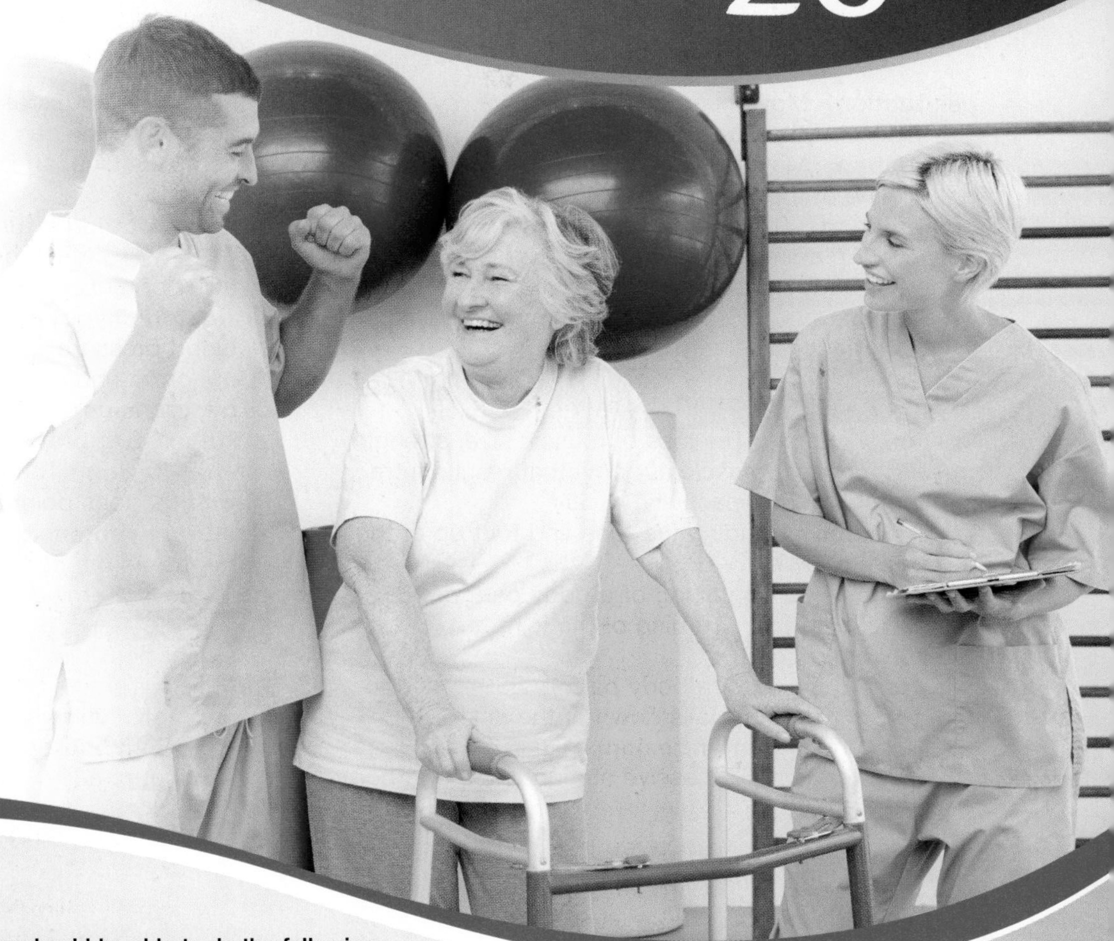

OBJECTIVES

After reading this chapter, the learner should be able to do the following:

- Describe bed rest.
- Describe the complications of bed rest and how to prevent them.
- Describe the devices used to support and maintain body alignment.
- Describe the purpose of a trapeze.
- Describe range-of-motion exercises.
- Describe how to help a falling client.
- Describe types of walking aids.
- Perform the procedures described in this chapter.

KEY TERMS

abduction Movement of a body part away from the midline of the body. *p. 539*
adduction Movement of a body part toward the midline of the body. *p. 539*
ambulation The act of walking. *p. 545*
brace An apparatus worn to support or align weak body parts or to prevent or correct problems with the musculo-skeletal system; also called **orthotic**. *p. 553*
contracture The lack of joint mobility caused by abnormal shortening of a muscle. *p. 535*
deconditioning The loss of muscle size, strength, and function (*muscle atrophy*) that results from immobility and inactivity. *p. 534*
dorsiflexion Bending the toes and foot up at the ankle. *p. 539*
extension Straightening of a body part. *p. 539*
external rotation Turning of the joint outward. *p. 539*
flexion Bending of a body part. *p. 539*
footdrop The foot falls down at the ankle (permanent **plantar flexion**). *p. 536*
hyperextension Excessive straightening of a body part. *p. 539*
immobility An excessive lack of exercise and activity, which can cause serious health complications, affecting every system in the body. *p. 535*
internal rotation Turning of the joint inward. *p. 539*
muscle atrophy A decrease in size or a wasting away of muscle. *p. 535*
orthostatic hypotension A drop in (*hypo*) blood pressure when the client stands up (*ortho* and *static*). Also known as **postural hypotension**. *p. 536*
orthotic See **brace**. *p. 553*
plantar flexion The foot (*plantar*) is bent (*flexion*) with the toes pointed away from the leg. *p. 539*
postural hypotension See **orthostatic hypotension**. *p. 536*
pronation Turning downward. *p. 539*
range of motion (ROM) Moving a joint to the extent possible without causing pain. *p. 538*
rotation Turning of the joint. *p. 539*
supination Turning upward. *p. 539*
syncope A brief loss of consciousness; fainting. *p. 536*

Being active is important for physical and mental well-being. Most people move about and function without help, but illnesses, surgery, injuries, pain, and aging can cause weakness and limit activity. Clients may be weakened by chronic illnesses, have to stay in bed for a long time, have permanent paralysis, or have progressive disorders (e.g., multiple sclerosis, Parkinson's disease, arthritis, muscular disorders—see Chapter 37), causing decreases in activity. Inactivity, whether mild or severe, affects not only the normal functions of all body systems but also the client's mental well-being.

Support workers can sustain injuries while assisting clients with exercise and activity. It is important that you practise proper body mechanics at all times (see Chapter 25). Choosing healthy lifestyle habits such as performing muscle stretches daily before assisting clients as well as paying attention to your posture and body mechanics at all times may decrease your own risk for injury.

Deconditioning is the loss of muscle size, strength, and function (*muscle atrophy*) that results from immobility and inactivity. Deconditioning can occur at any age—from infants to older adults; however, older clients become deconditioned more quickly. So, each client must be encouraged to be as active as possible. If a client cannot move without assistance, it is important that you assist the client to move in order to prevent permanent loss of joint function. Physiotherapists and occupational therapists are responsible for assessing the client's joint function and for suggesting exercises or mobility aids that can assist the client to regain muscle strength and function. The care plan tells you about the client's activity level and the exercises she is to perform.

To help promote exercise and activity, you need to understand the following:

- Bed rest
- How to prevent complications from bed rest
- How to help clients exercise

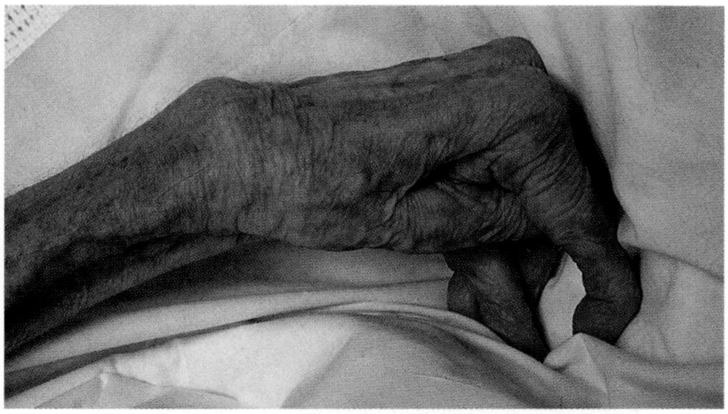

FIGURE 26–1 A contracture.

BED REST

Bed rest is ordered by the physician to treat a health problem and often also to do the following:

- Reduce physical activity
- Reduce pain
- Encourage rest
- Regain strength
- Promote healing

The activities allowed for each client will be specified in the care plan. Check with your supervisor if you have questions. The following types of bed rest are common:

- ***Strict bed rest.*** The client must remain in bed at all times and be assisted with all activities of daily living (ADLs) as needed. If the client is continent, he must use a bedpan or urinal.
- ***Bed rest with commode privileges.*** Some ADLs are allowed, such as self-feeding, oral hygiene, bathing, shaving, and hair care. The client can use the bedside commode for elimination needs (see Chapters 32 and 33); the care plan will state whether the client must receive assistance.
- ***Bed rest with bathroom privileges (bed rest with BRP).*** The client can use the bathroom for elimination needs.

Always ask your supervisor what *bed rest* means for each client.

Complications of Bed Rest and Immobility

Long-term bed rest and immobility can cause serious health complications, affecting every system in the body. **Immobility** is an excessive lack of exercise and activity. Pressure ulcers, constipation, fecal impaction, urinary tract infections, renal calculi (kidney stones), blood clots (thrombi), and pneumonia (infection of the lung) are some of the complications that can occur (see Chapter 37).

Contractures and muscle atrophy occur in the musculo-skeletal system. A **contracture** is the lack of joint mobility caused by the abnormal shortening of a muscle. ***Contractures form in as little as 48 to 72 hours if the muscle and joint have not been exercised!*** The contracted muscle becomes fixed into position, deformed, and unable to stretch (**FIGURE 26–1**). Contractures are not reversible. Common sites are the fingers, wrists, elbows, toes, ankles, knees, and hips. Contractures can also occur in the neck and spine. The person with a contracture suffers permanent deformity and disability. *Atrophy*, as defined in Chapter 21, is the decrease in size or the wasting away of tissue. **Muscle atrophy** is a decrease in size or a wasting away of muscle (**FIGURE 26–2**). These complications from lack of activity must be prevented to maintain normal body movement.

Orthostatic hypotension and blood clots (see Chapters 26 and 45) can occur from a lack of

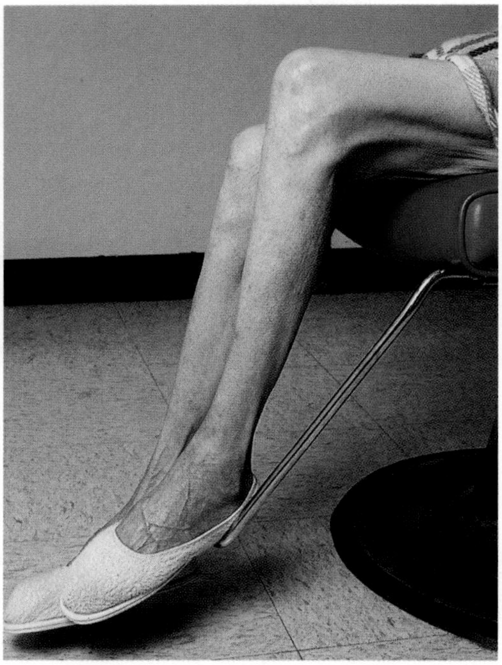

FIGURE 26–2 Muscle atrophy.

mobility. Orthostatic hypotension (or postural hypotension) is a drop in (*hypo*) blood pressure when the client stands up (*ortho* and *static*). When the client moves from lying or sitting to a standing position, the blood pressure drops, and the client experiences dizziness, weakness, and spots before the eyes, followed by syncope (fainting), which is a brief loss of consciousness. BOX 26–1 lists measures that prevent orthostatic hypotension, such as changing positions slowly.

You can help prevent complications from bed rest by providing good care and encouraging your client to move the limbs as much as possible, depending on the care plan. Make sure the client is in good body alignment. Reposition the client ***at least*** once every 2 hours, following the care plan (see Chapter 25). Also, help with range-of-motion (ROM) exercises, according to the care plan (see pp. 538–544).

Positioning

Body alignment and positioning are discussed in detail in Chapter 25. Supportive devices are often used to support and maintain the client in a certain position:

- ***Bed boards***—placed under the mattress (FIGURE 26–3) to prevent the mattress from sagging. They are usually made of plywood and are covered with canvas or other material. The two sections of the bed boards help raise the head of the bed and the foot of the bed.
- ***Footboards***—placed at the foot of mattresses (FIGURE 26–4) to prevent plantar flexion, which can lead to footdrop. In plantar flexion, the foot (*plantar*) is bent (*flexion*) with the toes pointed away from the leg. Footdrop occurs when the foot permanently falls down at the ankle (permanent plantar flexion). Footdrop is nonreversible. The footboard is placed in such a way that the soles of the feet are flush against it, and the feet are in good alignment, as in the standing position. Footboards also serve as bed cradles and keep top linens off the feet.
- ***Trochanter rolls***—prevent the hips and legs from turning outward (*external rotation*) (FIGURE 26–5 on page 538). They are made by folding sheets to the desired length and rolling them up. The loose end is placed under the client, from hip to knee, and the roll is tucked alongside the body. Pillows or sandbags also are used to keep the hips and knees in alignment.
- ***Hand rolls or hand grips***—prevent contractures of the thumb, fingers, and wrist. Commercial hand rolls are commonly available (FIGURE 26–6 on page 538). Foam rubber sponges, rubber balls, and finger cushions (FIGURE 26–7 on page 538) also are used.
- ***Splints***—keep the wrist, thumb, and fingers in normal position. They are usually secured in place with Velcro. Some have foam padding (FIGURE 26–8 on page 538).
- ***Bed cradles***—keep the weight of top linens off the feet (see FIGURE 24–7, on p. 472). The weight of top linens can cause footdrop and pressure ulcers.

Exercise

Exercise helps prevent contractures, muscle atrophy, and other complications of bed rest. Some exercise occurs with ADLs and from turning and moving in bed without assistance. However, additional exercises are needed for muscles and joints.

A trapeze is used for exercises to strengthen arm muscles. The trapeze is suspended from an overbed

BOX 26–1 Preventing Orthostatic Hypotension When Helping a Client From a Lying Position to a Standing Position

1. You may be requested to measure blood pressure (BP) (if allowed by your employer), pulse, and respirations in a lying position and then in a sitting position.* If no symptoms of a drop in blood pressure are reported, such as lightheadedness, proceed to the next step.
2. Position the client in Fowler's position. Raise the head of the bed slowly. If the bed cannot be raised, use pillows and backrests for positioning.
   - Ask the client if there is any weakness, dizziness, or spots before the eyes. Lower the head of the bed back to a flat position or remove the backrest if these symptoms occur. Report these symptoms to your supervisor.
   - You may be requested to measure BP (if allowed by your employer), pulse, and respirations.*
   - Keep the client in Fowler's position for a short while. Ask the client if there is any weakness, dizziness, or spots before the eyes. If not, proceed to the next step.
3. Help the client sit on the side of the bed with feet dangling over the edge (see Chapter 25).
   - Ask the client if there is any weakness, dizziness, or spots before the eyes. If any symptoms are reported, have your client lie back in the bed, and report the symptoms to your supervisor. If not, proceed to the next step.
4. Have the client continue to sit on the side of the bed for a short while.
5. Help the client stand up. Stay close to the client, and use good body mechanics.
   - Ask the client if there is any weakness, dizziness, or spots before the eyes. Help the client sit on the side of the bed if any of these symptoms occur. Report these symptoms to your supervisor.
   - You may be requested to measure BP (if allowed by your employer), pulse, and respirations.* If no symptoms are reported, proceed to the next step.
6. Help the client sit in a chair or walk, as directed by the care plan.
   - Ask the client if there is any weakness, dizziness, or spots before the eyes. If the client is walking, help the client sit down if symptoms occur. If no symptoms are reported, proceed to the next step.
7. Report all observations and complaints.

*Measure blood pressure, pulse, and respirations only if instructed (and allowed) to do so. Know your scope of practice and employer policy.

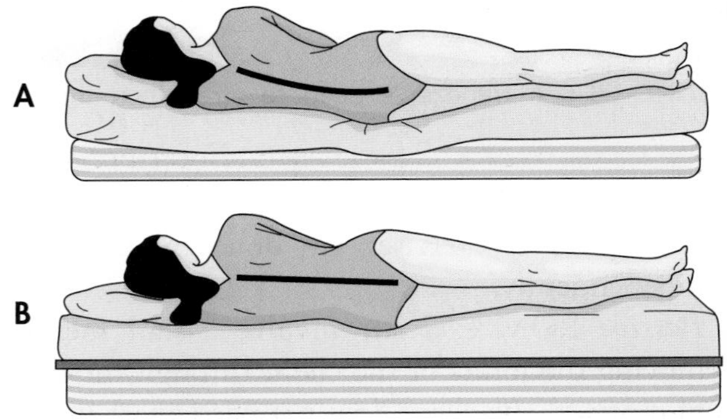

FIGURE 26–3 **A,** Mattress is sagging without bed boards. **B,** Bed boards are placed under the mattress, and there is no sagging.

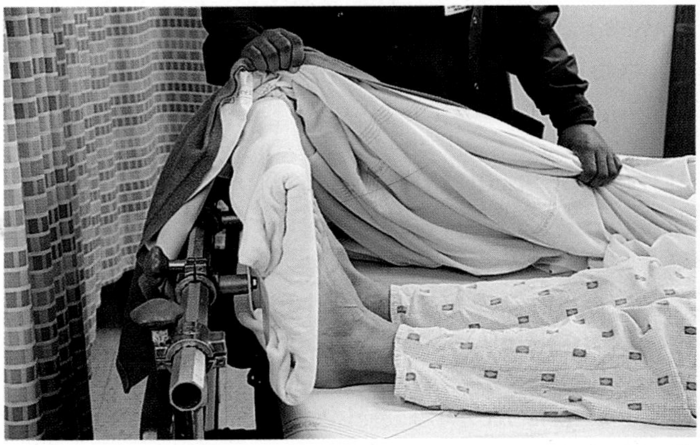

FIGURE 26–4 Footboard. Feet are flush against the board to keep them in normal alignment.

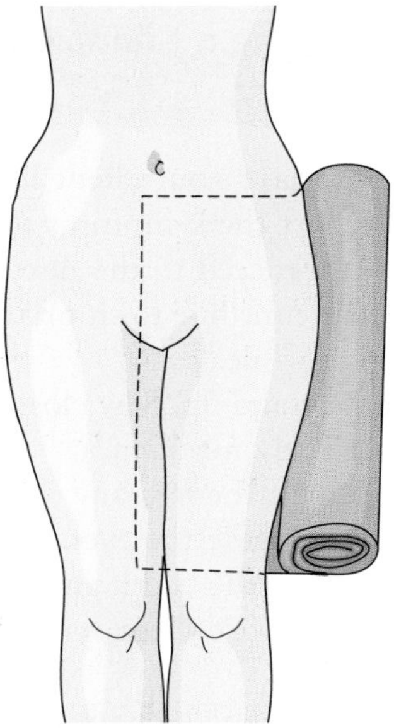

FIGURE 26–5 Trochanter roll made using a towel or sheet. It extends from the client's hip to the knee.

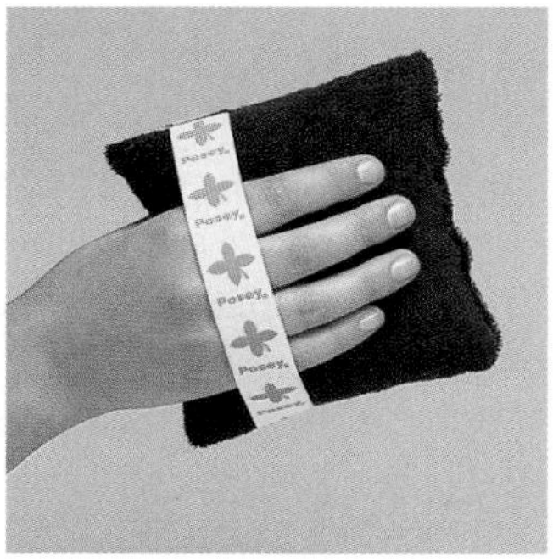

FIGURE 26–6 Hand grip. (**Source:** Image provided courtesy Posey Company, Arcadia, CA.)

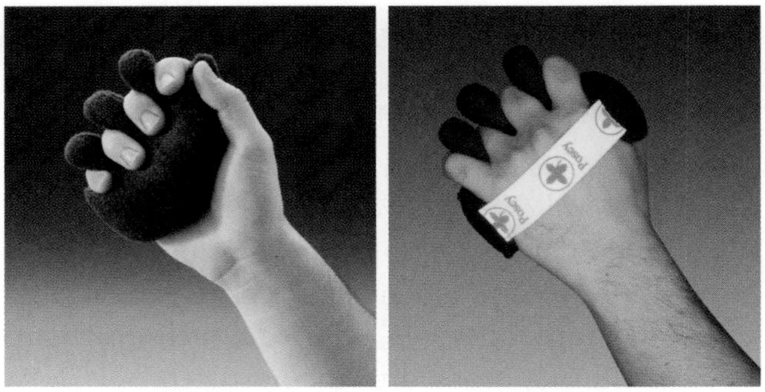

FIGURE 26–7 Finger cushion. (**Source:** Image provided courtesy Posey Company, Arcadia, CA.)

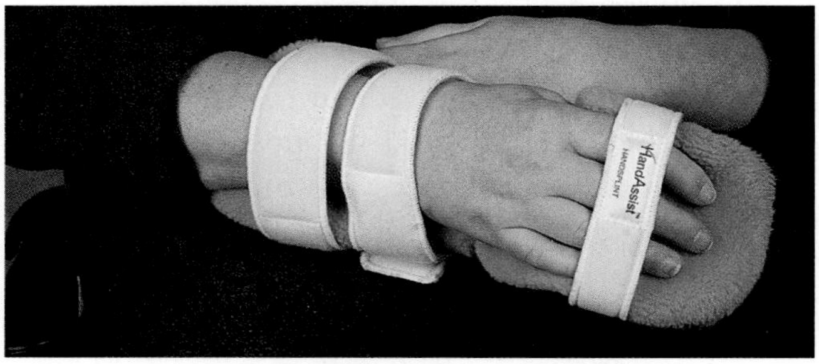

FIGURE 26–8 Splint.

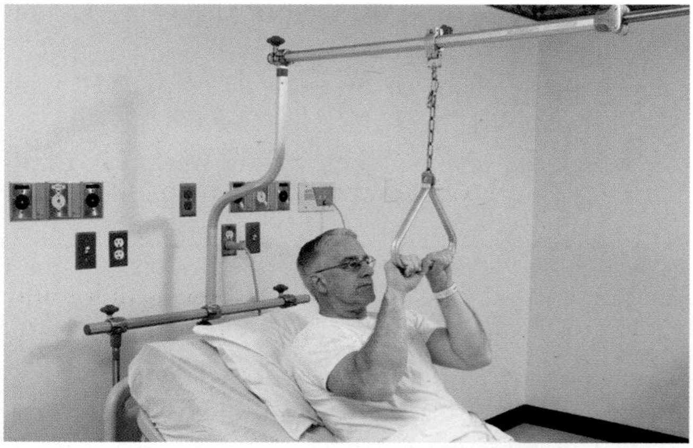

FIGURE 26–9 A trapeze is used to strengthen the arm muscles.

frame (FIGURE 26–9). The client grasps the bar with both hands to lift the trunk off the bed. The client can also use the trapeze to move up and turn in bed (see Chapter 25).

Range-of-Motion Exercises

Moving a joint to the extent possible without causing pain is the **range of motion (ROM)** of that joint. ROM exercises involve exercising the joints through their complete range of motion (BOX 26–2). Clients who need these exercises usually do them at least twice a day. ROM exercises are active, passive, or active–assistive. Music can help some clients to relax while ROM exercises are performed. It is important to ask your clients if they would like to have music played, which could relax them or motivate them.

- ***Active*** ROM exercises are done by the client independently.
- ***Passive*** ROM exercises involve a staff member moving the joints of the client through the range of motion. The client does not participate in joint movement.
- ***Active–assistive*** ROM exercises involve the client's participation as much as possible, with a support worker assisting in the exercises the client is not able to perform.

BOX 26–2 Joint Movements

Abduction—moving a body part away from the midline of the body
Adduction—moving a body part toward the midline of the body
Extension—straightening a body part
Flexion—bending a body part
Hyperextension—straightening a body part excessively
Dorsiflexion—bending the toes and foot up at the ankle
Rotation—turning the joint
Internal rotation—turning the joint inward
External rotation—turning the joint outward
Plantar flexion—bending the foot down at the ankle
Pronation—turning downward
Supination—turning upward

ROM exercises occur naturally during ADLs such as bathing, hair care, eating, reaching, and walking—all of which involve joint movements. Clients on bed rest and clients who have mobility loss from illness or injury, however, get very little activity. Therefore, their care plans usually call for ROM exercises. The care plan tells you which joints to exercise and whether the exercises are to be active, passive, or active–assistive. If you have questions, ask your supervisor (see the *Focus on Children: Play* and *Focus on Long-Term Care: Activity Programs* boxes).

ROM exercises can cause injury, such as muscle strain, joint injury, and pain, if not done properly. ***It is important to follow the client's care plan. Some ROM exercises (especially involving the neck) can cause serious client injury.*** Follow the guidelines in BOX 26–3 when performing or assisting with ROM exercises.

After performing ROM exercises with the client, report and record the following:

- The time the exercises were performed
- The joints exercised
- The number of times the exercises were performed on each joint
- Complaints of pain or signs of stiffness or spasm
- The degree to which the client took part in the exercises

FOCUS ON CHILDREN

Play

Any play activity promotes active ROM exercises in children. Examples include the following:

- Kicking a Mylar balloon or foam rubber ball
- Playing "pat-a-cake" and having the child clap, kick, jump, or do other motions
- Playing basketball using a wastebasket and a foam rubber ball or wadded paper
- Playing video games for finger and hand movements
- Playing with fingerpaints, clay, or playdough
- Having tricycle or wheelchair races
- Playing "hide and seek" by hiding a toy in the bed or room
- Colouring and painting

Always check the care plan for the child's activity limits. If you are still unsure, check with your supervisor.

Source: Adapted from Hockenberry, M.J., & Wilson, D. (2007). *Wong's nursing care of infants and children* (8th ed.). St. Louis, MO: Mosby.

BOX 26–3 Guidelines for Performing Range-of-Motion Exercises

- Exercise only the joints you are instructed to exercise.
- Expose only the body part being exercised.
- Use good body mechanics.
- Support the part being exercised.
- Move the joint slowly, smoothly, and gently.
- Do not force a joint beyond its present range of motion or to the point of pain.
- ***Perform range-of-motion exercises to the neck only if allowed by employer policy.*** In some facilities and agencies, only physiotherapists or occupational therapists do neck exercises because of the danger of neck injuries.

FOCUS ON LONG-TERM CARE

Activity Programs

Canada's provinces have long-term care legislation that requires facilities to have an assessment and care-planning process to prevent unnecessary reduction in a client's range of motion. Prevention involves active, active–assistive, or passive ROM exercises. Splints and braces are used if needed. The territories currently do not have this legislation.

In most provinces, for a long-term care facility to be licensed to operate, it needs to have activity programs in place. Recreational activities performed exercise the joints and muscles and stimulate the circulation. They also provide social opportunities and are mentally stimulating.

The activities must meet the interests and physical and psychosocial needs of each client. Facilities often arrange for bingo, movies, dances, exercise groups, gardening activities, shopping trips, museum trips, concerts, and guest speakers.

The right to personal choice is protected in all arrangements, so the client chooses which activities to take part in. Activities should promote physical, intellectual, social, spiritual, and emotional well-being, the last of which is promoted when the client attends activities of personal choice. Clients must not be forced to take part in activities that hold no interest for them.

Clients may need help getting to an activity and participating in it. As a support worker, you must provide assistance as necessary.

Activity ideas are always welcome from anybody. Clients may share ideas with you or tell you about favourite pastimes, or you may have your own ideas. Share these with the health care team so that they are given to the team that plans activities.

Performing Range-of-Motion Exercises

Advocate on behalf of the client's quality of life by promoting:

Dignity • Independence • Preferences • Privacy • Safety *(see BOX 1–4, on p. 17)*

PRE-PROCEDURE

1 Ensure that your own muscles are warmed up by performing ROM exercises on your own joints daily and before beginning this procedure. Practise good posture and body mechanics throughout this skill.
This may greatly reduce the risk for personal injury while providing client care.
Ask the client if he or she would like background music playing during the exercise.
2 Identify the client, according to employer policy.
3 Explain the procedure to the client.
4 Perform hand hygiene.
5 Obtain a **bath blanket or use the top sheet** to cover the client. Only the part of the body you are exercising should be exposed.
6 Provide for privacy.
7 Raise the bed to a comfortable working height. Follow the care plan for bed rail use.*
This is done to reduce the risk for back strain to the worker.

PROCEDURE

8 Lower the bed rail closer to you.
9 Place the client in the supine position.
10 Cover the client with a sheet. Fan-fold top linens to the foot of the bed.

Continued

Performing Range-of-Motion Exercises—cont'd

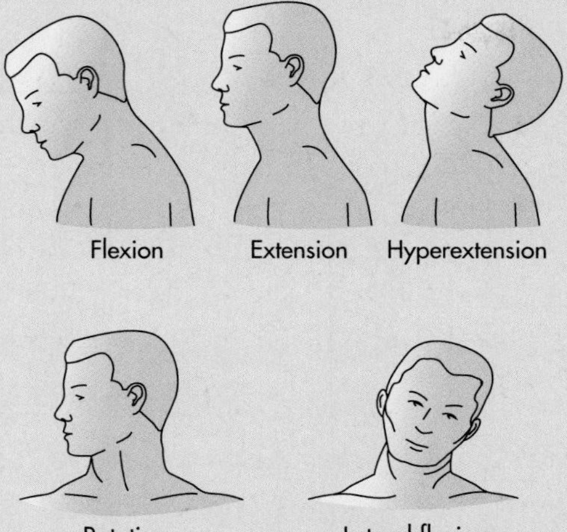

FIGURE 26–10 Range-of-motion exercises for the neck.

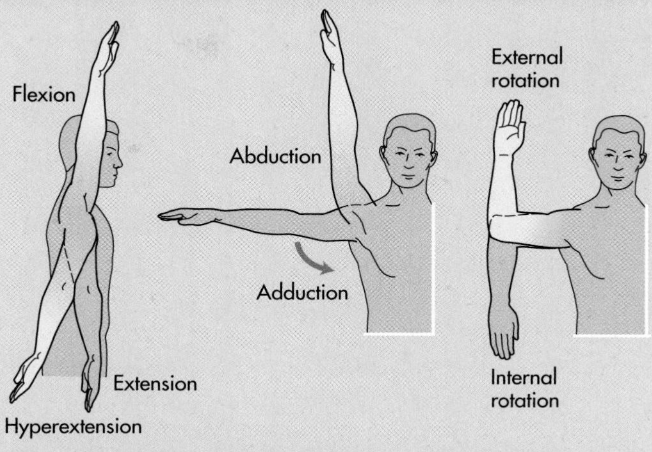

FIGURE 26–11 Range-of-motion exercises for the shoulder.

Fan-folded linens are easier to grasp and to straighten out than rolled-up linens.

11 Exercise the neck ***only if allowed by your employer and if your supervisor instructs you to do so*** (**FIGURE 26–10**). ***It is important to follow the client's care plan. Some ROM exercises (especially involving the neck) can cause serious client injury.***

Exercising the neck when it is not allowed can cause injury to your client.

- a Place your hands over the client's ears to support the head. Support the jaws with your fingers.
- b *Rotation*—turn the head from side to side.
- c *Lateral flexion*—move the head to the right and to the left. Stop if the client complains of discomfort.
- d Repeat *b* and *c* five times or the number of times stated on the care plan.

12 Exercise the shoulder (**FIGURE 26–11**):

Exercising each joint will reduce the risk for joint stiffening and loss of mobility.

- a Grasp the wrist with one hand. Grasp the elbow with your other hand.
- b *Flexion*—raise the arm straight in front and over the head.
- c *Extension*—bring the arm down to the side.
- d *Hyperextension*—move the arm behind the body. (Do this if the client sits in a straight-backed chair or is standing.)
- e *Abduction*—move the straight arm away from the side of the body.
- f *Adduction*—move the straight arm to the side of the body.
- g *Internal rotation*—bend the arm at the elbow. Place it at the same level as the shoulder. Move the forearm down toward the body.
- h *External rotation*—move the forearm toward the head.
- i Repeat *b* through *h* five times or the number of times stated on the care plan.

13 Exercise the elbow (**FIGURE 26–12**):

- a Grasp the client's wrist with one hand. Grasp the elbow with your other hand.
- b *Flexion*—bend the arm so the hand touches the same-side shoulder.
- c *Extension*—straighten the arm.
- d Repeat *b* and *c* five times or the number of times stated on the care plan.

14 Exercise the forearm (**FIGURE 26–13**):

- a *Pronation*—turn the hand so that the palm is down.
- b *Supination*—turn the hand so that the palm is up.

Continued

Performing Range-of-Motion Exercises—cont'd

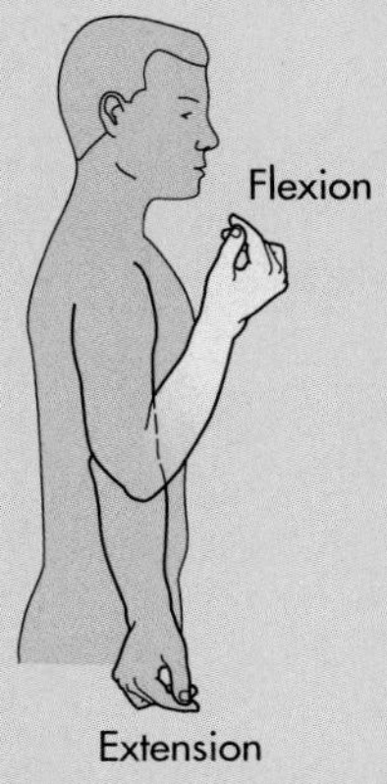

FIGURE 26–12 Range-of-motion exercises for the elbow.

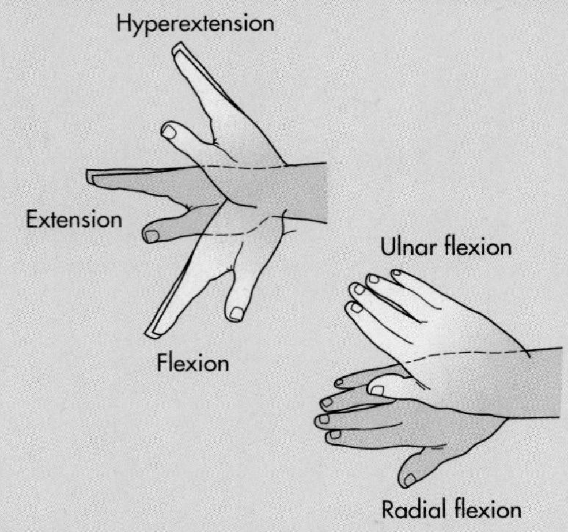

FIGURE 26–14 Range-of-motion exercises for the wrist.

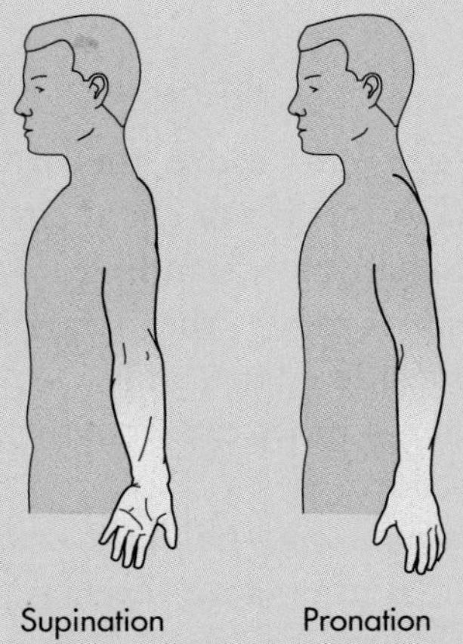

FIGURE 26–13 Range-of-motion exercises for the forearm.

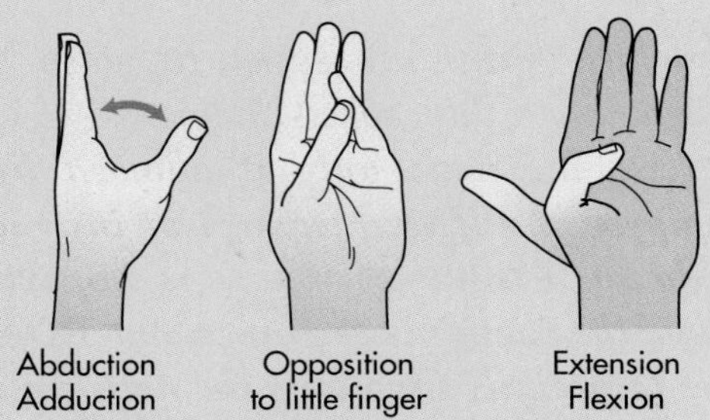

FIGURE 26–15 Range-of-motion exercises for the thumb.

   c Repeat *a* and *b* five times or the number of times stated on the care plan.

15 Exercise the wrist (FIGURE 26–14):
   a Hold the wrist with both hands.
   b *Flexion*—bend the hand down.
   c *Extension*—straighten the hand.
   d *Hyperextension*—bend the hand back.
   e *Radial flexion*—turn the hand toward the thumb.
   f *Ulnar flexion*—turn the hand toward the little finger.
   g Repeat *b* through *f* five times or the number of times stated on the care plan.

16 Exercise the thumb (FIGURE 26–15):
   a Hold the client's hand with one hand. Hold the thumb with your other hand.
   b *Abduction*—move the thumb out from the inner part of the index finger.
   c *Adduction*—move the thumb back next to the index finger.
   d *Opposition*—touch each fingertip with the thumb.
   e *Flexion*—bend the thumb into the hand.
   f *Extension*—move the thumb out to the side of the fingers.
   g Repeat *b* through *f* five times or the number of times stated on the care plan.

17 Exercise the fingers (FIGURE 26–16):
   a *Abduction*—spread the fingers and thumbs apart.
   b *Adduction*—bring the fingers and thumbs together.
   c *Extension*—straighten the fingers so that the fingers, hand, and arm are straight.

Continued

Performing Range-of-Motion Exercises—cont'd

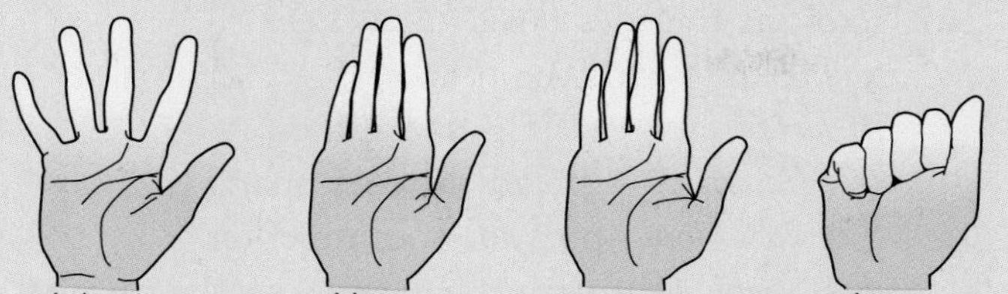

FIGURE 26–16 Range-of-motion exercises for the fingers.

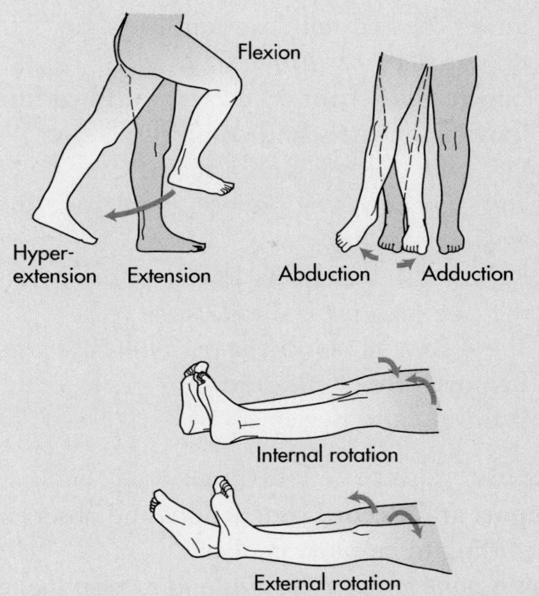

FIGURE 26–17 Range-of-motion exercises for the hip.

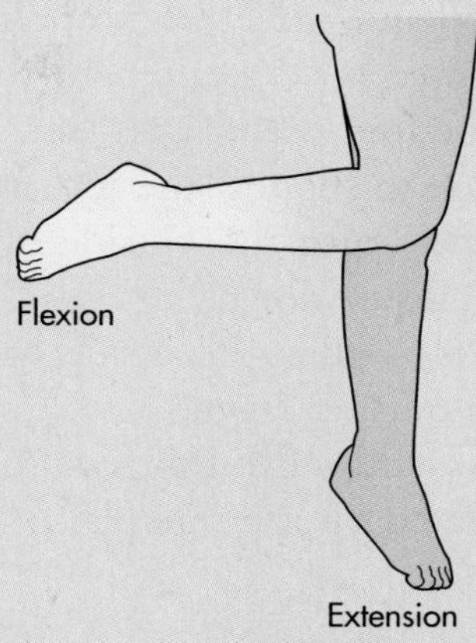

FIGURE 26–18 Range-of-motion exercises for the knee.

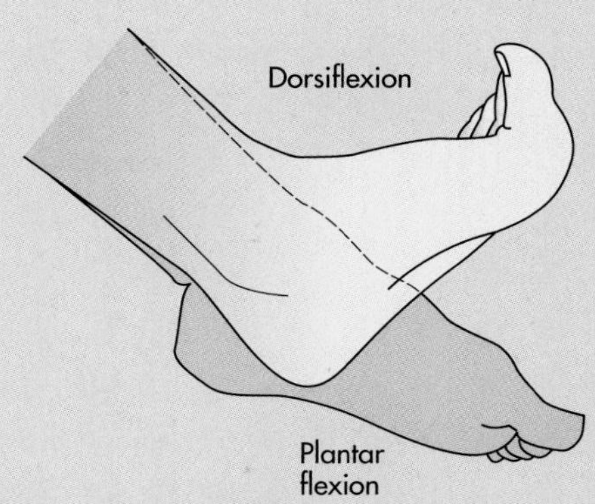

FIGURE 26–19 Range-of-motion exercises for the ankle.

- **d** *Flexion*—make a fist.
- **e** Repeat *a* through *d* five times or the number of times stated on the care plan.

18 Exercise the hip (**FIGURE 26–17**):
- **a** Support the leg. Place one hand under the knee. Place your other hand under the ankle.
- **b** *Flexion*—raise the leg.
- **c** *Extension*—straighten the leg.
- **d** *Abduction*—move the leg away from the body.
- **e** *Adduction*—move the leg toward the other leg.
- **f** *Internal rotation*—turn the leg inward.
- **g** *External rotation*—turn the leg outward.
- **h** Repeat *b* through *g* five times or the number of times stated on the care plan.

19 Exercise the knee (**FIGURE 26–18**):
- **a** Support the knee. Place one hand under the knee. Place your other hand under the ankle.
- **b** *Flexion*—bend the leg.
- **c** *Extension*—straighten the leg.
- **d** Repeat *b* and *c* five times or the number of times stated on the care plan.

20 Exercise the ankle (**FIGURE 26–19**):
- **a** Support the foot and ankle. Place one hand under the foot. Place your other hand under the ankle.
- **b** *Dorsiflexion*—pull the foot forward. Push down on the heel at the same time.
- **c** *Plantar flexion*—turn the foot down, or point the toes.

Continued

Performing Range-of-Motion Exercises—cont'd

d Repeat *b* and *c* five times or the number of times stated on the care plan.

21 Exercise the foot (**FIGURE 26–20**):
- a Continue to support the foot and ankle.
- b *Pronation*—turn the outside of the foot up and the inside down.
- c *Supination*—turn the inside of the foot up and the outside down.
- d Repeat *b* and *c* five times or the number of times stated on the care plan.

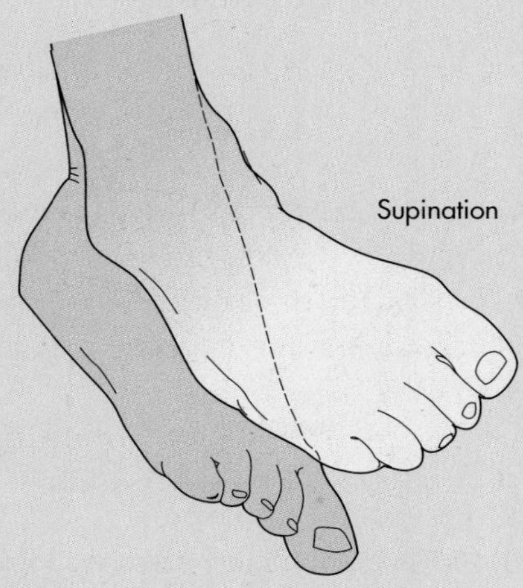

FIGURE 26–20 Range-of-motion exercises for the foot.

22 Exercise the toes (**FIGURE 26–21**):
- a *Flexion*—curl the toes.
- b *Extension*—straighten the toes.
- c *Abduction*—spread the toes apart.
- d *Adduction*—pull the toes together.
- e Repeat *a* through *d* five times or the number of times stated on the care plan.

23 Cover the leg.

24 Raise the bed rail, if used. Go to the other side. Lower the bed rail near you if it is up.

25 Repeat steps 12 through 22.

26 Ensure your client is covered with bed linens.

27 Provide for safety and comfort.

28 Place the call bell within reach.*
This is an easy, safe way for the client to contact staff, if necessary.

29 Return the bed to its lowest position. Follow the care plan for bed rail use.*
This is done to reduce the risk of the client falling.

30 Remove privacy measures.

31 Perform hand hygiene.

Report and Record your actions and observations according to employer policy.
This is done for legal reasons and to keep the rest of the health care team informed.

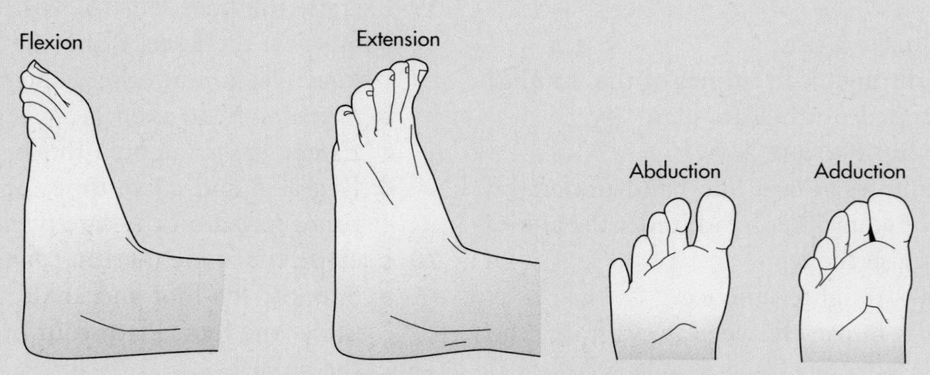

FIGURE 26–21 Range-of-motion exercises for the toes.

*Steps marked with an asterisk may not apply in community settings.

AMBULATION

Ambulation, the act of walking, helps prevent deconditioning if done regularly. A number of clients need help walking. Some clients become strong enough to walk independently, but some continue to need help, possibly even permanently.

After bed rest, activity is usually increased slowly and in steps. First, the client dangles the legs over the side of the bed. The next step is to sit in a bedside chair, followed by walking about in the room and then in the hallway. Ambulation is not a problem if complications (such as contractures and muscle atrophy) have been prevented by proper positioning and exercise.

Your facility may use a gait (transfer) belt when helping clients who are weak or unsteady (see **FIGURE 26–22** and Chapter 25). Encourage the client to use handrails along the wall for additional support. Always check the client for orthostatic hypotension.

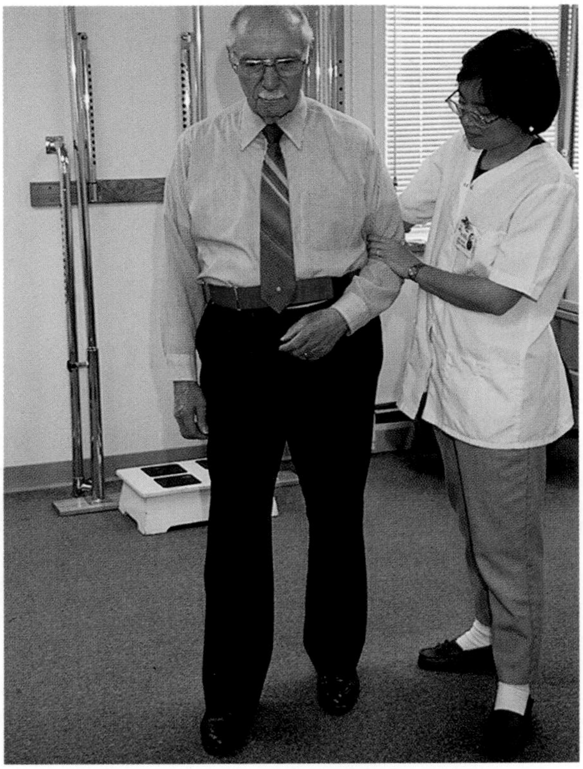

FIGURE 26–22 Assist with ambulation by walking slightly behind the client's side. Use a gait belt for the client's safety.

Before beginning the walk, remove any obstacles in the path. If necessary, place a chair nearby in case the client needs to rest. Also, make sure the client is wearing nonskid footwear.

If your client has suffered a cerebrovascular accident (CVA, or stroke) and has weakness or paralysis on one side of the body, the side of the client on which you walk will depend on the care plan, your employer's policy, and the walking environment. Generally, clients who have weakness on one side and are using a cane or handrails use the strong side for support while the support worker protects the weak side. If there are no handrails or walking aids, the support worker should walk on the weak side of the client to assist, walking slightly behind the client's side (**FIGURE 26–22**).

Encourage personal choices in walking. The client may want to walk outside and may prefer to walk at a particular time of day. The client may want to wait until a visitor arrives or leaves. Allow such choices whenever safe and possible and only with your supervisor's approval.

After helping the client with ambulation, report and record the following:

- How well the client tolerated the activity
- Any complaints of pain or discomfort
- The distance walked

Obesity and Lifestyle and Their Effect on Ambulation

People who are overweight subject their joints to increased wear, which in turn can contribute to the development of osteoarthritis (OA). The most common type of arthritis, OA causes the cartilage within the joints of the body to be worn away, resulting in pain and disfigurement in the joints (see Chapter 37). Obesity and a sedentary lifestyle are the main contributors to OA.[1] Excess weight puts stress on weight-bearing joints, such as knees and hips, and increases the risk for cartilage breakdown.[2] People who are overweight are encouraged to lose weight in order to reduce the load on their joints.

Helping the Client to Walk

123

Advocate on behalf of the client's quality of life by promoting:

Dignity • Independence • Preferences • Privacy • Safety

(see BOX 1–4, on p. 17)

PRE-PROCEDURE

1 Ensure that your own muscles are warmed up by performing ROM exercises on your own joints daily and before beginning this procedure. Practise good posture and body mechanics throughout this skill.
Warm-up exercises have been proven to reduce the chance of pain and personal injury while providing care.
2 Identify the client, according to employer policy.
3 Explain the procedure to the client.
4 Perform hand hygiene.
5 Collect the following supplies:
☐ **Robe and nonskid shoes**
These items help ensure that the client will not slip on the floor and that the client's body is covered.
☐ **Paper or sheet to protect bottom linens**
☐ **Gait (transfer) belt if used in your agency**
This helps prevent falls by providing a means to hold on to the client.
6 Provide for privacy.

PROCEDURE

7 Lower the bed to its lowest position. Lock the bed wheels. Lower the bed rail, if used.*
8 Fan-fold top linens to the foot of the bed.
Fan-folded linen is easier to grasp to cover your client than rolled-up linens at the end of the bed.
9 a Place paper or sheet on the bed.
This protects the bed linens from shoe soiling.
b Put the shoes on the client. It may be easier to put on shoes when your client is sitting on the side of the bed.
10 Help the client to dangle the legs (see the procedure *Helping the Client Sit on the Side of the Bed (Dangle the Legs)* on p. 508 in Chapter 25).
11 Help the client put on a robe if the client is not dressed.
12 Depending on your employer's policy, apply the gait belt (see the procedure *Applying a Transfer Belt* on p. 516 in Chapter 25).
13 Help the client stand up (see the procedure *Transferring the Client to a Chair or Wheelchair* on p. 517 in Chapter 25). If the client is wearing a gait belt, grasp it on each side. Alternatively, place your arms under the client's arms around to the shoulder blades. If the client is too weak to stand, safely seat the client back on the bed.
14 Stand at the client's side while the client gains balance. Hold the belt at the side and back, or have one arm around the client's back for support.
It is important to have a secure grasp on the client to help prevent a fall.
15 Encourage the client to stand erect with the head up and back straight.
This position helps improve the client's sense of balance.
16 Help the client walk. Walk to the side and slightly behind the client. Provide support with the gait belt (**FIGURE 26–22**), or have one arm around the client's back to support the client. Check the care plan regarding how to safely provide support.
17 Encourage the client to walk normally. The heel should strike the floor first. Discourage shuffling, sliding, or walking on tiptoes.

Continued

Helping the Client to Walk—cont'd

18 Walk the required distance if the client can tolerate the activity. Do not rush the client. As a support worker, you want to encourage any effort your clients make.
Discouraged clients may be less inclined to ambulate again.

19 Help the client return to bed:
- **a** Have the client stand at the side of the bed.
- **b** Pivot the client a quarter turn. The backs of the knees should touch the bed. It is important to know that if the client has a one-sided weakness (perhaps from a stroke), the client should always lead or pivot from the strong side.
- **c** Grasp the sides of the gait belt.
- **d** Lower the client onto the bed as you bend your knees. Remove gait belt and robe.
- **e** Help the client lie down (see the procedure *Helping the Client Sit on the Side of the Bed (Dangle the Legs)* on p. 508 in Chapter 25).

By helping to support the client while he slowly lowers himself to a seated position, you may prevent a fall.

20 Help the client to the centre of the bed.
This is done for the comfort of the client.

21 Remove shoes if they were not removed when the client was sitting on the side of the bed. Remove the paper from the bottom sheet if used.

POST-PROCEDURE

22 Provide for safety and comfort.

23 Place the call bell within reach.*
This provides an easy, safe way for the client to contact staff, if necessary.

24 Follow the care plan for bed rail use.*

25 Remove privacy measures.

26 Return the robe and shoes to their proper place.
This shows respect for your client's possessions.

27 Perform hand hygiene.

Report and Record your actions and observations, according to employer policy.
This is done for legal reasons and to keep the rest of the health care team informed.

*Steps marked with an asterisk may not apply in community settings.

Falls

A client may start to fall when standing or walking. If the client is weak, light-headed, or dizzy, fainting may occur. Falling may be caused by slipping or sliding on spills, waxed floors, or throw rugs or by wearing improper shoes (see Chapter 22).

When a client is falling, the support worker's instinct is to try to prevent the fall. However, trying to prevent a fall could cause greater harm. ***You could injure yourself and the client as you twist and strain to stop the fall.*** Or you could lose your balance, and both you and the client could fall, causing head, hip, and knee injuries to occur.

Instead, if a client starts to fall, ease the client to the floor. By doing so, you control the direction of the fall and also protect the client's head (see **FIGURE 26–23** on page 549).

Your response after the fall will depend on whether you work in a facility with help readily available or in a private home, where you will likely be working alone (see the *Focus on Home Care: When a Client Falls* box). If a client falls in a facility, do not move the client or allow the client to get up. Remain calm, and reassure the client. Call for a nurse to check the client for injuries, and, later, complete an incident report, as required by facility policy.

FOCUS ON HOME CARE

When a Client Falls

When working in a private home, you will not have a nurse present to help you if a client falls. Be aware of any procedures required by your employer in the case of a fall. Use the following as a guide.

If a client starts to fall, ease her to the floor (see the procedure *Helping the Falling Client*, below.). After the fall, check for the following signs:

- Pain or tenderness
- Swelling or bruising
- Inability to move a limb or difficulty moving a limb
- Bleeding
- Client report of having felt or heard a bone snap or pop

If you observe any of the above, or if you suspect the client has a head, neck, or back injury, ***do not move the client***. Call 9-1-1 and then your supervisor for help. Keep the client warm and calm, and stay with the client until help arrives.

If the client is unhurt and is able to assist, help her up. Follow these steps:

- Place a chair beside the client. Have the client use the armrests for support.
- Support the client's hips and assist her into a kneeling position, facing the chair.
- Have the client rest the forearms on the chair.
- Tell the client to lift one knee and place the foot on the floor. Assist as required.
- On the count of three, help the client push up, stand, and pivot into the chair, while holding on to the armrests.
- Once the client is in the chair, let her rest before assisting her up again.

Report the fall to your supervisor. Complete an incident report, according to employer policy.

Helping the Falling Client

123

Advocate on behalf of the client's quality of life by promoting:

Dignity • Independence • Preferences • Privacy • Safety *(see BOX 1–4, on p. 17)*

PROCEDURE

1 Stand with your feet apart. Keep your back straight.
A broad base of support will prevent you from losing your balance while performing this procedure.

2 Bring the client close to your body as quickly as possible. Use the gait belt if the client is wearing one. If not, wrap your arms around the client's waist. You can also hold the client under the arms (**FIGURE 26–23, A**).
This will ensure that the client does not fall forward on the face, and you can slide the client down your leg.

3 Move your leg so the client's buttocks rest on it.
*This position allows you to slide the client to the floor safely. Move your leg near the client (**FIGURE 26–23, B**).*

4 Lower the client to the floor, letting him slide down your leg. Bend at your hips and knees as you lower the client (**FIGURE 26–23, C**). Do not bend from the waist.
This helps prevent injury to you or the client.

5 After the fall:
   a If you are in a facility, call for a nurse. Stay with the client, and do not move.

Continued

Helping the Falling Client—cont'd

A

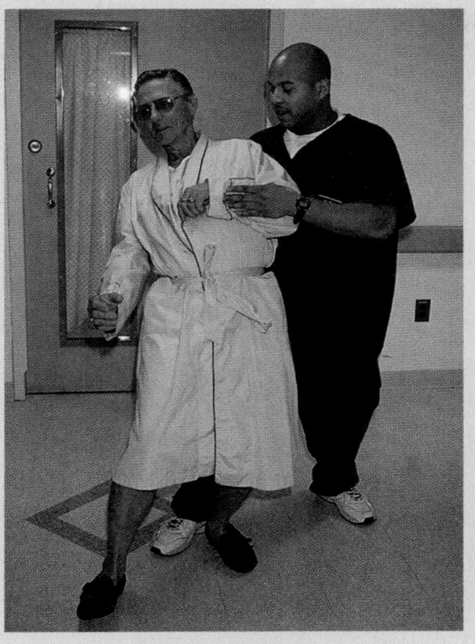

FIGURE 26–23 A

B

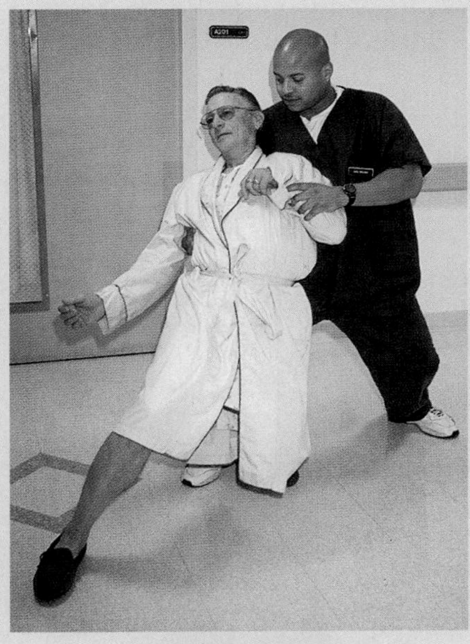

FIGURE 26–23 B

b If you are in a home care setting, check for obvious signs of injury. ***If there are obvious signs of injury, do not move the client; call 9-1-1, and then call your supervisor***. Keep the client warm and calm until help arrives.

C

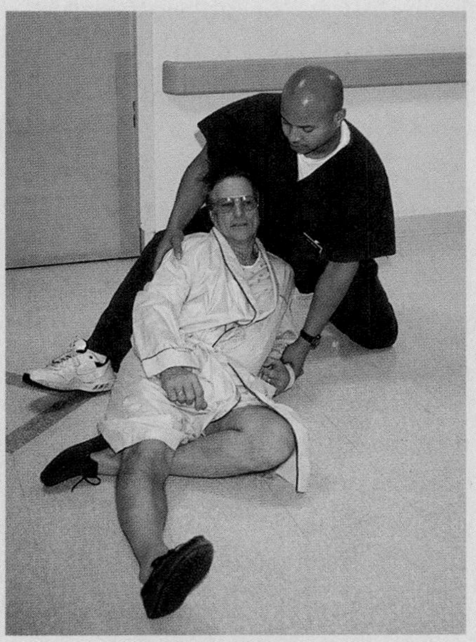

FIGURE 26–23 C

c The nurse will then assess if any injury has occurred to the client or to you.

d Many community agencies have policies against individual caregivers' helping clients off the floor unless the clients have the mobility to do so on their own.

Policies exist to prevent injuries or to reduce their severity.

Report and Record your actions and observations, according to employer policy. Include the following:

- ☐ How the fall occurred
- ☐ How far the client walked
- ☐ How activity was tolerated before the fall
- ☐ Any complaints before the fall
- ☐ The amount of assistance needed by the client while walking

This is done for legal reasons and to keep the rest of the health care team informed.

It is also important to complete an incident report and record the actions you took. See Figure 22-29 on page 412 for a sample incident report.

Walking Aids

Walking aids support the body and are ordered by the physician, nurse, or physiotherapist. The type ordered depends on the client's physical condition, the amount of support needed, and the type of disability.

Crutches

Crutches are used when the client cannot use one leg or when one or both legs need to gain strength. Some clients with permanent leg weakness use crutches, usually Lofstrand crutches (**FIGURE 26–24**), which are made of metal. A metal band fits around the forearm. Axillary crutches, made of wood or metal, extend from the underarm (*axilla*) to the ground (**FIGURE 26–25**). A regulated health care provider teaches the client to use crutches safely.

A client who needs crutches must learn to walk, climb upstairs and climb downstairs, and sit and stand using the crutches. Safety is important, as the client using crutches is at risk for falls. Follow these safety measures:

- Check the crutch tips. Report worn or torn crutch tips to your supervisor, and replace them according to policy. If the tips are wet, dry them with a towel or paper towels.
- Check crutches for flaws—wooden crutches for cracks and metal crutches for bends. All bolts must be tight.
- Make sure the client wears well-fitted, flat, nonskid street shoes.
- Ensure the client's clothing fits well. Loose clothing may get caught between the crutches and underarms. Loose clothing can also hang forward

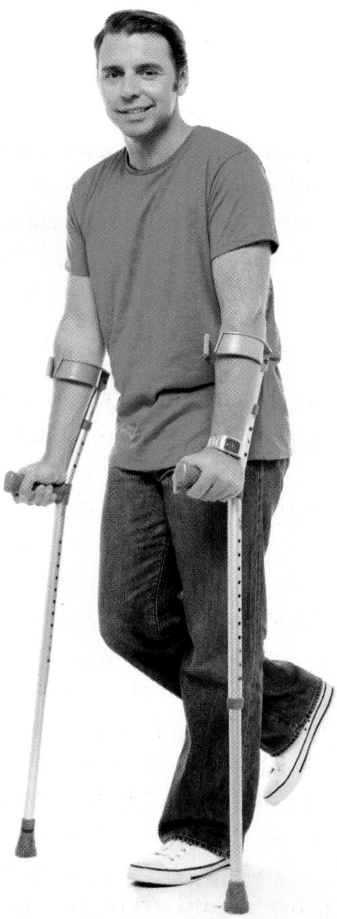

FIGURE 26–24 Lofstrand, or Canadian, crutches. (**Source:** stockyimages/Shutterstock.com)

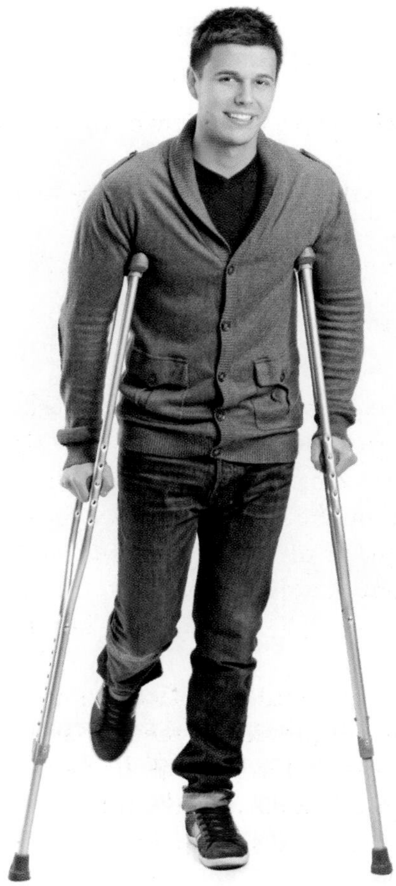

FIGURE 26–25 Axillary crutches. (**Source:** Ljupco Smokovski/Shutterstock.com)

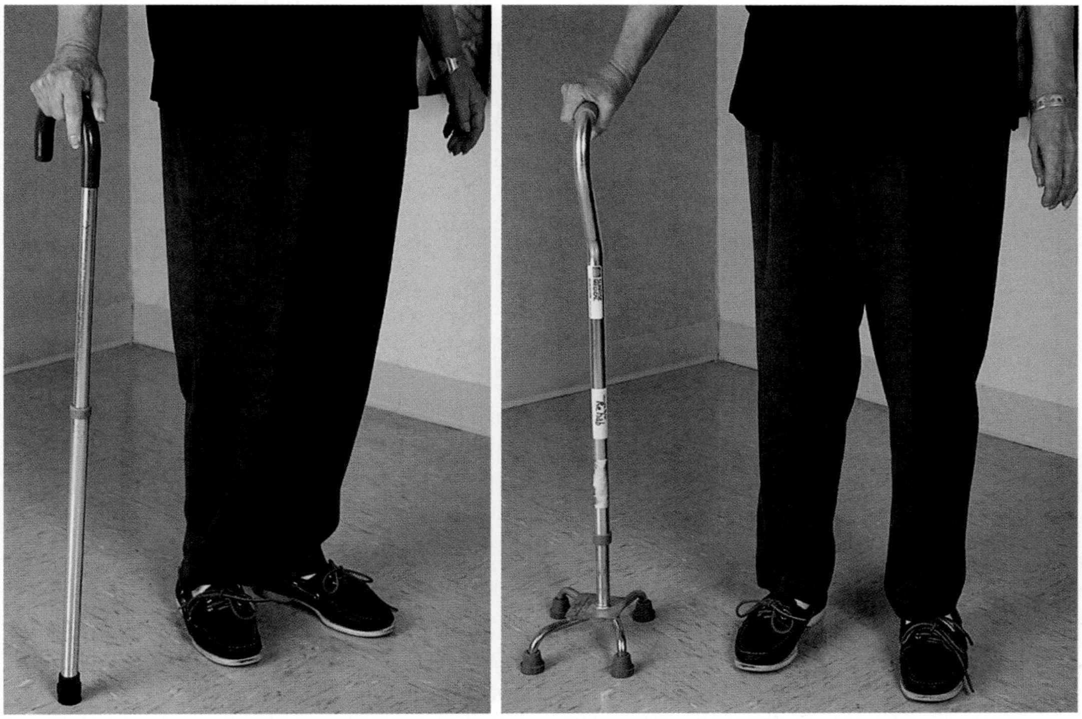

FIGURE 26–26 **A,** Single-tip cane. **B,** Four-point (quad) cane.

and block the person's view of the feet and crutch tips.

- Practise safety measures to prevent falls (see Chapter 22).
- Keep crutches within reach of the client when not in use.

Canes

Canes are used to help support a weak side of the body and to provide balance. Single-tip and four-point (quad) canes (**FIGURE 26–26**) are available. A cane is held on the *strong (unaffected) side* of the body. (For example, if the left leg is weak, the cane is held in the right hand.) Four-point canes give more support than single-tip canes do but are harder to move.

The cane tip should be placed about 15 to 25 cm (6 to 10 in.) to the side of the foot and about 15 to 25 cm (6 to 10 in.) in front of the foot on the strong side. The grip is level with the hip.

The person walks as follows:

1. The cane is moved forward 15 to 25 cm (6 to 10 in.) (**FIGURE 26–27, *A***).
2. The weak leg (opposite the cane) is moved forward even with the cane (**FIGURE 26–27, *B***).
3. The strong leg is brought forward and ahead of the cane and the weak leg (**FIGURE 26–27, *C***).

Walkers

A walker is a four-point walking aid (**FIGURE 26–28**). It gives more support than a cane does. Most people feel safer and more secure with a walker than with a cane. There are different kinds of walkers. The standard walker is picked up and moved about 15 to 20 cm (6 to 8 in.) in front of the client. The client then moves the weak leg and foot and then the strong leg and foot up to the walker (**FIGURE 26–29, *A* and *B***).

A wheeled walker has wheels on the front legs and rubber tips on the back legs (**FIGURE 26–30** on page 553). The client pushes the walker ahead about 15 to 20 cm (6 to 8 in.) and then walks up to it. The rubber tips on the back legs prevent the walker from moving while the client is walking or standing.

Baskets, pouches, and trays can be attached to walkers (**FIGURE 26–28**). The attachment is used to carry needed items. These help the client to be more

A B C

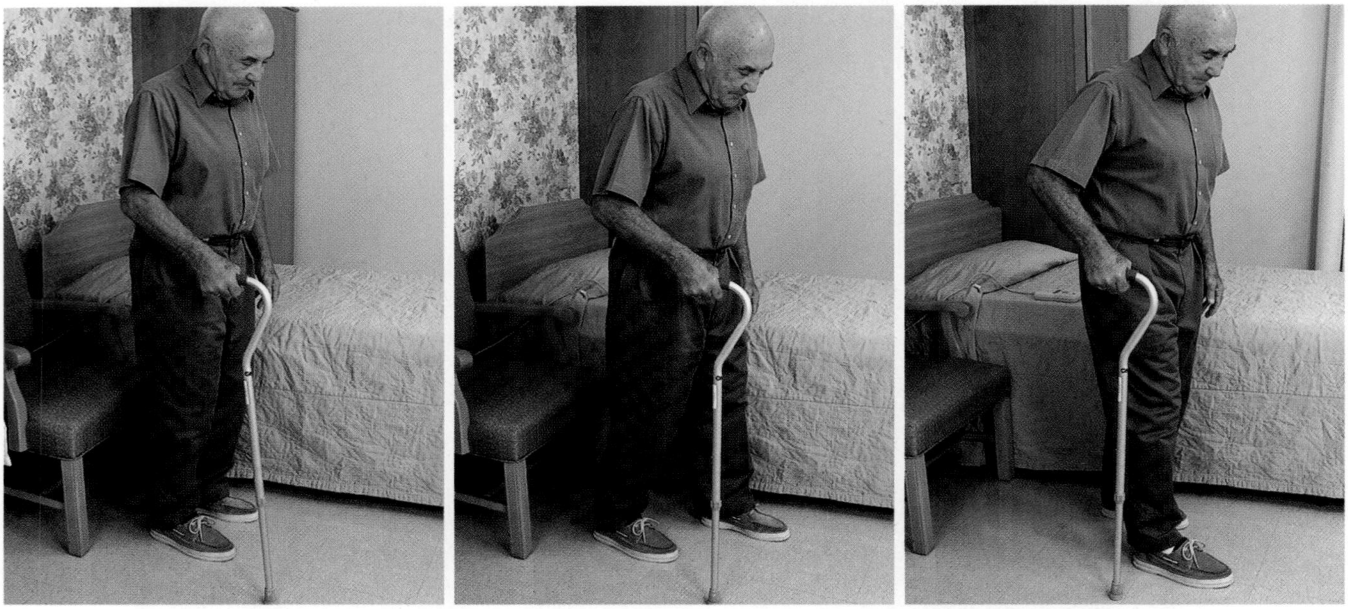

FIGURE 26–27 Walking with a cane. **A,** The cane is moved forward about 15 to 25 cm (6 to 10 in.). **B,** The leg opposite the cane (weak leg) is brought forward even with the cane. **C,** The leg on the cane side (strong leg) is moved ahead of the cane and the weak leg.

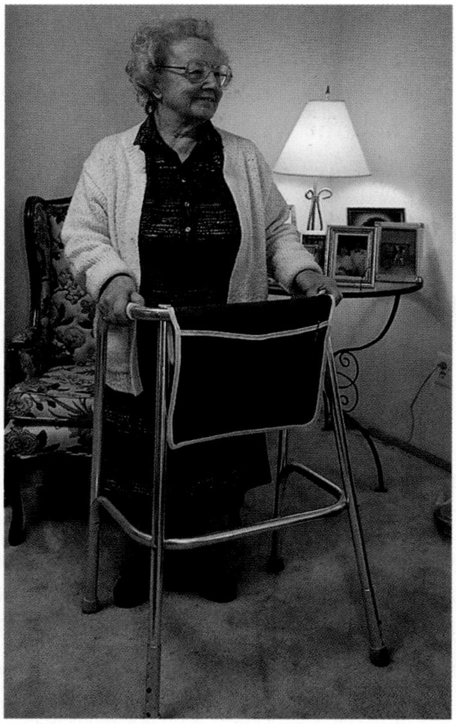

FIGURE 26–28 A walker. This walker has a pocket in the front designed to hold personal items.

A

B

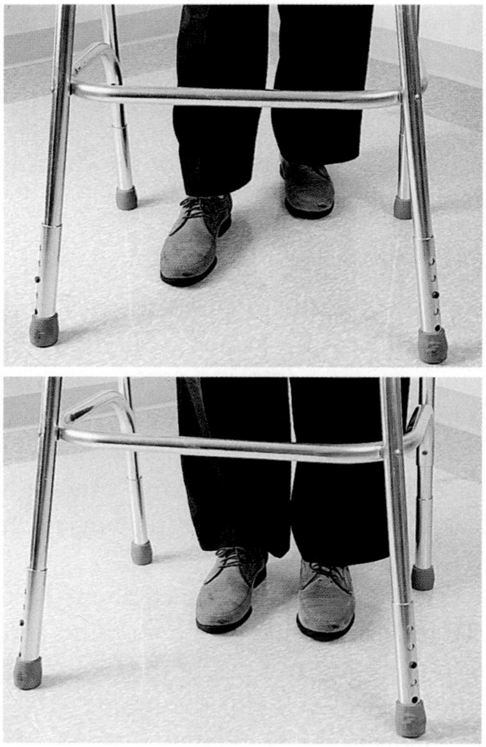

FIGURE 26–29 Walking with a walker. **A,** The walker is moved about 15 cm (6 in.) in front of the person. **B,** Both feet are moved up to the walker.

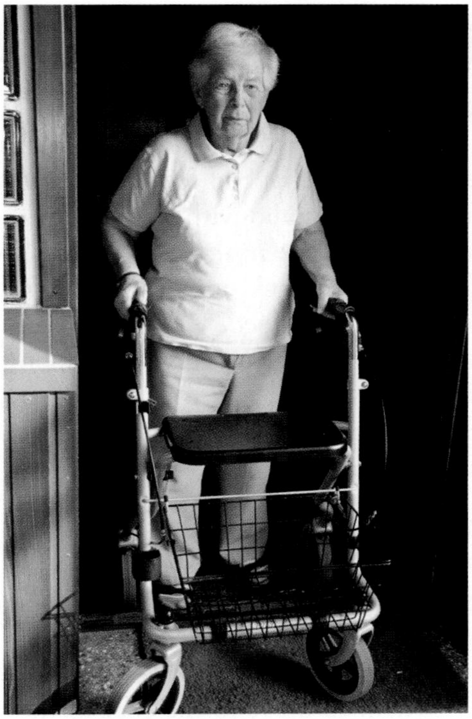

FIGURE 26–30 A woman using a wheeled walker. (**Source:** ©iStockphoto.com/SilviaJansen.)

independent and not have to rely on others. The attachment also keeps the hands free to grip the walker.

The client uses the walker for support when moving from a standing to a sitting position. Assist clients with walkers, as needed (**BOX 26–4**).

Braces

A **brace (orthotic)** is an apparatus—metal, plastic, or leather—worn to support or align weak body parts or to prevent or correct problems with the musculoskeletal system (see Chapter 37). A brace is applied over the ankle, knee, or back (**FIGURE 26–31**). An ankle–foot orthosis (AFO) is positioned in the shoe (**FIGURE 26–32**); then the foot is inserted, and the device is secured in place with a Velcro strap.

Skin and bony points under the braces should be kept clean and dry to prevent skin breakdown. Report redness or signs of skin breakdown (see Chapter 24) and any complaints of pain or discomfort. In facilities, the nurse assesses the skin under braces during every shift. The care plan tells you when to apply and remove a brace.

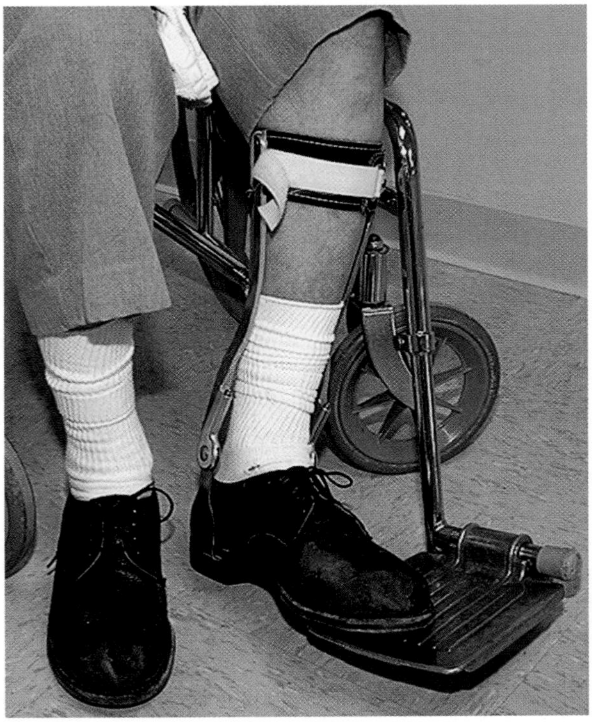

FIGURE 26–31 Leg brace.

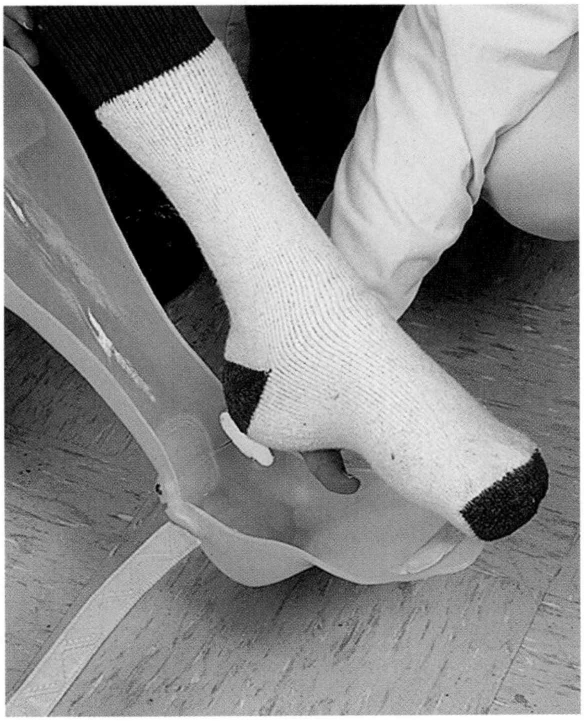

FIGURE 26–32 Ankle–foot orthosis.

BOX 26–4 Helping Clients With Walkers to Sit and Stand

Helping the Client Sit on a Chair, Wheelchair, or Toilet

- Lock the wheels of the wheelchair.
- Ask the client to stand with the back to the chair, wheelchair, or toilet.
- Ask the client to back up with the walker until the knees touch the seat.
- Ask the client to take one hand off the walker and to use that hand to reach and grasp the armrest or grab bar.
- Help the client slowly sit down. The buttocks should be at the back of the seat.
- If armrests or grab bars are not available, support the client as the client sits down. (Use a transfer belt if the client is weak or unsteady.)
- Move the walker away from the client.
- Support the client in the standing position.
- Place your hands under the client's arms and over the shoulder blades.
- Block the client's feet and knees with your feet and knees.
- Lower the client onto the seat slowly.

Helping the Client Sit on a Bed

- Use a transfer belt if the client is weak or unsteady.
- Raise the head of the bed to a sitting position.
- Ask the client to stand with the back to the bed. The client should be near the middle of the bed.
- Ask the client to back up with the walker until the knees touch the bed.
- Ask the client to reach for the bed with one hand. Assist as necessary.
- Help the client sit down slowly.
- Provide for comfort.

Helping the Client Move From Sitting to Standing

- Place the walker where the client can reach it with ease.
- Let the client position the walker.
- Ask the client to move to the edge of the seat or bed.
- Help the client rise to a standing position, as needed.
- Do not let the client pull himself up with the walker. He should push on the mattress or chair armrests and then transfer his hands to the walker.

CHAPTER REVIEW

KEY POINTS

- Being active is important for physical and mental well-being. Inactivity, whether mild or severe, affects not only the normal functions of all body systems but also the client's mental sense of well-being.
- Bed rest is ordered by a physician to reduce physical activity, reduce pain, encourage rest, regain strength, promote healing, or a combination of these.
- Complications of bed rest are contractures, atrophy, orthostatic hypotension, and syncope.
- A support worker must keep in mind important safety measures when moving a client from a lying position to sitting, from sitting to standing, and from standing to walking, and while using walking aids.
- Your role as a support worker may include providing range-of-motion exercises to your client to reduce the effects of bed rest and to maintain or improve the mobility of joints.
- The care plan and the supervisor or physiotherapist will give you instructions for the exercises.
- If your client starts to fall while walking, you must protect your client and yourself from injury.
- Walking aids include crutches, canes, walkers, and wheeled walkers, and as a support worker, you will need to know the purpose of each aid. Your client may tell you about any difficulties with the aid. Do not adjust any walking aids without direction from your supervisor.

CRITICAL THINKING IN PRACTICE

You are ambulating a resident in the hallway with a walker and gait belt. The resident says, "I feel dizzy." A chair is not nearby. You see a wheelchair at the nurses' station at the end of the hallway. What will you do? How might you use planning and teamwork to avoid this situation in the future?

REVIEW QUESTIONS

Answers to these questions are at the bottom of page 556.

Circle the BEST answer.

1. Ms. Porter is on bed rest. Which statement is true?
   A. She has orthostatic hypotension.
   B. Bed rest helps reduce pain and promotes healing.
   C. Everything will be done for her.
   D. Bed rest is not the cause of contractures.

2. Which helps prevent permanent plantar flexion?
   A. Bed boards
   B. A footboard
   C. Trochanter rolls
   D. Hand rolls

3. Which prevents the hip from turning outward?
   A. Bed boards
   B. A footboard
   C. A trochanter roll
   D. A leg brace

4. A contracture is:
   A. The loss of muscle strength as a result of inactivity
   B. The lack of joint mobility caused by the shortening of a muscle
   C. A decrease in the size of a muscle
   D. A blood clot

5. Passive range-of-motion exercises are performed by:
   A. The client
   B. A health care team member
   C. The client with the assistance of someone else
   D. The client with the use of a trapeze

6. ROM exercises are ordered for Ms. Porter. You should avoid doing one of the following:
A. Supporting the body part being exercised
B. Moving the joint slowly, smoothly, and gently
C. Forcing the joint through full range of motion
D. Exercising only the joints indicated by your supervisor

7. Flexion involves:
A. Bending the body part
B. Straightening the body part
C. Moving the body part toward the body
D. Moving the body part away from the body

8. You are getting a client ready to walk using a crutch. You should do the following:
A. Ensure the client wears loose clothing
B. Have the client wear slippers
C. Get any pair of crutches from physical therapy
D. Ensure that the bolts on the crutches are tight

9. A single-tip cane is used:
A. At waist level
B. On the strong side
C. On the weak side
D. On either side

Circle T if the answer is true, and circle F if the answer is false.

10. T F A single-tip cane and a four-point cane give equal support.

11. T F When a cane is used, the feet are moved first.

12. T F Mr. Jameel uses a walker. First, he moves the walker in front of him. Then, he moves his feet forward.

13. T F Mr. Jameel starts to fall. You should try to prevent the fall.

14. T F A client has a brace. Bony areas need protection from skin breakdown.

Answers: 1.B, 2.B, 3.C, 4.B, 5.B, 6.C, 7.A, 8.D, 9.B, 10.F, 11.F, 12.T, 13.F, 14.T

CHAPTER 27

Rehabilitation Care

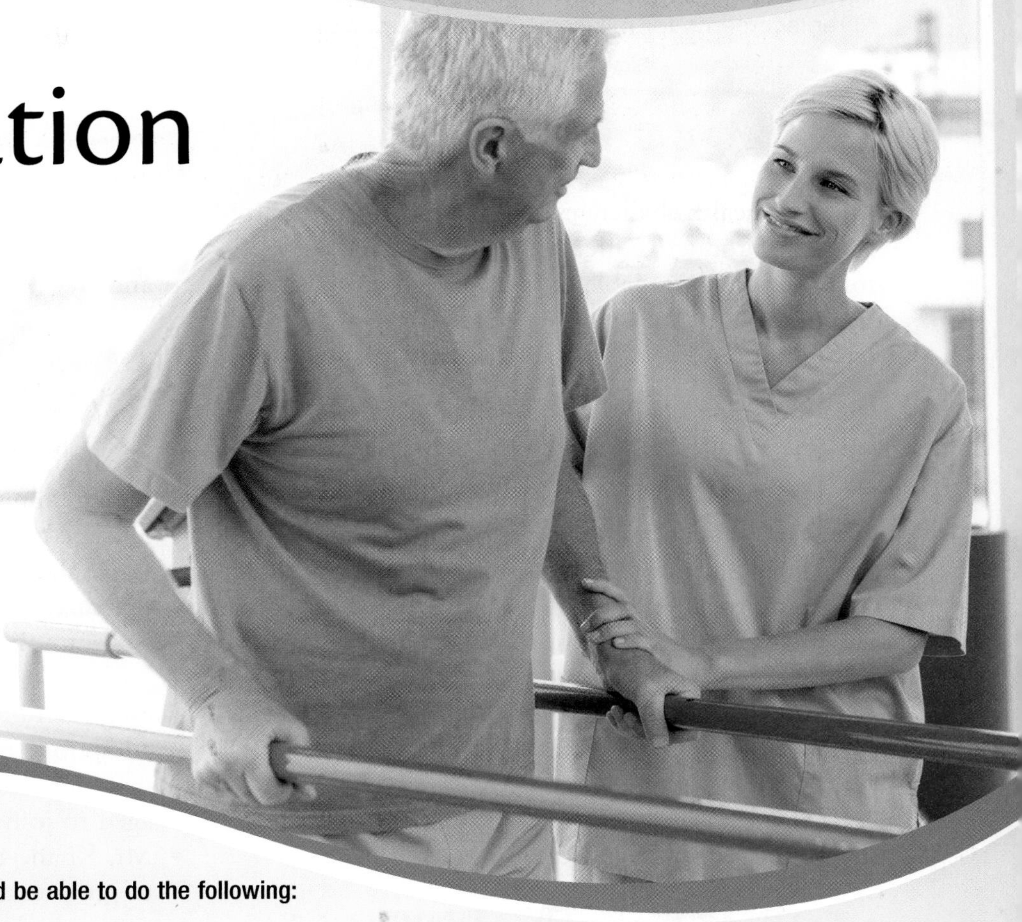

OBJECTIVES

After reading this chapter, the learner should be able to do the following:

- Describe the goals of rehabilitation.
- Explain how rehabilitation involves the whole client.
- Explain the family's role in the rehabilitation process.
- Explain the role of therapy and training in rehabilitation.
- Describe the rehabilitation settings.
- Explain the role of the rehabilitation team in the rehabilitation process.

KEY TERMS

prostheses (singular, *prosthesis*) Artificial replacements for missing body parts. *p. 561*

Injury or health challenges can affect a person's ability to lead a productive life. For example, after a stroke, some people are unable to walk or to communicate like they once could. Those people may benefit from rehabilitation care and restorative care services.

GOALS OF REHABILITATION

The goals of rehabilitation depend on the client's condition and circumstances. Rehabilitation may follow an acute injury or illness, or it may be part of the treatment for a persistent illness or disability. Rehabilitation can also maintain or slow the decline of functioning. For some clients, the goal is to return to work, and some others only want to be able to meet self-care needs and perform activities of daily living (ADLs). Most clients largely want to reduce their reliance on others and to become more independent. The following more specific goals are common:

- ***To restore function to former levels***. A full restoration of function is the goal for most clients with acute or temporary conditions. For example, a healthy client with a simple leg fracture aims for full recovery.
- ***To improve functional abilities.*** A return to former levels of functioning is not possible for some clients. They aim to improve their abilities to the best extent possible. For example, they may want to work on mobility skills or carrying out ADLs independently.
- ***To learn new skills.*** Some clients need to learn new skills to adjust to their disability or limitations. For example, Mr. Liptak's larynx was surgically removed because of cancer, and he is not able to speak anymore. His goal is to learn to communicate using, for example, sign language.
- ***To prevent further disability and illness.*** Complications that cause further disability and illness must be prevented. For example, immobility can lead to pressure ulcers or contractures, so proper skin care, exercise and activity, good alignment, and frequent repositioning are essential.

Consider the rehabilitation goals of the following clients:

- Chantal, 17, was in a car accident, which left her with hemiplegia (paralysis of one side of the body). She needs to maintain her current range of motion (ROM), adapt to a wheelchair, and perform self-care.
- Mr. Cunningham, 27, is addicted to cocaine. His goals include restoring healthy physical and psychological functions and preventing a relapse into addiction. He will learn how to avoid situations in which drugs are present, and he will be encouraged to join Narcotics Anonymous (NA).
- Mr. Khan, 49, has had a heart attack. His goal is to prevent another heart attack. His rehabilitation program should include counselling, which will recommend exercise, healthy eating, and stress management techniques.
- Mr. Egri, 68, had a stroke that resulted in hemiplegia and severe speech impairment. He needs to learn communication methods and to restore function. Prevention of another stroke through medication, exercises, and a healthy diet is a goal as well. His family needs to learn how to help with his care.
- Mrs. Boucher, 82, fractured her hip in a fall. Her goal is to remain in her own home. She needs to restore her ability to function at former levels. She also needs to take measures to prevent another fall (see the *Focus on Older Adults: Rehabilitation* box).

REHABILITATION SETTINGS

Many common health problems require rehabilitation services (**BOX 27–1**), which are offered

BOX 27–1 Common Health Problems Requiring Rehabilitation

- Acquired brain injury
- Alcoholism
- Amputation
- Brain tumour
- Burns
- Cerebral palsy
- Chronic obstructive pulmonary disease
- Mental illness
- Myocardial infarction (heart attack)
- Parkinson's disease
- Spinal cord injury
- Spinal cord tumour
- Stroke
- Substance abuse

FOCUS ON OLDER ADULTS

Rehabilitation

Rehabilitation often takes longer for older clients than for others. Age-related changes affect healing, mobility, vision, hearing, and other functions (see Chapter 21). Older clients often have chronic health problems that slow down their recovery. They are also at risk for injuries. Because older clients do not tolerate long or fast-paced programs, their rehabilitation is usually slow.

in most health care facilities and in the community:

- ***Hospitals.*** Most hospitals have rehabilitation units for inpatients and outpatients. Many programs in these units focus on brain injury and tumours, spinal cord injury, and stroke. Some hospitals offer cardiac and respiratory rehabilitation, and some have programs for complex medical and surgical conditions such as wounds and unstable diabetes.
- ***Specialized facilities.*** Some health care facilities focus on specific problems—for example, mental health disorder and substance abuse or addiction.
- ***Long-term care facilities.*** Most provide rehabilitation services similar to those found in hospitals. In some facilities, the term *restorative care* is used rather than *rehabilitation* because the care is provided by the client and family, nurses and support workers. (see p. 563).
- ***Community care.*** Home care services (see the *Focus on Home Care: Home Assessment* box) and adult day programs are offered as part of community care. A program for clients with brain injuries, for example, may teach life skills, social behaviour, and work techniques.

THE REHABILITATION PROCESS

Rehabilitation can be a short process; for example, a healthy client with a shoulder injury may need to do only a few simple exercises regularly for a few weeks until recovery is complete. However, rehabilitation is often a long, difficult process. The *Case Study: Rehabilitation Following a Brain Injury* box shows the rehabilitation process for a client who has experienced a serious brain injury.

The Rehabilitation Team

Rehabilitation requires a multidisciplinary team effort. Members of the team vary, depending on the client's needs. The team usually includes the client,

FOCUS ON HOME CARE

Home Assessment

After the rehabilitation team assesses the client's home (**BOX 27–2**), the case manager or occupational therapist discusses with the client and the family any safety risks and health hazards that have been identified. You may be asked to assist a member of the rehabilitation team to complete the assessment. If necessary, changes are made to make the home environment more appropriate for the client. The support worker should continue to be on the lookout for any safety risks during future contacts with the client and then gently suggest changes to the client or family to ensure a safe environment. If you identify any problems, you must report them to your supervisor.

BOX 27–2 Rehabilitation Team Home Review

Outdoors

- Where is the parking area located? What is the distance from the parking area to the door?
- Where is the mailbox?
- If the client has a vehicle, where is it parked?
- What is the width of car doors?
- Can the client turn the key?
- Can the client open and close doors?
- Are ramps needed?
- Are handrails needed?
- Are entrances well lit?
- Does the client have access to private or public transportation?
- Can the client operate a motor vehicle?
- What are the widths and heights of ramps and sidewalks, if any?

Indoors

- Are there any obstructions on floors?
- Are there steps in the house? Where are they located?
- How is furniture arranged?
- Can the client use the furniture?
- Where are telephones located?
- Can the client raise and lower windows?
- How are floors covered (wall-to-wall carpeting, tile, hardwood, throw rugs)?
- Can the client use a wheelchair throughout the house?
- Where is the fuse or circuit-breaker box located?
- Can the client control the heating?
- Are walkways, doors, and halls wide enough for the wheelchair (if the client is in a wheelchair)?
- Is there an elevator (if the client lives in an apartment or condominium building)?

Kitchen

- Does the client have access to the stove, sink, cupboards, storage areas, workspace, refrigerator, and other appliances?
- What is the height of the sink and countertops?
- Is there an open space under the sink to bring the wheelchair close to the sink (if the client is in a wheelchair)?
- Can the client turn faucets on and off?
- Can the client use the microwave oven?
- Can the client reach stove knobs?
- Are appliances arranged for the client's convenience?

Bathroom

- What are the heights of the sink, toilet, shower, and tub?
- Can the client reach the faucets?
- Can the client turn the faucets on and off?
- Is there space for using a wheelchair or other needed mobility devices?
- Can the client get into and out of the tub or shower?
- Are there grab bars by the toilet, shower, and tub?

Bedroom

- What is the height of the client's bed?
- Can the client access the closet? Can the client reach rods and shelves?
- Can the client transfer into and out of bed safely?
- How is furniture arranged?
- Does the furniture arrangement allow for the use of a wheelchair or other needed mobility device?
- Where is the nearest bathroom?

Safety

- Is the house number clearly visible and readable in case of an emergency?
- Do deadbolts and locks provide complete security? Can the client use the locks?
- Can the client see and talk to a visitor at the door without being seen?
- Are the steps, porch, and front door well lit?
- Are the steps, porch, and front door protected from rain, sleet, and snow?
- Is there a nonslip doormat?
- Can the client use the telephone?
- Are emergency telephone numbers kept close at hand?
- Can the client control the water temperature?
- Do electrical outlets have childproof covers?

Continued

BOX 27–2 Rehabilitation Team Home Review—cont'd

Safety—cont'd

- Where are the smoke detectors? Are they in working condition?
- Are rooms and hallways well lit?
- Can the client control indoor and outdoor lighting?
- Can the client exit the home quickly in an emergency?
- Is oxygen used in the home? Are safety measures in place?
- Does the client have access to the telephone, television, radio, and lights while in bed?
- Are space heaters used in the house? Are safety measures in place?
- Does the client have good judgement in regard to cooking and stove use?
- Are there fire extinguishers in the kitchen and close to any fireplaces?
- Is there a safe play area for children?
- Can the client safely dispose of blood, body fluids, secretions, and excretions?
- Is there a pest-free method of trash storage?

Source: Adapted from Hoeman, S.P. (1996). *Rehabilitation nursing: Process and application* (2nd ed.). St. Louis, MO: Mosby.

family members, physicians, nurses, occupational therapists, physiotherapists, support workers, and others—who all can help the client regain function and independence. The team meets often to discuss the client's progress, and changes are made in the rehabilitation care plan, as needed. The client and family attend the meetings whenever possible. Family members are key to the team.

All aspects of rehabilitation are interconnected. For example, following a stroke, Mr. Silva learns how to care for himself (physical health) and how to follow instructions (intellectual health), which increases his self-esteem (emotional health); family and friends visit often (social health), and his spiritual advisor visits every week (spiritual health).

The *Case Study: Rehabilitation Following a Brain Injury* box shows a rehabilitation team addressing all five dimensions of a client's health. The client's quality of life is central to care and treatment. The rehabilitation team encourages the client to control as many aspects of care as possible—being a key member of the rehabilitation team gives the client some control.

Role of the Family

Rehabilitation of clients also involves their family members, who need to learn about the illness, injury, or disability and how to care for their loved ones. Care often involves helping the client practise new skills. The family also learns new skills—for example, how to communicate with a spouse who has lost the ability to speak, how to cope with the behaviour of a teenager with a mental health disorder, or how to dress a child with physical disabilities. Counselling is provided, as needed, to help the family cope with changes affecting them. Families dealing with the rehabilitation of a member with a chronic health problem will need constant support from team members because the challenges to a normal family life can be overwhelming, and family members need to know that the team is listening to their concerns.

Therapy and Training

The professionals on the rehabilitation team choose the therapy and training needed to meet the client's goals. The client is taught how to improve a skill or how to perform a task and practises what was learned either independently or with a caregiver or a family member. You may be required to help clients practise skills or tasks.

The client's therapy and training may involve learning to use self-help devices. Specific equipment to meet the client's needs is obtained, and the client is taught how to use it:

- ***Prostheses.*** **Prostheses** are artificial replacements for missing body parts—for example, feet, knees, lower limbs, upper limbs, hands, breasts, and eyes. The goal for a prosthesis is to be like the missing body part in function and appearance. Artificial limbs are made from a variety of materials such as wood,

CASE STUDY Rehabilitation Following a Brain Injury

High school teacher Jeffrey Than, 34, was cycling to school when he was hit by a van. He sustained a severe blow to the head and broke several bones. After emergency care and surgery, he was placed in the intensive care unit (ICU). Because he had acquired a serious brain injury, he could not speak or recognize his family. After 10 days in the ICU, he was moved to the acute-care unit, where he stayed for 2 months.

Eventually Mr. Than was transferred to the hospital's rehabilitation unit, and 3 months later, he was discharged home. He received rehabilitation services at home and in the community for the next 6 months. During his long rehabilitation, Mr. Than's rehabilitation team worked with him and his family (see the chart below). The team's main goals were to help Mr. Than regain lost function and help the family learn new skills for his care.

Rehabilitation Team	Role
Mr. Than and his family	Made decisions regarding rehabilitation goals Were involved in every aspect of care Learned new skills and relearned old skills
Neurosurgeon	Led surgical team and aspects of rehabilitation after surgery
Orthopedic surgeon	Led surgical team and aspects of rehabilitation after surgery
Nurses	Coordinated and provided care at every stage
Specialist in rehabilitation medicine	Led and coordinated rehabilitation
Neuropsychologists	Evaluated thinking, memory, emotions, behaviour, and personality Planned behaviour-management treatment Headed adult day program
Case manager	Coordinated home care Arranged for adult day programs
Social workers	Provided counselling Headed adult day program
Occupational therapists	Assessed performance of ADLs Conducted home assessment prior to discharge Provided treatment, equipment, and devices to help client attain independence
Physiotherapists	Evaluated strength, flexibility, and balance Taught mobility exercises and equipment use
Speech–language pathologist	Tested speech and language function Taught communication strategies to the family
Family physician	Provided medical care after discharge
Support workers	Assisted with personal care and ROM exercises Assisted with household management Assisted with eating Helped with physiotherapy exercises Provided input at case conferences about Mr. Than's progress, changes in care, and any concerns Mr. Than expressed
Volunteers	Provided company to Mr. Than when the family was not around Assisted with household tasks

aluminum, and plastic. Most artificial limbs are powered by the client's muscles, either by muscles in the stump or by other nearby muscles, so a physiotherapist works with the client to strengthen these muscles. The client learns how to use and care for the prosthesis. As a support worker, you might help a client get used to wearing and using a prosthesis. You might also assist the client with care of the skin at the prosthesis site (see Chapter 37).

- ***Orthotics.*** An *orthotic* is an apparatus worn to support and align parts of the musculo-skeletal system and prevent or correct problems associated with it. Examples are splints, foot supports, and knee and back braces (see Chapter 26). The client learns how to put on, use, and care for the orthotic. You might help a client to put on an orthotic and practise moving or walking.
- ***Eating and drinking devices.*** These include glass holders, plate guards, and utensils with curved handles or cuffs (see Chapter 28).
- ***Self-care devices.*** These include electronic toothbrushes, combs, brushes, and sponges with long handles (FIGURE 27–1), as well as devices that help with dressing, cooking, writing, making phone calls, and performing other tasks (FIGURE 27–2).
- ***Devices to aid mobility.*** These include crutches, canes, walkers, and braces, as well as wheelchairs for some clients. If possible, clients in a wheelchair learn how to transfer themselves to and from the chair using a transfer board (FIGURE 27–3), which helps a person move from one seat to another. The client also learns to transfer to and from the bed, toilet, bathtub, sofas and chairs, and cars.
- ***Other equipment.*** Some clients need feeding tubes (see Chapter 29) or mechanical ventilation (see Chapter 41). Some of them are eventually weaned from the ventilator, but others must adapt to lifelong ventilation.

REHABILITATIVE CARE VERSUS RESTORATIVE CARE

Rehabilitative care is the process of restoring a person to the highest possible level of functioning through the use of therapy, exercise, and other methods. Restorative care, usually provided by nurses and support workers, aims to return clients to functioning at a higher capacity and being more independent through regaining their strength. Whereas more health care providers are on the team for a client in rehabilitative care, restorative care usually involves only the client and family, nurses, and support workers. Therapists and other professionals may be consulted as needed.

For clients who are too weak to perform ADLs, restorative care may involve measures that promote:

- Self-care
- Elimination
- Positioning

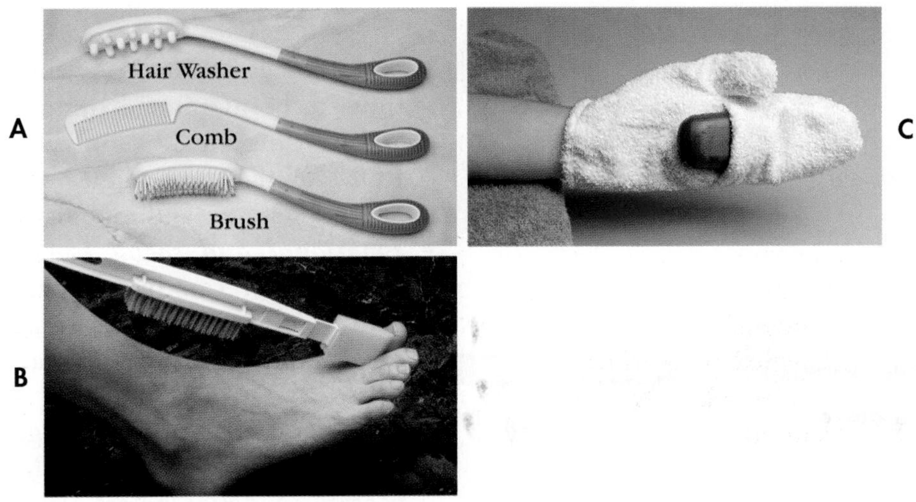

FIGURE 27–1 **A,** Long-handled combs and brushes for hair care. **B,** Long-handled brushes for bathing. **C,** Mitt with soap holder. (**Sources:** (for *A* and *B*) Courtesy of North Coast Medical, Gilroy, CA; (for *C*) Courtesy of ElderStore, Alpharetta, GA.)

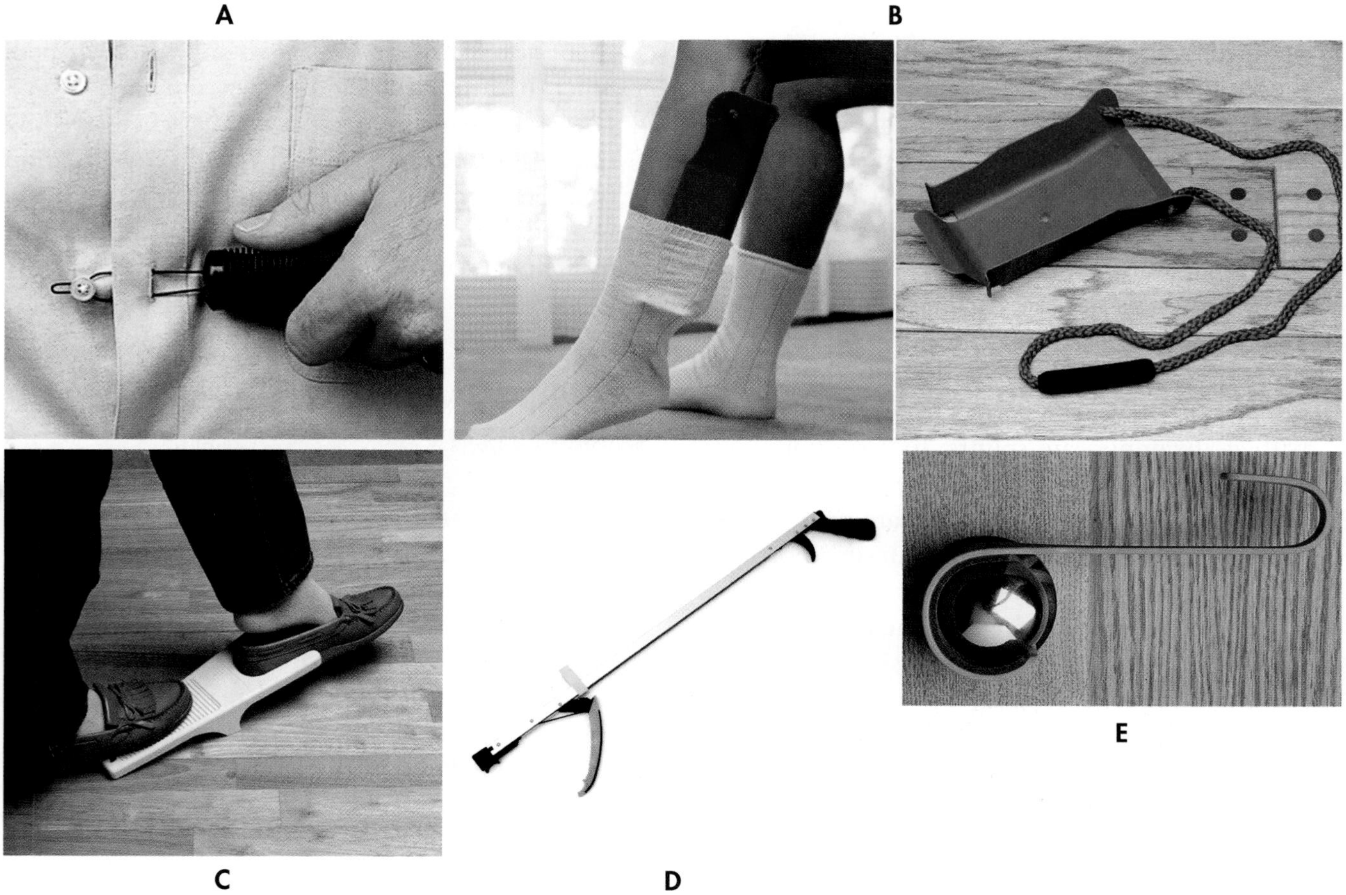

FIGURE 27–2 **A,** A button hook is used to button and zip clothing. **B,** A sock assist is used to pull on socks and stockings. **C,** A shoe remover is used to take off shoes. **D,** Reachers help retrieve items from high shelves. **E,** A doorknob turner increases leverage to help turn the knob. (**Sources:** (for *A, B, C,* and *E*) Courtesy of North Coast Medical, Gilroy, CA; (for *D*) Art Directors & TRIP/Alamy Stock Photo.)

- Mobility
- Communication
- Cognitive function
- Preventing unnecessary decline in function

Emphasis on the Whole Person

Illness and disability can affect a client's physical, emotional, social, intellectual, and spiritual health, so restorative care is aimed at the whole person. It addresses all dimensions of health, not only the physical.

- ***Physical health.*** The client's physical condition and ability to perform ADLs that were assessed by professionals during the rehabilitative process continue to be monitored by the client, the family, and all caregivers. Complications are prevented. ROM exercises are done. The client learns or relearns self-care and mobility skills.
- ***Emotional and social health.*** Emotional and social health can be assessed by professionals. Family counselling and assistance for re-entering the community and workplace are provided as needed.
- ***Intellectual health.*** Thinking, speech, memory, and organization are assessed. Measures to improve cognitive functioning are planned.
- ***Spiritual health.*** Counselling from spiritual advisors is provided as needed.

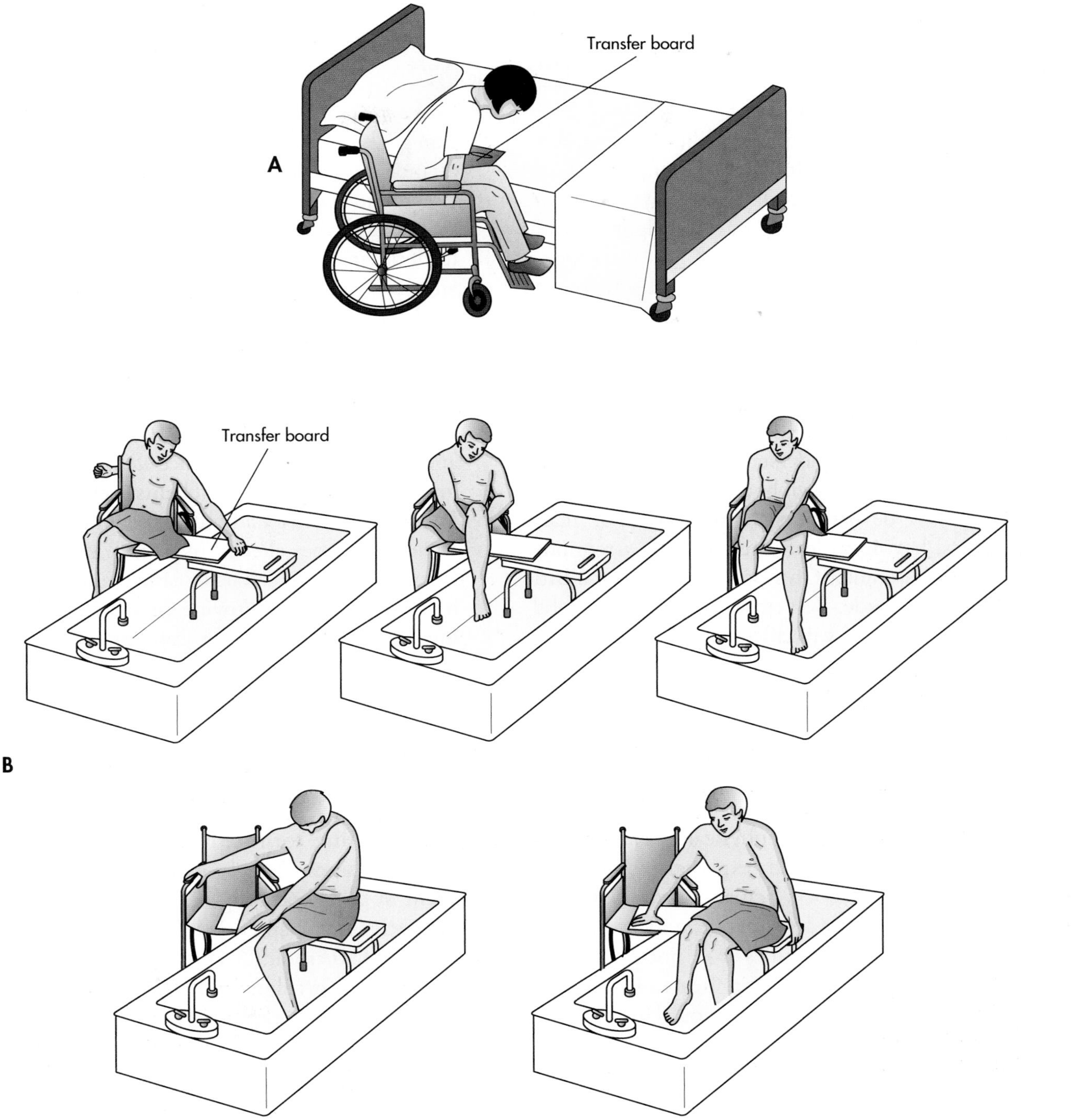

FIGURE 27–3 The client uses a transfer board. **A,** Transfer from a wheelchair to a bed. **B,** Transfer from a wheelchair to a bathtub.

ASSISTING WITH REHABILITATION AND RESTORATIVE CARE

As a support worker, you will encounter a number of clients undergoing some form of rehabilitation or restorative care, some of whom will be adjusting to overwhelming change. Rehabilitation is often slow and frustrating, as improvement may not be seen for weeks or months. Some clients improve quickly at first, but the pace of improvement may then slow, causing great frustration and hardship to clients, so you must be patient, supportive, and empathetic (see the *Providing Compassionate Care: Assisting With Rehabilitation and Restorative Care* box).

Providing Compassionate Care
Assisting With Rehabilitation and Restorative Care

- ***Dignity.*** Treat your clients with respect, and protect their right to dignity. Clients do not need your pity, but they do need encouragement and support. Focus on the positive by reminding them of their progress and highlighting their abilities and strengths. Provide emotional support and reassurance; when clients need someone to talk to, be a good listener.

  The process of regaining independence is often very slow, and you may grow impatient with your client when repeated explanations seem to have little or no result. Never show your impatience. Try to understand that having little control over one's own body movements or functions can be extremely frustrating. For many clients, having to learn new tasks is a reminder of their disability. Give praise when even a little progress is made. Remember that illness, disability, and fatigue can affect a client's ability to learn. Clients with brain injuries may have a particularly hard time learning new activities.

  Clients and family members faced with a condition that requires rehabilitation may experience a feeling of loss for the way their life may change. Emotional aspects of rehabilitation are interconnected with physical rehabilitation. Clients and families can experience all or some of these stages: shock, denial, anger, depression, reaction against independence, and acceptance. Clients and their families may not go through these steps at the same time. Reactions will vary, too, depending on the age of your client and the prognosis. Parents told that their child needs rehabilitation may react differently from an older person's family dealing with rehabilitation. Report your observations to your supervisor.
- ***Independence.*** Independence is a key rehabilitation goal. Encourage the client to perform ADLs as independently as possible. Do not rush the client, and allow him time to complete each task. Familiarize yourself with the client's self-help devices, and encourage the client to use them whenever necessary. When assisting the client, apply the methods developed by the rehabilitation team and practise with the client the tasks that must be performed. These methods will help you to guide and direct the client.
- ***Preferences.*** Ask clients about their preferences, and allow for personal choice *whenever possible*. Freedom of choice helps clients feel in control. Follow the client's daily routine and care plan.
- ***Privacy.*** Some clients may feel embarrassed to practise skills (such as eating and walking) in front of others. Provide privacy for practising skills, as well as for care procedures and elimination. Keep information about clients confidential.
- ***Safety***. Illness, disability, and fatigue increase the risk for accidents and injuries, so take the necessary measures to ensure safety (see Chapter 22). Never force clients to do more than they are able, and allow time for rest. Follow the care plan for safety measures needed for each client. Keep the client in good body alignment. Use safe transfer methods (see Chapter 25). Perform ROM exercises and turn and reposition the client as directed. Report signs and symptoms of complications such as pressure ulcers, contractures, elimination problems, and depression. In facility settings, make sure that the call bell and overbed table are placed on the client's unaffected side.

CHAPTER REVIEW

KEY POINTS

- Restorative care is client care that is usually provided by nurses and support workers. Its goal is to help a client regain strength and, in turn, independence and the ability to function at a higher capacity.
- Rehabilitation is the use of therapy, exercise, and other methods to restore a person to the highest possible level of functioning. Rehabilitation may be necessary due to an acute injury or illness (usually short-term), or it may be part of the treatment plan for a persistent illness or disability (often long-term). Rehabilitation can also maintain or slow the decline of functioning.
- Every client will have a different care plan and different team members involved, depending on the goals. As a support worker, you may be the person who has the most ongoing contact with your client, so your input into care conferences and your reports to your supervisor are vital.
- Therapy and rehabilitation are important to help clients reach their goal of independence. The care plan will establish your role in each step of rehabilitation.
- Family members are important members of the rehabilitation team. They need to learn about the illness, injury, or disability and how to care for their loved ones.
- A number of psychosocial elements could affect clients' reactions to their conditions.

CRITICAL THINKING IN PRACTICE

Mr. Lazar has right-sided weakness following a recent stroke. You are his support worker, assigned to help him with his care plan of restorative exercises after his discharge from the rehabilitation hospital. Today, Mr. Lazar is reluctant to participate in any of his usual exercises and, instead, has angrily told you to leave his house. He also said, "What is the point of doing all of this when I can't do it and it hurts to try?" You are unsure of what to do or say to him. Should you leave immediately, as he has asked you to? Should you call your supervisor?

REVIEW QUESTIONS

Answers to these questions are at the bottom of the next page.

Circle the BEST answer.

1. Which of the following is a common goal of rehabilitation?
   A. To restore function to former levels
   B. To prepare for surgery
   C. To prepare for relocation to a long-term care facility
   D. To prepare for chemotherapy
2. Rehabilitation is often slower for:
   A. Toddlers
   B. Adolescents
   C. Middle-aged adults
   D. Older adults
3. Which member of the rehabilitation team evaluates a client's strength and balance?
   A. The physiotherapist
   B. The occupational therapist
   C. The primary caregiver
   D. The speech therapist
4. The rehabilitation process addresses:
   A. What the client cannot do
   B. Only physical health
   C. The whole person
   D. Only emotional health
5. Rehabilitation takes place:
   A. Only in long-term care facilities
   B. Only in hospitals
   C. Only in specialized facilities
   D. In a variety of facility and community settings

Questions 6 to 9 relate to the following situation: Mr. Graziano, 72, has had a stroke and needs rehabilitation since his right side is paralyzed.

6. Mr. Graziano's personal care is:
   A. Done by him to the extent possible
   B. Done by you
   C. Postponed until he can use his right side
   D. Supervised by his physician

7. Mr. Graziano asks for some music to be played. You should:
   A. Tell him that music is not allowed
   B. Choose some music for him
   C. Ask him to choose some music
   D. Ask a therapist to choose some music

8. The call bell is on Mr. Graziano's right side. Since his right side is weak, you move it to the left side of the bed. You have provided compassionate care to Mr. Graziano by:
   A. Protecting him from abuse
   B. Providing for his safety
   C. Allowing personal choice
   D. Promoting his privacy

9. Mr. Graziano puts on his shirt using one arm. His progress is slow. You:
   A. Focus his attention on learning a new task
   B. Encourage him as he completes the task
   C. Ask him to sit down and rest
   D. Tell him he will learn the next task more quickly

Answers: 1.A, 2.D, 3.A, 4.C, 5.D, 6.A, 7.C, 8.B, 9.B

Chapter opener image: wavebreakmedia/Shutterstock.com

CHAPTER 28

Nutrition and Fluids

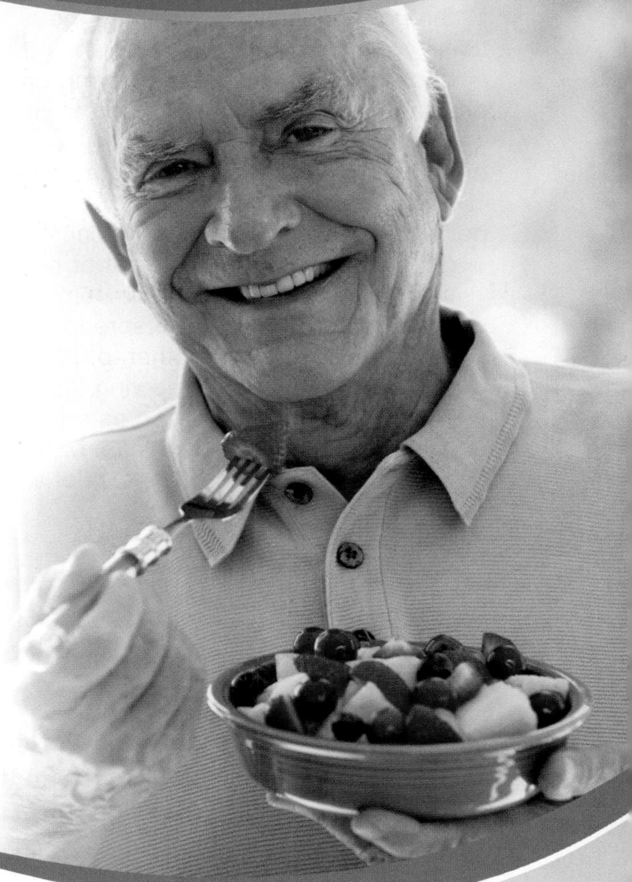

OBJECTIVES

After reading this chapter, the learner should be able to do the following:

- Describe the functions and major sources of protein, carbohydrates, fats, vitamins, minerals, and water.
- Explain the principles of *Eating Well With Canada's Food Guide* (or, simply, *Canada's Food Guide*).
- Explain the purpose of food labels.
- Explain how nutrient requirements change throughout the life cycle.
- Explain factors that affect eating and nutrition.
- Explain the role of the support worker in meal planning and preparation.
- Explain why food safety is important.
- Describe special diets.
- Explain the support worker's role in assisting clients to eat.
- Explain how to feed clients.
- Describe adult fluid requirements and the common causes of edema and dehydration.
- Describe the common special fluid orders.
- Explain the purpose of intake and output records.
- Perform the procedures described in this chapter.

KEY TERMS

absorption The process by which substances pass through the intestinal wall into the blood. *p. 570*
allergy A sensitivity to a substance that causes the body to react with signs or symptoms. *p. 578*
aspiration Inhalation of fluid or an object into the lungs. *p. 588*
calorie A unit of measure of the energy produced as the body burns food. *p. 571*
celiac disease Negative physical reaction to a gluten protein found in wheat or related grains such as barley, rye, and sometimes oats. *p. 587*
cross-contamination The spread of pathogens from one source to another. *p. 582*
daily value (DV) How a serving fits into the daily diet of an adult; expressed as a percentage based on recommended daily intake. *p. 579*
dehydration The excessive loss of water from body tissues. *p. 593*
foodborne illness An illness transmitted by contaminated food products. *p. 582*
gluten A protein that has come from wheat or related grains, such as barley, oats, rye, triticale, Kamut, or spelt. *p. 587*
ingestion The process of taking food and fluids into the body. *p. 570*
intake The amount of fluids taken in by the body. *p. 593*
nutrients Substances that are ingested, digested, absorbed, and used by the body. *p. 571*
nutrition Processes involved in the ingestion, digestion, absorption, and use of foods and fluids by the body. *p. 570*
output The amount of fluids lost by the body. *p. 593*

Food and water are necessary for life and health. The amount and quality of foods and fluids in the diet are important, as they affect a person's current as well as future health and well-being. For all age groups, a poor diet will affect physical and mental growth and function, increase the risk for disease, and slow healing. Poor physical and mental functioning increases the risk for accidents and injuries.

Food and drink contribute to social and emotional health also. Eating and drinking are part of social activity with family and friends (**FIGURE 28–1**). Many people need a friendly, social setting for meals; otherwise, they eat poorly.

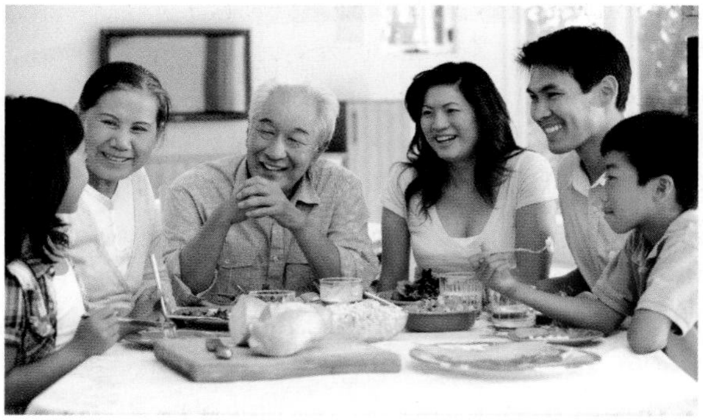

FIGURE 28–1 Meals are enjoyed when shared with family and friends. Source: © Creative stock | Dreamstime.com.

As a support worker, you will serve food and fluids to clients and assist them with eating. In home care, you may also prepare meals for clients. This chapter introduces you to the basics of nutrition.

BASIC NUTRITION

Nutrition refers to the processes involved in the ingestion, digestion, absorption, and use of foods and fluids by the body. **Ingestion** is the process of taking food and fluids into the body. *Digestion* is the process of physically and chemically breaking down nutrients so that they can be absorbed for use by the cells. **Absorption** is the process by which substances pass through the intestinal wall into the blood. Review the description of the digestive system in Chapter 17.

Good nutrition is needed for growth, healing, and the maintenance of body functions. Selected foods must provide a well-balanced diet and the correct amount of calories. A diet high in fat and calories can cause weight gain and obesity; if a person consumes fewer calories than needed, this results in weight loss. Those who follow *Eating Well With*

Canada's Food Guide will obtain all of the nutrients they need for a balanced diet.

Nutrients

Foods and fluids contain **nutrients**—substances that are ingested, digested, absorbed, and used by the body. Nutrients are grouped into proteins, carbohydrates, fats, vitamins, minerals, and water.

Proteins, fats, and carbohydrates give the body fuel for energy. The amount of energy provided by a nutrient is measured in calories. A **calorie** is a unit of measure of the energy produced as the body burns food. For example:

- 1 g of carbohydrate supplies the body with 4 calories
- 1 g of protein supplies the body with 4 calories
- 1 g of fat supplies the body with 9 calories

Protein

Protein is needed for tissue growth and repair. Protein sources include meat, fish, poultry, eggs, milk and milk products, cereals, beans, peas, and nuts. Animal products are the best sources of protein, so people who do not eat animal products must consume sufficient protein from plant sources, which are best eaten in combinations—for example, beans and rice. Protein deficiency can result in severe malnutrition. Children and older adults who do not eat properly are at the greatest risk.

Carbohydrates

Carbohydrates provide energy for the body and fibre for bowel elimination. Most carbohydrates come from plants. There are three main kinds of carbohydrates:

- ***Simple sugars*** are found in table sugar, fruits, and fruit juices.
- ***Starches*** are found in bread, pasta, rice, and potatoes.
- ***Fibre*** is found in bran, nuts, seeds, and raw fruits with skins. Fibre cannot be digested and passes through the intestines undigested.

During digestion, most carbohydrates (except fibre) are broken down into sugars, which are then absorbed into the bloodstream.

Fats

Fats provide energy, help the body to use certain vitamins, and add flavour to food. Some fat is necessary in the diet. Dietary fat that is not needed by the body (as with excess calories from all sources) is stored as body fat. There are three main types of dietary fat:

- ***Saturated fat*** is found in animal and dairy products (e.g., meat, butter, milk, and cheeses).
- ***Trans fat*** is found in margarine, shortening, store-bought cookies, cakes, pies, doughnuts, and fried foods. Trans fat is created when liquid oil is chemically altered to form a more solid substance. It is used to increase the flavour and shelf life of foods.
- ***Unsaturated fat*** is found in fish and many vegetable oils (e.g., canola oil and olive oil). Unsaturated fat is healthier than saturated fat and trans fat.

Vitamins

Vitamins are needed daily for normal function and growth, but they do not provide calories. Each vitamin is needed for specific body functions (TABLE 28–1)—for example, vitamin A is necessary for vision. Vitamins are an essential part of a healthy diet, and the lack of a specific vitamin may result in illness. All necessary vitamins can be obtained by following *Eating Well With Canada's Food Guide*. Vitamins A, D, E, and K are fat-soluble vitamins; excess doses of these vitamins are stored in the body and can cause complications. Vitamins C and B complex are called *water-soluble vitamins*; excess doses of these vitamins are excreted in urine. Older adults are at risk for developing vitamin deficiencies because the aging process affects the body's ability to absorb certain vitamins.

Minerals

Minerals are chemical substances found in both plant and animal foods. Each mineral is needed for specific body functions—for example, calcium and phosphorus are used to form strong bones and teeth. TABLE 28–2 lists the major functions and sources of minerals. All necessary minerals can be obtained by following *Canada's Food Guide*.

TABLE 28–1 Vitamins: Major Functions and Sources

	Major Functions	Sources
Vitamin A	Growth; vision; healthy hair, skin, and mucous membranes; resistance to infection	Liver, spinach, leafy green and yellow vegetables, yellow fruits, fish liver oils, egg yolk, butter, cream, whole milk
Vitamin B_1 (thiamine)	Muscle tone, nerve function, digestion, appetite, normal elimination, carbohydrate metabolism	Pork, fish, poultry, eggs, liver, breads, pastas, cereals, oatmeal, potatoes, peas, beans, soybeans, peanuts
Vitamin B_2 (riboflavin)	Growth, vision, protein and carbohydrate metabolism, healthy skin and mucous membranes	Milk and milk products, liver, leafy green vegetables, eggs, breads, cereals
Vitamin B_3 (niacin)	Protein, fat, and carbohydrate metabolism; nervous system function; appetite; digestive system function	Meat, pork, liver, fish, peanuts, breads and cereals, green vegetables, dairy products
Vitamin B_{12}	Formation of red blood cells, protein metabolism, nervous system function	Liver, meats, poultry, fish, eggs, milk, cheese
Folic acid	Formation of red blood cells, intestinal function, protein metabolism	Liver, meats, fish, poultry, leafy green vegetables, whole grains
Vitamin C (ascorbic acid)	Formation of substances that hold tissues together; healthy blood vessels, skin, gums, bones, and teeth; wound healing; prevention of bleeding; resistance to infection	Citrus fruits, tomatoes, potatoes, cabbage, strawberries, green vegetables, melons
Vitamin D	Absorption and metabolism of calcium and phosphorus; healthy bones	Fish liver oils, milk, butter, liver, exposure to sunlight
Vitamin E	Normal reproduction, formation of red blood cells, muscle function	Vegetable oils, milk, eggs, meats, cereals, leafy green vegetables
Vitamin K	Blood clotting	Liver, leafy green vegetables, egg yolk, cheese

Water

Water is the most important nutrient necessary for life. The body needs water for maintaining cell function, regulating body temperature, delivering nutrients, removing waste, and performing other body processes. Water enters the body through fluids and foods and is lost through urine and feces, through the skin as perspiration, and through the lungs with expiration. There must be a balance between the amount of fluid taken in and the amount lost. Death can result from inadequate water intake or from excessive fluid loss.

EATING WELL WITH CANADA'S FOOD GUIDE

Health Canada has developed guidelines to promote wise food choices among our diverse population (see **BOX 28–1**). *Eating Well With Canada's Food Guide* provides nutrition and healthy eating information

TABLE 28–2 Minerals: Major Functions and Sources

	Major Functions	Sources
Calcium	Formation of teeth and bones, blood clotting, muscle contraction, heart function, nerve function	Milk and milk products, leafy green vegetables, whole grains, egg yolk, dried peas and beans, nuts
Phosphorus	Formation of bones and teeth; use of proteins, fats, and carbohydrates; nerve and muscle function	Meat, fish, poultry, milk and milk products, nuts, egg yolk, dried peas and beans
Iron	Enabling of red blood cells to carry oxygen	Liver, meat, eggs, leafy green vegetables, breads and cereals, dried peas and beans, nuts
Iodine	Thyroid gland function, growth, metabolism	Iodized salt, seafood, and shellfish
Sodium	Fluid balance, nerve function and muscle function	Almost all foods
Potassium	Nerve function, muscle contraction, heart function	Fruits, vegetables, cereals, meats, dried peas and beans
Zinc	Growth process, healing process, immune system	Meat, poultry, whole grains, dried peas and beans, eggs

BOX 28–1 Creating Your Own Food Guide

To create a customized version of Canada's Food Guide, complete with your preferred food choices and physical activities, go to this link: http://healthycanadians.gc.ca/eating-nutrition/food-guide-aliment/my-guide-mon-guide/index-eng.php.

Remember that, in addition to eating right, exercise and activity (see Chapter 26) are an important part of a healthy lifestyle!

for all Canadians.[1] In addition to the English and French versions, the *Food Guide* has been published in 10 different languages, and these are available on Health Canada's website. These publications are great resources for support workers working with people of a variety of cultures!

Eating Well With Canada's Food Guide—First Nations, Inuit and Métis is a food guide tailored to include both traditional Indigenous foods and store-bought foods that are generally available and affordable across Canada. This publication is also available in Inuktitut, Ojibwe, Plains Cree, and Woods Cree.[2]

Healthy eating is needed for the following:

- To ensure a daily diet of the essential nutrients
- To promote health and an overall sense of physical and mental well-being
- To reduce the risk for health problems related to nutritional deficiencies

The *Food Guide* divides foods into four groups, each containing different foods and nutrients:

- ***Vegetables and fruit***—fresh, canned, frozen, and dried vegetables and fruits; fruit juices
- ***Grain products***—cereals, pasta, rice, and other foods made with flour
- ***Milk products***—milk (fresh, powdered, or evaporated), cream, cheese, yogourt, and ice cream
- ***Meat and alternatives***—fresh and canned meat, poultry, fish, eggs, beans, lentils, dried peas, nuts, peanut butter, and tofu

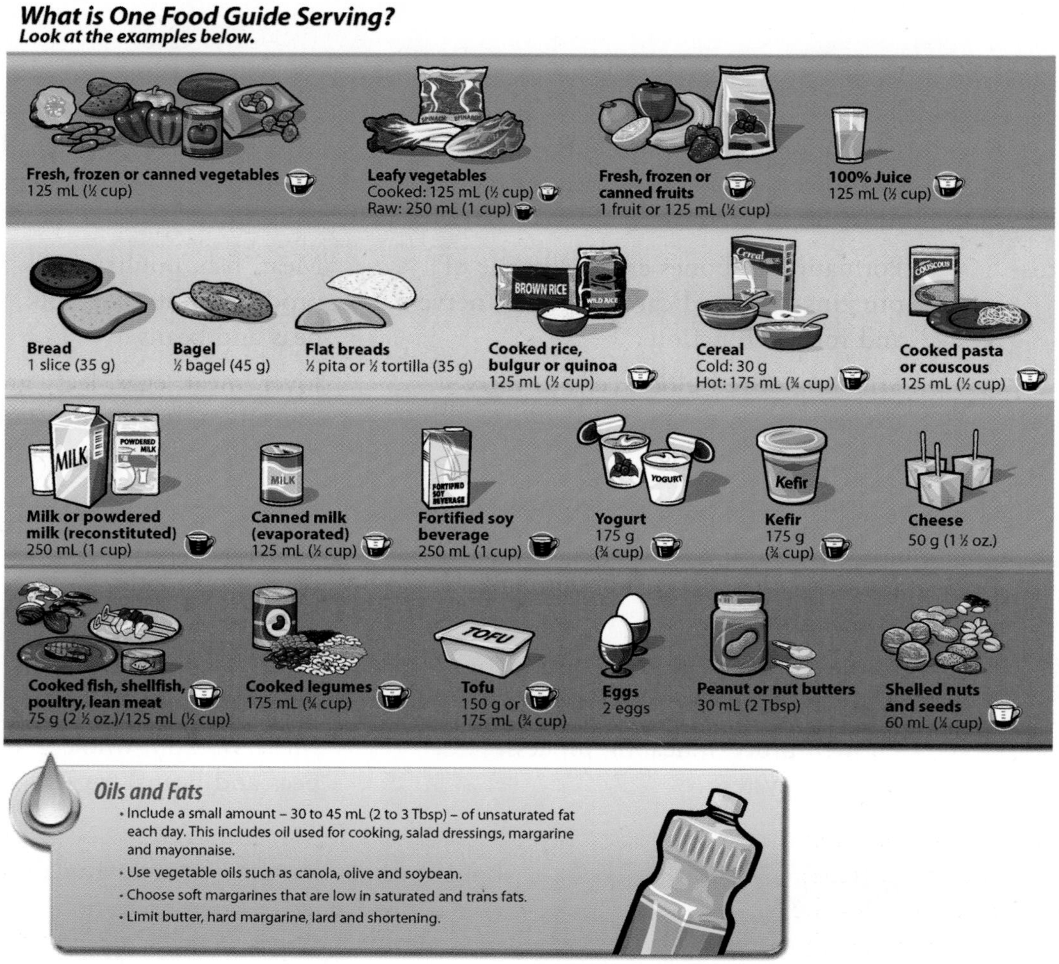

FIGURE 28–2 Single-serving sizes according to *Eating Well With Canada's Food Guide*. **Source:** *Eating Well with Canada's Food Guide*. Health Canada, 2011. Adapted and reproduced with permission from the Minister of Health, 2016.

A healthy diet contains foods from each food group. In the *Food Guide*, the four food groups are shown in a rainbow design. Single-serving sizes are recommended for each of the food groups (**FIGURE 28–2**). Most food servings should come from the green band, representing fruits and vegetables. Unfortunately, most Canadians eat too much fat. Eating more carbohydrates (whole bread, cereal, grains, vegetables, fruit, peas, beans, and lentils) helps reduce fat intake. Foods high in carbohydrates are filling, allowing a person to feel satisfied with smaller quantities of food.

The *Food Guide* recommends a small amount of oils and fats (e.g., oil for cooking, salad dressings, margarine, mayonnaise) be included in the diet—about 30–45 mL (2 to 3 tablespoons) of unsaturated fat per day. Vegetable oils (such as canola, olive oil, and soybean oil) and soft margarines that are low in saturated and trans fats are recommended. Butter, hard margarine, lard, and shortening should be used in limited amounts.

Diseases such as heart disease, high blood pressure, stroke, diabetes, osteoporosis, and certain cancers are related to diet and the kinds of foods eaten. Therefore, the goal and benefits of healthy eating are better overall health, lower risk of disease, and a healthy body weight. A person who eats well will have more energy, feel and look better, and have stronger muscles and bones.

Servings From the Food Groups

The number of servings a person needs depends on age and gender (**BOX 28–2**). Compared with adults,

BOX 28–2 Recommended Number of Food Guide Servings per Day

	Children			Teens		Adults			
Age in Years	**2–3**	**4–8**	**9–13**	**14–18**		**19–50**		**51+**	
Gender	**Girls and Boys**			**Females**	**Males**	**Females**	**Males**	**Females**	**Males**
Vegetables and fruit	4	5	6	7	8	7–8	8–10	7	7
Grain products	3	4	6	6	7	6–7	8	6	7
Milk and alternatives	2	2	3–4	3–4	3–4	2	2	3	3
Meat and alternatives	1	1	1–2	2	3	2	3	2	3

The chart above shows how many *Food Guide* servings you need from each of the four food groups every day.

Having the amount and type of food recommended and following the tips in *Canada's Food Guide* will help:

- Meet your needs for vitamins, minerals, and other nutrients
- Reduce your risk for obesity, type 2 diabetes, heart disease, certain types of cancer, and osteoporosis
- Contribute to your overall health and vitality

Source: *Eating Well with Canada's Food Guide*. Health Canada, 2011. Adapted and reproduced with permission from the Minister of Health, 2016.

young children have smaller appetites and need more calories for growth and development. Children have definite likes and dislikes, so they should be offered a variety of foods from the four food groups and small nutritious meals and snacks each day.

Women who are pregnant or breastfeeding need an extra two to three *Food Guide* servings each day. Women of childbearing age who plan to become pregnant or are breastfeeding need to take a multivitamin supplement containing folic acid every day. Adults over 50 years need to increase their intake of vitamin D and should take a daily vitamin D supplement of 400 international units (IU).

Vegetables and Fruits

Vegetables and fruits (including juices) provide carbohydrates, vitamins C and A, iron, and magnesium and are naturally low in fat. Eat at least one dark green vegetable (such as broccoli, romaine lettuce, or spinach) and one orange vegetable (such as carrots, sweet potatoes, or winter squash) each day. Try to prepare vegetables and fruits with little or no added fat, sugar, or salt. Many prepackaged or canned foods are high in sodium (salt). Fresh vegetables and fruits are more beneficial than juices. Frozen or canned fruit should be unsweetened as sweetened and syrupy products are high in sugar and calories.

Vegetables provide the best value when steamed, baked, or stir fried, and not deep fried, which can make vegetable preparations high in fat. For example, french fries are very high in fat compared with baked or boiled potatoes. Butter, oil, mayonnaise, salad dressing, sour cream, and sauces—toppings that are high in fat—are often added to vegetables. Small amounts of low-fat toppings help keep vegetable preparations low in fat.

Grain Products

It is recommended that at least half of the grain products consumed each day are those made from whole grain, such as whole grain bread, oatmeal, or whole wheat pasta. Eat a variety of whole grains such as barley, rice, oats, quinoa, or wild rice. Carbohydrates (especially fibre), protein, iron, thiamine, niacin, riboflavin, folic acid, iron, and zinc are the main nutrients in this group. Choose grain products that are low in fat, sugar, and salt. Enriched products are also recommended because of their higher content of iron and B vitamins (**BOX 28–3**).

BOX 28–3 Fortified and Enriched Foods

Food processing removes valuable nutrients from food. To replace losses or to enhance nutrient content, foods are *enriched* or *fortified*. In enriched foods—for example, wheat flour, cereal, and pasta—nutrients are replaced to their original level or higher. In fortified foods—for example, milk fortified with vitamin D—nutrients are added. Labels on products usually indicate whether a food has been fortified or enriched.

Milk Products

Milk and milk products are high in protein, calcium, carbohydrates, fat, riboflavin, and vitamins A and D. They are the richest source of calcium, which is needed to form and maintain strong bones. It is recommended that adults drink 500 mL (2 cups) of milk every day to get adequate vitamin D. Lower-fat milk products have less fat than whole-milk products and still provide the protein and calcium essential to a healthy diet. For example, one cup of skim milk has only a trace of fat, whereas 4% of the volume of whole milk is made up of butter fat. Choose products low in milk fat and butter fat. Skim, 1%, and 2% milk are healthy choices. Other low-fat foods in this group include cheeses made with skim milk, low-fat or nonfat yogourt, and ice milk, rather than ice cream.

If you do not drink milk, drink fortified soy beverages instead.

Meat and Alternatives

Protein, fat, thiamine, vitamin B_{12}, and iron are the main nutrients in the meat and alternatives group. The foods in this group vary in fat content. Wise choices of foods in this group help lower fat intake. Cold cuts and some luncheon meats are high in fat, so choose leaner meats, poultry, and fish. Chicken and turkey have less fat compared with veal, beef, pork, and lamb, and skinless chicken and turkey are even lower in fat. Veal is lower in fat compared with beef. Egg yolks have more fat compared with egg whites. Low-fat egg substitutes can be used for cooking and baking. Dried peas, lentils, and beans are recommended as meat alternatives, as they are low in fat and provide fibre and protein.

The method of cooking can help keep the fat in foods lower, as can trimming fat from meat and poultry. Baking, broiling, roasting, or microwaving is better than deep frying. Gravies and sauces also add fat.

Eat at least two servings of fish each week. Choose char, herring, mackerel, salmon, sardines, or trout.

Meat, poultry, and seafood are high in calories, so serving size is important. Restaurants frequently serve large portions of meat—for example, a 360-g (12-ounce) steak would equal four to six servings from this group.

NUTRITION THROUGHOUT THE LIFE CYCLE

Nutritional requirements differ throughout the life cycle of a person.

Infancy and Childhood

Infancy is a period of rapid growth and development. Babies can be either breastfed or bottle-fed. Breast milk provides the best source of nutrients and antibodies during the baby's first 6 months. Formula milk can provide adequate nourishment but lacks antibodies. The pediatrician or public health nurse usually provides guidance to parents on feed times for infants.

At 4 to 6 months, iron-fortified cereals are introduced, followed by puréed foods. Most babies are ready for "finger foods" and chopped foods at 10 months to 1 year. After the first year, the growth rate slows down.

As mentioned, children usually have strong likes and dislikes for foods, which can make meal planning a challenge. Regular meals and physical activity are important for them. ***Children under 4 years should not be given a low-fat diet, as fat is needed for brain development and energy.***

When you care for infants and children, your supervisor will provide instructions about their dietary requirements. Follow the care plan.

Adolescence

In both boys and girls, the biggest growth spurt after infancy occurs during puberty, and increased nutrients are needed for this rapid growth. Many adolescents, however, have unhealthy eating habits—for example, they may skip meals, consume only fast foods and soft drinks, diet, and drink alcohol. Poor eating habits can lead to eating disorders, iron deficiency, and poor health.

Young and Middle Adulthood

Nutritional requirements in young and middle adulthood depend on age, gender, body size, and activity levels. Unless extremely active, most adults have lower energy needs than adolescents, and energy needs continue to decline into the 40s and 50s. If calorie intake exceeds energy needs, adults gain weight. A healthy diet containing essential nutrients is, therefore, extremely important.

Pregnancy

Pregnant women and their developing fetuses require nutrient-rich food, about 500 additional calories per day.

Pregnant women are advised not to smoke, drink alcohol, or take drugs unless prescribed by a health care provider. Pregnant women who do not usually consume meat and dairy products need to discuss their diets with their physicians.

Health Canada suggests that pregnant and breastfeeding women increase folic acid, iron, and calcium intake. Low folic acid intake before and during pregnancy increases the risk for spinal cord and brain abnormalities in infants.

Late Adulthood

Older adults have wide variations in their health and nutritional status, as it is affected by emotional, social, and physical factors.

Many older adults are used to cooking for and eating with a family group. Preparing a meal for just one may hold no interest for them. As well, some older adults do not drive and may not be able to carry heavy grocery bags on public transit. They may not have family or friends nearby who can help them with shopping and meal preparation. Those with low incomes may avoid buying high-protein foods such as meat and cheese, which are usually expensive. Those living in long-term care facilities may not like the food that is served.

Physical changes related to aging, such as the following, can affect the nutrition of older adults both in the community and in a facility:

- Loss of teeth or poor-fitting dentures can affect the ability to chew and the desire to eat.
- Reduction of the number of taste buds may decrease the enjoyment of food.
- Decreased strength in and effectiveness of chewing and swallowing muscles may increase the risk of choking while eating.
- Vision, hearing, and perceptual problems may decrease meal enjoyment.
- Increased fatigue upon exertion may cause a reduced desire to continue eating.
- Impaired ability to feed oneself may decrease meal enjoyment.
- Decreased muscle strength and range of motion (ROM) may affect a person's ability to eat without assistance.
- Decreased saliva secretion may cause dysphagia—difficulty (*dys*) swallowing (*phagia*) (Chapters 17 and 21).
- Decreased peristalsis (common among older adults) can result in slower emptying of the stomach and colon, flatulence (gas), and constipation.
- Decreased secretion of digestive juices makes fried and fatty foods hard to digest and may cause indigestion.
- Nutrients are not absorbed as easily.
- Medications may have adverse effects such as nausea, constipation, and loss of appetite.

Older adults require certain foods to maintain their physical health. Because energy levels are usually lower in older adults, they require fewer calories to sustain body weight, but their nutritional requirements remain high. High-protein foods are needed for tissue growth and repair. Foods high in calcium help keep bones strong; high-fibre foods such as raw vegetables help avoid constipation, but they can be hard to chew and can cause indigestion. Foods providing soft bulk, such as cooked fruits and vegetables, are often preferred for older clients with constipation or chewing problems. Drinking more fluids may also aid digestion, kidney function, chewing, and swallowing.

Good oral hygiene and well-fitted dentures can help prevent irritation of gums and mouth sores and improve the ability to eat and taste.

FACTORS THAT AFFECT EATING AND NUTRITION

Nutrition and eating habits are affected by numerous factors; some of them begin during infancy and continue throughout life, whereas some others develop later:

- ***Personal choice.*** Likes and dislikes of certain foods are a matter of personal preferences that begin in childhood. They are influenced by the way foods taste, smell, and look and the way they are prepared.
- ***Allergies.*** An **allergy** is a sensitivity to a substance that causes the body to react with signs and symptoms. Common allergic reactions are swelling of the lips, throat, tongue, or face; skin rash; coughing or difficulty breathing; abdominal cramps; nausea; or diarrhea. In severe cases, *anaphylactic shock*—a life-threatening sensitivity to a substance that can be fatal—can occur. For some people, food allergies are just an annoyance, but for some others, avoiding certain foods is a matter of life and death. Nuts and shellfish cause the most severe reactions.
- ***Food intolerances.*** A food intolerance is a noticeable reaction to food, such as indigestion and diarrhea, but it does not involve the immune system and is not as serious as a food allergy. For example, lactose intolerance occurs in people who lack the enzyme lactase, which is needed to break down the sugar (lactose) in milk. Therefore, people who are lactose intolerant cannot digest milk.
- ***Culture.*** Culture influences dietary practices, food choices, and food preparation (see the *Respecting Diversity: Food Practices* box). The way food is cooked—frying, baking, smoking, and roasting food—or not cooked depends on cultural practices. The use of sauces and spices is also related to culture. Your employer will instruct you in food preparation for your client who may have special cultural dietary practices.
- ***Religion.*** Religious practices can often influence the selection, preparation, and eating of food. Members of a religious group may follow all, some, or none of the dietary practices of their faith. You need to be aware of and respect your clients' religious practices and special preparation.
- ***Finances.*** People with limited incomes often buy cheaper foods, so their diets may lack proteins and certain vitamins and minerals.
- ***Appetite.*** *Appetite* is the desire for food. When hungry, a person seeks food and eats until the appetite is satisfied. Aromas and thoughts of food can also stimulate the appetite. However, illness, medications, anxiety, pain, and depression, as well as unpleasant sights, thoughts, and smells, can cause lack of appetite.
- ***Illness.*** Appetite usually decreases during illness and during recovery from injuries, but nutritional needs increase. The body must fight infection, heal tissues, and replace blood cells and nutrients lost though vomiting and diarrhea. Some diseases and medications can cause a sore mouth, which makes eating painful. Loss of teeth affects chewing, especially protein foods. Illness makes preparing and serving meals difficult. Long-term care residents

---

Respecting Diversity

Food Practices

Food practices vary among cultures. For example, rice and beans are common protein sources in Mexico. Rice is also common in the Philippines, China, India, and Japan. A diet high in starch and fat is common in Poland. A low-fat, high-sodium diet is common in China. In some countries (such as India), beef is not eaten by most people.

As a support worker, you could have clients from a variety of cultures. Your employer will advise you of the dietary considerations for each.

Source: Adapted from D'Avanzo, C.E., & Geissler, E.M. (2007). *Mosby's pocket guide to cultural health assessment* (4th ed.). St. Louis, MO: Mosby.

---

need good nutrition to correct or prevent health problems; however, poor nutrition is common among this population.

- ***Aging.*** Factors that can affect the appetite of older adults are loss of teeth; poor-fitting dentures; vision, hearing, or perceptual problems; fatigue; and loss of control over their choices for meals (see the *Focus on Long-Term Care: Food and Quality of Life* box).

FOOD LABELS

Food labels are useful in planning a healthy diet and following special diets ordered by physicians, dietitians, or nurses. Nutrition labels are now mandatory on packaged food. Food labels have three components: a list of ingredients, nutrition facts, and nutrition claims.

List of Ingredients

Ingredient lists usually start with the major ingredient and list other ingredients in descending order. Use the list to compare two or more products. For example, Brand 1 may list wheat flour as the first ingredient, whereas Brand 2 may list bran first. Use the lists on food products also to check for ingredients that a client may be allergic to or have an intolerance to (see p. 578).

Nutrition Facts

The *Nutrition Facts Table* (**FIGURE 28–3**) contains information on calories and 13 nutrients, including fat, carbohydrates, and protein. **Daily value (DV)** shows how a serving fits into the daily diet of an adult and is expressed as a percentage based on recommended daily intake. Health Canada recommends the following daily intake of major nutrients:

- 60% of total calories per day should come from carbohydrates.
- 10% of total calories per day should come from protein.
- 30% (or less) of total calories per day should come from fat.
- 10% (or less) of total calories per day should come from saturated fat.

Nutrition Facts Per 125 mL (87 g)	
Amount	**% DV***
Calories 80	
Fat 0.5 g	**1 %**
Saturated 0 g + Trans 0 g	**0 %**
Cholesterol 0 mg	
Sodium 0 mg	**0 %**
Carbohydrate 18 g	**6 %**
Fibre 2 g	**8 %**
Sugars 2 g	
Protein 3 g	
Vitamin A	2 %
Vitamin C	10 %
Calcium	0 %
Iron	2 %
* DV = Daily Value	

3.6 cm x 7.7 cm = 27.7 cm^2

Valeur nutritive par 125 mL (87 g)	
Teneur	**% VQ***
Calories 80	
Lipides 0,5 g	**1 %**
saturés 0 g + trans 0 g	**0 %**
Cholestérol 0 mg	
Sodium 0 mg	**0 %**
Glucides 18 g	**6 %**
Fibres 2 g	**8 %**
Sucres 2 g	
Protéines 3 g	
Vitamine A	2 %
Vitamine C	10 %
Calcium	0 %
Fer	2 %
* VQ = valeur quotidienne	

3.6 cm x 7.7 cm = 27.7 cm^2

FIGURE 28–3 The *nutrition facts table.* (**Source:** © All rights reserved. *The Nutrition Facts Table*. Health Canada, 2008. Adapted and reproduced with permission from the Minister of Health, 2016.)

FOCUS ON LONG-TERM CARE

Food and Quality of Life

Food is important to a long-term care client's quality of life. Legislation ensures the following:

- Each client's dietary and nutritional needs are met.
- Nourishing, tasty, attractive, and well-balanced meals are served.
- Hot food is served hot, and cold food is served cold.
- Special diets are provided, as needed.
- Special eating utensils are provided (**FIGURE 28–4**) for clients whose hands, wrists, and arms may be affected by disease or injury; special eating utensils help the client to eat with minimum assistance.

In some long-term care facilities, clients can dine with guests—for example, spouses, partners, family members, or friends. The dietary department may provide the meal, or it may be brought by the visitor.

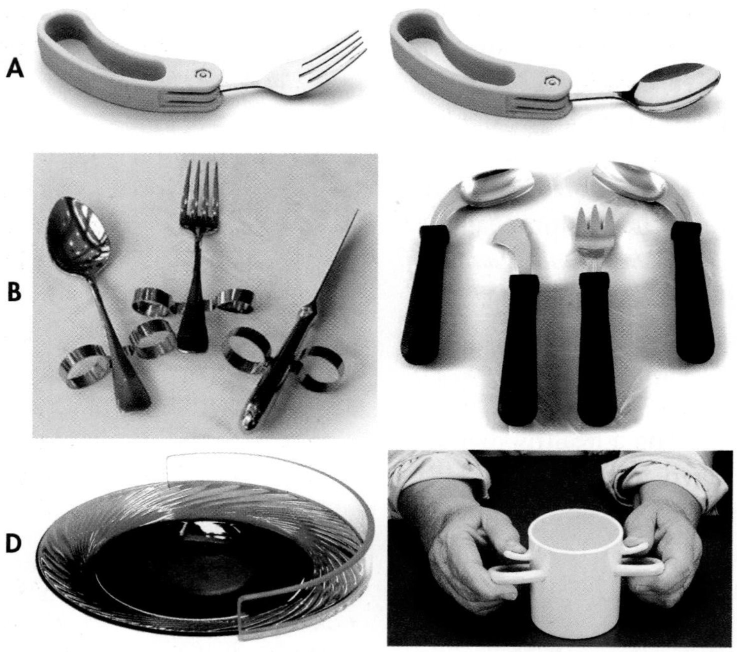

FIGURE 28–4 Eating utensils for clients with special needs. **A,** The curved fork and spoon fit over the hand. **B,** Special grips and swivel handles are helpful to some clients. **C,** Knives with rounded blades are rocked back and forth to cut food. Bent spoons and forks can be useful. **D,** Plate guards and rounded plates help keep food on the plate. **E,** Cups with double handles are easier for some clients to use. Courtesy of ElderStore, Alpharetta, GA.

Nutrition Claims

Manufacturers' nutrition claims about foods (such as "low in fat" or "high in fibre") must meet government requirements. The following diet-related health claims are allowed:

- A healthy diet low in sodium and high in potassium may reduce the risk for high blood pressure.
- A healthy diet adequate in calcium and vitamin D may reduce the risk for osteoporosis.
- A healthy diet low in saturated fat and trans fat may reduce the risk for heart disease.
- A healthy diet rich in vegetables and fruit may reduce the risk for some types of cancer.

It is always important to read the label! Some manufacturers will claim their products have "controlled (or decreased) fat," but this claim can be misleading as they have not indicated how much, if at all, the level of fat has decreased. Be careful of products labelled "controlled sugar" or "added sugar." Some foods labelled as "light" or "lite" or "fat-free" or even "sugar-free" may be higher in another ingredient, such as starches, thickeners, or sodium.

CAFFEINE INTAKE

Health Canada has been conducting research into caffeine consumption levels that can be recommended for various age groups. Its research has shown that consumption of 400 mg/day is not associated with any adverse effects in adults. For the majority of the adult population, small amounts of caffeine can help increase alertness and concentration. For some people, small or larger amounts of caffeine can cause insomnia, headaches, irritability, and nervousness.

For women who are pregnant, planning to become pregnant, or breastfeeding, the recommended intake is no more than 300 mg/day. If you asked your friends and family how much caffeine they consume in a day, they would probably count only the number of cups of coffee or tea they have. For example, they may say they generally have three coffees, but they do not specify if each cup is 240 mL (135 mg of caffeine),

480 mL, or 600 mL (595 mg of caffeine), and they do not add the caffeine from colas, chocolates, energy drinks, and over-the-counter medications.

Just one 600-mL cup of coffee contains more caffeine than the daily limit recommended for adults. How coffee is made also determines how much caffeine it contains. An average-sized 240-mL cup of instant coffee can contain as much as 106 mg of caffeine, whereas the same volume of roasted, ground, filter-dripped coffee contains 179 mg of caffeine. Even "decaffeinated" coffee contains caffeine. For example, a 240-mL cup of roasted, ground, filter-dripped decaffeinated coffee has 3 mg of caffeine, and the same volume of instant decaffeinated coffee contains 5 mg of caffeine.[3]

We know that caffeine has been identified in tea, coffee, chocolate, and some energy drinks. Certain herbs such as guarana and yerba mate that are added to energy drinks and bars also contain caffeine. Currently, these products are not required to identify the amount of caffeine added.

Recommended caffeine amounts for children are even less:

- 4–6 years: 45 mg/day
- 7–9 years: 62.5 mg/day
- 10–12 years: 85 mg/day

As a support worker, be aware of the amount of caffeine you are consuming and the amount your client is consuming, as too much caffeine can cause significant adverse effects.

Meal Planning and Preparation

Your role in meal planning and preparation depends on the care plan and on your client's needs. Most home care agencies expect clients' families to provide groceries and main meals. The case manager arranges for Meals on Wheels, if this service is available in your province or territory and if the family and client agree to use it. Meals on Wheels provides clients with their main meal of the day. You may need to prepare a light meal for a client—for example, toast for breakfast or a sandwich for lunch. Sometimes, you may have to prepare several meals and freeze them for future use. Occasionally, you may be required to plan menus and shop for groceries.

When preparing meals for clients, consider their dietary requirements, food preferences, eating limitations and eating habits.

- ***Dietary requirements.*** The care plan includes special diets, mealtime instructions, dietary practices, and food allergies and food intolerances. If there is no information in the care plan, ask your supervisor for guidance. A good cookbook is a helpful guide for planning and preparing meals.
- ***Food preferences.*** Many clients have strong food preferences and definite ideas about preparing meals. Follow the client's wishes. Never give clients food that they are not allowed. If you have concerns about a client's diet, speak with your supervisor.
- ***Eating and swallowing challenges.*** Follow the client's care plan to ensure that you consider the client's eating and swallowing limitations. Some clients may have difficulty holding regular cutlery and must have adaptive placements, plates, or cutlery. Some clients have swallowing difficulties that must be taken into consideration when their food is prepared (see p. 585). Clients who have difficulty seeing food on the plate may need your assistance to guide them (see pp.585–589).
- ***Eating habits.*** Clients may choose to have the main meal in the evening or at noon. Some clients eat several meals of the same size but never snack. Others snack between meals. Some clients eat the same things for breakfast and lunch every day.

Shopping for Groceries

You may be expected to shop for a client's food. Use shopping lists to remember needed items. If your client is on a special diet, read food labels carefully. The labels will tell you if the product is "diet," "low fat," and so on. Keep the list in one place, and encourage the client to add to it throughout the week. Add personal care items as needed. On shopping day, check and finalize the list.

Checking Expiry Dates

By law, expiry or "best before" dates must appear on products that have a limited shelf life. If stored properly, the product can be safely used before the date listed. There are three commonly used dates:

- ***Sell by date*** is the last recommended date of sale. Most products will keep for at least 3 days beyond this date.
- ***Best before date*** is the last date that the manufacturer will guarantee freshness.
- ***Expiry date*** is the last date that the product can be safely consumed.

Some products—for example, packaged meats and fish—contain only the date on which they were packaged. Select the products that were packaged most recently.

Handling Clients' Money

If you need to make food purchases for the client from a grocery store or convenience store, clients will usually provide cash. Always handle someone else's money carefully. You must be honest, efficient, and organized. Keep a separate wallet or purse for the client's money, change, and receipts. Use the receipts to total the money spent, and return the right amount of change to the client. Most employers have strict policies about handling clients' money. Be sure to follow these policies.

Following Recipes

Use a recipe to prepare meals. If necessary, consult a basic cookbook that has key terms. You may have to substitute ingredients if your client does not have an ingredient required for the recipe. For example, canola oil and margarine can usually be substituted for olive oil. Never substitute an ingredient without getting the client's permission and checking the care plan. Do not use a substitute ingredient if the client is on a special diet or has a food allergy or intolerance. Consult your supervisor for guidance.

Canada uses the metric system, which has quantities such as millilitres (mL) and grams (g). However, household units of measurement such as tablespoons or cups are also commonly used in recipes. TABLE 28–3 provides some common equivalents for metric units.

Food Safety

Food safety is an important consideration for all, because foodborne illnesses can cause serious illness or death. A **foodborne illness** is an illness caused by improperly cooked or stored food. Diarrhea, nausea, and vomiting are common signs and symptoms of a foodborne illness. Some people are at particularly high risk—for example, infants, children, older adults, people with chronic illnesses, and clients with weakened immune systems.

Pathogens are disease-causing microbes (see Chapter 23), which are commonly called *germs.* When pathogens are present in or on food, the food is said to be *contaminated.* Many foods naturally have pathogens in them in their raw state—for example, meat, fish, poultry, and eggs. When food is cooked properly, however, most pathogens are killed. However, raw food may spread pathogens to other, ready-to-eat foods—referred to as **cross-contamination**. For example, when fluids from raw chicken meat drip onto vegetables in the refrigerator, the vegetables become contaminated. If they are eaten before they are properly washed, they could cause illness.

It is usually hard to tell by sight, smell, or taste if something is contaminated. Safe food-handling practices and effective cooking can prevent cross-contamination and foodborne illnesses. Most pathogens thrive at room temperature, but they die at temperatures below 4°C (40°F) and above 60°C (140°F). Therefore, it is important to cook foods well and preserve them in the refrigerator. Never leave

TABLE 28–3 Approximate Equivalent Measurements

Liquids
1 cup = 250 millilitres (mL)
1 pint = 473 millilitres (mL)
1 quart = 1 litre (l)
½ teaspoon = 2.5 millilitres (mL)
1 teaspoon = 5 millilitres (mL)
1 tablespoon = 15 millilitres (mL)
Weights
1 ounce = 28 grams (g)
1 pound = 454 grams (g)

foods sitting out at room temperature for more than a few minutes.

If you prepare and serve meals to clients, you must know safe food-handling practices. Food safety training is a very educational course for all support workers to take and is available in most cities and towns. Observe safety practices when grocery shopping and when storing, cooking, reheating, and serving food (**BOX 28–4**).

SPECIAL DIETS

Physicians may order special diets for clients because of a nutritional deficiency or a disease, for the purpose of eliminating or decreasing certain substances in the diet, or for weight control (TABLE 28–4 on page 585). Special diets are common before and after surgery and for people with diabetes or an intolerance to gluten (p. 585). People with diseases of the heart, kidneys, gallbladder, liver, stomach, or intestines may receive special diets. Allergies, food intolerances, obesity, and other disorders also require special diets.

When a special diet is ordered, a nurse and dietitian work together to create a plan for meeting the client's nutritional needs. The plan takes into consideration the client's preferences, culture, religion, and food allergies and intolerances, as well as any eating problems such as dysphagia (see p. 585).

In facilities, the terms *regular diet, general diet,* and *house diet* mean that there are no dietary limits or restrictions. Two common special diets are the *sodium-controlled diet* and *diabetes meal planning.* Special diets can include special snacks i.e. high calorie & diabetic diets. between meal

The Sodium-Controlled Diet

The average amount of sodium found in the daily diet of a person is 3000 to 5000 mg, twice the daily amount required by the body. Healthy people excrete the excess sodium in the urine. Heart and kidney diseases, as well as some drugs and some complications of pregnancy, cause the body to retain the extra sodium.

Sodium causes the body to retain water. If there is too much sodium, tissues can swell with water, and excess fluid can build in the blood vessels, making the heart work harder. The extra workload for the heart can cause serious complications and even death. Restricting sodium in the diet helps the body retain less water, and less water in the tissues and blood vessels reduces the amount of work for the heart.

The physician may order sodium control (restriction) for the client. Many low-salt or salt-free foods are available in the market; use food labels to determine salt content.

- ***2000–3000-mg sodium diet***—called the *low-salt diet* or *no-added-salt diet.* Sodium restriction is mild, but all high-sodium foods are omitted. A minimum amount of salt is used for cooking, and salt is not added to foods at the table.
- ***1000-mg sodium diet***—sodium restriction is moderate. Food is cooked without salt, and foods high in sodium are omitted. Canned vegetables that are high in sodium due to canning are restricted in amount. Salt-free products such as salt-free bread are used. Diet planning is necessary.
- ***500-mg sodium diet***—sodium restriction is severe. Restrictions for the mild and moderate sodium diets are followed. In addition, vegetables high in sodium are omitted. Other restrictions are as follows: milk—1 cup per day; egg—1 per day; and meat—120 g (4 oz.) per day. Diet planning is essential.

Diabetic Diet

Diabetic diet meal planning is done for clients with diabetes. Type 1 diabetes is caused by the lack of insulin. Type 2 diabetes is caused by insulin resistance (see Chapter 37). In healthy people, the pancreas produces and secretes insulin, which enables the body to use the sugar consumed. In people who lack insulin, sugar builds up in the bloodstream rather than being used by cells for energy. Diabetes is usually treated with insulin or medication, diet, and exercise.

The dietitian and the client develop a meal plan together. Consistency is the key. The plan involves the following:

- ***The client's food preferences.*** It may be necessary to limit amounts or change the way food is prepared.

BOX 28–4 Guidelines for Safe Food Practices

Shopping

- Packaging should be secure. Do not buy packages that are ripped or have broken seals, and do not buy dented cans.
- Check the "best before" date. Do not buy expired items.
- Select refrigerated and frozen foods last. Do not buy items with ice crystals on the package.
- Put meats, poultry, and seafood in bags to avoid cross-contamination.

Food Storage

- Do not leave groceries in a warm car. Freeze or refrigerate items promptly.
- Store raw meat, poultry, and seafood in plastic bags on the bottom shelf of the refrigerator. This prevents their fluids from dripping onto other foods.
- Store leftovers in small, shallow containers in the refrigerator. Such containers allow rapid cooling and prevent the growth of pathogens. Cover the containers with lids, foil, or plastic wrap. Write on the containers the date you stored the leftovers.
- Do not refreeze food.

Food Preparation

- Wash your hands before and after preparing food. Wash your hands immediately before and after handling raw meat, poultry, seafood, or eggs to avoid cross-contamination of other foods.
- Do not cough or sneeze over food.
- Wear a hairnet.
- Wear gloves if you have cuts on your hands or wrists.
- Defrost foods in the refrigerator, in the microwave, or under cold running water. Do not defrost food at room temperature.
- Prevent contact between raw and ready-to-eat food.
- Wash vegetables and fruits to remove pathogens and pesticides.
- Discard food with expired "best before" dates. Discard food if it has mould on it. If in doubt about freshness, discard the product.
- Do not keep leftovers longer than 2 to 3 days.
- Use clean utensils to take food items from refrigerated containers.
- Rinse raw meats, poultry, and seafood before use. Wash the sink thoroughly (see Chapter 42).
- Avoid recipes that call for eggs not having to be cooked.
- Use different cutting boards for raw meats and poultry; seafood; cooked food; cheese; and washed fruits and vegetables. For added safety, cut raw meats, poultry, and seafood on disposable waxed paper placed on top of the board. Wash the cutting board thoroughly (see Chapter 42).
- Wash and dry the tops of cans to remove pathogens. Wash can openers to prevent pathogens from entering cans.
- Wash knives or scissors used to cut open food packages.
- Follow the guidelines for cleaning kitchens (see Chapter 42).

Cooking and Reheating Food

- Cook foods to at least their minimum safe temperature (TABLE 28–4). Cooking foods at the right temperature kills pathogens.
- Cook food thoroughly, especially meat, poultry, seafood, and eggs. Use a meat thermometer to determine if the meat is cooked. Eggs should be firm when eaten.
- Reheat sauces and gravies to a rolling boil.
- Stir and rotate food reheated in microwaves to prevent cold or hot spots.

Serving Food

- Serve food immediately after cooking it or removing it from the refrigerator. Remember, pathogens grow rapidly at room temperature.
- Serve food on a clean plate. Wash plates, platters, or containers used for raw meats, poultry, seafood, or eggs immediately after use.
- Use clean table linen, plastic mats, and eating surfaces.
- Do not use chipped or cracked dishes.

TABLE 28–4 Special Diets

Diet	Use	Foods Allowed
Clear-liquid: foods that are liquid at body temperature and that leave small amounts of residue; nonirritating and non–gas-forming	For postoperative care; acute illness; infection; nausea and vomiting; and in preparation for gastro-intestinal examinations	Water, tea, and coffee (without milk or cream); carbonated beverages; jelly; clear fruit juices (apple, grape, and cranberry); fat-free clear broth; hard candy, sugar, and popsicles
Full-liquid: foods that are liquid at room temperature or that melt at body temperature	Advance from clear-liquid diet postoperatively; for stomach irritation; for fever, nausea, and vomiting; and for people unable to chew, swallow, or digest solid foods	Foods on the clear-liquid diet, plus custard; eggnog; strained soups; strained fruit and vegetable juices; milk and milkshakes; strained, cooked cereals; plain ice cream and sherbet; pudding; yogurt
Mechanical soft: semi-solid foods that are easily digested	Advance from full-liquid diet; for chewing problems; gastro-intestinal disorders; and infections	All liquids; eggs (not fried); broiled, baked, or roasted meat, fish, or poultry that is chopped or shredded; mild cheeses (American, Swiss, cheddar, cream, and cottage); strained fruit juices; refined bread (no crust) and crackers; cooked cereal; cooked or puréed vegetables; cooked or canned fruit without skin or seeds; pudding; plain cakes and soft cookies without fruit or nuts
Fibre- and residue-restricted: food that leaves a small amount of residue in the colon	Diseases of the colon; diarrhea	Coffee, tea, milk, carbonated beverages, strained fruit juices; refined bread and crackers; creamed and refined cereal; rice; cottage and cream cheese; eggs (not fried); plain puddings and cakes; jelly; custard; sherbet and ice cream; strained vegetable juices; canned or cooked fruit without skin or seeds; potatoes (not fried); strained, cooked vegetables; plain pasta; *no raw fruits and vegetables*
High-fibre: foods that increase the amount of residue and fibre in the colon to stimulate peristalsis	Constipation and other gastro-intestinal disorders	All fruits and vegetables; whole wheat bread; whole grain cereals; fried foods; whole grain rice; milk, cream, butter, and cheese; meats

Continued

TABLE 28-4 Special Diets—cont'd

Diet	Use	Foods Allowed
Bland: foods that are mechanically and chemically nonirritating and low in roughage; foods served at moderate temperatures; no strong spices or condiments	Ulcers; gallbladder disorders; some intestinal disorders; after abdominal surgery	Lean meats; white bread; creamed and refined cereals; cream or cottage cheese; jelly, plain puddings, cakes, and cookies; eggs (not fried); butter and cream; canned fruits and vegetables without skin and seeds; strained fruit juices; potatoes (not fried); pastas and rice; strained or soft-cooked carrots, peas, beets, spinach, squash, and asparagus tips; creamed soups from allowed vegetables; *no fried foods*
High-calorie: calorie intake is increased to about 3000 to 4000; includes three full meals and between-meal snacks	For weight gain; some thyroid imbalances	Dietary increases in all foods; large portions of a regular diet with three between-meal snacks
Calorie-controlled: provides adequate nutrients while controlling calories to promote weight loss and reduction of body fat	For weight reduction	Foods low in fats and carbohydrates and lean meats; *avoid butter, cream, rice, gravies, salad oils, noodles, cakes, pastries, carbonated and alcoholic beverages, candy, potato chips, and similar foods*
High-iron: foods that are high in iron	Anemia; after blood loss; for women during the reproductive years	Liver and other organ meats; lean meats; egg yolks; shellfish; dried fruits; dried beans; leafy green vegetables; lima beans; peanut butter; enriched breads and cereals
Fat-controlled (low-cholesterol): foods low in fat and foods prepared without adding fat	Heart disease; gallbladder disease; disorders of fat digestion; liver disease; diseases of the pancreas	Skim milk or buttermilk; cottage cheese (no other cheeses allowed); jelly; sherbet; fruit; lean meat, poultry, and fish (baked, broiled, or roasted); fat-free broth; soups made with skim milk; margarine; rice, pasta, breads, and cereals; vegetables; potatoes
High-protein: aids and promotes tissue healing	Burns; high fever; infection; some liver diseases	Meat; milk, eggs, and cheese; fish and poultry; breads and cereals; leafy green vegetables
Sodium-controlled: a certain amount of sodium is allowed	Heart disease; fluid retention; liver disease; some kidney diseases	Fruits and vegetables and unsalted butter are allowed; adding salt at the table is not allowed; highly salted foods and foods high in sodium are not allowed; the use of salt in cooking may be restricted
Diabetes meal planning: the same amount of carbohydrates, protein, and fat are eaten at the same time each day	Diabetes	Determined by nutritional and energy requirements

- ***The calories needed.*** The same amount of carbohydrates, protein, and fat are eaten each day. The dietitian teaches clients, families, and other team members about portion control, food group regulations, and food substitutions.
- ***Eating meals and snacks at regular times.*** The client eats at the same time every day.

Gluten-Free Diet

Gluten is a protein that has come from wheat or related grains, such as barley, oats, rye, triticale, Kamut, or spelt. Gluten can also be introduced into a food if that food came into contact with gluten-contaminated items during manufacturing or distribution. Approximately 340 000 Canadians (or 1% of the population) cannot tolerate gluten.[4] **Celiac disease** is caused by a negative physical reaction to a gluten protein found in wheat or related grains such as barley, rye, and sometimes oats. The inflammation and destruction of the inner lining of the small intestine in celiac disease is caused by an allergic reaction to gluten in the diet.[4]

ASSISTING CLIENTS WITH EATING

A client's appetite and ability to eat can be affected by weakness and illness, odours, unpleasant equipment, an uncomfortable position, the need for oral hygiene, the need to eliminate, and pain. You can help control some of these factors by helping your clients prepare for meals:

- Assist with oral hygiene, elimination, and handwashing.
- Change clothing of and provide clean linens for clients who are incontinent.
- Be sure dentures, eyeglasses, and hearing aids are in place. Ensure that eyeglasses are clean and hearing aids are turned on.
- Help clients get to the dining room.
- Ensure a comfortable position for eating. Help clients transfer from beds to chairs or move to a sitting position in bed.

Making Meals Enjoyable

Some clients lose interest in eating because of illness or other factors. Small details can help a client enjoy a meal. Some of the following may not apply to clients on special diets. Check their individual care plans.

- ***Assist with menu choices.*** Help home care clients make choices from the Meals on Wheels menu. Help long-term care clients select a meal from the facility menu. If planning and preparing meals, involve the client in meal decisions.
- ***Make the setting attractive.*** In the client's home, let the client choose table linens and utensils.
- ***Serve hot meals immediately.*** Lukewarm meals lack appeal.
- ***Serve moderate portions.*** Some clients lose their appetite at the sight of too much food. Ask clients how much food they want. Place the desired amount on the plate.
- ***Make mealtimes social occasions.*** To avoid loneliness at mealtimes, encourage clients in long-term care facilities to dine with others. In home care settings, provide company to clients by staying with them while you do quiet tasks such as folding laundry.

Assisting Clients With Eating Problems

Changes resulting from aging, illness, and disabilities—such as chewing and swallowing problems, weakness, and vision loss—can cause eating problems.

Chewing Problems

Clients with chewing problems are served foods that provide soft bulk (see "Mechanical soft diet" in TABLE 28–4, p. 585). Purée foods with a food processor or blender. Follow the care plan. To help clients overcome chewing problems, do the following:

- Offer plenty of fluids
- Offer small mouthfuls
- Give the client time to chew

Swallowing Problems (Dysphagia)

Clients can have difficulty swallowing for many reasons. Certain medications (including chemotherapy) decrease saliva production, resulting in dry mouth. Clients with paralysis may have difficulty swallowing because their throat muscles are affected.

A swallowing assessment is completed by a speech pathologist, an occupational therapist, a physiotherapist, or a nurse who has received training in this assessment tool. Warning signs that your client is having difficulty swallowing include frequent clearing of the throat; a gurgling-sounding voice; delayed swallowing or holding of food in the mouth; multiple swallows for one bite; and trouble controlling food and saliva in the mouth.

Clients who have difficulty swallowing thin liquids often must drink thickened liquids. There are three common consistencies of thickened liquids[5]:

- ***Nectar-thickened or easily pourable***—consistency similar to thicker cream soup, or milkshake
- ***Honey-thickened or slightly thicker***—consistency similar to honey; pours very slowly
- ***Pudding-thickened***—will hold its shape when scooped; usually eaten with a spoon; similar to the consistency of pudding

A client who requires thickeners should not be given anything that melts, such as ice cream or ice cubes. Clients with dysphagia often do not get enough fluids, so it is important to offer fluids frequently throughout the day—every 2 hours or as per the care plan. Thickened liquids are considered part of a client's fluid intake.

Thick, soft, moist foods are served to clients who have problems swallowing. The care plan may include the following measures to help a client swallow:

- Help the client sit upright, leaning slightly forward.
- Ask the client to lower the chin while swallowing.
- Offer plenty of fluids.
- Give the client time to chew and swallow before offering more food.
- Ask the client to remain sitting for at least 30 minutes after the meal.

When feeding clients with swallowing problems, it is generally recommended that you give them one third of a teaspoon at a time. However, being fed such a small amount would involve many spoonfuls, which could tire the client. Follow the care plan regarding the amount you should feed at a time.

Clients with swallowing problems are at risk for choking and aspiration. **Aspiration** is the inhalation of fluid or an object into the lungs. If a client is unable to talk or cough, she may be choking, and you should call for help immediately. If no help is available, follow the emergency measures for choking (foreign-body airway obstruction) that you have been taught in your first-aid and CPR (cardiopulmonary resuscitation) course.

Weakness

Some clients are too weak to chew and swallow their food, and when they do not eat well, they become even weaker and have even less energy to eat. Never force a client to eat. If the client cannot eat, tell your supervisor. To encourage a client to eat, offer frequent, small, high-calorie meals, and serve nutritious drinks, including liquid dietary supplements. Soft foods that do not need much chewing are preferred. Follow the care plan, and do the following:

- Allow the client to rest before and after meals.
- Use the appropriate feeding utensils. For example, the Ministry of Health and Long-Term Care (MOHLTC) in Ontario requires that clients be fed using a teaspoon. Check with your supervisor and the client's care plan.
- Provide a straw to drink (if allowed) so the client does not need to lift the glass. Check with your supervisor and the client's care plan.
- Provide cups, glasses, and utensils that are light and easy to handle.

Vision Loss

Clients with vision loss are often keenly aware of food aromas and often can identify the foods served to them. Most of these clients can eat independently, with some guidance. To assist these clients to eat, do the following:

- Identify the location of foods and fluids on the tray or table.
- Use the numbers on a clock to identify the location of foods and fluids (**FIGURE 28–5**).
- Describe what you are offering if you are feeding the client.

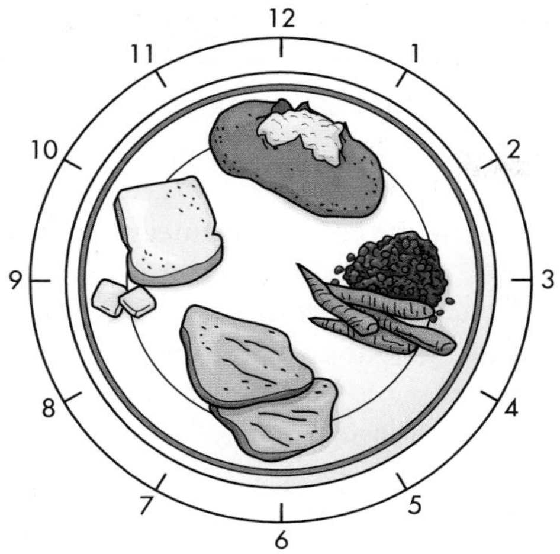

FIGURE 28–5 The numbers on a clock are used to help a client with vision loss locate food on a plate.

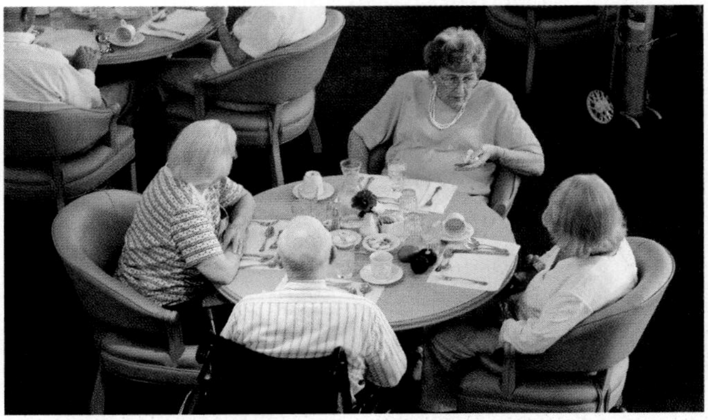

FIGURE 28–6 Clients enjoy a pleasant meal in the dining room. Source: © Dennis MacDonald/maXximages.com.

FOCUS ON LONG-TERM CARE

Dining Programs

Many long-term care facilities have special dining programs:

- ***Social dining***—clients eat in the dining room. Each table has four to six residents (FIGURE 28–6). Food is served as in a restaurant. Depending on the policy of the facility, agency, province, or territory, clients usually sit in the same place for each meal and are not moved except under special circumstances. They establish a relationship with the other clients at their table, and because this relationship is respected, their place is maintained. Follow the dining room seating plan posted in your facility dining room.
- ***Family dining***—food is placed in bowls and on platters, and clients serve themselves as they would at home.
- ***Assistive dining***—some facilities have circular or horseshoe-shaped tables. Clients who need assistance with eating are seated around the tables. In this arrangement, the support worker sits at the centre of the table and is able to feed as many as four clients. In Ontario, however, MOLTHC regulations indicate that a support worker can assist and feed a maximum of only two clients at a time. For this reason, circular or horseshoe-shaped tables are no longer used in Ontario. Follow the policy of your agency, facility, province, or territory for feeding clients.

Serving Meal Trays

Most clients in hospitals eat their meals in their rooms. However, long-term care clients are encouraged to eat in the dining room (see the *Focus on Long-Term Care: Dining Programs* box), but those who are too ill to move about eat in their rooms.

In most provinces and territories in Canada, clients in long-term care facilities must eat in the dining room unless they are ill. If a client wishes to eat in his room, a team conference to discuss the safety issues and risks of eating alone, especially if the client has dysphagia, must be scheduled and must involve the family, client, and staff. A staff member has to be with the client to supervise the meal. Follow your facility's policies.

Meals served in beds and bedrooms are delivered on trays, with the food served in containers that keep hot and cold foods at the correct temperature. Prepare clients for eating before meal trays arrive. Serve meal trays promptly so that food is served at the right temperature. Home care clients usually eat in the dining room or kitchen. If they are weak or ill, they may eat in bed or sitting in a chair in the bedroom.

Assisting a Client to Eat Meals From a Food Tray

123

Advocate on behalf of the client's quality of life by promoting:

Dignity • Independence • Preferences • Privacy • Safety *(see BOX 1-4, on p. 17)*

PRE-PROCEDURE

1 Identify the client, according to employer policy
This eliminates the possibility of mistaking one client for another.
2 Perform hand hygiene.
3 Prepare the client for the meal. Assist with handwashing.
4 If indicated in the client's care plan or if requested by your client, provide for privacy.
This ensures dignity for the client. However, most clients benefit from the social interaction that takes place at mealtime.
5 Make sure the tray contains everything needed. Make sure special utensils are included if needed.

PROCEDURE

6 Help the client to a sitting position.
This helps reduce the risk of choking.
7 Place the tray on the overbed table or other table.
8 Remove lids from dishes. Open milk cartons and cereal boxes, cut the meat, and butter the bread if indicated in the care plan (FIGURE 28–7).

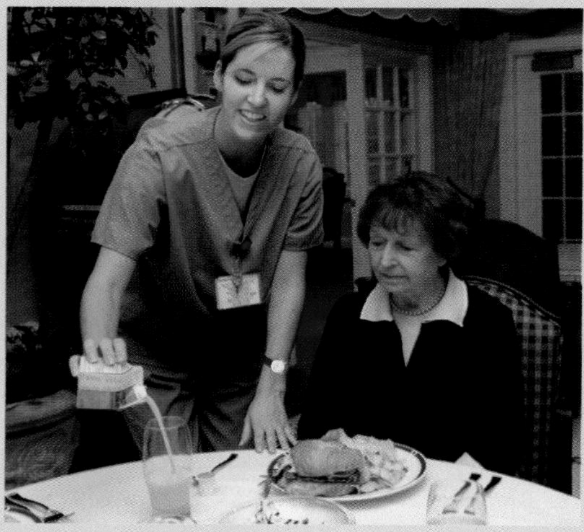

FIGURE 28–7 Open cartons and other containers for the client.

9 Place the napkin, clothes protector (if needed), and utensils within the client's reach.
10 Measure and record intake if ordered (see pp. 595–596). Note the amount and types of foods eaten.
11 Check for and remove any food in the client's mouth (pocketing). Wear gloves.
Pocketing food can lead to choking if kept in the mouth. Pocketing food indicates that the client has difficulty swallowing the food, which must be recorded and reported.
12 Remove the tray.
13 Assist with handwashing. Offer oral hygiene. Wear gloves for this step.
Handwashing decreases the risk for pathogen spread. Oral hygiene can stimulate saliva production, which can assist in chewing food and in digestion.
14 Clean any spills, and change soiled linen.
15 Help the client to return to bed if indicated.

POST-PROCEDURE

16 Provide for safety and comfort.
17 Place the call bell within reach.*
This provides an easy, safe way for the client to contact staff if necessary.
18 Follow the care plan for bed rail use.*
This helps ensure client safety.
19 Perform hand hygiene.

Report and Record your actions and observations, according to employer policy. Include the amount and kind of food eaten.
It is important to monitor the food intake of clients. Documentation is also done for legal reasons and to keep the rest of the health care team informed.

*Steps marked with an asterisk may not apply in community settings.

Assisting a Client With Eating

Some clients who cannot feed themselves because of weakness, paralysis, casts, and other physical limits need to be fed. Any client who needs to be fed may be at risk for swallowing difficulties or aspiration, so it is important that you pay close attention to the client. Needing to be fed can be difficult for the client to accept, so you need to be kind and supportive when feeding these clients (see the *Providing Compassionate Care: Assisting a Client With Eating* box).

Between-Meal Nourishments

Some special diets involve between-meal nourishments, such as crackers, milk, juice, a milkshake, cake, wafers, a sandwich, gelatin, and custard. Provide nourishments according to the care plan. Prepackaged nutritional liquid food supplements such as Ensure and Boost are meant only to be supplements and not meal replacements for an extended period, as they do not provide adequate nutritional balance. In home care settings, you may have to prepare the between-meal nourishments. In facilities, they are supplied to the unit. Provide eating utensils, a straw, and a napkin to the client. Follow the procedures for serving meals and feeding clients.

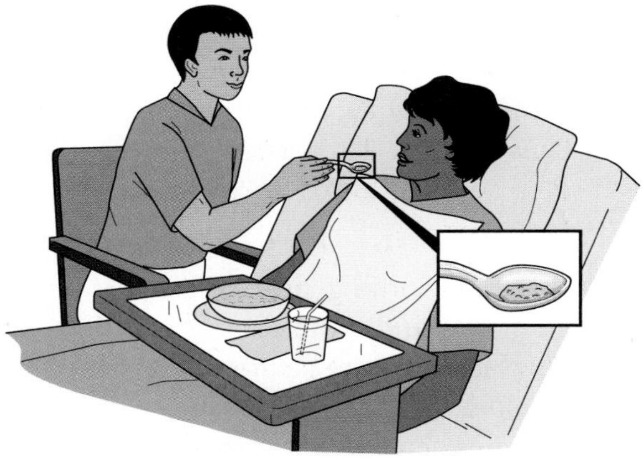

FIGURE 28–8 A teaspoon is used to feed a client.

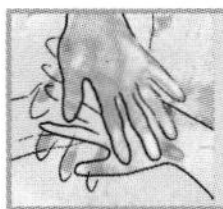

Providing Compassionate Care
Assisting a Client With Eating

- ***Dignity.*** Clients who cannot feed themselves may feel embarrassed, humiliated, or angry, and some clients can become depressed or resentful. Some of these clients may refuse to eat. Be gentle, patient, and encouraging, and ensure comfort. Sit facing the client, as it is more relaxing and shows that you have time for the client. Standing communicates that you are in a hurry, and clients should never be made to feel rushed. Clean up dribbles and spills in a tactful way to save the client from embarrassment.
- ***Independence***. Encourage the client to participate in some part of the meal, and allow the client to set the pace. The client may be able to gesture or nod to show preferences.
- ***Preferences.*** If the client wants to pray before eating, provide time and privacy for it. Describe the food on the tray, and ask the client the order in which foods and fluids should be served. Ask questions and use paraphrasing (see Chapter 5) to make sure that you understand the client's feelings and wishes. Engage the client in pleasant conversation.
- ***Privacy.*** Some clients do not like others to see them being fed. Be sensitive to your client's needs and feelings. Provide for privacy if desired by the client.
- ***Safety***. Follow the care plan. Use spoons, not forks, as they are less likely to cause injury. The spoon should be only one-third full (FIGURE 28–8) each time, as this portion is easy to chew and swallow. Some clients need even smaller portions. Sit facing the client so that you can immediately see signs of choking or any problems with eating, chewing, or swallowing. Give the client enough time to chew and swallow. Remember to offer fluids during the meal as they help with chewing and swallowing. Some clients may tend to fall asleep during their meals, which may pose a swallowing risk. Attempt to stimulate the client by gently stroking the cheek and addressing the client by name. If the client does not awaken, do not attempt to feed the client. Report your observations and record this situation in the appropriate manner.

Assisting the Client With Eating

123

Advocate on behalf of the client's quality of life by promoting:

Dignity • **I**ndependence • **P**references • **P**rivacy • **S**afety *(see BOX 1-4, on p. 17)*

PRE-PROCEDURE

1 Identify the client, according to employer policy.
2 Explain the procedure to the client.
3 Perform hand hygiene.
4 Prepare the client for mealtime. Assist with handwashing.
5 Provide for privacy only if requested by the client.
6 Help the client to a comfortable sitting position. Ensure the client is at a level that will not cause you risk for injury.
This helps prevent possible back injury to you and your client.
7 Place the tray on the overbed table or other table.

PROCEDURE

8 Drape a clothing protector across the client's chest and under the chin.
This keeps clothing cleaner and can prevent staining of clothing.
9 Prepare the food for eating.
Eating food in small pieces reduces the chances of choking.
10 Tell the client what foods are on the tray.
The client may indicate a food that is not preferred and, therefore, will not be eaten.
11 a Serve foods in the order the client prefers. Alternate between solid and liquid foods. Use a teaspoon for safety (see **FIGURE 28–8**). The amount of food in each spoonful should be enough for the client to sense the bulk in the mouth.
This stimulates chewing and swallowing.
b Allow time for chewing. Do not rush the client.
12 a Use straws if allowed in the care plan and if the client cannot drink out of a glass or cup. Use one straw for each liquid. Use a short straw if the client is weak.
b Some clients with dysphagia do not use straws. Instead, give thickened liquids with a spoon. Follow the care plan.
13 Talk with the client.
Mealtime should be treated as a relaxing social time. Clients will eat better if they are relaxed.
14 Encourage the client to eat.
15 Wipe the client's mouth with a napkin as soon as a spill occurs.
This helps ensure client dignity.
16 Note how much was eaten and which foods were eaten.
These are important observations to be recorded, as they will direct the next 24 hours of care for your client.
17 Measure and record intake if ordered.
18 Remove the tray.
19 Assist with oral hygiene (if in the care plan) and handwashing. Wear gloves for this step.

POST-PROCEDURE

20 Provide for safety and comfort.
21 Place the call bell within reach.*
This provides an easy, safe way for the client to contact staff if necessary.
22 Follow the care plan for bed rail use.*
This helps decrease the risk for falls.
23 Remove privacy measures.
24 Perform hand hygiene.

Report and Record your actions and observations, according to employer policy. Include the following:

- ☐ The amount of food eaten and the kind of food eaten
- ☐ Complaints of nausea or dysphagia
- ☐ Signs of aspiration

This is done for legal reasons and to keep the rest of the health care team informed.

*Steps marked with an asterisk may not apply in community settings.

Calorie Counts

For some clients, it is important to keep a record of calorie intake. A flow sheet is provided for this purpose, and you must note what the client ate and how much. For example, a client is served a chicken breast, a baked potato, green beans, a roll, pudding, and two pats of butter. You record on the form that the client finished all the chicken, half the potato, the roll, and one pat of butter but left the beans and the pudding. The care plans tell you which clients require calorie counts.

FLUID BALANCE

Harm, even death, can result from too much or too little water in the body, so fluid balance is essential for health. The amount of fluids taken in (**intake**) and the amount lost (**output**) must be equal. If fluid intake exceeds fluid output, tissues swell with water—a condition called *edema* (see Chapter 37). Edema is common in clients with heart and kidney diseases. **Dehydration** is a decrease in the amount of water in body tissues, which occurs when fluid output exceeds intake. Common causes are low fluid intake, vomiting, diarrhea, bleeding, excess sweating, and increased urine production.

Normal Fluid Requirements

An adult needs 1500 mL of water daily to survive. About 2000 to 2500 mL of fluid per day is needed for normal fluid balance, but water requirements increase in certain conditions—such as hot weather, exercise, fever, illness, and excessive fluid loss. Minimum water requirements vary with age (see the *Focus on Children: Fluid Requirements* and *Focus on Older Adults: Fluid Requirements* boxes).

FOCUS ON CHILDREN

Fluid Requirements

Infants and young children have more body water than do adults and, therefore, need higher fluid intake. Excessive fluid loss can quickly cause death in infants and children.

Special Orders

To maintain fluid balance in a client, the physician may specify the amount of fluid that a client can have in a 24-hour period. Common orders in the care plan are as follows:

- ***Encourage fluids.*** The client needs to drink more fluids. The order states the amount to ingest and provides a variety of allowed fluids. Fluids are kept within the client's reach and are offered regularly to clients who cannot feed themselves. Intake records are kept.
- ***Restrict fluids.*** Fluids are restricted to a specific amount. They are offered in small amounts and in small containers. The water pitcher is removed or kept out of sight. The client needs frequent oral hygiene, as it helps keep the mucous membranes of the mouth moist. Intake records are kept.
- ***Nothing by mouth (NPO).*** The client cannot eat or drink anything—*NPO* stands for the Latin term *nil per os,* meaning "nothing (*nil*) by (*per*) mouth (*os*)." Clients are usually NPO before and after surgery, before certain laboratory tests and X-ray procedures, and in the treatment of certain illnesses. Clients who are tube-fed may be NPO, in which case an NPO sign is usually posted above the bed and the water pitcher and glass are removed. Frequent oral hygiene is important, but you must ensure that the client does not swallow any fluid.

FOCUS ON OLDER ADULTS

Fluid Requirements

Older adults are at risk for diseases that affect fluid balance, such as heart disease, kidney disease, cancer, and diabetes. Many older adults also take medications that cause the body to lose fluids or retain water. Older adults are, thus, at risk for edema and dehydration.

Older adults may have a decreased sense of thirst. Their bodies need water, but they may not feel thirsty. Offer water often to your older clients.

Intake and Output Records

The physician or nurse may want a client's fluid intake and output measured, in which case you will have to keep intake and output (I&O) records. I&O records are used to evaluate fluid balance and kidney function and to plan medical treatment. They also are kept when the client has special fluid orders.

All fluids taken by mouth, as well as fluids given in IV therapy and tube feedings (see Chapter 29), are measured and recorded. The obvious fluids are measured—water, milk, coffee, tea, juices, soups, and soft drinks—as well as the fluid content in soft and semi-solid foods such as ice cream, sherbet, custard, pudding, jelly, and popsicles. Output measure includes urine, vomitus, diarrhea, and wound drainage.

Measuring Intake and Output

Intake and output are measured in millilitres (mL) or in cubic centimetres (cc). These metric-system measurements are equal in amount.

- 30 mL equals 1 ounce
- 500 mL is about 1 pint
- 1000 mL is about 1 quart

You need to know the serving size of bowls, cups, glasses, and other containers. The information may be on the I&O record or in the policy manual.

A container called a *graduate* is used to measure fluids, including leftover fluids, urine, vomitus, and drainage from suction (see Chapter 32). Similar to a measuring cup, the graduate is marked in millilitres or cubic centimetres as well as in ounces (**FIGURE 28-9**). Plastic urinals and kidney basins are also marked with measurements.

When intake or output is measured, the amount is recorded in the appropriate column on the I&O record (**FIGURE 28-10**). Amounts are totalled at the end of the shift and recorded on the client's chart. In facilities, totals are shared among staff during end-of-shift reporting.

Recording intake and output is ordered for many different reasons. As mentioned on pages 572 and 593, fluid (primarily water) balance is needed for health. Unequal intake and output amounts will alert the health care team to carry out interventions needed to correct the fluid balance.

The purpose of measuring I&O and how doing so can help are explained to the client. Some clients measure and record their intake themselves, and sometimes family members may help. For output measurement, the urinal, commode, bedpan, or specimen pan is used. Remind the client not to void in the toilet and not to put toilet tissue into the container that will be used for taking measurements.

Follow medical asepsis and Standard Practices when measuring intake and output.

Think About Safety

Guidelines for Feeding Clients

- To ensure client safety, check care plans to be aware of any food or liquid allergies or intolerances your clients may have.
- If you are working in a community setting and are expected to shop for the client's food, ensure that you check expiry dates on everything you buy.
- If you are preparing meals for your client, follow the client's recipes, and do not substitute ingredients without the permission of the client.
- When assisting a client with eating, follow the care plan, as your province or territory will have legislation that outlines the policy your facility or agency needs to follow.
- Clients with dysphagia will have special dietary needs to avoid choking. Follow the care plan.
- Notify your supervisor of any changes you have observed in your client's eating habits.

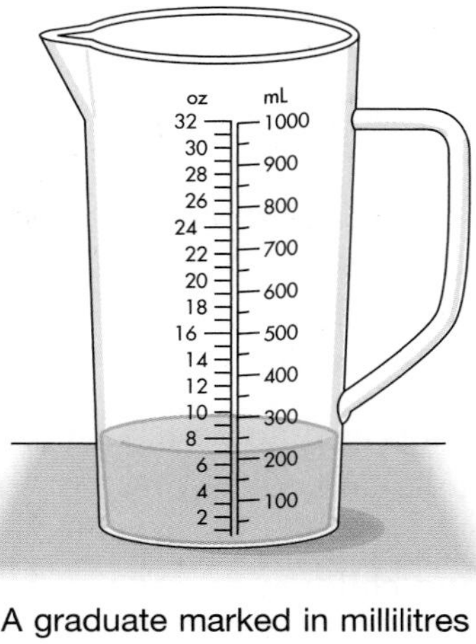

FIGURE 28-9 A graduate marked in millilitres and ounces.

CODE

O - Oral NG - Nasogastric
IV - Intravenous GT - Gastrostomy Tube

INTAKE

CODE

U - Urine
E - Emesis

OUTPUT

DATE	NIGHT	CODE	INIT.	DAY	CODE	INIT.	EVE	CODE	INIT.	24 HR TOTAL	NIGHT	CODE	INIT.	DAY	CODE	INIT.	EVE	CODE	INIT.	24 HR TOTAL

Initials		NURSE'S SIGNATURE	Initials		NURSE'S SIGNATURE	Initials		NURSE'S SIGNATURE	Initials		NURSE'S SIGNATURE
1			3			5			7		
2			4			6			8		

Name ______________________ Birthdate ______________

Admission Date ______________________ Medical Rec. # ______________

Physician ______________________

GSS #242

INTAKE & OUTPUT RECORD

Rev. 2-12-82

FIGURE 28–10 An intake and output record. Source: Sorrentino, S.A. (2000). *Mosby's textbook for nursing assistants* (5th ed., p. 384). St. Louis, MO: Mosby.

Measuring Intake and Output

123

Advocate on behalf of the client's quality of life by promoting:

Dignity • Independence • Preferences • Privacy • Safety *(see BOX 1-4, on p. 17)*

PRE-PROCEDURE

1 Identify the client, according to employer policy.
This eliminates the possibility of mistaking one client for another.

2 Explain the procedure to the client.

3 Perform hand hygiene.

4 Collect the following supplies:
- ☐ **I&O record**
- ☐ **Graduate**
- ☐ **Gloves**

5 Provide for privacy.

PROCEDURE

6 Put on gloves.

7 Measure intake as follows:
- a Pour remaining liquid in the serving container into the graduate.
- b Measure the amount at eye level, keeping the graduate level.

This helps ensure accurate measurement.
- c Check the consumed amount, as recorded on the I&O record.
- d Subtract the amount consumed from the full serving amount, and record the amount of intake.
- e Repeat steps *a* through *d* above for each liquid.
- f Total the intake amounts of all liquids.
- g Record the time and amount on the I&O record.

Intake and output recording monitors the client's food intake or fluid balance. This must be done for legal reasons and to keep the rest of the health care team informed.

8 Measure output as follows:
- a Pour fluid into the graduate used to measure output.
- b Measure the amount at eye level, keeping the graduate level.

9 Dispose of fluid in the toilet, taking care to avoid splashes.

10 Clean and rinse the graduate. Dispose of rinse into the toilet. Return the graduate to its proper place.

11 Clean and rinse the bedpan, urinal, kidney basin, or other drainage container. Discard the rinse into the toilet. Return the item to its proper place.

12 Remove gloves. Perform hand hygiene.

13 Record the amount on the I&O record.
Fluid intake is important in determining how the client's heart and kidneys are performing. Accuracy is essential.

14 Remove privacy measures.

POST-PROCEDURE

Report and Record your actions and observations, according to employer policy.
This is done for legal reasons and to keep the rest of the health care team informed.

CHAPTER REVIEW

KEY POINTS

- Foods and liquids contain nutrients, which are substances that are ingested, digested, absorbed, and used by the body. Our bodies need a certain amount of proteins, carbohydrates, fats, vitamins, minerals, and water each day.
- Health Canada's publication *Eating Well With Canada's Food Guide* promotes wise food choices. The *Food Guide* is available in English, French, and 10 other languages, and a tailored version is available for Indigenous people in Canada.
- Be aware of the amount of caffeine you and your clients consume daily. Too much caffeine can cause adverse effects.
- Nutritional requirements differ throughout a person's life cycle.
- Factors that can affect eating and nutrition are personal choices, allergies, food intolerances, culture, religion, finances, appetite, illness, and age.
- In the case of clients with type 1 diabetes, it is very important to record the intake for every meal and snack to ensure that their dietary intake is adequate for the amount of insulin they must take.
- Follow the care plan carefully, especially if you are to assist a client with eating.
- Recording intake and output is necessary when caring for a client who is ill. Harm, even death, can result from too much or too little water in the body.

CRITICAL THINKING IN PRACTICE

Mr. Lund has Parkinson's disease (see Chapters 36 and 37). This disease affects his movement, swallowing, and speech. When you try to feed him, he closes his mouth and shakes his head. He takes only small sips of thickened liquid. What do you do? What measures might be included in his care plan to meet nutrition and fluid needs?

REVIEW QUESTIONS

Answers to these questions are at the bottom of page 598.

Circle the BEST answer.

1. Nutrition is:
   A. Fats, proteins, carbohydrates, vitamins, minerals, and water
   B. The many processes involved in the ingestion, digestion, absorption, and use of foods and fluids by the body
   C. The *Canada's Food Guide* rainbow
   D. The balance between calories taken in and those used by the body

2. Protein is needed for:
   A. Tissue growth and repair
   B. Energy and fibre
   C. Body heat and the protection of organs from injury
   D. Improving the taste of food

3. *Eating Well With Canada's Food Guide* encourages:
   A. A low-carbohydrate diet
   B. A high-fat diet
   C. A low-fibre diet
   D. A low-fat diet

4. How many daily servings of grain product does the Food Guide recommend for women over 50 years of age?
   A. 5
   B. 6
   C. 4
   D. 3

5. Which food groups contain the most fat?
   A. Grain products and milk products
   B. Grain products and meat and alternatives
   C. Milk products and meat and alternatives
   D. Grain products and vegetables and fruit

6. The daily value (DV) is an amount that indicates:
- A. The number of calories an adult of average weight should consume daily
- B. Intake and output measured in millilitres (mL) or in cubic centimetres (cc)
- C. The nutrients in each meal served in hospitals and long-term care facilities
- D. A percentage of the recommended daily amount of a nutrient in a serving of food

7. Older adults:
- A. Have lower nutrient requirements than younger adults do
- B. Should eat a high-fat diet
- C. Should eat foods high in protein and calcium
- D. Should consume at least 3000 calories per day

8. Which of the following is an acceptable food safety practice?
- A. Washing your hands immediately after handling raw chicken
- B. Defrosting frozen chicken on the kitchen counter
- C. Cutting raw chicken and vegetables on the same cutting board
- D. Serving chicken that is crisp on the outside and pink on the inside

9. People with diabetes must:
- A. Restrict their intake of fluids
- B. Eat a diet high in saturated fat and protein
- C. Eat a high-fibre diet
- D. Eat the same amount of carbohydrates, protein, and fat each day

10. Which of the following is suggested for clients who are weak and fatigued?
- A. A straw for drinking liquids
- B. Large portions
- C. Foods that are high in calories
- D. Hard-to-chew foods

11. Adult fluid requirements for normal fluid balance are about:
- A. 1000 to 1500 mL daily
- B. 1500 to 2000 mL daily
- C. 2000 to 2500 mL daily
- D. 2500 to 3000 mL daily

12. A person is NPO. You should:
- A. Provide a variety of fluids
- B. Offer fluids in small amounts and small containers
- C. Remove the water pitcher and glass
- D. Prevent the person from having oral hygiene

Answers: 1.B, 2.A, 3.D, 4.B, 5.C, 6.D, 7.C, 8.A, 9.D, 10.C, 11.C, 12.C

Chapter opener image: Monkey Business Images/Shutterstock.com

CHAPTER 29

Enteral Nutrition and Intravenous Therapy

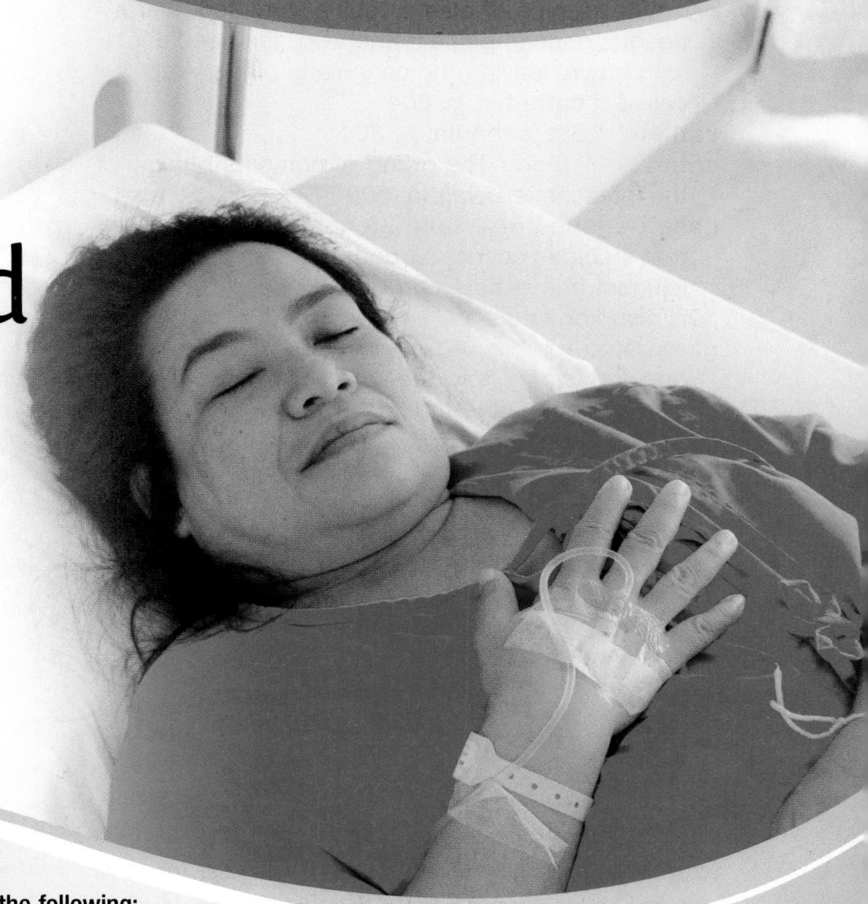

OBJECTIVES

After reading this chapter, the learner should be able to do the following:

- Explain the purpose of enteral nutrition and necessary comfort measures.
- Explain how to prevent aspiration and regurgitation.
- Identify the signs and symptoms of aspiration.
- Identify the solutions, equipment, and complications involved in intravenous (IV) therapy.
- Explain your role in ensuring the safety of clients receiving IV therapy.

KEY TERMS

cannula A type of plastic tubing threaded over a needle; once in place in the vein, the needle is withdrawn, leaving the cannula in place. Also called a **catheter**. *p. 604*

catheter See **cannula**. *p. 604*

enteral nutrition The giving of nutrients by way of the intestine (*enteral*). *p. 600*

gastro-jejunostomy tube A combination device that includes access to both the stomach and the jejunum (the middle part of the small intestine). It is also known as a *GJ-tube*. *p. 600*

gastrostomy tube A tube inserted through an opening (*stomy*) into the stomach (*gastro*). It is also known as a *G-tube*. *p. 600*

gavage Tube feeding. *p. 600*

infiltration Intravenous fluids' entering surrounding tissues. *p. 606*

intravenous (IV) therapy Fluids given through a needle or catheter inserted into a vein; also referred to as *IV*, *IV therapy*, and *IV infusion*. *p. 604*

jejunostomy tube A tube inserted into the intestines through an opening (*stomy*) into the middle part of the small intestine (*jejunum*). It is also known as a *J-tube*. *p. 601*

nasogastric (NG) tube A tube inserted through the nose (*naso*) into the stomach (*gastro*). It is also known as an *NG-tube*. *p. 600*

nasointestinal tube A tube inserted through the nose (*naso*) into the small intestine (intestinal). *p. 600*

ostomy A surgically created opening that is used to drain wastes or to feed the client. *p. 600*

percutaneous endoscopic gastrostomy (PEG) tube A tube inserted into the stomach (*gastro*) through a puncture wound (*stomy*) made through (*per*) the skin (*cutaneous*); a lighted instrument (*scope*) allows the physician to see inside the body cavity or organ (*endo*). *p. 601*

regurgitation The backward flow of food from the stomach into the mouth. *p. 603*

Clients may have special requirements in regard to nutrition and fluids. Because of illness, injury, or surgery, some clients have difficulty eating, drinking, chewing, or swallowing. For these clients, nutrition and fluids as well as medications are provided through tubes, as ordered by a physician. Only a qualified nurse or other professional administers the procedures. As a support worker, however, you care for clients who have had these procedures.

ENTERAL NUTRITION

People who cannot chew or swallow often require **enteral nutrition**, a nutritional formula delivered into the gastro-intestinal tract (*enteral*) through a feeding tube. **Gavage** is another term for tube feeding. Feeding tubes are used when food cannot pass normally from the mouth into the esophagus and then into the stomach. This need can arise due to cancers of the head, neck, and esophagus; trauma or surgery to the face, mouth, head, or neck; dysphagia caused by paralysis; and coma. As well, people with dementia who no longer know how to eat may require tube feedings. There are various types of feeding tubes:

- A **nasogastric (NG) tube** is inserted through the nose (*naso*) into the stomach (*gastro*) (**FIGURE 29–1**). A physician or a nurse performs the procedure.
- A **nasointestinal tube** is inserted through the nose (*naso*) into the small intestine (*intestinal*) (**FIGURE 29–2**). A physician or a nurse performs the procedure.
- A **gastrostomy tube** is inserted into the stomach. A surgically created opening (*stomy*) in the stomach (*gastro*) is needed for this procedure (**FIGURE 29–3**). It is also known as a *G-tube*.
- A **gastro-jejunostomy tube** is a combination device that includes access to both the stomach and the jejunum (the middle part of the small intestine). It is also known as a *GJ-tube*. Typically, tubes are placed into a G-tube stoma (a surgically created opening—see ***ostomy***), with a narrower long tube continuing through the stomach and small intestine. The GJ-tube is used if the client has a high risk for aspiration or when a tube cannot

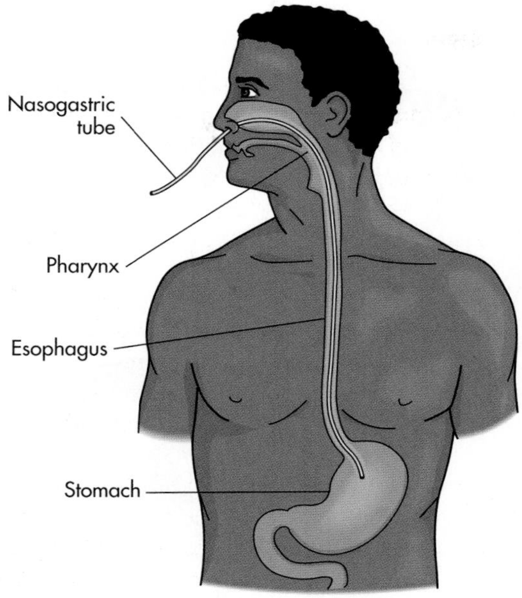

FIGURE 29–1 A nasogastric tube is inserted through the nose and esophagus into the stomach.

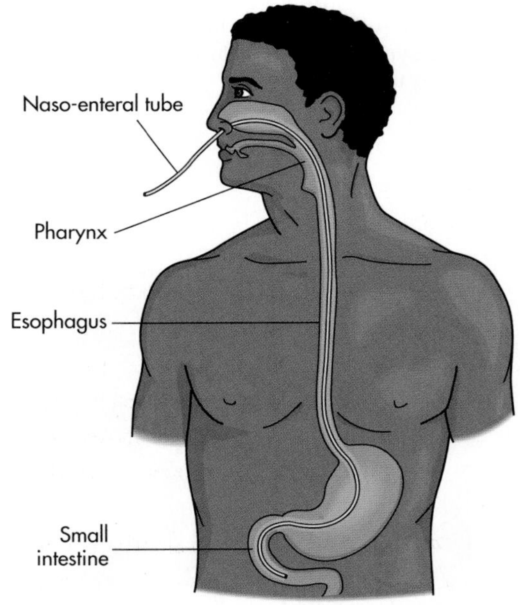

FIGURE 29–2 A nasointestinal tube is inserted through the nose into the duodenum or jejunum of the small intestine.

be placed into the client's stomach. It must be inserted by a physician in a hospital setting.

- A **jejunostomy tube** is inserted into the intestines. A surgically created opening (*stomy*) in the middle part of the small intestine (*jejunum*) is needed for this procedure (**FIGURE 29–4**). It is also known as a *J-tube*.

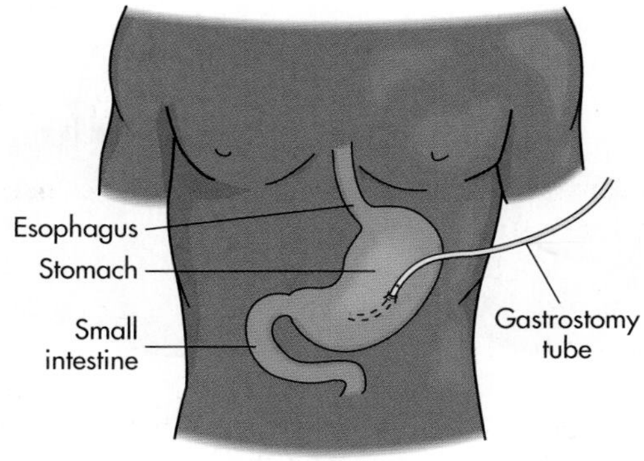

FIGURE 29–3 A gastrostomy tube.

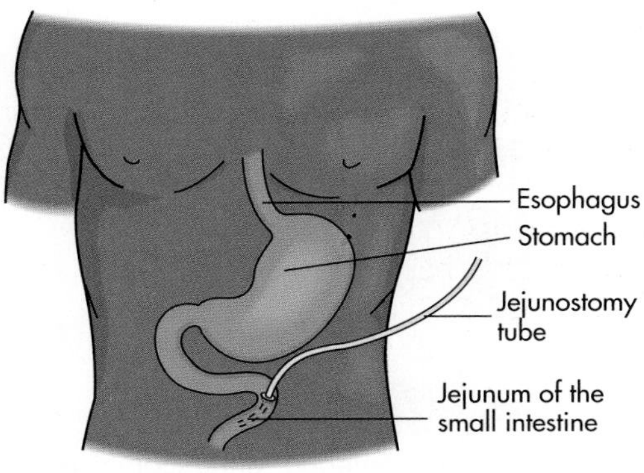

FIGURE 29–4 A jejunostomy tube.

- A **percutaneous endoscopic gastrostomy (PEG) tube** is a G-tube that is inserted with the use of an endoscope, which is a lighted instrument (*scope*) that allows the physician to see inside a body cavity or organ (*endo*), such as the stomach. The physician inserts the endoscope through the person's mouth and esophagus and into the stomach. A stab or puncture wound (*stomy*) is made through (*per*) the skin (*cutaneous*) and into the stomach (*gastro*). A tube is inserted into the stomach through the puncture wound (**FIGURE 29–5**).

Gastrostomy, jejunostomy, and PEG tubes are used for long-term enteral nutrition. An ostomy is a surgically created opening that is used to drain wastes or to feed the client. The ostomy may be temporary or permanent. In many facilities and agencies, it is the nurse who is responsible for running the formula through an enteral site. The physician orders the type of formula and the amount to be given to the client. Most formulas contain protein, carbohydrates, fat, vitamins, and minerals. Commercial formulas are

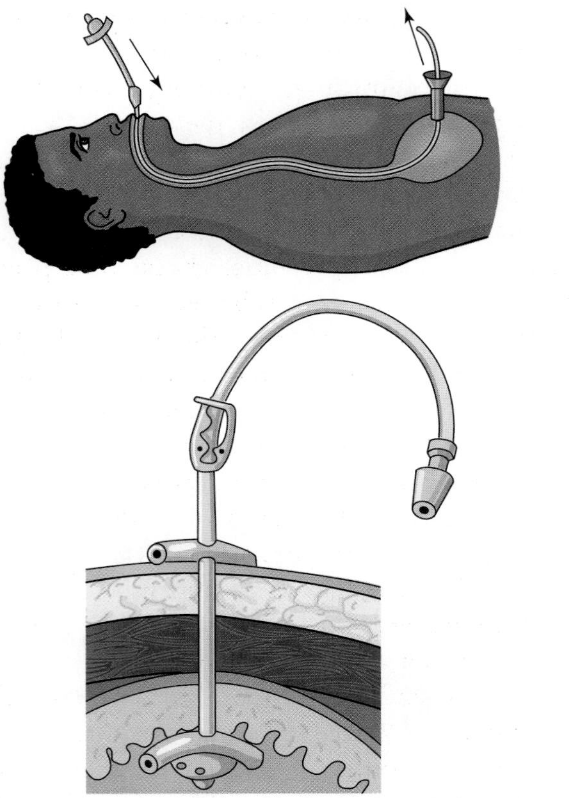

FIGURE 29–5 A percutaneous endoscopic gastrostomy tube.

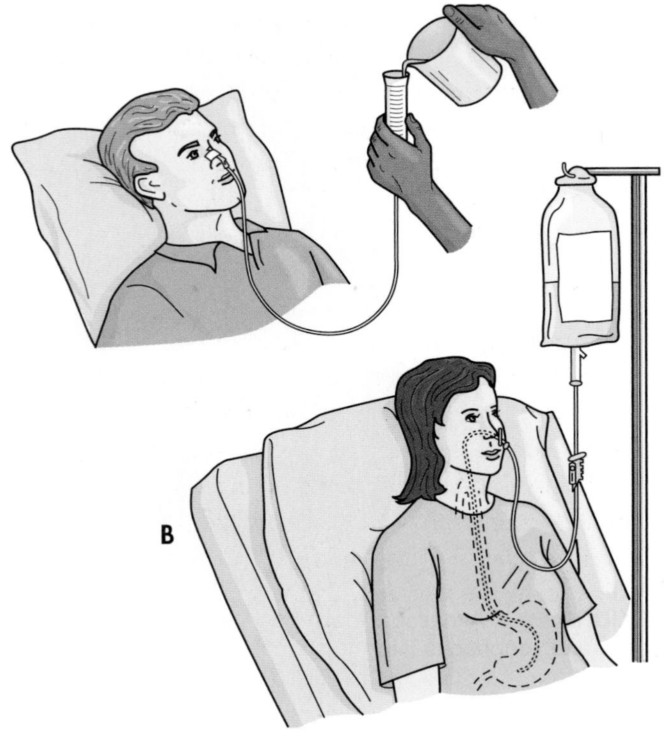

FIGURE 29–6 **A,** A tube feeding is given with a special calibrated volume syringe. **B,** Formula drips from a feeding bag into the feeding tube.

commonly used, or sometimes formulas are prepared by a facility's dietary department.

Scheduled and Continuous Feedings

The physician may order scheduled or continuous feedings. Scheduled feedings usually are given four times a day using a syringe, a rigid plastic container, or a feeding bag (FIGURE 29–6). Usually about 400 mL is given over 20 minutes during a scheduled feeding. The amount and rate are the same as those for regular meals. The physician will also specify how much water is to be given to the client each day, with the usual recommended amount being 2 000 mL/day.

Continuous feedings require electronic feeding pumps (FIGURE 29–7). Nasointestinal and jejunostomy tube feedings are always continuous.

Sometimes (depending on regional differences), continuous feedings are kept cold with ice chips around the container to prevent the growth of microbes. The formula warms to room temperature

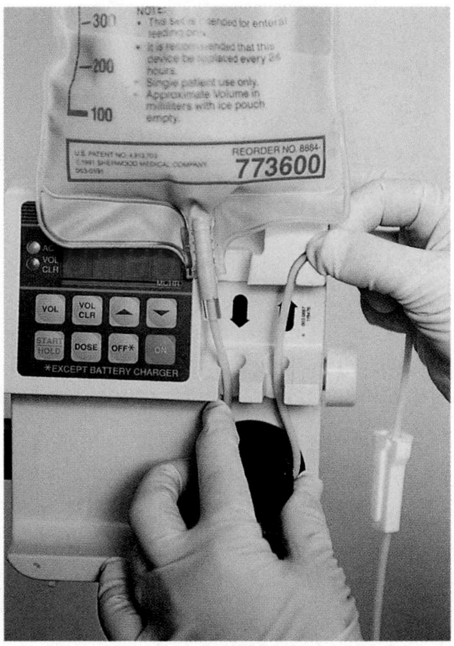

FIGURE 29–7 Feeding pump. (**Source:** Potter, P.A., & Perry, A.G. (2009). *Fundamentals of nursing: Concepts, process, and practice* (7th ed.). St. Louis, MO: Mosby.)

as it drips from the bag and passes through the connecting tubing to the feeding tube. Formula is given at room temperature, as cold fluids can cause stomach cramping. When the feeding is continuous, the nurse adds formula as needed (see the *Focus on Home Care: Enteral Nutrition* box).

Preventing Aspiration

Aspiration, which is the inhalation of fluid or an object into the lungs, is a major complication of nasogastric and nasointestinal tube feedings. Nasogastric and nasointestinal tubes pass through the esophagus and then into the stomach or small intestine. During insertion, the tube could accidentally slip into the respiratory tract, causing aspiration, which can cause pneumonia and even death. An X-ray is, therefore, usually taken after insertion to determine correct tube placement.

Coughing, sneezing, vomiting, suctioning, and poor positioning can move the tube out of place. A confused client can also move the feeding tube by pulling on it. The tube can move from the stomach or intestines into the esophagus and then into the airway. In a facility, a nurse checks tube placement before every scheduled tube feeding. In the case of continuous tube feedings, the nurse checks tube placement every 4 to 8 hours, depending on agency or facility policy. To do so, the nurse attaches a syringe to the tube and aspirates gastro-intestinal secretions. Then, the nurse measures the pH of the secretions. The pH readings will indicate if the tube has moved since the pH reading for stomach contents and intestinal contents differ.

With nasogastric, gastrostomy, and PEG tubes, aspiration can also occur from **regurgitation**, which is the backward flow of food from the stomach into the mouth. Delayed stomach emptying and overfeeding are common causes of regurgitation. To prevent regurgitation, the client should be in the sitting or semi-Fowler's position for the feeding and should remain in this position for 1 to 2 hours after the feeding to promote movement of the formula through the gastro-intestinal system and prevent aspiration. The left-side-lying position has to be avoided, as it prevents emptying of the stomach.

The risk for regurgitation is less with nasointestinal and jejunostomy tubes. Formula is given at a slow rate and passes directly into the small intestine. Remember that, during digestion, food passes slowly from the stomach to the small intestine and that the stomach can handle larger amounts of food at one time than the small intestine can.

FOCUS ON HOME CARE

Enteral Nutrition

As a support worker, you may provide home care to clients who are being fed via tubes, or in a facility, you may assist the nurse with a tube feeding.

You should take care never to:

- Insert feeding tubes
- Test the position of the tube
- Give the first dose of a tube feeding

However, some home care agencies do permit support workers to start the feeding pumps and pour formula into feeding bags or containers for gastrostomy tubes and jejunostomy tubes—but only if the tube has been established. These tasks are ***always*** delegated by a nurse. A home care nurse will teach you the task, either individually or in a course given by your agency. In most circumstances, you will need to be retrained to perform the task for each new client you work with, depending on the policy of your province, territory, agency, or facility. This process is needed to ensure competency in the delegated task. The person who teaches you the task has the responsibility of ensuring that the five rights of delegation (see Chapter 6) are being followed for the tube feeding.

Observations

Besides aspiration, which is the major risk, diarrhea, constipation, and delayed stomach emptying can also occur with tube feeding. Report the following immediately:

- Nausea
- Discomfort during the tube feeding
- Vomiting
- Diarrhea
- Distended (enlarged and swollen) abdomen

- Coughing
- Complaints of indigestion or heartburn
- Redness, swelling, drainage, odour, or pain at the ostomy site
- Elevated temperature
- Signs and symptoms of respiratory distress (see Chapter 41)
- Increased pulse rate
- Complaints of flatulence (see Chapter 33)

Comfort Measures

The client with a feeding tube is usually NPO (NPO stands for the Latin term *nil per os*, which means nothing by mouth). When dry mouth, dry lips, and sore throat cause discomfort, clients can suck on hard candy or chew gum, if allowed. Since one nostril is obstructed by the feeding tube, the client may breathe through the mouth, so frequent oral hygiene, lubricant for the lips, and mouth rinses are necessary. Sometimes, an ice bag applied externally to the throat can give relief for a sore throat. Give care as directed by your supervisor and the care plan.

Nasogastric and nasointestinal tubes can irritate and cause pressure on the nose. The nose and nostrils also are cleaned every 4 to 8 hours, depending on the policy of your agency or facility. To ensure that the tube does not exert pressure against the nostril, reposition the tube slightly away from the nostril. Sometimes, tubes alter the shape of the nostrils or cause pressure ulcers. Securing the tube using tape or a tube holder helps prevent these problems (**FIGURE 29–8**). Tube holders have foam cushions that prevent pressure on the nose and eliminate the need for retaping; frequent retaping can irritate the nose. The tube also is secured to the client's clothes with tape or by looping a rubber band around the tube and pinning the rubber band to the client's clothes with a safety pin. There should be some slack in the tubing to allow movement by the client, but a tube being too tight or too loose can cause displacement of the tube.

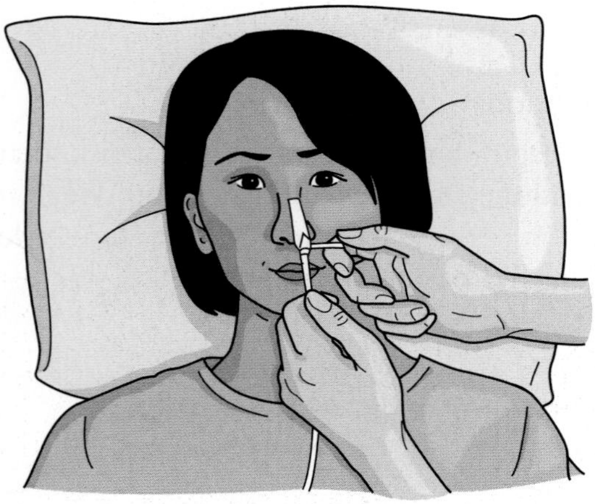

FIGURE 29–8 The feeding tube is taped to the nose.

INTRAVENOUS THERAPY

Intravenous (IV) therapy—also referred to as *IV* or *IV infusion*—involves giving fluids through a needle (such as a butterfly needle used on infants or children) or a cannula or catheter into a vein. A **cannula** (sometimes called a **catheter**) is plastic tubing threaded over a needle. Once the cannula or catheter is inserted into the vein, the needle is withdrawn. Physicians order IV therapy for the following purposes:

- To provide needed fluids when a client cannot take fluids by mouth
- To replace minerals and vitamins lost because of illness or injury
- To provide sugar for energy
- To administer medications and blood
- To provide *hyperalimentation*—the giving of a solution highly concentrated with nutrients

Think About Safety

Administering Food Through a Feeding Tube

Regurgitation is a risk when a client has a feeding tube, so ensure that your client is in the sitting or semi-Fowler's position while you are administering the feeding and that he remains in this position for 1 to 2 hours after the feeding. Follow the care plan.

The feeding tube should be pinned to your client's gown with enough slack to allow movement, but if it is too loose or too tight, the feeding tube could become dislocated.

Report any unusual signs or symptoms in the client to your supervisor immediately.

IV therapy is given in the hospital, outpatient care, subacute care, long-term care, and home care settings. Nurses are responsible for IV therapy—they start and maintain the infusion, according to the physician's orders, and also give IV medications and administer blood.

Central Intravenous Sites

The subclavian vein and the internal jugular vein—located close to the heart—are *central venous sites.* A physician inserts a long catheter—called a *central venous catheter* or *central line*—into a central vein. The catheter tip is then threaded into the superior vena cava or right atrium (**FIGURE 29–9, *A* and *B***). At times, the cephalic and basilic veins in the arm also are used for IV therapy. Catheters inserted into these sites are called *peripherally inserted central catheters (PICC)*. The catheter tip is threaded into the subclavian vein or the superior vena cava (**FIGURE 29–9, *C***). Only physicians and specially trained nurses can insert PICCs. The client is X-rayed after insertion of a central venous catheter or PICC to ensure proper placement.

Central venous sites are used to give large amounts of fluid and to administer long-term IV therapy. They also are used for IV medications that irritate the peripheral veins. Sometimes, surgery is necessary to insert a central venous catheter (see the *Focus on Home Care: Intravenous Therapy* box).

Assisting With Intravenous Therapy

The most common site for an IV is the client's lower arm or the back of the hand. Follow the safety measures in **BOX 29–1** to ensure you provide safe care. As a support worker, you help meet the hygiene and activity needs of clients who are receiving IV therapy, but you are *never* responsible for starting or maintaining IV therapy. A client who has an IV will also need the support worker's assistance to dress (see Chapter 31), and either the support worker or a nurse should teach the client how to ambulate safely with an IV line (see **FIGURE 29–10**). See the *Providing Compassionate Care: Enteral Nutrition and Intravenous Therapy* box.

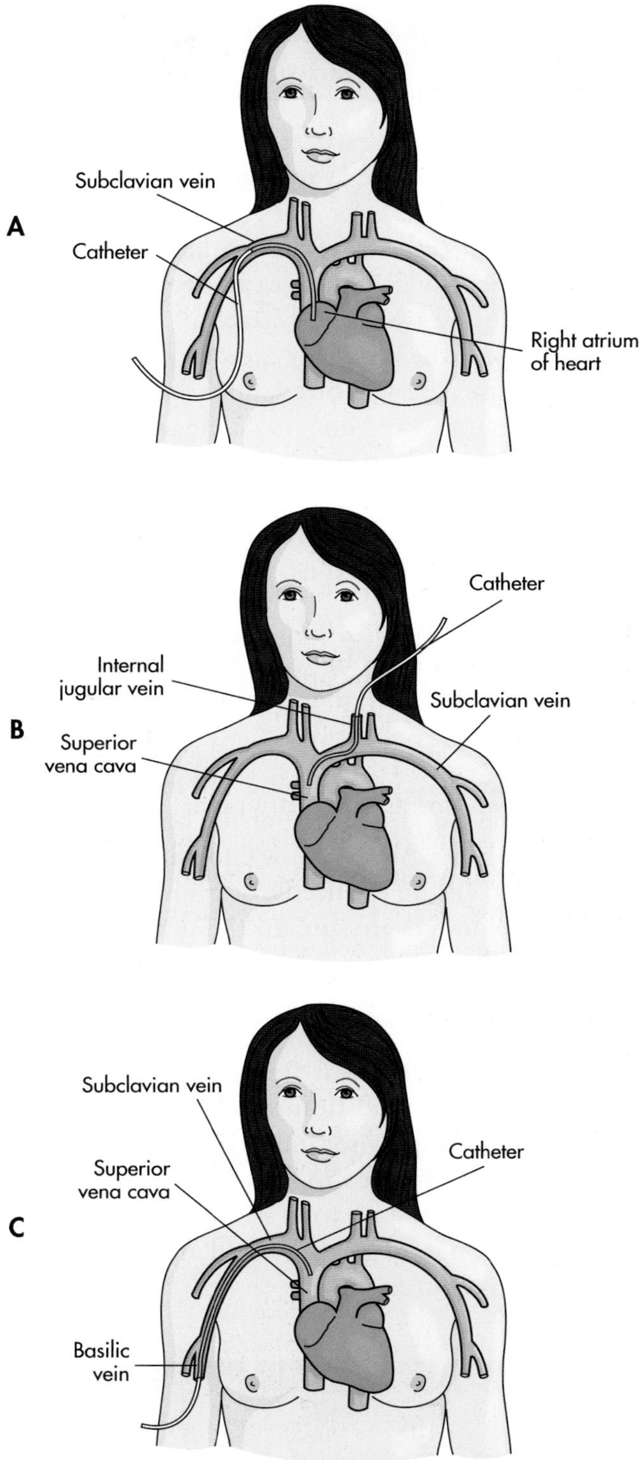

FIGURE 29–9 Central venous sites. **A,** Subclavian vein. The catheter tip is in the right atrium. **B,** Internal jugular vein. The catheter tip is in the superior vena cava. **C,** Basilic vein. The tip of the peripherally inserted central catheter is in the subclavian vein or the superior vena cava.

Report to nurse if IV is dripping too fast, too slow or not at all.

BOX 29–1 Safety Measures for Intravenous Therapy

- Follow Standard Practices.
- The position of the IV needle or catheter must be maintained. Do not move the needle, cannula, or catheter. If the needle or cannula is moved, it may come out of the vein; fluid will flow into the tissues (**infiltration**), or the flow will stop. If the needle or catheter becomes dislodged, the site will bleed; apply pressure with sterile gauze according to Standard Practices, and contact your supervisor immediately.
- Sometimes, the nurse may apply splints or restraints to prevent movement of the extremity (**FIGURE 29–10**) and, thus, the movement of the needle or cannula.
- Protect the IV bag, tubing, and needle or cannula when ambulating the client. Portable IV stands are rolled along next to the client (**FIGURE 29–11**).
- Assist the client with turning and repositioning. Move the bag to the side of the bed where the client is lying. Always allow enough slack in the tubing to ensure the needle or cannula does not dislodge due to pressure on the tube.
- Notify your supervisor immediately if bleeding occurs from the insertion site. Follow Standard Practices.
- Notify your supervisor immediately if there is any leaking of fluid from the IV site.
- Notify your supervisor immediately of any signs and symptoms listed in **BOX 29–2**.
- Always be aware of your scope of practice for your province or territory and the policies of your facility or agency.

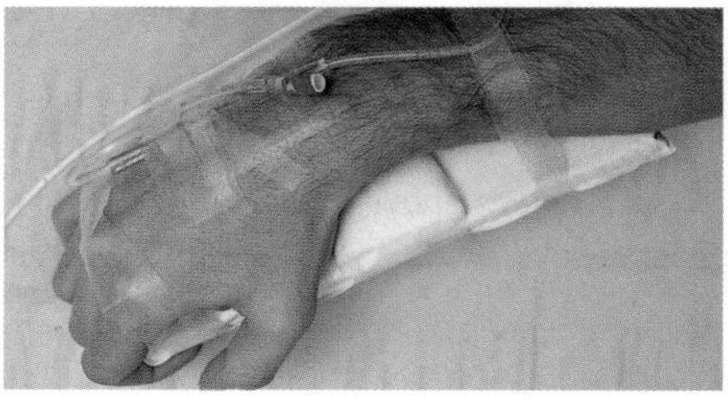

FIGURE 29–10 An armboard prevents movement at an IV site. (**Source:** Elkin, M.K., Perry, A.G., & Potter, P.A. (2007). *Nursing interventions and clinical skills* (4th ed.). St Louis: Mosby.)

FOCUS ON HOME CARE

Intravenous Therapy

Clients receiving IV therapy in their homes often have central venous catheters. The nurse teaches the client and family about administering IV medications and managing the catheter. Because these catheters or cannulas are inserted directly into a vein, you must be very careful when providing care. Ensure that you do not do anything around the insertion point that could dislodge the catheter. Report immediately any redness around the site. If a catheter falls out, apply pressure with sterile gauze until bleeding stops, and immediately inform your supervisor. If you are giving a tub bath to the client, ensure that the IV tubing is kept dry; if your client has a pump, it must be unplugged before the client enters the water. If your client is having a shower, keep the IV site dry by covering it with plastic wrap. Your supervisor will give you directions for care.

Complications can occur from IV therapy. Report at once if you see any of the signs and symptoms listed in **BOX 29–2**.

SUBCUTANEOUS INFUSION THERAPY

Many clients who receive palliative care or suffer from persistent pain may require frequent injections of pain medications to help reduce their pain. In many instances, the client may still be in pain in spite of having a topical pain patch. Numerous injections, however, may cause discomfort and possible infections or skin problems around the injection sites. To eliminate the need for frequent injections, some physicians order subcutaneous infusion therapy for their clients. Unlike an IV, in which a needle is inserted into the client's vein, a small needle is inserted into the client's subcutaneous tissue layer using Standard Practices. The needle tubing is then connected to an injection port, which is then securely taped into place onto the client's skin (see **FIGURE 29–12**). Pain medication can therefore be administered into the injection port instead of being injected into the skin.

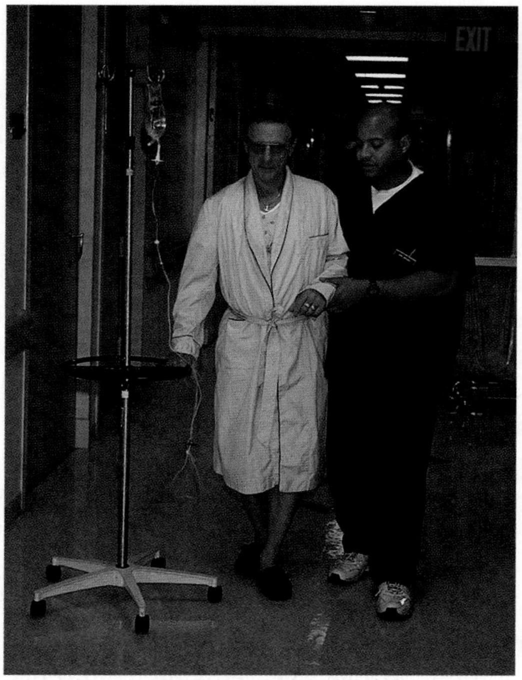

FIGURE 29–11 A portable IV stands allows the client to ambulate while on IV therapy. (**Source:** Elkin, M.K., Perry, A.G., & Potter, P.A. (2007). *Nursing interventions and clinical skills* (4th ed.). St Louis, MO: Mosby.)

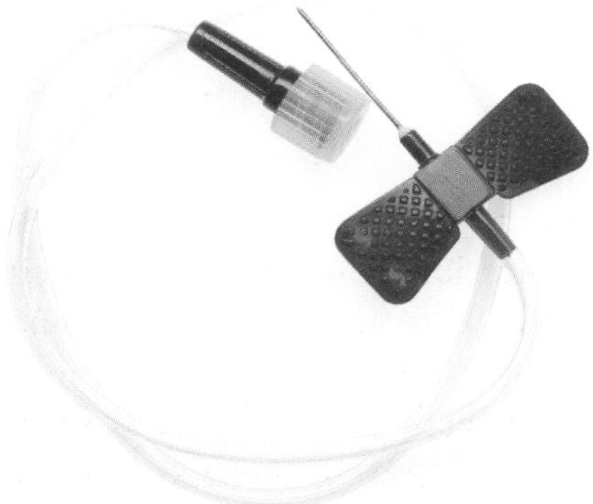

FIGURE 29–12 An example of a subcutaneous needle and injection port. Once inserted into the subcutaneous tissue, it must be securely taped in place. (**Source:** Andrew Rafalsky/ Shutterstock.com)

BOX 29–2 Signs and Symptoms of Intravenous Therapy Complications

As a support worker, you must report any of these signs or symptoms to your supervisor immediately.

Local—at the Intravenous Site

- Bleeding
- Puffiness or swelling
- Pale or reddened skin
- Complaints of pain at or above the IV site
- Hot or cold skin near the site
- Leaking of fluid from the site

Systemic—Involving the Whole Body

- Fever
- Itching
- Drop in blood pressure
- Tachycardia (pulse rate more than 100 beats per minute)
- Irregular pulse
- Cyanosis
- Changes in mental function
- Loss of consciousness
- Difficulty breathing (dyspnea)
- Shortness of breath
- Decreasing or no urine output
- Chest pain
- Nausea
- Confusion

In order for the medication to be effective, the position of the subcutaneous needle and injection port must be maintained. Do not attempt to move it. If the needle is moved, it may come out of the subcutaneous tissue, and, when injected, the pain medication will not be effective for pain relief. If the needle becomes dislodged, apply pressure with sterile gauze, according to Standard Practices, and contact your supervisor immediately.

Providing Compassionate Care

Enteral Nutrition and Intravenous Therapy

- ***Dignity.*** Clients who have to rely on feeding tubes to supply their nutrition may be embarrassed by their tube. Others may feel like an outcast when they are required to watch others eat when they are unable to. Report if the client is embarrassed about having their feeding while they have visitors; visiting hours can be arranged around the client's feeding times. Feeding tubes that are inserted into the client's nose should be taped in the most discreet way possible, perhaps using transparent tape or dressings.
- ***Independence.*** Encourage clients to be as independent as possible. If they are able to ambulate, provide a portable IV pole to hold the feeding bag so they can walk while receiving their feeding.
- ***Preferences.*** Encourage personal choices whenever possible. Allow clients receiving an enteral feeding to choose clothing that would cover their tubing dressing or stoma but also provide access for routine checking.
- ***Privacy***. Providing for privacy is important when checking the client's tubing site, especially if the client has tubing that enters into their abdominal area. Close the curtains or the door when inspecting the tubing or when the nurse is providing care to their dressing or stoma site.
- ***Safety***. To prevent regurgitation after an enteral feeding, ensure the client is in the sitting or semi-Fowler's position for the feeding. Keep the client in this position for 1 to 2 hours after the feeding as well to promote movement of the formula through the gastro-intestinal system and prevent aspiration. Avoid the left-side-lying position, which prevents emptying of the stomach.

CHAPTER REVIEW

KEY POINTS

- Some clients, because of illness, injury, or surgery, are not able to swallow, eat, or drink and need a feeding tube to provide nourishment and medications.
- Enteral nutrition feeding may be done through a nasogastric tube, a nasointestinal tube, a gastrostomy tube, a gastro-jejunostomy tube, a jejunostomy tube, or a percutaneous endoscopic gastrostomy tube.
- Feeding-tube formulas may be commercially prepared or prepared by the facility where the client is.
- The feeding tube can be moved out of place from coughing, sneezing, vomiting, suctioning, poor positioning, or the client pulling on the tube. The nurse checks on the position of the tubing, depending on your employer's policy.
- Aspiration is the major risk for clients with a feeding tube. Other symptoms to report immediately are nausea, discomfort, vomiting, diarrhea, distension, coughing, indigestion, respiratory distress, increased pulse rate, and complaints of flatulence.
- Physicians order IV therapy to provide needed fluids; to replace minerals, vitamins, or sugar; or to administer medication or blood.
- Sites used depend on the age of the client, the condition of the client, and the purpose of the IV therapy.
- As a support worker, you must be very careful when providing care to a client with an IV. You need to ensure that you do not move or dislodge the needle, catheter, or cannula. Re-insertion of an IV is painful for your client.
- As a support worker, you are never responsible for starting or maintaining IV therapy, but you must report immediately any of the signs and symptoms of IV therapy complications.

CRITICAL THINKING IN PRACTICE

Mrs. Stenson is receiving a continuous tube feeding. You hear her feeding pump alarm sound. You go to check on her. The head of her bed is flat and she says: "My mouth is dry." What do you do first? What do you do next? What can you do within your role limits? What does the nurse need to do?

REVIEW QUESTIONS

Answers to these questions are at the bottom of the next page.

Circle the BEST answer.

1. A gastrostomy tube is inserted into the:
 A. Small intestine
 B. Stomach
 C. Colon
 D. Nose

2. Which of the following is a common reason for tube feedings?
 A. Cancer of the lung
 B. Surgery to the mouth
 C. Chronic obstructive pulmonary disease (COPD)
 D. Pneumonia

3. Continuous feedings require:
 A. Electronic feeding pumps
 B. Intravenous (IV) bags
 C. Catheters
 D. Syringes

4. Aspiration is a major complication of:
 A. Hyperalimentation
 B. IV therapy
 C. Nasogastric and nasointestinal tubes
 D. Central venous catheters

5. A client with a feeding tube is usually:
 A. NPO
 B. On bed rest
 C. Allowed a regular diet
 D. In a coma

6. Care of a person who is NPO includes:
- A. Frequent oral hygiene
- B. Frequent repositioning of the client
- C. Lubrication of nostrils
- D. Frequent drinks of water

7. Which is a common IV site for adults?
- A. Back of the hand
- B. Upper arm
- C. Scalp
- D. Foot

8. A client is bleeding from an IV site. You should do everything *except:*
- A. Remove the IV catheter or needle
- B. Apply direct pressure
- C. Call your supervisor at once
- D. Use Standard Practices

9. Which is a sign of IV therapy complication?
- A. Swelling at the IV site
- B. Changes in appetite
- C. Frequent urination
- D. Constipation

Answers: 1.B, 2.B, 3.A, 4.C, 5.A, 6.A, 7.A, 8.A, 9.A

Chapter opener image: poramesstock/Shutterstock.com

CHAPTER 30

Personal Hygiene

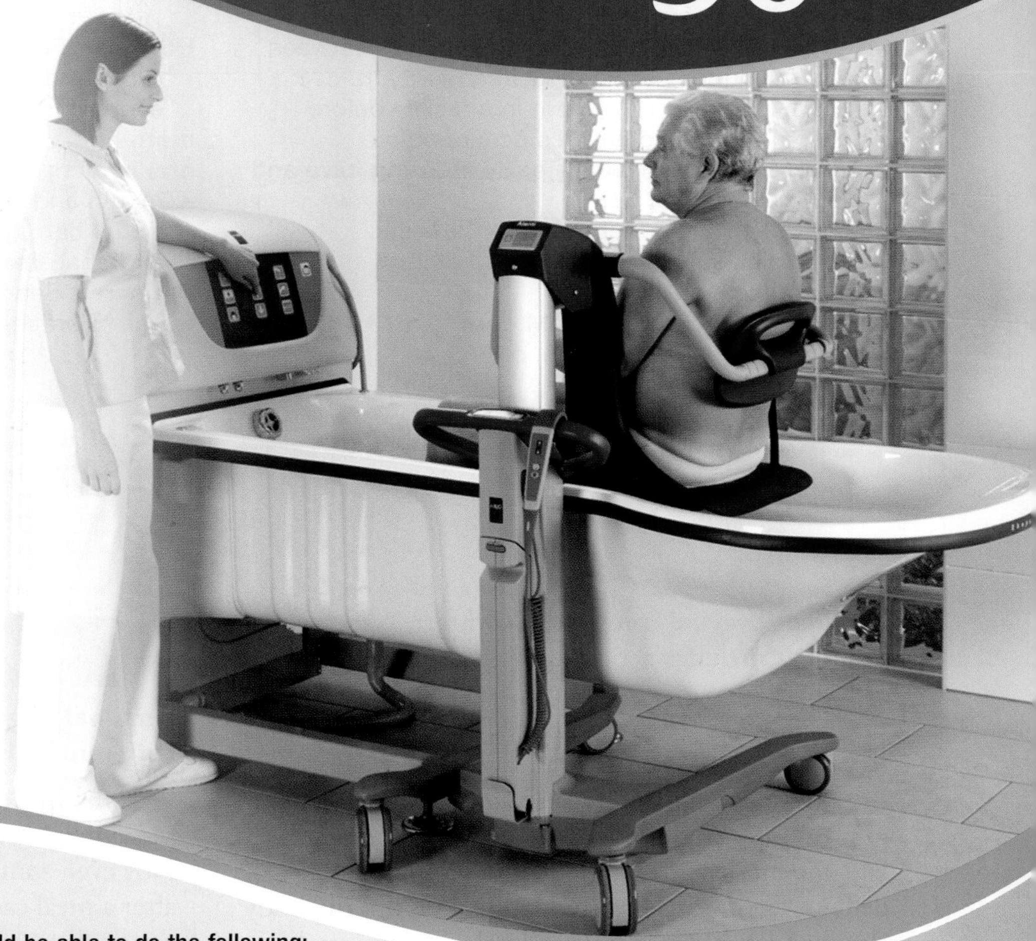

OBJECTIVES

After reading this chapter, the learner should be able to do the following:

- Explain the importance of personal hygiene.
- Describe oral hygiene and the observations to report.
- Describe the guidelines for bathing and the observations to report.
- Identify the safety precautions for clients taking tub baths or showers.
- Explain the purposes of a back massage.
- Identify the purposes of perineal care.
- Describe menstrual care.
- Perform the procedures described in this chapter.

KEY TERMS

afternoon care Routine care that occurs between lunch and the evening meal in a facility. *p. 613*
AM care Routine care given in a facility before lunch. AM care sometimes occurs before breakfast. Also known as **early morning care** and **morning care**. *p. 613*
biofilm A thin film that sticks to the teeth; it contains saliva, microbes, and other substances. *p. 613*
early morning care See **AM care**. *p. 613*
evening care See **HS care**. *p. 613*
HS care Routine care given in a facility at bedtime (*HS* stands for "hour of sleep"). Also known as **evening care** or **PM care**. *p. 613*
morning care See **AM care**. *p. 613*
oral hygiene Measures performed to keep the mouth and teeth clean; mouth care. *p. 613*
perineal care (pericare) Cleansing of the genital and anal areas. *p. 642*
PM care See **HS care**. *p. 613*
tartar Hardened biofilm on teeth. *p. 613*

Personal hygiene promotes comfort, safety, and health. It includes activities to clean the skin, teeth, mouth, genital area, and anus.

Good hygiene helps keep teeth, skin, and mucous membranes intact and healthy. When microbes enter the body through breaks in skin or mucous membranes, infections can result. Therefore, intact skin and mucous membranes are the body's first line of defence against disease. As well as keeping the body clean and healthy, personal hygiene prevents body and breath odours, promotes relaxation, and increases circulation.

Support workers often help clients with personal hygiene. Some clients need only minimal help, whereas some others may need hygiene care done for them. Illness, disability, and changes associated with aging affect a person's ability to practise hygiene. Many factors complicate hygiene and skin care, such as perspiration, elimination, vomiting, drainage from wounds or body openings, bed rest, and activity.

As well, culture and personal choice affect hygiene practices (see the *Respecting Diversity: Personal Hygiene Practices of Different Cultures* box). Most clients have established hygiene routines—for example, a bath at bedtime or in the morning, brushing teeth and washing face and hands on awakening, and so on. Usually, these and other hygiene measures are done before and after meals and at bedtime. The care plan lists what personal hygiene measures are needed for a client and when to provide them. You are required

Respecting Diversity

Personal Hygiene Practices of Different Cultures

Personal hygiene is very important to Hindus, as their religion requires at least one bath a day. However, some Hindus believe that bathing right after a meal can cause harm to the body. They also believe that eye injuries can occur from bathwater that is too hot. When preparing a bath, hot water can be added to cold water. However, cold water is not added to hot water. After bathing, the body is carefully dried with a towel.

In some Asian cultures, females are very modest, so as a support worker, you must ensure that a woman's body is covered as much as possible. Ask your client or her family how best to provide a bath while respecting the culture.

Muslims are taught to pray five times a day and need to wash their hands, feet, and mouth before each prayer.

Remember, not all individuals within a group follow every belief and practice of their culture and religion. Each client is unique.

Adapted from Giger, J.N. (2013). *Transcultural nursing* (6th ed.). St. Louis, MO: Mosby.

FOCUS ON LONG-TERM CARE

Daily Care

Facilities provide routine hygiene care at set times of the day. The amount of care given at each time and the terminology used vary from facility to facility, and each facility must adjust its procedures to address the various cultural needs of clients. The care plan will give you directions.

- **AM care** *(early morning care **or** morning care)*—routine care provided before lunch. Most clients are assisted to the bathroom, given a partial bath that includes perineal care, dressed, groomed, and provided mouth care before they go to the dining room for breakfast. If there is enough time, clients requiring a tub bath or shower would have one before breakfast. If there is not time, these clients might go to the dining room in their pyjamas or robe. The policies that dictate times when a client must be served breakfast and how the client must be dressed vary from province to province or from one facility to another. Some facilities allow clients to continue sleeping if they so desire and offer them a late breakfast. In other facilities, tub baths or showers are always given after breakfast.
- **Afternoon care**—routine care given after lunch and before the evening meal. Many clients like to have the afternoon care completed before naps, visiting time, or activity programs. Afternoon care usually includes assistance with going to the bathroom, oral hygiene, face washing, handwashing, and hair care.
- **HS care** *(evening care **or** PM care)*—care provided at bedtime. (*HS* stands for "hour of sleep.") HS care is aimed at relaxing the client and increasing comfort. It includes face washing, handwashing, oral hygiene, perineal care, back massages, and assistance with going to the bathroom. Bed linens and units are made neat and comfortable, and the client is helped into sleepwear.

Clients may feel frustrated, angry, or embarrassed because they need help with such personal care. Remember the priorities of support work when assisting with hygiene. Promote DIPPS—dignity, independence, preferences, privacy, and safety—to help the client feel more at ease during hygiene procedures (see the *Providing Compassionate Care: Assisting With Personal Hygiene* box).

to assist with personal hygiene whenever needed (see the *Focus on Long-Term Care: Daily Care* box). If you have questions, check with your supervisor.

ORAL HYGIENE

Oral hygiene (mouth care) keeps the mouth and teeth clean; prevents mouth odours, infections, and *cavities* (dental caries); increases comfort; and makes food taste better. It also prevents *periodontal disease* (gum disease, pyorrhea), which is an inflammation of the tissues around teeth. ***Oral care is an essential part of maintaining overall physical health and should never be overlooked!***

Poor oral hygiene allows the buildup of biofilm. **Biofilm**—which contains saliva, microbes, and other substances—is a thin film that sticks to teeth and leads to tooth decay or cavities. When biofilm hardens, it is called **tartar**. Tartar builds up at the gum line near the neck of the tooth, which leads to periodontal disease. Gums become red and swollen and bleed easily. As the disease progresses, bone is destroyed, and teeth become loosened, eventually resulting in tooth loss. The presence of bleeding gums during oral hygiene procedures is usually a sign of inflammation and usually means *more* mouth care is needed, not less.

Illness and disease often cause a bad taste in the mouth. Some medications and diseases cause a whitish coating on the mouth and tongue, and some others cause redness and swelling of the mouth and tongue. Dry mouth is a common result of oxygen administration, smoking, low fluid intake, mouth breathing, and anxiety. Some medications also cause dry mouth.

Providing Compassionate Care
Assisting With Personal Hygiene

- ***Dignity.*** Hygiene is a very personal and private matter. Most clients feel embarrassed that someone else needs to provide hygiene care for them, more so when the caregiver is of the opposite sex. Remember, personal hygiene is necessary for the client's health and well-being. Never show embarrassment or hesitation when assisting with hygiene procedures, as the client is likely to sense your discomfort. Talk to the client before and during the procedure. Let the client know what you will be doing. Listen to what the client has to say about the procedure, and address any concerns or questions. If appropriate, chat with the client about anything of interest. Your calm, professional manner will help put the client at ease. Minimizing exposure of the body during bathing promotes dignity.
- ***Independence.*** Allow and encourage clients to do as much self-care as possible. Sometimes, you only need to assist with a task. Give clients enough time to do what they can do independently. Check with your supervisor and the care plan to determine clients' abilities and limitations.
- ***Preferences.*** Clients usually have hygiene preferences and routines. Routines provide a sense of order and control. Clients have a say about when and how a hygiene procedure is done. Personal choice is allowed in such matters as bath times and products used. The care plan should reflect the client's preferences and cultural practices. If there is a conflict between the care plan and the client's wishes, inform your supervisor.
- ***Privacy.*** Protecting the client's privacy is very important when assisting with hygiene. All procedures must be done in a private area with minimal exposure of the client's body. Close doors, privacy curtains, and drapes before giving care. Ask family members or visitors to leave the room. If a family member or friend wants to help, the client must consent. Do not unnecessarily expose the client's body when assisting with the bath. Provide appropriate covers to clients when taking them to and from tubs or shower rooms.
- ***Safety.*** Some clients have skin that can be easily damaged. Always be gentle; never scrub the skin or use rough sponges or cloths. Make sure your fingernails are trimmed, and remove rings before giving skin care so as to prevent scratching or tearing the client's skin. Remember to wash your hands with soap and warm water before and after every procedure. Wear gloves when giving perineal care and oral care and any time you may have contact with blood, body fluids, secretions, or excretions. As well, gloves should be worn when you have cuts or rashes on your hands. Always check the water temperature before bathing the client.

Recent research is identifying a relationship between periodontal disease and other diseases. Scientists have found that bacteria that grow in the oral cavity can be aspirated into the lungs and cause respiratory diseases such as pneumonia. Periodontal disease can also increase a person's risk of heart disease. Some studies have shown that clients with oral disease are at greater risk for thickening of the carotid arteries, which leads to heart disease.

Your supervisor and the care plan will tell you the type of mouth care and assistance needed for the client. Oral hygiene is given to the client on awakening, after each meal, and at bedtime. Some medications may cause mouth dryness, which in turn, makes swallowing difficult. Some clients practise oral hygiene before meals in order to promote salivation and to improve the taste of their food.

When giving oral hygiene, you will come in contact with the client's mucous membranes. The mouth contains many microbes, so wear gloves and follow Standard Practices.

The gums may bleed

Equipment

For oral hygiene, a toothbrush, toothpaste, dental floss, and mouthwash are needed. Ensure that the toothbrush has soft bristles, and replace toothbrushes every 3 months. Use toothpaste that contains fluoride. Clients with dentures need a denture cleaner, a denture cup, and a denture brush or toothbrush. Use only products that are recommended for cleaning dentures to avoid damaging the dentures.

For clients with sore, tender mouths and for unconscious clients, sponge swabs are used for mouth care. However, be careful to always check that the foam pad is tight on the stick. If the foam pad comes off the stick, the client could choke on it. Lip moisturizers are often used to relieve dry lips.

Observations

It is important for you to observe the client's teeth and gums for signs of early problems, such as the following, and to report them promptly:

- Dry, cracked, swollen, or blistered lips
- Bleeding, swelling, or redness of the gums
- Presence of sores or white patches on the oral mucosa or tongue
- Presence of food or foreign objects on the tongue and in the mouth
- Missing or loose teeth (Remember that these can be a swallowing hazard!)
- Rough, sharp, or chipped areas on dentures
- Foul breath
- Difficulty swallowing or speaking (see Chapters 28 and 39)
- Complaints of pain or discomfort

Brushing Teeth

Most clients can perform oral hygiene procedures themselves, but in long-term care, the majority cannot perform them adequately. Others may need help gathering and setting up equipment. Encourage clients to be as independent as possible according to their abilities and their care plans. In the community, clients may choose to brush teeth in the bathroom, at the kitchen sink, or at the bedside.

You may have to brush the teeth of clients who are very weak or confused or who cannot use or move their arms. It can be difficult to provide mouth care to clients with dementia, but remember that even a small amount of mouth care is better than none. There is no consensus among dentists as to the proper brushing technique. Some recommend a circular motion, some the up-and-down motion, and others the side-to-side motion. All, however, agree that brushing should start at the gum line (see the *Focus on Children: Brushing Teeth* box).

FOCUS ON CHILDREN

Brushing Teeth

Children learn to brush their teeth around 3 years of age. However, they may not be thorough, so they may need help with brushing. Though older children can do a thorough job, it is often necessary to remind them to brush.

Brushing the Client's Teeth 123

Advocate on behalf of the client's quality of life by promoting:

Dignity • Independence • Preferences • Privacy • Safety *(see BOX 1–4, on p. 17)*

PRE-PROCEDURE

1 Identify the client, according to employer policy. *This eliminates the possibility of mistaking one client for another.*

2 Explain the procedure to the client.

3 Perform hand hygiene.

Continued

Brushing the Client's Teeth—cont'd

4 Collect the following supplies (your employer's procedures will confirm the equipment you will need):
- ☐ **Toothbrush**
- ☐ **Toothpaste**
- ☐ **Mouthwash (or solution specified in the care plan)**
- ☐ **Dental floss (if used)**
- ☐ **Lip moisturizer (if used)**
- ☐ **Water glass with cool water**
- ☐ **Straw**
- ☐ **Kidney basin or small bowl**
- ☐ **Face towel**
- ☐ **Paper towels**
- ☐ **Gloves**

By collecting all the necessary equipment beforehand, you will not have to leave your client's side and can eliminate wasting time and energy in obtaining the forgotten equipment.

5 Place paper towels on the overbed table (in facilities) or on a work area within easy reach. Arrange items on top of the paper towels.
This helps protect work areas.

6 Provide for privacy.

7 Raise the bed to a comfortable working height.

PROCEDURE

8 Lower the bed rail near you if it is up.*
This helps prevent back strain in the support worker.

9 Assist the client to a sitting or side-lying position facing you.
This helps prevent aspiration.

10 Place a towel over the client's chest.
This helps protect the client's clothing.

11 Adjust the overbed table so that you can reach it with ease.*

12 Put on gloves.

13 Apply toothpaste to the toothbrush.

14 Hold the toothbrush over the kidney basin or bowl. Pour some water over the brush.

15 Gently inspect the client's teeth, gums, and tongue. Note if there are any sores, white patches, swollen gums, or loose teeth.
Oral infections or loose teeth can cause serious health issues to the client. By noticing problems such as these and acting accordingly, you may reduce discomfort or serious health problems for the client.

16 Brush the client's teeth gently (**FIGURE 30–1**).

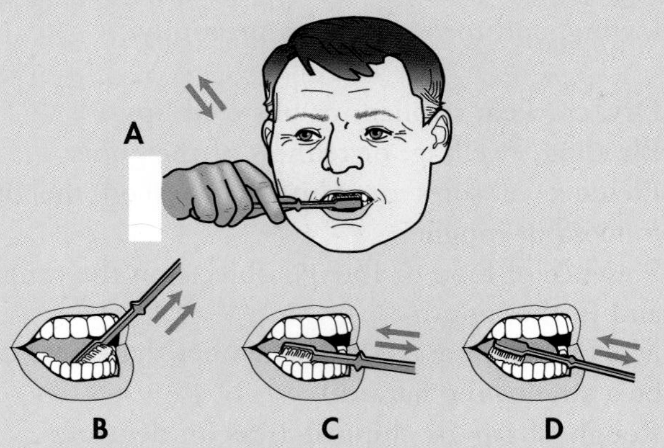

FIGURE 30–1 Brushing teeth. **A,** Position the brush at a 45-degree angle to the gums. Brush with short strokes. **B,** Position the brush at a 45-degree angle against the inside of the front teeth. Brush from the gum to the crown of the tooth with short strokes. **C,** Hold the brush horizontally against the inner surfaces of teeth. Brush back and forth. **D,** Position the brush on the biting surfaces of teeth. Brush back and forth.

Continued

Brushing the Client's Teeth—cont'd

17 Brush the client's tongue gently, if needed.
Dentists recommend brushing the tongue, but it can cause some clients to gag, so follow the care plan.
18 Allow the client to rinse the mouth with water. Hold the kidney basin or bowl under the client's chin. Repeat this step as needed. (**FIGURE 30-2**).
19 Floss the client's teeth (see the Procedure *Flossing the Client's Teeth* on p. 619). Follow the care plan.
20 Let the client use mouthwash or other solution. Hold the kidney basin or bowl under the client's chin.
This helps protect the client's clothing.
21 Remove the towel.
22 Remove and discard gloves. Perform hand hygiene.
23 Adjust the overbed table next to the bed.*

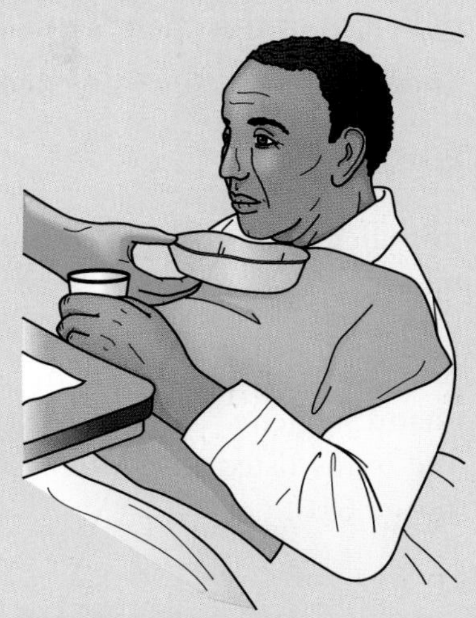

FIGURE 30-2 Hold a kidney basin under the client's chin.

POST-PROCEDURE

24 Provide for safety and comfort.
25 Place the call bell within reach.*
This provides an easy, safe way for the client to contact staff, if necessary.
26 Return the bed to its lowest position. Follow the care plan for bed rail use.*
This is done for the safety of your client.
27 Wear gloves for this step. Clean and return equipment to its proper place.
This makes it easier to find the next time it is needed.
28 Wipe off the overbed table or work area with paper towels. Discard the paper towels.
This helps prevent transfer of microbes.
29 Remove privacy measures.
30 Follow employer policies for handling dirty linen.
31 Perform hand hygiene.

Report and Record your actions and observations, according to employer policy.
This is done for legal reasons and to keep the rest of the health care team informed.

*Steps marked with an asterisk may not apply in community settings.

Assisting the Client to Brush Teeth at the Bedside

123

Advocate on behalf of the client's quality of life by promoting:

Dignity • Independence • Preferences • Privacy • Safety *(see BOX 1–4, on p. 17)*

PRE-PROCEDURE

1 Identify the client, according to employer policy.
This eliminates the possibility of mistaking one client for another.
2 Explain the procedure to the client.
3 Perform hand hygiene.
4 Collect the items listed in *Brushing the Client's Teeth* on page 616.
5 Place paper towels on the overbed table (in facilities) or on a work area that the client can easily reach from the bedside. Arrange items on top of paper towels.
6 Provide for privacy.
7 Raise bed to a comfortable working height.
Raising the bed will reduce your risk of back strain.

PROCEDURE

8 Lower the bed rail near you if it is up.
9 Position the client so that she can brush with ease.
This ensures client comfort and safety.
10 Place a towel over the client's chest.
This protects garments and linens from spills.
11 Adjust the overbed table in front of the client so that it is in a comfortable position for the client.*
12 Encourage independence by letting the client perform oral hygiene. This includes brushing teeth, rinsing the mouth, flossing, and using mouthwash or other solution. The client spits into the kidney basin or small bowl.
13 Inspect the tongue and gums for signs of redness, sores, swelling, or loose teeth.
It is important to use your observational skills as part of providing safe care to the client. Oral infections or loose teeth can cause serious health issues for the client.
14 Observe the client while she is brushing her teeth. If necessary, gently prompt or cue the client to brush all the teeth (see Chapter 36) and to spit whenever necessary.
Some clients may not be able to remember the mechanics of thorough tooth brushing initially but will remember if prompted or cued.
15 Remove the towel when the client is done.
16 Adjust the overbed table next to the bed.*

POST-PROCEDURE

17 Follow steps 24 through 31 in the procedure *Brushing the Client's Teeth* on page 617.

Report and Record your actions and observations, according to employer policy.
This is done for legal reasons and to keep the rest of the health care team informed.

*Steps marked with an asterisk may not apply in community settings.

Flossing

Flossing is a preventive measure. It removes plaque and tartar, which cause serious gum disease that leads to loosening and loss of teeth. Flossing also removes food lodged between teeth. It is usually done after brushing but can be done at other times—for example, after meals. If flossing is done only once a day, bedtime is the best time to floss.

You may be required to floss for clients who cannot do it themselves. Follow the care plan (see the *Focus on Children: Flossing* and *Focus on Older Adults: Flossing* boxes).

FOCUS ON CHILDREN

Flossing

Just like adults, preschoolers and older children need to floss. Older children can floss by themselves, but you need to floss for preschoolers. Older children need reminding and some supervision.

FOCUS ON OLDER ADULTS

Flossing

Flossing was not a common oral hygiene practice in the past, so some older adults may have never flossed their teeth. A client may refuse to floss or to let you do it. Respect the client's wishes. Inform your supervisor so that the client's care plan may be changed as needed.

Flossing the Client's Teeth

123

Advocate on behalf of the client's quality of life by promoting:

Dignity • Independence • Preferences • Privacy • Safety *(see BOX 1–4, on p. 17)*

PRE-PROCEDURE

1 Identify the client, according to employer policy.
This eliminates the possibility of mistaking one client for another.
2 Explain the procedure to the client.
3 Perform hand hygiene.
4 Collect the following supplies:
- ☐ **Kidney basin or small bowl**
- ☐ **Water glass with cool water**
- ☐ **Dental floss**
- ☐ **Face towel**
- ☐ **Paper towels**
- ☐ **Gloves**

By collecting all the necessary equipment beforehand, you will not have to leave your client's side and can eliminate wasting time and energy in obtaining the forgotten equipment.
5 Place paper towels on the overbed table (in facilities) or on a work area within easy reach. Arrange items on top of the paper towels.
This helps protect the overbed table or work area.
6 Provide for privacy.
7 Raise bed to a comfortable working height.
Raising the bed will reduce your risk for back strain.

PROCEDURE

8 Lower the bed rail near you if it is up.
9 Assist the client to a sitting or side-lying position facing you.
This helps prevent aspiration.
10 Place a towel over the client's chest.
This helps protect the client's clothing.
11 Adjust the overbed table so that you can reach it with ease.*
12 Put on gloves.
13 Break off a 45-cm (18-in.) piece of floss from the dispenser.
14 Hold the floss between the middle fingers of your hands (**FIGURE 30–3, *A***).
15 Stretch the floss with your thumbs.
16 Start at the upper back tooth on the right side. Work around to the left side.
17 Inspect the tongue and gums for signs of redness, sores, swelling, or loose teeth.
It is important to use your observational skills as part of providing safe care to the client.
18 Move the floss gently up and down between the teeth (**FIGURE 30–3, *B***).
19 Use a new section of floss after every second tooth.
20 Floss the lower teeth. Hold the floss with your index fingers (**FIGURE 30–3, *C***). Use up-and-down motions, and go under the gums, as for the upper teeth. Start on the right side. Work around to the left side.

Continued

Flossing the Client's Teeth—cont'd

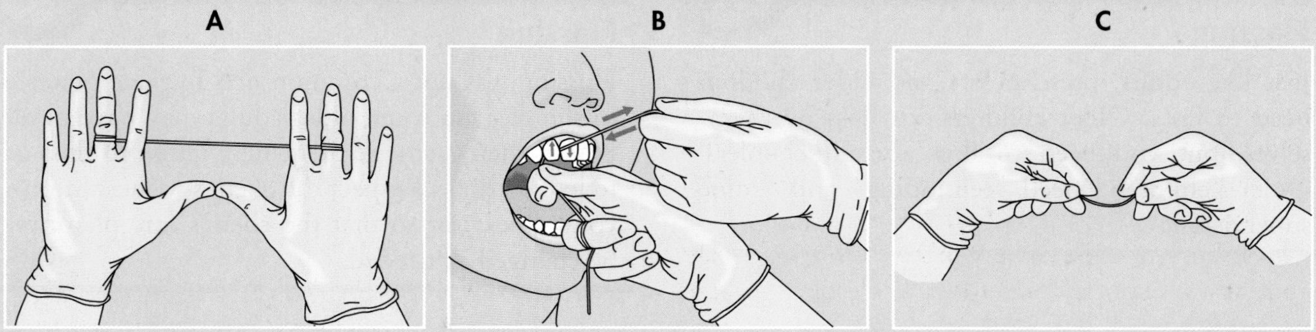

FIGURE 30–3 Flossing. ***A,*** Hold dental floss between the middle fingers to floss the upper teeth. ***B,*** Move floss up and down between teeth from the tip of the tooth to the gum line. ***C,*** Hold floss with the index fingers to floss the lower teeth.

21 Allow the client to rinse the mouth. Hold the kidney basin or bowl under the chin. Repeat rinsing as necessary.

22 Remove the towel.

23 Remove and discard gloves. Perform hand hygiene.

24 Adjust the overbed table next to the bed.*

POST-PROCEDURE

25 Follow steps 24 through 31 in the procedure *Brushing the Client's Teeth* on page 617.

Report and Record your actions and observations, according to employer policy.
This is done for legal reasons and to keep the rest of the health care team informed.

*Steps marked with an asterisk may not apply in community settings.

Mouth Care for an Unconscious Client

Unconscious clients need special mouth care procedures. They cannot eat or drink, they may breathe with their mouths open, and they may receive oxygen therapy (see Chapter 41), all of which cause mouth dryness and crusting on the tongue and mucous membranes. Oral hygiene helps keep the mouth clean and moist and prevents infection.

The care plan tells you what cleaning agent to use. Use sponge swabs to apply the cleaning agent. To prevent cracking of lips, apply a lubricant (check the care plan) to the lips after cleaning.

Unconscious clients usually cannot swallow and need to be protected from choking and aspiration (inhaling fluid or an object into the lungs), which increases the risk for pneumonia and death. To prevent aspiration, position the client on one side, with the head turned well to the side (FIGURE 30–4)

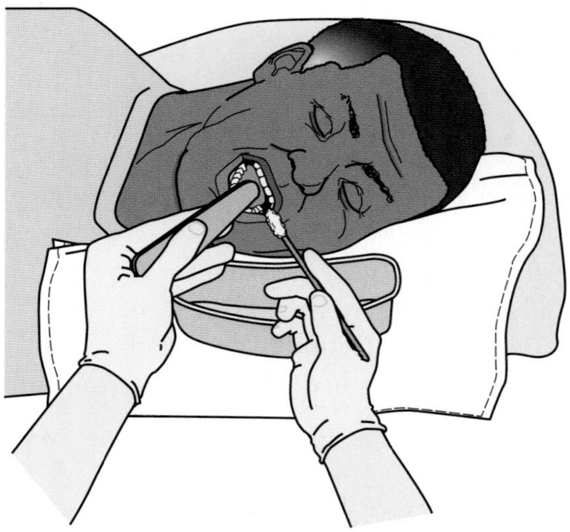

FIGURE 30–4 Turn the head of the unconscious client well to the side to prevent aspiration. Use a padded tongue blade to keep the client's mouth open while cleaning the mouth with swabs.

so that excess fluid runs out of the mouth, and when cleaning the mouth, use only a small amount of fluid. Sometimes, oral suctioning is needed (see Chapter 41).

Keep the client's mouth open with a padded tongue blade. If one is not available, make a padded tongue blade, as shown in **FIGURE 30–5**. Do not use your fingers to hold the client's mouth open, as the client could bite down on them. Remember, breaks in your skin from bites or any other reason will create a portal of entry for microbes and may become infected.

Unconscious clients cannot say anything or respond to what is happening, but some can hear. Always assume that unconscious clients can hear, and explain what you are doing step by step. Also, after completing care, tell the client that you are done and that you are leaving the room.

Check with your supervisor and the care plan for how often to do oral hygiene (usually at least every 2 hours) and what to use. Unconscious clients are also repositioned at least every 2 hours. Combining mouth care, skin care, and other comfort measures increases their comfort and safety.

A

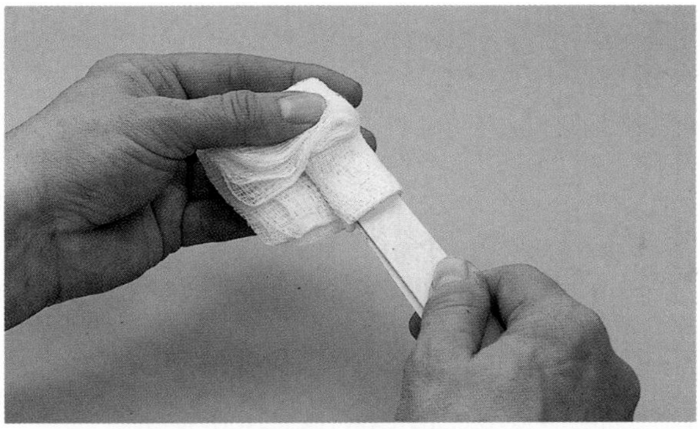

B

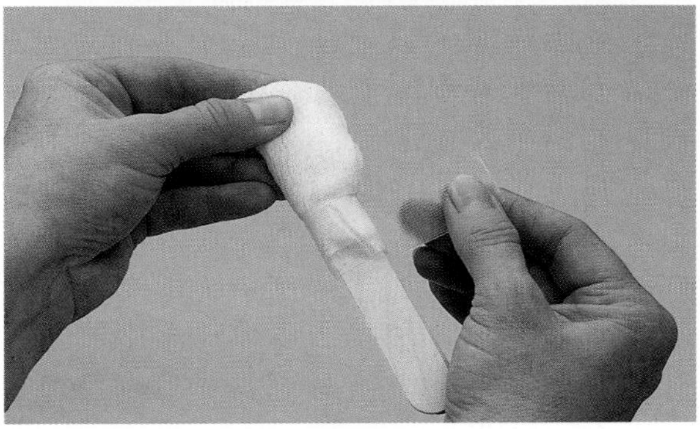

FIGURE 30–5 Making a padded tongue blade. **A,** Place two wooden tongue blades together, and wrap gauze around the top half. **B,** Tape the gauze in place.

Providing Mouth Care to an Unconscious Client 123

Advocate on behalf of the client's quality of life by promoting:

Dignity • Independence • Preferences • Privacy • Safety *(see BOX 1–4, on p. 17)*

PRE-PROCEDURE

1 Identify the client, according to employer policy.
This eliminates the possibility of mistaking one client for another.

2 Explain the procedure to the client.
Even though the client is unconscious, assume that the client can hear you.

3 Perform hand hygiene.

4 Collect the following, depending on your employer's procedures:
- ☐ **Cleaning agent (check the care plan)**
- ☐ **Sponge swabs**
- ☐ **Padded tongue blade**
- ☐ **Water glass with cool water**
- ☐ **Face towel**
- ☐ **Kidney basin or small bowl**
- ☐ **Lubricant for lips**
- ☐ **Paper towels**
- ☐ **Gloves**

5 Place paper towels on the overbed table (in facilities) or on a work area within easy reach. Arrange items on top of the paper towels.
This protects the overbed table or work area.

6 Provide for privacy.

7 Raise bed to a comfortable working height.
Raising the bed will reduce your risk for back strain.

Continued

Providing Mouth Care to an Unconscious Client—cont'd

PROCEDURE

8 Lower the bed rail near you if it is up.

9 Position the client in a side-lying position facing you. Turn his head well to the side.
This helps prevent aspiration of fluids, especially if the client has a diminished gag reflex.

10 Place a towel under the client's chin.
This helps protect the linen.

11 Place the kidney basin or bowl under the client's chin.
This helps catch any fluid spilled from the mouth.

12 Adjust the overbed table so that you can reach it with ease.*

13 Put on gloves.

14 Separate the upper and lower teeth with the padded tongue blade. Be gentle. Do not use force. If you force separation, you could fracture your client's jaw.

15 Inspect the tongue and gums for signs of redness, sores, swelling, or loose teeth.
It is important to use your observational skills as part of providing safe care to the client.

16 Clean the mouth with sponge swabs moistened with the cleaning agent (see **FIGURE 30–4**, on p. 620):
- **a** Clean the chewing and inner surfaces of teeth.

This helps reduce bacteria on teeth, gums, and the tongue.
- **b** Clean the outer surfaces of teeth.
- **c** Swab the roof of the mouth, insides of the cheeks, and the lips.
- **d** Swab the tongue.
- **e** Moisten a clean swab with water, and swab the mouth to remove the cleaning solution.

Leaving the cleaning solution in the mouth could cause irritation of the oral mucosa as well as be a risk for aspiration.
- **f** Place used swabs in the kidney basin or bowl.

17 Dry the client's mouth with the towel.
This helps prevent skin breakdown of the delicate skin around the mouth.

18 Apply lubricant to the lips.
This helps prevent cracking of the lips.

19 Remove the towel.

20 Remove gloves. Perform hand hygiene.

POST-PROCEDURE

21 Explain to the client that you are going to perform repositioning.
Your client may be able to hear you.

22 Reposition the client, and provide for safety and comfort.

23 Place the call bell within reach.*
Your client may recover consciousness and require assistance.

24 Return the bed to its lowest position. Follow the care plan for bed rail use.*
This is done for the safety of your client.

25 Clean and return equipment to its proper place.
This makes it easier to find the next time it is needed.

26 Discard disposable items. Wear gloves for this step.

27 Wipe the overbed table or work area with paper towels. Discard the paper towels.
This reduces the likelihood of pathogen spread.

28 Remove privacy measures.

29 Tell the client that you are leaving the room.
The client may be aware of your presence.

30 Follow employer policy for handling dirty linen.

31 Perform hand hygiene.

Report and Record your actions and observations, according to employer policy.
This is done for legal reasons and to keep the rest of the health care team informed.

*Steps marked with an asterisk may not apply in community settings.

Denture Care

Dentures are artificial teeth. A client may have a complete set of dentures or a partial set (see **FIGURE 30–6**). Mouth care is given and dentures are cleaned as often as natural teeth are. Dentures are very costly, so handle them carefully. They are slippery when wet and break or chip easily if dropped onto a hard surface (floor, sink).

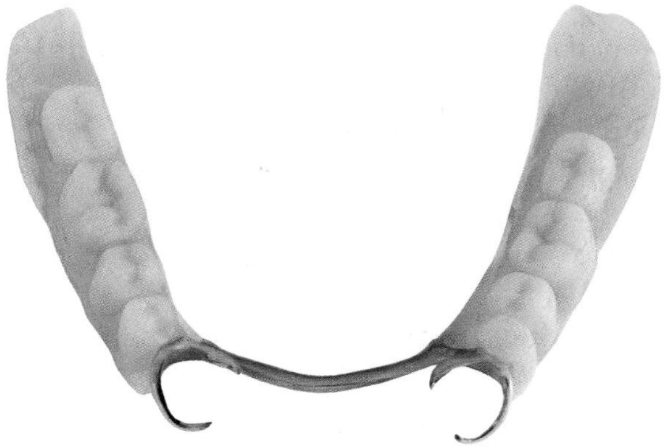

FIGURE 30–6 An example of a partial denture. The partial denture is held in place by metal hooks, which wrap around the client's own teeth. Proper brushing is necessary to ensure that food does not collect under or around the partial denture. (**Source:** MARGRIT HIRSCH/Shutterstock.com.)

The cleaning agent will have the manufacturer's instructions on how to use it and the water temperature required. Ensure that the dentures are soaked for the recommended time, as damage can occur if dentures are soaked in the cleansing agent for longer than recommended. Also, very hot water causes warping.

Depending on where you are employed, storage of dentures that are not going to be worn after cleaning varies. Some dentists and denturists recommend dentures be stored in a container and covered with water. If not covered with water, they can warp. Other dentists and denturists recommend storing them dry. Some clients remove their dentures at bedtime. Some clients do not wear their dentures all the time; they may wear them for eating and remove them after meals. Remind them not to wrap dentures in tissues or napkins, as there is a risk of their being discarded by mistake.

Most clients clean their own dentures, but some may need help to collect the cleaning items or to get to the bathroom. You are required to clean dentures only for those clients who cannot do it themselves.

Generally, clients do not like being seen without their dentures and remove them only for cleaning. After you have cleaned the dentures, return them to the clients as quickly as possible. Provide privacy for clients who clean their own dentures.

Providing Denture Care 123

Advocate on behalf of the client's quality of life by promoting:

Dignity • Independence • Preferences • Privacy • Safety *(see BOX 1–4, on p. 17)*

PRE-PROCEDURE

1 Identify the client, according to employer policy. *This eliminates the possibility of mistaking one client for another.*
2 Explain the procedure to the client.
3 Perform hand hygiene.
4 Collect the following:
- ☐ **Denture brush or toothbrush (soft bristle)**
- ☐ **Denture cup**
- ☐ **Denture cleaning agent**
- ☐ **Water glass with cool water**
- ☐ **Straw**
- ☐ **Mouthwash (or other specified solution)**
- ☐ **Kidney basin or small bowl**
- ☐ **Two face towels**
- ☐ **Paper towels**
- ☐ **Gauze squares**
- ☐ **Gloves**

5 Provide for privacy.

Continued

Providing Denture Care—cont'd

PROCEDURE

6 Lower the bed rail near you if it is up.
This helps prevent back strain.

7 Place a towel over the client's chest.
This helps protect the client's clothing.

8 Put on gloves.

9 Ask the client to remove dentures. Carefully place them in the kidney basin or bowl.
Dentures are delicate and expensive to replace. This helps prevent breakage.

10 If the client cannot remove dentures independently, remove them using gauze.
The gauze lets you get a good grip on slippery dentures.
  a Grasp the upper denture with your thumb and index finger (**FIGURE 30–7**).
  b Move the denture up and down slightly to break the seal. Gently remove the denture once the seal is broken. Place the denture in the kidney basin or bowl.
  c Remove the lower denture by grasping it with your thumb and index finger. Turn it slightly, and lift it out of the client's mouth. Place it in the kidney basin or bowl.

11 Raise the bed rail if used.

12 Take the kidney basin, denture cup, brush, and cleaning agent to the sink.

13 Line the sink with a towel, and fill it with water.
The towel will cushion the denture in case it falls and may prevent breakage.

14 Rinse dentures under warm running water. Return them to the denture cup.

15 Apply the cleaning agent to the brush.

16 Brush dentures as shown in **FIGURE 30–8**. Check for rough, sharp, or chipped areas on dentures.

17 Rinse dentures under running water. Use warm or cool water, as directed by the cleaning agent manufacturer.
Hot water can cause dentures to warp.

18 Place dentures in the denture cup.

19 Clean the kidney basin or bowl.

20 Bring the denture cup and kidney basin to the client.

21 Lower the bed rail if it is up.

22 Position the client for oral hygiene.

23 Assist the client to rinse with mouthwash or specified solution. Hold the kidney basin under the client's chin.
This helps protect the client's clothing.

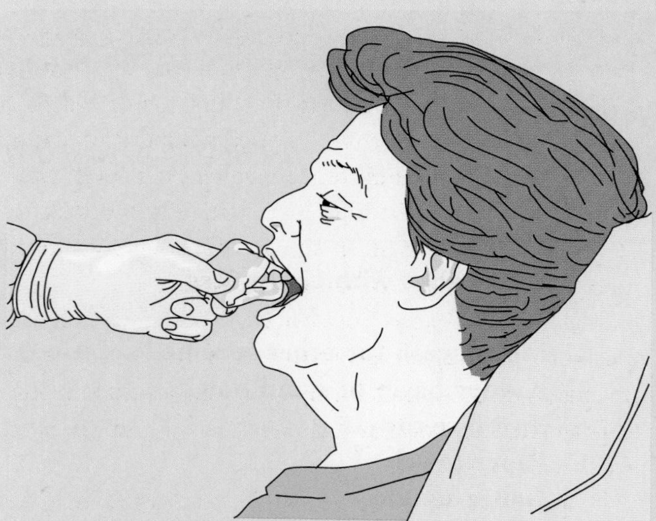

FIGURE 30–7 Removing the upper denture.

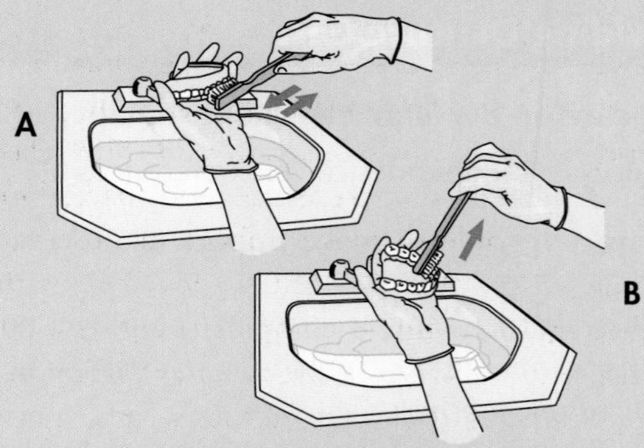

FIGURE 30–8 Cleaning dentures. **A,** Brush the outer surfaces of the upper denture with back-and-forth motions. Note that the denture is held over the sink, which is lined with a towel and filled halfway with water. **B,** Position the brush vertically to clean the inner surfaces of the denture. Use upward strokes.

Continued

Providing Denture Care—cont'd

24 Ask the client to insert dentures. If the client cannot do this, insert them in the following manner:

a Grasp the upper denture firmly with your thumb and index finger. Raise the upper lip with the other hand, and insert the denture. Use your index fingers to gently press on the denture to make sure it is securely in place. Be gentle to protect the denture from breakage and prevent injury to your client's mouth.

b Grasp the lower denture securely with your thumb and index finger. Pull down slightly on the lower lip, and insert the denture. Gently press down on it to make sure it is in place.

If the denture is not fitted properly, the client could choke.

25 Store dentures in a safe location if they are not going to be worn. Follow your employer's policy.

26 Remove the towel.

27 Remove gloves. Perform hand hygiene.

POST-PROCEDURE

28 Provide for safety and comfort.

29 Place the call bell within reach.*

This provides an easy, safe way for the client to contact staff if necessary.

30 Follow the care plan for bed rail use.*

31 Clean and return equipment to its proper place.

This makes it easier to find the next time it is needed.

32 Discard disposable items. Wear gloves for this step.

33 Remove privacy measures.

34 Follow employer policy for handling dirty linen.

35 Remove gloves and perform hand hygiene.

Report and Record your actions and observations, according to employer policy.

This is done for legal reasons and to keep the rest of the health care team informed.

*Steps marked with an asterisk may not apply in community settings.

BATHING

Bathing helps keep skin as well as the genital and anal areas clean by removing microbes, dead skin, perspiration, and excess oils. A bath is refreshing and relaxing, stimulates circulation, and exercises body parts. During baths, you are able to make important observations about clients, and you have time to get to know them.

A client may require a complete bath or a partial bed bath, a tub bath, or a shower, depending on the client's condition, self-care abilities, and personal choice. In facilities, bathing usually occurs after breakfast or the evening meal. The client's choice of bath time is respected whenever possible.

Bathing frequency is a matter of personal choice or employer policy. For example, some clients who live in their own homes may prefer to bathe daily, but in long-term care facilities, legislation may call for clients to have a complete bath once or twice a week and a partial bath daily and as needed. Besides personal choice, bathing frequency is affected by weather, physical activity, and illness. Bathing may need to be more frequent because of increased perspiration caused by high environmental temperatures or a fever. Some illnesses and dry skin may limit bathing to once every 2 or 3 days. Note that, in some cultures, only a family member is allowed to bathe a person.

Bathwater that is too hot can scald a frail, thin person. Many agencies, therefore, require two people to check each client's bathwater temperature using a digital thermometer and then record the temperature in the client's chart.

Guidelines to observe when assisting with bed baths, showers, and tub baths are listed in **BOX 30–1**. TABLE 30–1 on page 627 describes common skin care products (see the *Focus on Older Adults: Bathing* box).

BOX 30–1 Guidelines for Bathing Clients

- Follow the care plan for bathing method and skin care products. Allow personal choices whenever possible.
- Follow Standard Practices.
- Make sure the client fully understands the procedure before you begin. Talk with your supervisor if you are not sure that the client fully understands and agrees to the procedure.
- Collect all needed items *before* starting the procedure. For safety reasons, do not leave your client in the bathroom alone to collect any equipment.
- Provide for privacy. Close doors, shades, drapes, or privacy curtains.
- Cover the client for warmth and privacy.
- Eliminate drafts. Close doors and windows.
- Protect the client from falling.
- Use good body mechanics at all times (see Chapter 25).
- Protect the client from burns and scalds. Make sure water is not too hot, particularly for older adults. Check water temperature with a bath thermometer, the inside of your wrist, or your elbow. Water temperature for a complete bed bath is usually 43.3°C to 46.1°C (110°F to 115°F) for adults. However, older adults may need lower temperatures. Follow the care plan.
- Keep bar soap in the soap dish between lathering to prevent soapy water.
- Wash from the cleanest areas to the dirtiest areas.
- Encourage the client to help as much as is safely possible.
- Rinse the skin thoroughly to ensure that all of the soap is removed.
- Pat the skin dry to avoid irritating or breaking the skin. Never rub the skin.
- Dry under the breasts, between skin folds, in the perineal area, and between fingers and toes.
- Bathe skin thoroughly to wash off stool or urine if present. Follow Standard Practices.

FOCUS ON OLDER ADULTS

Bathing

Aging and soap cause dry skin, which is easily damaged. Therefore, older adults usually need a complete bath or shower only two times a week and partial baths on other days. When using soap, ensure thorough rinsing. Bar soaps should always be rinsed and placed where the bar can dry. Some older clients may bathe daily but not always use soap. Others may find that bath gels are easier to use than soaps.

Bath oils should never be added to tub baths, as they can increase the risk of a client slipping and falling. As well, the oil can cause irritation in the delicate mucous membranes of the urethra and vagina.

Special skin-cleansing products that do not require rinsing are now available. Follow the manufacturers' guidelines for use. Lotions applied after a bath can help keep skin soft and moisturized.

Observations

Observe the client's skin during bathing procedures. Report and record the following:

- The colour of the skin, lips, nail beds, and sclera (whites of the eyes)
- The location and description of rashes
- Dry skin
- Bruises or open skin areas
- Pale or reddened areas, particularly over bony parts
- Drainage or bleeding from wounds or body openings
- Swelling of feet and legs
- Corns or calluses on feet
- Skin temperature
- Complaints of pain or discomfort

The Complete Bed Bath

The *complete bed bath* involves washing the entire body while the client is still in bed. It is given to

TABLE 30–1 Common Skin Care Products

Type	Purpose	Considerations
Soaps	Clean the skin Remove oil, dirt, dead skin, skin oil, some microbes, and perspiration	Tend to dry and irritate the skin Dry skin is easily injured and causes itching and discomfort Skin must be rinsed well to remove all soap Not needed for every bath; plain water can clean the skin Plain water is often used for older adults and clients with very dry skin
Bath oils	Keep the skin soft and prevent drying	Some soaps contain bath oil Liquid bath oil can be added to bathwater Bath oils can cause showers and tubs to become slippery; safety precautions are necessary to prevent falls
Creams and lotions	Protect the skin from the drying effect of air and evaporation	Do not feel greasy but leave an oily film on the skin Should not contain alcohol because it will dry the skin Most are scented Lotion is used for back massage; applying lotion to bony points helps prevent skin breakdown Apply lotion to the back, elbows, knees, and heels after bathing Never apply to an area receiving radiation as the aluminum in the lotion could cause skin burns
Powders	Absorb moisture and prevent friction when two skin surfaces rub together	Not recommended by many agencies because their use encourages the growth of microbes If used, usually applied under the breasts, under the arms, in the groin area, and sometimes between the toes To apply powder, turn away from the client and sprinkle a small amount onto your hands or a cloth; apply in a thin, even layer Excessive amounts cause caking and crusts that can irritate the skin and allow microbes to grow Do not shake or sprinkle powder onto the client; inhaled powder can irritate the airway and lungs Should not be used near clients with respiratory diseases. Never use on an area that is receiving radiation, as the aluminum in the powder will cause skin burns Check the care plan before applying powder
Deodorants and antiperspirants	Deodorants mask and control body odours Antiperspirants reduce the amount of perspiration	Applied to the axillae (underarms) Should not be applied to irritated skin Are not a substitute for bathing

clients who cannot bathe themselves—clients who are unconscious, paralyzed, in casts or traction, or weak from illness or surgery.

Ask your supervisor about the client's ability to assist with the bath and about any activity or position limitations. Remember to follow Standard Practices. Also, remember to allow the client to make choices during the bath.

A bed bath is a new experience for many clients. Some may be embarrassed that another person can see their body, and some fear exposure and loss of privacy. Explain to the client how a bed bath is given and that you will cover the person's body for privacy. The bed bath procedure below applies to adults. Follow the adult procedure for bathing toddlers and older children. See Chapter 19 for bathing infants. Infants, young children, and older adults have fragile skin, so lower water temperatures must be used for them. Ask your supervisor or check the care plan for what water temperature to use. Always remember to test the bathwater before bathing a client.

Giving a Complete Bed Bath 123

Advocate on behalf of the client's quality of life by promoting:

Dignity • Independence • Preferences • Privacy • Safety *(see BOX 1–4, on p. 17)*

PRE-PROCEDURE

1 Identify the client, according to employer policy.
2 Explain the procedure to the client.
3 Offer the bedpan or urinal (see Chapter 32). Provide for privacy.
4 Perform hand hygiene.
5 Collect the following supplies:
   - ☐ **Wash basin**
   - ☐ **Soap**
   - ☐ **Bath thermometer, if available**
   - ☐ **Orange stick, nail file, or soft nail brush**
   - ☐ **Washcloth**
   - ☐ **Two bath towels and two face towels**
   - ☐ **Flat sheet**
   - ☐ **Clean gown, pyjamas, or clothing of the client's choice**
   - ☐ **Items for oral hygiene**
   - ☐ **Lotion**
   - ☐ **Powder**
   - ☐ **Deodorant or antiperspirant**
   - ☐ **Brush and comb**
   - ☐ **Other grooming items if requested by client**
   - ☐ **Paper towels**
   - ☐ **Gloves (Wear only when contact with blood, body fluids, secretions, or excretions is likely or when bathing the genital and rectal [perineal] areas.)**

6 Place paper towels on the overbed table (in facilities) or on a work area within easy reach. Arrange items on top of paper towels.
7 Close doors and windows.
This helps prevent drafts.
8 Provide for privacy.
9 Raise the bed to a comfortable working height.
This will reduce your risk for back strain.

PROCEDURE

10 Lower the bed rail near you if it is up. Remove the call bell.*
11 Provide oral hygiene if necessary (see the procedure *Brushing the Client's Teeth* on pp. 615–617).
12 Cover the client with the top sheet.
This ensures client warmth and privacy.
13 Lower the head of the bed until flat if the client can tolerate this position.* Ensure the client has at least one pillow.

Continued

Giving a Complete Bed Bath—cont'd

14 Raise the bed rail near you if bed rails are used. Fill the wash basin two thirds with water, and test the water by using a bathwater thermometer (**FIGURE 30–9**) to ensure that the water is a safe and comfortable temperature.

15 Place the basin on the overbed table or work area.

16 Lower the bed rail if it is up.

17 Help the client move to the side of the bed near you.

18 Place a bath towel over the client's chest.

19 Make a mitt with the washcloth (**FIGURE 30–10**), and use it for the entire bath.

20 Wash around the client's eyes with water. Do not use soap. Gently wipe from the inner part of the eye to the outer with a corner of the mitt (**FIGURE 30–11**).
Clean around the far eye first. Repeat this step to clean around the near eye, using a clean part of the mitt.
This helps prevent the transfer of possible microbes from one eye to the other.

21 Ask the client if you can use soap on the face.
Some clients do not want soap used on the face, as it can cause drying.

22 Wash the face, ears, and neck. Rinse and pat dry with the towel that is on the chest.

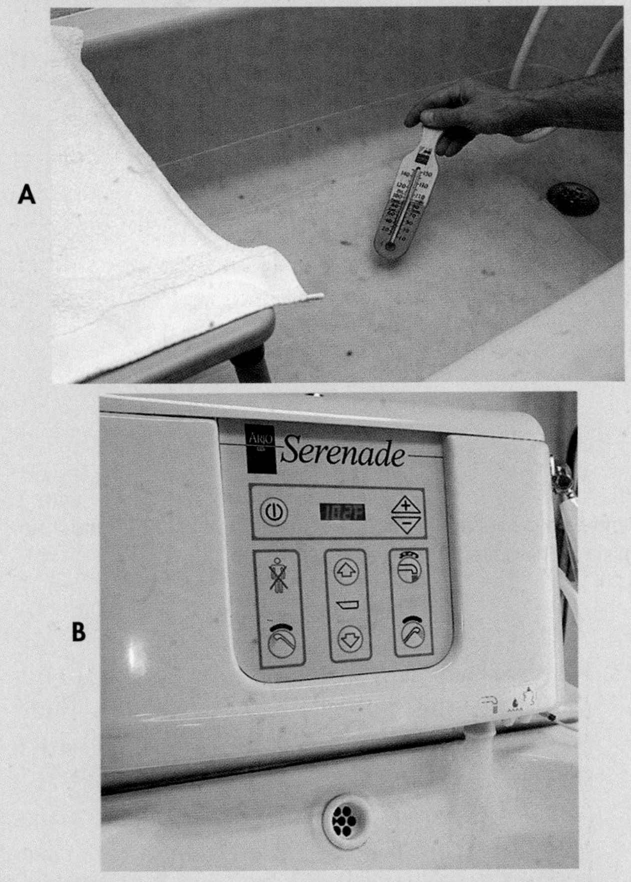

FIGURE 30–9 Measuring bathwater temperature. **A,** A bath thermometer is used to measure water temperature. **B,** The digital display shows water temperature.

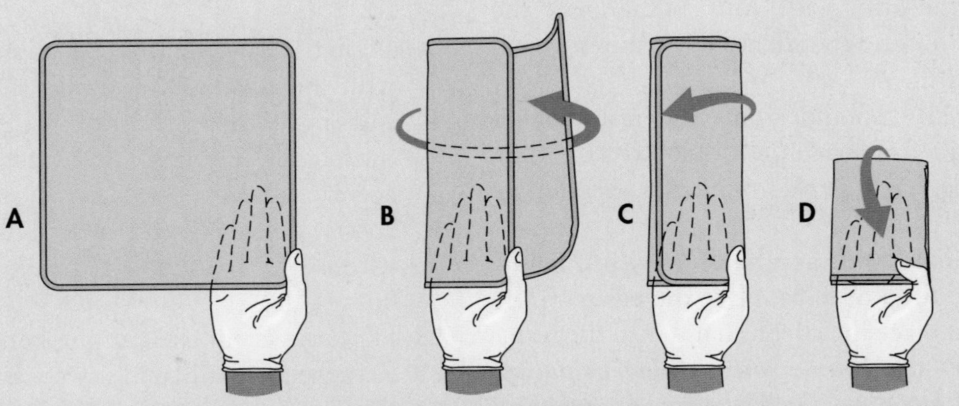

FIGURE 30–10 Making a mitted washcloth. **A,** Grasp the near side of the washcloth with your thumb. **B,** Bring the washcloth around and behind your hand. **C,** Fold the side of the washcloth over your palm as you grasp it with your thumb. **D,** Fold the top of the washcloth down, and tuck it under, next to your palm.

Continued

Giving a Complete Bed Bath—cont'd

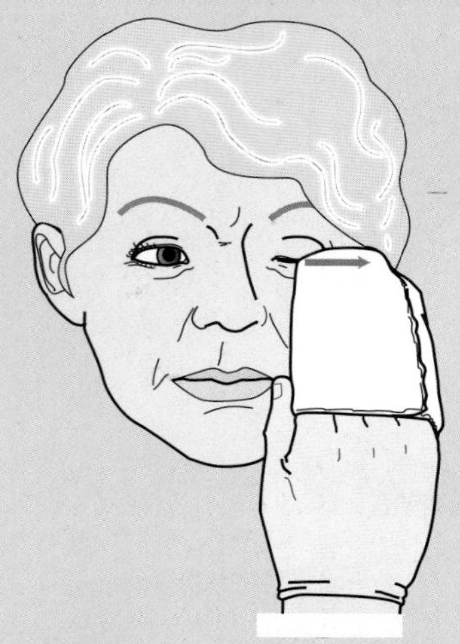

FIGURE 30–11 Wash around the client's eyes with a mitted washcloth. Wipe from the inner area to the outer area of the eye.

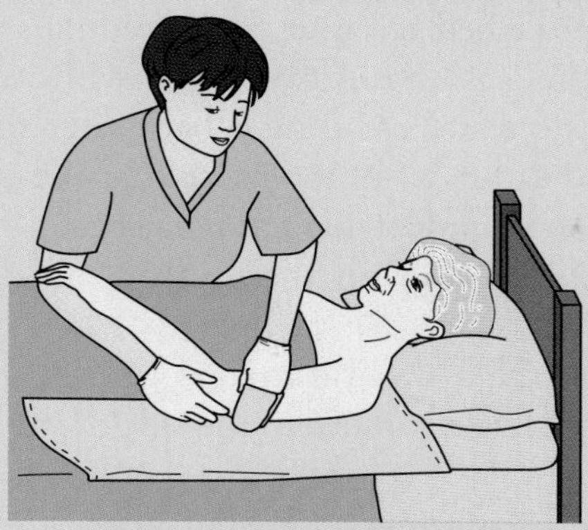

FIGURE 30–12 Wash the client's arm with firm, long strokes using a mitted washcloth.

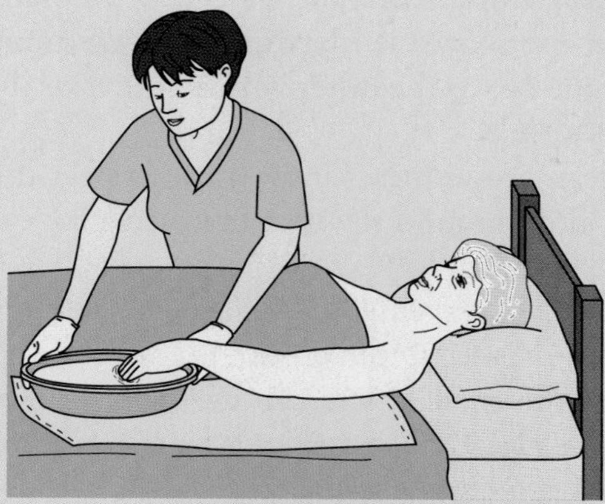

FIGURE 30–13 If the client's hands and nails are soiled with food or feces, place the wash basin on the bed (if allowed), and wash the client's hands in the wash basin.

23 Remove the client's garments, but take care not to expose the client. Keep the client's body, except the area you are washing, covered with a sheet.
Having waited until this time to remove garments helps the client feel less exposed and more comfortable with the bath.

24 Place a bath towel lengthwise under the client's far arm.
This helps protect the linen.

25 Support the arm, with your palm under the client's elbow and the client's forearm resting on your forearm.

26 Wash the arm, shoulder, and underarm (axilla) using long, firm strokes (FIGURE 30–12).
Using long, firm strokes increases circulation.
Rinse and pat dry.

27 If the client's hands and nails are visibly soiled with dried food or feces, place the basin on the towel, and place the client's hand into the water (FIGURE 30–13). ***Follow your employer's policy, as not all facilities allow placing the basin on the bed.***
Soaking is the only way to soften dried food or feces on hands and nails.
Wash the hand well, and clean under fingernails with the client's own orange stick, nail file, or soft nail brush. Ensure the wash basin is thoroughly cleaned afterwards according to agency policy.
Some agencies do not allow basins on the bed because if it spills on the floor, it creates a safety hazard.

28 Have the client exercise the hand and fingers.

29 Remove the basin, and dry the hand well. Cover the client's arm with the bath blanket.

30 Replace water in the basin if it is cooled, too soapy, or soiled. Repeat steps 24 to 29 for the near arm.

Continued

Giving a Complete Bed Bath—cont'd

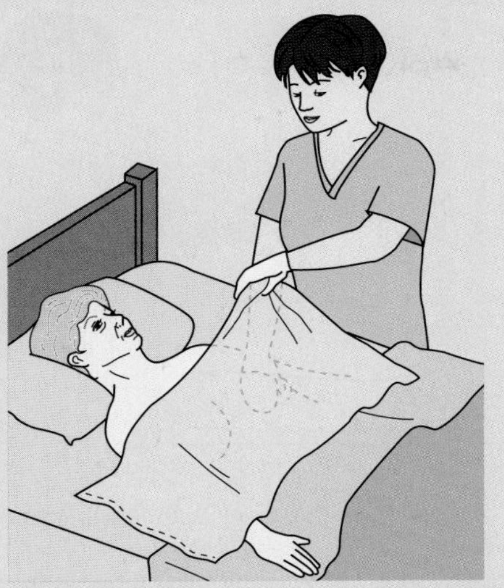

FIGURE 30–14 Place a bath towel horizontally over the chest area to avoid exposing the client's breasts. Lift the towel slightly to wash the breasts and chest and to observe skin condition.

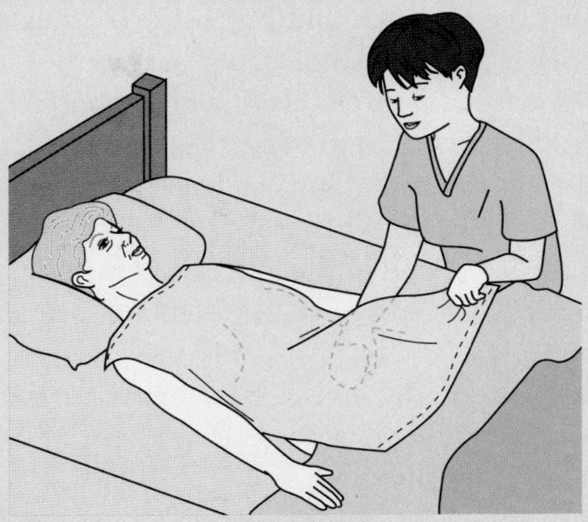

FIGURE 30–15 Turn the bath towel vertically to cover the breasts, abdomen, and pubic area. Lift the towel slightly to bathe the abdomen. Check the skin condition in abdominal folds.

31 Place a bath towel across the client's chest, and hold the towel in place. Pull the sheet from under the towel to the waist.

32 Lift the towel slightly, and wash the chest. While washing the chest and abdomen, observe the skin condition under the breasts, in the abdominal folds, and in the groin. Do not expose the client. Rinse and pat dry, especially under the breasts (FIGURE 30–14).
These areas can reveal the first sign of skin breakdown and will need special skin care, which will be directed by the care plan. Your observations and reporting of any changes will ensure that changes in skin condition will be addressed.

33 Turn the towel so that it is lengthwise over the chest and abdomen. Do not expose the client. Pull the sheet down to the pubic area.
This helps ensure privacy as much as possible.

34 Lift the towel slightly, and wash the abdomen (FIGURE 30–15). Rinse and pat dry.

35 Pull sheet up to the shoulders, covering both arms. Remove the towel.

36 If bed rails are used, raise the bed rail. Change soapy, soiled, or cooled water. Measure temperature as in step 14. Lower the bed rail when you return.

37 Uncover the far leg. Do not expose the genital area. Place a towel lengthwise under the foot and leg.

38 Bend the client's knee if it is comfortable for your client, and support the leg with your arm. Wash the leg with long, firm strokes. Rinse and pat dry.

39 Place the towel under the client's feet. Wash the client's feet.
If the client's feet are visibly dirty, and they need to soak in water to remove the dirt, it is usually safer and easier to wash them during a tub bath.

40 Use an orange stick, nail file, or soft nail brush to clean under toenails if necessary. If the client cannot bend the knee, wash the foot, carefully separating and washing between the toes. Rinse and pat dry.
Bacteria can grow in the area between toes if not dried properly.

41 Repeat steps 37 to 40 for the near leg.

42 If bed rails are used, raise the bed rail near you. Change the water. Measure temperature as in step 14. Lower the bed rail when you return.
This helps ensure the safety of the client.

43 Turn the client onto the side facing away from you. Keep the client covered with the bath towel or a sheet.

Continued

Giving a Complete Bed Bath—cont'd

44 Uncover the back and buttocks. Do not needlessly expose areas not being bathed.
This helps to keep the client warmer and respects the client's right to privacy. Place a towel lengthwise on the bed along the back.

45 Wash the back. Work from the back of the neck to the lower end of the buttocks. Use long, firm, continuous strokes (**FIGURE 30–16**). Rinse and dry well.

46 After the bath, give a back massage (see the procedure *Giving a Back Massage* on p. 641) if the client wants one.

47 Turn the client onto the back. Cover the client with the sheet.

48 If bed rails are used, raise the bed rail near you. Change the water to provide perineal care. Measure water temperature as in step 14. Lower the bed rail when you return.

49 Allow the client to wash the genital area, if able. Place the wash basin, soap, and towels within easy reach. Place the call bell (in facilities) within reach. Ask the client to call you when finished. Make sure the client understands what to do. Answer calls for assistance promptly.

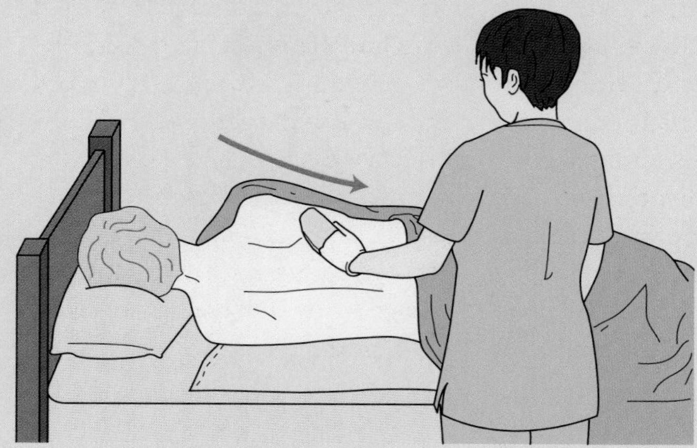

FIGURE 30–16 Wash the back with long, firm, continuous strokes. Note that the client is in a side-lying position. A towel placed lengthwise on the bed protects the linen from getting wet.

50 If the client cannot do perineal self-care, put on gloves, and provide perineal care for the client (see the procedures on pp. 642 and 646).

51 Apply deodorant or antiperspirant and lotion, as directed by the care plan or by the client.

52 Put clean garments on the client.

53 Comb and brush the hair (see Chapter 31).

54 Make the bed.

POST-PROCEDURE

55 Provide for safety and comfort.

56 Return the bed to its lowest position. Attach the call bell. Follow the care plan for bed rail use.*
This helps provide for client safety.

57 Empty and clean the wash basin. Return it and other supplies to their proper places.
This makes them easier to find the next time they are needed.

58 Wipe the overbed table or work area with paper towels. Discard the paper towels.

59 Remove privacy measures.

60 Follow employer policy for handling dirty linen.

61 Perform hand hygiene.

Report and Record your actions and observations, according to employer policy.
This is done for legal reasons and to keep the rest of the health care team informed.

*Steps marked with an asterisk may not apply in community settings.

Towel Baths

For a *towel bath,* usually an oversized towel is used so as to cover the client's body from neck to feet. The bath towel is saturated with a cleaning solution, which contains water, a cleaning agent, and a skin-softening agent. It also has a drying agent so that the client's body dries quickly. The towel bath is quick, soothing, and relaxing. Clients with dementia often accept this type of bath well. Your supervisor and the care plan will tell you when to use the towel bath. Follow employer policies and procedures.

Bag Baths

Bag baths are prepared commercially or by the employer. Eight to ten washcloths moistened with a cleaning agent that does not require rinsing are provided in a plastic bag. Before use, the washcloths are warmed in the microwave. Check with your supervisor and manufacturer's instructions for the microwave setting. A new washcloth is used for each body part, and the skin is air-dried, so towels are not needed.

The Partial Bath

The *partial bath* involves bathing the face, hands, axillae (underarms), back, buttocks, and perineal area. These areas develop odours or cause discomfort if they are not clean. Partial bed baths are given to clients who cannot bathe themselves. Some clients may be able to bathe themselves in the bed or at the bathroom sink (**FIGURE 30–17**). You will be required to assist them as needed, especially with washing the back.

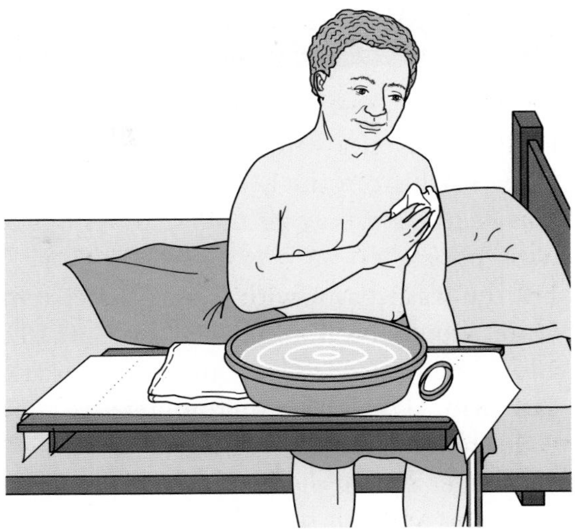

FIGURE 30–17 The client is bathing himself in bed. Necessary equipment is within his reach.

The guidelines for bathing and the considerations involved (see **BOX 30–1** on p. 626) also apply to partial bed baths.

Giving a Partial Bath 123

Advocate on behalf of the client's quality of life by promoting:

Dignity • Independence • Preferences • Privacy • Safety *(see BOX 1–4, on p. 17)*

PRE-PROCEDURE

1 Follow steps 1 through 8 in the procedure *Giving a Complete Bed Bath* (see p. 628). Put on gloves if that is your employer's policy.

PROCEDURE

2 Make sure the bed is in the lowest position.*
This is done for the safety of your client.

3 Assist with oral hygiene.

4 Remove the bedspread. Cover the client with the top sheet.
This is done to provide privacy.

Continued

Giving a Partial Bath—cont'd

5 Place paper towels on the overbed table (in facilities) or on a work area that the client can easily reach from the bedside.
This helps absorb water that splashes out of the wash basin.
6 Fill the wash basin with water. Water temperature should be 43.3°C to 46.1°C (110°F to 115°F) or as directed by your supervisor and the care plan. (Use a bath thermometer to measure water temperature.)
Bathwater can easily scald a person who is thin or frail or who has sensory challenges.
7 Place the basin on the overbed table or work area.
8 Position the client in Fowler's position. Or assist the client to sit at the bedside.
9 Adjust the overbed table so that the client can reach the basin and supplies.*
This helps ensure that the client is not reaching too far and risking falling.
10 Help the client undress. Respect cultural diversity when asking a client to undress.
11 Ask the client to wash easy-to-reach body parts. Explain that you will wash the back and other areas the client cannot reach.
12 Place the call bell within reach. Ask the client to use it if help is needed or when bathing has been completed.* If working in the community, assure the client that you will be outside the door and ask the client to call for assistance when needed.
13 Perform hand hygiene.
14 Leave the room if it is safe to do so. Stay within hearing distance and assure the client you will be available to help if needed. Return when the client calls for assistance. Knock before entering.
15 Change the bathwater. (Measure the bathwater temperature as in step 6.)
The water may be too cool, too soapy, or too soiled by now.
16 Raise the bed to a comfortable working height. Adjust the overbed table, as needed.*
This reduces your risk for back strain.
17 Ask the client to specify the parts that were self-washed. Wash and dry areas the client could not reach. The face, hands, underarms, back, buttocks, and genital and rectal areas (perineal area) are washed for the partial bath. Wear gloves for giving perineal care.
18 Give a back massage if the client agrees.
19 Apply deodorant or antiperspirant, as requested by the client.
20 Help the client put on clean garments.
21 Assist with hair care.
22 Assist the client to a chair (see the procedure *Transferring the Client to a Chair or Wheelchair* on p. 518). Otherwise, turn the client onto the side away from you.
23 Make the bed.
24 Return the bed to its lowest position.*
This helps ensure the safety of the client.

POST-PROCEDURE

25 Provide for safety and comfort.
26 Place the call bell within reach.*
This provides an easy, safe way for the client to contact staff if necessary.
27 Follow the care plan for bed rail use.*
28 Empty and clean the basin. Return the basin and supplies to their proper places.
This makes them easier to find the next time they are needed.
29 Wipe the overbed table or work area with paper towels. Discard the paper towels.
30 Remove privacy measures.
31 Follow employer policy for handling dirty linen.
32 Perform hand hygiene.

Report and Record your actions and observations, according to employer policy.
This is done for legal reasons and to keep the rest of the health care team informed.

*Steps marked with an asterisk may not apply in community settings.

Tub Baths and Showers

Some clients prefer tub baths, and others prefer showers. In both cases, falls and burns from hot water are risks, so ensuring safety is important (see the *Think About Safety: Safety Guidelines for Assisting Clients During Tub Baths and Showers* box). You must prevent slipping, falls, chills, and burns. *Give a tub bath or shower only if it is specified in the care plan.* Check with your supervisor and the care plan for special instructions.

Tub Baths

Many clients find tub baths relaxing, but they can cause a client to feel faint, weak, or tired. These risks are greater for clients who are on bed rest, so a bath should last no longer than 20 minutes.

In a facility, you will need to reserve the tub room for the client. Clean the tub before and after use to prevent the spread of microbes and infection, applying your knowledge of Workplace Hazardous Materials Information System (WHMIS).

Think About Safety

Safety Guidelines for Assisting Clients During Tub Baths and Showers

- Know the right water temperature. Check with your supervisor and the care plan. Usually, the optimal temperature is 40.5°C (105°F). Because of the risk for scalding injuries if the water is too hot, many agencies require two people to check each client's bathwater temperature using a digital thermometer and then record the bath or shower water temperature in the client's chart.
- Clean the tub or shower before and after use, as per WHMIS. This prevents the spread of microbes and infection.
- Dry the bathroom or shower room floor.
- Check hand rails, grab bars, hydraulic lifts, and other safety aids. They must be in working order.
- Place a bath mat in the tub or on the shower floor. The mat is not needed if there are nonskid strips or a nonskid surface.
- Cover the client for warmth and privacy during transport to and from the shower or tub room.
- Place needed items within the client's reach.
- Place the call bell (in facilities) within the client's reach. Show the client how to use the call bell in the shower or tub room.
- Have the client use safety bars when getting in and out of the tub or shower. The client must not use towel bars for support.
- Use good body mechanics when transferring clients to and from tubs and showers (see Chapter 25). If necessary, ask for help before beginning the transfer.
- Turn cold water on first and then the hot water. Turn hot water off first and then the cold water.
- Before the client gets into the shower, adjust water temperature and pressure to prevent chilling or burns. If a shower or bath chair is used, position the chair first.
- Fill the tub before the client gets into it.
- Measure the water temperature using a bath thermometer. Or use the digital display for showers and tub baths in facilities (see **FIGURE 30–9**).
- Keep the water spray directed toward the client during the shower to help keep the client warm.
- Avoid using bath oils, as they make tub and shower surfaces slippery.
- Keep the bar soap in the soap dish to prevent soapy water and to reduce the chance of slips and falls in the tub or shower.
- Do not leave weak or unsteady clients unattended in the tub or shower.
- Stay within hearing distance if the client can be left alone. Wait outside the door or shower curtain. You will be nearby if the client calls for you or has an accident.
- Drain the tub before the client gets out of the tub.

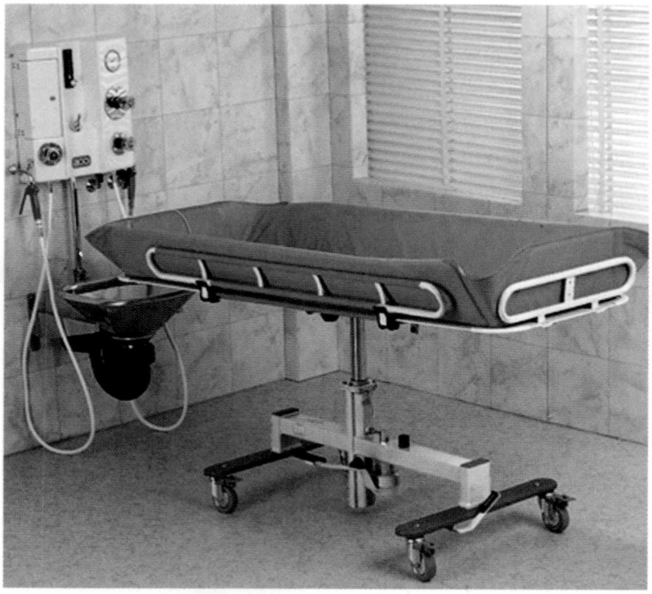

FIGURE 30–18 Portable tub. (Courtesy ArjoHuntleigh Inc.)

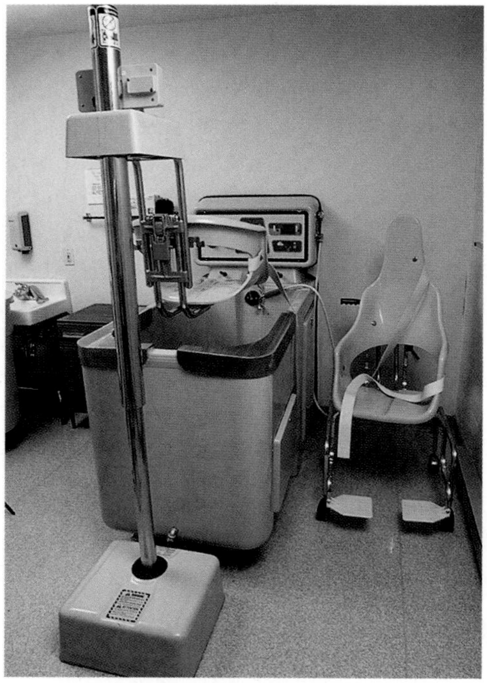

FIGURE 30–19 Whirlpool tub with a hydraulic lift.

Some facilities have portable tubs. The sides of them can be lowered to transfer the client from the bed to the tub (**FIGURE 30–18**) and raised after the transfer. The client is transported to the tub room in the portable tub. The tub is filled there, and the client is bathed in the usual manner. Remember to cover the client with a blanket for privacy and warmth during transfers and transports.

Whirlpool tubs have hydraulic lifts (**FIGURE 30–19**). The client is transported to the tub room in a special wheelchair or stretcher. The chair or stretcher is then lifted into the tub (**FIGURE 30–20**). The whirlpool action cleans the client's lower body, and you wash the upper body. Carefully wash under breasts, between skin folds, and in the perineal area. Dry the client after the bath. The whirlpool jets should be cleaned after each use, as per agency policy.

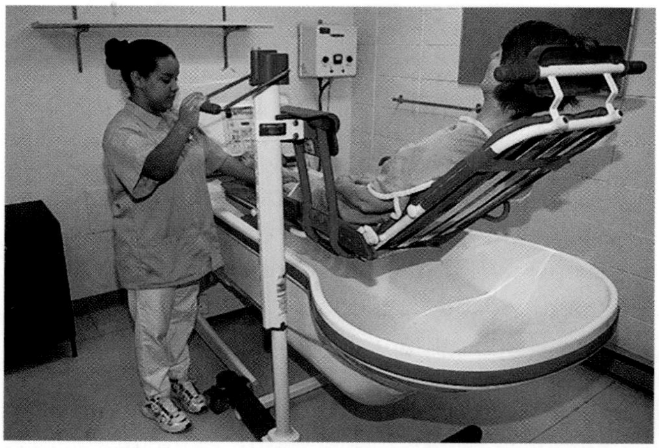

FIGURE 30–20 The stretcher and client are lowered into the tub. **(Note: There should always be two workers operating this mechanical device. Check your agency's policy.)**

In a client's home, the bathroom should be as safe as possible. Make sure that there is a rubber bath mat or nonskid strips on the tub or shower floor. Safety devices such as grab bars, transfer boards, and bath or shower chairs are helpful for some clients (**FIGURE 30-21**). The case manager and other members of the health care team arrange for these devices as needed. Make sure they are in place and used when necessary. Bring a straight chair into the bathroom so that the client can sit while the bath or shower is being prepared. Make sure that the bathroom is warm and well lit and the floor is free of clutter and water spills. Never leave a client unattended in the bathroom, so ensure that you are organized and have the necessary supplies for providing care.

Showers

Some facilities provide private baths or showers in the client's room. Other facilities have common baths or shower rooms that must be reserved before use. Shower rooms have shower stalls or shower cabinets (**FIGURE 30-22**). The client walks into the stall or cabinet or is wheeled in on a shower chair. An open part of the plastic seat lets water drain off the chair. The chair can be used to transport the client to and from the shower room. The wheels are locked during the shower to prevent the chair from moving.

The shower room may have more than one stall or cabinet. Protect the client's privacy. The client has the right not to be seen by others, so screen and cover the client properly, and close the door and the shower curtain.

Shower stalls and bathtub–shower units are common in most homes. If the client has to step into the bathtub to take a shower, make sure that safety bars are there for the client's use. Assist the client as needed with getting into and out of the shower.

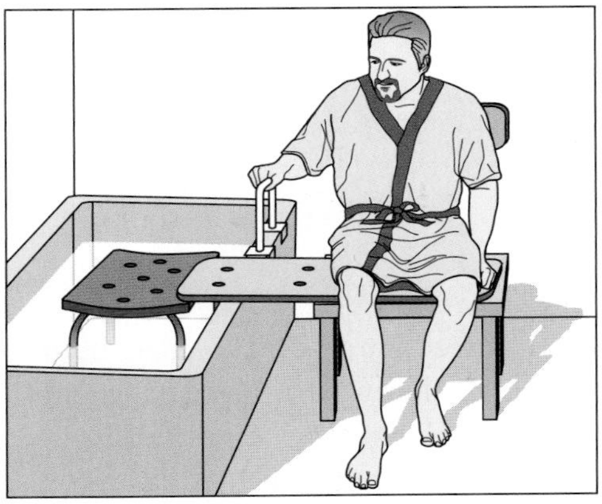

FIGURE 30–21 A client is using a transfer board, bath chair, and grab bar when taking a bath at home.

Home care clients can buy or rent a shower chair for home use, or a sturdy chair—for example, a sturdy lawn chair—can be used. The case manager will assist the client or family in finding a safe chair for shower use. Before every use, make sure the chair is steady and will not slide.

Turn on the water, and test its temperature before the client enters the shower. If the client can stand in the shower, encourage the client to use the grab bars, if available, for support during the shower. Like tubs, shower floors should have nonskid surfaces. If not, a rubber bath mat is used, but make sure the bath mat does not cover the drain. Never let weak or unsteady clients stand in the shower. They must use a shower chair. Contact your supervisor if you are concerned about the client's safety (see the *Focus on Children: Showers* box).

FOCUS ON CHILDREN

Showers

Many older children enjoy showers. Your supervisor will tell you how much help and supervision to give the child in your care. Remember, independence and privacy are important to older children.

A

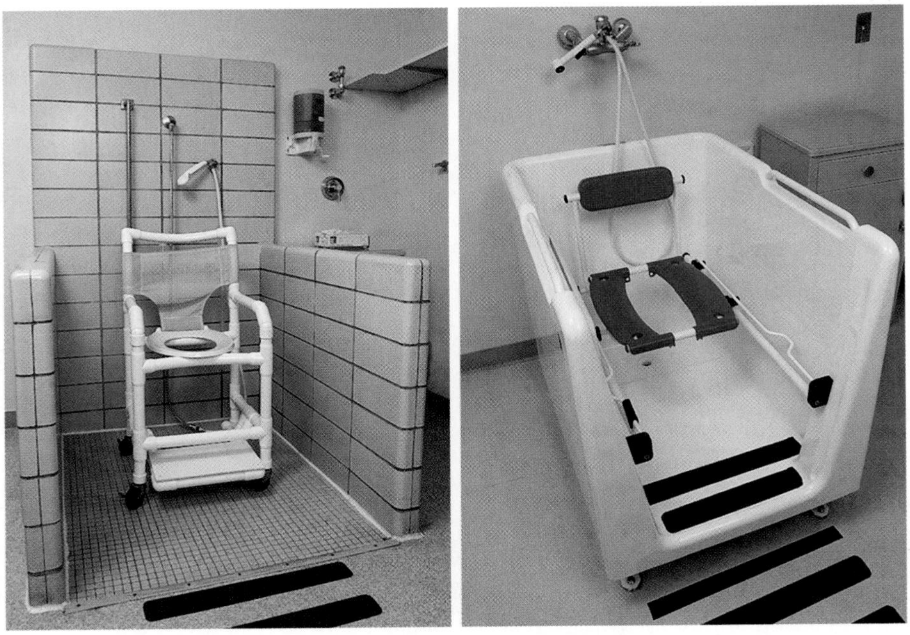

B

FIGURE 30–22 Common showers in facilities. **A,** Shower chair in a shower stall. **B,** Shower cabinet.

Assisting With a Tub Bath or Shower

123

Advocate on behalf of the client's quality of life by promoting:

Dignity • Independence • Preferences • Privacy • Safety *(see BOX 1–4, on p. 17)*

PRE-PROCEDURE

1 Reserve the bathtub or shower, according to employer policy.*
2 Identify the client, according to employer policy.
3 Explain the procedure to the client.
4 Perform hand hygiene.
5 Collect the following supplies:
- ☐ **Washcloth and two bath towels**
- ☐ **Soap**
- ☐ **Bath thermometer (for a tub bath), if available**
- ☐ **Straight chair (optional)**
- ☐ **Bath or shower chair (as necessary)**
- ☐ **Transfer board (if necessary)**
- ☐ **Clean garments**
- ☐ **Grooming items, as requested by the client**
- ☐ **Robe and nonskid footwear**
- ☐ **Rubber bath mat (if needed)**
- ☐ **Disposable floor mat (if needed)**
- ☐ **Gloves**

PROCEDURE

6 Place items in the bathroom or shower room. Use the space provided or a chair.
By collecting all the necessary equipment beforehand, you will not have to leave your client's side and can eliminate wasting time and energy in obtaining the forgotten equipment.
7 Clean the tub or shower.* Follow your employer's policy.
8 Place a rubber bath mat in the tub or on the shower floor. Make sure it does not block the drain.
This helps prevent slipping while also ensuring that the water can drain.
9 Place a bath mat on the floor in front of the tub or shower.
The bath mat provides a nonskid surface to help prevent falls in such a wet and slippery area.
10 Place the bath or shower chair in position. Lock the wheels. Position the transfer board if one is used.
This helps ensure client safety.
11 Put the *Occupied* sign on the door.*
12 Return to the client's room. Provide for privacy.
13 Help the client sit on the side of the bed.
14 Help the client put on a robe and nonskid footwear.
This provides privacy and safety for the client.
15 Assist the client to the bathroom or shower room. Use a wheelchair if necessary.
16 *For a tub bath:*
- a Have the client sit on the chair by the tub.
- b Fill the tub halfway with warm water (40.5°C, or 105°F, or a temperature that can be tolerated by the client) (**FIGURE 30–23**).
- c Measure water temperature with the bath thermometer, or check the digital display (see **FIGURE 30–9** on page 629).

For a shower:
- a Turn on the shower.
- b Adjust water temperature and pressure.

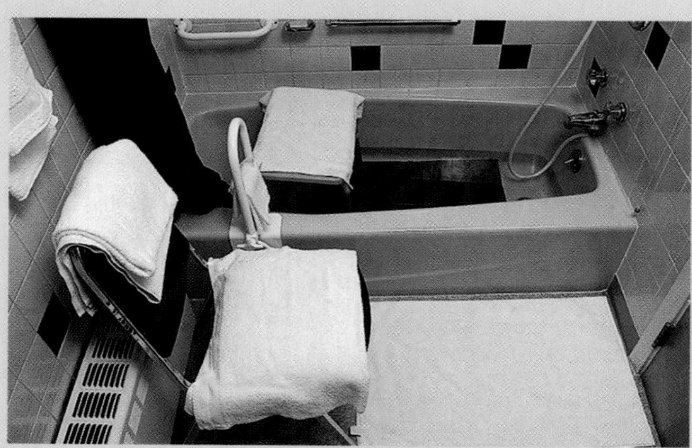

FIGURE 30–23 A bath mat is in the tub; the tub is filled halfway with water; a floor mat is in front of the tub; and a straight chair is next to the tub.

Continued

Assisting With a Tub Bath or Shower—cont'd

17 Help the client undress and remove footwear.
18 Assist the client into the tub or shower (see Chapter 25). Have the client use grab bars for support.
19 Assist with washing if necessary (a bath should last no longer than 20 minutes).
20 Place a towel across the chair.
21 Turn off the shower, or drain the tub. Cover the client while the tub drains.
This helps provide warmth and privacy.
22 Help the client out of the tub or shower and onto the chair. Encourage the client to use the grab bars.
This helps ensure client safety.
23 Help the client dry off by patting skin gently with the towel. Dry under breasts, between skin folds, around the perineal area, and between toes.
Ensuring that the client's skin is dry reduces the risk for skin breakdown.
24 Assist with applying lotion and other grooming items as needed.
25 Help the client dress and put on footwear.
26 Help the client return to the room. Assist the client into the bed or a chair.
27 Provide for privacy.
28 Give a back massage if the client returns to bed.
29 Assist with hair care and other grooming needs.

POST-PROCEDURE

30 Provide for safety and comfort.
31 Place the call bell within reach.*
32 Follow the care plan for bed rail use.*
33 Return to bathroom or shower room. Wearing gloves, remove soiled linen, discard disposable items, and clean the shower or tub using WHMIS.
34 Put the *Unoccupied* sign on the door.*
35 Return supplies to their proper places.
This makes them easier to find the next time they are needed.
36 Follow employer policy for handling dirty linen.
37 Perform hand hygiene.

Report and Record your actions and observations, according to employer policy.
This is done for legal reasons and to keep the rest of the health care team informed.

*Steps marked with an asterisk may not apply in community settings.

Dealing With Bathing Problems

Problems can arise when bathing a client. For example, the client may refuse the bath or be frightened by bathing procedures. The client may urinate or defecate during the procedure. You need to be prepared for these and other problems.

The Client Refuses the Bath

As with all procedures, the client has the right to refuse a bath. You cannot perform a bathing procedure without the client's informed consent. Sometimes, people feel too ill or too weak to bathe. Some are afraid of falling or getting chilled, and some may just be embarrassed. Listen carefully to the client to learn how you can provide reassurance. Did the client get cold during the last bath? If so, offer to raise the room temperature before you start. If the bathing area has a heat lamp, use it to provide extra warmth during bathing. Does the client think a bath is not needed? If so, remind the client that bathing promotes hygiene, comfort, and relaxation. If the client continues to refuse the bath, talk to your supervisor. Do not bathe clients against their wishes.

The Client Has Dementia

Clients with dementia are often frightened by bathing procedures. They do not understand what is happening or why and, therefore, may fear harm or danger. As a result, they may resist care, become agitated and combative, or shout at you and cry for help.

The guidelines in **BOX 30–1** on page 626 apply when you are bathing clients with dementia. The client's care plan lists measures to help the client through the bathing procedure. Such measures may include:

- Not rushing the client
- Using a calm, pleasant voice
- Diverting the client's attention (see Chapter 36)
- Calming the client and trying the bath again later

The Client Cannot Tolerate the Bathing Position

Some clients cannot sit or lie on their backs or sides for long periods due to disease, injury, surgery, or shortness of breath. You must adapt the procedure to meet the client's needs. For example, you may have to adapt your technique to accommodate whatever position the client finds most comfortable, scale down to a partial bath, or ask for help so that the client can be bathed quickly. Follow your supervisor's directions and the care plan.

The Client Urinates or Defecates

Some clients may have urinary or fecal incontinence (see Chapters 32 and 33). To try to avoid incontinence during the bath, toilet the client prior to every bed or tub bath. If a client urinates or defecates during a bed bath, put on gloves if you are not wearing them already. Turn the client away from you, and clean the client with toilet tissue and discard it in a bedpan. Change the soiled linens, and clean the bedpan. Remove your gloves, wash your hands, and put on clean gloves. Change the bathwater and washcloths to prevent contamination of other body areas.

If the client is taking a tub bath, drain the bath. Cover the client with a towel to prevent chilling. Help the client out of the tub. Remove stool with toilet tissue, and dispose of it in the toilet. Clean and refill the tub. Then help the client back into the tub. Use a clean washcloth for the bath. Remember to control your verbal as well as nonverbal reactions, taking care not to embarrass the client.

Hardened Secretions or Stool on the Client's Body

To remove hardened secretions or stool, use unscented lotion or petroleum jelly. Place some on a clean, damp washcloth or disposable cloth, as per your agency's policy. Gently clean the area. Repeat this step as needed. Do not rub or scratch. Doing so can irritate the skin and cause skin breakdown.

The Client Has an Erection

Privacy is important when a male client has an erection during the bath. If the client has dementia, he may not have conscious knowledge that he has an erection. Remain professional and calm and continue the bath, or tell him that you will give him some time alone if he would prefer. If you are uncomfortable with the client's erection, provide for safety, leave the room, and close the door. When you return, knock on the door before entering the room. Identify yourself, and ask if you can enter the room. Continue with the bath.

An erection is a normal reaction to physical contact, especially to the genital area. Try not to show any embarrassment. Remember, the client is probably embarrassed, too. A professional manner will help both of you.

THE BACK MASSAGE

The back massage (back rub) relaxes muscles and stimulates circulation. A massage is normally given after the bath and before bedtime. It should last 3 to 5 minutes. Observe the client's skin before giving the massage. Look for breaks, tears, bruises, reddened areas, and other signs of skin breakdown.

Application of lotion reduces friction during the massage. Before applying the lotion, warm it by placing the bottle in the bathwater, holding it under warm water, or rubbing some lotion between your hands.

The prone position is best for a massage. Older adults or people with a disability may find the side-lying position more comfortable. Use firm strokes, and always keep your hands in contact with the client's skin. After the massage, apply some lotion to the client's elbows, knees, and heels to keep the skin in those areas soft. These bony areas are most at risk for skin breakdown. Report any reddened areas or signs of skin breakdown at once.

Back massages as described in this procedure can be dangerous to some clients—for example, those with certain heart diseases, back injuries, back surgeries, skin diseases, and some lung disorders. Check with the care plan and your supervisor before giving back massages.

Giving a Back Massage

123

Advocate on behalf of the client's quality of life by promoting:

Dignity • Independence • Preferences • Privacy • Safety *(see BOX 1–4, on p. 17)*

PRE-PROCEDURE

1 Identify the client, according to employer policy.
2 Explain the procedure to the client.
3 Perform hand hygiene.
4 Collect the following supplies:
- ☐ **Bath blanket (if available)**
- ☐ **Bath towel**
- ☐ **Lotion**

5 Provide for privacy.
6 Raise the bed to a comfortable working height. *This helps reduce your risk for back strain.*

PROCEDURE

7 Lower the bed rail near you if it is up.
8 Position the client in the prone or side-lying position, with the client's back toward you.
9 Expose the back, shoulders, upper arms, and buttocks. Cover the rest of the body with the sheet.
10 Lay a towel on the bed along the back.
11 Warm the lotion between your hands. *Cold lotion can startle the client.*
12 Explain that the lotion may feel cool and wet. *This helps prepare the client.*
13 Apply lotion to the lower back area.
14 Stroke up from the buttocks to the shoulders. Then stroke down over the upper arms. Stroke up the upper arms, across the shoulders, and down the back to the buttocks. Use firm strokes. Keep your hands in contact with the client's skin. *Firm strokes encourage circulation and relax the client.* (**FIGURE 30–24**).
15 Repeat step 14 for at least 3 minutes, unless the client asks you to stop sooner.
16 Knead by grasping skin between your thumb and fingers. Be gentle, as skin can tear. Knead one side of the back, starting at the buttocks and moving up to the shoulder. Then knead down that side from the shoulder to the buttocks. Repeat on the other side of the back. (**FIGURE 30–25**).
17 Apply lotion to bony areas. Use circular motions with the tips of your index and middle fingers. Do not massage bony areas that are reddened (see Chapter 24).

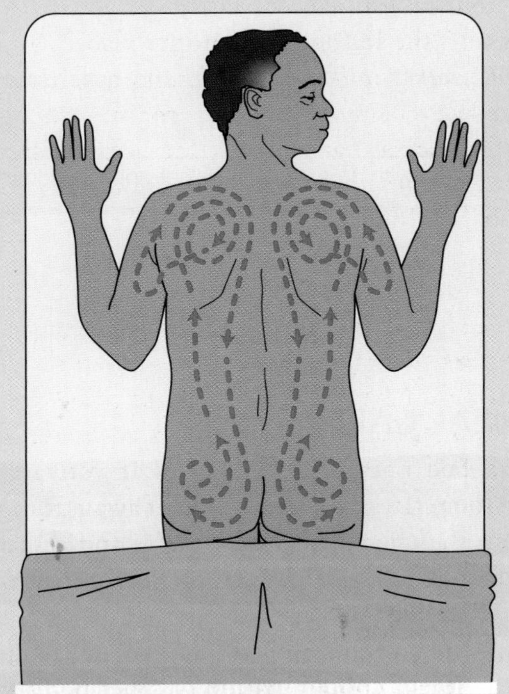

FIGURE 30–24 The client lies in the prone position for a back massage. Stroke upward from the buttocks to the shoulders, down over the upper arms, back up the upper arms, across the shoulders, and down the back to the buttocks.

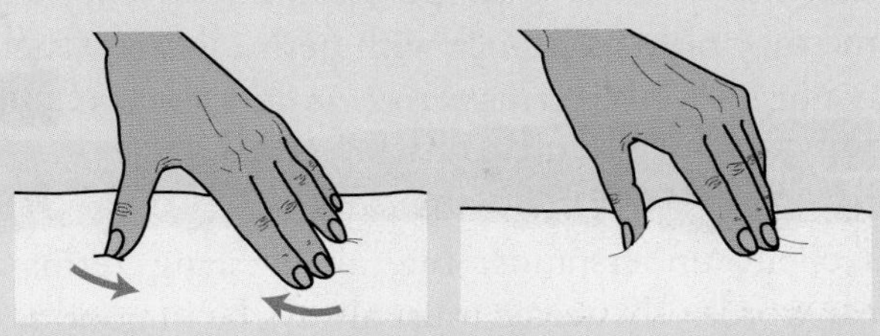

FIGURE 30–25 Kneading is done by grasping skin between the thumb and fingers.

Continued

Giving a Back Massage—cont'd

18 Use fast movements to stimulate and slow movements to relax the client.

19 Stroke with long, firm movements to end the massage. Tell the client that you are about to finish.

20 Cover the client. Remove the towel and bath blanket.

POST-PROCEDURE

21 Provide for safety and comfort.

22 Place the call bell within reach.*
This provides an easy, safe way for the client to contact staff if necessary.

23 Return the bed to its lowest position. Follow the care plan for bed rail use.*
This helps ensure client safety.

24 Return the lotion to its proper place.
This makes it easier to find the next time it is needed.

25 Remove privacy measures.

26 Follow employer policy for handling dirty linen.

27 Perform hand hygiene.

Report and Record your actions and observations, according to employer policy.
This is done for legal reasons and to keep the rest of the health care team informed.

*Steps marked with an asterisk may not apply in community settings.

PERINEAL CARE

Perineal care (pericare) involves cleaning the genital and anal areas, which provide a warm, moist, and dark place suitable for microbes to grow. Cleaning prevents infection, odours, and skin breakdown and promotes comfort.

Perineal care is done at least once every day during the bath. The procedure is also done whenever the area is soiled with urine or stool. Clients with certain disorders need perineal care more often. Your supervisor and the care plan tell you when the client needs perineal care.

Clients do their own perineal care if they can. Some may need assistance with perineal care. Clients may not know the terms *perineum* and *perineal.* Most understand terms such as *privates, private parts, crotch, genitals,* or the *area between the legs.* Use terms the client understands, but avoid slang terms or swear words. The terms must always be in good taste professionally.

Follow Standard Practices and medical asepsis when providing perineal care. Wear gloves. Work from the cleanest area to the dirtiest. The urethral area is the cleanest and the anal area the dirtiest, so clean from the urethra to the anal area. Clean around the perineum. When cleaning the perineum, use three strokes. Clean down the centre and then down each side. The perineal area is very delicate and easily injured. Use warm water, not hot water. Test the water temperature, according to employer policy. Use washcloths, towel wipes, or swabs, according to employer policy. Rinse the area thoroughly. Pat dry after rinsing to reduce moisture and to promote comfort.

When washing clients who have soiled themselves, wash the buttocks area first and then the anal area. Some clients with dementia may put their hands into their briefs or put their hands in the area you are cleaning. Wash their hands first and give them something—for example, a washcloth or a towel—to hang on to while you clean the area.

Report and record the following if observed when providing perineal care:

- Odours
- Redness, swelling, discharge, or irritation
- Complaints of pain, burning, or other discomfort
- Signs of urinary or fecal incontinence (see Chapters 32 and 33)
- Presence of hemorrhoids
- A male client's foreskin not retracting

FOCUS ON CHILDREN

Perineal Care

Children of all ages need perineal care. In children who wear diapers, the perineal area is often exposed to urine and stool. Inadequate wiping after urinating and defecating is a common problem in younger children. Older children may hesitate to clean the genital and anal areas.

Giving Perineal Care to a Female Client 123

Advocate on behalf of the client's quality of life by promoting:

Dignity • Independence • Preferences • Privacy • Safety *(see BOX 1–4, on p. 17)*

PRE-PROCEDURE

1 Identify the client, according to employer policy.
2 Explain the procedure to the client.
3 Perform hand hygiene.
4 Collect the following supplies:
- ☐ **Wash basin**
- ☐ **Soap or Peri Wash**
- ☐ **At least four washcloths**
- ☐ **Bath towel**
- ☐ **Flat sheet**
- ☐ **Bath thermometer**
- ☐ **Waterproof pad**
- ☐ **Gloves**
- ☐ **Paper towels**

5 Place paper towels on an overbed table (in a facility) or on a work area within easy reach from the bedside. Arrange items on top of the paper towels.
This helps to absorb any water that may splash out of the basin.
6 Provide for privacy.
7 Raise the bed to a comfortable working height.

PROCEDURE

8 Lower the bed rail near you if it is up.
9 Cover the client with a bath blanket. Fan-fold the top linen to the foot of the bed. The top sheet can be used if no bath blanket is available.
Fan-folded linen is easier to grasp and to straighten out than rolled-up linen.
10 Position the client on her back. Remove garments from the waist down.
11 Position waterproof pad under the client's buttocks.
This keeps the bottom sheet dry.
12 Drape the client as in **FIGURE 30–26**.
13 Raise the bed rail if used.
14 Fill the wash basin. Water temperature must be 40.5°C to 42.7°C (105°F to 109°F). Measure water temperature according to employer policy.
Water that is too hot can scald the client.
15 Place the basin on the overbed table or work area.
This helps prevent worker back strain.
16 Lower the bed rail if it is up.
17 Help the client flex her knees and spread her legs. If she cannot flex her knees, help her spread her legs as much as possible with her knees straight.
This helps expose the area.
18 Put on gloves.

Continued

Giving Perineal Care to a Female Client—cont'd

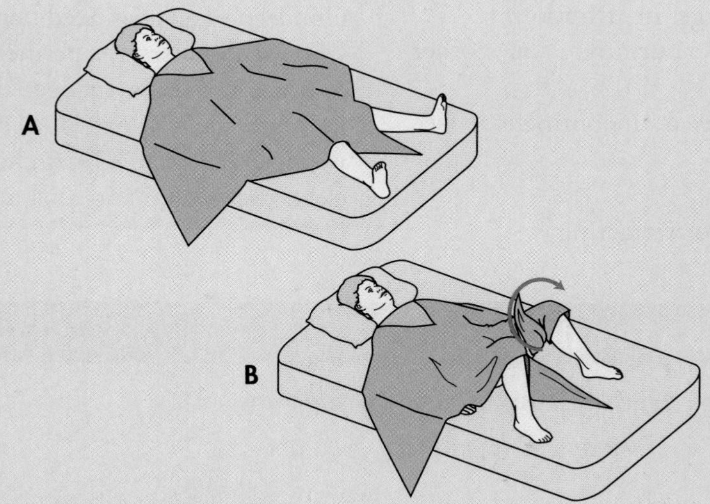

FIGURE 30–26 Draping for perineal care. **A,** Position the bath blanket in the shape of a diamond: one corner is at the neck, one corner is at each side, and one corner is between the client's legs. **B,** Wrap the corner of the blanket on either side of the client around the closest leg by bringing the corner under the leg, wrapping the corner around the leg and then tucking the corner under the hip.

19 Fold the corner of the bath blanket between the client's legs onto her abdomen.

20 Wet the washcloths. Squeeze out excess water from washcloths before using them.

21 Apply soap (if used) to a washcloth. Peri Wash is often used and does not require rinsing.

22 Separate the labia.

- **a** Wash the labia majora on the side closest to you. Repeat on the far side, using a different part of the cloth. Clean downward from top to bottom with one stroke (FIGURE 30–27).
- **b** Wash the labia minora in the same manner as above. Use a separate section of the cloth for each stroke.
- **c** Using a clean section of the cloth, wash down the middle, cleaning from the pubic area toward the rectal area in one stroke. Cleanse thoroughly around the clitoris and vaginal orifice.

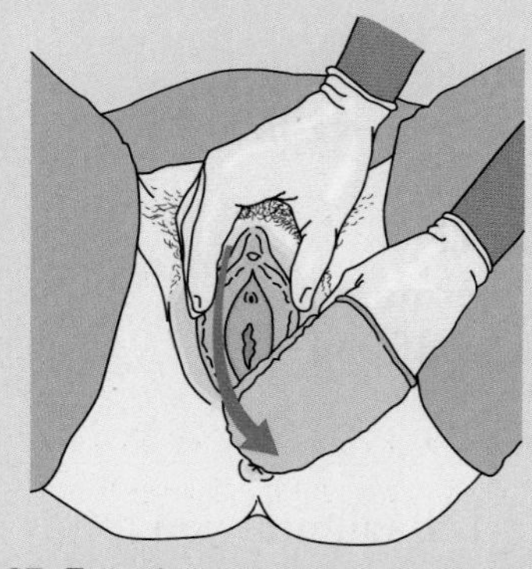

FIGURE 30–27 Female perineal care. Separate the labia with one hand. Use a mitted washcloth to cleanse between the labia with downward strokes.

23 Repeat steps 21 and 22 until the area is clean. Use a clean part of the washcloth for each stroke. Use more than one washcloth if needed.

24 Rinse the perineum with a clean washcloth. Separate the labia. Stroke in only one direction, from top to bottom. Go down the centre and then down each side. Repeat as necessary. Use a clean part of the washcloth for each stroke. Use more than one washcloth if needed. Clean from the cleanest area to the dirtiest area.
Washing in this way prevents introducing pathogens into the client's urethra or vagina.

25 Pat the area dry with the towel.
The skin in this area is delicate and easily irritated if rubbed.

Continued

Giving Perineal Care to a Female Client—cont'd

26 Fold the blanket back down between the client's legs.
This helps provide privacy.

27 Help the client lower her legs and turn onto her side away from you.

28 Apply soap to a washcloth.

29 Clean the rectal area. Separate buttocks and clean from the vagina to the anus with one stroke (**FIGURE 30–28**).
This helps prevent the transfer of pathogens from the anus to the vagina.

30 Repeat steps 28 and 29 until the area is clean. Use a clean part of the washcloth for each stroke. Use more than one washcloth if needed.

31 Rinse the rectal area with a washcloth. Stroke from the vagina to the anus. Repeat as necessary, using a clean part of the washcloth for each stroke. Use more than one washcloth if needed.
Ensuring that all of the soap is removed will help to prevent skin breakdown.

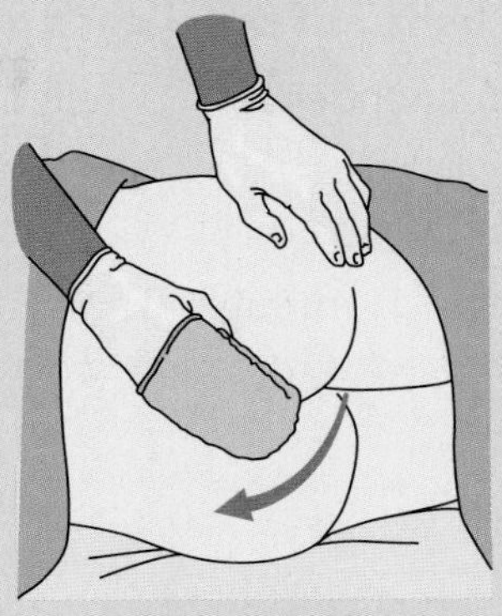

FIGURE 30–28 Cleaning the rectal area. Wipe from the vagina to the anus. The side-lying position allows thorough cleaning of the anal area.

32 Pat the area dry with the towel.

33 Remove the waterproof pad.

34 Remove gloves. Wash your hands.

POST-PROCEDURE

35 Provide for safety and comfort.

36 Cover the client.

37 Remove the bath blanket (if used).

38 Place the call bell within reach.*
This provides an easy, safe way for the client to contact the staff if necessary.

39 Return the bed to its lowest position. Follow the care plan for bed rail use.*

40 Empty and clean the wash basin.

41 Return the basin and supplies to their proper places.
This makes them easier to find the next time they are needed.

42 Wipe off the overbed table or work area with paper towels, and discard the paper towels.

43 Remove privacy measures.

44 Follow employer policy for handling dirty linen.

45 Perform hand hygiene.

Report and Record your actions and observations, according to employer policy.
This is done for legal reasons and to keep the rest of the health care team informed.

*Steps marked with an asterisk may not apply in community settings.

Giving Perineal Care to a Male Client

123

Advocate on behalf of the client's quality of life by promoting:

Dignity • Independence • Preferences • Privacy • Safety *(see BOX 1–4, on p. 17)*

PRE-PROCEDURE

1 Follow steps 1 through 21 in the procedure *Giving Perineal Care to a Female Client* on page 643.

PROCEDURE

2 Retract the foreskin if the client is uncircumcised and if the foreskin can be retracted (**FIGURE 30–29**).
Microbes and discharge can build up under the foreskin.
3 Grasp the penis.
4 Clean the tip using a circular motion. Start at the urethral opening, and work outward. Work from cleanest area to dirtiest area. The urethral opening is the cleanest (**FIGURE 30–30**). Repeat this step as necessary. Use a clean part of the washcloth each time.
5 Rinse the area with another washcloth.
Soap that remains on the skin can be drying and irritating.
6 Return the foreskin to its natural position.
7 Clean the shaft of the penis with firm downward strokes. Rinse the area.
8 Help the client flex his knees and spread his legs. If he cannot flex his knees, help him spread his legs as much as possible with his knees straight.
9 Clean the scrotum and rinse well. Observe for redness and irritation in the skin folds.
10 Pat dry the penis and scrotum.
Rubbing vigorously can be irritating to the delicate tissues and may cause the client to have an erection, which may embarrass him.
11 Fold the bath blanket back down between his legs.
12 Help him lower his legs and turn onto his side away from you.
13 Clean the rectal area (see steps 28 to 32 in the procedure *Giving Perineal Care to a Female Client*). Rinse and dry well.
14 Remove the waterproof pad.
15 Remove and discard the gloves. Perform hand hygiene.

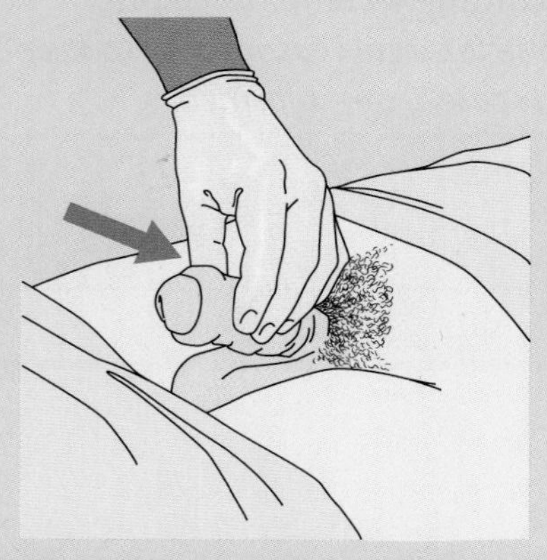

FIGURE 30–29 Male perineal care. Pull back the foreskin of the uncircumcised male. Return the foreskin to its normal position immediately after cleaning.

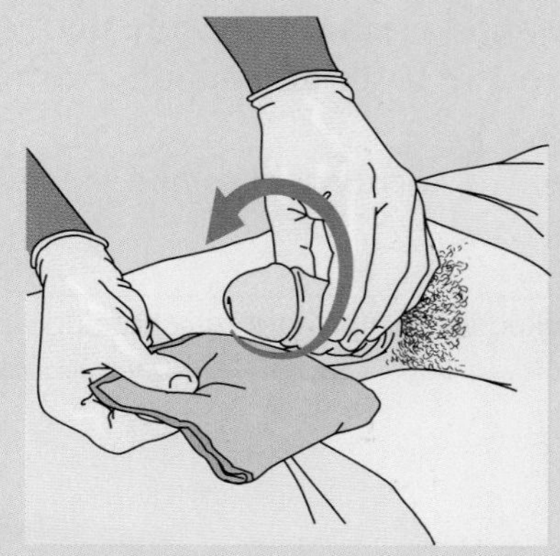

FIGURE 30–30 Clean the penis with circular motions starting at the urethra.

Continued

Giving Perineal Care to a Male Client—cont'd

POST-PROCEDURE

16 Follow steps 35 through 45 in the procedure *Giving Perineal Care to a Female Client.*

Report and Record your actions and observations, according to employer policy.
This is done for legal reasons and to keep the rest of the health care team informed.

MENSTRUAL CARE

Menstruation is a woman's monthly bleeding, when blood flows from the uterus through the vaginal opening (see Chapter 18). Sanitary pads absorb menstrual blood. Most menstrual periods last 3 to 5 days. Some clients need assistance with menstrual care, as they may be too ill or weak to change their sanitary pads.

Usually, women use disposable sanitary pads, which have adhesive strips that hold them in place in the woman's panties. Sanitary pads containing perfumes can irritate the skin and should be avoided. In some hospitals, female clients may use disposable sanitary pads that are held in place with reusable mesh panties.

Sanitary pads should be changed often. This promotes good hygiene and comfort and prevents odours and infection. Follow the care plan in regard to when to change the woman's sanitary pad. Frequency depends on the amount of menstrual flow. Usually, the pads need to be changed at least every 3 to 5 hours. However, they should be changed before they become soaked with blood.

Contact with the client's blood and mucous membranes is likely, so always wear gloves when removing or applying sanitary pads. Wash your hands, and help the client wash her hands after menstrual care. Dispose of sanitary pads according to employer policy. Also, follow employer policy for disposing of soiled mesh panties.

Record and report the following if observed while providing menstrual care:

- Odours
- Fever
- Redness, swelling, or irritation in the perineum
- Complaints of pain, burning, difficulty urinating, or other discomforts
- Heavy bleeding—for example, the sanitary pad becomes soaked within one hour of application (report this at once)
- Large number of blood clots on the pad (report this at once)

CHAPTER REVIEW

KEY POINTS

- Personal hygiene involves activities to clean the skin, teeth, mouth, genital area, and anus.
- Clients may feel embarrassed that they need help with these personal activities. Always ensure privacy and promote their dignity.
- Oral hygiene keeps the mouth and teeth clean; prevents mouth odours, infections, and cavities; increases comfort; and makes food taste better. Dental health is important as it can have an impact on general health.
- Bathing helps keep skin as well as the genital and anal areas clean by removing microbes, dead skin, perspiration, and excess oils. A bath is refreshing and relaxing, stimulates circulation, and exercises body parts. During the bath, you are able to make important observations about the client and note any changes.
- You will provide partial baths, complete bed baths, showers, and tub baths (involving different types of tubs), depending on your clients' needs and the equipment available to you.
- When providing perineal care to both females and males, always work from the cleanest area to the dirtiest area.

CRITICAL THINKING IN PRACTICE

You are a student in the clinical setting. You are helping a support worker position and turn a resident during perineal care. The support worker does not wear gloves, does not use a clean part of the washcloth for each stroke, and wipes from the back (bottom) to the front (top). What has the support worker done wrong? How can you correct the situation?

REVIEW QUESTIONS

Answers to these questions are at the bottom of the next page.

Circle T if the answer is true, and circle F if the answer is false.

1. T F Hygiene is needed for comfort, safety, and health.
2. T F Culture and personal choice affect hygiene practices.
3. T F Mrs. Lam's toothbrush has hard bristles. They are good for oral hygiene.
4. T F Unconscious clients are kept in the supine position for mouth care.
5. T F You use your fingers to keep an unconscious client's mouth open for oral hygiene.
6. T F Mr. Burnham has a lower denture. It is placed on a hard surface and washed in warm water.
7. T F Bath oils cleanse and soften the skin.
8. T F Powders absorb moisture and prevent friction.
9. T F Deodorants reduce the amount of perspiration.
10. T F The care plan says that Ms. Persaude can have a tub bath. You can allow her to take a 30-minute bath.
11. T F Weak clients can be left alone in the shower if they are sitting.
12. T F A back massage relaxes muscles and stimulates circulation.
13. T F Perineal care helps prevent infection.
14. T F The foreskin is returned to its normal position after cleaning.
15. T F Sanitary pads should be changed at least every 3 to 5 hours.

Circle the BEST answer.

16. When providing mouth care to an unconscious client, the client should be positioned:
A. On the back
B. On the side
C. Sitting up
D. On the stomach

17. What is the purpose of bathing?
A. Increasing circulation
B. Preventing odours and cleansing skin
C. Refreshing and relaxing the person
D. All of the above

18. Soaps do the following:
A. Remove dirt and dead skin
B. Remove pigment
C. Remove hair
D. Moisten the skin

19. Which action is correct when bathing Mrs. Smith?
A. Removing all of the covers
B. Rinsing her skin thoroughly to remove all of the soap
C. Washing from the dirtiest area to the cleanest area
D. Rubbing the skin dry

20. Water for Mr. Arnold's complete bed bath should be approximately:
A. 37.8°C (100°F)
B. 40.5°C (105°F)
C. 43.4°C (110°F)
D. 48.9°C (120°F)

21. You are going to give Mrs. Li a back massage. How long should it last?
A. 3 to 5 minutes
B. 1 to 2 minutes
C. 10 minutes
D. 6 to 7 minutes

Answers: 1.T, 2.T, 3.F, 4.F, 5.F, 6.F, 7.F, 8.T, 9.F, 10.F, 11.F, 12.T, 13.T, 14.T, 15.T, 16.B, 17.D, 18.A, 19.B, 20.C, 21.A

Chapter opener image: Courtesy ArjoHuntleigh Inc.

CHAPTER 31

Grooming and Dressing

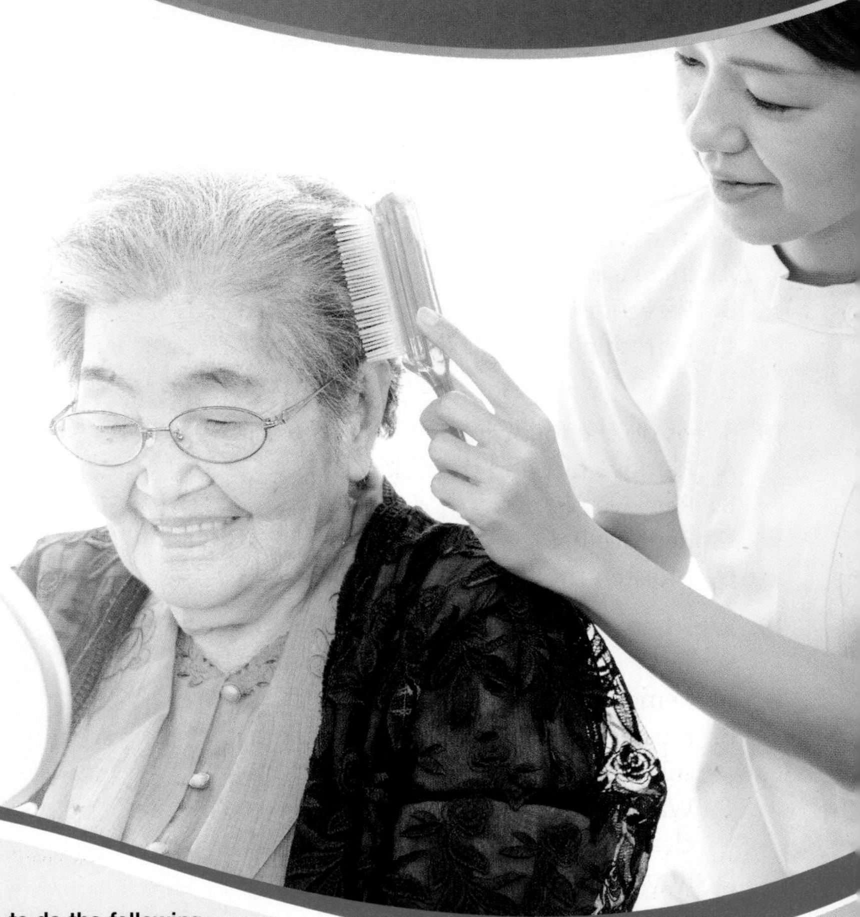

OBJECTIVES

After reading this chapter, the learner should be able to do the following:

- Explain the importance of hair care and shaving.
- Identify the factors that affect hair care.
- Explain how to care for matted and tangled hair.
- Describe how to shampoo hair.
- List the steps taken to shave a client.
- Explain why nail care and foot care are important.
- Describe how to dress and undress clients.
- Describe how to change an incontinence brief.
- Explain the purpose of elastic anti-embolic stockings and bandages and when to assist with them.
- Apply the procedures described in this chapter to clinical practice by providing culturally sensitive grooming.

KEY TERMS

alopecia Hair loss. *p. 651*

anti-embolic stockings Close-fitting, circular knitted, elastic stocking that are designed to prevent swelling in lower extremities or blood clots by increasing venous return to the heart. They are also called *compression stockings*, or *thromboembolic devices (TED)*. *p. 680*

dandruff Excessive amount of dry, white flakes that appear on the scalp, in the hair, or on the shoulders. *p. 652*

hirsutism Excessive and increased hair growth. *p. 652*

ingrown hair A hair that curls into the side wall of the hair follicle or into the skin surface, which causes the skin to become inflamed. Also known as **razor bumps**. *p. 661*

ingrown nails Toenails that grow inward at the side of the nail bed. *p. 664*

lice Small, insectlike parasites that live on the human body, most commonly on skin, hair, and the genital area. *p. 652*

parasite An organism that lives on or in another organism and derives its nutrients from it. *p. 652*

pediculosis Infestation with **lice**. *p. 652*

pediculosis capitis Infestation of the scalp (*capitis*) with lice. *p. 652*

pediculosis corporis Infestation of the body (*corporis*) with lice. *p. 652*

pediculosis pubis Infestation of the pubic (*pubis*) hair with lice. *p. 652*

podiatrist A physician who specializes in the evaluation and treatment of diseases of the foot. *p. 665*

razor bumps See **ingrown hair**. *p. 661*

Personal grooming—which involves having clean hair, nails, and clothes—is important not only to health care workers but to all people, whatever their nationality or culture. Good grooming not only helps promote emotional well-being and self-confidence but also helps prevent infection and increase comfort.

Clients' degree of attention in regard to their own grooming varies. Some are satisfied if their hair is just clean, whereas some others are very particular about the way it is washed and styled. Some clients may be content to have their hands just cleaned, but some others may want their nails to be cleaned, manicured, and polished as well. In regard to body hair, shaving and beard grooming are important to most men, and most women like to shave their legs and underarms. As well, most women who have facial hair would prefer to have this unwanted hair removed.

When you provide grooming care, keep in mind that it should be done in a considerate manner, respecting the client's dignity and right to privacy. Most workers understand that certain acts of grooming (such as shaving legs or underarms) need to be done in private for women, but they neglect to provide the same privacy when shaving a man's face!

HAIR CARE

How the hair looks and feels can affect a person's emotional well-being. People generally feel better about themselves when they are well groomed. Unfortunately, illness and disability can interfere with hair care, especially when clients are too ill to care for their hair themselves. It is the support worker's responsibility to assist with hair care (or any grooming for that matter) whenever needed, as stated on the client's care plan.

The care plan should address the individual client's hair care needs. Culture, personal choice, skin and scalp condition, physical and mental health, and self-care abilities should always be taken into consideration for providing hair care, and related information should be indicated on the client's care plan. Some common terms related to hair that may be used in care plans include the following:

- **Alopecia**—hair loss, which may be complete or partial. Male pattern baldness occurs due to aging or heredity. In women, hair thins with aging. Cancer treatments (radiation therapy to the head and chemotherapy) often cause alopecia in both men and women. Other causes include skin disease, stress, poor nutrition, pregnancy, some medications, and hormone changes. In many cases (but not all), the hair grows back once these issues have been resolved.

- **Hirsutism** (from Latin *hirsutus,* meaning "shaggy, hairy")—excessive and increased hair growth in women in locations where the occurrence of visible, coarse hair is normally minimal or absent (such as on the face or neck). It refers to a male pattern of body hair and is, therefore, usually a cosmetic and psychological concern. However, hirsutism may be a sign of a more serious medical problem, especially if it develops well after puberty.
- **Dandruff**—excessive amount of dry, white flakes on the scalp, in the hair, or on the shoulders. It often causes itching of the scalp and sometimes affects the eyebrows and ear canals as well. Medicated shampoos usually can solve the problem.
- **Pediculosis**—infestation with **lice**, which are small, insectlike parasites that live on the human body, most commonly on skin, hair, and the genital area. Lice (singular, *louse*) feed on human blood and lay their eggs on body hair and in clothing (**FIGURE 31–1**).

Lice do not cause dangerous infections but may carry pathogens that cause more serious diseases such as trench fever and typhus. Lice tend to be a problem primarily found in overcrowded areas or places that have inadequate bathing and laundry facilities, such as among the homeless or in military or refugee camps. All humans are equally at risk for infestation by lice, but older people are more prone to develop complications from it.

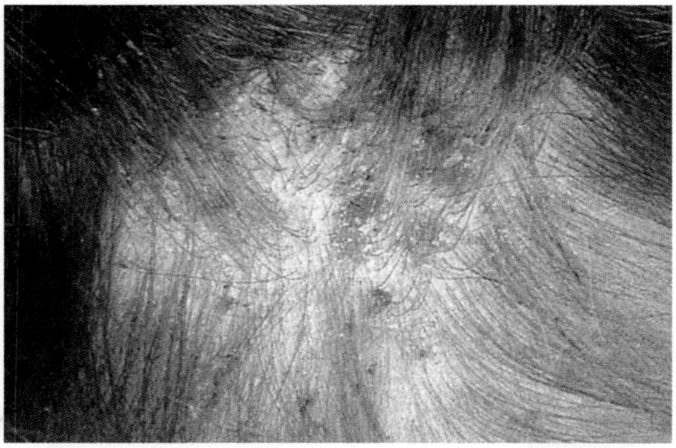

FIGURE 31–1 Pediculosis capitis. Note how the nits (eggs) attach themselves to the hair shafts. This client has been scratching the scalp, resulting in the reddened scalp areas evident in the photo. (**Source:** Habif, T.P. (1996). *Clinical dermatology: A guide to diagnosis and therapy* (3rd ed.). St. Louis, MO: Mosby.)

Lice are **parasites**, organisms that derive their nutrients from host organisms. Their bites cause severe itching in the affected body area. **Pediculosis capitis** is the infestation of the scalp (*capitis*) with lice, and **pediculosis pubis** is the infestation of the pubic (*pubis*) hair with lice. Both head lice and pubic lice attach their eggs to hair shafts. **Pediculosis corporis** is the infestation of the body (*corporis*) surfaces with lice.

Lice eggs (nits) attach to clothing and furniture and can easily spread to other people through clothing, furniture, bed linen, and physical contact, as well as by sharing of combs and brushes. They can be difficult to remove, but all lice and their eggs must be destroyed with due diligence.

Lice can be eradicated by using medicated shampoos, lotions, and creams (following manufacturers' directions carefully). Several applications of these products as well as manual removal of the nits are usually necessary. In addition, clients (and anyone they have shared items with) will need a thorough tub bath and must have their clothing and linens washed in hot water. Items that cannot be washed should be thoroughly vacuumed and placed in a sealed, airtight bag and stored for several weeks until the lice are destroyed. Report any signs of lice to your supervisor immediately, and follow your employer's policies.

Brushing and Combing Hair

Brushing and combing hair are part of the client's daily routine and is usually done in the morning (after the bath or shower) and at bedtime. However, assist with brushing and combing, as needed, during the day—for example, some clients may want their hair styled before visitors arrive.

Encourage clients to do their own hair care, and assist as needed. It is your responsibility to perform hair care for clients who cannot do it by themselves. Clients should be allowed to decide how to brush, comb, and style their hair (see the *Focus on Children: Grooming Preferences* box).

You should never cut a client's hair; only a professional barber or hairstylist should cut hair. Some facilities have barber shops or hair salons, where clients can have their hair shampooed, cut, and styled. Some hairstylists make visits to homes or long-term care (complex-care) facilities to provide their services.

Remember that people who have had chemical treatments (permanents ["perms"] or straightening) may have dry, somewhat brittle hair that is more prone to tangling, so it should be treated differently from unprocessed hair. Chemically treated hair should be brushed gently toward the hair ends, starting at the ends and working up toward the roots with each brush stroke. Chemically treated hair may get flattened during sleep, so it may need to be recombed or "fluffed up" after the client wakes up.

How to Brush or Comb Hair

Before giving hair care, you should place a towel over the client's shoulders to protect the client's clothing.

For a client who is unable to get out of bed, give hair care *before* changing the pillowcase. If it has to be done after a linen change, place a towel over the pillow or over the shoulders (if the client is in the sitting position) to collect falling hair, as hair on the client's clothing or pillowcase is unsightly and, in some situations, poses the risk of being inhaled or swallowed.

When brushing or combing hair, start at the scalp, and brush or comb to the hair ends (**FIGURES 31–2 AND 31–3**). Handle hair gently to avoid hurting the client or damaging the hair. Always brush slowly, never pulling or tugging at the client's hair. If you find that the client has matted or tangled hair, discuss with your supervisor what can be done. If you are directed to comb or brush through the matting and tangling, take a small section of hair near the ends, and gently comb or brush through to the ends. Work up to the scalp, brushing or combing in small sections, and eventually you will be able to brush or comb from the scalp to the hair ends. ***Never cut hair to remove tangles.***

Some Examples of Cultural Differences With Respect to Hair

The hair of Black people is extremely fragile, so you should be very gentle and careful to avoid unnecessary breakage and hair loss. Always use a wide-tooth comb or pick when combing the hair, and avoid fine-tooth combs because they tend to snag and pull out curly or kinky hair. If possible, use a good-quality, natural boar brush. Curly or kinky hair needs a lot of moisture, so you need to avoid drying products such as hairspray, mousse, or holding gels.[1]

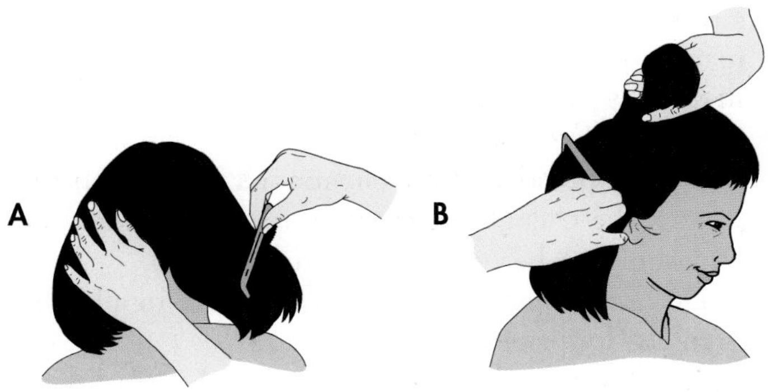

FIGURE 31–2 Parting hair. **A,** Part hair down the middle. Divide it into two sections. **B,** Then part each section into two smaller sections.

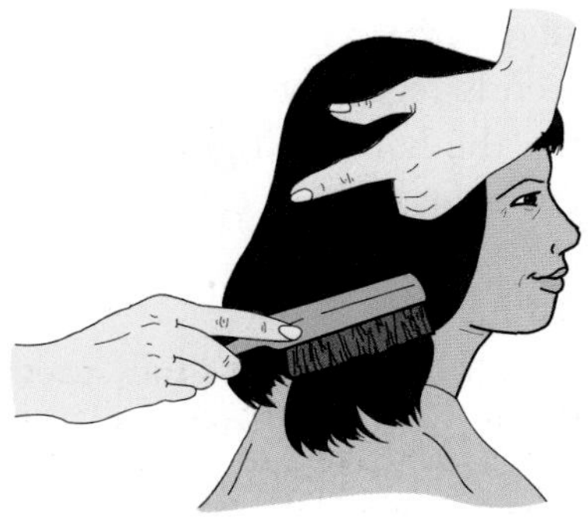

FIGURE 31–3 Brush hair by starting at the scalp. Brush down to the hair ends.

FOCUS ON CHILDREN

Grooming Preferences

Hairstyles are important to adolescents as well as other school-aged children. Do not make judgements about any child's hairstyle. Style hair in a manner that pleases both the child and the parents. Take care not to impose your hairstyle preferences on your client.

Black textured hair tends to produce less *sebum* (oily secretion created by the sebaceous gland) compared with the hair of White people. To add oil to dry hair, use products that contain moisturizers, such as leave-in conditioners and styling lotions.[1] Note that products that claim to be created for "curly hair" are not necessarily suitable for Black curly hair.

To groom any curly, coarse, and dry hair, use a wide-tooth comb, start at the neckline, comb the hair, and work higher, lifting and fluffing hair outward. Continue until you reach the forehead. Wetting the hair or applying a conditioner or petroleum jelly may make combing easier.[1]

The client may have certain practices or use special hair care products, and these should become part of the client's care plan. The client can guide you about these when you are giving hair care (see the *Respecting Diversity: Corn Braids* and *Respecting Diversity: Dreadlocks* boxes).

Women who wear hijabs need to take special care of their hair to keep it strong and healthy since the hair and scalp may not be regularly exposed to fresh air and vitamin D, absorbed through sunlight. To maintain hair health while respecting the client's need for privacy and dignity, here are a few tips:[2]

- Provide privacy for the client at all times. Consult with the client or her family to find out how to ensure that her preferences are respected.
- Do not tie hair up while it is wet. Try to allow it to air-dry prior to pulling it back.
- Try to get sunlight on the hair and scalp for at least a half hour each week.
- When possible, remove the hijab, underscarf, and hair tie, and run fingers through the hair and scalp to encourage circulation.
- Wash underscarves regularly.
- Trim hair ends regularly to get rid of split ends.
- Avoid tying the hair too tightly to prevent straining the hair roots, which can lead to hair loss.

Respecting Diversity

Corn Braids

Styling hair in corn braids is a common practice among some cultural groups. The braids are left intact even while shampooing. Remember that you should never do or undo braids without the client's consent, and consent may also be required by your supervisor. Some agencies have permission forms that the client has to sign, so know your agency's policy.

Caring for corn braids differs from caring for hair that is braided into a single large braid. If the client has a single braid, the braid should be undone each night, as the braid would cause discomfort if the client were to lie on it.

Respecting Diversity

Dreadlocks

Dreadlocks are coils of hair that are twisted, rubbed, or backcombed together in a specific way. They should not be combed out. Dreadlocks should be washed with a residue-free product; washing frequency depends on the client. If the client perspires considerably, frequent washing will reduce the salt buildup that sweat can produce on the client's scalp. For clients who do not perspire a lot, hair should be washed about once a week. The client's care plan will clarify the specifics of hair care.

Gently massaging the client's scalp for a few minutes each day will help to release natural oils from the sebaceous glands in the client's scalp. The client's care plan will specify the frequency and kind of care that is required.

Source: *Basic dreadlock care.* (2013). Retrieved from http://www.dreadhairstyles.com/D-Basic%20Dread%20Care.htm.

Who Can Cut a Client's Hair?

You should never cut a client's hair unless you have been specifically instructed to do so. In many long-term care facilities, the client (or the substitute decision maker) is required to sign a consent form giving permission for a haircut. Some facilities provide the option of an onsite salon where clients may pay to have their hair cut, washed, and groomed.

If you *must* cut a client's hair (e.g., to remove a section that is matted), ensure that proper consent has been obtained and details have been specified in the client's care plan. ***Only if absolutely necessary and when specified by your supervisor***, these steps should then be followed:

- Do not attempt to cut a client's hair if the client is agitated or noncooperative.
- Cut the smallest amount of hair possible to get rid of the matted hair.
- Make every attempt to ensure that the client's hair appears attractive. For instance, the haircut should not be lopsided and uneven, drawing attention to the client's hair.
- Use the correct type of hair shears (scissors). Never cut hair with scissors meant for other purposes, as they can tear the hair, causing discomfort to the client.

Observations to Make

Report and record the following if observed when brushing or combing:

- Scalp sores
- Flaking
- The presence of lice (check for tiny, white, oval-shaped specks in the hair; these are the nits, or egg cases)
- Patches of hair loss
- Very dry or very oily hair

Shampooing

The frequency of shampooing—once a week, two or three times a week, or every day—varies among clients, depending on such factors as the condition of the hair and scalp, hairstyle, and personal choice. Shampoo and hair conditioner products also involve personal choice (see the *Focus on Children: Shampooing* box).

Many clients need help with shampooing. If you are asked to assist a client, you should always keep in mind the client's personal preferences and need for privacy and safety. Whenever a client requests a shampoo, be sure to check the care plan for instructions regarding special care that is needed for that client's hair.

The shampooing method depends on the client's condition, safety factors, and personal choice (if permitted). Follow the care plan. Dry and style hair as quickly as possible after shampooing. If female clients want their hair curled or placed in hair rollers (rolling up) before it is dried, consult with your supervisor before doing it, as the client's family may prefer to use a hairdresser (see the *Focus on Long-Term Care: Shampooing* box).

Guidelines for shampooing are listed in **BOX 31–1**. Report and record the following observations after shampooing:

- Scalp sores
- Hair falling out in clumps
- How the client tolerated the procedure
- Any presence of lice

Shampooing During the Shower or Tub Bath

Clients who shower or bathe in a tub can usually be shampooed using a handheld shower nozzle. The client should tip the head back to keep shampoo and water out of the eyes. Support the back of the client's head with one hand, and shampoo with your other hand. Those who are not able to tip their head back should be assisted to lean forward and hold a folded washcloth over the eyes. Support the forehead with one hand as you shampoo with the other. Be sure that the client can breathe easily.

FOCUS ON CHILDREN

Shampooing

Oil gland secretion increases during puberty, so adolescents tend to have oily hair. Frequent shampooing is, therefore, necessary for them.

FOCUS ON LONG-TERM CARE

Shampooing

Shampooing is usually done once or twice weekly on a client's bath or shower day. If a female client has had her hair done in the hair salon, do not shampoo her hair. Protect her hair with a shower cap during the tub bath or shower.

BOX 31–1 Guidelines for Shampooing a Client's Hair

- Shampoo hair only if you are instructed to do it by your supervisor.
- Ask your supervisor, and check the care plan about what method to use (shampooing during the shower or tub bath, at the sink, or in bed).
- Check whether the client has position restrictions or limits. Remove hearing aids to prevent them from becoming wet and damaged.
- Return medicated shampoos to their proper storage place, or give them to your supervisor. Do not leave them at the client's bedside unless instructed to do so.
- Wear gloves and follow Standard Practices if the client has scalp lesions or head lice or if you have to use certain medicated shampoos. The client's care plan will specify if gloves are required.
- Check what water temperature to use. Usually, water temperature should be 40.5°C (105°F). Measure the water temperature, according to employer policy. ***Retest the water temperature frequently; in some facilities, it can cool down quickly.***
- Prevent shampoo from getting into the client's eyes by having the client hold a face towel or washcloth over the eyes.
- Cup your hand against the client's forehead when rinsing the hair to keep soapy water from running down the client's forehead and into the eyes.

Shampooing a Client's Hair at the Sink

Clients who can sit up may have their hair washed at a sink. However, they must be able to tilt the head forward or backward. Many older adults or people with disabilities have limited range of motion in their necks and upper backs, so you may not be able to use this method with them. It is your responsibility to follow the client's care plan.

For shampooing at a sink, the client can sit facing away from the sink or facing the sink. If the client uses a wheelchair, make sure the wheels are securely locked.

Facing the Sink

If the client chooses to sit facing the sink and the sink is low enough, follow these steps:

1. Have the client lean forward over the sink.
2. Place a towel over the shoulders.
3. Give the client a folded washcloth to hold over the eyes.
4. Wet and rinse the hair using a water pitcher or handheld nozzle.

Leaning Back

If the client prefers to lean back over the sink, follow these steps:

1. Place the chair or wheelchair so it faces away from the sink.
2. Place a folded towel over the sink edge to protect the neck (**FIGURE 31–4**).
3. Help the client tilt the head back over the edge of the sink.
4. Give the client a folded washcloth to hold over the eyes (**FIGURE 31–5**).
5. Wet and rinse the hair using a water pitcher or handheld nozzle.

Lying Down

If the client has to lie on a stretcher while the hair is shampooed at the sink, follow these steps:

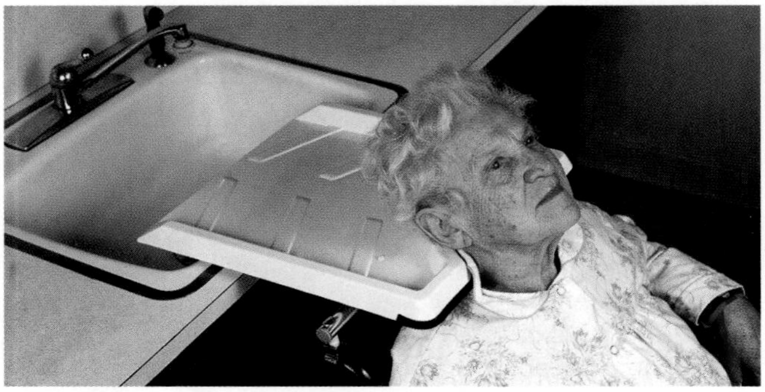

FIGURE 31–4 Shampooing at the sink. The wheelchair is in front of the sink, with its wheels locked in place. A wheelchair shampoo rinse tray may be useful. Note how the client's physical limitations were taken into account. Her head is resting on a rolled washcloth, allowing it not to be over-extended backward. (Courtesy of DeRoyal Industries Inc.)

1. Place the stretcher in front of the sink; lock the stretcher wheels, and apply the safety straps. Follow the care plan for side rail use.
2. Place a folded towel over the edge of the sink.
3. Help the client tilt the head over the edge of the sink.
4. Place a folded washcloth over the client's eyes (see **FIGURE 31–5A**).
5. Wet and rinse the hair using a water pitcher or handheld nozzle.

Assistive Devices

Assistive devices may make shampooing a client's hair easier. For example, you could use a plastic cape to drape over the client's shoulders and into the sink, or you may use a wheelchair shampoo rinse tray, which is made of plastic and clamps onto the back of the wheelchair, extending over the sink. The client's head rests directly on it. The water runs down the tray and into the sink (see **FIGURE 31–5**), and the tray's edges keep the water from spilling over the sides onto the floor.

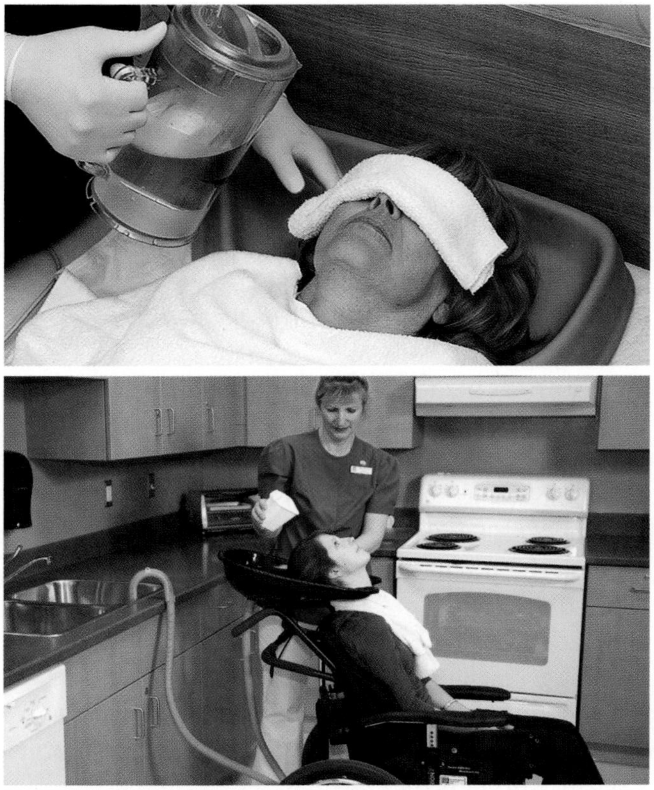

A

B

FIGURE 31–5 **A,** A shampoo tray is used when shampooing a client in bed. Keep the bedding dry by placing a waterproof pad or sheet of plastic covered with a towel underneath the client. The tray is directed to the side of the bed so that water drains into a collecting basin or bucket. The washcloth prevents water from splashing accidentally into the client's eyes; however, because the client cannot see what you are doing, you need to keep her informed of your actions at all times. **B,** A wash basin for use in the home. Note the drain that is designed to empty rinse water into the sink or a bucket on the floor. (**Source** (for *B*)**:** Brian Hillier.)

Shampooing in Bed

Clients who cannot tolerate sitting long enough to have their hair washed at the sink may have their hair shampooed while in bed. To begin, the client should be moved as close to the edge of the bed as possible to ensure that the client remains in proper body alignment and to help reduce the amount of stretching that you have to do. Place a folded cloth over the client's eyes when shampooing. Ask the client to assist in maintaining comfortable placement of the cloth since it may move during this procedure. Place a shampoo tray under the client's head to protect the linen and mattress from getting wet. The tray also drains the water into a basin placed on a chair next to the bed (see **FIGURE 31–5**). Use a water pitcher to wet and rinse the hair (see the *Focus on Home Care: Shampoo Trays* box).

FOCUS ON HOME CARE

Shampoo Trays

You can make a shampoo tray from a plastic shower curtain, a tablecloth, or even a plastic drop cloth used for painting. However, try to avoid using plastic garbage bags, as they slip and slide too easily and are not sturdy. To make a shampoo tray, first place the plastic under the client's head. To prevent water from spilling over the sides, make a raised edge by rolling up the plastic sheet around the edges. Place the ends of the plastic into the basin to direct the water into the basin. Check the care plan, and consult with your supervisor to confirm this option is best before starting the procedure.

Shampooing a Client's Hair in Bed

123

Advocate on behalf of the client's quality of life by promoting:

Dignity • Independence • Preferences • Privacy • Safety *(see BOX 1–4, on p. 17)*

PRE-PROCEDURE

1 Identify the client, according to employer policy.
This eliminates the possibility of mistaking one client for another.

2 Explain the procedure to the client.

3 Practise proper hand hygiene.

4 Collect the following supplies:
- ☐ **Two bath towels**
- ☐ **Face towel or washcloth**
- ☐ **Shampoo**
- ☐ **Hair conditioner (if requested by client)**
- ☐ **Bath thermometer**
- ☐ **Pitcher or nozzle (if needed)**
- ☐ **Shampoo tray (if needed)**
- ☐ **Basin or pail (if needed)**
- ☐ **Waterproof pad (if needed)**
- ☐ **Gloves (if needed)**
- ☐ **Comb and brush**
- ☐ **Hair dryer**

By collecting all the necessary equipment beforehand, you will not have to leave your client's side and can eliminate wasting time and energy in obtaining the forgotten equipment.

5 Arrange the items close at hand.
Planning ahead eliminates unnecessary steps and is less tiring for the client.

6 Provide for privacy. Practise proper hand hygiene.

PROCEDURE

7 Position the client as close to the edge of the bed as possible for the method you will use. Place the waterproof pad and shampoo tray under the head and shoulders, if needed.
Positioning the client close to you reduces your risk for back strain while washing hair.

8 Place a bath towel over the shoulders or over the pillow.
This protects the client's bedding and clothing.

9 Brush or comb hair to remove snarls and tangles.
It is easier to detangle dry hair than wet hair.

10 Raise the bed rail if used.
This decreases the risk of the client accidentally falling out of bed.

11 Obtain water. Water temperature should be about 40.5°C (105°F). Test temperature using a bath thermometer, according to your employer's policy. Allow the client to test the water temperature with the hand.
This ensures the client is comfortable with the water temperature and helps you avoid burning the client.

12 Lower the bed rail if used.

13 Put on gloves if needed.
Gloves are needed if the client has scalp problems of any kind.

14 Ask the client to hold a dampened face towel or washcloth over the eyes, making sure that it does not cover the nose or mouth.
A moistened cloth will not slip off as easily as a dry cloth would.

15 Use the pitcher or nozzle to wet the hair.
Shampoo will spread better and more evenly on wet hair.

16 Use a small amount of shampoo.
Too much shampoo is wasteful and difficult to rinse out of the hair. If left on the scalp, it can cause dryness and flakiness.

17 Work up a lather with both hands. Start at the hairline. Work toward the back of the head. If the client is leaning forward, start at the back of the head and work toward the hairline.
The hairline is usually the most oily or soiled area and should be lathered the longest.

Continued

Shampooing a Client's Hair in Bed—cont'd

18 Massage the scalp with your fingertip pads.
Massaging the scalp is relaxing for the client. Using fingertip pads will reduce the chances of scratching the scalp with your fingernails.

19 Rinse the hair.
Rinsing removes oil- and dirt-saturated shampoo.

20 Repeat steps 15 through 18.

21 Rinse the hair completely.
This ensures that no trace of shampoo is left in the hair or on the scalp.

22 Apply conditioner following the directions on the container.
Conditioners make the hair easier to comb.

23 Squeeze water from the client's hair.
This decreases drying time.

24 Cover the hair with a bath towel.
This helps remove excess water and keeps the client warm.

25 Dry the client's face with the towel.

26 Help the client raise the head if appropriate.
Many clients have weakened neck muscles. Assisting them will make the movement more comfortable for the clients and may decrease the risk for neck injury.

27 Rub the hair and scalp with the towel. Use the second towel if the first becomes wet.
This helps remove excess water and keeps the client warm.

28 Comb or brush hair to remove snarls and tangles.

29 Dry and style the hair as quickly as possible.
This helps prevent the hair from drying unstyled.

30 Remove gloves if used. Practise proper hand hygiene.

POST-PROCEDURE

31 Provide for safety and comfort.

32 Place the call bell within reach.*
This provides an easy, safe way for the client to contact staff if necessary.

33 Follow the care plan for bed rail use.*
This reduces the risk for client injury.

34 Remove privacy measures.

35 Clean and return equipment to its proper place.
This makes it easier to find for future use.

36 Discard disposable items.
Discarding used items decreases the risk for pathogen spread.

37 Follow employer policy for handling dirty linen.
Proper linen disposal will decrease the risk for pathogen spread.

38 Practise proper hand hygiene.

Report and Record your actions and observations, according to employer policy.
This is done for legal reasons and to keep the rest of the health care team informed.

*Steps marked with an asterisk may not apply in community settings.

SHAVING

Men shave for comfort and a sense of well-being. Women usually shave their legs and underarms, and some older women have coarse facial hair that they would like removed. You may be asked to remove unwanted hair in female clients by shaving, depilation (hair removal by tweezing or through chemical hair removers), or waxing. You must be aware of what your client's care plan has specified, and consult with your supervisor if you have any questions about the technique you should use.

Depending on their conditions, clients may prefer to shave themselves or may require your assistance. Shaving may be done at the sink, at the bedside, or in bed. You may need to use electric or manual shavers, depending on the client's condition, preference, and what is specified in the care plan (see the *Think About Safety: Guidelines for Shaving Clients* box).

Think About Safety

Guidelines for Shaving Clients

- While shaving a client, always follow Standard Practices, such as practising proper hand hygiene and wearing gloves.
- Because of the risk of transmitting pathogens (see Chapter 23) from one client to another, the same razors or shavers should not be used between clients. All clients should have their own razors and shavers.
- Follow the care plan for the type of shaver used for each client.
- Protect bed linens by placing a towel under the part that is being shaved. If you are shaving the client's face, place a towel over the client's shoulders to protect the clothing.
- Soften the client's facial hair before shaving by applying a warm, moist cloth onto the skin. If using a manual razor, use shaving cream (after applying the warm, moist cloth) to soften the skin and hair, making it easier to shave.
- Encourage the client to do as much as is safely possible.
- Stretch the skin taut, as needed.
- Shave in the direction of hair growth when shaving the face and underarms.
- When shaving the leg, shave up from the ankles, against the direction of hair growth.
- Rinse the shaved area completely.
- Shaving can potentially cut, nick, or irritate the skin. Ensure that you shave carefully and only after properly preparing the client's skin and hair.
- Follow Standard Practices to prevent contact with blood. Handle razor blades and disposable shavers extremely carefully to protect yourself from cuts; discard them in the sharps container (see Chapter 22).
- Apply direct pressure to nicks or cuts on the client (wear gloves).
- Report nicks, cuts, or skin irritation to your supervisor at once.
- Discard disposable razors and blades in the sharps container. Handle them carefully.
- Follow employer policy for disposing of sharps.
- If using an electric razor, make sure the shaver is in good working order before each use. Follow the safety rules for electrical equipment (see Chapter 22).

You may be given the following shaving instructions for certain clients:

- ***Manual shavers are generally not used on clients with dementia.*** However, some clients may be startled by the loud buzzing sound that an electric razor makes, or they may not be familiar with the type of razor you are using. These clients, therefore, may not understand what you are doing and may resist care and make sudden movements. It is important to introduce the razor to the client on every use, using a gentle and nonthreatening tone of voice and body language. Most agencies allow only the use of electric shavers for these clients because of the increased risk for the client to make sudden movements that could cause serious nicks and cuts.
- ***Manual shavers with open blades should never be used on clients receiving medications that slow down blood clotting (anticoagulants).*** In these clients, a nick or cut could cause serious bleeding. Electric shavers are preferable for clients taking these types of medications. If the client's care plan does not state what type of razor to use, it is important to ask your supervisor.
- ***Electric shavers are not used on clients receiving oxygen.*** A spark from the electric shaver could cause a fire.
- ***If an electric razor scratches the client's face, have the shaver repaired at once.*** Report and record the scratches; most agencies and facilities require that an incident report be completed.
- ***Never rinse out an electric razor under a running tap*** unless the manufacturer's instructions specify to do so. ***Electric razors should also never be immersed in water.***

Electric Shaver Maintenance

Simple cleaning routines performed on a regular basis help prolong the life of the electric shaver and can reduce skin irritation and the risk for injury to the client.[3]

- Many problems with electric shavers can be avoided by simply removing the cutting head and tapping the hair particles into a tissue after each use. Discard the tissue.
- Most electric shavers come with a cleaning brush, which also should be used after each shave to remove hair particles that cannot be removed by blowing on them.
- Some manufacturers advise spraying the shaver every week or so with a special spray to both lubricate and degrease the cutting blades.
- In addition, cutters and the foil surface should be replaced periodically (according to the manufacturer's directions).

Caring for Moustaches and Beards

Beards and moustaches need daily care to prevent food and mouth and nose drainage from collecting in the hair. Daily washing and combing usually are enough to keep beards and moustaches clean. Ask clients how they would like the beard or moustache groomed. ***Never trim or shave the beard or moustache without the client's consent.***

Shaving Legs and Underarms for Female Clients

The practice of shaving legs and underarms varies among cultures and individuals. Some women shave only the lower legs, whereas others shave to mid-thigh or the entire leg.

Female clients' legs and underarms should be shaved after the bath, when the skin is soft. To save time, collect the client's shaving items along with the bath items. When shaving, use soap and water or a shaving cream to work up a lather. Rinse the razor in a kidney basin, not in the bathwater. The guidelines in the *Think About Safety: Guidelines for Shaving Clients* box also apply when shaving the underarms and legs.

Pubic Hair

Pubic hair is found in the frontal genital area, in the crotch, and on the top insides of the legs. In most cases, pubic hair begins to appear within 3 years following puberty. With aging, a person will have less body hair, and the body hair may turn grey or white, much like the hair on the head. Many consider the care of pubic hair to be an important part of grooming, so they may choose to remove it. Some cultures, such as Muslim cultures, have rules that insist on the trimming or removal of pubic hair.

Hair removal of any kind, including that of pubic hair, can result in **ingrown hairs** (also known as **razor bumps**), which may be painful and red. An ingrown hair (**FIGURE 31–6**) does not grow straight

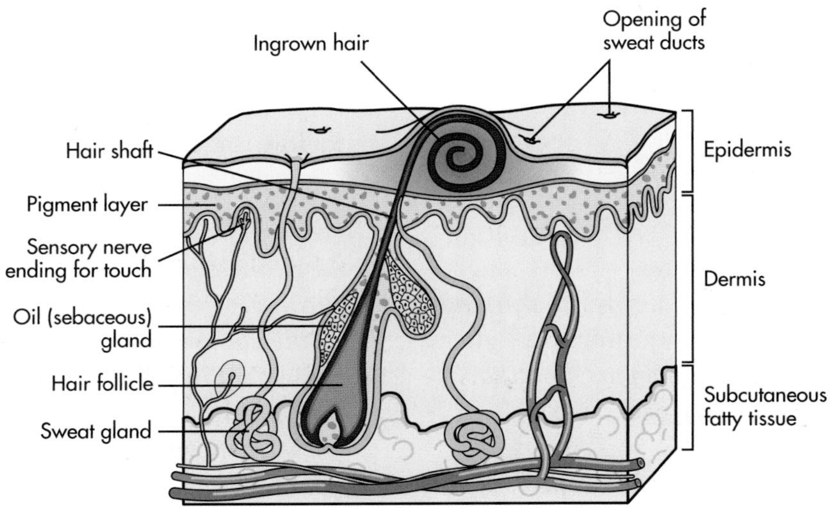

FIGURE 31–6 Ingrown hair.

out of the follicle opening. Instead, it curls into the side wall of the hair follicle or into the skin surface, causing the skin to become inflamed. This inflammation can result in the development of a pimple (such as a papule or a pustule) or a cyst (nodule), both of which are usually tender. The hair tip may continue to grow into the adjacent skin outside the follicle and may produce a larger and more inflamed area, which can produce permanent scarring or changes in the colour of the skin. If you observe any ingrown hairs, you should report and record them, according to your agency's policies.

As a support worker, you would rarely be asked to remove pubic hair. The pubic area is very delicate and can easily be nicked by razors or cut by sharp scissors. However, if you *are* required to, you should do it in a tactful, professional manner, ensuring that the client's rights to privacy and dignity are preserved at all times. The client's care plan would specify the steps involved in removing or trimming pubic hair.

Shaving a Client 123

Advocate on behalf of the client's quality of life by promoting:

Dignity • Independence • Preferences • Privacy • Safety *(see BOX 1–4, on p. 17)*

PRE-PROCEDURE

1 Identify the client, according to employer policy.
This eliminates the possibility of mistaking one client for another.
2 Explain the procedure to the client.
3 Practise proper hand hygiene.
4 Collect the following supplies:
- ☐ **Wash basin**
- ☐ **Bath towel**
- ☐ **Face towel**
- ☐ **Washcloth**
- ☐ **Blade razor or electric shaver, according to the client's care plan**
- ☐ **Mirror**
- ☐ **Shaving cream, soap, or lotion**
- ☐ **Shaving brush (optional)**
- ☐ **Aftershave lotion (men only)**
- ☐ **Tissues**
- ☐ **Paper towels**
- ☐ **Gloves**

It is important to plan thoroughly before starting any procedure. By collecting all the necessary equipment beforehand, you will not have to leave your client's side and can eliminate wasting time and energy in obtaining the forgotten equipment.

5 Arrange paper towels and supplies on the overbed table (in facilities) or on a work area within easy reach.
Arranging items will make it easier for you to work efficiently.
6 Provide for privacy. Practise proper hand hygiene.
7 Raise the bed to a comfortable working height. Follow the care plan for bed rail use.*

PROCEDURE

8 Fill the basin with warm water.
Warm water is used to rinse the client's skin and the manual razor. It is more comfortable than using hot or cold water, and it will soften the hair stubble.
9 Place the basin on the overbed table or work area.
10 Lower the bed rail near you if it is up.
11 Assist the client to the semi-Fowler's position if allowed. If this is not possible, assist the client to the supine position.
12 Adjust the lighting so you can see the client's face clearly.
The use of proper lighting will help prevent shaving errors.

Continued

Shaving a Client—cont'd

13 Place the bath towel over the chest. Allow the client to use a mirror.

14 Adjust the overbed table to allow for easy reach.*
This prevents worker back strain.

15 ***Method 1: Using a manual shaver:***
- **a** Affix the razor blade to the shaver tightly.
- **b** Wash the client's face. Do not dry.
- **c** Wet a washcloth or face towel with warm water. Wring it out.
- **d** Apply the washcloth or towel to the client's face for a few minutes.
- **e** Put on gloves.
- **f** Apply shaving cream with your hands or using a shaving brush.
- **g** Hold the client's skin taut with one hand.
- **h** Shave in the direction of hair growth. Use longer strokes on the larger areas of the face. Use shorter strokes around the chin and lips (FIGURE 31–7).

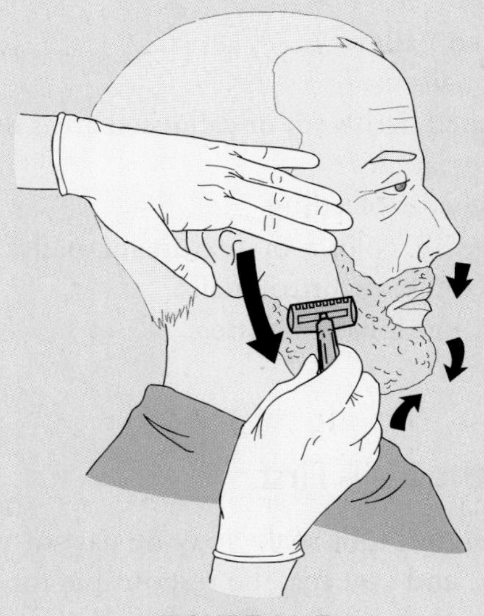

FIGURE 31–7

- **i** Rinse the razor frequently. Shake off excess water and lather.
- **j** Apply direct pressure to any area that bleeds.
- **k** Wash remaining shaving cream or soap from the client's face. Dry with a towel.

Some clients prefer the manual razor because they feel it gives them a closer shave. Check the care plan. Placing a warm, wet towel on the client's beard will soften it and make shaving easier. Shaving cream also lubricates the skin, softens the beard, and makes shaving easier.

16 ***Method 2: Using an electric shaver:***
- **a** Put on gloves.
- **b** Make sure the client's face is dry. Do not apply shaving cream or a warm cloth to the face. Hold skin taut with one hand.
- **c** Turn the razor on.
- **d** Place the razor over the hair growth. Move the razor back and forth or in a circular pattern.
- **e** Apply direct pressure to any area that bleeds.

An electric shaver is always used when the client is on certain medications or is prone to bleeding easily. Check your care plan.

17 Apply aftershave lotion if requested by the client.
This respects the client's need to feel better and smell nice.

18 Remove the towel and gloves. Practise proper hand hygiene.

19 Move the overbed table to the side of the bed.*
It is easier for the client to reach for items that may be on it.

POST-PROCEDURE

20 Provide for safety and comfort.

21 Place the call bell within reach.*
This provides an easy, safe way for the client to contact staff if necessary.

22 Return the bed to its lowest position. Follow the care plan for bed rail use.*
Lowering the bed will decrease the risk of the client falling.

Continued

Shaving a Client—cont'd

23 Clean and return equipment and supplies to their proper place. Discard disposable items. Wear gloves for this step.
24 Wipe off the overbed table or work area with paper towels. Discard paper towels properly.
25 Remove privacy measures.
26 Follow employer policy for handling dirty linen. *This decreases the risk for pathogen spread.*
27 Practise proper hand hygiene.

Report and Record your actions and observations, according to employer policy. In particular, report nicks or bleeding to your supervisor. *This is done for legal reasons and to keep the rest of the health care team informed.*

*Steps marked with an asterisk may not apply in community settings.

CARE OF NAILS AND FEET

Foot and nail care is a very important part of daily personal care to prevent infection, injury, and odours. Long or broken nails can scratch skin or snag clothing. Hangnails, **ingrown nails** (nails that grow in at the side), and nails torn away from the skin cause skin breaks, which can provide portals of entry for microbes and pathogens.

Feet are easily infected and injured. Dirty or moist feet, socks, and stockings harbour microbes and cause odours, and shoes and socks provide a warm, moist environment for the growth of microbes. Injuries occur from stubbing of toes, stepping on sharp objects, or being stepped on. Shoes that fit poorly can cause bunions, calluses, corns, blisters, or ingrown nails, all of which can be considerably painful. Infections or foot injuries are particularly serious in older adults and people with circulatory disorders. Poor circulation in the feet prolongs healing because it prevents white blood cells (WBCs) and oxygenated blood from entering that area. WBCs engulf and eat infected material, and oxygen provides the necessary energy for cells to function well. Diabetes and vascular disease are common causes of poor circulation, and gangrene and amputations are serious complications (see Chapter 37).

Important Things to Watch for

It is your responsibility to check the client's feet every day. Daily checking is especially important if the client has a circulatory disorder or diabetes or takes medications that affect blood clotting. Notify your supervisor if you observe any of the following:

- Very dry skin
- Foot odours
- Cracks or breaks in the skin, especially between the toes
- Ingrown nails
- Loose nails
- Reddened, irritated, or calloused areas on the feet, heels, or ankles
- Drainage or bleeding
- Change in colour or texture of nails, especially black, thick, or brittle nails
- Corns, bunions, or blisters

Soften the Nails First

Fingernail and foot soaks may be part of the client's care plan, and you may be responsible for providing them (see the procedure *Providing Nail and Foot Care* on p. 665). Generally, nails are easier to trim and clean when they have been softened. ***However, you should not cut a client's toenails immediately after soaking, as the tissue around the nail will be puffy from water absorption and more prone to nicks and cuts.*** Follow your agency's policies and the client's care plan for the right method to soften the client's nails. Some agencies advise the use of specific lotions for this purpose.

Tub baths are a good time for soaking feet and fingernails. If soaking is done at other times, the client can sit on the side of the tub and soak the feet. Make sure the client can step into and out of the tub. Otherwise, soak the feet in a basin. If it is comfortable, the client can soak the fingers in the sink or in a small basin or bowl. Usually, fingernail or foot soaks should last 15 to 20 minutes. Feet are easily burned, so you should check with your supervisor about the correct water temperature for foot soaks. ***You must be very careful when preparing soaks for people with decreased sensation or circulatory problems. They may not feel hot temperatures and are at risk for scalding or burning of their feet.***

Think About Safety

Important Points About Fingernail, Toenail, and Foot Care

Cut fingernails only if instructed to do so by your supervisor and the care plan. Nail clippers should be used to cut fingernails. ***Scissors are rarely used—know your agency's policy.*** When using clippers, use extreme caution to prevent damage to nearby tissue. Any equipment used for cutting nails should be discarded or thoroughly sanitized after each use, according to your agency's guidelines and policies.

Some employers do not allow support workers to cut or trim toenails under any circumstances, so you should always follow your employer's policy. Trimming and clipping toenails can easily cause injuries. If a client has a disease or illness that increases the risk for infection, you should know this. Support workers do ***not*** cut or trim toenails of the following clients:

- Clients with diabetes
- Clients with poor circulation to the legs and feet
- Clients who take medications that affect blood clotting
- Clients with very thick or ingrown nails
- Clients who are uncooperative or combative

FYI

If a client needs the toenails trimmed, tell your supervisor—never assume that you can go ahead and trim them yourself. If you are allowed to trim a client's toenails, always use either large straight nail clippers or specialized toenail clippers. In many areas, nurses or other health care workers who have specialized training in nail care can be contacted to provide nail care to a client. The client usually must pay a small fee for this service.

Also, support workers do not treat corns, bunions, or blisters, as these foot problems may require the care of a podiatrist. A **podiatrist** is a physician who specializes in the evaluation and treatment of diseases of the foot.

Providing Nail and Foot Care 123

Advocate on behalf of the client's quality of life by promoting:

Dignity • Independence • Preferences • Privacy • Safety *(see BOX 1–4, on p. 17)*

PRE-PROCEDURE

1 Identify the client, according to employer policy. *This eliminates the possibility of mistaking one client for another.*
2 Explain the procedure to the client.
3 Practise proper hand hygiene.
4 Collect the following supplies:
   - ☐ **Wash basin**
   - ☐ **Soap**
   - ☐ **Bath thermometer**
   - ☐ **Bath towel**

Continued

Providing Nail and Foot Care—cont'd

- ☐ **Face towel**
- ☐ **Washcloth**
- ☐ **Kidney basin**
- ☐ **Nail clippers (curved for hands and straight for feet)**
- ☐ **Nail file with sharp tip for cleaning under nails**
- ☐ **Lotion or petroleum jelly**
- ☐ **Paper towels**
- ☐ **Disposable bath mat**
- ☐ **Gloves**

It is important to plan thoroughly before starting any procedure. By collecting all the necessary equipment beforehand, you will not have to leave your client's side and can eliminate wasting time and energy in obtaining the forgotten equipment.

5 Arrange paper towels and other items on the overbed table (in facilities) or on a work area within easy reach.
Having easy reach makes items easier to grasp when needed.

6 Provide for privacy. Practise proper hand hygiene.

7 Help the client to a bedside chair. Place the call bell (in facilities) within reach.
This provides an easy, safe way for the client to contact staff if necessary.

PROCEDURE

8 Place the bath mat under the client's feet.
This eliminates the client's bare feet being on the cold floor.

9 Fill the wash basin. The care plan tells you what temperature to use. Measure the water temperature, according to employer policy.
This eliminates the risk of burning clients accidentally.

10 Place the basin on the bath mat.
The bath mat absorbs spills and helps prevent the wash basin from sliding.

11 Help the client remove shoes and socks.
Some clients become dizzy when bending over to untie shoes. Dizziness can lead to falls.

12 Help the client put the feet into the basin (**FIGURE 31–8**).

13 Adjust the overbed table or work area in front of the client. It should be low and close to the client.
This allows the client to reach the bedside table more easily.

14 To ensure the client does not get chilled, place a blanket around the shoulders if necessary. Most clients like their legs to be covered with a towel while their feet are soaking.
Soaking the feet and hands may quickly cool an older, frail client, and keeping them warm will promote comfort.

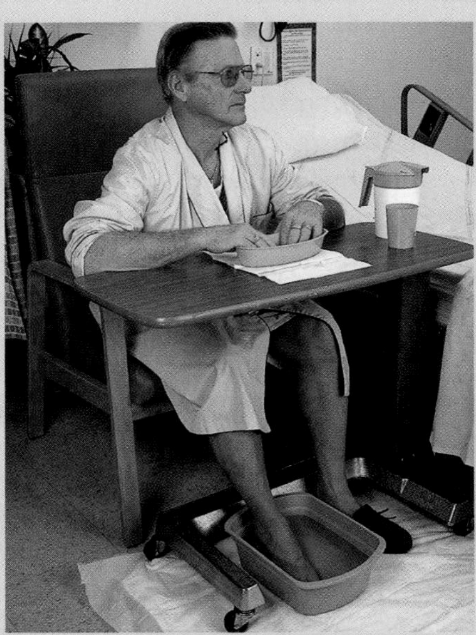

FIGURE 31–8 The feet soak in a foot basin, and the fingers soak in a kidney basin. Note the waterproof pad and facecloth under each which will absorb any splashed water.

15 For the fingernails:
If the client's nails are thick or visibly soiled, fill the kidney basin. Measure the water temperature, according to employer policy.
This eliminates the risk of burning clients accidentally. Soaking the fingernails may be the only way to soften hardened food or feces, which may be present under the client's fingernails.

Continued

Providing Nail and Foot Care—cont'd

16 Place the kidney basin on the overbed table or work area.

17 Put the client's fingers into the basin. Position the arms for comfort.
The client can easily become tired, stiff, and sore if not in a comfortable position.

18 Allow the feet and fingernails to soak for 10 to 15 minutes. Warm the water again as needed.
Soaking the nails will allow them to soften and make them easier to cut and file.

19 Remove the kidney basin. Thoroughly dry the client's hands, especially between the fingers.
Moisture left on fingers can cool the hands needlessly.

20 Put on your gloves.

21 Clean under the client's fingernails with the nail file tip. Use a towel to wipe the tip after each nail.
This removes accumulations of food bits or dirt from under the nails.

22 With nail clippers, clip the nails straight across so that the nails are even with or just below the tips of the fingers, according to the client's care plan and following your employer's policies (**FIGURE 31–9**).
Clipping them this way will help them be less likely to catch on clothing. ***Be careful not to accidentally cut the skin.***

23 Once the nails are dry and no longer soft, shape them with an emery board or nail file. File in one direction only.
Filing wet nails will leave the nails with jagged edges that can scratch skin or catch on clothing. Filing nails in a back-and-forth motion can damage the nail and cause discomfort for the client.

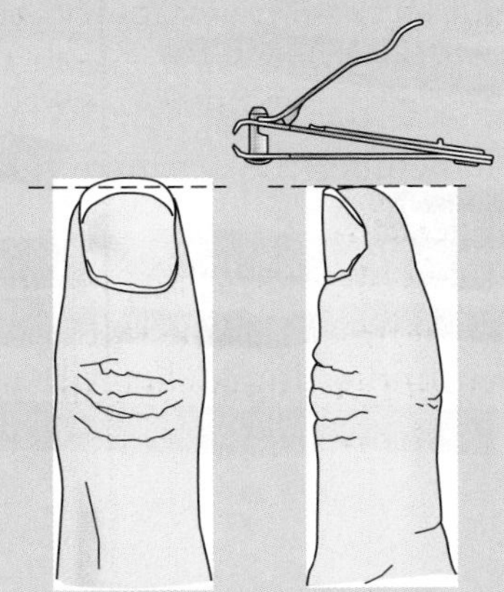

FIGURE 31–9

24 Move the overbed table aside, away from your working path.*

25 For the toenails:
It is always preferable to soak the client's feet in the bathtub while the client is being bathed. However, if the client's feet are very soiled or it is not possible to place the client in a tub, you may have to soak the client's feet in a basin. Wash the client's feet with soap and a washcloth. Wash between the toes. *Feet can trap bacteria, which can cause odour and infection. Using soap and water reduces bacteria and the accumulation of dead skin cells on the feet.*

26 Rinse the feet and between the toes.
Rinsing removes soil, dead skin cells, and soap residue from the skin.

27 Remove the feet from the basin. Dry thoroughly, especially between the toes.
Moist skin between the toes can harbour pathogens, leading to skin infections, which may be very difficult to cure and can lead to further health problems.

28 Clean under the toenails with a nail file edge.
This removes accumulations of dirt from under the nails.

29 ***Only if you are instructed*** to trim the client's toenails, perform steps 22 and 23, ensuring the client is safe and comfortable throughout the procedure.

30 Apply lotion or petroleum jelly to the tops and soles of the feet, but not between the toes. Warm the lotion before applying it by pouring a small amount into your hands and rubbing your palms together.
Lotion lubricates skin and prevents cracking.

31 Remove your gloves. Practise proper hand hygiene.

32 Help the client put on socks and shoes.
Some clients are at risk of falling if they bend over to do this themselves.

Continued

Providing Nail and Foot Care—cont'd

POST-PROCEDURE

33 Provide for safety and comfort.

34 Place the call bell within reach.*
This provides an easy, safe way for the client to contact staff if necessary.

35 Follow the care plan for bed rail use.*

36 Thoroughly clean, sanitize, and return equipment and supplies to their proper places. Discard disposable items. Wear gloves for this step.
Cleaning and sanitizing all reusable equipment will eliminate the risk for pathogen spread.

37 Remove privacy measures.

38 Follow employer policy for handling soiled linen.
This decreases the risk for pathogen spread.

39 Practise proper hand hygiene.

Report and Record your actions and observations, according to employer policy.
This is done for legal reasons and to keep the rest of the health care team informed.

*Steps marked with an asterisk may not apply in community settings.

CHANGING CLOTHING, INCONTINENCE BRIEFS, AND HOSPITAL GOWNS

Like everyone else, clients who live in the community or in long-term care (complex-care) facilities dress and undress at least once a day. Most clients wear clothes during the day and change into sleepwear at bedtime. Some are incontinent of urine or feces and must have their incontinence brief changed when necessary (see the procedure *Changing an Incontinence Brief* on p. 672). Clients who have incontinence may require more frequent changes of clothing. Some clients who have illnesses and cannot get out of bed choose to wear sleepwear and robes through the day. Clients who are hospitalized wear hospital gowns, especially if they are receiving intravenous (IV) therapy. Hospital gowns are put on and removed in a certain way when the client is receiving IV therapy (see the procedure *Changing the Gown of a Client With Intravenous Tubing* on p. 678).

Helping clients dress and undress is easier when the clients can move their arms and legs. Special techniques are required to safely, comfortably, and quickly dress and undress clients with arm or leg injuries or paralysis. Follow the guidelines in BOX 31–2 when dressing and undressing clients.

BOX 31–2 Guidelines for Changing Clients' Clothing or Hospital Gowns

- Provide for privacy. Practise proper hand hygiene. Do not expose the client.
- Encourage the client to do as much as possible.
- As much as possible, allow the client to choose what to wear. Make sure the right undergarments are chosen.
- Support the arm or leg when removing or putting on a garment.
- Put clothing on the *affected side* (the side affected by disease or disability) first. Never refer to the affected side as the "bad" side. When dressing a client, remember the acronym **DAF**—**D**ress **A**ffected side **F**irst.
- Remove clothing from the *unaffected* side (the side not affected by disease or disability) first. When undressing a client, remember the acronym **RUF**—**R**emove from **U**naffected side **F**irst.

Pay particular attention to clients' comfort when you are dressing them. Moving the joints can sometimes be very uncomfortable for the client, so you should always be organized, efficient, and as quick as possible. Never jerk or pull the client, which can be very uncomfortable and distressing.

When assisting a client with putting on socks and pants, put the client's socks on before putting the pants on. By dressing the client in this order, loose threads or the hem of the pants will not catch on the client's toes. Ensure that the client's socks go on smoothly and are not binding or bunched at the top.

Report and record the following observations after helping a client dress or undress:

- How much help was given
- How the client tolerated the procedure
- Any complaints from the client

Undressing a Client

123

Advocate on behalf of the client's quality of life by promoting:

Dignity • Independence • Preferences • Privacy • Safety

(see BOX 1–4, on p. 17)

PRE-PROCEDURE

1 Identify the client, according to employer policy. *This eliminates the possibility of mistaking one client for another.*
2 Explain the procedure to the client.
3 Practise proper hand hygiene.
4 Collect a **bath blanket** or **bedspread**.
5 Provide for privacy. Practise proper hand hygiene.
6 It may be easier to help a client undress while the client is sitting in a chair. However, ensure the client's privacy at all times. *If sitting in a chair, the client can lean forward more easily, and there are no bed linens that might get in the way.*
7 If the client must be dressed while in the bed, raise the bed to a comfortable working height.* *Raising the bed will reduce your risk for back strain. However, by lowering the head of the bed, it will be easier to slide the client up to a better position.*
8 Lower the bed rail (if it is up) on the client's affected side.
9 Place the client in the supine position. *This position is easiest for removing clothing.*
10 Cover the client with the bath blanket or bedspread. *This keeps the client warm and promotes privacy.* Fan-fold linens to the foot of the bed. *Fan-folding makes grasping and straightening linens easier than rolling them up would be.* Do not expose the client during the procedure.

PROCEDURE

11 Paying particular attention to the client's comfort, remove the back-opening garments as so:
   a Raise the client's head and shoulders (see Chapter 25), or turn the client onto the side away from you.
   b Undo buttons, zippers, ties, or snaps.
   c Bring the sides of the garment from the back to the client's sides (**FIGURE 31–10**).
   d Assist the client to the side-lying position to remove a back-opening garment. Tuck the far side of the garment under the client. Fold the near side onto the client's chest. (**FIGURE 31–11**).
   e Place the client in the supine position.
   f Slide the garment off the shoulder and arm. Remove the garment from the unaffected side first. (**FIGURE 31–12**).
   g Repeat the above step for the affected side.
   Removing garments from the unaffected side first allows the client to self-assist as much as possible and remain as independent as possible. Garment removal is easier when done in this order.

Continued

Undressing a Client—cont'd

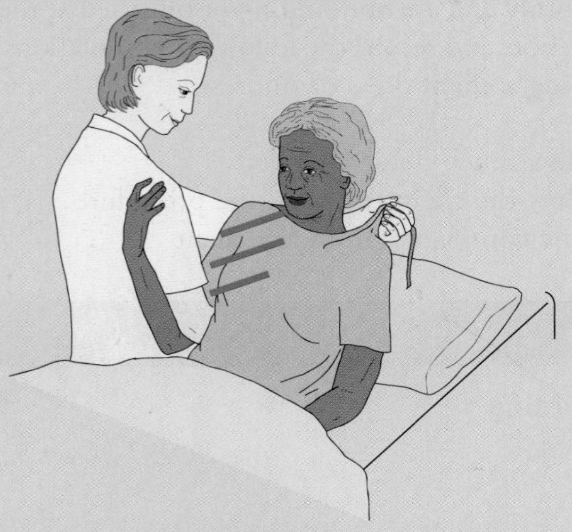

FIGURE 31–10

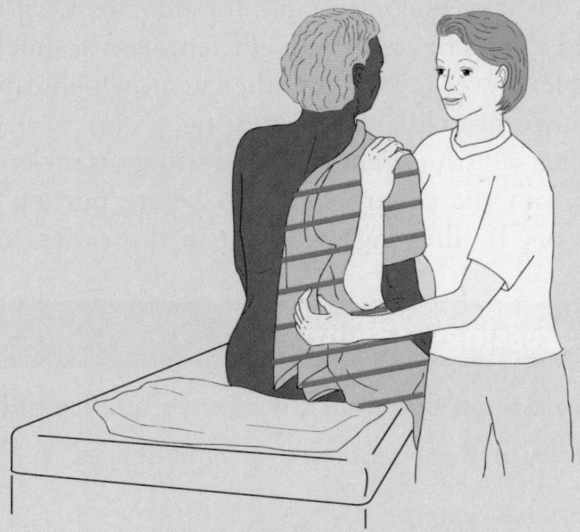

FIGURE 31–13

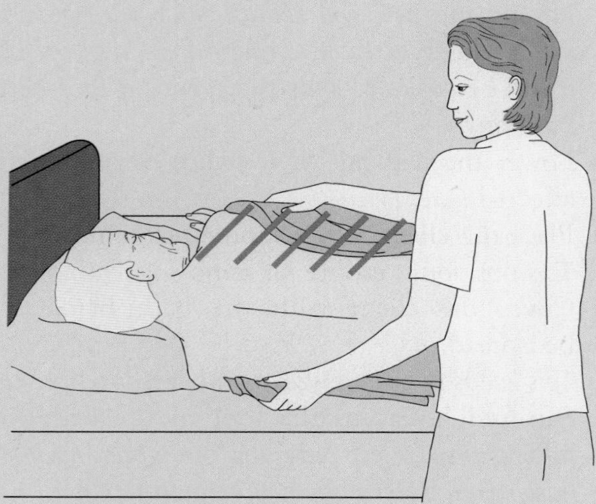

FIGURE 31–11

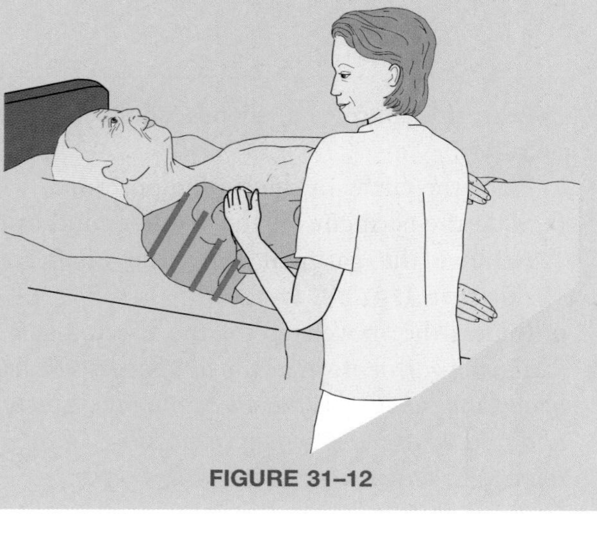

FIGURE 31–12

12 Paying particular attention to the client's comfort, remove front-opening garments as so:
- a Undo buttons, zippers, snaps, or ties.
- b Slide the garment off the shoulder and arm on the unaffected side.
- c Raise the client's head and shoulders. Bring the garment over to the affected side (FIGURE 31–13).
- d Lower the client's head and shoulders.
- e Remove the garment from the affected side.
- f If you cannot raise the client's head and shoulders:
  - i Turn the client toward you. Tuck the removed part of the garment under the client.
  - ii Turn the client onto the side facing away from you.
  - iii Pull the side of the garment out from under the client. Make sure that the client will not lie on it when supine.
  - iv Return the client to the supine position.
  - v Remove the garment from the affected side.

Garment removal is easier when done in this order.

Continued

Undressing a Client—cont'd

13 Paying particular attention to the client's comfort, remove pullover garments as so:
- **a** Undo any buttons, zippers, ties, or snaps.
- **b** Remove the garment from the client's unaffected side.
- **c** Raise the client's head and shoulders, or turn the client onto the side facing away from you. Bring the garment up to the client's neck (**FIGURE 31–14**).
- **d** Remove the garment from the affected side.
- **e** Bring the garment over the client's head.
- **f** Place the client in the supine position.

Pullover garments are usually the most difficult to remove. Starting with the client's unaffected side makes garment removal easier to manage and allows the client to maintain some independence by assisting with garment removal.

14 Paying particular attention to the client's comfort, remove pants or slacks as so:
- **a** Remove footwear.
- **b** Place the client in the supine position.
- **c** Undo buttons, zippers, ties, snaps, or buckles.
- **d** Remove the belt, if one is worn.
- **e** Ask the client to lift the hips and buttocks off the bed. Slide the pants down over the hips and buttocks (**FIGURE 31–15**).
- **f** Have the client lower the hips and buttocks.
- **g** If the client cannot lift the hips off the bed:
  - **i** Turn the client toward you in the side-lying position.
  - **ii** Slide the pants off the hip and buttock on the unaffected side (**FIGURE 31–16**).
  - **iii** Turn the client away from you onto the other side.
  - **iv** Slide the pants off the hip and buttock on the affected side (**FIGURE 31–17**).
- **h** Slide the pants down the legs and over the feet.

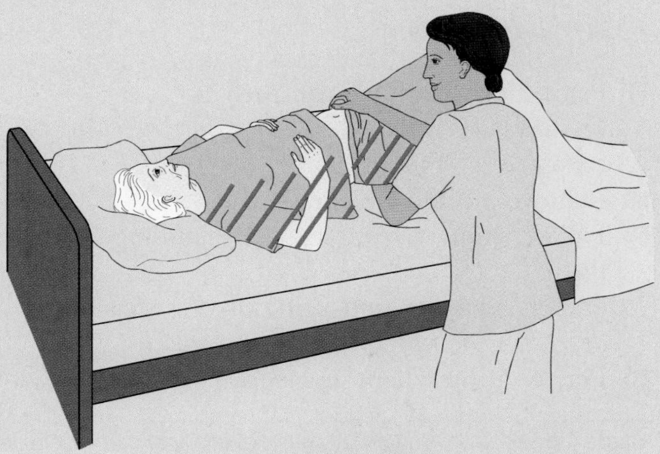

FIGURE 31–15

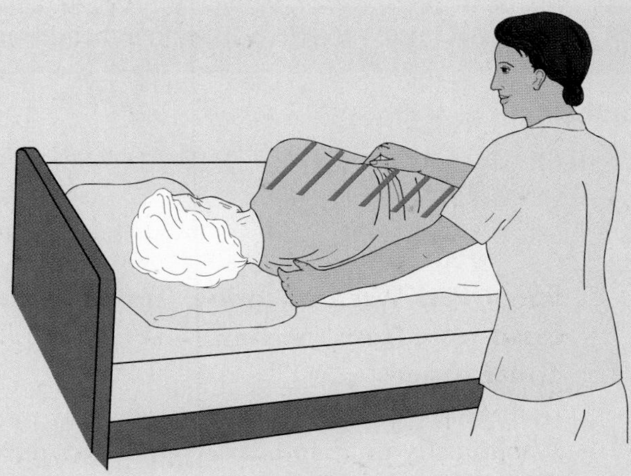

FIGURE 31–14

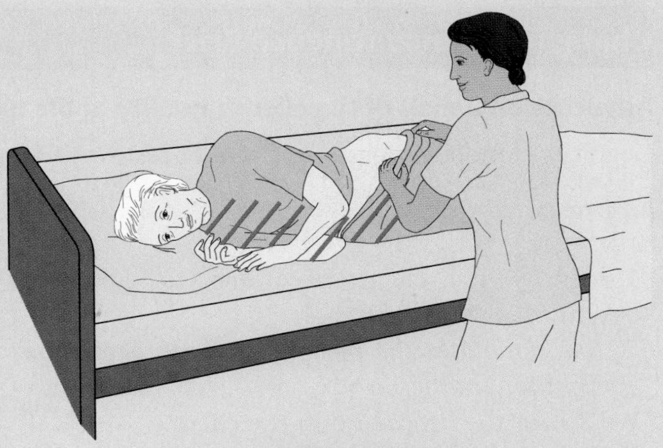

FIGURE 31–16

Continued

Undressing a Client—cont'd

15 Paying particular attention to the client's comfort, dress the client (see the procedure *Dressing a Client*, p. 675).
16 Help the client get out of bed if necessary. If the client will stay in bed, do the following:
  a Cover the client and remove the bath blanket or bedspread.
  b Provide for safety and comfort.
  c Return the bed to its lowest position. Follow the care plan for bed rail use.*

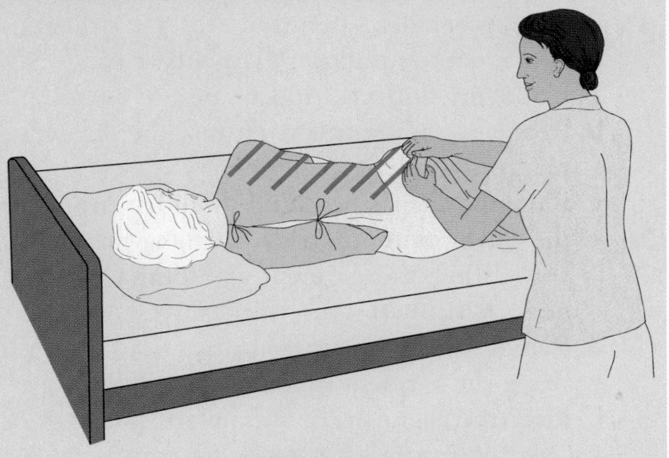

FIGURE 31–17

POST-PROCEDURE

17 Place the call bell within reach.*
This provides an easy, safe way for the client to contact staff if necessary.
18 Remove privacy measures.
19 Follow employer policy for handling soiled linen.
Proper handling and disposal of soiled linens decreases the risk for pathogen spread.
20 Practise proper hand hygiene.

Report and Record your actions and observations, according to employer policy.
This is done for legal reasons and to keep the rest of the health care team informed.

*Steps marked with an asterisk may not apply in community settings.

Changing an Incontinence Brief

123

Advocate on behalf of the client's quality of life by promoting:

Dignity • Independence • Preferences • Privacy • Safety *(see BOX 1–4, on p. 17)*

PRE-PROCEDURE

1 Identify the client, according to employer policy.
This eliminates the possibility of mistaking one client for another.
2 Explain the procedure to the client.
3 Perform hand hygiene.
4 Collect the following supplies:
  - ☐ **Wash basin**
  - ☐ **Soap or Peri Wash, as per agency policy**
  - ☐ **Spray Peri Wash or lotion (for softening dried feces from the skin)**
  - ☐ **Toilet paper**
  - ☐ **Bedpan or garbage bag**
  - ☐ **Washcloths or disposable wipes for perineal care, as per agency policy**
  - ☐ **Clean incontinence pad**
  - ☐ **Paper towels**
  - ☐ **Gloves**

Continued

Changing an Incontinence Brief—cont'd

It is important to plan thoroughly before starting any procedure. By collecting all the necessary equipment beforehand, you will not have to leave your client's side and can eliminate wasting time and energy in obtaining the forgotten equipment.

5 Place paper towels on the overbed table (in facilities) or on a work area within easy reach. Arrange items on top of paper towels.

6 Close doors and windows.
This helps prevent drafts.

7 Provide for privacy. Practise proper hand hygiene.

8 Raise the bed to a comfortable working height.
This will reduce your risk for back strain.

PROCEDURE

9 Lower the bed rail near you if it is up.
This helps prevent back strain. Remove the call bell.*

10 Cover the client with the top sheet.
This ensures client warmth and privacy.

11 Lower the head of the bed until flat.* Ensure the client has at least one pillow if the client can tolerate this position.

12 Raise the bed rail near you if bed rails are used. Fill the wash basin two thirds with water, and test the water using a bathwater thermometer (see **FIGURE 30–9**) to ensure that the water is a safe and comfortable temperature.

13 Place the basin on the overbed table or work area. If your agency does not use basins, you must obtain enough washcloths to provide perineal care to the client. You should have at least (a) one cloth that has been soaked, wrung out, and presoaped with soap or Peri Wash; (b) one wet cloth to be used to rinse the perineal area after it has been thoroughly washed; and (c) one dry towel for drying the client's skin thoroughly.

14 Lower the bed rail if it is up.

15 a Ensure that all the clothing is out of the way. Undo the tapes on either side of the brief.
b Put on gloves.

16 Turn the client onto the side facing away from you.

17 Place the bedpan or garbage bag on the client's bed next to you.

18 Gently remove the soiled brief from the front of the client, through the client's legs and then away from the back. If heavily soiled, begin to wipe the feces with toilet paper in long strokes away from the client's urethra.
Dried feces is difficult to remove and may irritate the skin. Peri Wash or lotion can soften the feces, making removal of it easier and less uncomfortable for the client.

19 Discard the soiled toilet paper into the bedpan or the garbage bag.
This helps protect the linen.

20 Roll up the soiled disposable brief and discard it into the bedpan or garbage bag.

21 Do not place soiled briefs or linens on the floor or on the client's overbed table.
Placing soiled linens on the floor or table will spread pathogens.

22 Wash the front genital area first by wiping in long strokes away from the urethra. Then wipe around the client's rectal area (see the procedures *Giving Perineal Care to a Female Client,* on p. 643, and *Giving Perineal Care to a Male Client,* on p. 646). Discard disposable wipe (if used) into plastic bag or bedpan. Place soiled cloths into wash basin.

23 Observe the client's skin for areas of redness or irritation.

24 Wipe the entire area using the soaped cloths until all visible incontinence is removed.

25 Rinse the entire area using the wet, unsoaped cloths to remove soap residue from the skin.
Soap residue can be drying and irritating to the skin. Peri Wash does not leave residue on the skin, so many agencies and facilities prefer it.

Continued

Changing an Incontinence Brief—cont'd

26 Dry area thoroughly with the dry towel.
Moist skin can harbour pathogens, which can cause skin infections.

27 Remove gloves.

28 Position the clean, fully-opened incontinence brief so that the lining of the brief is next to the client's skin. Make sure the tape tabs are at the back of the client. Note that the side of the brief is fan-folded on the side next to the client, with the adhesive strips at the top (**FIGURE 31–18, *A***). The client is ready to be rolled onto the brief for proper fitting.

29 Roll the client onto the back. Bring the front of the brief through the client's legs (**FIGURE 31–18, *B***).

30 Smooth the brief across the abdomen and fit a side of the brief around each of the legs. Fasten the bottom adhesive tabs on either side to the front of the brief (**FIGURE 31–18, *C***).

31 Gently pull the brief upward so the brief fits well in the groin and crotch area. Readjust the fastening tapes as needed to ensure a proper fit.

32 Tidy the bed linens.

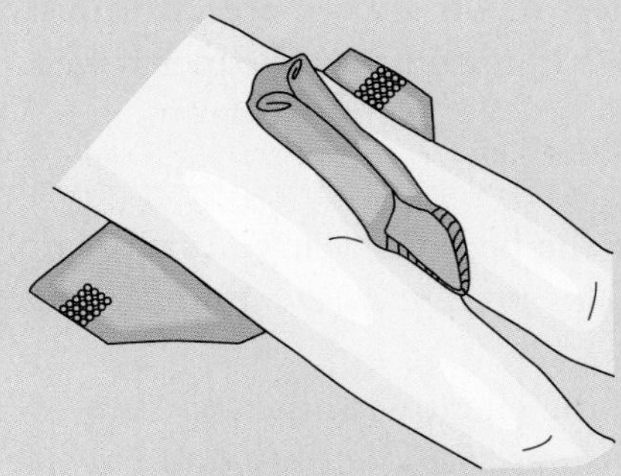

FIGURE 31–18 B

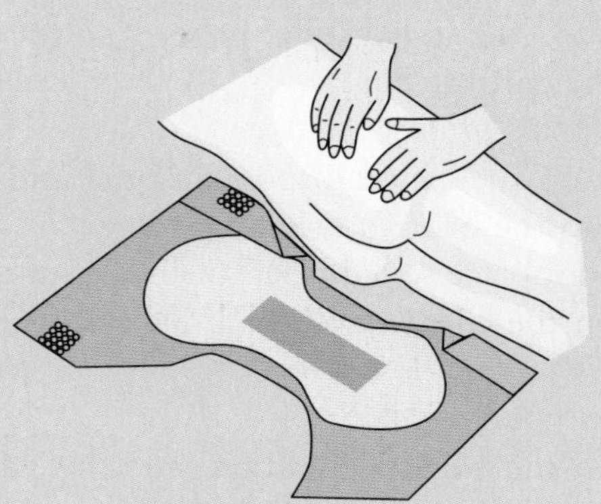

FIGURE 31–18 A

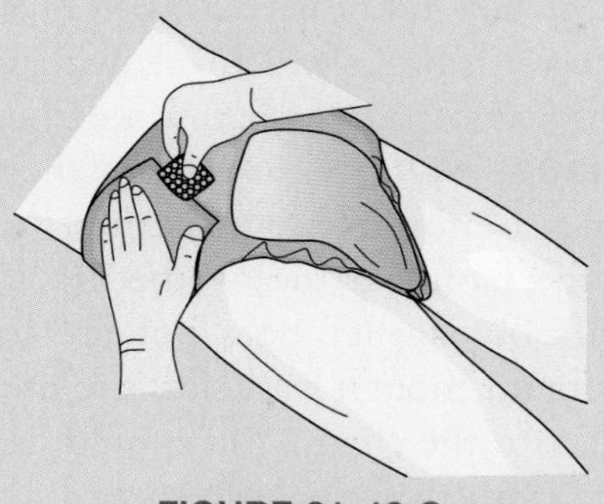

FIGURE 31–18 C

POST-PROCEDURE

33 Provide for safety and comfort.

34 Return the bed to its lowest position. Attach the call bell. Follow the care plan for bed rail use.*
This helps provide for client safety.

35 Empty and clean the wash basin. Return it and other supplies to their proper places.
This makes them easier to find the next time they are needed.

36 Wipe off the overbed table or work area with paper towels. Discard the paper towels.
This helps prevent the transfer of microbes.

37 Remove privacy measures.

38 Follow employer policy for handling dirty linen.

39 Perform hand hygiene.

Report and Record your actions and observations, according to employer policy.
This is done for legal reasons and to keep the rest of the health care team informed.

*Steps marked with an asterisk may not apply in community settings.

Dressing a Client

123

Advocate on behalf of the client's quality of life by promoting:

Dignity • Independence • Preferences • Privacy • Safety *(see BOX 1–4, on p. 17)*

PRE-PROCEDURE

1 Identify the client, according to employer policy.
This eliminates the possibility of mistaking one client for another.

2 Explain the procedure to the client.

3 Practise proper hand hygiene.

4 Collect a **bath blanket** or **bedspread** and **clothing** requested by the client.
By collecting all the necessary equipment beforehand, you will not have to leave your client's side and can eliminate wasting time and energy in obtaining the forgotten equipment.

5 Provide for privacy. Practise proper hand hygiene.

6 It may be easier to help the client undress while the client is sitting in a chair. However, ensure the client's privacy at all times.
If sitting in a chair, the client can lean forward more easily, and there are no bed linens that might get in the way.

7 If the client must be dressed in bed, raise the bed to a comfortable working height.*

8 Undress the client (see the procedure *Undressing a Client*, p. 669).

9 Lower the bed rail (if it is up) on the client's unaffected side.
The client would be better able to assist you from the unaffected side.

10 Place the client in the supine position.
This is the most comfortable position for the client for this procedure.

PROCEDURE

11 Cover the client with the bath blanket or bedspread. Fan-fold linens to the foot of the bed. Do not expose the client during the procedure.
This reduces the risk of the client becoming chilled or needlessly exposed.

12 Paying particular attention to the client's comfort, put on *back-opening* garments as so:

a Insert your hand into the sleeve from the wrist cuff, and gently grasp the client's hand.
Grasping the client's hand and guiding it through the sleeve of the garment will make getting dressed easier and will minimize the risk of the client's fingers getting caught in the garment's sleeve.

b Slide the garment onto the arm and shoulder of the affected side, pulling the client's hand through the sleeve.
By following these steps, you save time and energy for both the client and you, and the client is less likely to become tired.

c Bring the sides of the garment to the back.

d Turn the client toward you:

i Bring one side of the garment to the client's back (**FIGURE 31–19, *A***).

ii Turn the client away from you.

iii Bring the other side of the garment to the client's back (**FIGURE 31–19, *B***).

iv Fasten buttons, snaps, ties, or zippers.

v Place the client back into the supine position.

13 Put on the *front-opening* garments as so:

a Slide the garment onto the arm and shoulder on the affected side by grasping the client's hand through the garment's sleeve.

Continued

Dressing a Client—cont'd

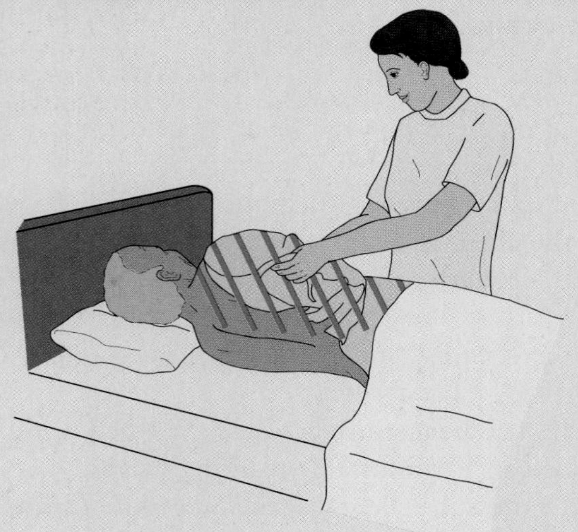

FIGURE 31–19 A

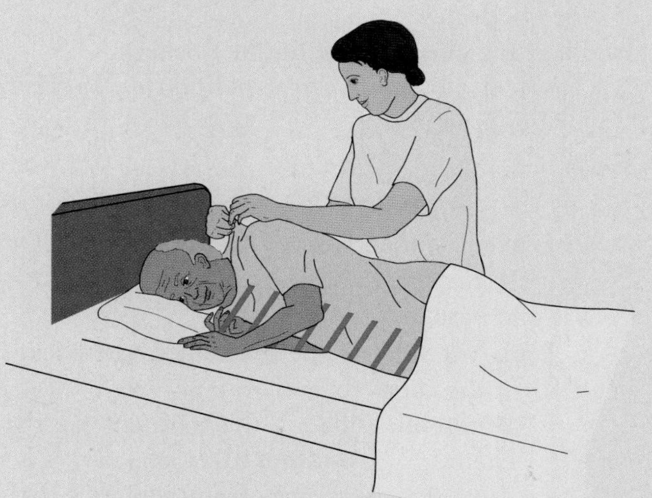

FIGURE 31–19 B

b If the client can assist you, raise the client's head and shoulders. Bring the side of the garment around to the back. Help the client lie down. Slide the garment onto the arm and shoulder of the unaffected side.

c If the client is not able to raise the head and shoulders:
  i Turn the client toward you.
  ii Tuck the garment under the client.
  iii Turn the client away from you.
  iv Pull the garment out from under the client.
  v Turn the client back to the supine position.
  vi Slide the garment over the arm and shoulder of the unaffected side.

d Fasten buttons, snaps, ties, or zippers.

14 Paying particular attention to the client's comfort, put on *pullover* garments as so:
  a Place the client in the supine position.
  b Bring the neck of the garment over the head.
  c Slide the arm and shoulder of the garment onto the client's affected side by gently grasping the client's hand through the client's sleeve.
  d Raise the client's head and shoulders.
  e Bring the garment down.
  f Slide the arm and shoulder of the garment onto the unaffected side.
  g If the client is not able to raise the head and shoulders off the bed:
    i Turn the client toward you.
    ii Tuck the garment under the client.
    iii Turn the client away from you.
    iv Pull the garment out from under the client.
    v Place the client in the supine position.
    vi Slide the arm and shoulder of the garment onto the unaffected side.
  h Fasten buttons, snaps, ties, or zippers.

15 Paying particular attention to the client's comfort, put socks and footwear on the client.
It is important to ensure comfort measures such as (a) ensuring that toes are not caught in the sock's fibres, (b) eliminating bunching, and (c) eliminating twisting.

Continued

Dressing a Client—cont'd

16 Paying particular attention to the client's comfort, put pants or slacks on the client as so:
   a Slide the pants over the feet and up the legs.
   b Ask the client to raise the hips and buttocks off the bed.
   c Bring the pants up over the buttocks and hips.
   d Ask the client to lower the hips and buttocks.
   e If the client is not able to raise the hips and buttocks:
      i Turn the client onto the unaffected side.
      ii Pull the pants over the buttock and hip on the affected side.
      iii Turn the client onto the affected side.
      iv Pull the pants over the buttock and hip on the unaffected side.
      v Place the client in the supine position.
   f Fasten buttons, ties, snaps, zipper, and belt buckle.

17 If the client has a urinary catheter and leg bag (see Chapter 32), ensure that the catheter tubing is not kinked or pulling.
Kinked or stretched urinary tubing could lead to pain and injury to the client. If urine is not able to drain properly, there is an increased risk for urinary tract infection.

18 Help the client get out of bed. If the client stays in bed, do the following:
   a Cover the client. Remove the bath blanket or bedspread.
   b Provide for safety and comfort.
   c Return the bed to its lowest position. Follow the care plan for bed rail use.*

POST-PROCEDURE

19 Place the call bell within reach.*
This provides an easy, safe way for the client to contact staff if necessary.

20 Remove privacy measures.

21 Follow employer policy for handling soiled linen.
Proper handling and disposal of soiled linen decrease the risk for pathogen spread.

22 Practise proper hand hygiene.

Report and Record your actions and observations, according to employer policy.
This is done for legal reasons and to keep the rest of the health care team informed.

*Steps marked with an asterisk may not apply in community settings.

Changing Hospital Gowns

Hospitalized clients wear hospital gowns, especially when they are receiving IV therapy. Some facilities and agencies have special gowns for IV therapy that have openings along the sleeve and close with ties, snaps, or Velcro, but many facilities and agencies still use standard hospital gowns. If your client is wearing a special gown for IV therapy, use the procedure for changing gowns described below.

If the client has an IV pump that controls the infusion and is wearing a standard hospital gown, ***do not use this procedure***. To avoid pulling on the IV, the client is usually dressed with the arm with the IV line outside the sleeve.

Changing the Gown of a Client With Intravenous Tubing

123

Advocate on behalf of the client's quality of life by promoting:

Dignity • Independence • Preferences • Privacy • Safety *(see BOX 1–4, on p. 17)*

PRE-PROCEDURE

1 Identify the client, according to employer policy.
This eliminates the possibility of mistaking one client for another.
2 Explain the procedure to the client.
3 Practise proper hand hygiene.
4 Collect a **clean gown** and **a bath blanket** or bedspread.
It is important to plan before starting any procedure. By collecting all the necessary equipment beforehand, you will not have to leave your client's side and can eliminate wasting time and energy in obtaining the forgotten equipment.
5 Provide for privacy.
6 Practise proper hand hygiene.
7 Raise the bed to a comfortable working height.*

PROCEDURE

8 Lower the bed rail near you if it is up.*
9 Position the client in a supine position. Cover the client with a bath blanket or bedspread. Fan-fold other linen to the foot of the bed.
This prevents the rest of the bed from getting wet if the IV tubing accidentally comes apart.
10 Untie the gown. Free the parts that the client is lying on.
This procedure will be easier to perform if the client is not lying on clothing.
11 Remove the gown from the arm with no IV tubing.
It is easier to start with this arm.
12 Gather up the sleeve of the arm with the IV tubing. Slide it over the IV site and tubing. Remove the arm and hand from the sleeve.
This reduces the risk of the client's sleeve catching on the IV tubing. (**FIGURE 31–20, *A***).
13 Keep the sleeve gathered. Slide your arm along the tubing to the bag (**FIGURE 31–20, *B***).
14 Remove the IV bag from the pole. Slide the bag and tubing through the sleeve (see **FIGURE 31–20, C**). Do not pull on the tubing. Keep the bag above the client.
Pulling on the tubing could dislodge the IV catheter from the client's arm.

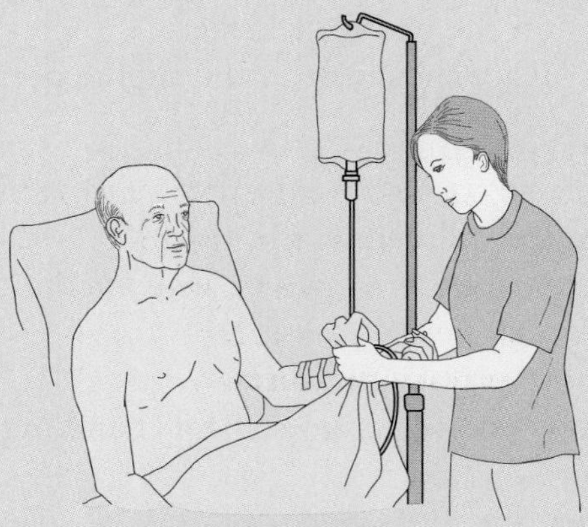

FIGURE 31–20 A

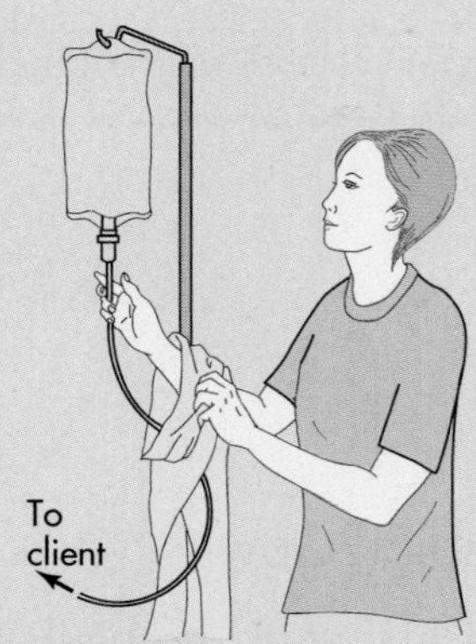

FIGURE 31–20 B, Slip the gathered sleeve along the IV tubing to the bag.

Continued

Changing the Gown of a Client With Intravenous Tubing—cont'd

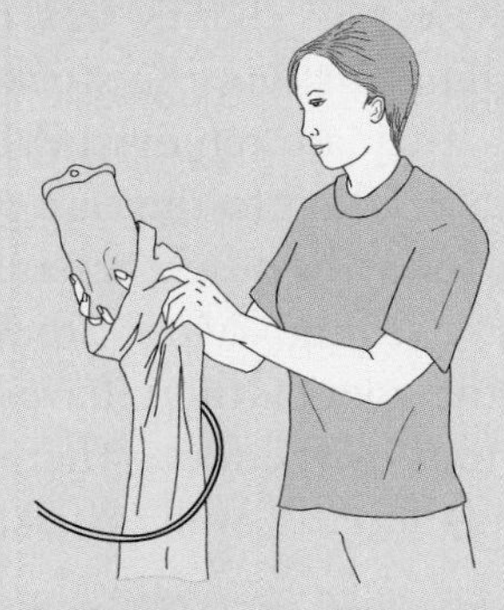

FIGURE 31–20 C, Remove the IV bag from the pole and pass it through the sleeve.

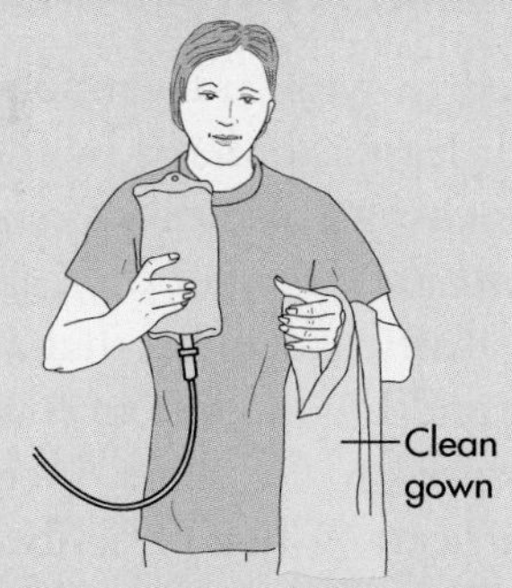

FIGURE 31–20 D, Slip the gathered sleeve of the clean gown over the IV bag.

15 Hang the IV bag on the pole.
The IV bag needs to be higher than the client's heart, or the IV fluid will not infuse properly.

16 Gather the sleeve of the clean gown that will go on the arm with the IV infusion.
Gathering the sleeve will make it easier to put it on the client.

17 Remove the bag from the pole. Slip the gathered sleeve of the clean gown over the IV bag at the shoulder part of the gown (see **FIGURE 31–20, *D***). Hang the bag. It is important that the IV apparatus is not disconnected or the tubing twisted or caught on anything.
This eliminates the risk of dislodging the IV needle from the client's arm.

18 Slide the gathered sleeve over the tubing, hand, arm, and IV site. Then slide it onto the shoulder.
By gathering the sleeve, you are able to perform this part in one easy step.

19 Put the other side of the gown on. Fasten the back by rolling the client onto the side. Return the client to a supine position.

20 Cover the client. Remove the bath blanket or bedspread if no longer needed.

POST-PROCEDURE

21 Provide for safety and comfort.

22 Return the bed to its lowest position. Follow the care plan for bed rail use.*
This reduces the risk for client injury.

23 Place the call bell within reach.*
This provides an easy, safe way for the client to contact staff if necessary.

24 Remove privacy measures.

25 Follow employer policy for handling soiled linen.
Proper handling and disposal of soiled linens decrease the risk for pathogen spread.

26 Practise proper hand hygiene.

Report and Record your actions and observations according to employer policy. (In facilities, ask your supervisor to check the flow rate.)
This is done for legal reasons and to keep the rest of the health care team informed.

*Steps marked with an asterisk may not apply in community settings.

APPLYING ELASTIC ANTI-EMBOLIC STOCKINGS AND BANDAGES

Some clients need to wear anti-embolic stockings or bandages on their legs, as ordered by their physicians. **Anti-embolic stockings**, also called *compression stockings* or *thromboembolic devices* (*TED*), are close-fitting, circular, knitted, elastic stockings that are designed to prevent swelling and blood clots in lower extremities by exerting pressure on the veins, increasing venous blood flow to the heart. When prescribed, these stockings must be applied as part of the client's daily dressing routine. Clients with circulatory disorders and heart disease and those on bed rest are at risk for blood clots. A blood clot (*thrombus*) can form in deep leg veins, break loose, travel through the bloodstream, and lodge in a distant vessel. If the clot lodges in the lungs, severe respiratory problems or death can result.

Applied incorrectly, anti-embolic stockings can harm the client. Therefore, you may be asked to apply them only on clients in stable condition. It is your responsibility to know and follow your employer's policy, the stocking manufacturer's instructions, and the client's care plan.

Applying Anti-Embolic Stockings

Anti-embolic stockings come in a variety of sizes and lengths (thigh-high or knee-high). The care plan lists the correct size to use. Stockings are applied in the morning before the client gets out of bed, as, otherwise, the client's legs can swell from sitting or standing, making the stockings very difficult to put on. They are removed every 8 hours for 30 minutes or according to the care plan. The client lies in bed whenever the stockings are off to prevent the legs from swelling. Most stockings have an opening near the toes. Others have an opening at the top or bottom of the foot. The opening is used to check circulation as well as skin colour and temperature.

The client usually has two pairs of stockings. One pair is washed while the client wears the other pair. Wash the stockings by hand with a mild soap, and then hang them to dry.

Make sure that the stockings are smooth, not bunched up or binding, and without twists, creases, or wrinkles after you apply them. Bunching, binding, or twisting stockings can affect circulation, and creases and wrinkles can cause skin breakdown. Report and record the following observations after applying elastic stockings:

- Skin colour and skin temperature
- Leg and foot swelling
- Signs of skin breakdown
- Complaints of pain, tingling, or numbness

Applying Anti-Embolic Stockings 123

Advocate on behalf of the client's quality of life by promoting:

Dignity • Independence • Preferences • Privacy • Safety *(see BOX 1–4, on p. 17)*

PRE-PROCEDURE

1. Identify the client, according to employer policy.
   This eliminates the possibility of mistaking one client for another.
2. Explain the procedure to the client.
3. Practise proper hand hygiene.
4. Collect **anti-embolic stockings** in the correct size and length and **utility gloves**.
   Anti-embolic stockings that are too tight will constrict the client's blood circulation. If the stockings are too large, they will not be effective at improving venous blood supply back to the heart.
5. Provide for privacy.
6. Practise proper hand hygiene.
7. Raise the bed to a comfortable working height and lower the head of the bed.*
   Raising the bed will reduce your risk for back strain. Lowering the head of the bed will make it easier to slide the client up to a better position.

Continued

Applying Anti-Embolic Stockings—cont'd

PROCEDURE

8 Lower the bed rail near you if it is up.
It is too difficult to work over a raised bed rail.
9 While the client is still in bed, place the client in the supine position.
These types of stockings should be applied before the client gets out of bed, before the blood has had a chance to collect in the feet.
10 Fan-fold the top linen toward the client's thighs, exposing the client's legs.
This exposes only the areas that you need access to.
11 a Apply the utility gloves.
Wearing gloves makes anti-embolic stockings easier to apply and to smooth out.
b Turn the stocking inside out down to the heel (**FIGURE 31–21, *A***).
This prevents the stocking from bunching, tearing, or twisting.
12 Slip the foot of the stocking over the toes, foot, and heel (see **FIGURE 31–21, *B***).

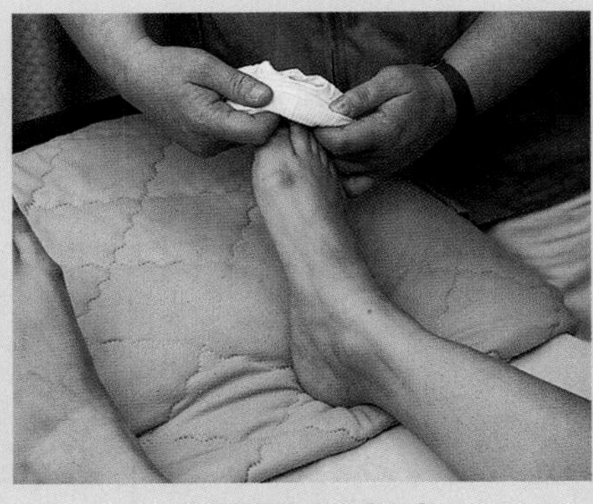

FIGURE 31–21 A

13 Grasp the stocking top. Slip it over the foot and heel. Pull it up the leg. It turns right side out as it is pulled up. The stocking must be even and snug (see **FIGURE 31–21, *C***).
14 Remove twists, creases, bunching, or wrinkles.
These could decrease the effectiveness of the stocking and can cause harm to the client.
15 Repeat steps 11b through 14 for the other leg.

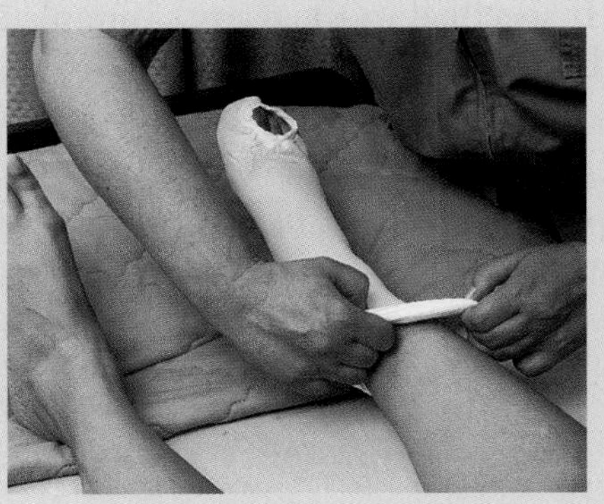

FIGURE 31–21 B

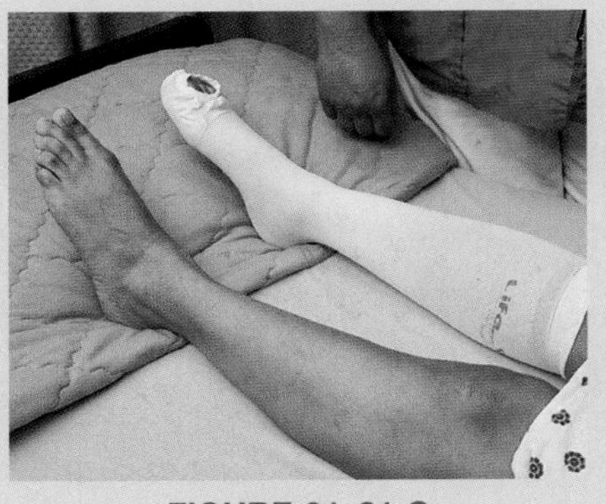

FIGURE 31–21 C

POST-PROCEDURE

16 Cover the client.
17 Provide for safety and comfort.
18 Place the call bell within reach.*
This provides an easy, safe way for the client to contact staff if necessary.
19 Return the bed to its lowest position. Follow the care plan for bed rail use.*
This reduces the risk for client injury.
20 Remove privacy measures.
21 Practise proper hand hygiene.

Report and Record your actions and observations, according to employer policy.
This is done for legal reasons and to keep the rest of the health care team informed.

*Steps marked with an asterisk may not apply in community settings.

Applying Elastic Bandages

Elastic bandages are applied to the upper or lower extremities and have the same purposes as anti-embolic stockings; they may also hold dressings in place.

The bandage is applied from the lower (distal) part of the extremity to the top (proximal) part. Your supervisor and the care plan will tell you which area to bandage and the proper width of the bandage to use for that client. If the roll of bandage is not long enough to cover the part, another roll of bandage may be added.

Elastic bandages are removed every 8 hours for 30 minutes. If specified in the client's care plan, bandages may be washed in mild soap and water, rinsed well, patted dry, and then hung up to dry overnight. Cleaning properly is especially important if the client perspires on the bandage or has soiled the bandage in any way.

Follow these guidelines when applying elastic bandages:

- Use the correct length and width.
- Position the body part in good alignment.
- Face the client during the procedure.
- Expose fingers or toes, if possible, to allow circulation checks.
- Apply the bandage with firm, even pressure.
- Make sure the bandage is firm and snug. It must not be tight, as a tight bandage can affect circulation.
- Check the colour and temperature of the extremity every hour.
- Reapply a loose, wrinkled, moist, or soiled bandage.

Report and record the following observations after applying elastic bandages:

- Skin colour and skin temperature
- Swelling in the leg and foot
- Signs of skin breakdown
- Complaints of pain, tingling, or numbness

Applying Elastic Bandages 123

Advocate on behalf of the client's quality of life by promoting:

Dignity • Independence • Preferences • Privacy • Safety *(see BOX 1–4, on p. 17)*

PRE-PROCEDURE

1 Identify the client, according to employer policy.
This eliminates the possibility of mistaking one client for another.
2 Explain the procedure to the client.
3 Practise proper hand hygiene.
4 Collect the following supplies:
☐ **Elastic bandage**, as directed by the care plan
☐ **Tape or metal clips** (unless the bandage has Velcro)
It is important to plan thoroughly before starting any procedure. By collecting all the necessary equipment beforehand, you will not have to leave your client's side and can eliminate wasting time and energy in obtaining the forgotten equipment.
5 Provide for privacy.
6 Practise proper hand hygiene.
7 Raise the bed to a comfortable working height.*
This reduces the risk for client injury.

Continued

Applying Elastic Bandages—cont'd

PROCEDURE

8 Lower the bed rail near you if it is up.
9 Help the client to a comfortable position. Expose the part you will bandage.
10 Make sure the area is clean and dry.
If the area that is to be bandaged is moist, it can harbour pathogens and cause a skin infection in the bandaged area.
11 Hold the bandage so that the roll is up. The loose end must be on the bottom (**FIGURE 31–22, *A***).
This makes properly applying the bandage easier.
12 Apply the bandage to the smallest part of the wrist, foot, ankle, or knee.
13 Make two turns around the part (**FIGURE 31–22, *B***).
This holds the bandage securely in place.
14 Make overlapping spiral turns in an upward direction. Each turn overlaps about two thirds of the previous turn (**FIGURE 31–22, *C***).
Applying the bandage in this manner will encourage blood flow to be returned to the heart. Applying it incorrectly can cause swelling of the hand or foot.
15 Apply the bandage smoothly with firm, even pressure. The bandage must be snug but not tight.
The bandage is designed to be applied this way.
16 Secure the bandage in place with Velcro, tape, or a clip. Ensure that the bandaged area does not put pressure on the clip.
Pressure on the clip can cause an injury to the underlying tissues.
17 Check the fingers or toes for coldness or cyanosis (bluish colour). Ask the client about any pain, itching, numbness, or tingling. Report and record any abnormal observations. Remove the bandage if you note any, and report your observations to your supervisor.
These are signs that blood circulation to the extremities is decreased because the bandage is too tight. If the bandage is not removed and the area checked immediately, serious problems may occur.

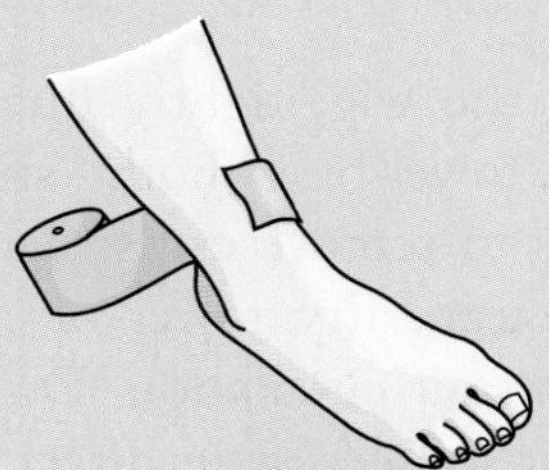

FIGURE 31–22 A

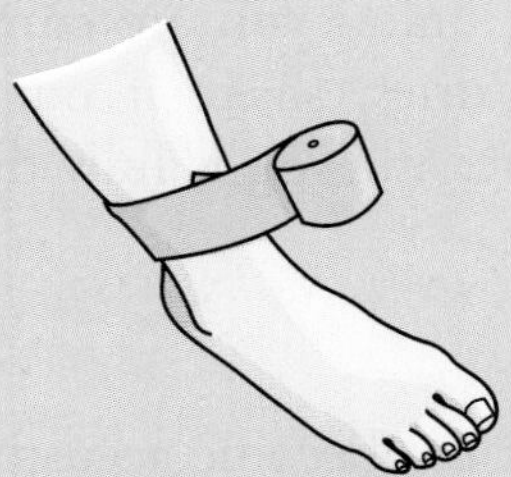

FIGURE 31–22 B

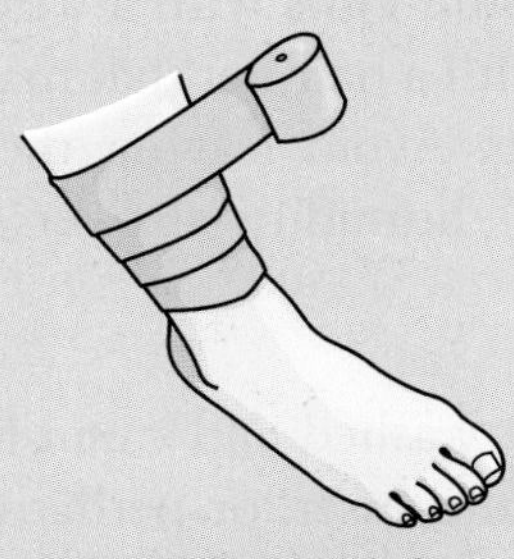

FIGURE 31–22 C

POST-PROCEDURE

18 Follow steps 16 through 21 of the *Applying Anti-Embolic Stockings* procedure on page 680.

Report and Record your actions and observations, according to employer policy.
This is done for legal reasons and to keep the rest of the health care team informed.

*Steps marked with an asterisk may not apply in community settings.

COMPASSIONATE CARE

When helping with grooming and dressing, remember to focus on the whole client rather than only on the task. Promote the client's dignity, independence, preferences, privacy, and safety (see the *Providing Compassionate Care: Assisting Clients With Grooming and Dressing* box).

Care of Wigs

Wigs are worn for a variety of reasons. Some Orthodox Jewish married women remove all their hair and wear only a head covering, while some others wear a wig to cover their hair. Some clients may have lost their hair due to natural aging or as a result of chemotherapy treatments for cancer. Some clients may be bald from birth, and some others may have become bald after an illness or an injury to their scalp.

Whatever the reason, people—both men and women—may wear wigs for warmth, modesty, or body image. Wigs can be very expensive, so it is important to care for them properly so that they are kept clean, attractive, and comfortable. When caring for a client's wig, you should follow the maintenance steps in the client's care plan. Below are some tips on maintenance.[4]

Storage

After removing the wig, keep it on a wig stand (or head form) to maintain the shape. Smooth out straight hair or fluff curls with a wire brush or pick. Cover the wig with a hair net that maintains the style without matting. Avoid leaving the wig near heat (radiators, vents), humidity (showers), or dusty areas.

Washing

Wigs are usually washed and cared for by the client (or family), a hairdresser, or perhaps even by representatives from the store that sells specialty items such as wigs or mastectomy prosthetics. ***Because wigs can be very expensive to replace, it is important to check your agency's policies before washing a client's wig. Some agencies do not allow support workers to wash a client's wig or hairpiece.*** Shampooing frequency depends on wearing frequency. Generally, a wig should be washed after every 6 to 8 uses in warm climates or after every 12 to 15 uses in cooler ones. However, if the client is especially active, uses heavy hairspray, or lives in an especially humid climate or in one with poor air quality, the wig should be washed about once a week to remove excess perspiration and dirt.

Before washing, smooth out a straight-hair wig or fluff a curly-hair wig gently and completely with a wire brush or pick. Add a capful of wig shampoo or baby shampoo to a basin of cool (never hot) water. Immerse the wig gently and soak for 2 minutes. Rinse well by swishing in clean, cool water. Gently squeeze out excess water without twisting the wig. For extra shine and softness, apply wig conditioner and leave it on for 5 minutes. Rinse again in clean, cool water. Gently squeeze out excess water without twisting the wig.

Drying

After washing the wig, tightly finger-squeeze each curl. Gently towel-blot both straight-hair and curly-hair wigs to remove excess water. Let the wig air-dry on a clean, dry towel or on a wire head form that allows air circulation. Do not set the wig stand near heat sources or in direct sunlight. Never use blow-dryers or other heat appliances on synthetic wigs. Also, be sure not to comb, brush, or pick a wet wig unless you are completely restyling it. As the wig dries, shake it out periodically for fast drying. Once the wig is fully dry, style it in the normal manner.

Wearing

Once the client has become accustomed to the wig, the wig can be worn for daily activities. Advise the client to avoid blasts of heat on synthetic wigs—for example, when quickly opening an oven door.

Providing Compassionate Care

Assisting Clients With Grooming and Dressing

- ***Dignity.*** Being clean and well groomed helps the client maintain dignity. People often feel good about themselves when they have a neat appearance and are wearing clean clothing. When assisting with grooming, handle the client's hygiene products, shaver, hair dryer, brush and comb, perfumes, and other personal care items carefully. When handling clothing, take care not to break zippers, tear clothing, lose buttons, or cause other damage. Treat the client's property with care and respect. If damage occurs, notify your supervisor.
- ***Independence.*** Encourage the client to be as independent as possible. Provide assistance only when needed. Like other activities of daily living (ADLs), dressing and undressing stimulate circulation and increase muscle strength and flexibility. They also increase the client's confidence and self-esteem. Sometimes, allowing clients to do what they can for themselves requires patience and understanding. Give the client extra time to dress and undress independently.

  If the client has self-care devices, encourage their use. Self-care devices that promote independence with dressing and undressing include the following:
  - Button hooks (see **FIGURE 27–2, *A***, on p. 564)
  - Sock pullers (see **FIGURE 27–2, *B***)
  - Shoe removers (see **FIGURE 27–2, *C***)
  - Pantyhose aids
  - Trouser pulls
  - Pant clips
- ***Preferences.*** Encourage personal choices whenever possible. Clients will have their own grooming practices. Do not impose your standards on clients. Ask clients how they want their hair styled, what hair or shaving products they use, and what clothing they want to wear.
- ***Privacy.*** Providing for privacy is important when dressing and undressing the client. Do not expose the client when you are performing the procedures described in this chapter. Also, provide privacy when assisting with grooming.
- ***Safety.*** Remember to dress the affected side first (DAF) and remove clothing from the unaffected side first (RUF). Also, remember to check clients with elastic (anti-embolic) stockings and bandages frequently. Check for signs of reduced circulation, swelling, or skin breakdown. Report your observations to your supervisor. This information is needed to provide complete care to the client.

CHAPTER REVIEW

KEY POINTS

- Good grooming promotes comfort, a positive sense of well-being, and self-confidence while preventing infection.
- The client should be invited to participate in all grooming activities to promote the client's sense of independence. Follow the care plan carefully at all times.
- Safety of the client and the worker should always be a priority in all grooming activities.
- The support worker must observe for any problems in the client's hair or scalp and report any abnormal findings to the appropriate supervisor.
- Brushing, combing, and shampooing hair are necessary in order to maintain healthy and shiny hair. The support worker should be respectful of a client's styling preferences.
- Only a professional barber or stylist should cut a client's hair, not the support worker.
- When shampooing hair, keep in mind that many older clients and those with disabilities have limited range of motion in their necks and upper backs. Shampooing methods should, therefore, be chosen mindfully.
- When shaving a client, you should always first check the client's care plan in case the client has a bruising or bleeding problem.
- Support workers should be aware of a client's potential foot and nail problems and should report them immediately to the appropriate supervisor. Foot and nail care should be performed with any such problems in mind.
- When undressing or dressing a client or changing an incontinence brief, support workers should follow the DIPPS principles.
- Elastic bandages or anti-embolic stockings can cause circulation problems if they are applied improperly. All steps need to be carefully followed to prevent these issues.

CRITICAL THINKING IN PRACTICE

Mr. Risk has very long, thick, and curling toenails and very foul-smelling feet. You would like him to feel better, so you would like to provide foot care. Is foot care within your scope of practice as a support worker? What is (or is not) allowed? How would you find out if you are unsure?

REVIEW QUESTIONS

Answers to these questions are at the bottom of the next page.

Circle the BEST answer.

1. Mr. Lee has alopecia. This is:
   A. Excessive body hair
   B. Dry, white flakes on the scalp
   C. An infestation of lice
   D. Hair loss
2. When brushing hair that is not matted or tangled, start at:
   A. The forehead, and brush backward
   B. The hair ends
   C. The scalp, and brush toward the hair tips
   D. The back of the neck, and brush forward
3. Brushing is important to keep the hair:
   A. Soft and shiny
   B. Clean
   C. Free from lice
   D. Long
4. Mr. Lee wants his hair washed. You should:
   A. Wash his hair during his shower
   B. Wash his hair at the sink
   C. Shampoo him in bed
   D. Follow the care plan
5. When shaving Mr. Lee with a blade razor, you need to do the following:
   A. Remove any existing beard or moustache
   B. Moisten the beard before shaving to soften it
   C. Shave perpendicular to the direction of hair growth
   D. Shave when the skin is dry

6. Mr. Lee is nicked during shaving. Your first action should be to:
   A. Practise proper hand hygiene
   B. Apply direct pressure
   C. Tell your supervisor
   D. Apply a bandage

7. When shaving a man's face, you should shave:
   A. Left to right, from one side to another
   B. Right to left, from one side to another
   C. Up to down from chin to neck
   D. Down to up from neck to chin

8. Fingernails are cut with:
   A. Toenail clippers
   B. Scissors
   C. A nail file
   D. Nail clippers

9. You should never attempt to trim nails on clients who are:
   A. Alert and oriented
   B. Diabetic
   C. Paralyzed
   D. Awake

10. Anti-embolic stockings are used to:
   A. Bring down swelling in the legs
   B. Improve the appearance of the legs
   C. Exert pressure on the veins
   D. Reduce circulation

11. Anti-embolic stockings are applied:
   A. Before the client gets out of bed
   B. When the client is standing
   C. After the client's shower or tub bath
   D. Before the client goes to sleep

12. When applying an elastic bandage:
   A. The body needs to be in good alignment
   B. The fingers or toes are covered
   C. It is applied from the largest to the smallest part of an extremity
   D. It is applied from the upper to the lower part of the extremity

13. When dressing a client who has hemiplegia (paralysis) on the right side, you should place the client's right arm inside the sleeve:
   A. First
   B. Last
   C. Not place her arm in a sleeve
   D. You should not be dressing clients with hemiplegia.

Circle T if the answer is true, and circle F if the answer is false.

14. T F You can shave a client's beard and moustache if you think he would be more comfortable without facial hair.
15. T F When dressing a client, you should dress the unaffected side first.
16. T F Clothing is removed from the unaffected side first.
17. T F The client chooses what to wear.
18. T F Wigs should never be washed. They should only be dry-cleaned.

Answers: 1.D, 2.C, 3.A, 4.D, 5.B, 6.B, 7.D, 8.D, 9.B, 10.C, 11.A, 12.A, 13.A, 14.F, 15.F, 16.T, 17.T, 18.F

CHAPTER 32

Urinary Elimination

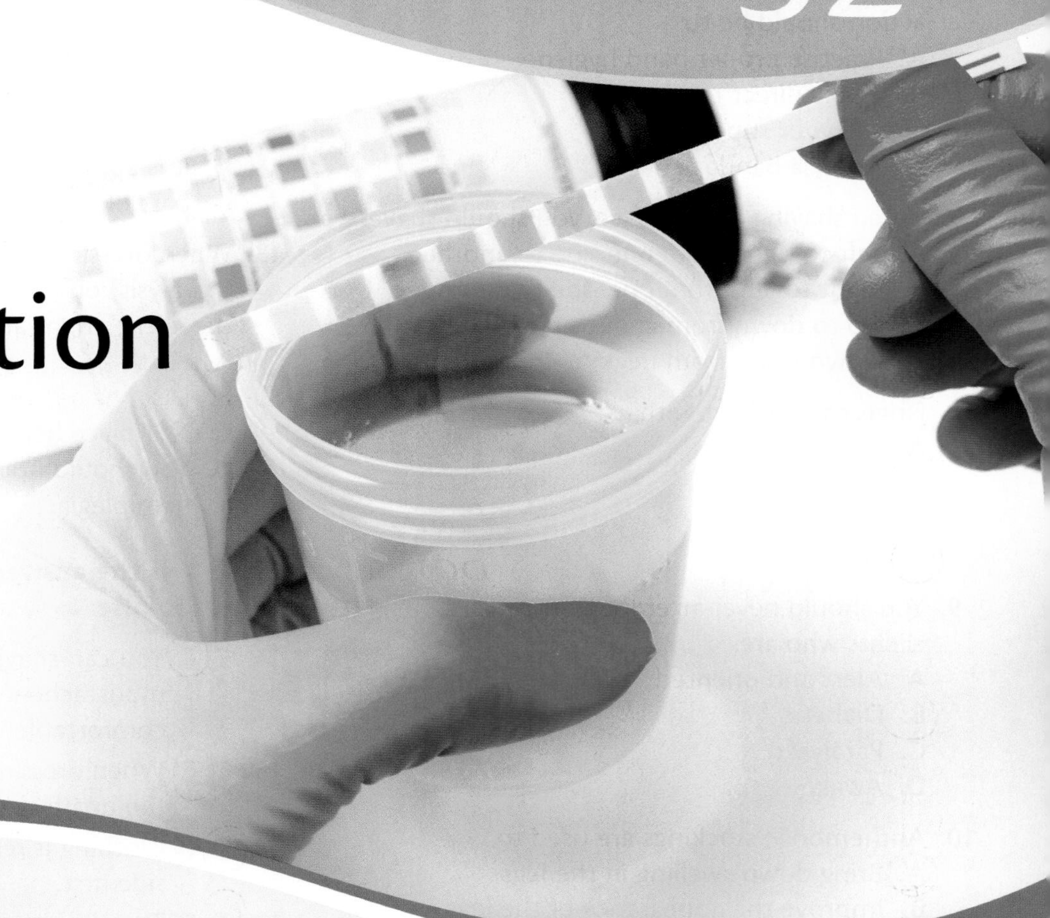

OBJECTIVES

After reading this chapter, the learner should be able to do the following:

- Identify the characteristics of normal urine.
- Describe the guidelines for maintaining normal urinary elimination.
- List the observations to make about urine.
- Describe urinary incontinence and the care required.
- Explain why catheters are used.
- Explain the differences among straight, in-dwelling, suprapubic, and condom catheters.
- Describe the guidelines for caring for clients with in-dwelling catheters.
- Describe the methods of bladder training.
- Describe the guidelines for collecting urine specimens.
- Explain how to care for a client with a ureterostomy.
- Apply the procedures described in this chapter to clinical practice properly.

KEY TERMS

catheterization The process of inserting a catheter. *p. 702*
condom catheter A sheath that slides over the penis; tubing connects the catheter and drainage bag. *p. 713*
dysuria Painful or difficult (*dys*) urination (*uria*). *p. 692*
Foley catheter See **in-dwelling catheter**. *p. 702*
fracture pan A small, thin, rimmed bedpan that is about 1 cm deep at one end. Also called a slipper pan. *p. 691*
functional incontinence Urinary incontinence caused by physical conditions or environmental barriers that prevent the client from reaching the toilet in time. *p. 700*
glucosuria Glucose, a type of sugar (*glucos*) in the urine (*uria*). *p. 720*
hematuria Blood (*hemat*) in the urine (*uria*). *p. 692*
ileal conduit An artificial bladder made out of a section of the ileum. *p. 724*
in-dwelling catheter A tube (plastic, latex, or other material) that is inserted into the bladder through the urinary meatus and urethra. A balloon within the catheter that is inflated after insertion prevents the catheter from slipping out of the bladder. Also known as a **Foley** or **retention catheter**. *p. 702*
ketones A by-product of fatty acid metabolism. *p. 721*
micturition See **urination**. *p. 690*
oliguria Scant amount (*olig*) of urine (*uria*)—usually less than 500 mL in 24 hours. *p. 692*
overflow incontinence The leaking of urine when the bladder is too full. *p. 700*
polyuria The production of abnormally large amounts (*poly*) of urine (*uria*). *p. 692*
reflex incontinence The loss of urine at predictable intervals. *p. 700*
retention catheter See **in-dwelling catheter**. *p. 702*
slipper pan See **fracture pan**. *p. 691*
stoma A surgically created opening from a portion of the body cavity to the outside environment. *p. 724*
straight catheter A catheter that is inserted to drain the bladder and is then removed. *p. 702*
stress incontinence The leaking of urine during exercise and certain movements. *p. 700*
suprapubic catheter A catheter that is surgically inserted into the bladder through the abdomen. *p. 702*
ureterostomy An artificial opening (*stomy*) between the ureter (*uretero*) and the abdomen. *p. 724*
urge incontinence The loss of urine in response to a sudden, urgent need to void. *p. 700*
urinary frequency The need to urinate at frequent intervals. *p. 692*
urinary incontinence The inability to control the passage of urine from the bladder; the loss of bladder control. *p. 692*
urinary urgency The need to void immediately. *p. 692*
urination The process of emptying urine from the bladder. Also known as micturition or voiding. *p. 690*
voiding See **urination**. *p. 690*

Eliminating waste is one of the important functions of the body. The body's waste products are removed through various body systems—digestive, respiratory, integumentary, and urinary. The digestive system gets rid of solid wastes from the body; the lungs get rid of carbon dioxide; the skin sweats, thus getting rid of water and other substances; and the urinary system removes waste products from blood (which come from body cells after breaking down and metabolizing food for energy) and maintains the body's water balance (see Chapter 17 to review the urinary system).

When assisting a client with elimination, you may be exposed to urine or stool (feces) directly or indirectly—for example, on linen and clothing that are soiled with these bodily fluids. Protect yourself and your client by following the rules of medical asepsis and Standard Practices (see Chapter 23). Follow the infection control precautions in **BOX 32–1** when assisting with elimination.

NORMAL URINATION

The healthy adult excretes about 1 500 mL (millilitres) of urine a day. Factors such as age, disease, the amount and kinds of fluid ingested, dietary salt, and medications affect urine production. Some

BOX 32–1 Transmission-Based Practices When Assisting With Elimination

- Perform hand hygiene before and after wearing gloves.
- Wear gloves whenever there is a risk for contact with urine, feces, secretions, or mucous membranes—for example, when doing the following:
  - Assisting clients who have diarrhea, urinary incontinence (p. 701), or fecal incontinence (see Chapter 33)
  - Handling or cleaning bedpans, urinals, commodes, toilets, or bathroom floors
  - Handling soiled clothing or linens
  - Changing incontinence products
  - Measuring clients' output
  - Collecting specimens
- Change gloves between procedures on the same client, as the gloves may be contaminated. For example, change gloves after giving perineal care and before cleaning an in-dwelling catheter.
- Remove contaminated gloves before touching a clean surface. For example, remove soiled gloves before raising the bed rails.
- Remember that soiled incontinence briefs should never be placed on the floor. Placing briefs on the floor is both unhygienic (see Chapter 23) and a source of offensive odour. If you cannot leave the client while you are changing incontinence briefs, you should place the soiled briefs at the foot of the bed (never on the floor!), ensure the client's safety and privacy, and then discard the briefs into the proper container. Ensure that the lid is placed on the container for odour control.
- Wear a protective apron or gown if there is a chance that you might be sprayed or splashed with blood, body fluids, secretions, or excretions—for example, when you are emptying bedpans or commodes.
- Cover bedpans and tightly cap urinals when carrying them. Dispose of body wastes immediately and carefully to avoid splashing. If splashing occurs, clean the area immediately. Clean and disinfect bedpans, urinals, and commodes immediately after use.
- Place soiled disposable materials in leak-proof plastic bags. Seal them tightly. Immediately discard the bags, according to employer policy.
- Place soiled linen and clothing in a leak-proof plastic bag. Launder it as soon as possible, according to employer policy. In a client's home, wash soiled linen separately from other laundry.

substances such as coffee, tea, alcohol, and some medications increase urine production. A diet high in salt causes the body to retain water; when water is retained, less urine is produced.

Urination, **micturition**, and **voiding** all mean the process of emptying urine from the bladder. The amount of fluid intake, personal habits, and available toilet facilities, as well as activity, work, and illness, affect frequency of urination. People usually void at bedtime, after getting up, and before meals. Some people void every 2 to 3 hours, and some others void less frequently. The need to void at night causes sleep disturbance in many people. You should be aware that although many of the clients in facilities are incontinent of urine, ***incontinence is not a normal part of aging***.

Clients may need help with urinary elimination. When assisting a client with toileting, follow the Transmission-Based Practices (see BOX 32–1). Some clients may need help getting to the bathroom, and others may use bedpans, urinals, or commodes. Follow the guidelines listed in BOX 32–2 to help maintain normal elimination. Remember that it is your responsibility to follow the client's care plan when assisting with urinary elimination.

Observations to Make About Urine

Urine normally appears pale yellow, straw-coloured, or amber and is clear with no particles. A faint odour is normal. Observe urine for colour, clarity, odour, amount, and particles.

Some foods normally affect urine colour. Red food dyes, beets, blackberries, and rhubarb will make urine look red, and carrots and sweet potatoes cause bright yellow coloration. Certain medications also cause changes in urine colour. Asparagus causes a change in the odour of urine.

BOX 32–2 Guidelines for Maintaining Normal Elimination

- Practise medical asepsis, and follow Standard Practices.
- Provide fluids as instructed by the care plan.
- Monitor the client's normal voiding routines and habits. Check with your supervisor and the care plan.
- Help the client to the bathroom when the request is made, or provide a commode, bedpan, or urinal. The need to void may be urgent, so be considerate of that.
- Help the client assume a normal position for voiding if possible. Women sit or squat, and most men stand.
- For the client's comfort, warm the bedpan or urinal under warm water.
- Cover the client for warmth and privacy.
- Ensure privacy. Pull the curtain around the bed, close room and bathroom doors, and pull drapes or window shades. Leave the room if the client can be left alone.
- To ease the discomfort of clients who feel embarrassed about voiding with others close by, tell them that running sink water, flushing of the toilet, or sounds from the TV or radio mask urination sounds.
- Remain nearby if the client is weak or unsteady.
- Place the call bell (in facilities) and toilet tissue within reach.
- Allow enough time to void; do not rush the client. However, do not allow the client to lie on a bedpan for a long time, as it may cause skin excoriation (irritation) or pressure ulcers.
- Promote relaxation. Some people like to read during elimination.
- If the client has difficulty initiating urination, you might try placing the client's fingers in some warm water or wrapping a warm blanket around the client.
- Provide thorough perineal care as needed.
- Assist with proper hand hygiene after voiding by providing a wash basin, soap, washcloth, and towel.
- Assist the client to the bathroom or offer the bedpan, urinal, or commode at regular times in case the client is too embarrassed or too weak to ask.

Report to your supervisor if you observe urine that looks or smells abnormal (TABLE 32–1). Do not discard the urine, but cover it with a labelled paper towel, and keep it in the client's bathroom or in the soiled utility room until your supervisor can observe it or gives you permission to dispose of it.

Report complaints of urgency, burning on urination, or dysuria—painful or difficult (*dys*) urination (*uria*)—usually caused by urinary tract infection (UTI). Refer to BOX 32–3, on page 693, for some common causes of UTIs.

Bedpans

Bedpans are used for clients who are not able to get out of bed. Female clients use bedpans for voiding and bowel movements, and male clients use them only for bowel movements. Bedpans are made of plastic, stainless steel, or even sometimes a biodegradable cardboard. Stainless steel bedpans are often cold, so it is best to warm up the bedpan before use by holding it under warm running water. Wipe it dry with a paper towel.

With your supervisor's permission, you can lightly dust the bedpan rim with talcum powder to avoid the bedpan's sticking to the client's skin after use. ***Powder should not be used if a urine specimen is needed.*** You may also want to protect the bed and linen by placing a waterproof pad or incontinence pad under the bedpan before use.

A **fracture pan**—commonly called a **slipper pan**—has a thinner rim and is only about 1 cm deep

TABLE 32–1 Common Urinary Elimination Problems

	Definition	Causes
Dysuria	Painful or difficult (*dys*) urination (*uria*)	Urinary tract infection, trauma, urinary tract obstruction
Hematuria	Blood (*hemat*) in urine (*uria*)	Kidney disease, urinary tract infection, trauma
Nocturia	Frequent urination (*uria*) at night (*noct*)	Increased perfusion to kidneys when lying down, resulting in increased urine production; excessive fluid intake; kidney disease; disease of the prostate; congestive heart failure
Oliguria	Scant amount (*olig*) of urine (*uria*)—usually less than 500 mL in 24 hours	Inadequate fluid intake, shock, burns, kidney disease, heart failure
Polyuria	The production of abnormally large amounts (*poly*) of urine (*uria*)	Medications, excessive fluid intake, diabetes, hormone imbalance
Urinary frequency	The need to urinate at frequent intervals	Excessive fluid intake, bladder infections, pressure on the bladder, medications
Overflow incontinence	The leaking of urine when the bladder is too full	Weak bladder muscles, resulting in incomplete emptying of the bladder; blockage or obstruction; neurological conditions such as diabetic neuropathy, multiple sclerosis, and spinal cord injuries
Urinary incontinence	Inability to control the passage of urine from the bladder	Trauma, disease, urinary tract infections, reproductive or urinary tract surgeries, aging, fecal impaction, constipation, not getting to the bathroom in time
Urinary urgency	The need to void immediately	Urinary tract infection, fear of incontinence, full bladder, stress

Adapted from Birchenall, J., & Streight, E. (1997). *Mosby's textbook for the home care aide* (p. 262). St. Louis, MO: Mosby.

at one end (**FIGURE 32–1**). The smaller end is placed under the buttocks (**FIGURE 32–2**). Fracture pans are used by the following:

- Clients in casts
- Clients in traction
- Clients with limited back motion
- Clients with fragile bones or painful joints
- Clients who have had a hip fracture

Follow medical asepsis and Standard Practices when handling bedpans and their contents. Bedpans must be thoroughly cleaned after each use. Follow employer policy.

BOX 32–3 Common Causes of Urinary Tract Infections

The urinary system is structured to prevent infections, but occasionally (or frequently in some people), people do get UTIs. UTIs can occur when bacteria enter the urinary tract through the urethra, the body's urine portal to the outside.

One type of UTI, specifically infection of the bladder (*cystitis*), is more common in women than men because the distance between the urethral opening to the anus is shorter in women, as is the distance from the urethral opening to the bladder.

Another type of UTI, infection of the urethra (*urethritis*), can occur when bacteria from the gastro-intestinal system and anus are spread to the urethra, usually through sexual practices. Both men and women can get infections of the urethra.

In seniors, UTIs can be caused by inadequate emptying of the bladder, sometimes because of blockages in the urinary tract, neurological causes (such as stroke), certain medications, or the presence of a urinary drainage catheter that has introduced hostile bacteria into the bladder.

Ways to Prevent UTIs

For all people:

1. Ensure proper hydration. Water will keep urine diluted. Also drink antioxidant drinks such as cranberry or blueberry juice.
2. Empty the bladder at regular intervals.
3. Provide good perineal care after each voiding and especially after each bowel movement.
4. Follow agency or facility guidelines for care of catheters.
5. Avoid unnecessary urinary catheterizations.

For women:

6. Wipe from front to back.
7. Urinate soon after sex to clear out bacteria that may have entered the urethra.
8. Do not use douches, sprays, or powders that can alter the normal flora in the vaginal area.
9. Avoid bubble baths, bath oils, and other perfumed products that can irritate the urethra.
10. Wear breathable fabrics and loose-fitting clothing that allow the vaginal area to stay dry.

Sources: MediResource Inc. (n.d.). *Urinary tract infections: The facts.* Retrieved from http://bodyandhealth.canada.com/channel_condition_info_details.asp?disease_id=234&channel_id=2015&relation_id=28996; Saskatchewan Infection Prevention and Control Program. (2013). *Guidelines for the prevention and treatment of urinary tract infections (UTIs) in continuous care settings*. Retrieved from http://www.ipac-canada.org/IPAC-SASKPIC/UTI%20Guidelines%2019April2013.pdf; MediResource C-Health. (n.d.). *7 ways to help prevent UTI*. Retrieved from http://chealth.canoe.ca/channel_section_details.asp?text_id=5717&channel_id=7&relation_id=24636.

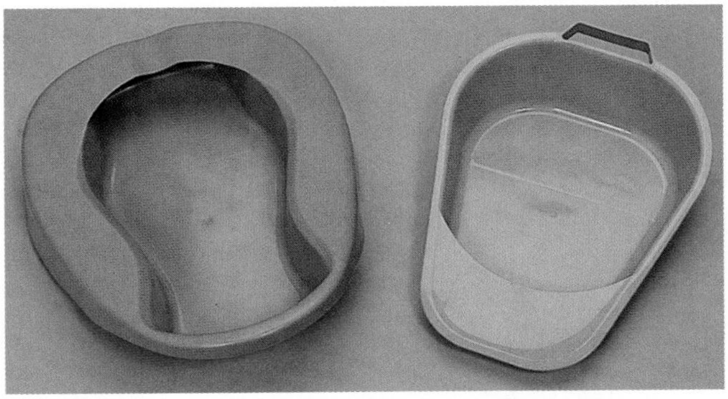

FIGURE 32–1 The regular bedpan and the fracture pan.

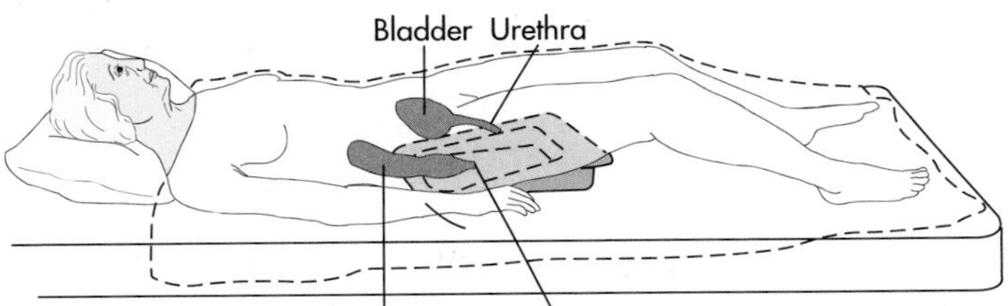

FIGURE 32–2 A client positioned on a fracture pan. The smaller end is placed under the buttocks.

Giving the Bedpan

123

Advocate on behalf of the client's quality of life by promoting:

Dignity • Independence • Preferences • Privacy • Safety *(see BOX 1–4, on p. 17)*

PRE-PROCEDURE

1 Identify the client, according to employer policy.
This eliminates the possibility of mistaking one client for another.

2 Explain the procedure to the client.

3 Provide for privacy.

4 Practise proper hand hygiene. Put on gloves.

5 Collect the following supplies:
- ☐ **Bedpan**
- ☐ **Bedpan cover (or paper towels)**
- ☐ **Toilet tissue**
- ☐ **Extra gloves**

By collecting all the necessary equipment beforehand, you will not have to leave your client's side and can eliminate wasting time and energy in obtaining the forgotten equipment.

6 Arrange equipment on the chair or bed.
Avoid placing heavily contaminated items on the overbed table since food is served on it. It is important to plan thoroughly before starting any procedure.

PROCEDURE

7 Warm and dry the bedpan, if necessary.
These steps convey concern for the client's comfort.

8 Lower the bed rail near you if it is up.

9 Place the client in the supine position, keeping the bed as flat as possible. You may use pillows to raise the client's head and shoulders.
Placing the client in this position makes bedpan placement and removal easiest.

10 Fold the top linens and the client's gown out of the way. Keep the lower body covered.
This helps ensure privacy.

11 Ask the client to flex the knees and raise the buttocks by pushing against the mattress with the feet.
This helps elevate the client's buttocks for easier bedpan placement.

12 Slide your hand under the lower back, and help raise the buttocks.
This assists the client in raising the buttocks.

13 Slide the bedpan under the client (**FIGURE 32–3**).

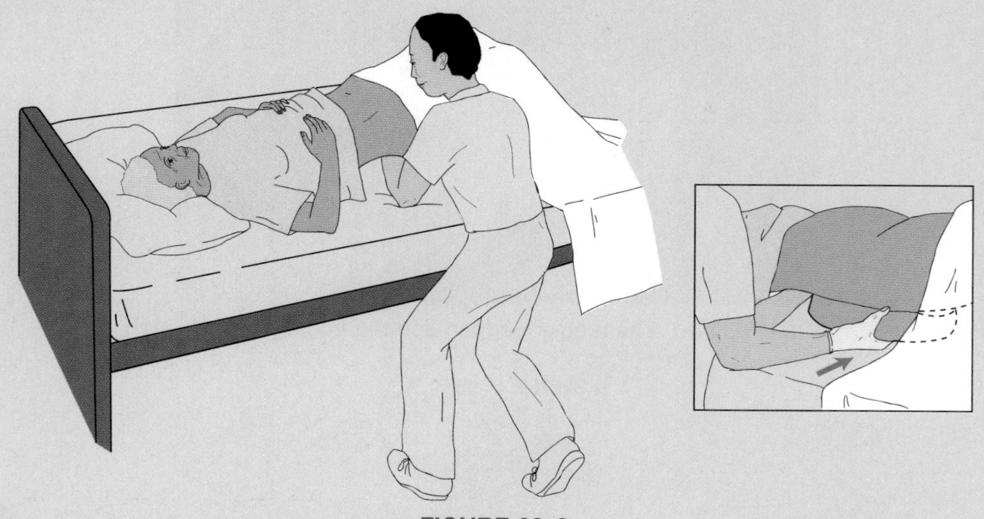

FIGURE 32–3

Continued

Giving the Bedpan—cont'd

14 If the client cannot assist in getting on the bedpan:
  a Turn the client onto the side away from you.
  b Place the bedpan firmly against the buttocks (FIGURE 32–4, *A*).
  c Push the bedpan down and toward the client (see FIGURE 32–4, *B*).
  d Hold the bedpan securely. Turn the client onto the back.
  e Make sure the bedpan is centred and under the client.

15 Cover the client.

16 Raise the head of the bed so that the client is in the sitting position. If the bed is not adjustable, assist the client into the sitting position, using pillows for support.
The sitting position allows easier evacuation of bladder and bowel.

17 Make sure the client is correctly positioned on the bedpan so that the urethra and anus are directly over the opening (FIGURE 32–5).
This is to ensure the urine will land in the bedpan and not run off onto the bed.

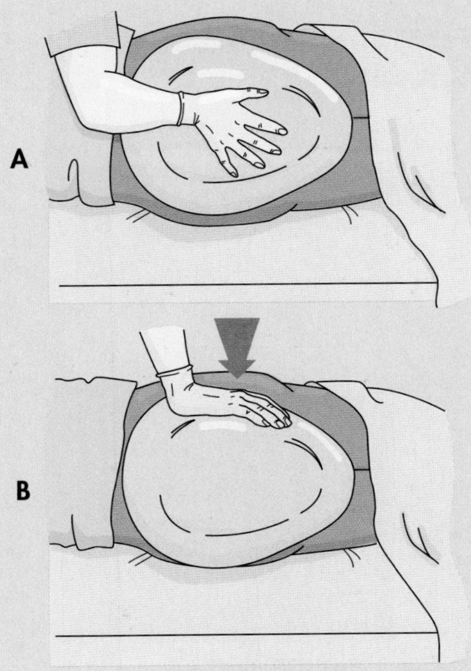

FIGURE 32–4

18 Raise the bed rail if used.

19 Place the toilet tissue and call bell (in facilities) within reach.
This provides an easy, safe way for the client to contact staff if necessary.

20 Ask the client to call when done or if help is needed.
This reduces the risk for client injury.

21 Practise proper hand hygiene.

22 Leave the room, and close the door.
Most clients find it easier to use the bedpan when privacy is respected.

23 Return when the client calls. Knock before entering.

24 Practise proper hand hygiene. Put on gloves.

25 Raise the bed to a comfortable working height. Lower the bed rail (if used) and the head of the bed.* Or remove the pillows, and place the client in the supine position.
Raising the bed will reduce your risk for back strain. Lowering the head of the bed will make it easier to remove the bedpan safely without spilling its contents.

26 Ask the client to raise the buttocks, and remove the bedpan. If the client cannot raise the buttocks, hold the bedpan securely, and turn the client onto the side facing away from you.

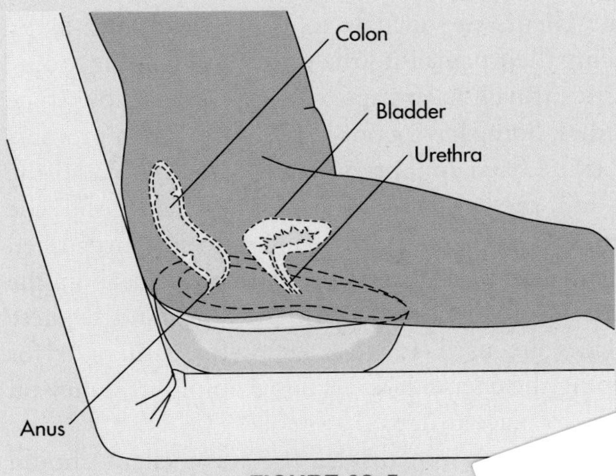

FIGURE 32–5

Giving the Bedpan—cont'd

27 Clean the genital area if the client cannot do so. Clean from the front (urethra) to the back (anus) with toilet tissue, using a fresh tissue for each wipe. Provide perineal care.
Perineal care is important to prevent skin infection and irritation. It also helps the client feel refreshed.

28 Cover the bedpan and take it to the bathroom. Remember to lower the bed and raise the bed rail (if used) before leaving the bedside.
Covering the contents of the bedpan helps contain odours and respects the client's right to privacy.

29 Note the colour, amount, and character of urine or stool.
The support worker needs to report accurate observations to the supervisor.

30 Empty the bedpan into the toilet and rinse the bedpan with cold water. Clean it with a disinfectant.

31 Remove soiled gloves. Practise proper hand hygiene.

32 Put bedpan and lid away.
This makes them easier to locate the next time they are needed.

33 Help the client practise proper hand hygiene.

POST-PROCEDURE

34 Provide for safety and comfort.

35 Place the call bell within reach.*
This provides an easy, safe way for the client to contact staff if necessary.

36 Follow the care plan for bed rail use.*

37 Remove privacy measures.

38 Follow employer policy for disposing of soiled linen.

39 Practise proper hand hygiene.

Report and Record your actions and observations, according to employer policy.
This is done for legal reasons and to keep the rest of the health care team informed.

*Steps marked with an asterisk may not apply in community settings.

Urinals

Male clients use urinals to void (**FIGURE 32–6**) by placing their penis into the urinal and voiding. Some plastic urinals have caps at the top and hook-type handles. Some have a one-way spout, which prevents the urine from spilling out. The urinal hooks to the bed rail, the back of a chair, or any place within the client's reach that is sturdy enough to support a filled urinal. The urinal should ***never*** be placed on the client's overbed table, bedside table, or stand, as these surfaces are used as work areas, for eating, or for keeping the client's items. Follow employer policy on where to place urinals.

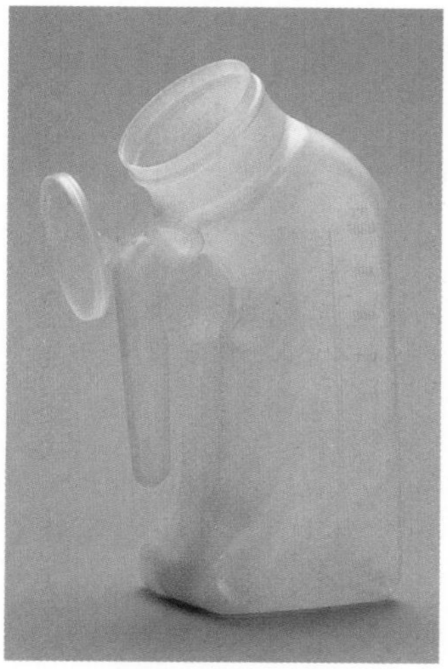

FIGURE 32–6 A urinal.

While using the urinal, the male client should stand (the best position for bladder emptying), sit on the side of the bed, or lie in bed. For some clients who cannot stand without the support of one or two people, you may have to place and hold the urinal for them.

Remind clients to cap the urinal after voiding if there is a cap, to prevent urine from spilling. You should also remind clients to hang used urinals on bed rails or the backs of chairs and to call you when their urinals need emptying. Follow medical asepsis and Standard Practices when handling urinals and their contents. A filled urinal spills easily, causing safety hazards. Also, it may be embarrassing for the client to have the filled urinal around. You should always empty urinals promptly and rinse and clean them thoroughly (in the same manner as bedpans) after each use to prevent odours and the buildup and spread of microbes.

Providing a Urinal to a Male Client 123

Advocate on behalf of the client's quality of life by promoting:

Dignity • Independence • Preferences • Privacy • Safety *(see BOX 1–4, on p. 17)*

PRE-PROCEDURE

1 Provide for privacy.

2 Determine if the client will stand, sit, or stay in bed.
The client must be able to urinate safely.

3 Practise proper hand hygiene. Put on gloves.

PROCEDURE

4 Give the client the urinal if he is in bed. Remind him to tilt the bottom down.
This prevents urine spills.

5 If the client is going to stand:
 a Help him sit on the side of the bed.
 b Help him put on nonskid footwear.
 c Help him stand. Provide support if he is unsteady.
 d Give him the urinal.
This reduces the risk for client injury.

6 Position the urinal if necessary. Position his penis in the urinal if he cannot do so.
Positioning the urinal properly prevents spillage while the client urinates.

7 Provide for privacy.

8 Place the call bell within reach.*
This provides an easy, safe way for the client to contact staff if necessary.

9 Ask the client to call when he is done or if he needs help.
This reduces the risk for client injury.

10 Remove gloves. Practise proper hand hygiene.

11 Leave the room, and close the door.

12 Return when the client calls for you. Knock before entering.

13 Practise proper hand hygiene. Put on gloves.

14 Close the cap on the urinal if there is one. Take the urinal to the bathroom.
The cap is placed on the urinal to prevent spilling the urine.

15 Note the colour, amount, and character of the urine.

16 Empty the urinal in the toilet, rinse it with cold water, and clean it with disinfectant.
This decreases the risk for pathogen spread.

17 Return the urinal to its proper place.
This allows easy access the next time it is needed.

18 Remove gloves. Practise proper hand hygiene. Put on clean gloves.

19 Help the client wash his hands.

20 Remove gloves. Practise proper hand

Providing a Urinal to a Male Client—cont'd

POST-PROCEDURE

21 Provide for safety and comfort.
22 Place the call bell within reach.*
This provides an easy, safe way for the client to contact staff if necessary.
23 Follow the care plan for bed rail use.*
24 Remove privacy measures.
This reduces the risk for client injury.
25 Follow employer policy for soiled linen.
This decreases the risk for pathogen spread.
26 Practise proper hand hygiene.

Report and Record your actions and observations, according to employer policy.
This is done for legal reasons and to keep the rest of the health care team informed.

*Steps marked with an asterisk may not apply in community settings.

Commodes

A commode is a portable chair or wheelchair with an opening for a bedpan or container, which allows a normal position for elimination (see FIGURE 25–28, p. 521). Some commode chairs have wheels so that they can be moved. Clients who are unable to walk to the bathroom often use commodes. The commode arms and back provide support and help prevent falls. The bedpan or container should be cleaned after each use, as with the regular bedpan, following Standard Practices. If a specimen is not required, placing a small amount of water in the commode container or bedpan will allow for easier cleaning after use.

For clients who cannot sit unsupported on the toilet, a commode may be wheeled into the bathroom and positioned over the toilet, without the bedpan or container in place. Clients who are able to walk to the bathroom but need extra support, therefore, have privacy and safety during elimination. It is your responsibility to ensure that the commode wheels are locked and that the commode is positioned correctly over the toilet.

In some cases, the client may be lowered onto a commode chair, which is then wheeled into the bathroom and positioned over the toilet. To prevent injury to the client, you must ensure that the client's buttocks do not rub against the toilet while you are positioning the commode chair over it. In addition, you must ensure that the commode chair's wheels are locked so that they do not roll. Securing the wheels helps stabilize the client and prevent falls.

Clients should never be tied or restrained to a commode. While commodes are very useful, they can tip easily, so clients who cannot sit up on their own should not be placed on a commode. The longest time a client should be on a commode chair is 20 to 30 minutes.

Helping the Client to the Commode

123

Advocate on behalf of the client's quality of life by promoting:
Dignity • Independence • Preferences • Privacy • Safety *(see BOX 1–4, on p. 17)*

PRE-PROCEDURE

1 Explain the procedure to the client.
2 Provide for privacy.
3 Practise proper hand hygiene. Put on gloves.
4 Collect the following:
- ☐ **Commode**
- ☐ **Toilet tissue**

Continued

Helping the Client to the Commode—cont'd

- ☐ **Cover or bath blanket (if one is available)**
- ☐ **Several pairs of gloves**
- ☐ **Transfer belt (optional)**

By collecting all the necessary equipment beforehand, you will not have to leave your client's side and can eliminate wasting time and energy in obtaining the forgotten equipment.

PROCEDURE

5 Bring the commode next to the bed. Remove the cushion, and lift the container lid.
Planning ahead will reduce the need for unnecessary steps, will reduce time, and will be safer for the client.

6 Help the client sit on the side of the bed.
This will reduce the risk for client injury.

7 Help the client put on a robe and nonskid footwear.
Nonskid footwear reduces the risk for client injury.

8 If necessary, assist the client to the commode. Use a transfer belt if needed.
The transfer belt allows you to grasp the client more securely, thereby ensuring client safety.

9 Cover the client with a cover or bath blanket (if one is available).
This helps ensure warmth.

10 Place the call bell (in facilities) and toilet tissue within reach.
Placing the call bell within reach provides an easy, safe way for the client to contact staff if necessary.

11 Ask the client to call when done or if help is needed. (Stay with the client if necessary. Be respectful. Provide as much privacy as possible.)

12 Remove gloves. Practise proper hand hygiene.

13 Leave the room, and close the door.

14 Return when the client calls. Knock before entering.

15 Practise proper hand hygiene. Put on gloves.

16 Help the client clean the genital area, as needed. Remove gloves. Practise proper hand hygiene.

17 Help the client back to the bed. Remove the client's robe and footwear. Follow the care plan for bed rail use.*
This ensures the client's safety.

18 Put on clean gloves. Remove and cover the commode container. Clean the commode.

19 Take the container to the bathroom.

20 Check urine and stool for colour, amount, and character.
These are important observations and should be later reported, according to your agency's policies.

21 Empty in the toilet and clean and disinfect the container.
This reduces bedpan odour and the risk for contamination.

22 Return the container to the commode and the commode to its proper place. Return other supplies to their proper places.
This makes them easier to find the next time they are needed.

23 Remove soiled gloves. Practise proper hand hygiene. Put on clean gloves.

24 Help the client with handwashing.

25 Remove gloves. Practise proper hand hygiene.

POST-PROCEDURE

26 Provide for safety and comfort.

27 Place the call bell within reach.*
This provides an easy, safe way for the client to contact staff if necessary.

28 Follow the care plan for bed rail use.*

29 Remove privacy measures.

30 Follow employer policy for handling soiled linen.
This decreases the risk for pathogen spread.

31 Practise proper hand hygiene.

Report and Record your actions and observations, according to employer policy.
This is done for legal reasons and to kee[illegible] the health care team informed.

*Steps marked with an asterisk may not apply in community settings.

URINARY INCONTINENCE

Urinary incontinence—the loss of bladder control—may be temporary or permanent. The different types of incontinence are as follows:

- **Stress incontinence**—the leaking of urine during exercise and certain movements. Urine loss is small (less than 50 mL). Often called *dribbling*, it occurs with laughing, sneezing, coughing, lifting, or other activities. Late-in-life pregnancy and obesity are other causes. The problem is common in women, as pelvic muscles weaken due to pregnancies and aging.
- **Urge incontinence**—the loss of urine in response to a sudden, urgent need to void. The client cannot get to a toilet in time. Urinary frequency, urinary urgency, and nighttime voidings are common. Causes include UTIs, nervous system disorders, bladder cancer, and an enlarged prostate.
- **Overflow incontinence**—the leaking of urine when the bladder is too full. The client feels as though the bladder is never completely empty and experiences only dribbling or a weak urine stream. Diabetes, enlarged prostate, and some medications are causes.
- **Functional incontinence**—the loss of urine that occurs when the client has bladder control but cannot get to the toilet in time. Immobility, restraints, unanswered calls for help, lack of a call bell within reach, confusion, disorientation, difficulty removing clothing, and not knowing where to find the bathroom are all causes of functional incontinence.
- **Reflex incontinence**—the loss of urine at predictable intervals. Urine is lost whenever the bladder becomes full, even when the client does not feel the need to void. Nervous system disorders and injuries are common causes.

Sometimes incontinence results from surgery to the intestinal, rectal, or reproductive system. The presence of more than one type of incontinence is called *mixed incontinence*.

Problems Related to Urinary Incontinence

Incontinence is embarrassing for the client. Clothing and linens get wet, odours develop, and the client is usually cold and uncomfortable. The client can develop skin irritation, skin breakdown, and infection. The urge to urinate can be so strong that some clients may rush to the washroom and sustain injury by slipping or falling on the way.

You can minimize incontinence by ensuring the client has the opportunity to urinate regularly—for example, before and after each meal, before and after activities, and before going to sleep and upon wakening. Incontinence can affect clients' pride, dignity, and self-esteem and cause them to avoid participating in activities, going out, or visiting with others out of fear of being incontinent in public. These clients need your support, understanding, and compassion.

Check with your supervisor and consult the care plan for the best ways to meet the client's needs. Care measures depend on the type of incontinence. The client's care plan may include some of the measures listed in BOX 32–4. ***It is essential that you provide frequent, proper skin care and change the client into clean, dry garments after each episode. Promptly changing wet bed linens is also essential, and failure to do so is considered a form of neglect.*** Other clients may need bladder training (p. 714), and some clients require catheterization to control incontinence.

For clients with uncontrolled urinary incontinence, a variety of incontinence products are available, and the most suitable product for each client is selected by a nurse, the client, or the client's family. In addition, some clients use garment protectors or incontinence pads (FIGURE 32–7).

Stress for the Caregiver

Caring for people with incontinence can be stressful. Some family members who are caregivers cannot cope with problems associated with incontinence and often seek long-term care for the client. As a professional caregiver, even you may find caring for these clients stressful, as they may need frequent care that includes changing wet garments and linens and giving skin care. Do not lose patience. The client's needs are great, and your role is to meet these needs. If you find yourself becoming short-tempered and impatient, discuss it with your supervisor immediately. Remember, the client has the right to be free from abuse, mistreatment, and neglect. The incontinence is beyond the client's control and is not

BOX 32–4 Care Measures for Clients With Urinary Incontinence

- Record the client's voidings, including both episodes of incontinence and successful use of the toilet, commode, bedpan, or urinal.
- Answer all calls for assistance promptly. The client may have an urgent need to void.
- Promote normal urinary elimination (see **BOX 32–2**, on p. 691).
- Promote normal bowel elimination (see Chapter 33).
- Encourage urination at scheduled intervals.
- Monitor the client's bladder training program.
- Encourage the client to wear clothing that is easy to remove. Incontinence can occur as the client is trying to deal with buttons, zippers, and undergarments.
- Encourage the client to do pelvic muscle exercises, as directed by the care plan.
- Help prevent UTIs:
  - Encourage adequate fluid intake, as directed by the care plan.
  - Encourage the client to wear cotton undergarments.
  - Provide perineal care, as needed (see Chapter 30). Keep the perineal area clean and dry.
  - Decrease fluid intake before bedtime (the client's *daily* fluid intake is usually not restricted, however).
- Provide proper skin care (see Chapter 30).
- Provide dry garments and linens.
- Observe for signs of skin breakdown (see Chapter 24).
- Use incontinence products (sometimes called "briefs"), as directed by the care plan (see Chapter 31). Follow manufacturer's instructions. Remove them when they become wet and discard or wash them (depending on the type of product and the manufacturer's instructions).
- While changing a client's incontinence products, do not place the soiled brief on the floor, as doing so will spread pathogens. Dispose of the soiled item directly into the proper container.
- For clients who are catheterized, follow employer policy for securing the catheter tubing to the client's leg. Many agencies use an adhesive strip to prevent the tubing from being pulled and the injury that could result (see **FIGURE 32–12**, on p. 704).

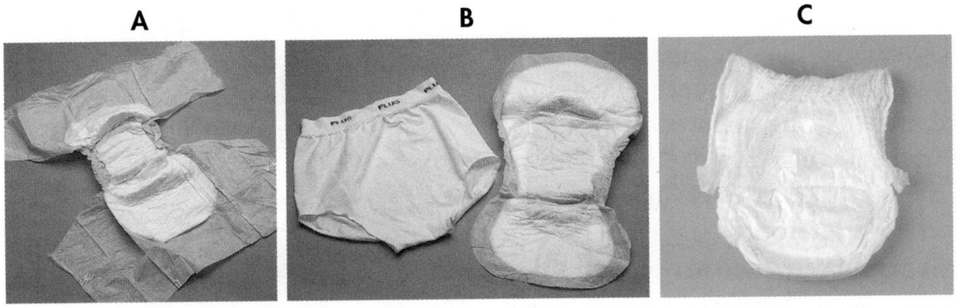

FIGURE 32–7 Garment protectors. **A,** Complete incontinence brief. **B,** Pant liner which adheres to undergarment. **C,** Pull-on incontinence brief. (**Source** (for C): holohololand/iStock/Thinkstock)

something he or she chooses to let happen. Showing kindness, empathy, understanding, and patience is very important.

Incontinence Pads

Incontinence pads help keep bed linen dry. Some facilities (mainly hospitals) use disposable incontinence pads, and some others use multi-purpose items as both transfer sheets and incontinence pads, since these items have two layers of padding and a waterproof backing. Incontinence pads are placed over the bottom sheet from the client's head to mid-thigh (see Chapter 25, p. 498). Fluid passes through the first layer and is absorbed by the lower layer. When the pad becomes wet or soiled, change it and any bed linen, and place them directly into linen hamper, according to your employer's policies. Just placing a dry incontinence pad over wet bed linen to save time could be considered neglect.

CATHETERS

A *catheter* is a tube (plastic, latex, or other material) used to drain or inject fluid through a body opening. A *urinary catheter* is a tube that is inserted into the bladder to drain urine. Catheter insertion (**catheterization**) is done by a nurse or physician or even by the client if the client learns how to do it.

Occasionally, a physician might order a client to be catheterized after the client has voided to determine how much urine is left in the bladder. A client who was catheterized for 300 mL but voided only 200 mL would need medical treatment for inadequate emptying of the bladder and urinary retention.

- A **straight catheter** is a tube that drains the bladder and is removed after one use. It is inserted through the urethra into the bladder.
- An **in-dwelling catheter** (also called a **retention** or **Foley catheter**) is a tube (plastic, latex, or other material) that is inserted into the bladder through the urinary meatus and urethra (FIGURE 32–8). A balloon within the catheter is inflated after insertion, preventing the catheter from slipping out of the bladder (FIGURE 32–9). Tubing connects the catheter to the drainage bag.
- A **suprapubic catheter** is a catheter that is surgically inserted through the abdomen, above the pubic bone, into the bladder. It is a type of in-dwelling catheter; that is, it is left in the bladder and is attached to a drainage bag with tubing. Suprapubic catheters may be used in clients needing long-term catheterization or after certain types of surgeries. The insertion site (the opening on the abdomen) and the tubing must be cleaned daily with soap and water and covered with dry gauze. Follow the care plan and your assignment sheet.

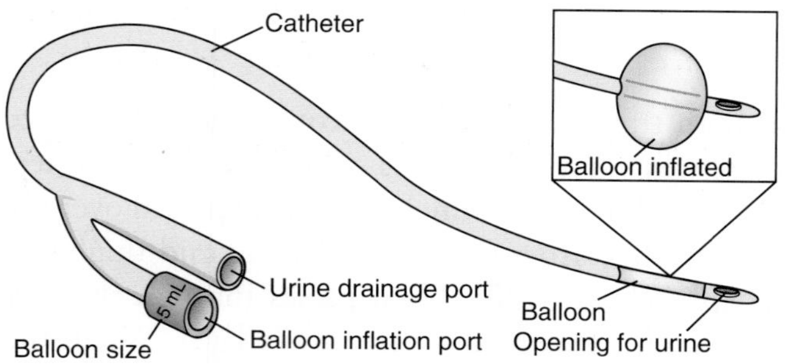

FIGURE 32–8 Parts of an in-dwelling catheter (retention or Foley catheter).

Purposes of Catheters

- Catheters often are used before, during, and after surgery to keep the bladder empty. Catheterization reduces the risk of accidental bladder injury during surgery, and after surgery, it prevents the pressure on nearby organs that a full bladder could cause.
- Catheters allow hourly urinary output measurements in clients with critical illnesses.
- Catheters are the last resort for managing incontinence, since they do not treat the cause of incontinence, and the risk of infection is high. However, some clients have wounds and pressure ulcers that must be protected from contamination by urine.
- Clients who are extremely weak or have disabilities and are unable to use the bedpan, commode, or toilet—for example, those who are dying—can be

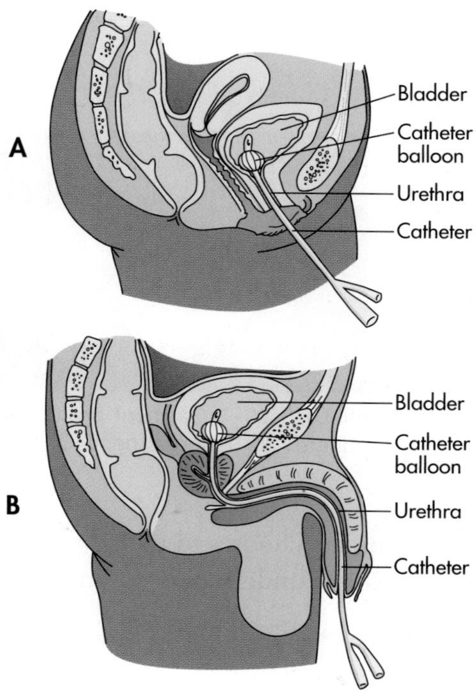

FIGURE 32–9 **A,** In-dwelling catheter in the female bladder. The inflated balloon at the top prevents the catheter from slipping out through the urethra. **B,** In-dwelling catheter with the balloon inflated in the male bladder.

made more comfortable by having incontinence managed by a catheter.

- Catheters have diagnostic uses such as collecting sterile urine specimens and measuring residual urine. For such purposes, the catheter is inserted *after* the client has voided.

As a support worker, you will be required to care for clients with in-dwelling catheters. Follow the guidelines listed in the *Think About Safety: Guidelines for Caring for Clients With In-Dwelling Catheters* box on page 705 to promote comfort and safety.

Giving Catheter Care

123

Advocate on behalf of the client's quality of life by promoting:

Dignity • Independence • Preferences • Privacy • Safety *(see BOX 1–4, on p. 17)*

PRE-PROCEDURE

1 Identify the client according to employer policy.
This eliminates the possibility of mistaking one client for another.
2 Explain the procedure to the client.
3 Practise proper hand hygiene.
4 Collect the following:
- ☐ **Items for perineal care** (see p. 643)
- ☐ **Gloves**
- ☐ **Bed protector or incontinence pad**
- ☐ **Cover or bath blanket** (if one is available)

By collecting all the necessary equipment beforehand, you will not have to leave your client's side and can eliminate wasting time and energy in obtaining the forgotten equipment.
5 Provide for privacy.
6 Raise bed to a comfortable working height*
Planning ahead will reduce time and needless effort and can ensure client safety.

PROCEDURE

7 Lower the bed rail near you if it is up.*
8 Put on gloves.
9 Cover the client with a cover or bath blanket if one is available. Fan-fold the top linen to the foot of the bed.
This ensures privacy for the client and helps keep the client warm.
10 Drape the client for perineal care (see **FIGURE 30–26**, on p. 644).
Draping exposes only the area that needs to be exposed for perineal care, helping to preserve the client's dignity and need for privacy.
11 Fold back the cover or bath blanket to expose the genital area.
12 Place the bed protector under the buttocks. Ask the client to flex the knees and raise the buttocks off the bed.
Bed protectors help keep the bedding clean and dry.
13 Give perineal care (see the procedures *Giving Perineal Care to a Female Client*, on p. 643, and *Giving Perineal Care to a Male Client*, on p. 646).
This removes any soiling or lint from the perineal area, which might be a source of irritation or infection.
14 Apply soap to a clean, wet washcloth.
15 Separate the labia (female), as in **FIGURE 30–27**, on p. 644. Or retract the foreskin (uncircumcised male), as in **FIGURE 30–29**, on p. 646. Check for the presence of crusts, abnormal drainage, or secretions.
16 Hold the catheter near the meatus (insertion point).
This prevents the risk of accidentally tugging on the catheter and injuring the client.

Giving Catheter Care—cont'd

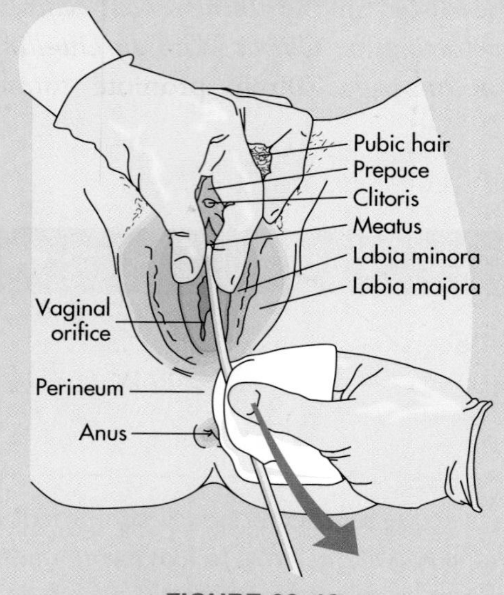

FIGURE 32–10

17 Clean the catheter from the meatus down the catheter about 10 cm (4 in.) (**FIGURE 32–10**). Clean downward, away from the meatus with one stroke. Do not tug or pull on the catheter. Repeat as needed with a clean area of the washcloth. Use a clean washcloth if needed.
Cleaning this way brings pathogens away from the urinary meatus, reducing the risk for infection.
18 Rinse the catheter.
19 Secure the catheter. Coil and secure tubing (**FIGURE 32–11**).
A secured catheter is less likely to cause injury if pulled or tugged.
20 Remove the bed protector.
21 Cover the client. Remove the cover or bath blanket (if one was used).
22 Remove gloves. Practise proper hand hygiene.

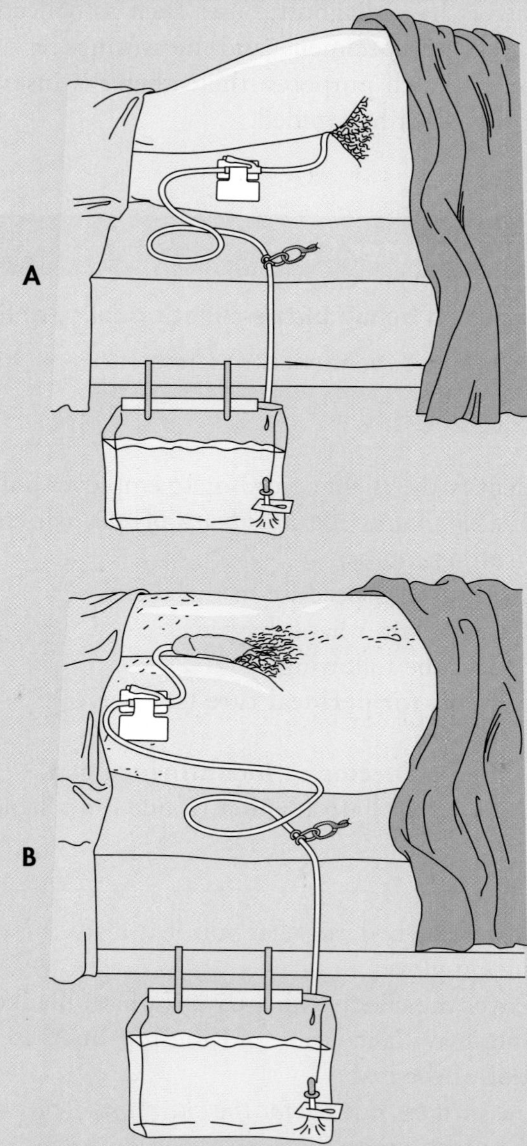

FIGURE 32–11 **A,** The drainage tubing is secured to the female client's thigh to prevent it from being pulled. Enough slack is left on the catheter to prevent friction at the urethra. **B,** The catheter is secured to the male client's upper thigh, leaving enough slack so that the client's penis is not being pulled.

POST-PROCEDURE

23 Provide for safety and comfort.
24 Place the call bell within reach.*
This provides an easy, safe way for the client to contact staff if necessary.
25 Return the bed to its lowest position. Follow the care plan for bed rail use.*
This reduces the risk for client injury.

Continued

Giving Catheter Care—cont'd

26 Clean and return equipment to its proper place. Discard disposable items.
This makes it easier to locate equipment the next time it is needed.

27 Remove privacy measures.

28 Follow employer policy for handling soiled linen.
This reduces the risk for pathogen spread.

29 Practise proper hand hygiene.

Report and Record your actions and observations, according to employer policy.
This is done for legal reasons and to keep the rest of the health care team informed.

*Steps marked with an asterisk may not apply in community settings.

Think About Safety

Guidelines for Caring for Clients With In-Dwelling Catheters

- Follow the rules of medical asepsis and Standard Practices.
- Make sure urine flows freely through the catheter or tubing. Tubing should not have kinks, and the client should not lie on the tubing.
- When the client is being moved, the catheter tube must remain slack, never taut or pulled.
- Make sure the catheter is connected to the drainage tubing. If the catheter and drainage tube become disconnected, follow your facility's policy to cleanse the drainage tube cap and reattach it.
- Urine provides the ideal environment for the growth of microbes. If the drainage bag is at a higher level than the bladder, urine can flow back into the bladder, and an infection can develop. ***Keep the drainage bag below the level of the bladder*** to prevent urine from flowing backward into the bladder.
- If the client is in bed, attach the drainage bag to the bed frame; if in a chair, attach it to the back of the chair. ***Never attach the drainage bag to the bed rail because the drainage bag would be higher than the level of the bladder if the bed rail is raised.***
- Move the drainage bag to the side of the bed to which the client will be turned. You must remember to move the drainage bag before turning the client.
- Do not let the drainage bag rest on the floor because microbes on the floor can contaminate the system.
- Coil the drainage tubing on the bed. Secure it to the bottom linen (**FIGURE 32–11**). Use a clip, tape, or a safety pin and rubber band, according to your employer policy. Tubing must not loop below the drainage bag.
- In women, secure the catheter to the inner thigh, as in **FIGURE 32–11, *A***, and in men, secure it to the thigh (see **FIGURE 32–11, *B***) to prevent excessive movement of the catheter and reduce friction at the insertion site. Secure the catheter with tape or another device, as ordered by the care plan to prevent the catheter from pulling on the urethral opening. ***Many agencies and facilities do not tape the catheter to the client, as some adhesive tapes can be irritating to the client's skin. Always check your client's care plan and your employer's policy.***
- Check for leaks at the site where the catheter connects to the drainage bag. Report any leaks immediately.
- Provide catheter care, if ordered, once or twice a day. It includes cleaning the part of the tube that extends outside of the body. Catheter care helps prevent bladder or urethral infections (see the

Continued

Think About Safety—cont'd

procedure *Giving Catheter Care*, on p. 703). Some employers consider it sufficient to provide only perineal care. However, catheter care is sometimes needed after fecal elimination and when there is vaginal drainage. Follow the care plan.

- Provide perineal care daily, after bowel movements, and when vaginal drainage is present. Follow the care plan.
- Empty the drainage bag at the end of the shift or at intervals specified in the care plan. Measure and record the amount of urine (see the procedure *Emptying a Urinary Drainage Bag*, on p. 709). Report increases or decreases in the amount of urine.
- Use a clean, dry measuring container to measure each client's urine.
- Do not let the drain or the drainage bag touch any surface. Wipe the end of the drainage spout with an antiseptic wipe each time after draining the bag.
- Immediately report any complaints of pain, burning, urge to urinate, or irritation. Also report the colour, clarity, and odour of urine and the presence of particles.
- Encourage fluid intake, as instructed by the care plan.
- Always check the care plan before changing a client's in-dwelling catheter bag to a leg bag. Changing from one bag to another places the client at risk for a urinary infection. If it *is* in the client's care plan, proper aseptic technique should be practised at all times.

Source: MyHealth Alberta. (2014). When you have an Indwelling catheter: After your visit. Retrieved from https://myhealth.alberta.ca/alberta/pages/When-you-have-an-indwelling-catheter-after-your-visit.aspx.

Changing a Drainage Bag to a Leg Bag 123

Advocate on behalf of the client's quality of life by promoting:

Dignity • Independence • Preferences • Privacy • Safety *(see BOX 1–4, on p. 17)*

PRE-PROCEDURE

1. Identify the client, according to employer policy.
   This eliminates the possibility of mistaking one client for another.
2. Explain the procedure to the client.
3. Practise proper hand hygiene.
4. Collect the following:
   - ☐ **Gloves**
   - ☐ **Drainage bag and tubing**
   - ☐ **Antiseptic wipes**
   - ☐ **Bed protector**
   - ☐ **Sterile cap and catheter plug**
   - ☐ **Catheter clamp**
   - ☐ **Paper towels**
   - ☐ **Bedpan**
   - ☐ **Cover or bath blanket** (if one is available)

   By collecting all the necessary equipment beforehand, you will not have to leave your client's side and can eliminate wasting time and energy in obtaining the forgotten equipment.
5. Arrange paper towels and equipment on the work area.
   It is important to plan thoroughly before starting any procedure.
6. Provide for privacy.

Continued

Changing a Drainage Bag to a Leg Bag—cont'd

PROCEDURE

7 Have the client sit on the side of the bed.
This position facilitates drainage into the bladder.

8 Put on gloves.

9 Help the client lie back down. Raise the bed to a comfortable working height.*
This reduces your risk for back injury.

10 Cover the client with a cover or bath blanket (if one is available). Expose the catheter and drainage tubing. Place the bed protector under the leg.
Covering keeps the client warm and respects privacy.

11 Clamp the catheter. The clamp is applied to the catheter, not to the drainage tubing (**FIGURE 32–12**).
This prevents urine from draining out of the bladder from the catheter into the drainage tubing.

12 Let urine drain from below the clamp site into the drainage tubing.
This empties the lower end of the catheter.

13 Open the antiseptic wipes. Set them on the paper towels.
Arranging items allows for easier access.

14 Open the package with the sterile cap and plug (**FIGURE 32–13**). Set the package on the paper towels. Do not let anything touch the sterile cap or plug.
Keeping the sterile items on a sterile field prevents them from becoming contaminated.

15 Open the package with the leg bag drainage tubing, and attach the drainage bag to the bed frame.
Attaching the drainage bag to the bed frame keeps it off the floor, where it can become contaminated, but keeps it handy for reconnecting.

16 Disconnect the catheter from the drainage tubing. Do not let anything touch the ends.
Touching can contaminate the ends of the tubing and could lead to UTI.

17 Remove the cap from the leg bag drainage tubing. Do not let anything touch the ends.
Both ends need to remain sterile or clean. Contamination of them can lead to a serious UTI.

18 Insert the end of the catheter into the leg bag drainage tubing.

19 Place the sterile cap on the end of the drainage bag tubing (**FIGURE 32–14, *A***). If you contaminate the tubing end, wipe it with an antiseptic wipe. Do so before you put the sterile cap on.
The drainage tubing system should be kept sterile to prevent urine from becoming contaminated, which could lead to serious bladder infection.

20 Remove the clamp from the catheter.
This allows the urine to drain from the bladder.

21 Loop the tubing, and secure it to the client's leg (**FIGURE 32–14, *B***).
Securing it reduces the risk of its being tugged and causing injury to the client.

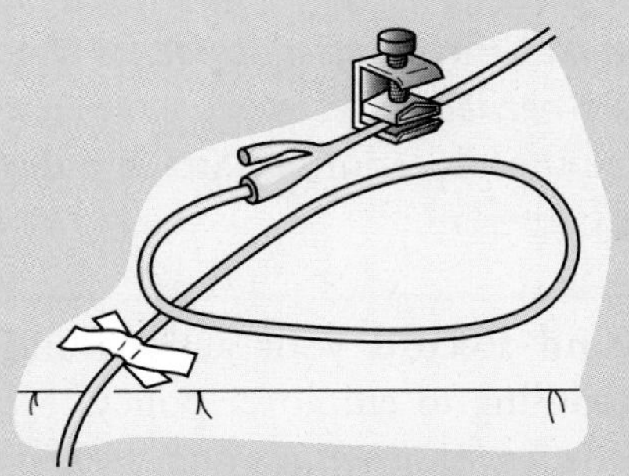

FIGURE 32–12

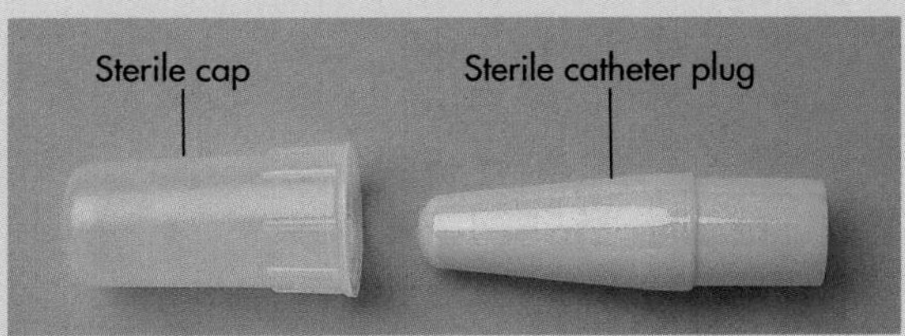

FIGURE 32–13 Sterile cap and sterile catheter plug. The inside of the cap is sterile. It is inserted into the catheter. Touch only the end of the plug.

Continued

Changing a Drainage Bag to a Leg Bag—cont'd

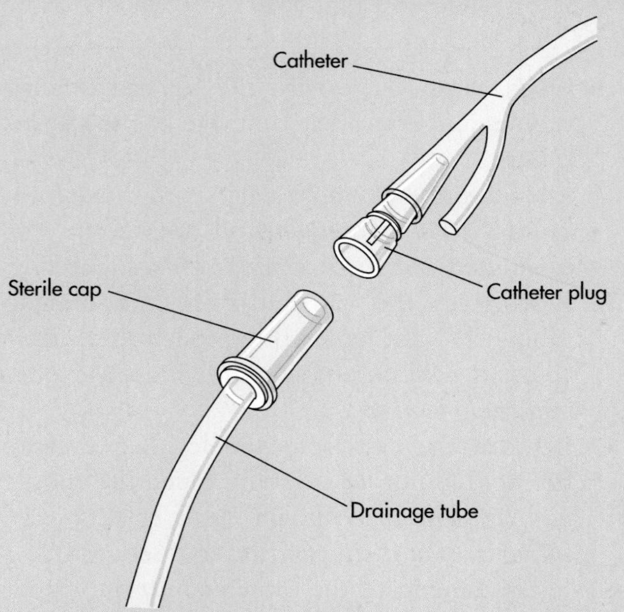

FIGURE 32–14 A, Sterile catheter plug inserted into the end of the catheter. A sterile cap is on the end of the drainage tube.

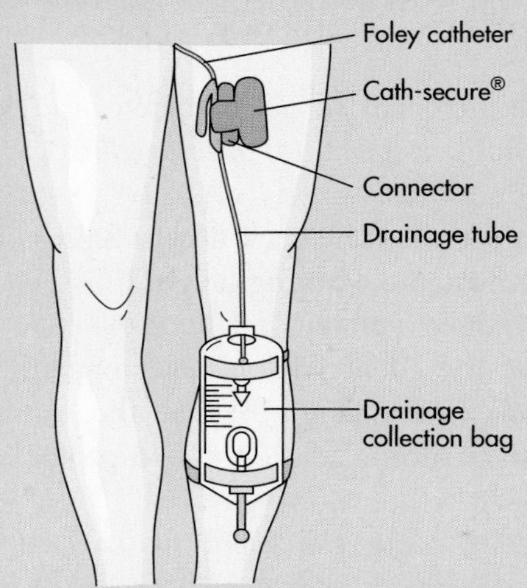

FIGURE 32–14 B, A catheter leg bag in place. The catheter tubing should never pull in the client's urethra. In this image, tape is used to secure the catheter to the client's leg. Many agencies do not allow the use of tapes to secure catheters in place as they sometimes cause skin irritation.

22 Remove the drainage tubing from the bed. Place it in the bedpan.
This is done in case the tubing leaks urine.
23 Remove and discard the bed protector. Place in the hamper if it is washable.
24 Cover the client. Remove the cover or bath blanket (if one was used).
This keeps the client warm and respects privacy.
25 Take the bedpan to the bathroom.
26 Drain the drainage bag into a measuring cup, make a note of the measurement, empty the measuring cup into the toilet (see the procedure *Emptying a Urinary Drainage Bag*, on p. 709), and rinse out the measuring cup. Record the amount if required by agency policy.
Actions and observations should be recorded and reported for legal reasons and to keep the rest of the health care team informed.

POST-PROCEDURE

27 Remove gloves. Practise proper hand hygiene.
28 Provide for safety and comfort.
29 Place the call bell within reach.*
This provides an easy, safe way for the client to contact staff if necessary.
30 Return the bed to its lowest position. Follow the care plan for bed rail use.*
31 Remove privacy measures.
32 Discard the drainage tubing and bag or clean the bag, according to employer policy.
This decreases the risk for pathogen spread.
33 Return the bedpan and other supplies to their proper places.
This makes them easier to locate the next time they are needed.
34 Reverse the procedure to attach a drainage bag to the catheter.

Report and Record your actions and observations, according to employer policy.
This is done for legal reasons and to keep the rest of the health care team informed.

*Steps marked with an asterisk may not apply in community settings.

Emptying a Urinary Drainage Bag 123

Advocate on behalf of the client's quality of life by promoting:

Dignity • Independence • Preferences • Privacy • Safety *(see BOX 1–4, on p. 17)*

PRE-PROCEDURE

1 Identify the client, according to employer policy.
This eliminates the possibility of mistaking one client for another.
2 Explain the procedure to the client.
3 Practise proper hand hygiene.
4 Collect the following:
☐ **Graduate (measuring container)**
☐ **Gloves**
☐ **Paper towels**
By collecting all the necessary equipment beforehand, you will not have to leave your client's side and can eliminate wasting time and energy in obtaining the forgotten equipment.
5 Provide for privacy.

PROCEDURE

6 Put on gloves.
7 Place paper towels on the floor. Place the graduate on top of the paper towel.
This decreases the risk for pathogen spread.
8 Position the graduate under the drainage bag drain.
This allows the graduate to collect urine.
9 Open the clamp on the drainage bag, and direct the drain into the graduate.
10 Allow all the urine to drain into the graduate. Do not let the drain touch the graduate (**FIGURE 32–15**).
This helps prevent the graduate from becoming contaminated.
11 Close the clamp securely. Wipe the drain tip with an antiseptic wipe as per your agency policy, and position the drain tip properly (see **FIGURE 32–12**, on p. 707).
The clamp prevents urine from leaking out.
12 Measure the urine.
13 Remove and discard the paper towel.
14 Dispose of the urine in the toilet.
Do not drain the urine down the sink. Doing so would contaminate the sink and may cause odours to escape from the sink drain.
15 Rinse the graduate, and dispose of the rinse water in the toilet.
16 Return the graduate to its proper place.
This makes it easier to locate the next time it is needed.

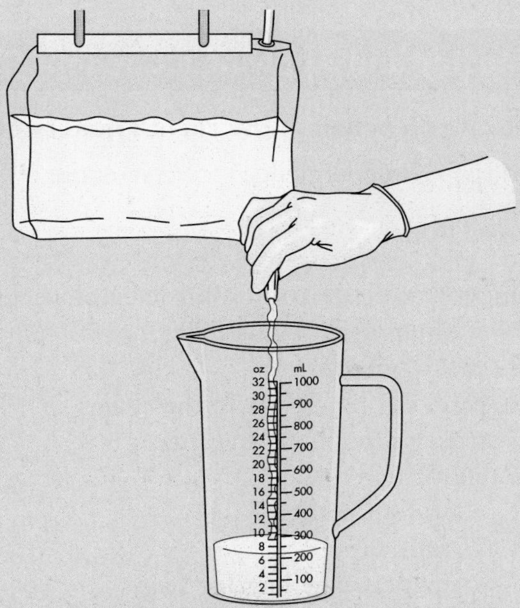

FIGURE 32–15 (**Source:** Potter, P.A., & Perry, A.G. (2009). *Fundamentals of nursing: Concepts, process, and practice* (7th ed.). St. Louis, MO: Mosby.)

17 Remove gloves. Practise proper hand hygiene.
18 Record the time and amount on the intake and output (I&O) record (see Chapter 28).
Actions and observations should be recorded and reported for legal reasons and to keep the rest of the health care team informed.

Continued

Emptying a Urinary Drainage Bag—cont'd

POST-PROCEDURE

19 Remove privacy measures.

Report and Record your actions and observations, according to employer policy. (**FIGURE 32–16**). *This is done for legal reasons and to keep the rest of the health care team informed.*

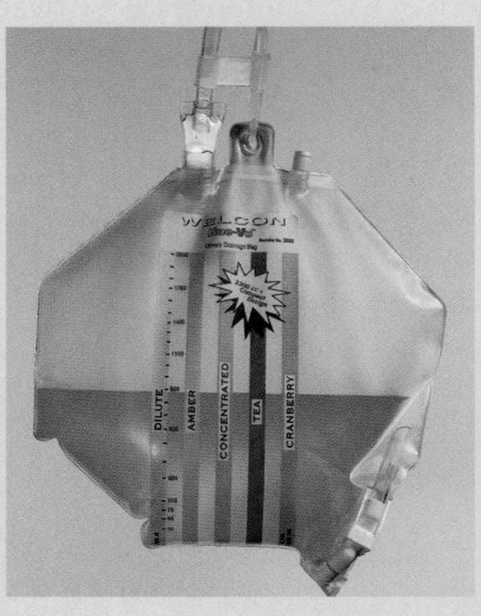

FIGURE 32–16 This urinary drainage bag has a comparison chart for the urine colour. (**Source:** Courtesy of Welcon, Inc., Fort Worth, TX.)

Removing and Applying a Condom Catheter

123

Advocate on behalf of the client's quality of life by promoting:

Dignity • **I**ndependence • **P**references • **P**rivacy • **S**afety *(see BOX 1–4, on p. 17)*

PRE-PROCEDURE

1 Identify the client, according to employer policy. *This eliminates the possibility of mistaking one client for another.*

2 Explain the procedure to the client.

3 Practise proper hand hygiene.

4 Collect the following:

- ☐ **Condom catheter**
- ☐ **Elastic tape**
- ☐ **New drainage bag/leg bag**
- ☐ **Cap for the drainage bag**
- ☐ **Basin of warm water**
- ☐ **Soap**
- ☐ **Towel and washcloths**
- ☐ **Cover or bath blanket (if one is available)**
- ☐ **Gloves**
- ☐ **Bed protector**
- ☐ **Paper towels**

By collecting all the necessary equipment beforehand, you will not have to leave your client's side and can eliminate wasting time and energy in obtaining the forgotten equipment.

5 Place paper towels on the work area. Arrange equipment on top of the paper towels.

6 Provide for privacy.

7 Raise the bed to a comfortable working height.* *This reduces your risk for back injury.*

PROCEDURE

8 Lower the bed rail near you if it is up. *It is easier than reaching over a raised bed rail.*

9 Cover the client with a cover or bath blanket (if one is available). Lower the top linen to the knees.

10 Ask the client to raise the buttocks off the bed, or turn the client onto the side facing away from you. *This allows you to slide the bed protector under the client.*

Continued

Removing and Applying a Condom Catheter—cont'd

11 Slide the bed protector under the client's buttocks.
This helps prevent soiling of the bedding.

12 Have the client lower the buttocks, or turn the client onto the back.

13 Secure the drainage bag to the bed frame (not the bed rail), or have a leg bag ready. Close the drain.
If bed rails are raised, urine can drain back into the bladder, leading to UTI.

14 Expose the genital area. Expose only what you need to see.
Exposing only what you need to see respects the client's privacy.

15 Put on gloves.

16 Remove the condom catheter:
- **a** Remove the tape. Roll the sheath off the penis.
- **b** Disconnect the drainage tubing from the condom. Cap the drainage tube.
- **c** Discard the tape and condom.

Discarding the old condom will reduce the risk for pathogen spread.

17 Provide perineal care (see the procedure *Giving Perineal Care to a Male Client*, on p. 646). Observe the penis for skin breakdown or irritation.
Perineal care reduces buildup of dried secretions around the urinary meatus.

18 Remove the protective backing from the condom.
This exposes the adhesive strip.

19 Hold the penis firmly. Roll the condom onto the penis. Leave a 2.5-cm (1-in.) space between the penis and the catheter end (FIGURE 32–17).

20 Secure the condom with elastic tape. Apply tape in a spiral (see FIGURE 32–17). Do not apply tape completely around the penis.
Applying tape in a spiral manner prevents cutting off circulation to the penis.

21 Connect the condom to the new drainage tubing. Coil excess tubing on the bed (see FIGURE 32–11, on p. 704), or attach a leg bag.
Using a new bag whenever a condom catheter is changed reduces the risk for pathogen spread to the client. Proper tubing positioning allows urine to drain out of the bladder and away from the penis. If allowed to collect around the penis, old urine can cause skin irritation.

22 Remove the bed protector.

23 Remove gloves. Practise proper hand hygiene.

24 Cover the client. Remove the cover or bath blanket (if one was used).

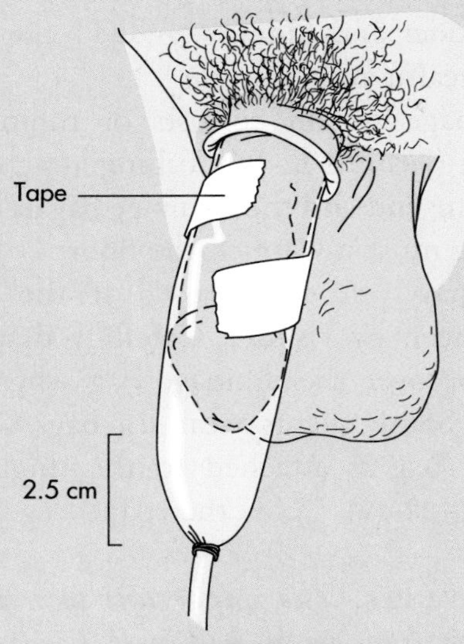

FIGURE 32–17

POST-PROCEDURE

25 Provide for safety and comfort.

26 Place the call bell within reach.*
This provides an easy, safe way for the client to contact staff if necessary.

27 Return the bed to its lowest position. Follow the care plan for bed rail use.*
This reduces the risk for client injury.

28 Remove privacy measures.

29 Practise proper hand hygiene. Put on clean gloves.

30 Measure and record the amount of urine in the bag. Clean or discard the drainage bag, according to employer policy.
Cleaning or discarding equipment in a correct manner reduces the risk for pathogen spread.

31 Discard disposable items.

Continued

Removing and Applying a Condom Catheter—cont'd

32 Clean and return the wash basin and other equipment to their proper places.
This makes them easier to locate the next time they are needed.

33 Remove gloves. Practise proper hand hygiene.

Report and Record your actions and observations, according to employer policy.
This is done for legal reasons and to keep the rest of the health care team informed.

*Steps marked with an asterisk may not apply in community settings.

Drainage Systems

A closed drainage system is used for in-dwelling catheters (including suprapubic catheters) so that nothing enters the system from the catheter to the drainage bag. The urinary system must remain sterile; otherwise, infection can occur when microbes enter the drainage system and travel up the tubing or catheter into the bladder and kidneys. A UTI can threaten the client's health and even life.

The drainage system consists of tubing and a drainage bag (**FIGURE 32–18**). Tubing attaches to the catheter at one end and the drainage bag at the other end. The bag must not touch the floor.

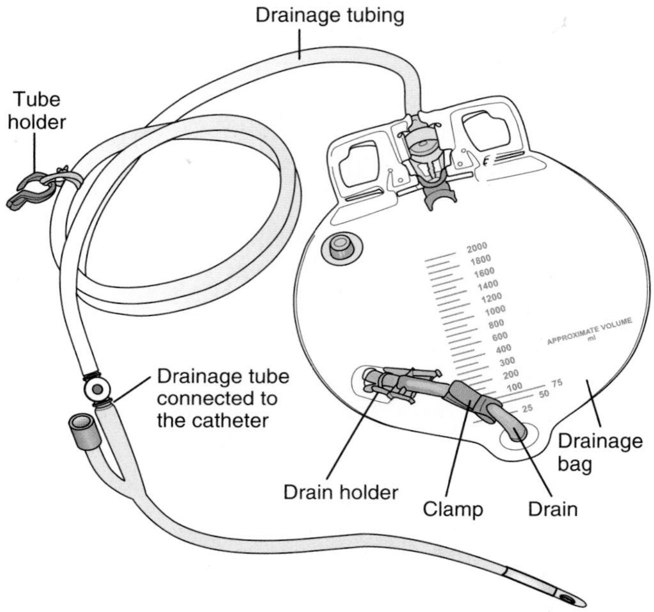

FIGURE 32–18 Parts of a urine drainage system.

Clients may feel embarrassed if the drainage bag can be seen by visitors. Carefully drape a bed sheet or robe over the drainage bag when visitors are present. Some clients wear leg bags when not in bed. The bag is attached to the thigh or calf (see **FIGURE 32–19**), and the pant leg or robe covers it.

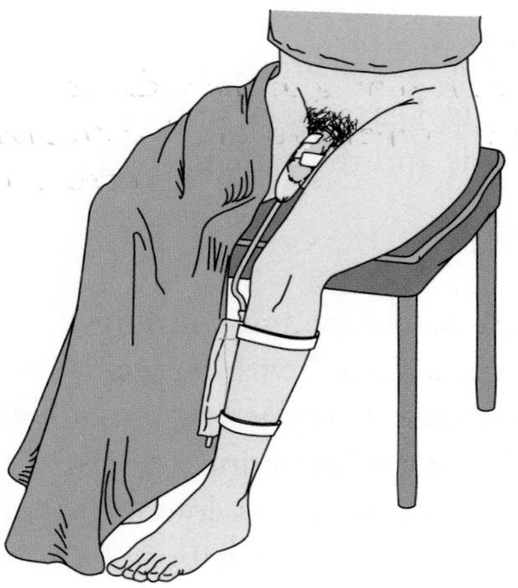

FIGURE 32–19 A condom catheter attached to a leg bag.

As stated earlier, ***it is important to never hang the drainage bag on a bed rail because when the bed rail is raised, the bag is at a higher level than the bladder***. When the client walks, the bag must remain at a lower level than the bladder.

Measuring Urine Drainage

The urine drainage bag is emptied at routine times, according to your agency's policy. If you are responsible for this task, follow the guidelines to measure the urine from a drainage bag:

- Always follow Standard Practices when handling any bodily fluids.
- Follow the procedure *Emptying a Urine Drainage Bag* to empty the bag.
- Never use the measurements marked on the drainage bag to measure the amount of urine collected. These measurements are often inaccurate and unreliable.
- Place the see-through graduated cup or measuring cup on a flat surface to read the urine measurement. Look at the measurement as close to eye level as possible. Holding the measuring cup in the air will result in inaccurate measurements.
- After you have obtained your urine measurement, discard the urine down the toilet or bedpan flusher. Do not pour the urine into a sink drain, as it would contaminate the sink and produce an unpleasant odour.
- Rinse and wash out the measuring cup, according to your agency's policy.

Accidental Disconnection

Sometimes drainage systems are disconnected accidentally. If that happens, reattach the catheter, and inform your supervisor immediately. Do not touch the ends of the catheter or tubing. To reattach the catheter, do the following:

- Wash your hands, and put on gloves.
- Wipe the end of the tube and the end of the catheter with antiseptic wipes, as per your employer's policy. Use a separate wipe for the tube end and for the catheter end (see **FIGURE 32–10** on page 704).
- Do not put the ends down. Do not touch the ends after you clean them.
- Connect the tubing to the catheter.
- Discard the wipes into a biohazard plastic bag.
- Remove the gloves, and practise proper hand hygiene.

Leg bags are replaced by drainage bags when the client returns to bed. Some employers do not allow support workers to replace leg bags with drainage bags, as the risk of infection is high. You must be formally trained, supervised, and monitored to do this task. If you are delegated this task, be sure to follow employer policies and procedures.

You will have to open the drainage system that was previously closed, while taking care to prevent microbes from entering the system. Review the principles of surgical asepsis in Chapter 23. Drainage bags are emptied according to the care plan. Usually this task is completed at the following times:

- At the end of each shift
- When replacing a leg bag with a drainage bag
- When replacing a drainage bag with a leg bag
- When a leg bag is becoming full

In many instances, you will be required to measure the amount of urine that is in the drainage bag prior to emptying it, a task called *measuring output* (see p. 596 for a description of how to measure intake and output [I&O]).

Report and record the following:

- The amount of urine measured
- The colour, clarity, and odour of urine
- Particles in the urine
- Complaints of pain, burning, irritation, or the need to urinate
- Drainage system leaks

The Condom Catheter

Condom catheters—also called *external catheters* and *urinary sheaths*—are often used for male clients with urinary incontinence. A **condom catheter** is a soft sheath that slides over the penis and is held in place with elastic tape. *This tape can cause irritation to the penis, so many agencies no longer use condom catheters.* Tubing connects the condom catheter and the drainage bag; leg bags are often used for male clients (**FIGURE 32–19**).

Wash the penis thoroughly with soap and water, and dry it before applying the condom catheter. Follow the manufacturer's instructions for application. A new condom catheter is usually applied daily or every few days. Follow the care plan.

Elastic tape secures the catheter in place. Use the elastic tape packaged with the condom catheter. Some condom catheters come with the elastic tape already lining the catheter. The elastic tape expands according to penis size so as to allow blood flow to the penis. ***Never use adhesive tape to secure condom catheters. Since adhesive tape does not expand, blood flow to the penis would be cut off, harming the penis.*** Follow medical asepsis and Standard Practices when removing and applying condom catheters.

Report and record the following:

- Reddened or open areas on the penis
- Swelling of the penis
- Colour, clarity, and odour of the urine
- Particles in the urine

BLADDER TRAINING

Bladder training programs have been developed for clients with urinary incontinence. Some clients need bladder training after removal of an in-dwelling catheter. After having an in-dwelling catheter for some time, they may have lost muscle tone in the bladder, so the bladder may no longer be able to stretch sufficiently to hold urine. These clients may have urinary incontinence until bladder tone is restored. Control of urination is the goal of the bladder training program, which would be part of the client's care plan. You are required to assist with bladder training, as directed by your supervisor and the care plan.

There are two basic methods of bladder training:

1. The client uses the toilet, commode, bedpan, or urinal at scheduled times. The client is given 15 or 20 minutes to initiate voiding. The guidelines for maintaining normal urination (see p. 691) are followed. The normal position for voiding is assumed if possible. Privacy is important. Help the client relax, and provide encouragement. These techniques can help the client succeed.
2. The client has a catheter. The catheter is clamped to prevent urine from draining out of the bladder (see **FIGURE 32–12**, on p. 707). Usually, the catheter is clamped for 1 hour at first, and eventually it is clamped for 3 to 4 hours at a time. Urine drains from the bladder when the catheter is unclamped. When the catheter is removed, you will encourage the client to void every 3 to 4 hours or as directed by your supervisor and the care plan.

COLLECTING URINE SPECIMENS

Urine specimens (samples) are collected for urine tests. Physicians use test results to make a diagnosis or evaluate treatment. Follow the guidelines in **BOX 32–5** when collecting specimens.

The Random Urine Specimen

The random urine specimen is collected for a urinalysis. No special measures are needed, and the specimen is collected at any time. Often, clients can collect the specimen themselves, but clients who are weak or very ill will need assistance.

It is difficult to collect any type of urine specimen from very old adults and very young children, and especially from people who are unable to follow instructions—for example, clients who have dementia or a severe mental health disorder. Your supervisor will have suggestions on how you may successfully obtain specimens from these clients, while ensuring that their rights to dignity and privacy are respected.

There is 3 types of urine specimens: Random, midstream & 24-hour.

BOX 32–5 Guidelines for Collecting Urine Specimens

- Explain the procedure to the client thoroughly and ensure cooperation.
- Follow the rules of medical asepsis and Standard Practices. Wear gloves when collecting specimens.
- Use a clean container for each specimen.
- Use a container appropriate for the specimen.
- Label the container accurately. Write on it the client's full name, address or room and bed number, date, and the time the specimen was collected. If preprinted labels are used, place a label on the container.
- Do not touch the inside of the container or lid.

Continued

BOX 32–5 Guidelines for Collecting Urine Specimens—cont'd

- Collect the specimen at the time specified.
- Ask the client not to defecate during specimen collection. The specimen must not contain feces.
- Ask the client to dispose of used toilet tissue in the toilet and to ensure that the specimen does not contain tissue.
- Put the lid on the specimen container.
- Place the specimen container in a plastic bag for transportation. In a facility, take the specimen and requisition slip to the laboratory or storage area. In community settings, follow your supervisor's instructions for storing the specimen. Tell the client or family members where the specimen is stored. Follow your supervisor's instructions for sending the specimen to the laboratory.
- Urine specimens must be kept cool and should be tested within 2 to 4 hours unless a preservative has been added to the specimen container. Note that nearly all 24-hour collection bottles contain a preservative, and it is important ***not*** to pour that out.
- **Report and record** the following observations:
  - Difficulty in obtaining the specimen
  - Colour, clarity, and odour of urine
  - Particles in urine
  - Complaints of pain, burning, urgency, dysuria, or other problems

Collecting a Random Urine Specimen

123

Advocate on behalf of the client's quality of life by promoting:

Dignity • Independence • Preferences • Privacy • Safety *(see BOX 1–4, on p. 17)*

PRE-PROCEDURE

1 Identify the client, according to employer policy. *This eliminates the possibility of mistaking one client for another.*
2 Explain the procedure to the client.
3 Practise proper hand hygiene.
4 Collect the following:
   - ☐ **Bedpan and cover, urinal, or specimen pan** (FIGURE 32–20)
   - ☐ **Specimen container and lid**
   - ☐ **Label**
   - ☐ **Gloves**
   - ☐ **Plastic bag**

   By collecting all the necessary equipment beforehand, you will not have to leave your client's side and can eliminate wasting time and energy in obtaining the forgotten equipment.

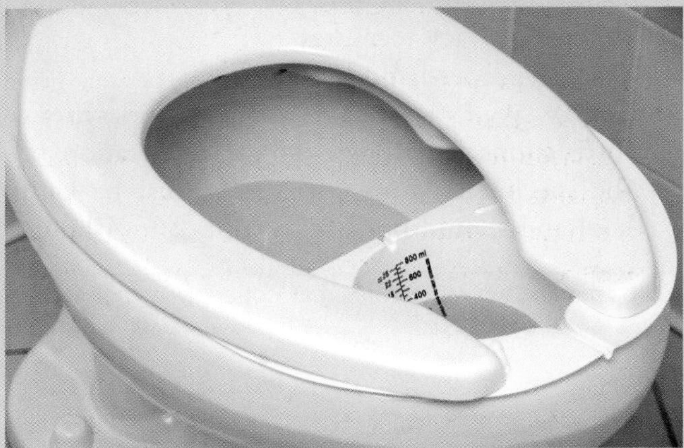

FIGURE 32–20 The specimen pan is placed on the rim of the toilet. It has graduated markings for measuring urine. (**Source:** Rob Byron/Shutterstock.com)

Continued

Collecting a Random Urine Specimen—cont'd

PROCEDURE

5 Label the container.
Proper labelling will reduce the risk of misplacing the specimens.
6 Put the container and lid in the bathroom.
7 Provide for privacy.
8 Put on gloves.
9 Ask the client to urinate in the receptacle (the bedpan, urinal, or specimen pan). Remind the client to put toilet tissue into the wastebasket or toilet, not in the bedpan or specimen pan.
Putting toilet paper in the bedpan will make the urine specimen unusable.
10 Take the receptacle to the bathroom.
This provides privacy and limits odours to one location.
11 Measure the urine if I&O is ordered.
12 Pour about 120 mL (4 oz.) of urine into the specimen container. Dispose of excess urine.
13 Place the lid on the specimen container. Put the container in a plastic bag.
The plastic bag reduces the risk of splashing and pathogen transfer.
14 Clean and return the receptacle to its proper place.
This makes it easier to locate the next time it is needed.
15 Help the client with handwashing.
16 Remove gloves. Practise proper hand hygiene.

POST-PROCEDURE

17 Provide for safety and comfort.
18 Place the call bell within reach.*
This provides an easy, safe way for the client to contact staff if necessary.
19 Follow the care plan for bed rail use.*
This reduces the risk for client injury.
20 Remove privacy measures.
21 Practise proper hand hygiene.
22 Follow your agency's policy or supervisor's instructions for storage and transportation of the specimen. Urine specimens must be kept cool and should be tested within 2 to 4 hours unless a preservative has been added to the specimen container. Note that nearly all 24-hour collection bottles contain a preservative, and it is important ***not*** to pour that out.

Report and Record your actions and observations, according to employer policy.
This is done for legal reasons and to keep the rest of the health care team informed.

*Steps marked with an asterisk may not apply in community settings.

The Midstream Specimen

The midstream specimen is also called a *clean-voided specimen* or a *clean-catch specimen*. The perineal area is cleaned before any voiding begins so as to reduce the number of microbes in the urethral area. The client starts to void into the toilet, bedpan, urinal, or commode. Then the stream is stopped, and a sterile specimen container is held in position. The client voids into the container until the required amount of specimen is obtained.

Stopping the stream of urine midway is hard for many people. You may need to hold the container in place and collect the specimen after the client starts to void.

Collecting a Midstream Specimen

123

Advocate on behalf of the client's quality of life by promoting:

Dignity • Independence • Preferences • Privacy • Safety *(see BOX 1–4, on p. 17)*

PRE-PROCEDURE

1 Identify the client, according to employer policy.
This eliminates the possibility of mistaking one client for another.

2 Explain the procedure to the client.

3 Practise proper hand hygiene.

4 Collect the following:

- ☐ **Clean-voided specimen kit (with antiseptic solution)**
- ☐ **Label**
- ☐ **Disposable gloves**
- ☐ **Sterile gloves (if not in the kit)**
- ☐ **Bedpan, urinal, or commode if needed**
- ☐ **Plastic bag**
- ☐ **Antiseptic wipe as per your facility policy**
- ☐ **Supplies for perineal care**

By collecting all the necessary equipment beforehand, you will not have to leave your client's side and can eliminate wasting time and energy in obtaining the forgotten equipment.

PROCEDURE

5 Provide for privacy.

6 Label the container.
Proper labelling reduces the risk of losing the specimen.

7 Put on gloves, and provide perineal care. Remove gloves. Practise proper hand hygiene.

8 Open the sterile kit. Use sterile technique (see Chapter 23).

9 Put on the sterile gloves.
Sterile gloves do not contain pathogens. Pathogens getting into the specimen could alter the test results.

10 Pour the antiseptic solution over the cloth intended for perineal care.

11 Open the sterile specimen container. Do not touch the inside of the container or lid. Set the lid down so that the inside is up.
Touching the inside cap could contaminate it.

12 *For a female: Clean the perineum with the cloth intended for perineal care:*

- a Spread the labia with your thumb and index finger. Use your nondominant hand.

This hand is now contaminated. It must not touch anything sterile.

- b Clean down the urethral area from front to back. Use a clean corner of the cloth intended for perineal care for each stroke.

By using clean corners with each stroke, you reduce the risk of contaminating the area with pathogens.

- c Keep the labia separated to collect the urine specimen (steps 14 to 17).

13 *For a male: Clean the penis with the cloth intended for perineal care:*

- a Hold the penis with your nondominant hand.
- b Clean the penis starting at the urethral opening. Use the cloth intended for perineal care and clean in a circular motion.
- c Keep holding the penis until the specimen is collected (steps 14 to 17).

This hand is now contaminated. It must not touch anything sterile.

14 Ask the client to void into the toilet, bedpan, commode container, or urinal. This beginning stream will be discarded.
Urine that first exits the urethra may be contaminated with normal flora and other pathogens. Voiding flushes the urethra of these pathogens.

Continued

Collecting a Midstream Specimen—cont'd

15 Hold the specimen container to collect the stream of urine. For a female, keep the labia separated, if possible.
Labia could contaminate the urine specimen. Urine that is collected after that first stream is considered to be sterile.
16 Collect about 30 to 60 mL of urine (1 to 2 oz.).
17 Remove the specimen container before the client stops voiding.
Urine at the end of the voiding may contain pathogens washed from the urethra and the urinary meatus.
18 Let go of the labia or penis.
19 Allow the client to finish voiding into the toilet, bedpan, commode container, or urinal.
20 Put the lid on the specimen container. Touch only the outside of the container or lid.
This helps avoid the risk of contaminating the specimen.
21 Wipe the outside of the container with an antiseptic wipe, as per your facility policy.
22 Place the container in a plastic bag.
The plastic bag reduces the risk for pathogen transfer in case the outside of the container were to become contaminated.
23 Provide toilet tissue after the client finishes voiding.
24 Remove and empty the bedpan, commode container, or urinal.
25 Clean the bedpan, urinal, or commode container and other items. Return the equipment to its proper place.
This makes it easier to locate the next time it is needed.
26 Remove gloves. Practise proper hand hygiene.
27 Help the client with handwashing.
28 Repeat proper hand hygiene.

POST-PROCEDURE

29 Follow steps 17 through 22 in the procedure *Collecting a Random Urine Specimen* on page 715.

Report and Record your actions and observations, according to employer policy.
This is done for legal reasons and to keep the rest of the health care team informed.

The 24-Hour Urine Specimen

For a 24-hour urine specimen, all urine voided during a 24-hour period is collected. The collected urine is kept chilled on ice or refrigerated during the collection period (**FIGURE 32–21**) to prevent the growth of microbes. A preservative is added to the collection container for some tests.

The client's first voiding of the day of collection is discarded. *All* of the urine voided during the next 24 hours is then collected. The client and staff must have a clear understanding of the procedure and the test period. In home care settings, the client and primary caregiver will need to collect some of the specimen on their own. As the support worker, make sure they understand what needs to be done. Contact your supervisor if they are unsure. Follow the guidelines for collecting urine specimens.

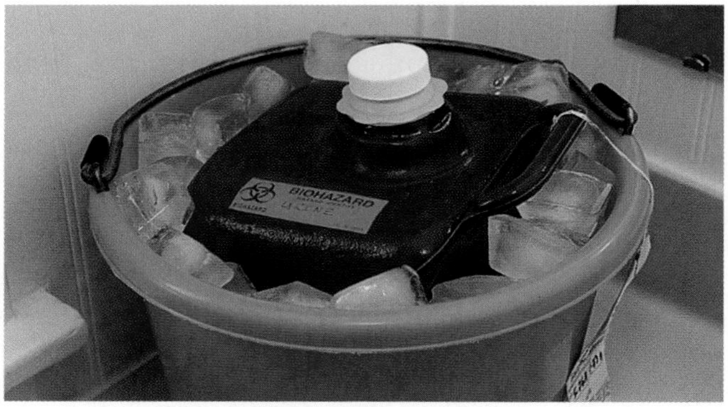

FIGURE 32–21 To preserve the 24-hour urine specimen, the urine container may be stored in a bucket of ice. There is usually a preservative supplied in the specimen container, which should be kept in the container and not poured out. (**Source:** Birchenall, J., & Streight, E. (1997). *Mosby's textbook for the home care aide* (p. 315). St. Louis, MO: Mosby.)

Collecting a Specimen From an Infant or Child

If a specimen is needed from an infant or a child who is not toilet trained, a collection bag is applied over the urethra. A parent or a staff member will assist you in the bag's application if the child is agitated. This procedure may also be adapted for clients who are in wheelchairs or who are incontinent.

Collecting a Urine Specimen From an Infant or Child 123

Advocate on behalf of the client's quality of life by promoting:

Dignity • Independence • Preferences • Privacy • Safety (see BOX 1–4, on p. 17)

PRE-PROCEDURE

1 Identify the child, according to employer policy
This eliminates the possibility of mistaking one client for another.
2 Explain the procedure to the child and the parents.
3 Practise proper hand hygiene.
4 Collect the following:
- ☐ **Collection bag**
- ☐ **Wash basin**
- ☐ **Cloth intended for perineal care**
- ☐ **Bath towel**
- ☐ **Two diapers, one with a 2.5-cm (1-in.) hole cut into it over the area of the child's urethra**
- ☐ **Specimen container**
- ☐ **Gloves**
- ☐ **Plastic bag**
- ☐ **Scissors**

By collecting all the necessary equipment beforehand, you will not have to leave your client's side and can eliminate wasting time and energy in obtaining the forgotten equipment.

PROCEDURE

5 Provide for privacy.
6 Remove and dispose of the diaper.
The worn diaper is considered contaminated.
7 Clean the perineal area with the cloth intended for perineal care. Use a new corner for each stroke. Rinse and dry the area.
This reduces the risk of contaminating the urine sample.
8 Practise proper hand hygiene.
9 Position the child on the back. Flex the child's knees, and separate the legs.
This is the best position for you to fix the urine collection bag on the child.
10 Remove the adhesive backing from the collection bag.
11 Apply the disposable collection bag to the perineum (**FIGURE 32–22**). Do not cover the anus. Urine collects in the bag for a specimen.
The anal area is considered contaminated.

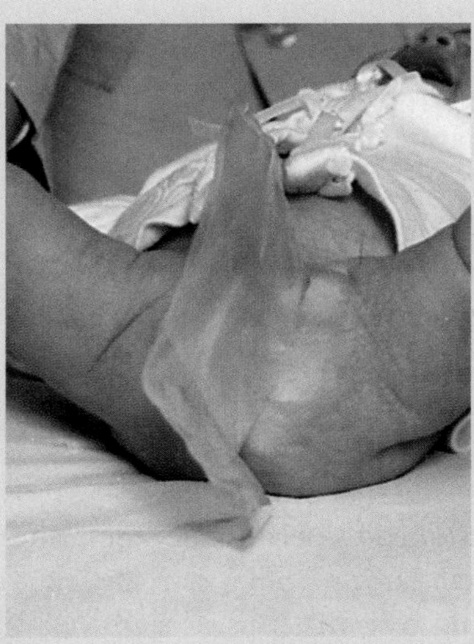

FIGURE 32–22 (**Source:** Hockenberry, M.J., & Wilson, D. (2011). *Wong's nursing care of infants and children* (9th ed.). St. Louis, MO: Mosby.)

Continued

Collecting a Urine Specimen From an Infant or Child—cont'd

12 Put a new diaper on the child.
13 Pull the collection bag through a 2.5-cm (1-in.) hole in the bottom of the diaper.
This allows you to observe the bag to see if the client has voided.
14 Practise proper hand hygiene.
15 Raise the head of the crib if allowed. This helps urine to collect in the bottom of the bag.
Urine that is allowed to stay on the client's skin can irritate the delicate skin tissue.
16 Raise the crib rail.
This reduces the risk for client injury.
17 Check the bag periodically to see if the child has voided. (Wear gloves, and provide for privacy.)
The urine specimen should be collected as soon as possible after voiding.
18 Provide for privacy if the child has urinated.
19 Put on gloves.
20 Lower the crib rail.
21 Remove the diaper.
22 Remove the collection bag gently.
23 Press the adhesive surfaces of the bag together, or transfer the urine to the specimen container through the drainage tab.
24 Clean the perineal area, rinse, and dry well.
This is done to remove old urine, which can irritate the delicate skin.
25 Put a new diaper on the child.
26 Remove gloves. Practise proper hand hygiene.

POST-PROCEDURE

27 Provide for safety and comfort. Raise the crib rail.
28 Remove privacy measures.
29 Write the requested information on the specimen container. Place the container in the plastic bag.
Specimen containers should be properly labelled to reduce the risk of losing them.
30 Clean and return the equipment to its proper place. Discard disposable items. (Wear gloves for this step.)
This makes equipment easier to locate the next time it is needed.
31 Practise proper hand hygiene.
32 Follow your supervisor's instructions for storage and transportation of the specimen.
This helps reduce the risk of spoiling the specimen.

Report and Record your actions and observations, according to employer policy.
This is done for legal reasons and to keep the rest of the health care team informed.

TESTING URINE

You may be asked to perform simple urine tests—for example, measuring pH, glucose, ketones, and blood—using reagent strips. Ensure that the reagent strips are not outdated by checking the expiry date on the container. Straining urine for stones is another simple test. A physician orders the type and frequency of urine tests, and you must ensure accuracy when performing the tests. Promptly report the results, according to employer policy.

- ***Testing pH***—Urine pH measures indicate whether urine is acidic or alkaline. Changes in normal pH (4.6 to 8.0) occur due to illness, foods, and medications. A routine urine specimen is needed.
- ***Testing for glucose and ketones***—In clients with diabetes, the pancreas does not secrete enough insulin (see Chapter 37), which is needed by the body to use sugar for energy. If not used by the body, sugar builds up in the blood, and some of it will appear in urine. **Glucosuria** means glucose, a type of sugar (*glucos*, *glycos*), in urine (*uria*). The

client with diabetes may also have **ketones** in the urine. Ketones appear in urine because of the rapid breakdown of fat for energy, which happens when the body cannot use sugar. Testing is usually done four times a day: 30 minutes before each meal (ac) and at bedtime (hs). The physician uses the test results to regulate the client's medication and diet.

To test for glucose and ketones, follow the instructions printed on the side of the reagent bottle. (See "Using Reagent Strips" below.)

- ***Testing for blood***—Normal urine is free of blood. Injury and disease can cause blood (*hemat*) to appear in urine (*uria*), a state called *hematuria*. Sometimes, blood can be seen in urine, and at other times it is not visible (*occult*), so a routine urine specimen is needed.

Using Reagent Strips

Reagent strips are chemically treated "dipsticks." They have different sections that change colour as a reaction to urine. To use a reagent strip, dip the strip into the urine specimen, wait the specified length of time, and compare the colour on the strip with the colour chart on the bottle (**FIGURE 32–23**). You will probably need a watch or a clock to keep track of the time, according to the instructions. Instructions vary, depending on the test. Your supervisor will tell you how to perform the urine test that has been ordered by the physician. Read the manufacturer's instructions before you begin. Always check the date on the container. Do not use the product past its expiry date.

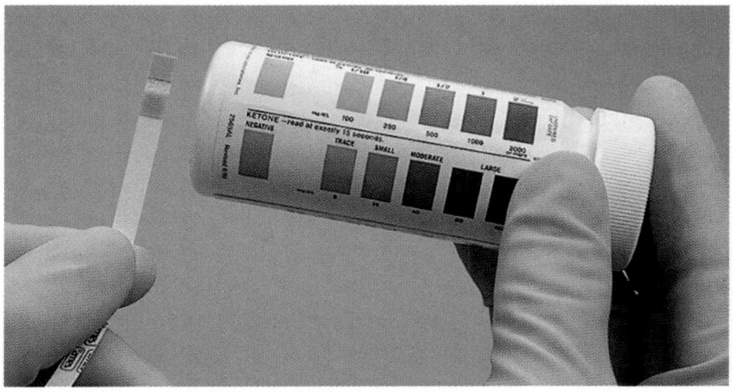

FIGURE 32–23 Reagent strip for glucose and ketones.

Testing Urine With Reagent Strips

123

Advocate on behalf of the client's quality of life by promoting:

Dignity • Independence • Preferences • Privacy • Safety *(see BOX 1–4, on p. 17)*

PRE-PROCEDURE

1 Practise proper hand hygiene.
2 Put on gloves.
3 Collect the following:
- ☐ **Urine specimen (check with your supervisor for method to obtain)**
- ☐ **Reagent strip, as ordered**
- ☐ **Gloves**

By collecting all the necessary equipment beforehand, you can eliminate wasting time and energy in obtaining the forgotten equipment.

PROCEDURE

4 Remove a strip from the bottle. Recap the bottle immediately. The cap must be on tight.
The cap prevents air and moisture from spoiling the expensive reagent strips.

5 Dip the reagent strip into the specimen.
The reagent strip cannot work without first being immersed in the urine.

6 Remove the strip after the correct amount of time (follow manufacturer's instructions).
It is important to follow manufacturer's instructions to get the proper results.

7 Tap the strip gently against the specimen container.
This helps remove excess urine.

Continued

Testing Urine With Reagent Strips—cont'd

8 Wait the required length of time (follow manufacturer's instructions).

9 Compare the colour on the strip with the colour chart on the bottle. Read the results.
This will provide the information that you require.

10 Discard disposable items and the specimen according to employer policies.

POST-PROCEDURE

11 Clean and return equipment to its proper place.
This makes it easier to locate the next time it is needed.

12 Remove gloves. Practise proper hand hygiene.

Report and Record the results and other observations, according to employer policy.
This is done for legal reasons and to keep the rest of the health care team informed.

Straining Urine

Stones (*calculi*) can develop in the kidneys, ureters, or bladder. Stones vary in size—some are the size of a pinhead; others are the size of an orange. Stones that cause severe pain and damage to the urinary system may require surgical removal. Some stones exit the body through urine. When the care plan calls for the client's urine to be strained, all the urine is poured through a disposable strainer. If any stones are found, they are sent to the laboratory for examination.

Straining Urine 123

Advocate on behalf of the client's quality of life by promoting:

Dignity • Independence • Preferences • Privacy • Safety (see BOX 1–4, on p. 17)

PRE-PROCEDURE

1 Identify the client, according to employer policy.
This eliminates the possibility of mistaking one client for another.

2 Explain the procedure to the client. Also, explain that the urinal, bedpan, commode, or specimen pan is used for voiding.

3 Practise proper hand hygiene.

4 Collect the following:
- ☐ **Strainer and 10 × 10 cm (4 × 4 in.) gauze**
- ☐ **Specimen container**
- ☐ **Urinal, bedpan, commode, or specimen pan**
- ☐ **Two labels stating that all urine has been strained**
- ☐ **Gloves**
- ☐ **Plastic bag**

By collecting all the necessary equipment beforehand, you will not have to leave your client's side and can eliminate wasting time and energy in obtaining the forgotten equipment.

Continued

Straining Urine—cont'd

PROCEDURE

5 Arrange items in the client's bathroom. Place the specimen pan in the toilet (see FIGURE 32-20, on p. 715).
Placing it in the bathroom provides privacy for the client.
6 Place one label in the bathroom. Place the other near the bed.
Labels are reminders for the client and for the staff.
7 Put on gloves.
8 Offer the bedpan or urinal, or assist the client to the bedside commode or bathroom.
This allows the client to empty the bladder so the test can begin with a fresh sample.
9 Provide for privacy.
10 Tell the client to call you after voiding.
11 Remove gloves. Practise proper hand hygiene.
12 Return when the client calls you. Knock before entering the room.
13 Practise proper hand hygiene. Put on gloves.
14 Place the strainer or gauze over the specimen container.
15 Pour urine into the specimen container. Urine passes through the strainer or gauze (FIGURE 32-24).
16 Discard the urine.
The urine specimen is not required anymore.

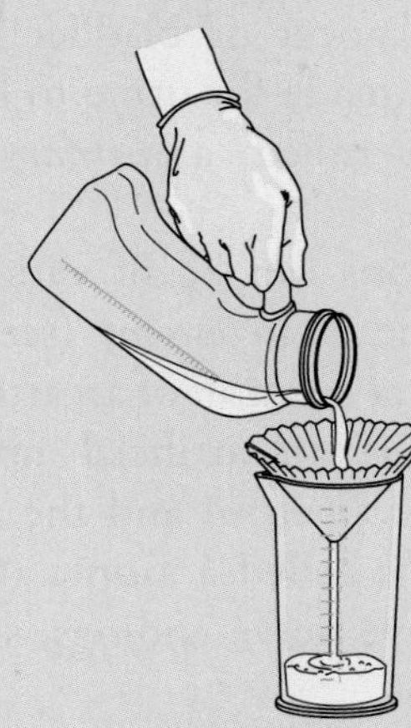

FIGURE 32-24

17 Place the strainer or gauze in the container if any crystals, stones, or particles appear.
The strainer or gauze will catch the crystals, stones, or particles.
18 Provide perineal care if needed.
Perineal care reduces the risk for odours, skin irritation, and pathogen spread.
19 Clean and return equipment to its proper place.
This makes it easier to locate the next time it is needed.
20 Remove soiled gloves. Practise proper hand hygiene.
21 Help the client with handwashing.
22 Repeat proper hand hygiene.

POST-PROCEDURE

23 Provide for safety and comfort.
24 Place the call bell within reach.*
This provides an easy, safe way for the client to contact staff if necessary.
25 Follow the care plan for bed rail use.*
This reduces the risk for client injury.
26 Remove privacy measures.
27 Label the specimen container with the requested information. Put the container in the plastic bag. (Wear gloves for this step.)
28 Practise proper hand hygiene.
29 Follow your agency policies or your supervisor's instructions for storage and transportation of the specimen.
This reduces the risk of spoiling the specimen.

Report and Record your actions and observations, according to employer policy.
This is done for legal reasons and to keep the rest of the health care team informed.

*Steps marked with an asterisk may not apply in community settings.

THE CLIENT WITH A URETEROSTOMY OR AN ILEAL CONDUIT

The bladder is sometimes surgically removed as part of treatment for cancer or bladder injuries. Since provision must be made for urine to leave the body, a new pathway—called a *urinary diversion*—is created.

Urinary diversions can be of various types. The most common one is an *ostomy* (see Chapter 29), which is the surgical creation of an artificial opening. A **ureterostomy** is an artificial opening (*stomy*) between the ureter (*uretero*) and the abdomen. The artificial opening is called a **stoma** (FIGURE 32–25). Stomas do not have nerve endings, so they are not painful.

Some clients may have an **ileal conduit**, an artificial bladder fashioned out of a section of the ileum (part of the small intestine). Urine drains from the ureters into the newly created artificial bladder and then through the stoma.

An ostomy appliance (which some call a "pouch") is applied over the stoma. The ostomy appliance is a disposable plastic bag that adheres to the skin around the stoma and that urine drains into. The ostomy appliance is replaced any time it leaks, as leaking urine can cause skin irritation, skin breakdown, and infection. Leaks also often cause clients to worry about odours and embarrassing wetness. Immediately after this type of surgery, the client will receive care from a nurse, but you may be required to care for clients with long-standing ureterostomies. The client assists with care as much as possible.

It is your responsibility to provide good skin care to the client with a ureterostomy. These clients are at risk for skin breakdown around the stoma, caused by the draining urine and by the adhesive of the ostomy appliance. You need to report and record changes in the client's skin around the stoma.

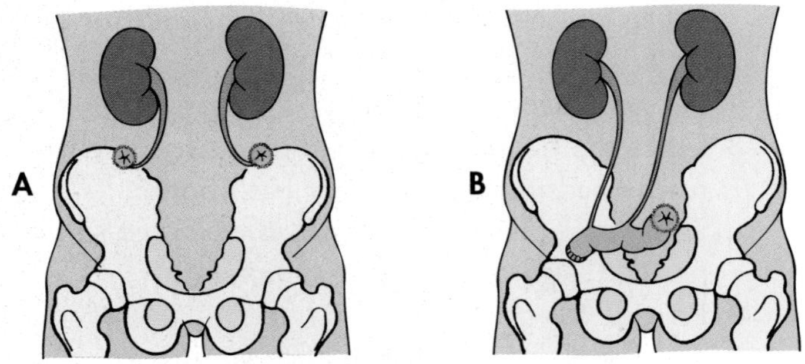

FIGURE 32–25 Ureterostomies. **A,** Both ureters are brought through the skin onto the abdomen. The client has two stomas, one for each ureter. **B,** The ileal conduit. A small section of the small intestine is removed and one end sutured closed to form an artificial bladder, or neobladder. The other end is brought through the skin onto the abdomen to form a stoma. The ureters are attached to this part of the small intestine, and urine collects in the newly created artificial bladder and drains through the stoma. (**Source:** Beare, P.A., & Myers, J.L. (1998). *Principles and practices of adult health nursing* (3rd ed.). St. Louis, MO: Mosby.)

Changing a Ureterostomy Pouch

123

Advocate on behalf of the client's quality of life by promoting:

Dignity • Independence • Preferences • Privacy • Safety *(see BOX 1–4, on p. 17)*

PRE-PROCEDURE

1 Identify the client, according to employer policy. *This eliminates the possibility of mistaking one client for another.*
2 Explain the procedure to the client.
3 Practise proper hand hygiene.
4 Collect the following:
- ☐ **Clean pouch with skin barrier**
- ☐ **Skin barrier (if not part of pouch)**
- ☐ **Pouch clamp, clip, or wire closure**
- ☐ **Clean ostomy belt (if used)**
- ☐ **Four to eight 5 × 5 cm (2 × 2 in.) gauze squares**
- ☐ **Adhesive remover**
- ☐ **Cloth for applying adhesive remover**
- ☐ **Bedpan with cover**
- ☐ **Waterproof pad**
- ☐ **Cover or bath blanket (if one is available)**
- ☐ **Toilet tissue**
- ☐ **Wash basin**

Continued

Changing a Ureterostomy Pouch—cont'd

- ☐ **Bath thermometer**
- ☐ **Soap or cleansing agent, according to the care plan**
- ☐ **Pouch deodorant**
- ☐ **Paper towels**
- ☐ **Gloves**
- ☐ **Disposable bag**

By collecting all the necessary equipment beforehand, you will not have to leave your client's side and can eliminate wasting time and energy in obtaining the forgotten equipment.

5 Arrange the paper towels on the work area. Place the items on paper towels.
Planning ahead reduces wasted steps and exhausting the client.

6 Provide for privacy.

7 Raise the bed to a comfortable working height.*

PROCEDURE

8 Lower the bed rail near you if it is up. (*Note:* This procedure can be performed while the client is sitting on the toilet, provided that the client is able to sit without assistance for a length of time and that the position is preferred by the client and the support worker.)

9 Cover the client with a cover or bath blanket (if one is available). Fan-fold the linen to the foot of the bed.
This ensures client warmth and privacy.

10 Place the waterproof pad under the client's buttocks.
This is done to absorb any urine or water that may drip while performing this procedure.

11 Put on gloves.

12 Disconnect the pouch from the belt. Remove the belt.

13 Remove the pouch by gently pushing the skin down and away from the skin barrier (if it is separate). Place the pouch in the bedpan.
Being gentle reduces the risk of causing injury to the stoma or surrounding skin and provides a more comfortable experience for the client.

14 Place one or two gauze squares over the stoma.
The gauze absorbs any urine that may leak out during this procedure.

15 Wipe around the stoma with toilet tissue or a gauze square. Place soiled tissue in the bedpan. Discard gauze squares into the disposable bag.

16 Apply adhesive remover on a piece of cloth. Clean around the stoma to remove any remaining skin barrier. Clean from the stoma outward.
Always wipe from clean to dirty.

17 Cover the bedpan, and take it to the bathroom. (If bed rails are used, raise them before leaving the bedside.*)
Covering the bedpan keeps its contents private and reduces odours.

18 Measure the urine. Report any abnormality in the urine. Empty the pouch and bedpan into the toilet. Note the colour, clarity, and odour of the urine. Put the pouch in the disposable bag.
Actions and observations should be recorded and reported to keep the rest of the health care team informed and for legal reasons.

19 Remove gloves. Practise proper hand hygiene. Put on clean gloves.

20 Fill the wash basin with warm water. (Measure the temperature of the water with a bath thermometer. Check the care plan for the correct temperature to use.) Place the basin on the work area on top of paper towels. Lower the bed rail near you if it is up.

21 Clean the skin around the stoma with water and soap or another cleansing agent as per your facility policy. Rinse and pat dry.
This decreases the risk for pathogen spread.

22 Observe the stoma and the skin around the stoma. Report any skin irritation or breakdown.
Urine collecting around the stoma could cause skin irritation and soreness.

23 Apply the skin barrier if it is a separate device.
There are a variety of appliance styles. The care plan will tell you what appliance and equipment to use.

Continued

Changing a Ureterostomy Pouch—cont'd

24 Put a clean ostomy belt on the client (if a belt is worn).
The belt helps secure the appliance while it is being worn.

25 Add deodorant to the new pouch.
The deodorant helps reduce the odour associated with urine.

26 Remove adhesive backing on the pouch.

27 Remove the gauze square that was used to absorb the urine from the stoma. Discard it into the disposable bag.

28 Centre the pouch over the stoma, with the drain pointing downward (**FIGURE 32–26**).
Point the drain downward so the urine can drain away from the stoma.

29 Press around the skin barrier. Apply gentle pressure from the stoma outward.
This ensures that the pouch is sealed to the skin.

30 Maintain pressure for 1 to 2 minutes.
This helps the backing to warm to body temperature and the seal to be activated.

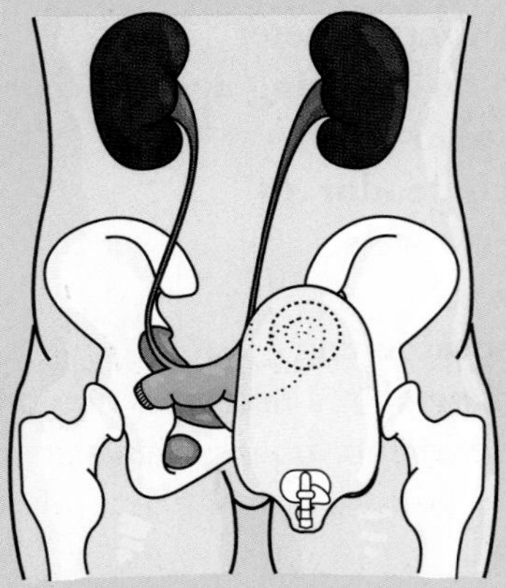

FIGURE 32–26 Ureterostomy pouch.

31 Connect the belt to the pouch (if a belt is worn).
The belt helps the appliance to be secured.

32 Remove the waterproof pad.

33 Remove gloves. Practise proper hand hygiene.

34 Cover the client.

POST-PROCEDURE

35 Provide for safety and comfort.

36 Place the call bell within reach.*
This provides an easy, safe way for the client to contact staff if necessary.

37 Return the bed to its lowest position. Follow the care plan for bed rail use.*
This reduces the risk for client injury.

38 Remove privacy measures.

39 Clean the bedpan, wash basin, and other equipment. Put on gloves for this step.
This decreases the risk for pathogen spread.

40 Return equipment to its proper place.
This makes it easier to find the next time it is needed.

41 Discard the disposable bag, according to employer policy. Follow employer policy for handling soiled linen.
This decreases the risk for pathogen spread.

42 Remove gloves. Practise proper hand hygiene.

Report and Record your actions and observations, according to employer policy.
This is done for legal reasons and to keep the rest of the health care team informed.

*Steps marked with an asterisk may not apply in community settings.

COMPASSIONATE CARE

Elimination is a very personal and private act. Be sensitive to the client's feelings of embarrassment or discomfort. You should try to make the client feel better about accepting your help. Tell your supervisor if the client refuses care. It is your responsibility to promote the client's dignity, independence, preferences, privacy, and safety (see the *Providing Compassionate Care: Assisting Clients With Elimination* box.)

Providing Compassionate Care
Assisting Clients With Elimination

- ***Dignity.*** Never do anything to increase the client's embarrassment. Always be encouraging and positive when providing care. Do not show disgust at the sights or odours associated with elimination and ostomy care. Remember that your nonverbal behaviours and expressions reveal your feelings. For example, do not wrinkle your nose or grimace while you are assisting the client. Never refer to incontinence products as *diapers*, as this term can humiliate the client.
- ***Independence.*** Respond promptly to all requests for help with elimination, as the need may be urgent. Believe clients when they ask for help, even if they just used the toilet, bedpan, urinal, or commode. Your prompt response gives the client some sense of control.
- ***Preferences.*** Respect the client's preferences, whenever possible. For example, some male clients may want to use the urinal sitting up, and some others may prefer to do it lying down.
- ***Privacy.*** Provide as much privacy as possible. Lack of privacy may inhibit the client and interfere with elimination. Pull privacy curtains and close doors, shades, and drapes. Ask visitors or family members to step out of the room. If allowed by the care plan, leave the room after assisting the client to the bathroom or providing a bedpan, urinal, or commode. Or, to be immediately available, stand just outside the door, stand on the other side of the privacy curtain, or stay by the client's side but look away if safe to do so. Ask your supervisor for advice on ways to protect the client's privacy.
- ***Safety.*** Do not leave clients who are weak or dizzy. If you can leave the client and a call bell is available, make sure it is always within reach. Stay close enough so that you can hear the client's call for help. Remember to follow Standard Practices.

CHAPTER REVIEW

KEY POINTS

- The body's waste products are removed through the digestive, respiratory, integumentary, and urinary systems. The urinary system removes waste products from blood and maintains the body's water balance.
- *Urination*, *micturition*, and *voiding* all mean the process of emptying urine from the bladder.
- The amount of fluid intake, personal habits, and available toilet facilities, as well as activity, work, and illness, affect urinary frequency.
- Urinary incontinence is not a normal part of aging.
- Urine should be observed for colour, clarity, odour, amount, and particles. It normally is clear, has no particles, and appears pale yellow, straw-coloured, or amber. A faint odour is normal.
- Some foods naturally affect urine colour. Certain medications also cause changes in urine colour. Some foods such as asperagus will change the odour of urine.
- Report to your supervisor if you observe urine that looks or smells abnormal. Report complaints of urgency, burning on urination, or dysuria (painful or difficult urination), usually caused by a UTI.
- You should be familiar with the various common urinary problems.
- You should be familiar with the types and causes of urinary incontinence.
- Clients with urinary incontinence need frequent, proper skin care and should be changed into clean, dry garments after each episode. Promptly changing wet bed linen is also essential; failure to do so is considered a form of neglect.
- You should know the following procedures associated with urinary care: (1) assisting a female client to void in a bedpan, (2) assisting a male client with using a urinal, (3) assisting a client to use a commode chair, (4) providing catheter care for clients with in-dwelling catheters, (5) providing catheter care for a male client with a condom catheter, (6) obtaining urine specimens, (7) testing urine, (8) straining urine, and (9) changing a ureterostomy pouch.

CRITICAL THINKING IN PRACTICE

Mrs. Riley has a urinary catheter. She tells you: "I feel like I have to pee, and I feel pressure down there." She points to her lower abdomen. There is no urine in her drainage bag. Is this normal? What do you do?

REVIEW QUESTIONS

Answers to these questions are at the bottom of the next page.

Circle the BEST answer.

1. Which of the following statements is true?
   A. Urine normally has a foul odour.
   B. A client normally voids about 1 500 mL a day.
   C. Urine is normally cloudy and amber or brown in colour.
   D. Micturition usually occurs after going to bed and before rising.
2. Which will help normal elimination?
   A. Helping the client assume a supine position for urination
   B. Talking to the client while the client is trying to void
   C. Helping the client to the bathroom or commode or providing the bedpan or urinal as soon as requested
   D. Always staying with the client who is using a bedpan
3. The best position for using a bedpan is:
   A. Fowler's position
   B. The supine position
   C. The prone position
   D. The side-lying position
4. After using the urinal, the male client should:
   A. Put the urinal on the bedside stand
   B. Hook the urinal to his bed rail
   C. Put the urinal on the overbed table
   D. Empty the urinal

5. Urinary incontinence:
- A. Is permanent
- B. Requires urine tests
- C. Requires good skin care
- D. Is always treated with an in-dwelling catheter

6. Which of the following is your responsibility when supporting Mrs. Jones, who has an in-dwelling catheter?
- A. Hook the drainage bag to the bed rail
- B. Keep the drainage bag below the level of her bladder
- C. Hide the tubing by placing it underneath the client
- D. Try to comfort her by saying that her urge to void is all in her head

7. Mr. Powers has a condom catheter. You should apply elastic tape:
- A. Completely around the penis
- B. To the inner thigh
- C. To the abdomen
- D. In a spiral fashion

8. The goal of bladder training is to:
- A. Remove the catheter
- B. Allow the client to walk to the bathroom
- C. Gain voluntary control of urination
- D. Heal the stoma

9. When collecting a random urine specimen into a bedpan, you should do the following:
- A. Label the bedpan with the requested information
- B. Wash the client's perineum first with antiseptic soap
- C. Collect the specimen at the time specified
- D. Allow the client to use toilet tissue and then place it in the bedpan

10. The perineum is cleaned before collecting:
- A. Random specimens
- B. Midstream specimens
- C. 24-hour urine specimens
- D. Random and 24-hour urine specimens

11. A 24-hour urine specimen involves:
- A. Collecting all urine voided by a client during a 24-hour period
- B. Collecting a random specimen every hour for 24 hours
- C. Not allowing the client to urinate for 24 hours
- D. Testing the urine for glucose and blood

12. Straining of urine is done to find:
- A. Hematuria
- B. Stones
- C. Nocturia
- D. Urgency

13. Which of the following should you do for the client who has a ureterostomy?
- A. Pull off the adhesive ostomy appliance every hour
- B. Tape the ostomy appliance down whenever it leaks
- C. Report any changes in the skin around the stoma
- D. Provide incontinence briefs

Answers: 1.B, 2.C, 3.A, 4.B, 5.C, 6.B, 7.D, 8.C, 9.C, 10.B, 11.A, 12.B, 13.C

Chapter opener image: Alexander Raths/Shutterstock.com

CHAPTER 33

Bowel Elimination

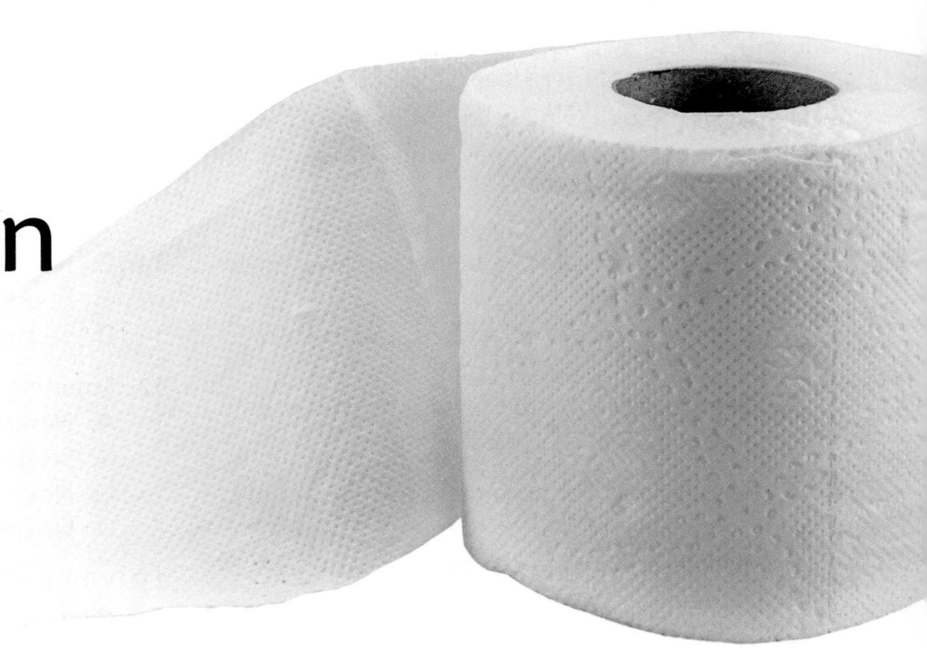

OBJECTIVES

After reading this chapter, the learner should be able to do the following:

- Describe normal stools and the normal pattern and frequency of bowel movements.
- List the observations to make about bowel movements.
- Identify the factors that affect bowel elimination.
- Describe common bowel elimination issues.
- Describe the measures that promote comfort and safety during defecation.
- Describe bowel training.
- Explain why enemas are given.
- Know the common enema solutions.
- Describe the comfort and safety measures for giving enemas.
- Explain the purpose of rectal tubes.
- Describe how to care for a client with an ostomy pouch.
- Explain why stool specimens are collected.
- Perform the procedures described in this chapter.

KEY TERMS

colostomy An artificial opening (*stomy*) between the colon (*colo*) and the abdominal wall. p. 739
constipation A condition in which bowel movements are less frequent than usual; the stool is hard, dry, and difficult to pass. p. 733
defecation The process of excreting feces from the rectum through the anus; bowel movement. p. 731
diarrhea The frequent passage of liquid stools. p. 734
enema The introduction of fluid into the rectum and lower colon. p. 736
fecal impaction The prolonged retention and accumulation of feces in the rectum. p. 734
fecal incontinence The inability to control the passage of feces and gas through the anus. Also known as *anal incontinence*. p. 735
feces The semi-solid mass of waste products in the colon. p. 731
flatulence The excessive formation of gas in the stomach and intestines. p. 735
flatus Gas or air from the stomach or intestines passed through the anus. p. 735
hemorrhoids Swollen veins in the anal canal. p. 734
ileostomy An artificial opening (*stomy*) between the ileum (small intestine; *ileo*) and the abdominal wall. p. 740
melena Dark, tarry stools containing decomposing blood. p. 744
stool Excreted feces. p. 731
suppository A cone-shaped, solid medication that is inserted into a body opening. p. 736

Like urinary elimination, bowel elimination—the excretion of wastes from the digestive system—is a basic physical need (see Chapter 17). Many factors affect bowel elimination—for example, privacy, personal habits, age, diet, exercise and activity, fluids, and medications. Problems related to any of these factors may occur easily and then interfere with elimination. As a support worker, you are required to assist clients by promoting normal bowel elimination. Bowel elimination problems and treatments for them may be uncomfortable, frustrating, embarrassing, and humiliating for the client. Be sensitive and offer emotional support (see the *Providing Compassionate Care: Assisting Clients With Elimination* box on p. 727). Follow Standard Practices and the infection control guidelines listed in **BOX 23–7** on page 445.

NORMAL BOWEL MOVEMENTS

Foods and fluids that are partially digested in the stomach are called *chyme*, and these pass from the stomach into the small intestine and enter the large intestine (large bowel or colon), where the fluids are absorbed. Chyme thus becomes more solid in consistency. Once it is in the colon, this semi-solid mass of waste products is referred to as **feces**.

Feces move through the intestine by *peristalsis*—the alternating contraction and relaxation of intestinal muscles. Feces move through the colon to the rectum, where they are stored until they are excreted from the body. **Defecation** (bowel movement, or BM) is the process of excreting feces from the rectum through the anus. **Stool** is another term for excreted feces.

On average, people have a bowel movement every day or every 2 to 3 days. Some people have two or three bowel movements a day. People defecate at different times—for example, after breakfast or in the evening. Many older adults expect to have a bowel movement every day, and the slightest irregularity causes them concern. Reassurance from all team members can help relieve their anxiety.

Stools are normally brown in colour from bile that is produced in the liver and is important to the digestive process (see Chapters 17 and 28). However, some medications, such as some iron-replacement meds, or health challenges, such as bleeding in the stomach, small intestine, or both, will cause the stools to appear black or *tarry* (black, unformed, and sticky, similar to tar); bleeding in the lower colon or rectum or eating beets will make the stools appear red. A diet that contains a lot of green vegetables can cause green stools. Various diseases and infections can cause clay-coloured, white, pale brown, orange, or green stools.

Stools are normally soft, formed, moist, and shaped like the rectum. They have a characteristic odour, which is caused by bacterial action in the intestines. Normal flora bacteria are necessary for stools to form. Certain foods (for example, eggs, onions, and garlic) can cause odours in the stools. Medications (such as some multivitamins) can also cause stools to be foul-smelling.

Observations

Whether you work in the community or in a facility, it is essential that you accurately record your client's bowel movements during your shift so that your team can decide if adjustments in diet or medications are necessary. It is important for the support worker to know the client's regular bowel routine and to adhere to the routine whenever possible. For example, if the client prefers to use the commode chair for a bowel movement, help the client to do so.

Your careful observations about the client's stools are important for the care-planning process. Observe the stool for the following: colour, amount, consistency, odour, shape, and size. When you observe abnormal stools and if you work in a facility, ask a nurse to observe the bowel movement. Also report any abnormalities in bowel movement frequency and complaints of pain.

FACTORS AFFECTING BOWEL MOVEMENT

Normal defecation, as gauged by frequency, consistency, colour, and odour of stools, can be affected by many factors:

- ***Privacy.*** Like urination, defecation is a private act. Lack of privacy deters many people from defecating despite having the urge. Clients who ignore the urge to defecate because others are present can become constipated. Odours associated with defecation can be embarrassing.
- ***Personal habits.*** Many clients routinely have a bowel movement after breakfast, as food in the stomach may stimulate the bowels to move. Some do relaxing activities—for example, drinking a hot beverage, reading a book or newspaper, or taking a walk—which make defecation easier.
- ***Diet.*** A well-balanced diet and bulk are needed to promote regular bowel movements. High-fibre foods such as fruits, vegetables, and whole grain cereals and breads leave a residue that provides needed bulk. However, many people do not eat enough fruits and vegetables. Some clients refuse to eat fruits and vegetables, thinking they will not be able to digest them. For adults who do not have teeth or have poorly fitting dentures, chewing some foods can be difficult. Bran, prunes, and juices help prevent constipation, but some other foods can cause either diarrhea or constipation; for example, milk causes constipation in some people and diarrhea in others. Other foods, including chocolate, can cause similar reactions. Spicy foods can irritate the intestines, resulting in frequent stools or diarrhea. Gas-forming foods such as onions, beans, cabbage, cauliflower, radishes, and cucumber stimulate peristalsis, and increased peristalsis results in defecation. But many people avoid gas-forming foods because they cause stomach ache or bloating.
- ***Fluids.*** Stool consistency depends on the amount of water absorbed in the colon. The amount of fluid ingested, urine output, and vomiting can affect stool consistency. Feces become hard and dry when large amounts of water are absorbed by the colon and when fluid intake is poor. Hard, dry feces move through the intestines at a slower rate, resulting in constipation. Drinking 6 to 8 glasses of water every day promotes regular bowel movement. Warm fluids—coffee, tea, hot cider, and warm water—increase peristalsis.
- ***Activity.*** Exercise and activity maintain overall muscle tone, which can stimulate peristalsis. Irregular elimination and constipation often occur due to inactivity and bed rest resulting from disease, surgery, injury, and aging. The care plan lists comfort and safety measures to meet the client's elimination needs. The actions in **BOX 33–1** are routinely practised to promote comfort and safety during defecation.
- ***Medications.*** On the one hand, medications can prevent constipation or control diarrhea; on the other hand, some medications can cause diarrhea

BOX 33–1 Promoting Comfort and Safety During Defecation

- Assist the client to the toilet or commode, or provide the bedpan, as soon as the client requests it.
- To promote privacy, assist the client to the bathroom, or wheel the client into the bathroom on the commode if possible. Position the commode over the toilet. Be cautious when transporting clients on commodes, as these normally have small wheels that make them difficult to manoeuvre over uneven surfaces. They also may not have safety belts to prevent the client from tipping forward. Be aware of the safety measures you need to take. Smaller clients and male clients who have a pendulous scrotum are at risk of having their buttocks or scrotum rubbed or pinched between the commode seat and the toilet bowl.
- Provide for privacy. Ask visitors or family members to leave the room. Close doors, pull privacy curtains, and close window curtains, blinds, or shades.
- Make sure the bedpan is warm.
- Position the client in the normal sitting position.
- Cover the client for warmth and privacy.
- Allow enough time for defecation. Do not rush the client.
- Place the call bell (in facilities) and toilet tissue within the client's reach.
- Stay around if the client is weak or unsteady.
- Leave the room if the client can be left alone. Stay within hearing distance.
- Provide perineal care.
- Dispose of stools promptly to reduce odour and prevent the spread of microbes.
- Assist the client with handwashing after elimination.
- If the client has fecal incontinence, follow the care plan, which will tell you when to assist with elimination.
- Follow Standard Practices.

or constipation as adverse effects. Medications for pain relief often cause constipation. Antibiotics, which are normally prescribed to fight or prevent infection, often cause diarrhea. Diarrhea occurs when the antibiotics kill normal flora (bacteria that are always present) in the large intestine.

- ***Aging.*** As people age, feces tend to pass through the intestines at a slower rate, resulting in constipation. However, older people who are active and eat a well-balanced diet may not suffer from constipation. While older clients may lose bowel control, this loss of control is not a normal consequence of aging. Some older adults may not completely empty the rectum and will need to defecate again 30 to 45 minutes after the first bowel movement.
- ***Disability.*** Some clients with disabilities are not able to control their bowel movements and defecate whenever feces enter the rectum. Such clients need a bowel training program (see p. 735), with the goal of having a bowel movement at the same time each day.

COMMON PROBLEMS

Common problems that affect normal bowel movement include constipation, fecal impaction, diarrhea, fecal incontinence, and flatulence.

Constipation

Constipation is a condition in which bowel movements are less frequent than usual, and the stool is hard, dry, and difficult to pass, causing the client to strain to have a bowel movement. Clients may complain of abdominal discomfort, a feeling of fullness, or increased gas (*flatus*). Stools could be large or marble sized. Large-sized stools cause pain as they pass through the anus. Constipation occurs when feces move through the intestine slowly, allowing more time for water absorption in the colon. Common causes of constipation include a low-fibre diet, ignoring the urge to defecate, decreased fluid intake, inactivity, medications, aging, and certain diseases.

A client may be too embarrassed to tell you about the constipation. If you note that the client is having fewer bowel movements than normal, inform your supervisor. If a client is prone to constipation, it is important to keep a record of its frequency.

Common measures used to prevent or relieve constipation include changing the diet (increasing fibre, increasing fluids) and encouraging physical activity. The physician may order medications or enemas for prolonged constipation. **Hemorrhoids**, which are swollen veins in the anal canal, are often associated with constipation and straining at bowel movements, as well as other causes, such as pregnancy.

As a support worker, you play a very important role in preventing constipation in your clients by ensuring adequate activity, fluids, and privacy. Prevention of constipation is much better than treatment. It is essential to accurately record your client's bowel movements during your shift to enable team members to recognize and treat constipation in a timely manner.

Fecal Impaction

Fecal impaction is the prolonged retention and accumulation of feces in the rectum. Feces become hard or puttylike in consistency and grow increasingly so as more water is absorbed. The constipated stool can form a large solid mass or several small, hard masses. Fecal impaction results if constipation is not relieved. Once the feces are impacted, the client will be unable to defecate easily without intervention. If left untreated, a fecal impaction can lead to complete bowel obstruction, which will require surgery.

The client may try many times to defecate. If a client shows any of the following signs or symptoms of a fecal impaction, report it at once:

- Abdominal discomfort, which can be severe or cause swelling or both
- Cramping
- A feeling of fullness or pain in the rectum
- Nausea or vomiting; vomitus that smells like stool
- Fever
- Increased urge or decreased ability to urinate
- Liquid feces seeping from the anus. Seepage may look like diarrhea but is, in fact, liquid feces passing around the hardened fecal mass.

A physician or nurse performs a digital (finger) exam to check for impaction. In Alberta, support workers' competencies include rectal touch, which is done by inserting a lubricated, gloved finger into the rectum and feeling for a hard mass. The client may feel uncomfortable after the procedure. The physician may order medications and enemas to remove the impaction, and on occasion, the physician or nurse may remove the fecal mass manually with a gloved finger, a process called *digital removal of an impaction*.

Diarrhea

Diarrhea is the frequent passage of liquid stools. Feces move through the intestines rapidly, thereby reducing the time for fluid absorption in the colon. The need to defecate is urgent, and some clients may not be able to get to a bathroom in time. Abdominal cramping, nausea, and vomiting may also occur.

Causes of diarrhea include infections, certain medications, foods that irritate the stomach, and pathogens in food and water. Diet and medications reduce peristalsis and stop the diarrhea.

Skin breakdown and pressure ulcers are a risk because of liquid feces and frequent wiping with toilet tissue. Products such as *barrier creams* are often applied to the anal area after each cleaning. It is important to follow your employer's policies regarding the application of any topical product (see Chapter 43). When a client has diarrhea, as a support worker, you need to do the following:

- Assist with the client's elimination needs promptly
- Dispose of stools promptly to prevent odours and the spread of microbes
- Provide good skin care, as directed by your agency's or facility's policies

Fluid lost through diarrhea must be replaced so as not to lead to *dehydration*—the excessive loss of water from tissues. Signs and symptoms of dehydration include *oliguria* (scant amount of urine), dark urine, pale or flushed skin, dry skin, coated tongue, cracked lips, sunken eyes, thirst, weakness, dizziness, and confusion. Falling blood pressure and increased pulse and respirations are serious signs, which may precede death. The care plan tells you how to meet the client's

FOCUS ON CHILDREN

Dehydration

The bodies of infants and young children contain large amounts of water. Infants and children are at risk for dehydration, and death from dehydration can occur quickly in them. Report any liquid or watery stool immediately. Note the number of wet diapers in 24 hours. Infants wet less when dehydrated. Fewer than six wet diapers in 24 hours may indicate that an infant is dehydrated. Report any concerns immediately.

FOCUS ON OLDER ADULTS

Dehydration

Older adults are at risk for dehydration, as the amount of body water decreases with aging. Diarrhea is, therefore, very serious in older adults, and any signs of diarrhea should be reported immediately, as death can result from unrecognized and untreated dehydration.

Pathogens often cause diarrhea, so preventing the spread of infection is important. Always follow Standard Practices when you come into contact with stools.

fluid needs. The physician orders intravenous fluids in severe cases (see the *Focus on Children: Dehydration* and *Focus on Older Adults: Dehydration* boxes).

Fecal Incontinence

Fecal incontinence (or *anal incontinence*) is the inability to control the passage of feces and gas through the anus due to intestinal and nervous system diseases, injuries, fecal impaction, diarrhea, and some medications. Fecal incontinence can also occur because of delayed requests for help to use the bathroom, commode, or bedpan.

Clients with mental health disorders, dementia, or cognitive disorders (see Chapters 35 and 36) may not recognize the urge to *defecate*, and as a result, some may soil themselves, the furniture, and the walls. In such situations, a common problem support workers encounter is resistance to care, making washing and changing the client difficult. Follow the client's care plan. Also, talk to your supervisor if you have problems providing care to a client who has been incontinent of stool and is resisting care.

Flatulence

Gas and air are normally found in the stomach and intestines and are expelled through the mouth (*eructating*, or belching) and the anus. Gas and air passed through the anus are called **flatus**. **Flatulence** is the excessive formation of gas or air in the stomach and intestines. Common causes are as follows:

- Swallowing air while eating and drinking, especially when chewing gum, eating quickly, drinking through a straw, and drinking carbonated beverages (peope who are tense or anxious also tend to swallow large amounts of air when drinking)
- Bacterial action in the intestines
- Gas-forming foods (onion, beans, cabbage, cauliflower, radishes, cucumber)
- Constipation
- Bowel and abdominal surgeries
- Medications that decrease peristalsis

If flatus is not expelled, the intestines distend; that is, they swell or enlarge due to the pressure of the gases. Abdominal cramping or pain (sometimes severe), shortness of breath, a swollen abdomen, belching, and burping can occur. "Bloating" is a common complaint. Exercise, walking, and the left-side-lying position often produce flatus, which will relieve the bloating. Physicians may order enemas, medications, or rectal tubes to relieve flatulence.

BOWEL TRAINING

Bowel training is the process of establishing a regular fecal elimination pattern. It has two goals:

1. To gain control of bowel movement
2. To prevent fecal impaction, constipation, and fecal incontinence

The urge to defecate is usually felt after a meal, often after breakfast. The client's usual time of day for a bowel movement is noted on the care plan, and the use of the toilet, commode, or bedpan should be offered at this time. Factors that promote elimination are part of the care plan and bowel training program. These include a high-fibre diet, increased fluids, warm fluids, activity, and privacy. Your supervisor will tell you about a client's bowel training program.

The physician may order a suppository to stimulate defecation. A **suppository** is a cone-shaped, solid medication that is inserted into a body opening. It eventually dissolves at body temperature. Suppositories are preferred over enemas as they are usually more comfortable for the client. A nurse inserts a rectal suppository into the rectum, or it can be self-applied by the client, and you may assist as needed (see Chapter 43). It takes time for the suppository to dissolve and work in the body, but a bowel movement typically occurs after about 30 minutes.

ENEMAS

An **enema**—the introduction of fluid into the rectum and lower colon—is ordered by physicians to remove feces and to relieve constipation or fecal impaction. Clients with severely limited mobility or who are paralyzed are at risk for these problems. Enemas also are ordered to clean the bowel of feces before certain surgeries or X-ray procedures. Sometimes, enemas are ordered to relieve excessive flatulence and intestinal distension and constipation.

Enemas are usually safe procedures, and, often, clients can give themselves enemas at home. However, enemas are invasive and involve inserting a tube into a body opening, so they can be dangerous for any adult and are more so for those with certain heart and kidney diseases. Therefore, giving an enema is a controlled act, meaning the authority to perform it should usually be delegated to you by a nurse (see Chapter 6). If you are delegated to perform an enema, you first must answer the following questions:

- Do your provincial or territorial laws and employer's policies allow you to perform the procedure?
- Do you have the necessary education and training?
- Have you reviewed the procedure with a nurse?
- Is a nurse available to answer questions and to supervise you?

If having an enema is part of the client's activities of daily living (ADLs), this task is exempted from being considered a controlled act. However, ***permission for you to give an enema must always be in your employer's policy.***

The Commercial Enema

Commercial enemas stimulate and distend the rectum and cause defecation. They are often ordered to relieve constipation, specifically when complete cleansing of the bowel is not needed.

Manufacturers prepare and package the commercial enema so that it is ready to administer. Children should be given only the amount of enema stated in their care plan (see *Focus on Children: Normal Saline Enemas*). The solution is usually administered at room temperature. To give the enema, squeeze the sides of the bottle with enough pressure to push the enema contents into the client's rectum. As the bottle empties, roll it up from the bottom. Do not release pressure on the bottle, as that would cause the solution to be drawn from the rectum back into the bottle.

Encourage the client to retain the solution until the urge to defecate is felt. The enema usually takes 5 to 10 minutes to take effect, but some people may immediately feel the urge to defecate; others may become incontinent of stool. It is, therefore, very important to have all your equipment on hand prior to performing the procedure. Remaining in Sims' position on the left side may help the client to retain the enema longer.

FOCUS ON CHILDREN

Normal Saline Enemas

Only normal saline enemas (0.9% sodium chloride) are used in children because children are at particular risk for electrolyte imbalance. The amount of enema solution varies for infants and children. If you are delegated to give an enema to a child, your supervisor will give you the necessary instructions.

Giving a Commercial Enema to an Adult

123

Advocate on behalf of the client's quality of life by promoting:

Dignity • Independence • Preferences • Privacy • Safety *(see BOX 1–4, on p. 17)*

PRE-PROCEDURE

1 Identify the client, according to employer policy.
This eliminates the possibility of mistaking one client for another.
2 Explain the procedure to the client.
3 Perform hand hygiene.
4 Collect the following supplies:
- ☐ **Commercial enema**
- ☐ **Bedpan, commode chair, or clean incontinence briefs** (if the client is incontinent of stool) (*Note:* If the client's care plan indicates the client can use a toilet, try to ensure that it is not occupied at the time of the procedure so that the client can use it after the enema is given).
- ☐ **Waterproof pad**
- ☐ **Water-soluble lubricating jelly**
- ☐ **Toilet tissue**
- ☐ **Gloves**
- ☐ **Robe and nonskid footwear**
- ☐ **Sheet**
- ☐ **Bag or container to place toilet tissue into**

By collecting all the necessary equipment beforehand, you will not have to leave your client's side and can eliminate wasting time and energy in obtaining the forgotten equipment.

5 Provide for privacy.
6 Raise the bed to a comfortable working height if your client is in an adjustable bed.*
This reduces your risk for back strain.
7 Read the directions for how to safely administer the enema.
This is important to prevent the risk for injury to the client and to maximize the effectiveness of the enema.

PROCEDURE

8 Lower the bed rail near you if it is up.
This reduces your risk for back strain.
9 Cover the client with a sheet. Fan-fold the top linen to the foot of the bed.
This provides warmth and helps your client feel more comfortable. A fan-folded sheet is easier to grasp and to straighten out than a rolled-up sheet would be.
10 Position the client in Sims' position on the left side, with right knee bent.
This allows the solution to follow the natural curve of the colon and rectum as it flows downward and will improve the retention of the solution.
11 Put on gloves.
12 Place the waterproof pad under the client's buttocks.
This protects the bed linen.
13 Expose the anal area.
This helps you observe where you will be inserting the tubing.
14 Position the bedpan near the client.
This is done in the event your client is not able to retain the enema.
15 Remove the cap from the enema tip. Check the tip for adequate lubricant. Add lubricating water-soluble jelly to coat the tip if necessary.
Tips may dry with the passage of time. The lubricant allows for easier insertion of the tube into the rectum and reduces the chance of injury.
16 Expel excess air by gently squeezing the container.
Air can cause distension.
17 Separate the buttocks to see the anus.

Continued

Giving a Commercial Enema to an Adult—cont'd

18 Ask the client to take a deep breath through the mouth.
This helps the client relax.

19 Gently insert the enema tip 5 cm (2 in.) into the rectum as the client exhales (**FIGURE 33–1**). Be gentle if hemorrhoids are present.
Insertion of the tube can be painful if hemorrhoids are present. Exhaling assists the sphincter to relax.
Stop if the client complains of pain, you feel resistance, or bleeding occurs. If bleeding occurs, notify the nurse immediately.
Bleeding in the rectum may indicate a dangerous health concern and should, therefore, be reported immediately.

20 **a** Squeeze the sides of the enema with enough pressure to push the enema contents into the client's rectum.
b As the bottle empties, roll up the bottle from the bottom. Release pressure on the bottle after removing the tip from the rectum.
Gentle release avoids trauma to the mucosa.

21 Put the empty bottle into the box, tip first.
The tip could be contaminated with stool and microorganisms.

22 Help the client onto the bedpan and raise the head of the bed; help the client into a sitting position; or help the client to the bathroom or commode. If the client remains in bed, raise the bed rail, if used. If the client gets up, ensure a robe and nonskid footwear are worn. The bed should be in the lowest position.
An upright, sitting position facilitates defecation by gravity.

23 Place the call bell (in facilities) and toilet tissue within reach. Remind the client not to flush the toilet.
The call bell provides an easy, safe way for the client to contact staff if necessary. Not flushing the toilet allows you to observe the colour and amount of stool or urine excreted.

24 Discard disposable items following agency policies for disposal of items.

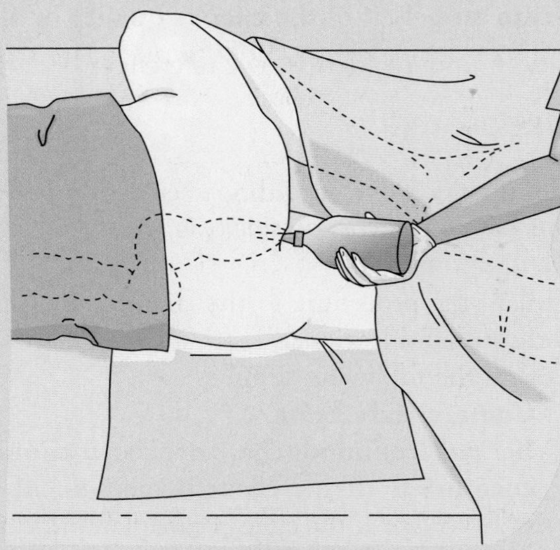

FIGURE 33–1

25 Remove gloves. Perform hand hygiene.
Feces can spread pathogens, so always use gloves when there is any chance of contact.

26 Leave the room if the client can be left alone. Stay within hearing distance.
Clients may become weak after this procedure and may need your assistance.

27 Return when the client calls. Knock before entering.

28 Perform hand hygiene. Put on gloves.

29 Lower the bed rail if it is up.
This helps prevent worker back strain.

30 Observe results of the enema for amount, colour, consistency, and odour. Follow your employer's policy on reporting the results. In some facilities, support workers call their supervisor to observe the results. In a community setting, you will need to report the effectiveness of the enema, depending on your agency's policies.
This determines the effectiveness of the enema. Abnormal results can indicate illness or health problems.

31 Help the client clean the perineal area.
This provides comfort for your client and can prevent breakdown of the skin around the anus.

Continued

Giving a Commercial Enema to an Adult—cont'd

32 Remove the bed protector.
33 Follow your employer's policies to empty, clean, and disinfect the bedpan or commode. Flush the toilet.
34 Return equipment to its proper place.
This makes it easier to find the next time it is needed.
35 Remove gloves. Perform hand hygiene.
36 Help the client with handwashing. Wear gloves if necessary.
37 Replace the top linen and sheet.

POST-PROCEDURE

38 Provide for safety and comfort.
39 Place the call bell within reach.*
This provides an easy, safe way for the client to contact staff if necessary.
40 Return the bed to its lowest position. Follow the care plan for bed rail use.*
41 Remove privacy measures.
42 Follow employer policy for handling soiled linen and used supplies. Wear gloves for this step.
43 Perform hand hygiene.

Report and Record your actions and observations, according to employer policy.
This is done for legal reasons and to keep the rest of the health care team informed. Any abnormal observation can indicate illness or health problems.

*Steps marked with an asterisk may not apply in community settings.

RECTAL TUBES

A nurse inserts a rectal tube into the rectum to relieve flatulence and intestinal distension. Flatus then is passed with less effort or straining.

The rectal tube is a flexible tube which is usually inserted 10 cm (4 in.) into the adult rectum. It is left in place for only 20 to 30 minutes at a time so as not to irritate the rectum. It can be re-inserted every 2 to 3 hours.

The tube may be connected to a flatus bag or to a water container. These tools are used primarily for clients who have skin breakdown and are experiencing an abnormal frequency of loose stools. The bag inflates as gas passes into it. If the tube is connected to a water container, the water bubbles as gas passes through the tube into the water. For this system, the rectal tube is attached to connecting tubing, which is placed in the water container.

Feces may be expelled along with flatus. If a flatus bag is not used, the open end of the tube is placed in a folded, waterproof pad.

THE CLIENT WITH AN OSTOMY

Sometimes, surgical removal of part of the intestines is necessary as part of the treatment for cancer, diseases of the bowel, or trauma (such as stab or bullet wounds). Following the surgery, an *ostomy*—the surgical creation of an artificial opening (*stoma*)—is sometimes needed (see Chapters 29, 31, and 32). The client wears a pouch over the stoma to collect feces and flatus.

Colostomy

A **colostomy** is the surgically created opening (*stomy*) between the colon (*colo*) and the abdominal wall. Part of the colon is brought out onto the abdominal wall, and a stoma is created. Feces and flatus pass through the stoma instead of through the anus. Colostomies may be permanent or temporary. The colostomy is permanent if the diseased part of the colon has been removed. A temporary colostomy may be created during surgery to give the diseased or injured

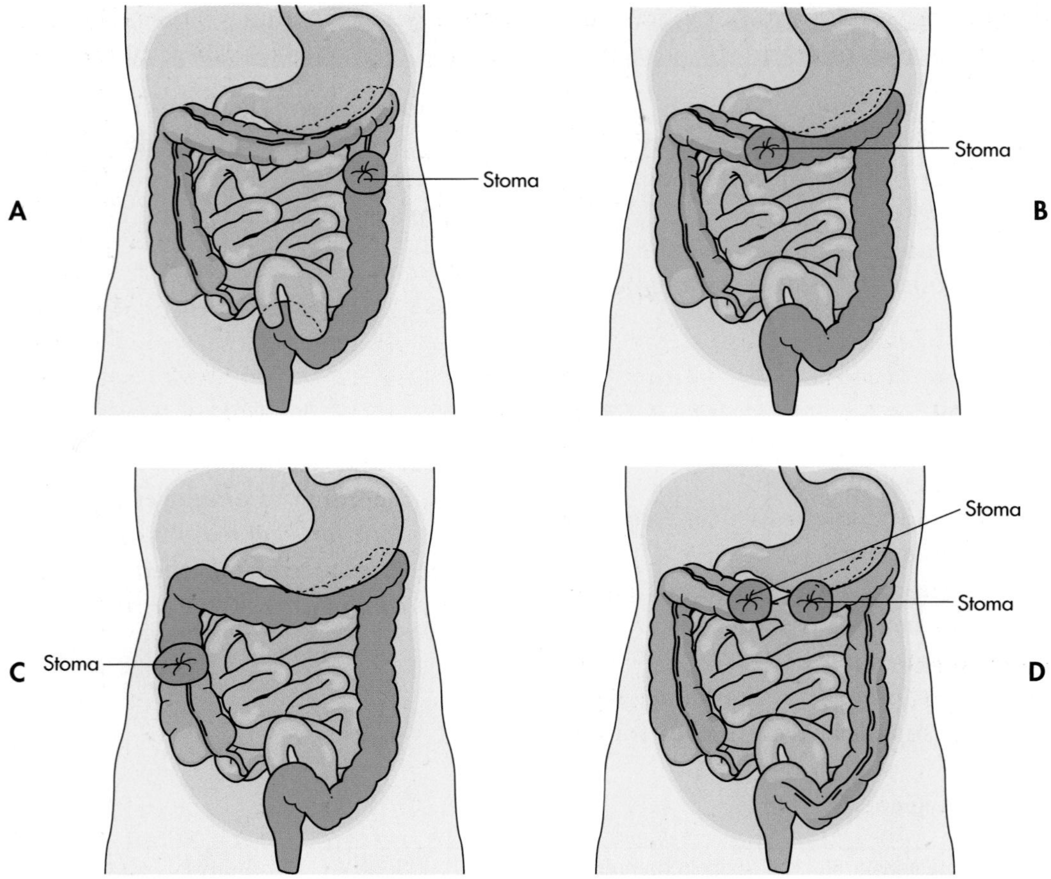

FIGURE 33–2 Colostomy sites. *Shading* shows the part of the bowel that was surgically removed. **A,** Descending colostomy. **B,** Transverse colostomy. **C,** Ascending colostomy. **D,** Double-barrel colostomy—two stomas are created: one for the excretion of feces and the other for the administration of medicine into the bowel to help it heal. This type of colostomy is usually temporary.

bowel time to heal if the colon does not require removal. Eventually, another surgery would reconnect the bowel.

Stomas usually appear pink, but some can appear red and "angry." Both are, in fact, healthy stomas. Some support workers may needlessly worry that touching or cleaning a red stoma would cause pain. A stoma's appearing dusky or blue-tinged could indicate a bowel obstruction, which can be life threatening and must be reported.

The location of the colostomy depends on the site of colon disease or injury (**FIGURE 33–2**). Stool consistency is affected by the nature of the surgery and ranges from liquid to formed stools. The more colon that remains to absorb water, the more solid and formed the stools will be. If the colostomy is near the beginning of the colon, stools will be liquid, whereas the colostomy near the end of the large intestine results in formed stools.

Feces can irritate the skin, so skin care is essential to prevent skin breakdown around the stoma. Skin is washed and dried whenever the pouch is removed, and a skin barrier is applied around the stoma. The skin barrier prevents feces from coming into contact with the skin. The skin barrier may be part of the pouch or a separate device.

Ileostomy

An **ileostomy** is the surgically created opening (*stomy*) between the ileum (small intestine [*ileo*]) and the abdominal wall. Part of the ileum is brought out onto the abdominal wall, and a stoma is created. The entire colon is removed. As a result, water is not absorbed, and liquid feces drain constantly from the ileostomy that has a pungent odour.

Feces in the small intestine is very acidic and contains digestive juices that are extremely irritating to the skin. The ileostomy pouch must fit well so that feces do not touch the skin to avoid excoriation and breakdown. Good skin care is essential.

Ostomy Pouches

The pouch has an adhesive backing that is applied to the skin (**FIGURES 33–3** through **33–5**). Clients who have had a colostomy for many years may have the pouch attached to a belt. Many pouches have a drain at the bottom that is closed with clips, clamps, or wire closures. The drain is opened to empty the pouch of feces and also when the bag balloons or bulges with flatus. The drain is wiped with toilet tissue before it is closed.

The pouch is changed every 3 to 7 days and whenever it leaks. Some clients want the pouch changed daily or whenever it becomes soiled. There are two

Change in the morning

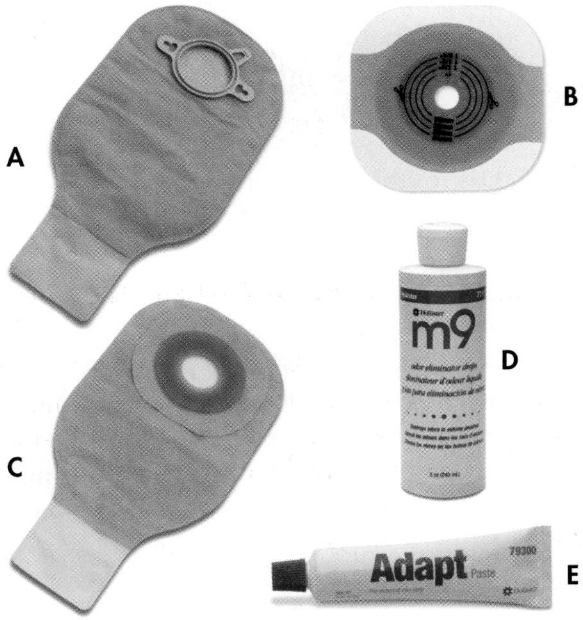

FIGURE 33–3 Ostomy equipment. **A,** Two-piece detachable system. The pouch opening is already precut by the manufacturer to fit the size of the flange on the skin barrier. **B,** Skin barrier. **C,** One-piece pouch with skin barrier attached. The bottom of the pouch will be closed with either a hook and loop strip or a plastic clip (not shown). **D,** Odour eliminator drops. **E,** Paste. (**Source:** Images courtesy of Hollister Incorporated, Libertyville, IL.)

pouch systems commonly used: (1) a two-part system and (2) an all-in-one system. In the two-part system, frequent pouch changes should not damage the skin, as the appliance would not be changed but just the bag. In an all-in-one system, the skin could be damaged by frequent changes. Many clients are able to manage their ostomy pouches without help.

Children of different ages, even premature infants, can have ostomies for a variety of reasons. If changing a child's ostomy pouch is assigned to you, pay particular attention to the delicate skin surrounding the stoma and report any abnormal observations immediately.

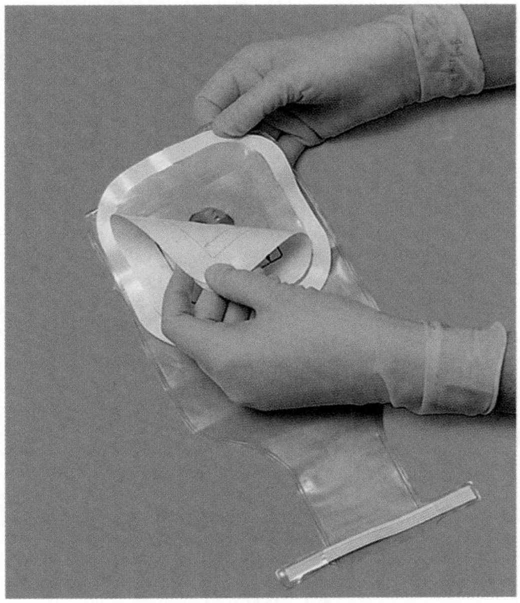

FIGURE 33–4 Preparing an ostomy pouch. (**Source:** Potter, P.A., & Perry, A.G. (2005). *Fundamentals of nursing* (6th ed., p. 1413). St. Louis, MO: Mosby.)

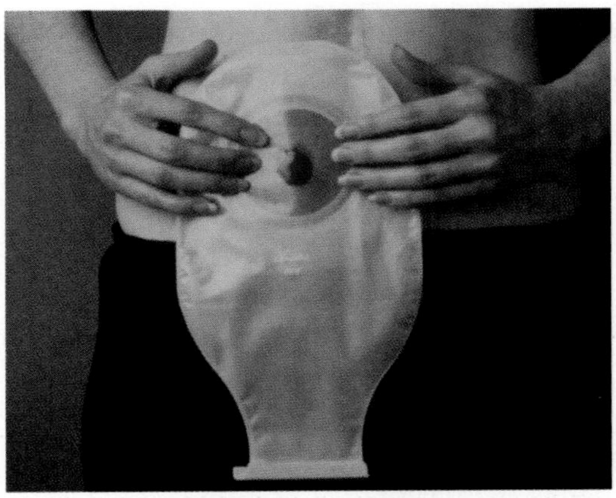

FIGURE 33–5 Applying a one-piece pouch. (**Source:** Potter, P.A., & Perry, A.G. (2005). *Fundamentals of nursing* (6th ed., p. 1414). St. Louis, MO: Mosby.)

Odours can be prevented by the following:

- Good hygiene
- Emptying the pouch regularly
- Avoiding gas-forming foods
- Placing deodorants into the pouch (as per the care plan)

The client can wear normal clothes when using an ostomy pouch. However, tight undergarments can prevent feces from entering the pouch. Also, any bulging of the pouch from feces and flatus can be seen through tight clothes.

Peristalsis increases after eating, so stomas are usually inactive before breakfast; that is, expulsion of feces is less likely at this time. If the client prefers to shower or bathe with the pouch off, it is best done before breakfast. Showers and baths are delayed 1 or 2 hours after applying a new pouch so as to give the adhesive backing on the pouch time to stick to the skin.

Do not flush pouches down the toilet. Follow employer policy for disposing of used pouches.

Changing an Ostomy Pouch

123

Advocate on behalf of the client's quality of life by promoting:

Dignity • Independence • Preferences • Privacy • Safety *(see BOX 1–4, on p. 17)*

PRE-PROCEDURE

1 Identify the client, according to your employer's policies.
This eliminates the possibility of mistaking one client for another.
2 Explain the procedure to the client.
3 Perform hand hygiene.
4 Collect the following supplies:
- ☐ **Clean pouch with skin barrier**
- ☐ **Skin barrier, as ordered (if not part of pouch)**
- ☐ **Pouch clamp, clip, or wire closure**
- ☐ **Clean ostomy belt (if used)**
- ☐ **Four to eight gauze squares**
- ☐ **Adhesive remover**
- ☐ **Cotton balls or cloths**
- ☐ **Bedpan with cover**
- ☐ **Waterproof pad**
- ☐ **Bath blanket**
- ☐ **Toilet tissue**
- ☐ **Wash basin**
- ☐ **Bath thermometer**
- ☐ **Graduated measuring container (for measuring liquid stool, if needed)**
- ☐ **Soap or cleansing agent, according to the care plan**
- ☐ **Pouch deodorant**
- ☐ **Paper towels**
- ☐ **Gloves**
- ☐ **Disposable bag**

By collecting all the necessary equipment beforehand, you will not have to leave your client's side and can eliminate wasting time and energy in obtaining the forgotten equipment.
5 Arrange paper towels on a work area. Place items on top of paper towels.
6 Provide for privacy.
7 Raise bed to a comfortable working height.*

PROCEDURE

8 Lower the bed rail near you if it is up.
This reduces your risk for back strain.
9 Cover the client with a sheet. Fan-fold the linen to the foot of the bed.
This ensures client warmth and privacy, and a fan-folded sheet is easier to grasp and to straighten out than a rolled-up sheet.
10 Place the waterproof pad under the client's buttocks.
This protects the linen.
11 Put on gloves.
12 Disconnect the pouch from the belt if one is worn. Remove the belt. Observe any redness in the area, and record and report to your supervisor.

Continued

Changing an Ostomy Pouch—cont'd

13 Remove the pouch gently. Gently push the skin down and away from the skin barrier. Place the pouch in the bedpan.
Gentle removal prevents skin tearing. Pushing the skin down gently assists in removal.

14 Wipe around the stoma with toilet tissue or a gauze square. This removes mucus and feces. Place soiled tissue in the bedpan.
Feces on the skin can lead to skin irritation, infection, or even ulceration.

15 Moisten a gauze square with adhesive remover. Clean around the stoma to remove any remaining skin barrier. Clean from the stoma outward.
This decreases the chance of skin breakdown in this area.

16 Cover the bedpan, and take it to the bathroom. (If bed rails are used, raise them before leaving the bedside.) *This reduces odour around your client.*

17 Measure the feces if directed by the care plan.

18 Note the colour, amount, consistency, and odour of feces. If the feces is abnormal, report and show it to the appropriate person. Then, empty the pouch and bedpan into the toilet. Put the pouch in the disposable bag.
Abnormal feces can indicate health problems in your client.

19 Remove gloves. Perform hand hygiene. Put on clean gloves.

20 Fill the wash basin with warm water. (Measure the temperature of water with a bath thermometer. Check the care plan for correct temperature.) Place the basin on top of the paper towels on the work surface. Lower the bed rail near you if it is up.
Water that is too hot could burn the sensitive skin around the stoma.

21 Using soap or other cleansing agents, clean the skin around the stoma with water. Rinse and pat dry.
If not removed as soon as possible, feces can cause the skin to break down very quickly. Moist skin can harbour pathogens, leading to skin breakdown.

22 Observe the stoma and skin around the stoma. Report any irritation or skin breakdown.

23 Apply the skin barrier if it is a separate device.
This protects the skin.

24 Put a clean ostomy belt on the client (if a belt is worn and changed daily).
Some clients do not change the belt daily. The care plan will tell you what the client has requested.

25 Add deodorants to the new pouch. Some pouches have deodorant packages already inside. Check the care plan.

26 Remove adhesive backing on the pouch.

27 Centre the pouch over the stoma. The drain points downward and is secured with a clip. The bag is emptied from the bottom.

28 Press around the skin barrier so that the pouch seals to the skin. Apply gentle pressure from the stoma outward.
This prevents leakage and ensures a good seal.

29 Maintain pressure for 1 to 2 minutes.
This ensures a good seal.

30 Connect the belt to the pouch (if a belt is worn).
This ensures that the appliance is secure.

31 Remove the waterproof pad.

32 Remove gloves.

33 Perform hand hygiene.

34 Cover the client.

POST-PROCEDURE

35 Provide for safety and comfort.

36 Place the call bell within reach.*
This provides an easy, safe way for the client to contact staff if necessary.

37 Return the bed to its lowest position. Follow the care plan for bed rail use.*

38 Remove privacy measures.

Continued

Changing an Ostomy Pouch—cont'd

39 Clean the bedpan, wash basin, and other equipment. Put on gloves for this step.

40 Return equipment to its proper place.
This makes it easier to find the next time it is needed.

41 Discard the disposable bag, according to employer policy. Follow employer policy for soiled linen.

42 Remove gloves. Perform hand hygiene.

Report and Record your actions and observations, according to employer policy.
This is done for legal reasons and to keep the rest of the health care team informed.

*Steps marked with an asterisk may not apply in community settings.

STOOL SPECIMENS

When internal bleeding is suspected, feces are checked for blood. Stools are also analyzed to identify fat, microbes, parasites (worms), and other abnormal contents. The guidelines for collecting stool specimens are the same as those for collecting urine specimens (see Chapter 32). Follow Standard Practices.

The stool specimen must not be contaminated with urine. Some tests require warm (fresh) stools. The specimen is taken to the laboratory immediately for such tests.

Testing Stools for Blood

Blood can appear in stools for many reasons, including ulcers, colon cancer, and hemorrhoids. Often, blood in stools is clearly visible. Bright red blood could be from hemorrhoids or cuts or abrasions in the anal area and can usually be seen if bleeding is low in the gastro-intestinal (GI) tract. Stools are black and tarry (**melena**) if there is bleeding in the stomach or upper GI tract. When reporting blood in the stool, you must describe the colour, as it may be an important clue when investigating the source.

Sometimes, bleeding may occur in very small amounts, which will be difficult to detect just by observing the stools. So, stools are tested for the presence of *occult* (*hidden* or *unseen*) *blood*, often done to screen (test) for colon cancer.

Numerous types of tests are available. Follow the manufacturer's instructions for the test ordered, and follow Standard Practices. The care plan and your assignment sheet will tell you when to collect the specimen. Many factors can affect the test results—for example, eating red meat. Therefore, the client cannot eat red meat for 3 days before the test. Bleeding from hemorrhoids or menstrual periods also affects test results.

Collecting a Stool Specimen

123

Advocate on behalf of the client's quality of life by promoting:
Dignity • Independence • Preferences • Privacy • Safety *(see BOX 1–4, on p. 17)*

PRE-PROCEDURE

1 Identify the client, according to employer policy.
This eliminates the possibility of mistaking one client for another.

2 Explain the procedure to the client.

3 Perform hand hygiene.

4 Collect the following supplies:
- ☐ **Bedpan and cover or bedside commode**
- ☐ **Urinal (or bedpan with cover) for voiding**

Continued

Collecting a Stool Specimen—cont'd

- ☐ **Specimen pan for the toilet or commode**
- ☐ **Specimen container and lid**
- ☐ **Tongue blade**
- ☐ **Disposable bag**
- ☐ **Gloves**
- ☐ **Toilet tissue**
- ☐ **Laboratory requisition slip**
- ☐ **Plastic bag**

By collecting all the necessary equipment beforehand, you will not have to leave your client's side and can eliminate wasting time and energy in obtaining the forgotten equipment.

5 Label the container.

6 Provide for privacy.

PROCEDURE

7 Ensure that your client is wearing a robe and nonskid footwear when using the bathroom. Assist the client onto the bedpan or a commode if the client does not use the bathroom.

8 Ask the client to void. Provide the bedpan, commode, or urinal if the client does not use the bathroom. Empty and clean the device. Wear gloves.
The presence of urine can interfere with the test results, and you need to wear gloves, as feces can spread pathogens.

9 Place the specimen pan under the toilet seat if the client uses the bathroom.
The specimen will be collected from the pan.

10 Ask the client not to put toilet tissue in the bedpan, commode, or specimen pan. Provide a disposable bag for toilet tissue.
Tissue can alter specimen results.

11 Place the call bell (in facilities) and toilet tissue within reach. Raise or lower bed rails, according to the care plan.*
This provides an easy, safe way for the client to contact staff if necessary.

12 Perform hand hygiene, and leave the room if safe to do so. Stay within hearing distance.
Staying nearby allows you to hear if your client calls for assistance.

13 Return when the client calls. Knock before entering. Perform hand hygiene.

14 Lower the bed rail near you if it is up.
This reduces your risk for back strain.

15 Put on gloves. Provide perineal care if needed.

16 Use a tongue blade to take about 30 mL (2 tablespoons) of feces from the bedpan, commode, or specimen pan to the specimen container (FIGURE 33–6).
Take the sample from the middle of a formed stool. If required by employer policy, take stool from two different areas on the specimen.

A B

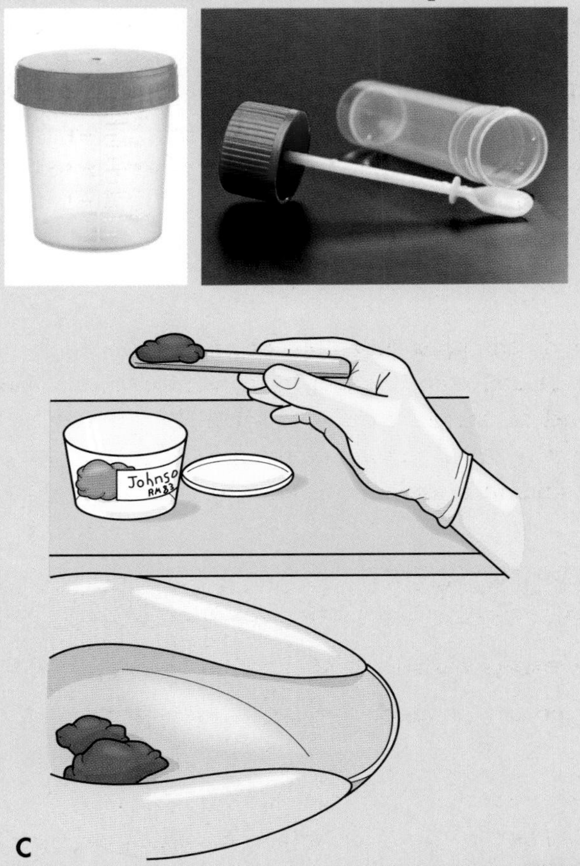

C

FIGURE 33–6 **A,** Stool specimen container. **B,** Stool specimen container with spoon. **C,** Collecting a stool specimen. (**Source:** *(for A)* © Can Stock Photo Inc./RidvanArda *(for B)* luchschen/iStock/Thinkstock)

Continued

Collecting a Stool Specimen—cont'd

17 Put the lid on the specimen container. Do not touch the inside of the lid or container. Place the container in the plastic bag.
This prevents accidental spillage.

18 Wrap the tongue blade in toilet tissue and dispose of it, according to your employer's policy.
This decreases the risk for pathogen spread.

19 Empty, clean, and disinfect the equipment, following agency policies.

20 Remove gloves. Perform hand hygiene.

21 Return equipment to its proper place.
This makes it easier to find the next time it is needed.

22 Assist the client with handwashing. Wear gloves if needed.

POST-PROCEDURE

23 Provide for safety and comfort.

24 Place the call bell within reach.*
This provides an easy, safe way for the client to contact staff if necessary.

25 Return the bed to its lowest position. Follow the care plan for bed rail use.*
This reduces the risk for client injury.

26 Remove privacy measures.

27 Follow your supervisor's instructions for specimen storage and transportation.

28 Perform hand hygiene.

Report and Record your actions and observations, according to employer policy.
This is done for legal reasons and to keep the rest of the health care team informed.

*Steps marked with an asterisk may not apply in community settings.

CHAPTER REVIEW

KEY POINTS

- Each client will have different patterns and frequency of bowel movements, and it is important that you report to your supervisor any changes in your client's normal routine, colour, amount, odour, shape, size, or frequency of stools.
- Always follow Standard Practices when you come into contact with feces, as it may contain pathogens.
- A number of factors can affect bowel movements—for example, lack of privacy, personal habits, diet, fluids, activity, medications, aging, and disability.
- Constipation, if not treated, can lead to fecal impaction; if fecal impaction is not treated, it can lead to a bowel obstruction, which is a very serious condition.
- Fluids lost through diarrhea, vomiting, or both must be replaced, or dehydration—which can be a very serious condition in infants, children, and older adults—can result. Accurate reporting and recording of the frequency and amount of the stools and vomitus you observe is very important so that your supervisor can adjust the care plan to replace the fluids lost. ***This is a very important role, as you, as the support worker, most closely observe how much fluid the client is losing.***
- Bowel training can help your client gain control of bowel movements and develop a regular pattern of elimination, which will prevent fecal impaction, constipation, and fecal incontinence.
- Administering enemas is a delegated act, which you must be taught by a nurse.
- Dealing with all aspects of bowel elimination with your clients can be very embarrassing for them, so always remember the DIPPS principles.

CRITICAL THINKING IN PRACTICE

A client shares a bathroom with a roommate. You respond to the client's call light. He says he needs to have a bowel movement urgently. The bathroom is occupied. What do you do?

REVIEW QUESTIONS

Answers to these questions are at the bottom of the next page.

Circle the BEST answer.

1. Which of the following is true?
   A. Most people have a bowel movement every day or every 2 to 3 days.
   B. Stools are normally black and runny.
   C. Diarrhea occurs when feces move slowly through the intestines.
   D. Constipation results when feces move through the large intestine rapidly.
2. The prolonged retention and accumulation of feces in the rectum is called:
   A. Constipation
   B. Fecal impaction
   C. Diarrhea
   D. Fecal incontinence
3. Which will promote comfort and safety for your client having a bowel movement?
   A. Not asking visitors to leave the room
   B. Helping the client assume a sitting position
   C. Not warming the bedpan if used in bed
   D. Telling the client to hurry
4. Bowel training is aimed at:
   A. Gaining control of bowel movements and developing a regular elimination pattern
   B. Ostomy control
   C. Preventing diarrhea
   D. Preventing bleeding
5. Which statement about ostomies is true?
   A. Good skin care around the stoma is essential.
   B. Deodorants cannot control odours.
   C. The client does not wear a pouch.
   D. Feces are always liquid.

6. A client wears an ostomy pouch. It is usually emptied:
   A. Every 4 to 6 hours
   B. Every morning
   C. Every 3 to 7 days
   D. When feces are present

7. Black, tarry stool is called:
   A. Melena
   B. Feces
   C. Hemostool
   D. Occult blood

Answers: 1.A, 2.B, 3.B, 4.A, 5.A, 6.D, 7.A

Chapter opener image: nuwatphoto/Shutterstock.com

CHAPTER 34

Beds and Bed Making

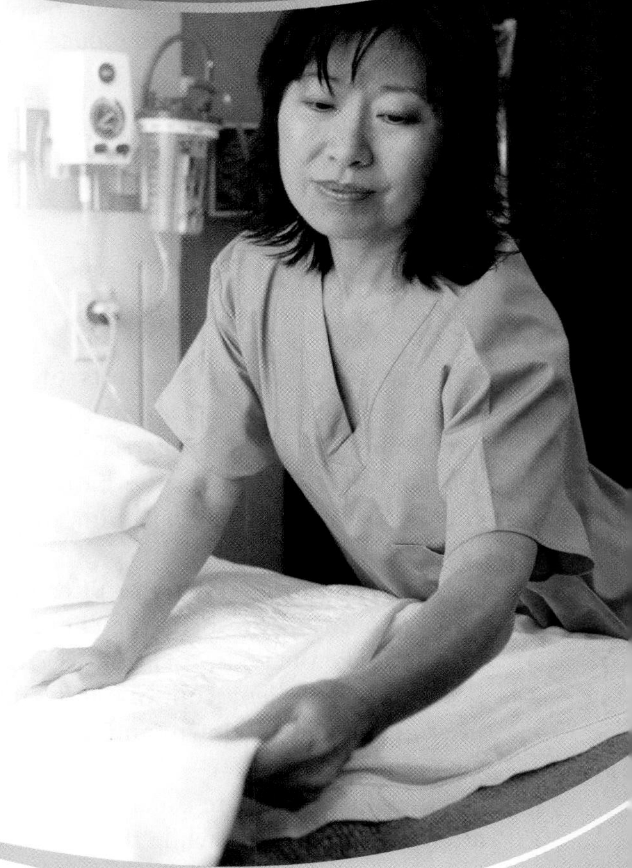

OBJECTIVES

After reading this chapter, the learner should be able to do the following:

- Identify the basic bed positions.
- Describe how to handle linen according to the rules of Standard Practice.
- List the types of bed linens used when making a client's bed.
- Describe safety measures for bed making.
- Describe the differences between open and closed beds.
- Demonstrate the procedures described in this chapter.

KEY TERMS

alternating pressure mattress A special type of mattress that has alternating areas of pressure of air, gel, or water baffles to reduce the risk for pressure sores. *p. 750*

fitted sheet A sheet (usually with elastic edges) tailored to fit a particular size of mattress. *p. 758*

incontinence pad A pad placed in the centre of the bed on top of the bottom sheet to protect the bedsheets from body fluids. Also called *absorbent pad* or *soaker pad*. *p. 755*

Clients spend varying amounts of time in bed—some are on complete bed rest and never get out of bed; some clients are on partial bed rest (getting up only to stretch or go to the bathroom); and some clients spend their waking hours out of bed, using the bed only to rest or sleep.

It is important to know the different types of beds, how to position the beds for clients' comfort, and how to make the beds. A clean, dry, and wrinkle-free bed promotes client comfort and safety and helps prevent skin breakdown and pressure ulcers (see Chapter 24).

In facilities, beds are usually made in the morning after clients' baths or while they are taking a shower or are out of the room. Clients usually like their beds made and rooms cleaned before visitors arrive. In private homes, beds are made according to the care plan and the client's preferences.

Linen must be straightened whenever it is loose or wrinkled and at bedtime. Check linen for crumbs after meals, and remove crumbs. Linen should be changed whenever it becomes wet, soiled, or damp. Follow Standard Practices when changing linen soiled with blood, body fluids, excretions, or secretions.

THE BED

Many home care clients use their regular beds. Hospital beds are used in hospitals and long-term care facilities, as well as in some homes, by home care clients. Many hospital beds have at least partial bed rails (see Chapter 22 for a discussion of bed rails and their use). Remember, bed rails have many safety hazards and can be a form of restraint. Raise and lower them only as directed by your supervisor and the care plan.

Regular Beds

In clients' homes, you will see twin-, double-, queen-, and king-sized beds, as well as waterbeds, sofa sleepers, cots, and recliners. Also, a number of private homes have motorized and electrically adjusted beds. Clients receiving palliative care in the community often have hospital-type beds.

Regular beds cannot be raised. The lower the bed, the more you will have to bend and reach when giving care or making the bed, so use good body mechanics to protect your back (see Chapter 25).

A good mattress is neither too hard nor too soft. A poor-quality mattress may not provide the needed support or comfort and could harm the client's back or skin. If you have concerns about a client's mattress, tell your supervisor. Many clients who are thin or bedridden, or who require frequent repositioning, are prone to skin breakdown and pressure ulcers. An **alternating pressure mattress** is a special mattress that has alternating areas of pressure of air, gel, or water baffles to reduce the risk for pressure sores (see *Focus on Safety: Alternating Pressure Mattresses and Side Rails*).

Hospital Beds

Hospital beds have electrical or manual controls and can be raised horizontally to give care, reducing bending and reaching. The lowest horizontal position lets the client get out of bed with ease (**FIGURE 34–1**) and is also necessary as a safety measure for the

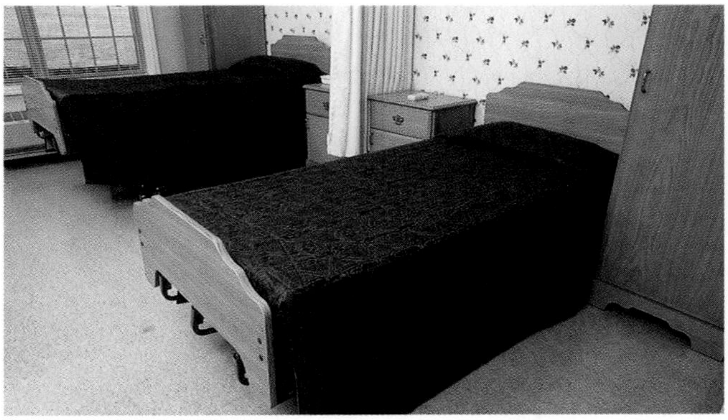

FIGURE 34–1 One bed is in the highest horizontal position, and the other is in the lowest horizontal position.

FOCUS ON SAFETY

Alternating Pressure Mattresses and Side Rails

The air, gel, or water baffles in an alternating pressure mattress reduce the risk for pressure sores. It is important when making a bed with an alternating pressure mattress to ensure that layers of bed linens do not reduce the effectiveness of the baffle action. Most manufacturers recommend that incontinence pads of any type *not* be used, and some recommend that even a bottom sheet not be used. If they can be used, ***bottom sheets should not be tucked under the mattress as they would be with a regular mattress.*** Instead, they should be allowed to hang down at the sides. If the client needs to be repositioned, a slider sheet (or slider sheet system) designed for this use should be used (see Chapter 25). Bottom sheets that cannot be tucked in can be a source of wrinkles (and pressure areas) under the client's fragile skin. It is, therefore, important to pull and straighten the sheet under the client whenever the client is repositioned.

Any client using an alternating pressure mattress should be checked frequently. There have been reported cases of clients who have died as a result of being wedged between the air mattress and the bed frame.[1] Bed rails also can cause injury to the client who is on an alternating pressure mattress. Always follow the client's care plan regarding their use and regularly monitor any client who has side rails. Refer to Chapter 22 for a discussion on side rail safety.

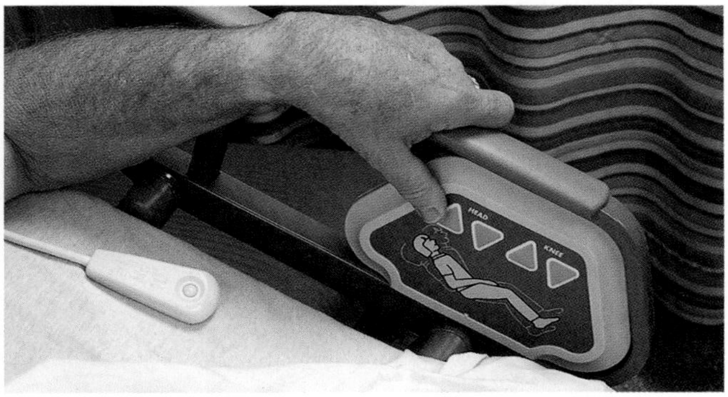

FIGURE 34–2 Controls for an electrically operated bed.

client. The head of the bed can be kept flat or raised to varying degrees for the client's comfort.

Most hospital beds are electrically controlled. Controls are on a side panel, on the bed rail, or on a panel at the foot of the bed (FIGURE 34–2), and clients are taught how to safely use the controls. Clients are advised of the risks associated with having the bed in the high position. They are also advised of any position limitations or restrictions.

Most electrically controlled beds can be "locked" into any position to prevent the client from raising or lowering the head or foot of the bed. Clients restricted to certain positions—for example, clients with dementia—may need to have their beds locked. You must also be alert to potential dangers if children, confused clients, or clients with impaired cognition or altered levels of consciousness have easy access to the controls. Follow the care plan, and check with your supervisor.

Manually operated beds are also still in use in some facilities and homes. These beds have cranks at the foot of the bed (FIGURE 34–3)—the left crank raises or lowers the head of the bed; the right crank adjusts the knee portion; and the centre crank raises or lowers the entire bed. The cranks are pulled out and up for use, and after use they should be pushed in and turned down. Cranks in the "up" position are safety hazards, as anyone walking past could bump into them.

Hospital beds should always be left in their lowest position for the safety of the client. Raise the bed only immediately before giving care and when making the bed. As soon as you have finished, return the bed to its lowest position. Never leave the client alone when the bed is raised.

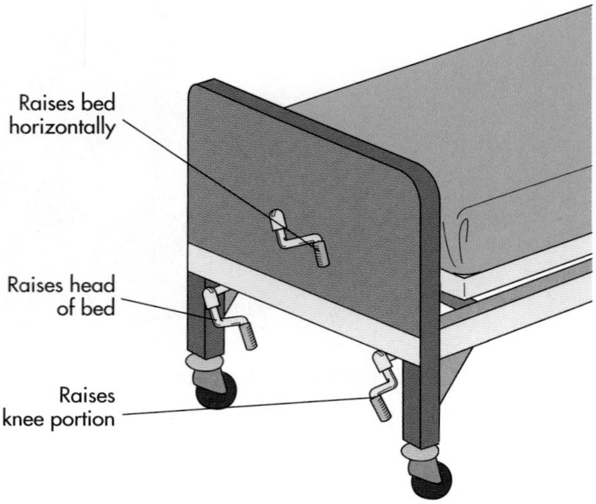

FIGURE 34–3 Manually operated hospital bed.

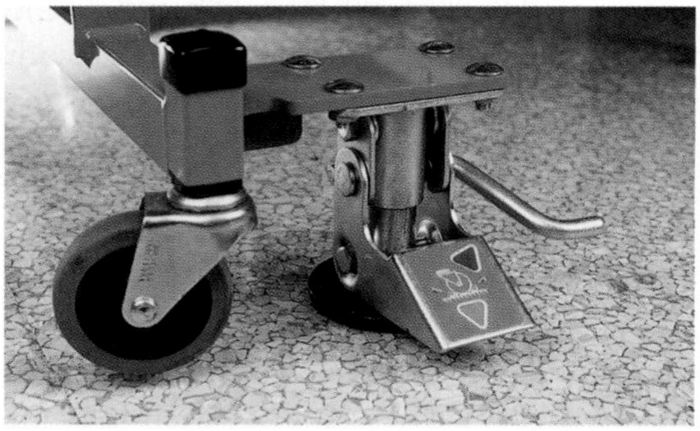

FIGURE 34–4 Lock on a bed wheel. (**Source:** Sorrentino, S.A. (2004). *Assisting with patient care* (2nd ed., p. 148). St. Louis, MO: Mosby.)

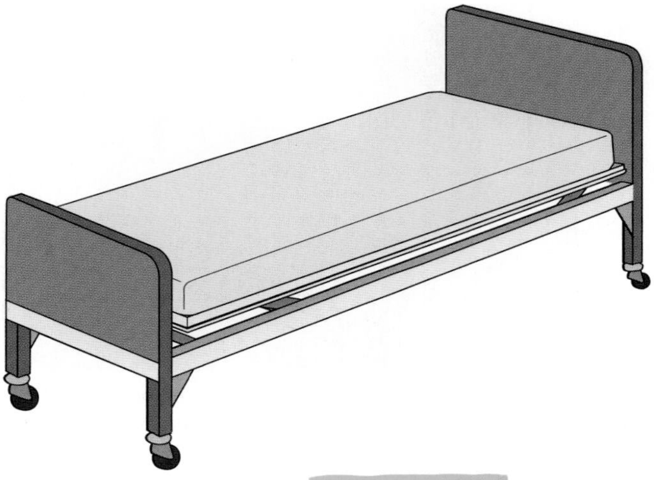

FIGURE 34–5 Flat bed position.

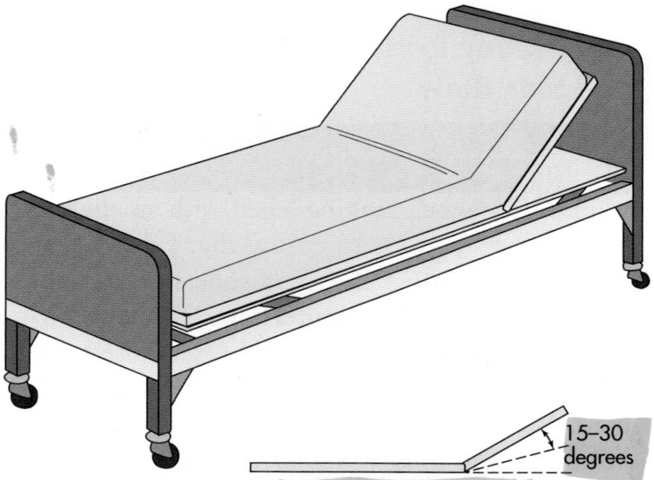

FIGURE 34–6 Low Fowler's position.

Hospital bed legs have wheels that let the bed move easily. Some beds have wheels that can be locked to prevent the bed from moving (FIGURE 34–4). Other beds have different locking mechanisms. Make sure bed wheels are locked at all times unless you are moving the bed to another location. Ensure that bed rails are up if moving a client in the bed within your facility. You or the client could be injured if the bed moves during any care or transfer.

Bed Positions

There are several basic bed positions: the flat position, Fowler's positions (low, semi-, and high Fowler's), the Trendelenburg position, and the reverse Trendelenburg position.

- ***Flat position***—the usual sleeping position. The flat position is also used after a spinal cord injury or surgery for cervical traction and to deliver care (FIGURE 34–5).
- ***Low Fowler's position***—a semi-sitting position in bed. The head of the bed is elevated by 15 to 30 degrees, or the client is propped up with a backrest or pillow (FIGURE 34–6).
- ***Semi-Fowler's position***—a semi-sitting position in bed. The head of the bed is raised by 30 to 45 degrees (FIGURE 34–7). The client can also be propped up with a backrest or pillows. The foot of the bed may be raised at the knee so that the client does not slide down in bed. However, raising the knee portion can interfere with leg circulation. Check with the care plan and your supervisor before positioning a client in the semi-Fowler's

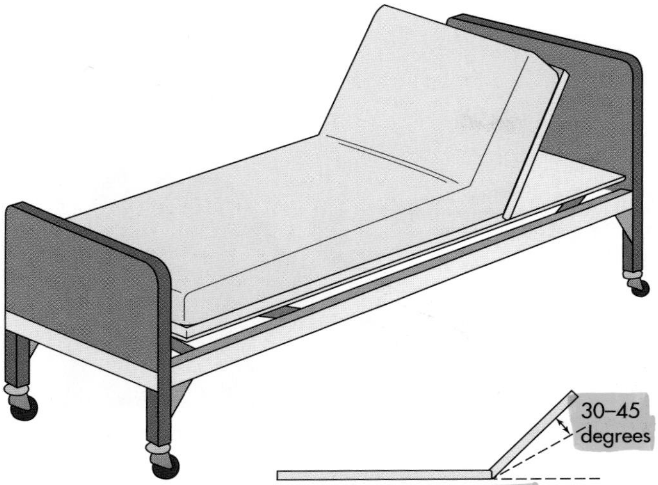

FIGURE 34–7 Semi-Fowler's position.

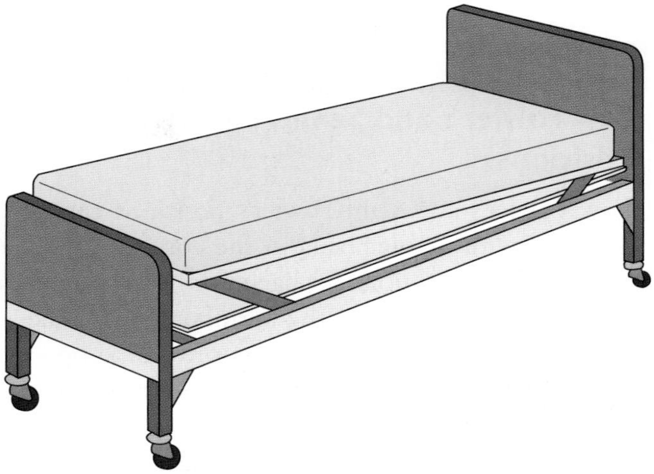

FIGURE 34–9 Trendelenburg position.

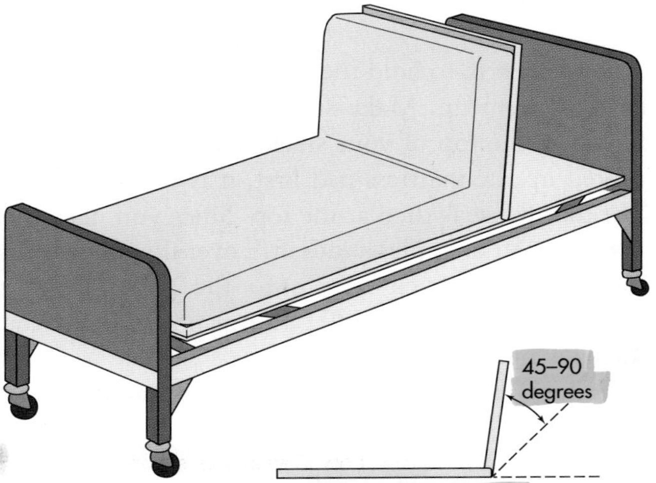

FIGURE 34–8 High Fowler's position.

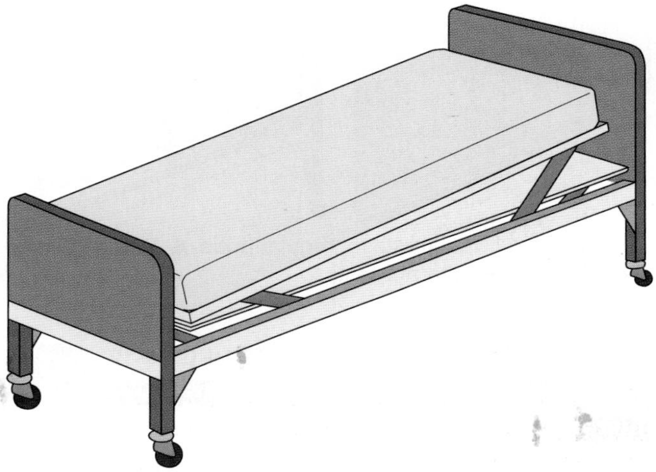

FIGURE 34–10 Reverse Trendelenburg position.

position (see the *Focus on Home Care: Low Fowler's and Semi-Fowler's Positions* box).

- ***High Fowler's position***—a semi-sitting position in bed. The head of the bed is elevated by 45 to 90 degrees (FIGURE 34–8). However, clients are not often placed above a 60-degree sitting position, as they are too uncomfortable at that angle. Clients who must eat while in bed are placed in a high Fowler's position to reduce the risk for choking and aspiration. Once the meal is finished, the client can then be returned to the semi-Fowler's position.
- ***Trendelenburg position***—the head of the bed is lowered, and the foot of the bed is raised (FIGURE 34–9). Blocks are placed under the legs at the foot of the bed, or the entire bed frame is tilted. This position requires a physician's order and is used for postural drainage.
- ***Reverse Trendelenburg position***—the opposite of the Trendelenburg position. The head of the bed is raised, and the foot of the bed is lowered (FIGURE 34–10). Blocks are put under the legs at the head of the bed, or the entire bed frame is tilted. This position requires a physician's order and is used to promote gastric emptying.

LINEN

When handling linen and making beds, follow the rules of Standard Practices. Perform hand hygiene before collecting clean linen. Your uniform is considered dirty, so you must always hold linen away

FOCUS ON HOME CARE

Low Fowler's and Semi-Fowler's Positions

Low Fowler's and semi-Fowler's positions can be achieved with regular beds in the community by using a combination of backrests and pillows (FIGURE 34–11). Check the headboard to make sure it is sturdy, as it needs to provide support when the client leans against it. Large, sturdy sofa pillows are useful if a backrest is not available.

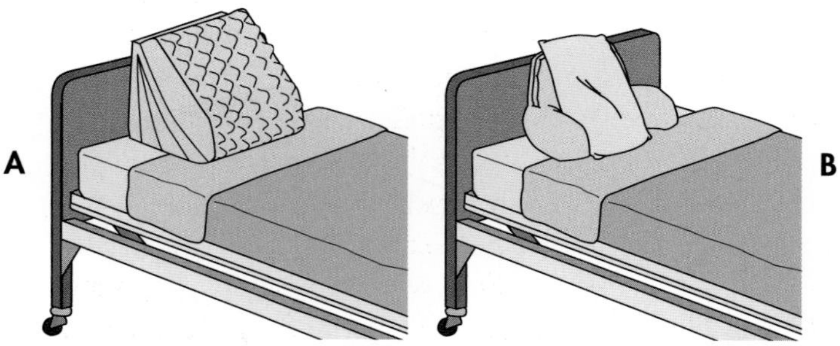

FIGURE 34–11 Backrests for regular beds. **A,** Wedge pillow. **B,** Sturdy pillow with armrests.

from your body and uniform (FIGURE 34–12). Never shake linen in the air, as doing so could spread microbes. Clean linen should be placed on a clean surface. ***Never put clean or soiled linen on the floor.*** If clean linen accidentally touches the floor, put it in the laundry. If you are changing the linens in a semi-private room or a room with four beds, remember that linens for one client should be placed only on *that client's* furniture, not on another client's furniture. Take into the room only the linens you will need. If you find you have taken extra linens into the room, do not place them back in the linen room or on the linen cart—leave them in the client's room. The linens can then be used the next time linens are changed.

Collect required linen in the reverse order you will use it:

- Pillowcase(s)
- Bedspread (if used)
- Blanket or comforter (if used)
- Top sheet (flat or fitted)
- Incontinence pad (if used)

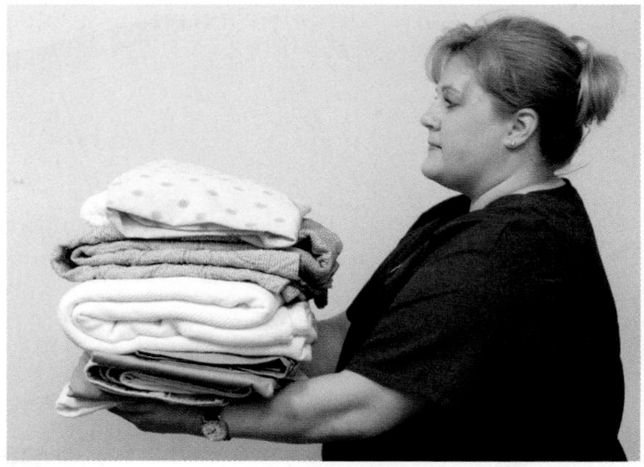

FIGURE 34–12 Hold linen away from your body and uniform.

- Bottom sheet (flat or fitted)
- Mattress pad (if used)

Use one arm to hold the linens and the other hand to pick them up. Make sure the item you will use first is at the top of your stack. For example, if you picked up the mattress pad first, it is at the bottom. The pillowcase is then at the top. Since you need the mattress pad first, place your arm over the pillowcase; then turn the stack over onto the arm with the pillowcase (FIGURE 34–13). The arm that held the linens is now free.

Follow Standard Practices when removing used linen. Used linen is considered dirty (contaminated with microbes). Wear gloves when handling linen soiled with blood, body fluids, secretions, or excretions. Also, check the linen for misplaced personal belongings—dentures, hearing aids, eyeglasses, watches, or jewellery—that clients may leave in their beds. Watch for stray needles in the linen, especially when clients self-medicate.

Remove each piece of linen separately. Roll the linen away from you. The side that touched the client is then inside the roll. The side that has not touched the client is outside (FIGURE 34–14).

Immediately place used linen in a laundry container or a special linen bag. Remove the bag from the client's room. Never place soiled linen on the floor, as it contributes to the spread of pathogens. Follow employer policy regarding soiled linen (see Chapter 23).

How often linen is changed varies among work settings (TABLE 34–1 on page 756). Follow the care plan and your employer's policy. ***In all settings, linen is changed when wet, damp, or soiled.***

A turning pad (or turning sheet) is a small pad placed over the middle of the bottom sheet. It is used to turn and move the client in bed (see **FIGURE 34–20**, on p. 760). If the client's care plan calls for an **incontinence pad** to protect the bed, many agencies and facilities use washable incontinence pads as turning pads (see *Focus on Home Care: Incontinence Pads*). Turning pads prevent pain, skin damage, and bone and joint damage by protecting the client's skin from friction and shearing when the client is moved in bed. A turning pad is also known as a *sliding pad* or *transfer sheet* in some facilities. In some settings where turning pads are unavailable—and only if necessary for brief use—flat sheets are folded into the size of a turning pad and used as a turning pad. However, it should never be left under the client, as the increased bulk of the folded sheet can cause pressure areas under the client.

In most facilities throughout the country, no-lift policies exist for the safety of the client and the health care worker. For this reason, turning pads are never referred to as *lift pads* in these facilities. If your employer has a no-lift policy, you should never attempt moving or lifting the client without checking first with your supervisor.

Most facilities use either reusable or disposable incontinence pads. Follow your facility's policy. Check your provincial or territorial legislation and

A

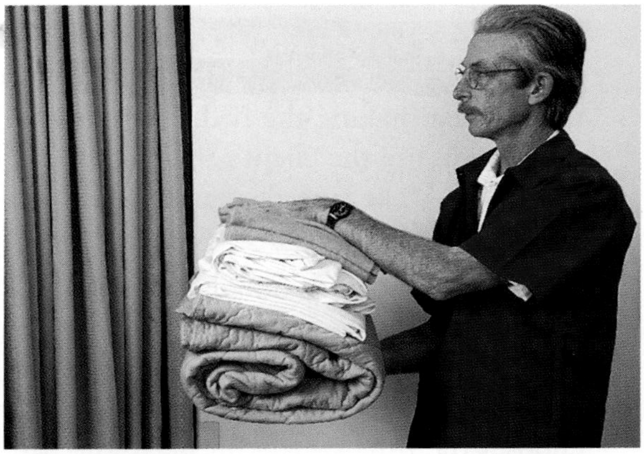

B

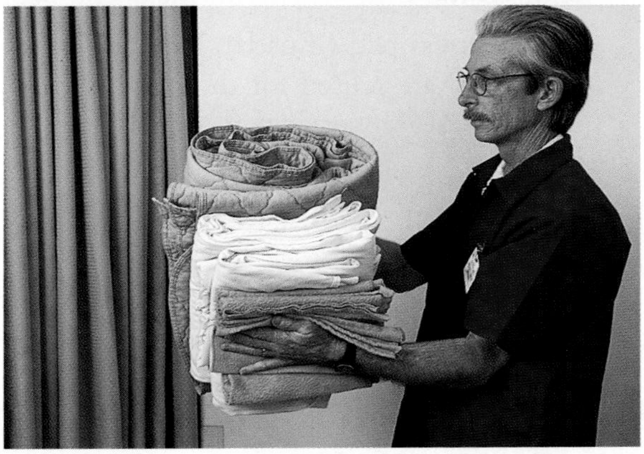

FIGURE 34–13 Collecting linen. **A,** Place your arm over the top of the linen stack. **B,** Turn the linen stack over onto your arm. Note that the linens are held away from the body.

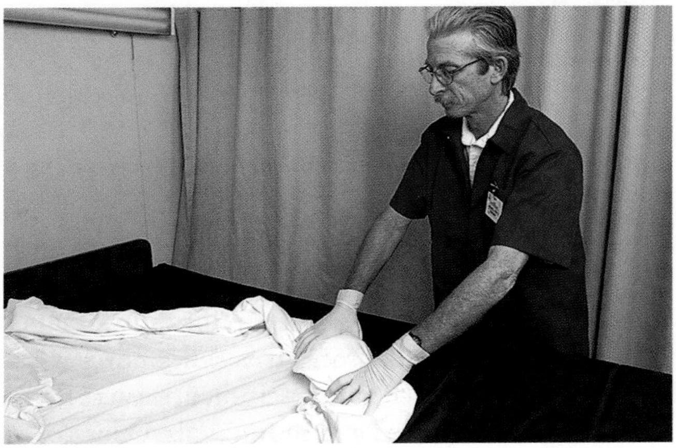

FIGURE 34–14 Roll dirty (used) linen away from you.

FOCUS ON HOME CARE

Incontinence Pads

Medical supply stores sell disposable or washable waterproof pads, which are used as incontinence pads. Disposable waterproof pads should never be used as a turning pad since they will tear if used for this purpose. Washable incontinence pads, however, are usually strong enough to be used for turning most clients.

The case manager discusses the need for these items with the client and family. Some clients place plastic mattress protectors on their beds, but these protectors do not protect the bottom linens (bottom sheet and mattress pad). Never use plastic garbage bags or dry-cleaning bags, as these are not strong enough to protect the linens and mattress. As well, they slide easily and can move out of place, and the danger of suffocation is great if the client's movements result in the bag covering the client's nose and mouth. Again, your supervisor and the care plan will tell you what is safe to use for the client.

TABLE 34–1 Linen Changes in Different Settings

Setting	How Often	Special Considerations
Home care	Usually weekly When wet, damp, or soiled	Follow the client's preferences for linen choice. For example, some clients want extra blankets. Others do not want any blankets.
Long-term care	Usually weekly. Pillowcases, top sheets, and bottom sheets may be changed twice a week When wet, damp, or soiled	Some clients bring their own bedspreads, pillows, blankets, or quilts from home. Use them when making the bed. Remember, these items are the client's property. Handle with care. Make sure they are labelled with the client's name. If the facility uses coloured linens, let the client choose what colour to use. Also, let the client decide how many pillows or blankets to use. If possible, the client also chooses the time when you make the bed.
Hospitals	Varies depending on the hospital's policy When a client is discharged When wet, damp, or soiled	The mattress pad (if used), blanket, and bedspread are reused for the same client unless they are wet or very wrinkled.

your facility's policies regarding the use of incontinence pads.

BED MAKING

Your job as a support worker will include making beds. No matter what type of bed you make, safety and medical asepsis are important. Follow Standard Practices. **BOX 34–1** lists the guidelines for bed making (also see the *Focus on Children: Crib Safety* box).

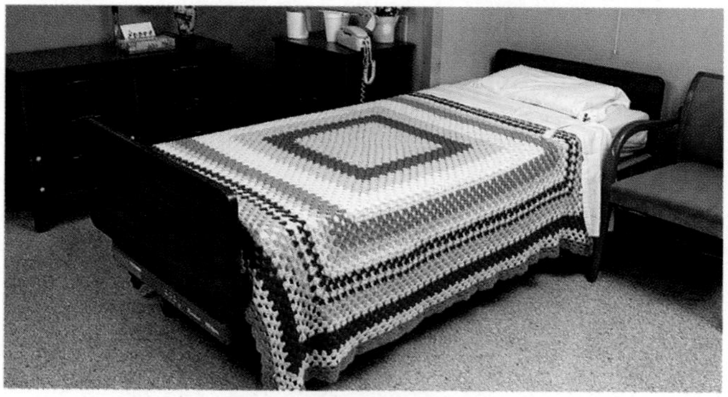

FIGURE 34–15 A closed bed. (**Source:** Sorrentino, S.A., & Gorek, B. (2003). *Mosby's textbook for long-term care assistants* (4th ed., p. 277). St. Louis, MO: Mosby.)

The Closed Bed

A *closed* bed is made when the bed is expected to be unoccupied for several hours or days. The top linen is pulled up, and the bedspread is neatly pulled over the pillow. In some facilities, the pillow is placed on top of the bedspread (**FIGURE 34–15**). A closed bed is usually made when the client is up for most or all of the day. Clean linen is used as needed.

In facilities, after a client is discharged, the bed frame and mattress are cleaned and disinfected. A closed bed is then made and kept ready for a new client.

BOX 34–1 Guidelines for Bed Making

- Use good body mechanics at all times.
- Follow the rules of medical asepsis.
- Follow Standard Practices.
- Make the bed according to the client's wishes and the care plan. If the client's wishes are unsafe, tell your supervisor.
- Have a bag bin ready for disposal of soiled linen. Follow employer's policies.
- Perform hand hygiene before handling clean linen and after handling dirty linen.
- Bring enough linen to the client's room.
- Do not use torn linen.
- Never shake linen in the air. Shaking linen spreads microbes, lint, and dust.
- Hold linen away from your uniform. Dirty linen as well as clean linen must not touch your uniform.
- Never put used, soiled linen or clean linen on the floor. Handle and dispose of linen according to employer policy (see Chapter 23).
- Linen must be straightened whenever loose or wrinkled and at bedtime.
- Make one side of the bed, as much as possible, before going to the other side. This practice saves time and energy.
- Change wet, damp, or soiled linen right away to help prevent breakdown of your client's skin.
- Manually operated beds have handles used to position the beds. The handles are pulled out during use. Ensure that after use, the handles are pushed in and turned down as anyone walking past could bump into them.
- Hospital beds have wheels that let the bed move easily. Make sure the bed wheels are locked when giving bed care or transferring your client to or from the bed.
- Clients are advised of the risks associated with having the bed in high positions. They are also advised of any position limitations or restrictions.

FOCUS ON CHILDREN

Crib Safety

Cribs, crib linen, mattresses, other linen, and bumper pads all pose many dangers to infants, as they can lead to strangulation and suffocation. Report any safety hazard to your supervisor. Always follow these safety rules:

- The crib mattress must be firm. A soft mattress can cover the baby's nose and mouth, causing suffocation.
- The mattress must fit snugly in the crib frame. The baby's head could get caught between the frame and the loose mattress and cause strangulation.
- The space between the mattress and crib sides should be no more than 3 cm. Only two adult fingers should fit in the space. If more than two fingers fit, the mattress is too small.
- The mattress must be at least 65 cm (34 in.) lower than the top of the crib rails to protect the baby from falling out of the crib. The mattress should be lowered even more when the baby can stand in the crib.
- Plastic garbage bags and dry-cleaning bags must not be used to protect the mattress.
- Bumper pads are no longer recommended for use in cribs, as they pose a risk for strangulation of the baby.
- Do not tuck blankets and top sheets under the mattress, as the baby can get caught in them.
- Do not place pillows, fluffy comforters, stuffed toys, or heavy blankets in the crib when the baby is in it, as these items can cause suffocation.
- Check linens for loose threads or stitching, and trim any found as loose stitching can cause strangulation.
- The space between the side bars should be no more than 6 cm.
- Cribs manufactured before 1986 do not meet regulations and must not be used.

Making a Closed Bed 123

Advocate on behalf of the client's quality of life by promoting:

Dignity • Independence • Preferences • Privacy • Safety *(see BOX 1–4, on p. 17)*

PRE-PROCEDURE

1 Perform hand hygiene.
2 Collect the following supplies:
- ☐ **Clean linen**
- ☐ **Mattress pad (if used)**
- ☐ **Bottom sheet (flat or fitted sheet)**
- ☐ **Incontinence or turning pad (if used)**
- ☐ **Top sheet**
- ☐ **Blanket or comforter (if used)**
- ☐ **Bedspread (if used)**
- ☐ **Two pillowcases (may be only one, depending on facility policy)**
- ☐ **Gloves**
- ☐ **Laundry bag (follow employer policy for disposal of dirty linen)**

By collecting all the necessary equipment beforehand, you can eliminate wasting time and energy in obtaining the forgotten equipment.

PROCEDURE

3 Place linen on a clean surface.
4 Place laundry bag near the bed if this option is available in your facility. (Follow employer policy for disposal of dirty linen.)
5 Make sure to remove all the linen. Clean the bed and the bed frame if the client has been discharged.
6 Raise the bed to a comfortable working height.*
Raising the bed will reduce the risk for back strain.
7 Put on gloves if handling linen soiled with blood, body fluids, secretions, or excretions.
This decreases the risk for pathogen spread.
8 Remove dirty linen. Roll each piece away from you, and place it in the laundry bag.
This decreases the risk for pathogen spread.
9 Remove and discard gloves. Perform hand hygiene.
10 Move the mattress to the head of the bed.
This ensures comfort for your client.
11 Put the mattress pad (if used) on the mattress. Make sure the pad is even with the top of the mattress.
The pad provides comfort to your client.
12 Place the bottom sheet on the mattress pad:
  a Unfold it lengthwise.
  b Place the centre crease in the middle of the bed (see **FIGURE 34–16**) with the large hem at the top and the small hem at the bottom and the hem stitching facing downward. If using a **fitted sheet** (one tailored to fit the mattress—usually with elasticized corners), place the top of the sheet over the mattress on your side of the bed.
  Ensuring the hem stitching faces downward helps reduce irritation of your client's skin.
  c Position the lower edge of the sheet so that it is even with the bottom of the mattress. If using a fitted sheet, pull the sheet over the bottom corner.

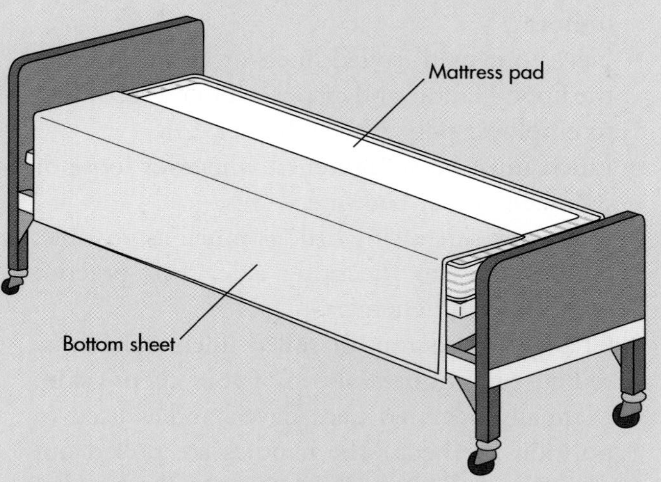

FIGURE 34–16 The bottom sheet is on the bed with the centre crease in the middle. The lower edge of the sheet is even with the bottom of the mattress.

Continued

Making a Closed Bed—cont'd

13 Open the sheet. Fan-fold it toward the other side of the bed (**FIGURE 34–17**).
This helps reduce back strain when you go to the other side of the bed.

14 Tuck the top of the sheet under the mattress. Make sure the sheet is tight and smooth.
This helps reduce irritation of your client's skin.

15 If using a flat bottom sheet, mitre the top corners of the sheet (**FIGURE 34–18**). If using a fitted bottom sheet, pull all remaining corners under the mattress.

16 Pull the bottom sheet tight so that there are no wrinkles.
This helps reduce irritation of your client's skin. (**FIGURE 34–19**).

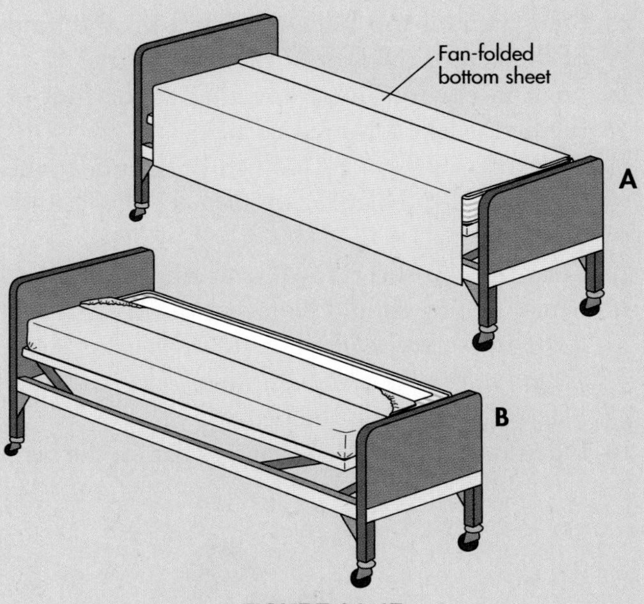

FIGURE 34–17

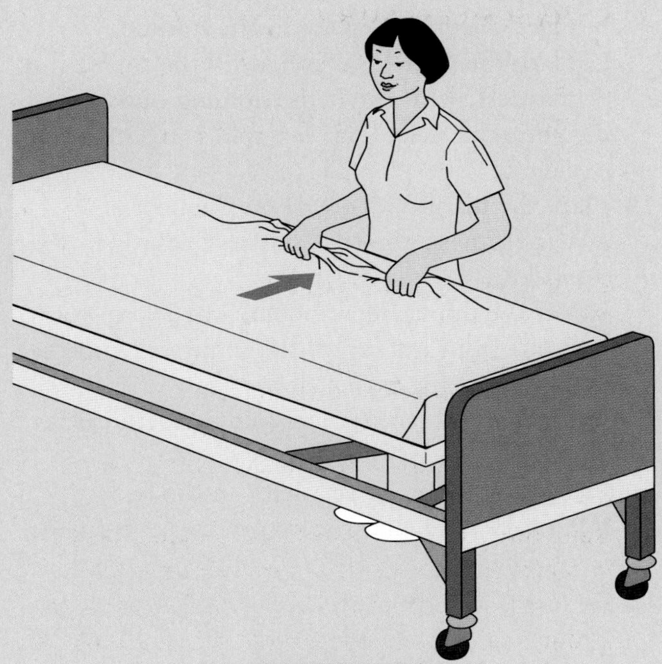

FIGURE 34–19

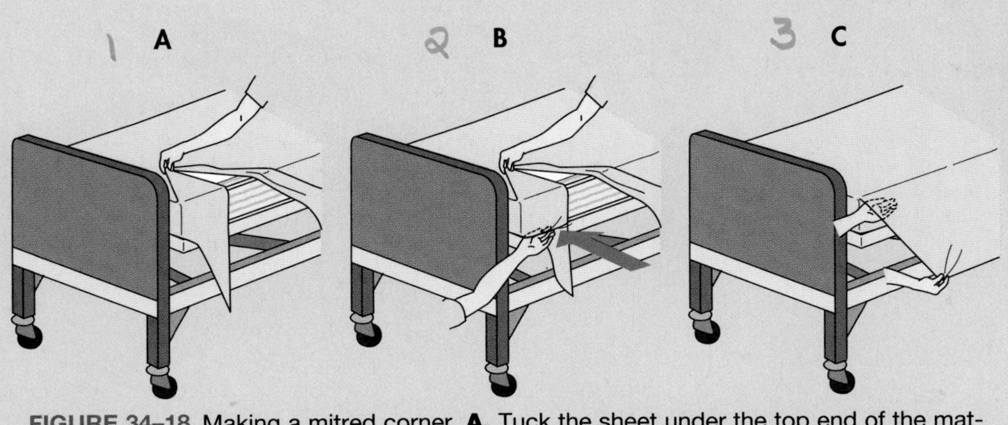

FIGURE 34–18 Making a mitred corner. **A,** Tuck the sheet under the top end of the mattress. Raise the side of the sheet onto the mattress. **B,** Tuck the remaining portion of the sheet under the mattress. **C,** Bring the raised portion of the sheet off the mattress.

Continued

Making a Closed Bed—cont'd

17 Place an incontinence pad or turning pad (if used) in the centre of the bottom sheet (**FIGURE 34–20**). Many agencies and facilities use the incontinence pads to turn the client (see Chapter 25).
These can be used to keep the bottom sheet clean or to make turning the client easier.

18 Put the top sheet on the bed:
- a Unfold it lengthwise.
- b Place the centre crease in the middle.
- c Place the wide hem even with the top of the mattress, with the hem stitching outward.
- d Open the sheet, and fan-fold it to the other side.

19 Place the blanket (if used) on the bed:
- a Unfold it so that the centre crease is in the middle.
- b Put the upper hem about 15 to 20 cm (6 to 8 in.) from the top of the mattress, with the hem stitching facing downward.
- c Open the blanket. Fan-fold it to the other side.

20 Place the bedspread (if used) on the bed:
- a Unfold it so that the centre crease is in the middle.
- b Place the upper hem even with the top of the mattress.
- c Open and fan-fold the bedspread to the other side.
- d Make sure the bedspread facing the door is even and covers all the top linen.

21 Tuck in all the top linens (including blanket and bedspread, if used) together at the foot of the bed. The bedding should be smooth and tight. Make a mitred corner.

22 Go to the other side of the bed.

23 Straighten all top linens. Work from the head of the bed to the foot of the bed.

24 Tuck in the top linens together at the foot of the bed. Make a mitred corner.

25 Turn the top hem of the bedspread under the top hem of the blanket to make a cuff (**FIGURE 34–21**).

26 Turn the top sheet down over the spread. The hem stitching should be facing down.
If the bedspread is to cover the pillow, tuck the spread under the pillow at the pillow's bottom.

27 Place the pillow on the bed.

28 Open the pillowcase so that it is flat on the bed.

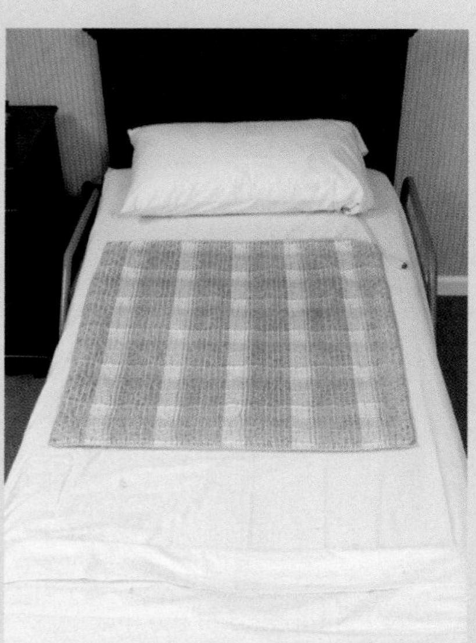

FIGURE 34–20

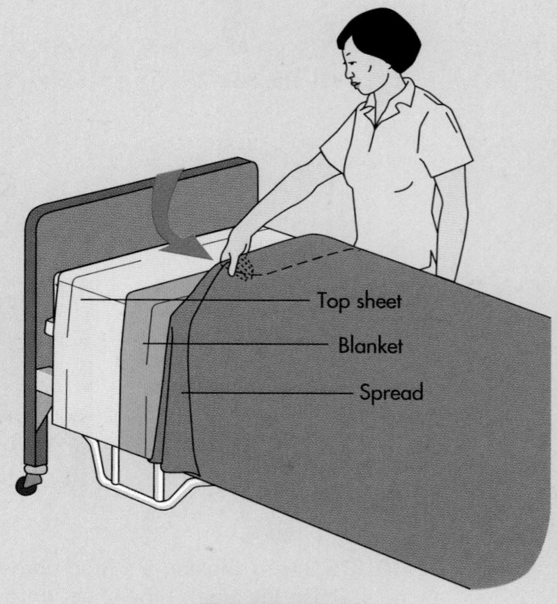

FIGURE 34–21

Continued

Making a Closed Bed—cont'd

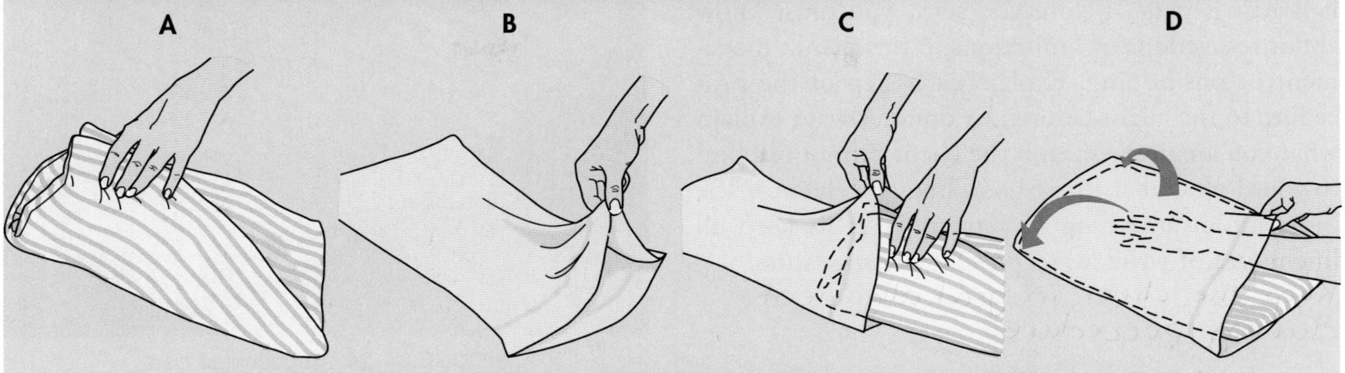

FIGURE 34–22 Putting a pillowcase on a pillow. **A,** Grasp the corners of the pillow to form a "V." **B,** The pillowcase is flat on the bed; the pillowcase is opened with the free hand. **C,** The "V" end of the pillow is guided into the pillowcase. **D,** The "V" end of the pillow falls into the corners of the pillowcase.

29 Put the pillow in the pillowcase (**FIGURE 34–22**). Fold the pillowcase edges under together, and tuck them in next to the pillow.
This prevents the pillow from slipping out.

30 Place the pillow on the bed. The open, tucked end should be away from the door and the seam of the pillowcase toward the head of the bed.

POST-PROCEDURE

31 Attach the call bell to the bed.*
This provides an easy, safe way for the client to contact staff, if necessary.

32 Lower the bed to its lowest position. Lock the bed wheels.*

33 Follow your employer's policies as to where you put clean leftover linens in your client's room.

34 Remove the laundry bag from the room (if your facility has laundry bags in clients' rooms). Follow employer policy for care of dirty linen.

35 Perform hand hygiene.

*Steps marked with an asterisk may not apply in community settings.

The Open Bed

An *open* bed is made shortly before the bed is to be occupied. Top linens are folded back so that the client can get into bed easily (**FIGURE 34–23**). An open bed is made when the client is out of bed only for a short time, or it is made just before the client goes to bed.

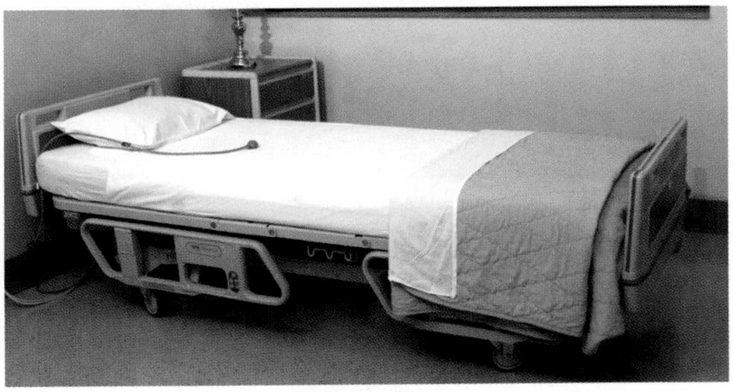

FIGURE 34–23

The Occupied Bed

An *occupied* bed is made while the client is still in the bed (**FIGURE 34–24**) because the client cannot get

out of bed for reasons of illness or injury. Mechanical lifts may be used to lift the client out of the bed while it is being made. Before you start, you must know about restrictions or limitations in the client's movement or positioning. Explain each step of the procedure to the client before it is done. Always explain what you are doing even if the client cannot respond to you. Remember to use good body mechanics. The most important thing to remember is to keep all linens free of wrinkles to prevent pressure sores.
Keep the client in good alignment during procedure.

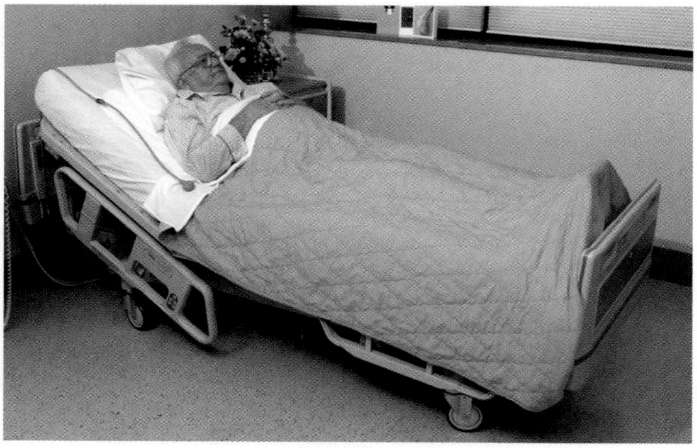

FIGURE 34–24 An occupied bed.

Making an Open Bed

Advocate on behalf of the client's quality of life by promoting:

Dignity • Independence • Preferences • Privacy • Safety *(see BOX 1–4, on p. 17)*

PROCEDURE

1 Perform hand hygiene.
2 Collect linens for a closed bed, depending on your employer's policy.
3 Make a closed bed (see *Making a Closed Bed*, pp. 758–761).
4 Fan-fold top linens to the foot of the bed (see **FIGURE 34–23**).
5 Attach the call bell to the bed.*
This provides an easy, safe way for the client to contact staff if necessary.
6 Lower the bed to its lowest position.*
This reduces the risk for client injury or falls.
7 Follow your employer's policy regarding where clean linen is stored in the client's room.
8 Follow employer policy for care of dirty linen.
9 Perform hand hygiene.

*Steps marked with an asterisk may not apply in community settings.

Making an Occupied Bed

Advocate on behalf of the client's quality of life by promoting:

Dignity • Independence • Preferences • Privacy • Safety *(see BOX 1–4, on p. 17)*

PRE-PROCEDURE

1 Identify the client, according to employer policy.
This eliminates the possibility of mistaking one client for another.
2 Explain the procedure to the client.
3 Perform hand hygiene.
4 Collect the following supplies:
- ☐ **Laundry bag (if available)**
- ☐ **Clean linen** (see *Making a Closed Bed*, pp. 758–761)

Continued

Making an Occupied Bed—cont'd

By collecting all the necessary equipment beforehand, you will not have to leave your client's side and can eliminate wasting time and energy in obtaining the forgotten equipment.

5 Place linen on a clean surface.

6 Provide for privacy.

7 Remove the call bell.*

8 Place the laundry bag (if available in your facility) near the bed or follow your employer's policy.

9 Raise the bed to a comfortable working height. Follow the care plan for bed rail use.*

Raising the bed will reduce your risk for back strain.

10 Lower the head of the bed. It should be as flat as possible. Lower the bed rail near you if it is up.*

PROCEDURE

11 Put on gloves when handling linens soiled with blood, body fluids, secretions, or excretions.

12 Loosen top linen at the foot of the bed.

13 Remove the bedspread and blanket separately. Fold them as shown in **FIGURE 34–25** if you will reuse them. Place each over a chair.

14 Leave the top sheet on your client to provide warmth and privacy.

15 Slide the mattress to the head of the bed.

16 Position the client on the side of the bed opposite to where you will begin changing the bed. Adjust the pillow for comfort and ensure that side rails are up (if available).

17 Loosen old bottom linen from the head of the bed to the foot of the bed.

18 Fan-fold old bottom linens one at a time toward the client. Start with the old incontinence pad (if used) (**FIGURE 34–26**). If the incontinence pad is heavily soiled, remove the pad or roll it tightly to contain the soiling.

19 Cleanse the client's buttock and genital area if necessary. (See the procedure *Giving a Complete Bedbath* on page 628 of Chapter 30.)

20 Place a clean incontinence pad over the old incontinence pad. Fan-fold toward the client, tucking it next to the client, preventing further contact between the wet or soiled incontinence pad and the client's skin.

If the client is left to lie on a wet or soiled incontinence pad, skin breakdown can occur.

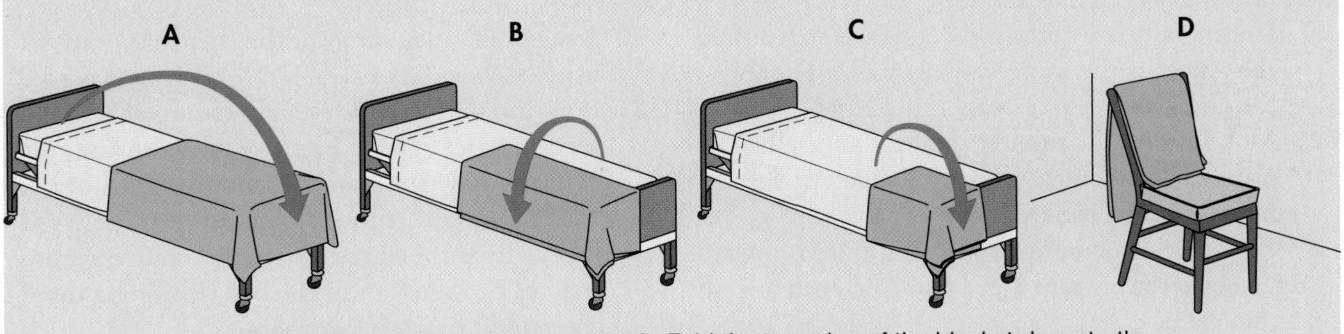

FIGURE 34–25 Folding linens for reuse. **A,** Fold the top edge of the blanket down to the bottom edge. **B,** Fold the blanket from the far side of the bed to the near side. **C,** Fold the top edge of the blanket down to the bottom edge again. **D,** Place the folded blanket over the back of a straight chair.

Continued

Making an Occupied Bed—cont'd

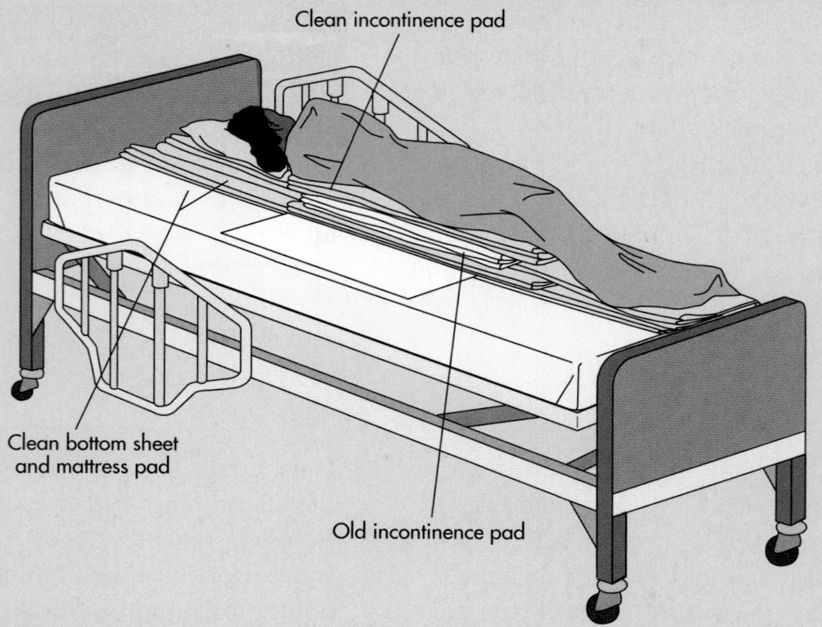

FIGURE 34–26 The linens are fan-folded towards the client. For safety's sake, never leave the bedside when the client is lying this close to the edge of the bedrail. (**Source:** Potter, P.A., & Perry, A.G. (2009). *Fundamentals of nursing* (rev. 7th ed., p. 900). St. Louis, MO: Mosby.)

21 If your facility uses a mattress pad on the bed, unfold it lengthwise, with the centre crease in the middle.

22 If using a flat bottom sheet, place the clean sheet on the mattress pad (if used) or on the mattress, with the hem stitching away from the client. Unfold the sheet so that the crease is in the middle and the small hem is even with the bottom of the mattress.
If using a fitted bottom sheet, place and unfold the sheet in the same way as with a flat sheet, but fit the sheet one corner at a time.

23 Make a mitred corner at the head of the bed (if using a flat sheet). Tuck the sheet under the mattress from the head to the foot.

24 Pull the clean incontinence pad (if used) toward you over the bottom sheet. Fan-fold both toward the client.

25 Raise the bed rail if it was used. Go to the other side, and lower the bed rail.*
This reduces the risk for client injury.

26 Explain to the client that the client will roll over a bump. Assure the client that there is no risk for a fall.

27 Help the client turn to the other side. Adjust the pillow for the client's comfort.

28 Remove the soiled incontinence pad and loosen bottom linen. Remove one piece at a time, and place each piece in the laundry bag (if available), or follow your employer's policy for care of dirty linens.

29 Remove and discard gloves if they were worn. Wash your hands.

30 Straighten and smooth the mattress pad (if used).

31 Pull the fan-folded clean bottom sheet and incontinence pad toward you, ensuring the client is now on a smooth, lump-free surface. Make a mitred corner at the top if using a flat sheet. Tuck the sheet under the mattress from the head to the foot of the bed. If using a fitted sheet, pull over each corner.
A smooth, tight foundation reduces the chance of skin irritation and discomfort.

32 Pull the incontinence pad tightly toward you.

33 Place the client in the supine position in the centre of the bed. Adjust the pillow for comfort.

Continued

Making an Occupied Bed—cont'd

34 Put a clean top sheet on the bed. Unfold it lengthwise. The crease is in the middle, and the large hem is even with the top of the mattress. Hem stitching is on the outside.
This helps decrease skin irritation.
35 Ask the client to hold on to the clean top sheet so that you can remove the old top sheet from beneath. If the client is unable to help, tuck the clean top sheet under the client's shoulders. Remove the old top sheet.
36 Place the blanket (if used) on the bed. Unfold it so that the crease is in the middle and it covers the client. The upper hem should be 15 to 20 cm (6 to 8 in.) from the top of the mattress.
37 Place the bedspread (if used) on the bed. Unfold it so that the centre crease is in the middle and it covers the client. The top hem is even with the mattress top.
38 Turn the top hem of the bedspread under the blanket to make a cuff.
39 Bring the top sheet down over the bedspread to form a cuff.
40 Go to the foot of the bed.
41 Make a toe pleat using the top linens. Make a 5-cm (2-in.) pleat across the foot of the bed. The pleat is about 15 to 20 cm (6 to 8 in.) from the foot of the bed.
This allows circulation in the client's feet.
42 Lift the mattress corner with one arm. Tuck all top linens under the mattress together. Make a mitred corner.
43 Raise the bed rail if it was used. Go to the other side, and lower the bed rail.*
44 Straighten and smooth top linens.
45 Tuck the top linens under the mattress. Make a mitred corner.
46 Change the pillowcase(s).
47 Raise the head of the bed to a level appropriate for the client, or use pillows to position the client.

POST-PROCEDURE

48 Provide for safety and comfort.
49 Place the call bell within reach.*
This provides an easy, safe way for the client to contact staff, if necessary.
50 Lower the bed to its lowest position. Follow the care plan for bed rail use.*
51 Follow your employer's policy for care of soiled linen.
52 Remove privacy measures, as needed.
53 Perform hand hygiene.

*Steps marked with an asterisk may not apply in community settings.

CHAPTER REVIEW

KEY POINTS

- The basic bed positions are the flat position, Fowler's positions, the Trendelenburg position, and the reverse Trendelenburg position. The care plan will tell you which position to place the client in. The client's position depends on his or her condition.
- The linens required for bed making and the frequency of linen changes will vary among health care settings. Follow your employer's policies.
- Clean linen must be held away from your uniform to prevent transfer of microorganisms, and dirty linen must be removed with gloves and placed into the receptacle approved by your employer.
- A *closed* bed is made when the bed is expected to be unoccupied for a while; the top linens are pulled up, with the top sheet folded over the bedspread into a cuff or the bedspread pulled neatly over the pillows, as per facility policy. An *open* bed is made shortly before the bed is to be occupied; top linens are folded back so that the client can easily get into bed. An *occupied* bed is made with the client in it.
- One of the most important concepts in this chapter to remember is that the bottom sheet, next to your client's skin, needs to be wrinkle free to prevent skin irritation, which can lead to skin breakdown of buttocks, ankles, and elbows and to bedsores.
- Use good body mechanics to reduce your chance of injury when making a bed.

CRITICAL THINKING IN PRACTICE

You need to give a person a bath in bed (Chapter 30) and change linens. The person must remain in bed. Which type of bed will you make? Will you change linens or give the bath first? While changing linens, identify when you need to apply and remove gloves and practise hand hygiene.

REVIEW QUESTIONS

Answers to these questions are at the bottom of the next page.

Circle the BEST answer.

1. A hospital bed:
   A. Cannot be raised or lowered
   B. Cannot be controlled by the client
   C. Usually has bed rails
   D. Is kept in the highest position at all times
2. The Trendelenburg bed position:
   A. Is a semi-sitting position
   B. Has the head of the bed lowered, and the foot of the bed raised
   C. Is a flat position for sleeping
   D. Has the head of the bed raised, and the foot of the bed lowered
3. Which of the following requires a linen change?
   A. Soiled linen
   B. Loose linen
   C. Linen after the client has had an afternoon nap
   D. Wrinkled linen
4. When handling linen:
   A. Put dirty linen on the floor
   B. Hold linen away from your body and uniform
   C. Shake linen to remove crumbs
   D. Take the extra linen to another client's room
5. The client has an alternating pressure mattress. Which is true?
   A. It is the preferred mattress type for any client at risk for pressure sores.
   B. The bottom sheet must be tightly tucked in under the mattress.
   C. It should be protected with several layers of bottom sheets and incontinence pads.
   D. It poses no risk to a client when it is being used.

6. The client's care plan calls for a disposable waterproof pad to be placed on the client's bed. Which is true?
   A. Dry-cleaning bags should never be used for this purpose.
   B. The pad should be placed under the bottom sheet.
   C. The client's consent is needed.
   D. Disposable pads are strong enough to be used to turn the client.

7. The following are crib safety rules. Which one is true?
   A. Bumper pads should remain in the crib until the baby moves to a bed.
   B. The mattress must fit snugly in the crib frame.
   C. Plastic garbage bags and dry-cleaning bags may be used to protect the mattress.
   D. Pillows, fluffy comforters, and heavy blankets are safe to use when the baby is in the crib.

8. An open bed is made:
   A. When the bed will be unoccupied for a period
   B. Shortly before the bed is to be occupied
   C. With the client in it
   D. So that a client can be moved to or from a stretcher

9. When making an occupied bed, you should:
   A. Cover the client with a clean top sheet
   B. Remove all pillows
   C. Lower both bed rails before beginning
   D. Fan-fold top linens to the foot of the bed

Answers: 1.C, 2.B, 3.A, 4.B, 5.A, 6.A, 7.B, 8.B, 9.A

CHAPTER 35

Mental Health Disorders

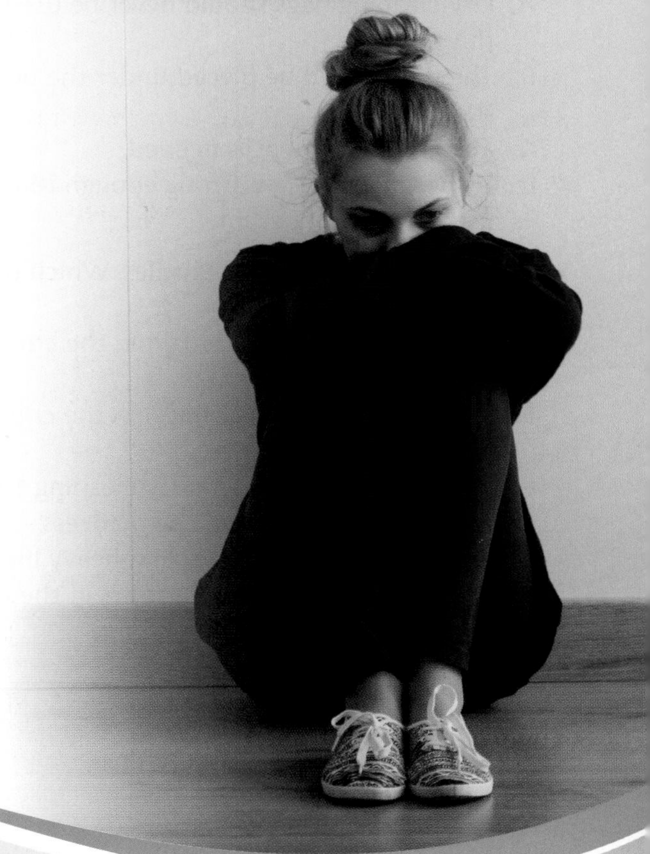

OBJECTIVES

After reading this chapter, the learner should be able to do the following:

- Describe the effects of mental health disorders on everyday life.
- List factors that may contribute to mental health disorders.
- Describe the stigma experienced by people with mental health disorders.
- Describe the effect of mental health disorders on families.
- Explain the importance of DIPPS when supporting clients with mental health disorders and their families.
- Understand how culture can influence the interpretation and treatment of mental illness.
- Define the following disorders and describe how to support clients with these disorders:

  Schizophrenia spectrum
  Depressive
  Trauma and stressor-related
  Feeding and eating
  Suicidal behaviour
  Substance-related and addictive
  Bipolar and related
  Anxiety
  Obsessive–compulsive and related
  Sleep–wake
  Disruptive, impulse-control, and conduct
  Personality

KEY TERMS

acquired brain injury (ABI) Damage to brain tissue caused by disease, medical condition, accident, or violence. Also known as **traumatic brain injury**. *p. 776*

affect A person's feelings, emotions, and moods and the way the person demonstrates them. *p. 781*

amenorrhea Absence of at least three consecutive menstrual periods as normally expected to occur. *p. 788*

anxiety A vague, uneasy feeling in response to stress. *p. 783*

anxiety disorders A group of mental health disorders whose main symptom is **anxiety**, with fears and worries so disproportionate to the situation as to affect normal functioning. *p. 783*

bipolar and related disorders A group of related brain disorders that cause unusual shifts in a person's mood, energy, and ability to function. *p. 779*

clinical depression See **major depressive disorders**. *p. 781*

compulsion The uncontrollable urge to perform an act. *p. 786*

conduct disorder A disorder that causes the person to repeatedly violate the personal or property rights of others and the basic expectations of society. *p. 794*

delusion A fixed, false belief that is not based on reality. *p. 778*

depressive disorders A group of disorders in which the client has sad, empty, or irritable moods accompanied by physical and thought changes that are severe enough to affect the client's ability to function. *p. 781*

detoxification A process of allowing an abused substance to exit the body naturally or of removing the substance from the body medically; the person being detoxified may go into **drug withdrawal**. *p. 796*

***Diagnostic and Statistical Manual of Mental Disorders*, fifth edition (*DSM-5*)** A manual published by the American Psychiatric Association that is used throughout North America to classify mental health disorders. *p. 772*

disruptive, impulse-control, and conduct disorder Disorders in which the client displays difficult, disruptive, aggressive, or antisocial behaviours. *p. 793*

drug tolerance The state at which the body gets accustomed to a substance, causing the individual to need larger and larger amounts of it to experience the same effect. *p. 795*

drug withdrawal A physical reaction that occurs when a person abusing a substance stops taking it. *p. 795*

emotional illness See **mental health disorder**. *p. 770*

feeding and eating disorders Altered body image perceptions that lead to disturbances in eating behaviours and an abnormal concern with body weight and shape. *p. 787*

hallucination Seeing, smelling, hearing, tasting, or feeling something that is not real. *p. 778*

major depressive disorder A state of mind in which a person has severe feelings of worthlessness, self-blame, sadness, disappointment, and emptiness that last for weeks and interfere with the person's ability to perform activities of daily living; also known as **clinical depression**, although this term is not used anymore by physicians. *p. 781*

mental disorder See **mental health disorder**. *p. 770*

mental health A state of mind in which a person copes with and adjusts to the stressors of everyday living in socially acceptable ways. *p. 770*

mental health disorder A disturbance in a person's ability to cope with or adjust to stress, affecting the person's thinking, mood, or behaviours and impairing functioning; also known as **mental illness**, **mental disorder**, **emotional illness**, or **psychiatric disorder**. *p. 770*

mental illness See **mental health disorder**. *p. 770*

obsession A persistent thought or desire. *p. 786*

obsessive–compulsive and related disorders Mental health disorders characterized by recurrent obsessions and compulsions that interfere with a person's daily life and relationships. *p. 786*

panic An intense and sudden feeling of fear, anxiety, terror, or dread for no obvious reason. *p. 783*

paranoia Extreme suspicion about a person or a situation. *p. 778*

personality disorders A group of disorders involving rigid and socially unacceptable behaviours. *p. 796*

psychiatric disorder See **mental health disorder**. *p. 770*

psychosis A mental state in which a person's perception of reality is impaired. *p. 778*

psychotherapy A form of therapy in which a client explores thoughts, feelings, and behaviours with help and guidance from a mental health specialist. *p. 774*

reactive depression A term that some health care providers use to describe normal reactions, such as feelings of loss and sadness in response to what a person has just experienced. *p. 781*

remission A period when the signs and symptoms of a disease lessen or disappear. *p. 779*

repression The keeping from the conscious mind of (or "burying of") unpleasant or painful thoughts. *p. 772*

schizophrenia spectrum disorders An extremely complex group of mental health disorders characterized by delusions, hallucinations, disturbances in thinking, and withdrawal from social activity. *p. 778*

sleep–wake disorders Conditions in which repetitive disturbed sleep patterns lead to distress and impairment in that person's daytime functioning. *p. 790*

substance-related and addictive disorder The deliberate misuse of and inability to stop the abuse of prescription medications, illegal drugs, alcohol, or other substances. *p. 795*

suicidal behaviour disorder A disorder whose main trait is recurrent thoughts about or a preoccupation with ending one's own life. *p. 791*

traumatic brain injury See **acquired brain injury (ABI).** *p. 776*

Mental health disorders can affect all dimensions of a person's life—physical, emotional, spiritual, social, and intellectual. As a support worker, you will care for and support clients and family members with physical health problems, mental health problems, or both. This chapter discusses many common mental health disorders that you may have seen in people you know or may have experienced personally.

There may be no relationship between a client's physical and mental health problems, but in some clients, physical problems can result from mental health problems or the reverse. To be able to provide care to your clients and their families while ensuring dignity, respect, and compassionate care, you need to understand what they are experiencing and be aware of your own attitude toward mental health and mental illness. Be sensitive to the feelings of your clients and their families (see the *Providing Compassionate Care: Supporting Clients With Mental Health Disorders* box on the next page). This chapter describes many of the most common mental health disorders that affect Canadians.

MENTAL HEALTH AND MENTAL HEALTH DISORDERS

A **mental health disorder**, which can be caused by a combination of genetic, biological, personality, and environmental factors, is a disturbance in a person's ability to cope with or adjust to stress; as a result, the person's thinking, mood, and behaviours are affected, and functioning is impaired. Twenty percent of Canadians (one in five) will personally experience a mental health disorder during their lifetime.[1] Mental health disorders affect people of all ages, cultures, and educational and income levels. Many people may be uncertain whether they have a mental health disorder (see **BOX 35–1** on page 772). The onset of most mental health disorders occurs during adolescence or young adulthood. The terms **mental illness**, **mental disorder**, **emotional illness**, and **psychiatric disorder** all refer to *mental health disorder*.

Mental health is a state of mind in which a person copes with and adjusts to the stressors of everyday living in socially acceptable ways. It is influenced by three factors: (1) inherited characteristics, (2) childhood nurturing, and (3) life circumstances. With good mental health, a person can cope with life's problems and challenges and can "bounce back," or recover, from difficult situations.

People who are mentally healthy may feel anxiety, sadness, grief, and loneliness from time to time, but they can handle normal amounts of stress and are able to express and control their emotions appropriately. They feel capable and competent, know their own needs, can form stable and satisfying relationships, and lead an independent life.

Impact of Mental Health Disorders

More than one million Canadians currently live with a severe or persistent mental health disorder. Even if not affected personally, most Canadians in their lifetime will have a family member, friend, or co-worker affected by a mental health disorder, ailment, or addiction.[1]

The statistics regarding mental health disorders are staggering:[1]

- Twenty percent of Canadians will personally experience a mental health disorder during their lifetime.
- Schizophrenia affects 1% of the population in Canada.
- Anxiety disorders affect 5% of the population.
- About 8% of adults in Canada will experience a major depressive disorder in the course of their lives.
- Suicide rates in some Indigenous communities are among the highest in the world: five to seven times higher than the national average for First Nations youth and 11 times the national average for Inuit youth.
- Anxiety disorders are the most common of all mental health issues. It is estimated that 1 in 10 Canadians is affected by them.

Mental health disorders are costly to the individual, the family, the community, and the health care system. In 2004, it was estimated that for people with schizophrenia, the total costs of health care, supportive care, and other related care had reached $6.85 billion. The total economic cost for people with all other types of mental health disorder would make that figure considerably higher.[1]

Today, 86% of hospitalizations for mental health disorders in Canada occur in general hospitals. In Canada, diagnosed mental illness is responsible for one third of the total number of hospital days each year, and the estimated cost of mental health

Providing Compassionate Care
Supporting Clients With Mental Health Disorders

- ***Dignity.*** Treat clients with mental health disorders as you would any other client. Show respect, and promote dignity. Do not label them—for example, it is not acceptable to say that a client is "a schizophrenic" or "a drug addict." It is acceptable to say that the client "has schizophrenia" or "has a substance-dependence disorder."

  Be patient and understanding. Do not patronize (talk down to) the client. Do not feel offended or hurt by the client's remarks or actions. Remember, the client may have difficulty relating to others. Be accepting of the client and help her feel good about herself. Treat the client as a valued, worthy individual.
- ***Independence.*** Clients with mental health disorders have the right to autonomy. They should be encouraged to be as independent as is safely possible. People with mental health disorders are impaired in some areas but are rarely impaired in all areas. For example, a client with schizophrenia usually has no problems with ambulation.
- ***Preferences.*** Allow clients to make choices in their care, according to the care plan. Having options gives them a greater sense of control. Feelings of loss of control can cause some people with mental health disorders to become withdrawn, so encourage clients to express their wishes, likes, and dislikes.
- ***Privacy.*** Discuss the client only with the health care team. Respect the client's and the family's right to confidentiality and privacy.
- ***Safety.*** Stress, fatigue, and physical illness make mental health disorders worse and may trigger episodes. Observe the client carefully for any signs of stress or illness, and report such signs at once. Remember also that clients with mental health disorders may be more likely to fall or injure themselves if they are unable to focus on their surroundings. Provide a calm, stress-free, and safe environment. The client's care plan will list activities and situations that should be avoided. Follow the safety guidelines in Chapter 22. For guidance on handling abusive situations, see Chapter 16.

BOX 35–1 How Do I Know if I Have a Mental Health Disorder?

Most people, at one time or another, have asked themselves this question: "Are my problems or symptoms getting in the way of my life?" If you think the answer is yes, then you may have a mental health disorder.

The ***Diagnostic and Statistical Manual of Mental Disorders*, fifth edition (*DSM-5*)**, published by the American Psychiatric Association, is used throughout North America to classify mental health disorders. The manual states that you may have a mental health disorder if what you feel is severe enough to cause "clinically significant distress or impairment in [your] social, occupational, or other important areas of functioning."

People with a mental health disorder experience a disturbance in their ability to cope with or adjust to stress. They may have an alteration in their thinking, mood, or behaviour or in some combination of these aspects. They may feel high levels of distress and fear and often have trouble coping with everyday life. They may have difficulties keeping a job, staying in school, forming strong family and social relationships, and performing daily routines. People with mental health disorders often behave differently from what is considered "normal," and their thinking, mood, or behaviours may be affected or impaired, with symptoms ranging from mild to severe.

If you think that you may have a mental health disorder, you should have yourself thoroughly evaluated by your doctor as soon as possible. When you see your doctor, you should describe how you are feeling as completely as you can. Your doctor may then take a complete medical history and examine you for any physical conditions that might be contributing to your condition. The doctor may also advise you to refrain from drinking alcohol; to avoid taking any nonprescribed medications or drugs; to eat properly, reducing sugar and caffeine intake; to get plenty of exercise; and to get at least 8 hours of sleep.

If you still feel that you have a mental health disorder after making these changes to your lifestyle, your doctor may then prescribe medications, propose another course of treatment, or refer you to a mental health professional. Remember that it is always best to seek treatment as early as possible!

disorders and addictions to the Canadian economy is about $18 billion each year. It is estimated that by 2020, depressive illnesses will become the second leading cause of disease burden worldwide and the leading cause in developed countries such as Canada, representing a global cost of hundreds of billions of dollars.[2]

Causes of Mental Health Disorders

The causes of mental health disorders are complex, as there are numerous contributing factors, including the following:

- ***Biological factors***. Chemical imbalances in the body can cause mental health disorders. Some disorders run in families, which suggests that they can be inherited (passed from parent to child).
- ***Childhood experiences.*** Childhood traumas or conflicts, particularly when memories of them are repressed, can cause mental health disorders. **Repression** means the keeping from the conscious mind of (or "burying of") unpleasant or painful thoughts. For example, a client who was sexually abused during childhood has no recollection of the abuse.
- ***Social and cultural factors.*** These include poverty, discrimination, and social isolation.
- ***Stressful life events.*** Although stress is a fact of everyday life, too much stress can cause serious health concerns, especially if it is not dealt with in a healthy-lifestyle manner. Family situations and workplace pressures can be stressful. Change is also stressful (see Chapter 7), especially when associated with loss (such as the death of a loved one or a divorce), and can lead to physical and mental health issues.

- ***Poor physical health or disability***. People with serious illnesses, injuries, or disabilities are at risk for certain mental health disorders.

Supporting Clients and Their Families

It is now known that mental health disorders can be treated successfully in the vast majority of circumstances. Until the 1960s, many people with chronic or severe mental health disorders lived in psychiatric facilities. Today, only those who are severely ill live in facilities. Unfortunately, a few people with mental health disorders end up living on the streets, as they are too ill to hold a job or apply for financial assistance, may fear receiving treatment, or are not aware of their own illness.

Most people with mental health disorders are able to live in the community, where they may be offered treatment and assistance with life skills and employment. For example, once depression is recognized, help can make a difference for 80% of people who are affected, allowing them to get back to their regular activities.[1] People with chronic or moderately severe mental health disorders are able to live in their homes, in group homes, or in assisted-living facilities, depending on their needs. Support workers provide valuable care and support to clients with mental health disorders and to their families in a wide variety of settings.

The Importance of DIPPS

While you are caring for and providing support to a person with a mental health disorder, your actions should always focus on respect and acceptance of the client and the family. Remember the principles of DIPPS (see the *Providing Compassionate Care: Supporting Clients With Mental Health Disorders* box on page 771). BOX 35–2 lists the principles that govern health care workers' care and support for clients with mental health disorders and for their families.

Mental health disorders affect people in different ways, and people with mild disorders tend to have

BOX 35-2 Principles of Mental Health Care

1. ***Follow the care plan.*** Tell your supervisor if support measures are not working.
2. ***Do no harm.*** Provide a safe, comfortable setting for the client. You need to provide both safe care and protection from harm at all times. A safe, quiet, and neat setting can calm the client. You should remember to act as the client's advocate whenever necessary.
3. ***Accept each client as a whole person***. You should be accepting of the client and refrain from making any judgements.
4. ***Be patient and supportive.*** Speak calmly; avoid speaking in a loud or sharp tone of voice.
5. ***Develop mutual trust.*** Remember to *do what you say you will do.* Being on time, providing the care as promised, and explaining all procedures will promote trust and reduce your client's anxiety.
6. ***Explore behaviours and emotions.*** Many clients will share with you what they are feeling and thinking if they trust you and if you take the time to listen to them.
7. ***Observe the client carefully.*** Observe for any changes in the client's behaviour, mood, and thinking, such as signs and symptoms of fatigue, stress, anxiety, fear, and frustration, as well as signs and symptoms of illness. Report and record all of your observations, according to employer policy.
8. ***Encourage responsibility.*** Taking responsibility for their own actions helps clients build self-worth, dignity, and confidence.
9. ***Encourage effective adaptation.*** Clients who are mentally stressed may behave in socially unacceptable ways or may be harmful to themselves or others. It is often your responsibility to intervene when this behaviour happens and to help clients find better ways of coping.
10. ***Provide consistency.*** Maintaining a routine promotes a sense of control. Consistency and reliability of your care will also provide security and stability for the client. This will, in turn, help reduce the client's stresses and anxieties.

fewer problems than those with more pronounced mental health issues. Severe mental health disorders, however, almost always cause distress not only to the affected individuals but to their families as well. The individuals with the disorder may be unable to function, and their behaviours may become disruptive at times. The support worker often provides the needed reassurance and support to these clients and also to their families.

Because they might have been exposed to negative attitudes in the past, your clients and their families may be particularly sensitive to any verbal or nonverbal signs that indicate disapproval of them or *stigmatization* of people with mental health disorders. Therefore, you need to pay particular attention to your body language and verbal language and should make every attempt to convey to them that you are respectful, nonjudgemental, and accepting of their behaviours (see Chapter 5 for a discussion of ways to communicate acceptance and respect).

Team Approach

The care-planning process aims at addressing the needs of clients with mental health disorders, including their physical, safety, and emotional needs, and usually requires input from various members of the health care team. The physician may order medications, depending on the client's disorder, signs, and symptoms, as a number of mental health disorders can be controlled effectively with medication.

The health care team may include a family physician, nurse, occupational therapist (who helps the person learn or relearn skills for the performance of life tasks), social worker (who provides assistance such as helping a client resolve employment problems), support worker, and one or more of the following mental health specialists:

- ***Psychiatrists***—physicians who specialize in mental health disorders and who can prescribe medications for treatment.
- ***Psychologists and psychotherapists***—health care providers educated in treatments for mental health disorders that do not involve prescribing medications.
- ***First Nations and Inuit mental health providers***—elders, healers, and cultural counsellors, who are vital parts of many First Nations and Inuit mental health services, and other members of a treatment or mental health and wellness staff, who assist clients and provide services to First Nations and Inuit people and communities. Some practitioners use exclusively traditional First Nations or Inuit healing methods or both.

Treatment of mental health disorders often involves **psychotherapy**, which is a form of therapy in which a client explores thoughts, feelings, and behaviours with help and guidance from a mental health specialist. The various forms of psychotherapy include the following:

- ***Psychoanalysis***—explores the unconscious conflicts and reasons behind the person's mental health issues.
- ***Behaviour therapy***—attempts to change behaviour by using various techniques. The focus is on the behaviour, not on the underlying reasons for the behaviour.
- ***Group therapy***—a group of people who meet regularly to discuss their problems under the guidance of a mental health specialist.
- ***Family therapy***—family members meet regularly with a mental health specialist to discuss their problems.

Stigma of Mental Health Disorders

Chapter 4 included a discussion about how some people feel uncomfortable or fearful in the company of people who have illnesses and disabilities. They may stare or avoid eye contact and may treat these people differently from others who are well or appear able-bodied. This altered treatment is commonly faced by people with mental health disorders, who are often discriminated against because of a lack of understanding of mental health disorders. Some people fear being with a person with a mental health disorder; they do not know what to expect and may believe that the person is dangerous. Some may blame people with mental health disorders for their problems. Such attitudes lead people to avoid and exclude those with mental health disorders, often causing them to feel ashamed, rejected, and isolated.

Stigma is shame or social disgrace associated with a particular circumstance, quality, or person, such as "the stigma of a mental health disorder." A report from the Mental Health Commission of Canada stated that for individuals with mental health disorders, stigma is a major reason for not seeking treatment, taking prescribed medication, or attending counselling.[3] It also stated that stigma affects men more than it does women and also influences the person's successful reintegration into the family or into society in general. The stigma extends to the workplace, with employers often having concerns about the person's ability to function at the level of other employees. Although it is against current human rights legislation to openly discriminate against people with mental health disorders, many employers still do.

The Canadian Alliance for Mental Illness and Mental Health (CAMIMH) is an organization that represents mental health professionals and individuals concerned with mental health. The main goal of the CAMIMH is to prevent stigma and discrimination against people with mental health disorders. Through educational programs, the organization promotes greater understanding and acceptance of people with mental health disorders.[4]

As a support worker, you must remember that all clients (and their families) have the right to caring, nonjudgemental support and the right to be treated with dignity and respect, as stressed throughout this textbook.

Effect on the Family

Family members of clients with mental health disorders must make difficult decisions about care, treatment, and housing. They may feel anxious about an uncertain future, and the financial burden of caring for a loved one who is ill may be significant. Some family members may feel guilty and blame themselves for the illness, and some others may be at risk for depression themselves.

Family members are also affected by the stigma of mental health disorders. Friends and acquaintances who feel uncomfortable may not offer their time or social support. One woman described how differently people reacted to her husband's physical illness than to her son's mental health disorder: "When my husband had cancer, neighbours and friends were very kind. The phone rang constantly with offers to help. People brought over meals and sent flowers and cards. When my son was diagnosed with schizophrenia, everything was different. Nobody called. Nobody asked how we were doing. They pretended everything was fine. We felt very much alone."

Culture and Its Influence on Mental Health Disorders and Treatment

The need for understanding cultural differences among clients receiving support care has been emphasized repeatedly in this book. As stated in Chapter 10, *culture* is not limited to ethnic background but can extend to any group of interacting individuals who share similar learned characteristics, such as families, groups of friends, or even people who have shared similar experiences in the past. Culture has a profound influence on understanding mental health disorders and their treatments. People in one culture may not find it hard to seek medical attention for their mental health disorder, while people in another culture may see it as a sign of weakness. Similarly, some family members may refuse to acknowledge a loved one's mental health disorder, whereas others may readily be open about it. Some cultures distrust traditional medicine and prefer to consult their local healer for herbal treatments or other remedies.

Interpretations of the signs and symptoms of what some call "mental illness" vary greatly from culture to culture and even from person to person. What may be appropriate behaviour in one culture or group of people may be considered "insanity" in another. For example, someone who has lived through severe poverty might be afraid or hesitant to throw anything away, even items such as rubber bands or paper clips; some, in contrast, may consider keeping these things odd behaviour (see the *Supporting Mrs. Hill: The Effect of Past Experiences* box on the next page). Understanding your clients' cultural background before caring for them will help you show respect for their cultural differences and preferences as you provide care. Make sure that you follow the DIPPS principles.

Refugees

It is important to understand the unique status of refugees. *Refugees* are people who had to escape from their former country, leaving their homes and families behind, to seek safe shelter elsewhere. Many refugees have seen or experienced imprisonment,

Supporting Mrs. Hill: The Effect of Past Experiences

After falling and breaking her hip in her backyard, followed by a lengthy hospitalization and rehabilitation, Anabelle Hill, 85, was finally discharged home for supportive care. As her support worker, Tina was assigned to assist Mrs. Hill with her daily bath and with leg exercises. On Tina's first visit to Mrs. Hill's home, she noticed the house seemed clean but overfull, with items everywhere. In the kitchen, there were boxes of empty plastic containers, egg crates, and items such as string, all neatly sorted and packed. Tina also noticed that Mrs. Hill used a handkerchief when she blew her nose, did not own any paper towels, and used clean, rewashed rags instead of toilet tissue.

Trying to be helpful, Tina politely offered to put the boxes of items at the curbside for recycling. Mrs. Hill became upset and told her that it was "unnecessary to throw everything away." Later, when Tina talked to her supervisor about what she saw, the supervisor told Tina that many people who had been very poor during the Great Depression tended to keep items that seemed useless to others and suggested that Mrs. Hill may be one of those people.

The next time Tina went to Mrs. Hill's house, she asked Mrs. Hill about her experiences during the Depression. Tina found out that Mrs. Hill's family was homeless during that time and that they all survived by begging for food and living in a deserted shed on someone's farm. Tina began to understand Mrs. Hill's insistence on reusing items that Tina would have just thrown away. Tina then remembered another client who had also had many boxes of used items in his home and who had also survived a similar experience.

torture, murder of loved ones, extreme hunger, and poverty. They must learn to cope with life in a new country, learn new customs and a new language, and adjust to the new country's laws. Because of their particularly difficult circumstances, many refugees have a higher incidence of depression, anxiety, and stress and may be distrustful of the support care they are receiving. Some of your clients may exhibit some of these effects of having had terrible experiences in their countries of origin or as soldiers in wars. As a support worker, you should know when to report your observations to your supervisor (see *Supporting Mr. Awondo: How Past Traumatic Events can be Triggers* on p. 786 for an example of the changes that occurred when a support worker reported his client's behaviours to his supervisor).

Providing Care and Support for Clients With Mental Health Disorders

There are different types of mental health disorders, and this chapter briefly addresses the most common of these, paying particular attention to the role of the support worker caring for clients with these disorders and for their families. Common mental health disorders addressed in this chapter include acquired brain injuries; schizophrenia spectrum disorders; bipolar and related disorders; major depressive disorders; anxiety disorders; trauma and stressor-related disorders; obsessive–compulsive and related disorders; feeding and eating disorders; sleep–wake disorders; suicidal behaviour disorder; disruptive, impulse-control, and conduct disorders; substance-related and addictive disorders; and personality disorders. Disorientation, delirium, and dementia, which are conditions and mental health disorders of particular significance in older adults, are discussed in Chapter 36.

ACQUIRED BRAIN INJURIES

An **acquired brain injury (ABI)** is any type of sudden injury or illness that causes temporary or permanent damage to the brain. It is also called **traumatic brain injury**. An ABI can be the result of some kind of trauma to the head through a fall, collision, assault, concussion, stroke, tumour, or lack of oxygen or of an illness such as meningitis. ABI is the fourth leading cause of disability in Canada, and more than 50,000 Canadians sustain a brain injury each year.[5] Young adults are at greatest risk for acquiring a brain injury.[6] Many people who live with ABI are mislabelled, misdiagnosed, and misunderstood. This situation may lead to an increased risk for frustration, anxiety, or depression in the client (see *Supporting Greg Wood: How an ABI Can Affect Behaviour* on the next page).

An ABI will affect both the client and the family. Family members of clients with ABI may be required to provide long-term care and may even need to alter their own retirement plans. Families must learn to adjust if the clients have mood swings and periods of anger or depression or if they can no longer contribute to the family income as they used to. Clients with ABI may require ongoing physiotherapy, speech therapy, occupational therapy, or even psychotherapy, depending on the cause and extent of their injury.[7]

Symptoms of Acquired Brain Injury (ABI)

Many people with ABI have problems associated with the following:[5]

- Attention and concentration
- Memory
- Orientation to person, place, or time
- Decision making
- Problem solving
- Learning new ideas

Physical symptoms of ABI may include:

- Headache
- Fatigue
- Dizziness
- Uneven gait/walking
- Nausea
- Visual disturbances (such as blurred vision)
- Seizures
- Changes in sleep patterns
- Changes in eating patterns
- Loss of one or more senses, such as sight or hearing

Clients with ABI may exhibit the following behavioural changes:

- Depression
- Anxiety
- Irritability
- Emotional or impulse-control difficulties
- Decreased initiative or motivation

Supporting Clients With Acquired Brain Injury

While providing support to clients with acquired brain injury, keep the following in mind:[8]

- ***Follow clients' care plans in reassuring them that what they are experiencing is a result of brain injury.*** Clients with ABI may have forgotten about the injury that occurred but may be aware that they feel "different" from before. One goal of the health care team is to teach and to reinforce information about the reasons for their symptoms. Doing so will help to reduce the fear and anxiety clients may now feel.
- ***Encourage clients to establish routines and structure in daily tasks.*** Being able to establish a routine when carrying out everyday tasks such as bathing, dressing, eating, or toileting will reinforce a sense of accomplishment and self-esteem. It can also reduce anxieties resulting from trying to decide what to do.
- ***Encourage clients to set both long-term and short-term goals.*** Goals help the client with ABI to focus on a specific task and can motivate the client to work toward reaching the goals. Goals should always be realistic and achievable. If a certain goal is not achieved, the client may need to be supported to accept the failure and to try again.
- ***Ensure that clients' adaptive devices are within reach.*** If a client must use an adaptive device (such as a wheelchair, memory aid, or picture board) to assist with ambulation or communication, it should be easy for the client to reach and use.
- ***Encourage clients to "put the past behind them."*** A client who focuses on lost abilities may refuse to participate in rehabilitation activities. Although this reaction is normal for a short period, if

prolonged, it may prevent the client from reaching her full potential.

- ***Follow the steps in "Supporting Clients With Anxiety Disorders," on page 785, and "Supporting Clients With A Depressive Disorder," on page 783, if directed to do so by your supervisor.***
- ***Observe for and report signs indicating alcohol or substance use.*** The client with ABI who is feeling depressed may wish to drink alcohol or to take recreational drugs or substances and may lack the ability to reason that these substances may be harmful.

Supporting Greg Wood: How an ABI Can Affect Behaviour

Greg Wood is an athletic 18-year-old high school student who had a promising career as a hockey player. During a hockey game, Greg was tripped by another player, causing him to fall face-first on the ice. Although he had a helmet on, he lost consciousness for an hour. He was taken to the hospital and diagnosed with a concussion. In the 6 months following this accident, Greg suffered daily headaches and dizziness and was unable to go to school or to skate, even for short periods. He frequently yelled at his parents and younger sister, and he punched several holes in his bedroom wall. Because his parents did not wish to leave Greg by himself while they were at work, they hired a support worker to stay with him during the day and to make his meals.

One day, Sam, his support worker, noticed that Greg smelled of beer and that he was unsteady on his feet. Sam found several empty beer bottles in the bathroom next to the shower. When Sam asked Greg about them, Greg began to swear and throw books across the room at Sam, almost hitting him. Sam reported the event to his supervisor. At the end of Sam's shift, Greg began to cry and apologized to him. Greg told Sam that his hockey teammates did not come over anymore because he seemed so "different" from how he was before.

SCHIZOPHRENIA SPECTRUM DISORDERS

Schizophrenia spectrum disorders, which affect 1% of Canadians, are extremely complex mental health disorders characterized by symptoms such as delusions, hallucinations, disorganized speech (such as frequently becoming incoherent), grossly disorganized behaviours, and reduced or even dazed emotional expressions.[9] These disorders affect a person's ability to function in all aspects of life, including work, school, social life, family relationships, and self-care. Although there are many theories for the cause or causes of schizophrenia, a dominant theory proposes the existence of a biochemical imbalance in those affected.[10] It is also believed that substance and drug abuse may trigger underlying genetic vulnerabilities in some people.[9] People with schizophrenia spectrum disorders display one or more of the following:

- **Psychosis**—a mental state in which a person's perception of reality is impaired.
- **Delusions**—false beliefs that are not based on reality.
- ***Delusions of grandeur***—false and exaggerated beliefs about the importance, talent, or wealth of oneself. For example, a woman believes she is a goddess or the prime minister.
- ***Delusions of persecution***—false beliefs about being mistreated, abused, or harassed. For example, a man believes that his neighbour wants to kill him.
- **Hallucination**—seeing, hearing, tasting, smelling, or feeling things that are not real. For example, the person may see faces and hear voices that are not really there.
- **Paranoia**—extreme suspicion about a person or a situation. For example, a person may imagine being watched, followed, or controlled by someone else and may have delusions of persecution.

Without treatment, a person with schizophrenia suffers severe mental impairment. The person has problems relating to others; responses are inappropriate; and communication is disturbed. The person may ramble in speech or repeat what others say. Sometimes, the person's speech cannot be understood.

Some people with schizophrenia may have one severe psychotic episode that lasts for a month or more. Most suffer signs and symptoms throughout their lives but may have periods of **remission**, when the signs and symptoms of the disease lessen or disappear.

Some people with schizophrenia have frightening hallucinations and hear voices ordering them to harm themselves or others, and some may have friendly, peaceful hallucinations. Others may have very disorganized thoughts and speech. Some people with severe schizophrenia withdraw (stay away) from others and the world and may sit alone for hours without moving, speaking, or responding.

Supporting Clients With Schizophrenia Spectrum Disorders

- Focus on one task or activity at a time so as to help the client to focus.
- Be aware of your nonverbal communication. Avoid body language and facial expressions that could be considered threatening.
- Do not argue with the client about a delusion or hallucination not being real; it is real to the client. You can suggest gently to the client that the delusion is not real.
- Do not pretend that the delusion or hallucination is real. Comfort the client, and show empathy. Tell your supervisor if your client is having a delusion or hallucination.
- Use distractions to avoid disturbing the client. For example, play music, or take the client for a walk.

BIPOLAR AND RELATED DISORDERS

Bipolar and related disorders, also known by its street name *manic-depressive illness*, are a group of related brain disorders that cause unusual shifts in a person's mood, energy, and ability to function, different from the normal ups and downs that everyone goes through. About 1% of Canadians will experience this disorder.[1] Like diabetes or heart disease, bipolar and related disorders are long-term illnesses that must be carefully managed throughout a person's life. A manic episode is diagnosed if elevated mood occurs with three or more of the other symptoms of mania most of the day, nearly every day, for 1 week or longer. If the person's mood is irritable, four additional symptoms must be present for the diagnosis.

A client with bipolar disorder has emotional lows (depression) and emotional highs (mania) and thoughts, moods, and behaviours that swing from normal to grandiose and then to depressed. These symptoms can result in damaged relationships, poor job or school performance, and even suicide. Bipolar disorder is, however, treatable, and with proper treatment, those with this disorder can lead full and productive lives.

Bipolar disorder tends to run in families. Signs and symptoms can range from mild to severe and typically develop in late adolescence or early adulthood. However, some exhibit the first symptoms during childhood, and others, late in life. It is often not recognized as an illness, and some of the affected may suffer for years before it is properly diagnosed and treated. Children and adolescents can also develop bipolar disorder; it is more likely to occur in children of parents who have the disorder themselves. Unlike many adults with bipolar disorder, whose episodes tend to be more clearly defined, children and young adolescents with the disorder often experience very fast mood swings between depression and mania many times within a day. Children with mania are more likely to be irritable and prone to destructive tantrums than to be overly happy and elated. Mixed symptoms also are common in youths with bipolar disorder. Older adolescents who develop the illness may have the more classic, adult-type episodes and symptoms.

Bipolar disorder in children and adolescents can be hard to distinguish from other issues, such as drug abuse, that occur in these age groups and have similar symptoms. As with any illness, effective treatment depends on accurate diagnosis. Children or adolescents with emotional and behavioural symptoms should be carefully evaluated by a mental health professional. Most people with bipolar disorder—even those with the most severe forms—can achieve substantial stabilization of their mood swings and related symptoms with proper treatment. Because bipolar disorder is a recurrent illness, those affected need long-term preventive treatment.

The symptoms of bipolar and related disorders usually occur in three phases: (1) the acute phase (when the symptoms are escalating), (2) the continuation phase (when the symptoms are still visible and the client is usually being treated), and (3) the maintenance phase (when the client's acute symptoms have subsided). In most cases, the disorder is much better controlled if treatment is continuous than if it is periodical. However, even when there are no breaks in treatment, mood changes can occur and should be reported immediately to the doctor, who may be able to prevent a full-blown episode by making timely adjustments to the treatment plan. Working closely with the doctor and communicating openly about treatment concerns and options can contribute significantly to treatment effectiveness.

Signs and Symptoms of Mania (or a Manic Episode)

- Increased energy, activity, and restlessness
- Excessive "high"; overly good, euphoric mood
- Extreme irritability
- Racing thoughts and very fast talking, jumping from one idea to another
- Distractibility, inability to concentrate
- Little need for sleep
- Unrealistic beliefs in one's abilities and powers
- Poor judgement
- Spending sprees
- A prolonged period of behaviour that is different from usual
- Increased libido (sex drive)
- Abuse of drugs, particularly cocaine, alcohol, and sleep medications
- Provocative, intrusive, or aggressive behaviour
- Denial that anything is wrong

Supporting Clients With Bipolar and Related Disorders

The support worker can assist in keeping a chart of daily mood symptoms, treatments, sleep patterns, and life events to help the client and the family to better understand and cope with the illness. See TABLE 35–1 for a description of phases of treatment

TABLE 35–1 Phases of Treatment of Bipolar and Related Disorders and the Role of the Support Worker

Phase	Period	Goal of Treatment	Your Role
Acute treatment: Symptoms are beginning to escalate	6–12 months	To reduce symptoms and inappropriate behaviours	Observe for changes in the client's behaviour Report these changes to your supervisor Provide a safe, secure, consistent environment for the client
Continuation: Symptoms are still evident, but they are beginning to decrease with treatment	4–9 months	To prevent relapses into distressing emotional states	Observe the client for any signs or symptoms of depression or mania (see BOX 35-3) Report these to your supervisor
Maintenance: The client does not have acute symptoms	Indefinite	To prevent recurrences, as some clients think they are "cured" and stop taking their medication	Same as above

BOX 35-3 Signs and Symptoms of Depression

- Fatigue and lack of interest
- Inability to experience pleasure
- Feelings of uselessness, hopelessness, and helplessness
- Decreased sexual interest
- Increased dependency
- Anxiety
- Slow or unreliable memory
- Paranoia
- Agitation
- Focus on the past
- Thoughts of death and suicide
- Difficulty completing ADLs
- Changes in sleep patterns
- Poor grooming
- Withdrawal from people and interests
- Muscle aches, abdominal pain, and headaches
- Nausea and vomiting
- Dry mouth
- Loss of appetite
- Weight loss

of bipolar and related disorders and the role of the support worker.

- During depression:
  - Follow the guidelines for major depression.
- During manic periods:
  - Provide a calm environment without too many distractions.
  - Encourage periods of rest.
  - Encourage self-care; assist as required.
  - Do not argue; arguing could irritate the client.

DEPRESSIVE DISORDERS

Depressive disorders are a group of disorders in which the client has sad, empty, or irritable moods accompanied by physical changes and thought changes *that are severe enough to affect the client's ability to function.* These disorders include major depressive disorder, persistent depressive disorder, premenstrual dysphoric disorder, substance/medication-induced depressive disorder, and depressive disorder due to another medical condition.

Most people feel depressed at one time or another—for example, after the loss of a loved one, the loss of a job, or any other major negative event in life. Grief is a normal and natural feeling that all people experience during their lives (see Chapter 46 for a discussion of the normal stages of grief and loss). Feelings of loss and sadness are *normal reactions* to recent experiences and are sometimes referred to as **reactive depression**. This sort of depression is different from a **major depressive disorder** (which is sometimes called **clinical depression**).

Major Depressive Disorder

Major depressive disorder consists of severe feelings of worthlessness, self-blame, sadness, disappointment, and emptiness that last weeks. The physical and emotional effects of depression interfere with the person's ability to perform the activities of daily living (ADLs). Sleeping, eating, working, studying, and emotional **affect** (expression), are affected. A person with depression may think about or attempt suicide. Major depressive disorder may occur only once, brought on by a stressful event such as the death of a loved one, a divorce, or a job loss, or may recur throughout a person's life and at any age. Once depression is recognized, medical intervention can make a difference for 80% of people who are affected, allowing them to get back to their regular activities.[1] Depression is, unfortunately, common among older adults (see the *Focus on Older Adults: Depression* box on the next page). For signs and symptoms of depression, see BOX 35-3.

Major depressive disorder is usually treated by any (or a combination) of the following:

- ***Psychotherapy***—a form of therapy in which a person explores thoughts, feelings, and behaviours with help and guidance from a mental health specialist.
- ***Drug therapy***—medications prescribed by a doctor. Street drugs, abuse of over-the-counter (OTC) medication, and alcohol interfere with the helping action of many medicines and, therefore, will usually be discouraged.

- ***Electroconvulsive therapy (ECT)***—a short-term treatment that alters brain chemicals. Before ECT, clients are administered anesthesia to put them in a dreamlike state and medications to relax their muscles. An electrical current is then briefly sent to the brain through electrodes placed on the client's temples, which cause a seizure. It is not known exactly how ECT works, but it is believed that it alters brain chemicals, serotonin, endorphins, and adrenalin.

Seasonal Affective Disorder

Seasonal affective disorder (*SAD*) is a type of depression that occurs each year at the same time, usually starting in fall or winter and ending in spring or early summer. It is common in colder regions, where people tend to spend the majority of their winter months indoors. Signs and symptoms may be mild to severe (see **BOX 35–3**), and the condition is often mistaken for major depression. The treatment, however, may be different—SAD is usually treated with *phototherapy*, which involves exposure to light from a box containing white fluorescent light tubes.

Other Types of Depressive Disorders

The following disorders do not fit within the categories but may affect some clients:

- ***Disruptive mood dysregulation disorder (DMDD).*** Much worse than temper tantrums, DMDD begins in children under the age of 10 years of age and is characterized by severe and recurrent temper outbursts that are exceedingly

FOCUS ON OLDER ADULTS

Depression

Depression is common in older adults, in part because they experience many losses—death of family members and friends and diagnoses of medical conditions that lead to a loss of health, loss of body functions, and loss of independence. Other factors that may trigger depression in older adults include the following:

- Loneliness
- Loss of a beloved pet
- Poor nutrition
- Overuse, underuse, or misuse of prescribed medications
- Adverse effects of some medications
- Loss of control over finances
- Loss of memory

Depression in older adults is often overlooked or misdiagnosed. Many will not admit to feeling depressed but will instead complain of having many aches and pains; others may be agitated and irritable. An older client with depression may be thought to have dementia (see Chapter 36), so the depression goes untreated. Ways to reduce the likelihood of depression in older adults include the following:

- Ensuring the client has adequate nourishing food and water
- Ensuring the client has regular bowel movements
- Ensuring the client has regular medical checkups by a family physician or nurse practitioner
- Ensuring the client takes medications correctly
- Ensuring the client avoids excessive use of OTC medications or alcohol
- Providing support and encouraging involvement with others
- Providing opportunities for physical activity
- Providing opportunities to be outside in the fresh air and sunlight
- Providing opportunities to interact with pets
- Providing opportunities for stimulation of the senses
- Providing opportunities to interact with reminiscence groups
- Providing situations that allow the client to feel wanted and needed

out of proportion in length and severity for the situation.

- ***Persistent depressive disorder***. Persistent depressive disorder is diagnosed when a client has a depressed mood most of the day for at least 2 years plus at least four of the following symptoms: poor eating (or overeating), insomnia or sleeping for long periods of time, low energy or fatigue, low self-esteem, poor concentration, feelings of hopelessness.
- ***Premenstrual dysphoric disorder***. At least five of the following symptoms appear in the week prior to each menstrual period and then are minimized or absent in the week after each period: mood swings, irritability, depressed moods, anxiety or tension, decreased interest in usual activities, difficulty concentrating, and a sense of feeling out of control.
- ***Substance/medication-induced depressive disorder***. Unexplained depressed mood or extreme lack of interest in all or most activities after becoming intoxicated, after withdrawing from intoxication, or after exposure to a medication.

Supporting Clients With a Depressive Disorder

- ***Show that you enjoy being with the client.*** Listen to your client. Show an interest in the client's life.
- ***Know that most clients who have never been diagnosed with depression do not know that they are depressed.*** Many clients will not say they are depressed because they are not familiar with the symptoms.
- ***Do not minimize the client's problems***. Do not say, "Cheer up" or "Snap out of it." Such statements suggest that the client is exaggerating the problem and has control over it.
- ***Be positive.*** One positive experience may encourage further positive experiences.
- ***Encourage rest.*** It can refresh the client and improve energy.
- ***Encourage proper nutrition***. Maintaining normal blood sugar and energy levels is important.
- ***Encourage activity and social interactions.*** They can improve the client's outlook and sense of well-being. However, do not tire the client with activities.
- ***Be alert for warning signals of suicidal intent*** (**BOX 35–4**). Report any signals to your supervisor at once.
- ***Provide a safe, secure, stable environment.*** Clients with depression may feel less control over their environments but will be comforted by a feeling of safety.
- ***Follow the care plan.*** The care plan may state, for example, that the client may not have access to medication bottles but may take medications *from a dosette or blister-packaged container only* (see Chapter 43).
- ***Ensure safety.*** Sharp items, belts, cords, or items similar to these may be locked away if the client is voicing intentions of suicide.
- ***Encourage normal activities***. The client should be encouraged to do their ADLs or be assisted as needed—for example, with bathing, preparing meals, and taking in adequate fluids. These measures can maintain the body's homeostasis and prevent other health issues.

ANXIETY DISORDERS

Anxiety disorders are a group of mental health disorders whose main symptom is extreme anxiety, with fears and worries so disproportionate to the situation as to affect normal functioning. **Anxiety** is a vague, uneasy feeling in response to stress. Anxiety disorders affect about 5% of the Canadian population.[1] Most begin in childhood and tend to continue if not treated, and they are twice as likely to affect women as men.[9] An anxious person feels a sense of dread, danger, or harm. Some amount of anxiety is normal, but clients with anxiety disorders experience extreme anxiety. Many anxiety disorders can be treated with medication, and clients will generally notice a reduction of symptoms as long as they take their medications continuously. The main types of anxiety disorders are discussed in this chapter.

Panic Disorder

Panic is an intense and sudden feeling of fear, anxiety, terror, or dread for no obvious reason. The physical symptoms of fear (shortness of breath, racing heart, sweat) escalate very quickly when a client has a *panic*

BOX 35-4 Warning Signs of Suicidal Intent

It is important to understand that suicidal feelings and actions are symptoms of an illness that can be treated. While some suicide attempts are carefully planned over time, others are impulsive acts that have not been thought through.

Warnings signs of suicidal intent include the following:

- Signs and symptoms of depression
- Repeated expressions of hopelessness, helplessness, or desperation
- Expressions of interest in killing oneself
- Having a plan for suicide, such as taking pills or hanging oneself at a specific place and time
- Loss of interest in friends, hobbies, or previously enjoyed activities
- Giving away prized possessions or putting personal affairs in order
- Telling someone else about final wishes
- A change in personality or mood—for example, sudden and unusually happy behaviour after a period of depression
- A change in appearance—for example, a person who is usually well groomed is untidy and unwashed
- Failure to recover from a loss or crisis
- A sudden tendency to take big risks
- Refusing to eat, drink, or take medications

If you are feeling suicidal or know someone who is, take the following actions:

- Call a doctor, emergency room, or 9-1-1 right away to get immediate help.
- Make sure you (or the suicidal person) are not left alone.
- Prevent access to large amounts of medication, weapons, or other items that could be used for self-harm.

With proper treatment, suicidal feelings can be overcome.

Source: Canadian Mental Health Association. (2015). *Suicide Awareness.* Retrieved from http://edmonton.cmha.ca/mental_health/suicide-awareness/.

attack. Many clients experience symptoms that are similar to those of a heart attack (e.g., chest pains).

Clients who wonder if they have panic disorder should ask themselves the following questions:

- Do I have sudden bursts of fear for no reason?
- Do I feel physically unwell when they happen?
- Are there times when, for no reason, I experience chest pains, a racing heart, dizziness, sweating, stomach problems, nausea, and a feeling of loss of control?
- Do I fear at those times that I am dying or going crazy?

Panic attacks can happen anytime, anywhere, and without warning. Clients who have panic attacks may live in fear of having another attack and may avoid places where they experienced an attack in the past. For some clients, fear takes over their lives, and they are not able to leave their homes.

Panic disorder is more common in women than in men. It usually starts in young adulthood, often during times of excessive stress. Panic disorder can last for months or years.

The treatment for panic disorder includes teaching the client to recognize and change thinking patterns before they lead to a panic attack, as well as medications prescribed by a doctor.

Phobic Disorder

Phobia means fear, panic, or dread. A person with a phobic disorder has intense fear of a particular thing or situation. Often, phobias occur after an event—for example, a fear of flying may develop after a person hears reports of a recent plane crash. Clients who struggle with phobias often feel embarrassed and stupid because they know their fear is exaggerated. Common phobias include *agoraphobia* (fear of open, crowded, public places) and *claustrophobia* (fear of small, enclosed places). Symptoms of phobic disorder include the following:

- Excessive worry
- Sleep disruption from worrying
- Fatigue or irritability
- Difficulty concentrating
- Physical symptoms such as increased sweating, heavy breathing, irregular heartbeats (palpitations), dizziness, faintness, muscle pain or tension, and even diarrhea from interference with digestion

Other Types of Anxiety Disorders

The following anxiety disorders do not fit within the categories above but may affect some clients:[9]

- ***Separation anxiety disorder.*** Persistent and excessive worrying about losing major attachment figures (such as parents or significant others), which can result in the client's reluctance to leave the house to separate from them or in nightmares about losing them.
- ***Selective mutism.*** A condition that lasts for a month or more in which the client experiences consistent inability or extreme reluctance to speak in a specific social situation, despite being able to speak in other situations.
- ***Social anxiety disorder.*** Severe distress or feelings of anxiety involving one or more social situations in which the client may be exposed to criticism or rejection, lasting for more than 6 months.

Supporting Clients With Anxiety Disorders

- ***Avoid situations that are known to cause anxiety.*** For example, if a client is afraid of small, closed spaces, keep the person away from these.
- ***Avoid discussing subjects that cause anxiety.*** Keep the conversation on other subjects.
- ***Provide comfort during periods of anxiety.*** Stay with the client who is extremely anxious or is having a panic attack. Use touch to reassure the client if appropriate. Offer limited, clear choices to make decision making easier so as not to induce further stress. Report the situation to your supervisor.

Trauma and Stressor-Related Disorders

Trauma and stressor-related disorders are anxiety disorders that can develop after an individual has experienced or witnessed a major trauma. Any traumatic event such as war, fires, accidents, burns, torture, kidnapping, concentration camps, incest, or violent crimes can overwhelm the normal psychological coping mechanisms of the person witnessing or experiencing these events.

Post-traumatic stress disorder (PTSD) is a trauma and stressor-related disorder that can occur in people of all ages, races, cultures, and genders. Signs and symptoms include the following:

- Vivid nightmares of the traumatic event(s)
- Feeling of nervousness, edginess
- Avoidance of *triggers* that recall memories of traumatic event
- Difficulty concentrating or sleeping
- Feelings of loss of control

PTSD symptoms fall into three categories. People with PTSD will have at least one symptom in each of these categories:[11]

1. Reliving or re-experiencing the trauma
2. Attempts to avoid thoughts, situations, or people that are reminders of the trauma
3. Increased anxiety or arousal, including being constantly on guard for danger, and being easily startled

Survivors with PTSD are more likely to experience substance abuse, phobias, chronic pain, poor concentration, sleep disturbances, and extreme anxiety. Some survivors with PTSD might become easily angered, whereas others may feel overwhelming guilt because others have died and they have survived. The client in *Supporting Mr. Awondo: How Past Traumatic Events can be Triggers* on the next page fits the description of someone living with PTSD.

Post-Traumatic Stress Disorder in Children

Children who have experienced traumatic events may develop fear of the dark, fear of being alone, separation anxiety, nightmares, stomach aches, or headaches. They are often afraid to talk to their

Supporting Mr. Awondo: How Past Traumatic Events Can Be Triggers

Jesus Awondo, 44, single, fled to Canada 20 years ago from a South American country. Two weeks ago, at work, he fell from a scaffold and broke numerous bones in his body. After being discharged from hospital, he was cared for at home by Bob, a support worker. Bob came to Mr. Awondo's house every day to assist him with his ADLs.

While caring for him, Bob noticed that Mr. Awondo usually fell asleep after his bed bath but never had a quiet sleep. Yesterday, while he was sleeping, Mr. Awondo started to scream, mumble loudly, and try to swing his cast-covered arms around in the air. When Mr. Awondo woke up, Bob told him about what he had observed.

Mr. Awondo said that in his home country, he had watched his wife and child being killed with machetes by the local drug gangs. He had been bound, gagged, and placed in a cage, where rats were allowed to crawl on him. He told Bob that he had frequent nightmares about these events, and since his injury at work, his nightmares had increased in their duration and frequency. Bob reported the event to his supervisor, who arranged for Mr. Awondo's doctor to see him at his home. Mr. Awondo's medical treatment was then changed and resulted in Mr. Awondo sleeping more peacefully at night, in spite of an occasional nightmare.

parents about the events for fear of upsetting them.[12]

Post-Traumatic Stress Disorder in Older Adults

The signs and symptoms of PTSD in older adults are often the same as those in children. Many older adults may have been traumatized when they were much younger, and extreme changes in their lives may trigger PTSD symptoms—for example, deaths of friends and family members or sudden loss of daily social contact. In long-term care facilities, rough treatment or a feeling of a loss of control when receiving care may trigger symptoms of PTSD in clients.[12]

Supporting Clients With Post-Traumatic Stress Disorder

As a support worker, you should be aware of the following:

- As with all clients, treat the client with PTSD according to the DIPPS principles.
- Personal care should be provided in a gentle manner that is respectful of the client's right to privacy.
- Clients should be given the opportunity to verbalize or reminisce about their experiences.
- Clients may have witnessed traumatic events in their past, and PTSD may be triggered at any time.
- Change in a client's willingness to be toileted, dressed, undressed, bathed, or fed may be a clue that the client has PTSD. Such a reaction should be reported to the supervisor immediately and always be documented.

OBSESSIVE–COMPULSIVE AND RELATED DISORDERS

Obsessive–compulsive and related disorders are mental health disorders characterized by recurrent obsessions and compulsions that interfere with a person's daily life and relationships.[9] An **obsession** is a persistent thought or desire, and a **compulsion** is the uncontrollable urge to perform an act. The obsession may be violent in nature and is usually disturbing to the person; the person may try to ignore the obsessive thought or deal with it by repeating an act over and over again. Examples of common obsessions include the following:

- Fearing that one's thoughts will cause someone harm
- Ruminating about (being preoccupied with) hurting someone

As the support worker caring for a client with obsessive–compulsive disorder (OCD), if you observe repeated behaviours, you should report them to your supervisor. You should be aware that the client performs these behaviours to help relieve stress, and the person may not be able to stop without feeling extremely stressed and anxious.

Example of common compulsions include the following:

- Repeatedly washing hands, bathing, or cleaning household items
- Checking things several times a day—for example, checking if the stove is off, the windows are locked, and so on
- Repeating a name, phrase, or tune
- Preoccupations with throwing things away that have little value, or the opposite, excessive hoarding

Hoarding Disorder

Hoarding disorder is defined as a persistent anxiety and distress in parting with possessions or animals, regardless of their actual value. This behaviour can lead to health problems for the client due to the accumulation of dust, mould, or excrement; cramped living conditions; and strained relationships with significant others. About 75% of clients who have hoarding disorder also have an anxiety disorder.

Other Obsessive–Compulsive and Related Disorders

- ***Body dysmorphic disorder***—preoccupation with perceived flaws in one's own body that are not observable to others.
- ***Trichotillomania (hair pulling) disorder***—the need to pull out one's hair, resulting in hair loss. This hair pulling causes significant personal and social distress.[9]
- ***Excoriation (skin-picking) disorder***—the need to recurrently pick one's own skin, resulting in skin lesions. This skin-picking causes significant personal and social distress.
- ***Substance/medication-induced obsessive–compulsive and related disorder***—body-related repetitive behaviours that are triggered by exposure, intoxication, or exposure of a substance or medication.

Supporting a Client With Obsessive–Compulsive and Related Disorders

- ***Show that you enjoy being with the client.*** Listen to the client. Show an interest in the client's life.
- ***Do not minimize the client's problems.*** Clients with OCD usually understand that their experiences do not make sense. Trying to argue over one's obsessions or compulsions does not help anyone.
- ***Be positive.*** One positive experience may encourage further positive experiences.
- ***Encourage rest.*** It can refresh the client.
- ***Avoid "helping" behaviours around OCD.*** Helping behaviours, such as ensuring a client avoids things that cause anxiety can make practising healthy coping skills harder for a client in the long run. Instead, you may be more helpful to the client if you focus on the feelings behind the behaviours.
- ***Provide a safe, secure, stable environment.*** Signs of OCD can be more difficult to manage during times of stress—and even happy occasions can be stressful. Recognize when a client may need extra support and try to plan ahead.
- ***Follow the care plan.*** The care plan may state that the client cannot have access to medication bottles but that the person may take medications *from a dosette or blister-packaged container only* (see Chapter 43).
- ***Encourage normal activities.*** The client should be encouraged to do ADLs and be assisted as needed with bathing, preparing meals, and taking in adequate fluids. These measures can maintain the body's homeostasis and prevent other health issues.
- ***Recognize accomplishments.*** Remember that for the client with OCD, every small step toward managing OCD behaviour can take a lot of courage and hard work.

FEEDING AND EATING DISORDERS

Feeding and eating disorders are altered body image perceptions that lead to disturbances in eating behaviours and an abnormal concern about body weight and shape. These occur mainly in teenage girls and young women and can be life threatening.

One reason younger women are particularly vulnerable to feeding and eating disorders is their tendency to go on strict diets to achieve an "ideal" figure. Others especially at risk for feeding and eating disorders include athletes, actors, dancers, models, and TV personalities for whom thinness has become a professional requirement. Some affected individuals recover, but some do not. The two most common eating disorders are *anorexia nervosa* and *bulimia nervosa*.

Feeding and eating disorders are not the same as the anorexia clients in a long-term care facility may have. Feeding and eating disorders usually occur in young people and may signal a much deeper, more complex psychological problem, whereas an older adult may refuse to eat because of a fear of choking, a sick feeling, depression, or a dislike for the texture or taste of the food.

People who have an ongoing preoccupation with food and weight, even when they are thin, often benefit from exploring their thoughts and relationships with help and guidance from a therapist. Early diagnosis and treatment helps ensure the most successful outcome. Some clients can be treated as outpatients, but others may need hospitalization to correct a dangerously low weight and food bingeing behaviours. The most effective strategies for treatment have been weight restoration to within 10% of normal—weight gain of 2.2 to 6.6 kg (1 to 3 lb.) per week is considered safe and desirable—and individual, family, and group therapies. Fortunately, most of the complications experienced by clients with anorexia nervosa are reversible once their normal weight is restored. However, clients with bulimia nervosa may suffer permanent damage to their bodies, especially to their teeth because of enamel wear or to their throats and esophagus due to their frequent purging. For these clients, proper oral and dental care must be emphasized.

Anorexia Nervosa

Anorexia nervosa is a serious, complex, and often chronic, life-threatening feeding and eating disorder defined by three key features:[13]

- A refusal to maintain minimal body weight within 15% of an individual's normal weight
- An intense fear of gaining weight
- A distorted body image of being "fat" or "ugly"

Like all feeding and eating disorders, anorexia nervosa tends to occur around puberty but can develop during any major life change. Anorexia nervosa predominately affects adolescent girls and young women, although it also occurs in men and older women. Some women with this illness have **amenorrhea** (absence of at least three consecutive menstrual periods as normally expected to occur) as a result.

Personality traits common in persons with anorexia nervosa are low self-esteem, social isolation (which usually occurs after behaviours associated with anorexia nervosa begin), and perfectionism. These clients tend to be good students and excellent athletes. It seems clear (although not to the client) that focusing on weight loss and food allows the client to ignore other problems that are too painful or seem impossible to resolve. The satisfaction of achieving control over weight and food becomes very important, even though the rest of the person's life may be chaotic and emotionally painful.

Generally, a doctor who specializes in eating disorders should make the diagnosis and rule out other physical disorders. Other psychiatric disorders such as depression and OCD can occur along with anorexia nervosa. In addition, some people will engage in recurrent binge eating and purging episodes. Starvation, weight loss, and related medical complications can result in death. In fact, anorexia nervosa has the highest mortality rate (6%) among all psychiatric conditions.

People with anorexia nervosa ignore hunger and thus control their desire to eat. This desire is frequently masked by cooking for others or hiding food in personal spaces. Obsessive exercising may accompany the starving behaviour, which may mislead others into thinking that the person is healthy.

Signs and Symptoms of Anorexia Nervosa

- Obsession with food and weight
- Refusal to maintain minimal normal body weight
- Thoughts of looking fat in spite of being bone-thin

- Brittle nails and hair
- Dry and yellow skin
- Cessation (stoppage) of menstruation
- Depression
- Frequent complaints of feeling cold (because body temperature drops)
- Lanugo fine hair, usually on a newborn) on the body
- Strange eating habits such as cutting food into tiny pieces
- Refusal to eat in front of others
- Preparing elaborate dishes for others but not eating them
- Abuse of laxatives and enemas to rid the body of food
- Abuse of diuretics (drugs that cause the kidneys to produce large amounts of urine, through which extra fluid in the body is lost, causing weight loss)

Causes

Feeding and eating disorders tend to run in families, with female relatives most often affected—for example, a girl has a 10 to 20 times higher risk of developing anorexia nervosa if she has a sibling who has the disease. Behavioural and environmental influences, as well as stressful events, are likely to increase the risk for feeding and eating disorders.

Anorexia Nervosa's Effects on the Body

- Damage to vital organs such as the heart and brain
- Irregular heart rhythms or heart failure
- Calcium loss from bones, which can become brittle and prone to breakage

The worst outcome for people with anorexia is starving themselves to death.

Bulimia Nervosa

Bulimia nervosa is a psychological feeding and eating disorder that is characterized by episodes of binge eating followed by inappropriate methods of weight control (purging). *Binge eating* is a compulsion in which an individual eats a much larger amount of food than most people would in a similar situation—sometimes up to 20,000 calories at a time—during periods of uncontrolled, impulsive, or continuous eating. Binge eating is not a response to intense hunger but is usually a response to depression, stress, or low self-esteem. During a binge-eating episode, the individual experiences a loss of control, which is followed by a short-lived calmness and later self-loathing. The cycle of overeating and purging usually becomes an obsession and is repeated often.

The foods binged on are usually considered "comfort foods"—sweet foods that are high in calories or smooth and soft foods such as ice cream, cake, and pastry. An individual may binge anywhere from twice a day to several times daily.

People with bulimia nervosa can look perfectly normal. Most of them are of normal weight, but some may be overweight. Women with bulimia tend to be high achievers. It is often difficult to recognize bulimia because bingeing and purging are done in secret and those with the condition often deny having it.

Currently, the causes of bulimia are not definitely known but are generally thought to be similar to those that trigger anorexia nervosa.

Signs and Symptoms of Bulimia Nervosa

- Eating uncontrollably
- Purging
- Strict dieting
- Fasting
- Vigorous exercising
- Vomiting or abusing laxatives or diuretics in an attempt to lose weight
- Vomiting blood
- Using the bathroom frequently after meals
- Preoccupation with body weight
- Depression or mood swings; feeling "out of control"
- Swollen glands in neck and face
- Heartburn
- Bloating
- Indigestion
- Constipation
- Irregular menstrual periods
- Dental problems
- Sore throat
- Weakness and exhaustion
- Bloodshot eyes
- Compulsive exercising
- Excessive concern about shape and weight

Bulimia Nervosa's Effects on the Body

- Erosion of tooth enamel because of repeated exposure to acidic gastric contents through vomiting
- Dental cavities; sensitivity to hot or cold food
- Swelling and soreness in the salivary glands (from repeated vomiting)
- Stomach ulcers
- Rupture of the stomach and esophagus
- Disruption in the normal bowel release function
- Electrolyte imbalance
- Dehydration
- Irregular heartbeat
- A greater risk for suicidal behaviour
- Decreased libido (sex drive)

Pica

Pica is a feeding and eating disorder defined as persistently eating substances without nutritional value for a period of at least a month. Clients who have been diagnosed with pica have been reported to put in their mouth and/or eat a wide variety of nonfood substances, such as clay, dirt, sand, stones, pebbles, hair, feces, lead, laundry starch, vinyl gloves, plastic, pencil erasers, ice, fingernails, paper, paint chips, coal, chalk, wood, plaster, light bulbs, needles, string, cigarette butts, wire, and burnt matches.[14]

Although pica is more common in children, it is the most common feeding and eating disorder in clients with developmental disabilities. Depending on what is eaten, pica may not be harmful, may cause some problems (such as chipped teeth), or may cause life-threatening problems such as intestinal obstructions.

Causes of Pica

Nutritional deficiencies such as iron deficiency anemia and zinc deficiency may cause pica. Pica may also be caused by poor diet, malnutrition, starvation, developmentally poor judgement, or obsessive–compulsive disorder.

Supporting Clients With Feeding and Eating Disorders

People can and do recover from eating disorders. These points may assist you when supporting someone with a feeding and eating disorder:

- ***Be patient.*** Do not be surprised by your client's reaction of anger to or denial of your presence. There is a lot of shame and pain associated with having a feeding and eating disorder.
- ***Be compassionate.*** Feeding and eating disorders are a complex problem, and food and body weight issues are only symptoms of deeper problems.
- ***Be encouraging.*** Encourage these client to see themselves as more than their feeding and eating disorders. Do so by talking about other aspects of their lives and interests that are unrelated to food.
- ***Be nonjudgemental.*** Do not blame or shame the client. Avoid commenting on the client's looks—even if you are trying to compliment the client, comments about weight and appearance only reinforce the client's obsession with body image and weight.
- ***Be positive.*** Avoid negative statements about behaviours. Find neutral, comfortable places and times to discuss issues.
- ***Prevent the client from eating nonfood substances.*** Clients with pica should be prevented from continuing to eat nonfoods so that medical problems, such as nutritional deficiency or lead toxicity, can be diagnosed. Medical treatment for the client may vary according to the severity of the cravings and the cause of the pica and may include psychosocial therapy or medications.
- ***Report to your supervisor if you hear vomiting or see evidence of food refusal.*** Ask your supervisor for guidance on ways to deal with these symptoms appropriately.

SLEEP–WAKE DISORDERS

Sleep–wake disorders are conditions in which repetitive disturbed sleep patterns lead to distress and impairment in the affected person's daytime functioning. Sleep is absolutely essential for an individual's normal, healthy functioning. Scientists and medical professionals do not fully understand this complex physiological phenomenon. It is not clear exactly why the body requires sleep, although inadequate sleep can have severe detrimental effects on health.

Studies have shown that sleep is essential for normal immune system function to maintain the ability to fight disease and sickness, for normal nervous system function, and for the ability to function both physically and mentally. In addition, sleep is necessary for learning and for normal, healthy cell growth. Sleep–wake disorders are generally classified into 10 conditions:[9]

1. Lack of sleep (e.g., *insomnia disorder*)
2. Breathing-related sleep disorders (e.g., *obstructive sleep apnea*, a medical condition)
3. Hypersomnolence disorder (e.g., excessive sleep)
4. Narcolepsy, a medical condition
5. Circadian-rhythm sleep–wake disorders
6. Nightmare disorder
7. Nonrapid eye movement (NREM) disorder
8. Rapid eye movement (REM) disorder
9. Willis–Ekbom disease (restless legs syndrome)
10. Substance/medication-induced sleep disorder

In most cases, sleep disorders can be easily managed once they are properly diagnosed. Insomnia, which occurs more often in women and older adults, is the most common sleep disorder.

The amount of sleep that a person needs to function normally depends on several factors. Infants sleep most of the day (about 16 hours); teenagers usually need about 9 hours of sleep a day; and adults need an average of 7 to 8 hours of sleep a day. Although older adults require about as much sleep as younger adults do, they usually sleep for shorter periods and spend less time in the deep stages of sleep. About 50% of adults over the age of 65 have some type of sleep disorder, although it is not clear whether it is a normal part of aging or a result of medications that older adults commonly use.

Both REM and deep sleep are essential parts of the normal sleep cycle. Sleepwalking and bedwetting occur during deep sleep, and dreams occur during REM sleep, when the muscles of the body stiffen, eyes move, heart rate increases, breathing becomes more rapid and irregular, and blood pressure rises.

Supporting Clients With Sleep–Wake Disorders

- Instruct the client to avoid foods and medicines that alter the balance of chemicals that affect sleep. Caffeine, for example, can cause insomnia (lack of sleep). Antidepressant medications can cause loss of REM sleep. Smoking and alcohol can cause loss of REM sleep and deep sleep.
- If the client appears to have periods of not breathing at all, or if the client wakes up with a headache every morning, sleep apnea should be suspected. Encourage the client to seek medical attention, as sleep apnea is a medical disorder that must be treated. The client might also benefit from sleeping on the side, with a pillow between the knees.
- Clients with problems of sleeping too much should see the doctor for a physical checkup to rule out narcolepsy, which is a medical condition.
- You should observe, report, and record how long the client is sleeping during each stage of sleep. Make a note of the client's use of prescription or nonprescription drugs or alcohol, which might be causing any sleep problems.

SUICIDAL BEHAVIOUR DISORDER

Suicidal behaviour disorder is a disorder in which one has recurrent thoughts or a preoccupation with ending one's own life. Suicide—to kill (*caedere*) oneself (*sui*)—is a common cause of death in both males and females from adolescence through middle age, although it has also been found to be the cause of death among some school-aged children and older adults.[15] People with mental health disorders are at high risk for suicide. People who attempt suicide view life as unbearable and may believe that their families and friends are better off without them.

Suicide accounts for 24% of all deaths among 15- to 24-year-olds and 16% among 25- to 44-year-olds and is one of the leading causes of death in both men and women from adolescence to middle age.[1] The mortality rate due to suicide among men is four times the rate among women, although, statistically, women attempt suicide more often than men do. Men tend to use violent means to kill themselves (e.g., hanging, firearms), so their attempts are often fatal. Women usually choose less violent means (e.g., taking an overdose of pills), so many survive their attempts.

Attempted suicide is a sign of a serious mental health issue, and the person attempting suicide needs to seek professional care and be put on a suicide prevention program. Any child or adolescent who has suicidal feelings, talks about suicide, or attempts suicide should be taken seriously and should receive immediate help from a mental health specialist (see the *Focus on Older Adults: Suicide* box).

Risk Factors That May Lead to Suicidal Intent or Behaviour

Certain risk factors may trigger suicidal intent or behaviour:

- Mental health disorder, especially depression, bipolar disorder, or schizophrenia
- A history of abuse
- A family history of suicide
- The suicide of a friend
- A prior suicide attempt
- A major crisis such as the loss of a relationship, family problems, loss of position in society, and work, money, or legal problems
- Pressure to succeed
- Isolation
- Early losses in life
- Sexual identity issues
- Feelings of deep hopelessness and helplessness
- Recent diagnosis of a life-threatening illness
- Substance abuse

For older adults, risk factors might also include the following:[16]

- Personality factors, such as personality disorders, emotional instability, rigid personality, and poor coping skills

FOCUS ON OLDER ADULTS

Suicide

Did you know that older adults over the age of 85 have the highest suicide rate of any group in Canada?[17] Older adults are at risk for suicide because they experience many losses, including the deaths of family members and friends, loss of physical health, and loss of cognitive (mental) abilities. Depression is common in older adults (see the *Focus on Older Adults: Depression* box, on p. 782). According to the Canadian Medical Association, recent research indicates that the suicide rate is climbing among older-adult men; right now across Canada, about 31 of every 100,000 older adults, especially those over 85 years old, kill themselves. Most of them are white males, and most die through violent means.

Some older adults choose suicide to avoid loneliness. For others, the loss of independence, such as losing their driver's licence, or a serious illness makes suicide seem better than the threat of prolonged suffering or the thought of causing hardships for their families.

Important Questions to Ask the Older Adult You Suspect to Be Suicidal[18]

Ask about the person's feelings:

- Do you feel tired of living?
- Have you been thinking about ending your life?
- Have you been thinking about suicide?

Ask about a suicide plan:

- Have you thought of specific ways to end your life?
- Have you given your possessions away?
- Have you asked someone to help you end your life or join you in death?
- Have you collected pills in order to take an overdose?
- Have you started to put a suicide in action?

Ask about the person's reasons to live:

- What has kept you from harming yourself?
- Who or what makes life so worth living that you would not harm yourself?

As with any person who speaks of suicide, the older adult with suicidal intentions should be carefully monitored and should be given medical treatment as soon as possible.

- Medical illness, such as chronic pain; sensory impairment
- Negative life events, such as loss or financial difficulties
- Functional impairment, such as a loss of independence or problems performing ADLs

Supporting Clients Who Have Suicidal Intent

- If a client talks about suicide, take the person seriously.
- Tell your supervisor at once.
- Do not leave the client alone.
- Encourage the client to talk. Having a conversation gives your supervisor time to get help and also shows the client that you care. Be a good listener.
- Do not minimize the client's concerns. Do not make comments such as "You shouldn't have such thoughts," "Things will work out," or "Look on the bright side."
- In a home care setting, stay with the client until help arrives. Your supervisor may send a nurse, a case manager, or emergency personnel to help the client.

DISRUPTIVE, IMPULSE-CONTROL, AND CONDUCT DISORDERS

Disruptive, impulse-control, and conduct disorders are disorders in which the clients display difficult, disruptive, aggressive, or antisocial behaviours; these disorders are often associated with physical or verbal injury to self, others, or objects or with violating the rights of others. These behaviours can appear in several forms and can be defensive, premeditated, or impulsive. They are grouped into three types: (1) angry/irritable mood, (2) argumentative/defiant behaviour, and (3) vindictiveness. Clients with dementia may display aggressive behaviours (see Chapter 36), but those behaviours are not premeditated and are merely responses to the environment.

Oppositional Defiant Disorder

Clients with *oppositional defiant disorder* (ODD) repeatedly engage in a pattern of defiant, disobedient, and hostile behaviour toward authority figures, beginning in childhood. This behaviour goes beyond acceptable misbehaviour for the given child's age and continues for at least 6 months.

Symptoms of Oppositional Defiant Disorder in Clients:

- Resistance or stubbornness toward taking direction from others
- Unwillingness to compromise
- Frequent anger or resentfulness
- Frequent cruel or revenge-seeking behaviours
- Frequent arguments with, talking back to, or challenging of authority
- Irritable, resentful, or negative attitude
- Provoking others, which comes across as mean, spiteful, or rude behaviours
- Displaying temper tantrums or outbursts
- Always blaming others or denying responsibility
- Repeated trouble at school
- Few or no friends

Intermittent Explosive Disorder

The client with intermittent explosive disorder has recurrent behavioural outbursts, indicating a failure to control aggressive impulses. The outburst may be verbal or physical, and the anger is caused by the inability to cope mentally with a situation. If your clients (or others you know) have persistent problems with anger, they may have important underlying issues that they have not yet resolved—for example, a perceived loss of control in their values being met. They also may be using ineffective emotional coping methods. Many of the calming methods that a person uses to help deal with negative emotions can help when dealing with the person's anger as well, such as taking a deep breath and walking away to "cool down." These outbursts usually have social, financial, or legal consequences. Sometimes support workers have to learn to manage their own anger, as well (**BOX 35–5**).

Symptoms of Intermittent Explosive Disorder

- Intentional behaviours that cause physical or emotional harm to others
- Frequent impulsive actions
- Frequent irritability

BOX 35-5 Dealing With Your Own Anger

- ***Understand the hurt and fear underlying the anger.*** Remember that anger stems from fear and a sense of helplessness, such as a feeling that you are losing control of a situation. The real threat may not be the surface issue (e.g., someone being late to the movie) but the underlying issue (e.g., not being important to someone you love or being mistreated). Identifying emotions of fear and hurt will open the door to recognizing and dealing with underlying issues.
- ***Develop empathetic understanding.*** If you choose to decrease your anger at someone, the first step is to make every effort to see the situation from the other person's point of view. You might begin by asking for an explanation of that person's perspective and then try to understand that person's situation, point of view, and the reasons for that person's beliefs and behaviour. Not having empathetic understanding is usually the major hurdle to getting control of anger. "Forgiving is not forgetting; it is remembering and letting go."[19]
- ***Assume the best intentions (whenever possible).*** Try to assume the best intentions in others until there are repeated indications for other motives.
- ***Understand that sometimes "life is not fair."*** There is nothing "fair" about some people being born into happy, prosperous families and living prosperous, long, happy lives, while other people are born into miserable situations and die young after leading a life filled with suffering. This discrepancy is part of reality, and it is pointless to get angry about it. Make the most of what you have.
- ***Do not hold on to anger for motivation.*** Do you want to do something just to punish the person you are angry with or to "get even"? Holding on to anger or hurt can only hurt you! Wait until you have calmed down, and then talk to the person, stating reasons for your actions calmly. This course of action is much more effective than giving punishment out of anger!
- ***Examine underlying expectations of other people.*** Unfulfilled expectations can lead to anger. What are your expectations of yourself and of others for a given situation? Are you expecting more than is realistic from this person in this particular situation? People are who they are, and one of the root causes of anger is not accepting people (or events) as they are.
- ***Choose happiness instead of anger.*** People who habitually choose anger over happiness lead frustrated, angry lives—not happy lives. Remind yourself of this fact to get more control of your anger. Say to yourself, "Self, why choose anger when you can choose thoughts that produce happiness?"

- Frequent outbursts of anger
- Attempts to provoke others or retaliate against behaviours of others

Conduct Disorder

Clients with **conduct disorder** repeatedly violate the personal or property rights of others and society. This disorder usually begins in childhood with less severe behaviours such as lying and shoplifting and then progresses to more severe behaviours such as burglary or auto theft, as the client develops increased strength, cognitive abilities, and sexual maturity. The causes of this disorder vary but may include severe family dysfunction with exposure to constant or aggressive bickering between parents, limited financial and emotional resources, instability, disturbances of family values, peer rejection, and poor performance in school.

Symptoms of Conduct Disorder in Clients

- Bullying, threatening, or intimidating others
- Engaging in antisocial behaviours
- Having a problem with authority figures
- Frequently starting fights
- Using weapons or tools capable of causing serious physical harm to people or property
- Being physically cruel to animals or people

- Stealing while confronting a victim (e.g., mugging, purse snatching, armed robbery)
- Using physical violence toward others (in the form of rape, assault, murder, etc.)
- Destruction of property (such as starting fires or breaking windows)
- Frequently "conning," manipulating, or telling lies to obtain things and favours or to avoid debts or obligations
- Staying out at night despite parents' curfew rules (before the age of 13)
- Repeatedly running away from home, or running away from home for a lengthy period
- Abusing alcohol or drugs

Supporting Clients With Disruptive, Impulse-Control, and Conduct Disorders

- Remember that as a support worker, you must accept clients in a caring, nonjudgemental way. Clients with disruptive, impulse-control, and conduct disorders may lack insight into their feelings and not be able to deal with them in the moment.
- When approaching the client, maintain a safe distance between the two of you. A client who feels threatened may strike out at you.
- Ensure that you keep an open pathway to an exit in case the client's actions become aggressive.
- Avoid doing anything that might escalate the situation. For example, do not touch the client.
- If clients are verbally aggressive but not physically aggressive, try to determine the cause of their anger. Determine if they are cold, hungry, in pain, or frightened about something.
- Try to understand the client's anger in the cultural context. Some men, for example, would rather yell and scream than admit that they are frightened or in pain.
- You do have the right to ask the client to speak to you politely as a professional. Do not yell back, but remain calm and professional yourself.
- Most employers that provide support services to clients with anger management issues will offer (or encourage you to take on your own) courses such as "Managing Disruptive Behaviours" so that you can learn to deal with aggressive clients in a nonconfrontational manner.
- If the client is verbally aggressive, your main concern is your safety and the safety of others. You should leave the situation and immediately call your supervisor. If the client is threatening to harm you physically, you should get to a safe place and call the police immediately. Refer to the section "Managing Challenging or Responsive Behaviours" in Chapter 36, on page 827.
- Identifying clients' important life values and understanding their lack of confidence in their ability to be happy may help you to overcome clients' anger. With approval from your supervisor, gently inform clients that they need to realize that anger is a choice they have made and that it is not helpful to blame others (or themselves). For some clients, remaining angry can simply be the easiest way out.
- Encourage the client to find new ways to think about a situation. Remind the client that making oneself happy requires skillful effort and mental control.

SUBSTANCE-RELATED AND ADDICTIVE DISORDERS

A **substance-related and addictive disorder** is the deliberate misuse of and inability to stop the abuse of prescription medications, illegal drugs, alcohol, or other substances. These disorders tend to result in problems in relationships and work. Abused substances affect the central nervous system—some have a calming or depressing effect, whereas others have a stimulating effect on the mind and on thinking. Many are also *mood altering*—that is, after taking the substance, users may feel happy, self-confident, and relaxed—but some drugs cause hallucinations, an exaggerated sense of one's own abilities, or an emotional or aggressive state. People with this disorder may show evidence of tolerance and withdrawal. **Drug tolerance** occurs when the person needs larger and larger amounts of the substance to experience the same effect. **Drug withdrawal** is a physical reaction that occurs when the person stops taking the substance. Signs and symptoms of withdrawal, which can be severe, may include depression, agitation, abdominal cramps, nausea, diarrhea, and painful muscle spasms.

Some people with addiction turn to criminal acts to support their habit. Without treatment, death is a risk; common causes of death are overdoses, suicide, and diseases contracted from using contaminated needles.

Treatment for substance-related and addictive disorder depends on the substance being abused. People who have abused any type of drugs, alcohol, or a combination of these will need **detoxification**—a process of allowing an abused substance to exit the body naturally or of removing the abused substance from the body medically. The person being detoxified usually goes into drug withdrawal, and usually requires hospital care. Almost all treatment programs involve psychotherapy with mental health professionals who help clients manage their issues.

Alcohol Use Disorder (AUD)

Alcohol is abused more than any other substance. Signs and symptoms of alcohol abuse include intoxication (drunkenness), memory problems, difficulty concentrating, tremors, and loss of interest in family and friends. These clients are at risk for liver, pancreas, and heart problems. Many people who abuse alcohol have poor nutrition, and many are also addicted to nicotine (cigarettes), so they are at risk for lung disease and certain cancers. Women who drink during pregnancy can give birth to a baby with fetal alcohol spectrum disorder (see Chapter 19).

The *DSM-5* divides alcohol use disorder into mild, moderate, and severe subcategories. These subcategories are based on the extent of people's alcohol use, their cravings for alcohol, and the extent to which alcohol has disrupted their lives.[9]

For most people, exceeding even two drinks a day can do significant harm. Women who have more than 10 drinks a week have higher rates of cancer and other problems than do women who drink less.[20] Men who have more than 15 drinks a week also have higher rates of alcohol-related problems.[20] Some people drink every day, and some go for days or weeks without drinking and then drink a great deal within a short period. People who have mental health disorders, are under stress, or are lonely may turn to alcohol to feel better. Older adults who live alone are at risk for alcohol abuse.

People with alcohol problems may be emotional, aggressive, and abusive, and their families are at risk for abuse and other problems. Some people who are "happy drunks" or the "life of the party" may not be violent toward others, but they certainly put their own health at risk, and if they drink and drive, they risk killing themselves and others on the road.

The main treatment is to avoid drinking. Groups such as Alcoholics Anonymous (AA) help people with drinking cessation. Individual and family counselling is often needed as part of the treatment.[21]

Supporting Clients With Substance-Dependence Disorders

- ***Report suspicions of substance abuse at once.*** You may smell alcohol on a client's breath, or you may observe that a client's medication is running out more quickly than it should. This information is confidential. Do not discuss the matter with anyone but your supervisor.
- ***Avoid confrontation.*** If you think a client is abusing a substance, do not argue. Tell your supervisor of the situation immediately. Do not discuss the matter with anyone else.
- ***Never buy alcohol, drugs, or other substances for clients.*** Purchasing alcohol, drugs, or other substances for clients is unethical. Report any such requests from clients to your supervisor.

PERSONALITY DISORDERS

Personality disorders are a group of disorders involving rigid and socially unacceptable behaviours that are not expected from a person of that culture. A personality disorder is identified by a pervasive pattern of experience and behaviour that is abnormal with respect to any two of the following: thinking, mood, personal relations, and the control of impulses. Individuals with personality disorders have problems relating to others. They may be demanding, hostile, manipulative, inflexible, maladaptive, and antisocial. Because of their behaviours, people with personality disorders are not able to function well in society.

Most personality disorders that begin as problems in personal development and character peak during adolescence. Personality disorders are not illnesses in a strict sense, as they do not disrupt emotional, intellectual, or perceptual functioning. However, those with personality disorders often live a life that is not positive, proactive, or fulfilling. As such, personality disorders are also associated with failure to reach one's potential.

In order to heal, individuals must first have the desire to change in order to break through the enduring pattern of a personality disorder. They must also gain insight into their inner experiences (e.g., severe or repeated trauma during childhood, such as abuse) and their behaviours. Healing is possible when individuals choose to take control of and are committed to changing their lives. Support systems (e.g., therapy, self-help groups, friends, family, medication) are usually necessary for full treatment of people with a personality disorder.

According to the *DSM-5*, some of the main types of personality disorders are the following:

- ***Antisocial personality disorder***—a lack of regard for the moral or legal standards in the local culture or a marked inability to get along with others or abide by societal rules. People with this disorder are sometimes called *psychopaths* or *sociopaths*.
- ***Avoidant personality disorder***—marked social inhibition, feelings of inadequacy, and extreme sensitivity to criticism.
- ***Borderline personality disorder***—lack of identity; rapid changes in mood; intense, unstable interpersonal relationships; impulsiveness; and lack of stability in the way one reacts to things and in self-image.
- ***Dependent personality disorder***—an extreme need for other people, to the point of being unable to make any decisions or take an independent stand. People with this disorder also have a fear of separation, behave in a submissive manner, and lack decisiveness and self-confidence.
- ***Histrionic personality disorder***—exaggerated, almost theatrical, and often inappropriate displays of emotional reactions in everyday behaviour. People with this disorder shift their emotional expressions suddenly and rapidly.
- ***Narcissistic personality disorder***—general lack of empathy for others, a need to be admired by others, an inability to see the viewpoints of others, and hypersensitivity to the opinions of others.
- ***Obsessive–compulsive personality disorder***—perfectionism and inflexibility. People with this disorder are preoccupied with uncontrollable patterns of thought and action.
- ***Paranoid personality disorder***—a marked distrust of others, including the belief, without reason, that others are exploiting, harming, or trying to deceive. People with this disorder have an overall lack of trust and believe that others are betraying them and that there are hidden meanings in messages.
- ***Schizoid personality disorder***—a very limited range of emotion, both in expression of and in experiencing emotions. People with this disorder are indifferent to social relationships.

Common Signs and Symptoms of Personality Disorders

- Self-centredness that manifests itself through a "me first," self-preoccupied attitude
- Lack of individual accountability that results in a victim mentality and blame of others, society, and the universe for one's problems
- Lack of perspective taking and empathy
- Manipulative and exploitative behaviour
- Unhappiness, depression, and other mood and anxiety disorders
- Vulnerability to other mental health disorders such as obsessive–compulsive tendencies and panic attacks
- Distorted or superficial understanding of self and of others' perceptions; an inability to see one's own objectionable, unacceptable, disagreeable, or self-destructive behaviours or the issues that may have contributed to the personality disorder
- Being socially maladaptive, changing the rules of the game, introducing new variables, or otherwise influencing the external world to conform to one's own needs

Supporting Clients With Personality Disorders

- Remember that as a support worker, you must accept clients in a caring, nonjudgemental way. Clients with personality disorders may lack insight into their feelings and not be able to deal with them in the moment.
- Speak to your client in a factual, professional manner.

- Provide care and support as specified in the client's care plan, in a respectful, efficient manner.
- All staff members need to deal with the client in as consistent a manner as possible; otherwise, the client may attempt to play one staff member against another, creating havoc in a unit in a facility.
- ***Just as you would with any other client in any other setting***, refrain from giving your home phone number, email address, or information about your private life to the client to avoid any misunderstanding that doing so constitutes an invitation to private correspondence.
- As with any client in any setting, do not accept gifts, money, or other items from your client. Doing so might be misinterpreted by your client as a sign of affection or special treatment.
- Consult with the client's family members or close friends for ways to successfully deal with that person.

CHAPTER REVIEW

KEY POINTS

- Mental illness can be caused by a combination of genetic, biological, personality, and environmental factors. It is a disturbance in a person's ability to cope with or adjust to stress, affecting the person's thinking, mood, and behaviours and impairing the person's functioning.
- Mental health is a state of mind in which a person copes with and adjusts to the stressors of everyday living in socially acceptable ways. It is influenced by three factors: (1) inherited characteristics, (2) childhood nurturing, and (3) life circumstances.
- When caring for a person with a mental health disorder, you should follow the 10 principles outlined in **BOX 35–2**, on page 773.
- Caring for a person with a mental health disorder usually involves a team approach.
- Culture has a profound influence on understanding mental health disorders and their treatments.
- Acquired brain injury (ABI) is a sudden injury to the brain (e.g., concussion, lack of oxygen, infection) that causes temporary or permanent damage.
- Schizophrenia spectrum disorder is an extremely complex mental health disorder characterized by delusions, hallucinations, disturbances in thinking, and withdrawal from social activity.
- Bipolar and related disorders are brain disorders that cause unusual shifts in a person's mood, energy, and ability to function.
- Anxiety disorders (e.g., panic disorder, phobic disorder) are a group of mental health disorders in which fears and worries disproportionate to a situation affect a person's normal function.
- Depressive disorders are a group of disorders in which the client has sad, empty, or irritable moods accompanied by thought changes. These disorders impair the client's ability to function.
- Depression in older adults is often overlooked or misdiagnosed, sometimes as dementia. Many older adults do not admit to feeling depressed but, instead, complain of having aches and pains; others may be agitated and irritable.
- Trauma and stressor-related disorders are anxiety disorders that can develop after an individual has experienced or witnessed a major trauma (e.g., war, fire, accident, violent crime). Post-traumatic stress disorder (PTSD) is one type of trauma disorder. It can occur in people of all ages, races, cultures, and genders.
- Obsessive–compulsive and related disorders are mental health disorders characterized by recurrent obsessions and compulsions that interfere with a person's daily life and relationships.
- Feeding and eating disorders (e.g., anorexia nervosa, bulimia nervosa, pica) are caused by altered body image perceptions that lead to disturbances in eating behaviours and an abnormal concern about body weight and shape.
- Sleep–wake disorders are conditions in which repetitive disturbed sleep patterns lead to distress and impairment in daytime functioning.
- Suicidal behaviour disorder is diagnosed when a person has recurrent thoughts or a preoccupation with ending one's own life.
- Health care workers need to be aware of the warning signs of suicidal intent (both in young people and in older adults) and know what to do if they suspect suicidal intent.
- Disruptive, impulse-control, and conduct disorders are defined by clients' display of difficult, disruptive, aggressive, or antisocial behaviours, resulting in physical or verbal injury to self, others, or objects or in a violation of the rights of others.
- A substance-related and addictive disorder is the deliberate misuse of and inability to stop the abuse of prescription medications, illegal drugs, alcohol, or other substances, as well as the resulting problems in relationships and work.
- A personality disorder is identified by a pervasive pattern of experience and behaviour that is abnormal with respect to any two of the following: thinking, mood, personal relations, and the control of impulses. Because of their behaviours, people with personality disorders are not able to function well in society or relate well to others.

CRITICAL THINKING IN PRACTICE

You are a support worker working for a home care agency. Today, you noticed that one of your clients smelled of alcohol and slurred his words. During his care, he told you that he wanted to kill himself and that he had a gun in the house and knew "how to use it." What should you do? What are your responsibilities in this situation? How can you ensure your safety?

REVIEW QUESTIONS

Answers to these questions are at the bottom of page 802.

Circle the BEST answer.

1. Which of the following is true?
   A. People with mental health disorders usually create their own problems.
   B. Chemical imbalances in the body can cause mental health disorders.
   C. Treatment for mental health disorders might include physiotherapy and medication.
   D. Most people with mental health disorders should be hospitalized.

2. Mr. Mueller sees a psychologist. Together, they explore the unconscious conflicts and underlying reasons for Mr. Mueller's problems. This kind of psychotherapy is:
   A. Psychoanalysis
   B. Occupational therapy
   C. Behaviour therapy
   D. Group therapy

3. Mrs. Paré is afraid of catching a disease and washes her hands hundreds of times a day. Mrs. Paré likely has a(n):
   A. Panic disorder
   B. Phobic disorder
   C. Anorexia nervosa
   D. Obsessive–compulsive disorder

4. Mr. Lau has a bipolar and related disorder. This means he:
   A. Has delusions
   B. Is hostile
   C. Is very suspicious
   D. Has severe mood swings

5. Which *best* describes how culture can impact mental health? Culture:
   A. Can dictate the way that the brain reacts to traumatic events
   B. Can influence the way a person's behaviours are interpreted
   C. Can predict the presence of mental health disorders in people
   D. Has no effect on mental health disorders

6. Which of the following might have the biggest impact on whether or not 10-year-old Mike develops a mental health disorder in the future? Mike:
   A. Has been abused
   B. Eats a balanced diet and gets 8 hours of sleep a night
   C. Has a parent who suffers from major depression
   D. A and C

7. Shira, 15, has lost 30 pounds. She is terrified of becoming fat, even though she is extremely thin. She avoids food. Shira likely has:
   A. Bulimia nervosa
   B. Repression
   C. Anorexia nervosa
   D. Claustrophobia

8. Mrs. Alam has a major depressive disorder. You should avoid:
   A. Showing her that you care
   B. Telling her how lucky she is
   C. Encouraging periods of rest
   D. Encouraging activity and social interactions

9. A client with a major depressive disorder suddenly seems happy. She asks you to leave early because she is expecting friends. You should:
   A. Leave as requested
   B. Leave as soon as the friends arrive
   C. Call your supervisor to report the situation
   D. Stay until you are scheduled to leave

10. You are supporting a client with a bipolar and related disorder, who is in the manic phase of the illness. You should:
A. Offer limited choices
B. Direct her to clean her house
C. Provide a stimulating environment
D. Get her to become tired so that she will fall asleep

11. Your client, who you meet with at a day program for older adults, complains that she has not been able to sleep for weeks. Before reporting this, you should:
A. Ask her more about her lifestyle
B. Advise her to get a new mattress
C. Ask her if she is depressed
D. Tell her that *you* never get enough sleep

12. Mrs. Smith, an older woman who has just been admitted to a long-term care facility, tells you that she hopes that she "will die soon." Before notifying your supervisor, you should:
A. Tell her that she will get used to her new environment soon
B. Introduce her to other residents on her ward
C. Not respond, but observe her for signs of depression
D. Ask questions that will allow her to elaborate on why she feels this way

13. Zaid, 16, who used to be a soccer star in his high school, failed to make the soccer team last week. He tells his sister that she can have all of his electronic gadgets, and she then told you. What should you do?
A. Watch what he does next
B. Talk to his friends about this
C. Offer him money for the gadgets
D. Notify your supervisor immediately and suggest his sister stay with him till help arrives

14. Mr. Wilder is a World War II veteran. How might going to his local branch of the Legion help him deal with the new feelings of depression he has?
A. It will give him a chance to talk openly about the horrors of war that he never talked about before.
B. It will give him an opportunity to talk to other people his age.
C. It will provide a stimulating environment and give him somewhere to go.
D. All of the above.

15. Kathy, 19, has schizophrenia. She usually insists on having her MP3 player and headphones on all day because, she says, she likes to listen to music. Today, you realize that the headphones are not attached to her player. Before notifying your supervisor, you should:
A. Take her headphones away from her
B. Point out this fact and reattach them
C. Ask her to remove her headphones
D. Talk to her to try to find out if she is having hallucinations

16. Kathy says giant insects are climbing up the wall. She is terrified. You see nothing on the wall. You should:
A. Insist that Kathy is seeing things
B. Pretend you also see the insects
C. Offer Kathy comfort and report the hallucination
D. Leave Kathy alone and call for help

17. You are supporting a client in the home, and you discover several half-empty bottles of gin in her bathroom cupboard. You should:
A. Replace the gin with water
B. Notify your supervisor
C. Point them out to your client
D. Ask her to breathe on you so that you can smell her breath

18. Which of the following is true? People with a substance-related and addictive disorder:
A. Can overcome their addictions
B. Have only themselves to blame
C. Can be addicted only to street drugs
D. Will not experience withdrawal symptoms from prescription medications

19. The client who you are supporting in the community asks for your home phone number. You should:
A. Give her only your cellphone number
B. Give her your friend's phone number
C. Give a false number so that she cannot call you
D. Explain that you do not give out your phone number to clients

20. You are supporting a client in his own home who is recovering from neurosurgery. His care plan says that he has an addiction to drugs and alcohol. You should:
A. Go through his cupboards looking for alcohol
B. Refuse to care for him because you do not drink
C. Provide respectful care that is stated in his care plan
D. Tell him about the time you got "wasted" last week to make him feel comfortable with you

21. You are newly employed as a support worker at a group home for adult male clients who are recovering from addictions. One day, while you are in the kitchen observing some of the clients making pancakes, in another room, a fight over the television remote breaks out between two of the newly admitted clients. You enter the room just as Bob punches Juan in the nose. Being the first worker at the scene, what should you do first?
A. Get your supervisor to deal with this.
B. Separate the two clients and talk to them separately.
C. Grab both by their arms and shout at them, "Quit this, now!"
D. Instruct them to clean the mess they made, and observe them while they do this.

Answers: 1.B, 2.A, 3.D, 4.D, 5.B, 6.D, 7.C, 8.B, 9.C, 10.A, 11.A, 12.D, 13.D, 14.D, 15.D, 16.C, 17.B, 18.A, 19.D, 20.C, 21. You should separate the two clients and talk to them separately. Begin with Bob, the aggressor. You should speak in a firm but soft voice that is both professional and friendly. Never grab an aggressive client, as doing so might increase the client's anger. Distance yourself so that you are just beyond arm's length in case the client tries to hit you. By separating the two from each other and from other clients, you can help defuse this situation. Try to discuss ways that they can deal with their issues in a nonconfrontational manner. After they calm down, you can try role-playing with them to reinforce what you have discussed.

Chapter opener image: Photographee.eu/Shutterstock.com

CHAPTER 36

Disorientation, Delirium, and Dementia

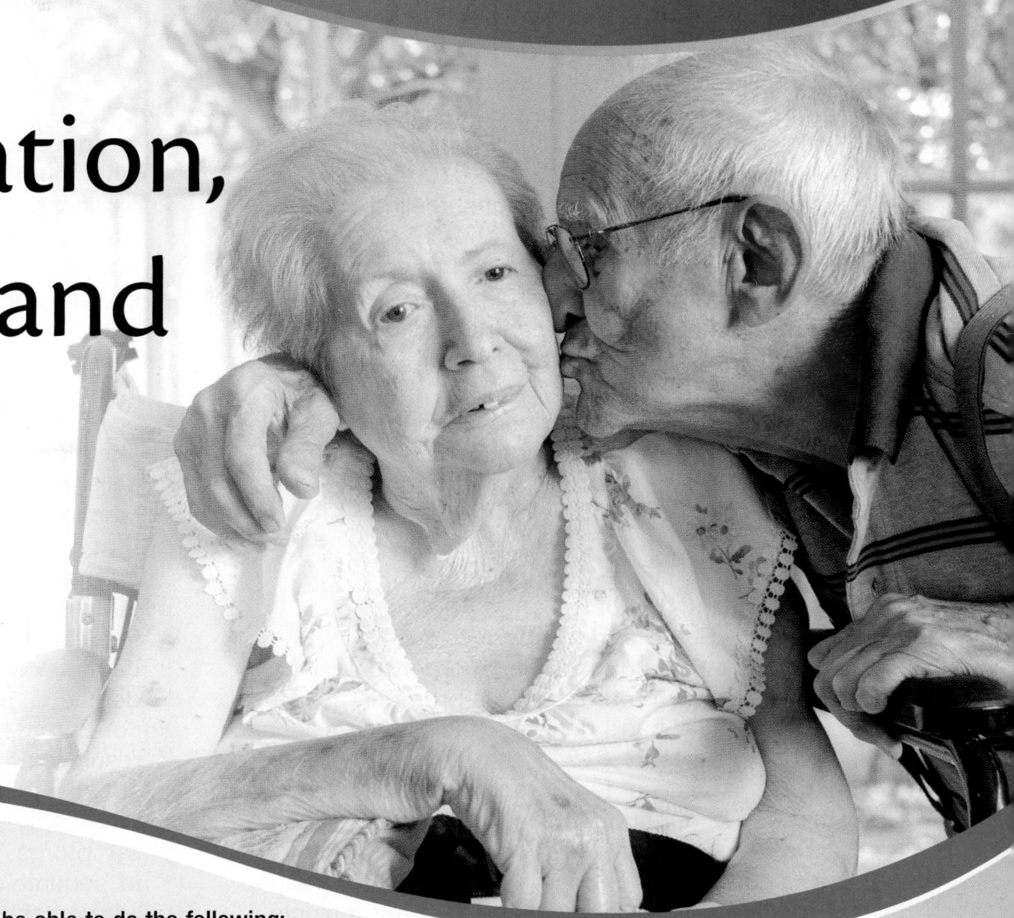

OBJECTIVES

After reading this chapter, the learner should be able to do the following:

- Describe disorientation, delirium, and dementia and their causes.
- Differentiate between normal and abnormal mental changes related to aging.
- List measures that help clients who are disoriented.
- Differentiate among disorientation, delirium, and dementia.
- Describe dementia and its signs and symptoms.
- Explain why depression is often associated with dementia.
- List different forms of and causes of dementia.
- Describe the common stages of dementia.
- Describe how to support a client with dementia.
- List examples of challenging or responsive behaviours and possible causes.
- Describe how caring for family members with dementia can affect primary caregivers.
- Apply the principles learned in this chapter to the care and support of clients with disorientation, delirium, or dementia.

KEY TERMS

Alzheimer's disease and related dementias (ADRD) A progressive, degenerative disease that gradually destroys nerve cells (neurons) in most areas of the brain and causes thinking and memory to become seriously impaired; the most common form of dementia. *p. 810*

apathy An absence of emotional feeling, which appears as indifference. *p. 807*

apraxia Impairment of the skilled motor system, resulting in the loss of being able to perform learned, purposeful movements, including activities of daily living (bathing, brushing teeth, and so on). *p. 809*

cognitive function Brain function involving the memory, thinking, reasoning, understanding, judgement, and behaviour functions of the brain. *p. 805*

cognitive impairment The loss of the ability to remember, think, reason, understand, or live independently. *p. 805*

confusion See **disorientation**. *p. 805*

cueing Providing of prompts in order to assist a client to complete a task. This prompting can be in the form of hand gestures, facial expressions, or verbal phrases. *p. 818*

delirium A state of temporary mental disorientation that can occur suddenly. *p. 806*

dementia A general term that describes the progressive loss of brain functions, which include cognitive and social functions. It is not a single disease but a group of illnesses that involve memory, behaviour, learning, and communication. Dementia is categorized as being either a mild or major **neuro-cognitive disorder**, depending on its symptoms. *p. 808*

disorientation Mental confusion, or an impaired ability to recall people, time, or places as a result of (or any combination of) physiological changes to the brain, disease process, or substance-induced factors. Also known as **confusion**. *p. 805*

euphoria An exaggerated or abnormal expression of physical or emotional well-being that is not based on reality or truth. *p. 807*

Gentle Persuasive Approaches (GPA) A program designed to train direct care providers in techniques to handle and reduce difficult responsive behaviours (e.g., grabbing, biting, and hitting) that are associated with dementias such as Alzheimer's disease to prepare the care providers for vulnerable care situations and for avoiding potential workplace injury. *p. 829*

hoarding Collecting things and putting them away in a guarded manner. *p. 833*

neuro-cognitive disorder A significant decline in attention, functioning, learning, memory, language, deliberate motor movement, and social functioning. *p. 808*

primary dementia Dementia that does not result from any other disease. *p. 810*

pseudo-dementia False (*pseudo*) dementia. Pseudo-dementia occurs when severe depression causes cognitive changes that mimic dementia. *p. 814*

secondary dementia Dementia that occurs as a result of a physical disease, ingestion of damaging substances, or injury. *p. 810*

sundowning A condition in which the signs, symptoms, and behaviours of dementia increase at bedtime or during hours of darkness. *p. 830*

validation therapy A type of therapy for people with dementia that focuses on empathy and advocates accepting the affected person's perception of reality. *p. 828*

Wernicke–Korsakoff syndrome A brain disorder that is caused by lack of thiamine (vitamin B1); affects the nervous system, including the brain; and is usually associated with heavy alcohol consumption over a long period. *p. 813*

Chapter 35 discussed mental health disorders, most of which involve changes in the brain's function—which usually occur in late childhood or early adulthood—due to chemical imbalances or lifestyle choices. This chapter addresses the changes in behaviour that take place over time as the brain is affected by aging, illness, or, again, lifestyle. Although some changes in the nervous system, including the brain, occur normally with aging (**BOX 36–1**), some other changes are caused by disease. This chapter addresses disorientation, delirium, and dementia.

The section on "Managing Challenging or Responsive Behaviours" near the end of this chapter describes some of the behaviours exhibited by people with

BOX 36–1 Normal Changes in the Nervous System Associated With Aging

- Brain cells are lost.
- Nerve conduction slows.
- Response and reaction times are slower.
- Reflexes are slower.
- Vision and hearing decrease.
- Taste and smell decrease.
- Touch and sensitivity to pain decrease.
- Blood flow to the brain is reduced.
- Changes in sleep patterns occur.
- Mild word-finding problems occur.

dementia and suggests ways that caregivers can safely and respectfully support clients who demonstrate these disruptive and responsive behaviours.

You should be aware that ***disorientation, delirium, and dementia are NOT a normal part of aging.*** The reasons a person may develop disorientation, delirium, or dementia are discussed in this chapter.

Diseases that affect the brain can affect **cognitive function** (the term *cognitive* relates to brain or mind). Cognitive functioning involves the following functions of the brain:

- Memory
- Thinking
- Reasoning
- Ability to understand
- Judgement
- Behaviour

Loss of cognitive function affects all dimensions of a person's life. The state of having lost the ability to remember, think, reason, understand, or live independently is referred to as **cognitive impairment**.

DISORIENTATION

Disorientation, also called **confusion**, is the term for an impaired ability to recall people, time, or places as a result of (or any combination of) physiological changes to the brain, disease process, or substance-induced factors. In most circumstances, ***disorientation is a symptom of an underlying medical condition*** such as depression, electrolyte imbalance, or even a brain tumour. The word *disorientation* is a generic descriptive term, and refers *only* to the client's disturbed orientation to people, time, or places. Disorientation can occur suddenly (such as after ingesting too much alcohol) or over a long period (such as when it is associated with a mental health disorder). Disorientation is usually more common in older adults but can also occur in younger people. Disorientation can be *reversible* or *not reversible*, depending on its causes.

Disorientation that is permanent is caused by physical changes to the structure of the brain and is called *nonreversible dementia*. Dementia is the main focus of this chapter. Disorientation that is *reversible* can occur during hospitalization or in other unfamiliar surroundings or when clients are in pain, have electrolyte imbalance, or are suffering from lack of sleep.

Disorientation that occurs suddenly and usually without warning is called *delirium* and is also discussed later in this chapter. Delirium can be caused by an infection in the body (such as a urinary tract infection [UTI]), an extreme lack of sleep, an electrolyte imbalance (from a bout of influenza, for example), certain drugs, a combination of prescription and over-the-counter medications, or a toxic amount of these drugs. ***It is important that people who experience sudden disorientation without a known cause be seen by a physician. For example, sudden disorientation resulting from a stroke needs to be treated medically within hours, or else it could result in permanent cognitive, mental, or physical disorders or even death.***

People with disorientation often exhibit behaviour changes and may be angry, restless, depressed, or irritable. Some disoriented people may behave aggressively. Other signs and symptoms of disorientation include the following:

- Anxiety
- Tremors
- Hallucinations (p. 831)
- Delusions (p. 831)

- Decline in level of consciousness
- Disorganized thinking and speech
- Attention problems

Causes of Disorientation

- UTI (one of the main causes)
- Alcohol intoxication
- Low blood sugar
- Head trauma or head injury
- Concussion
- Fluid and electrolyte imbalance
- Nutritional deficiencies, particularly niacin, thiamine, vitamin C, or vitamin B_{12}
- Fever
- Sudden drop in body temperature (hypothermia)
- Low levels of oxygen (e.g., from chronic lung disorders)
- Medications
- Infections
- Brain tumour
- Certain physiological illnesses, especially in older adults (see Chapter 37)
- Certain mental health illnesses such as clinical depression or schizophrenia (see Chapter 35)
- Sleep deprivation (loss)
- Seizures

Diagnosing Disorientation, Delirium, and Dementia

People with ongoing disorientation that has come on gradually (over weeks, months, or years) need to see a doctor to have the problem evaluated. The doctor will perform a physical examination and ask questions to determine if the client has any of the following signs or symptoms of disorientation:

- Getting days and nights mixed up
- Being awake during usual sleep time
- Not recognizing people
- Not knowing where one is
- Not knowing the date and time
- Not answering simple questions appropriately
- Having persistent feelings of disorientation or repeated episodes of disorientation
- Having disorientation that is rapidly getting worse
- Having disorientation that comes and goes

In addition, the doctor will ask about other conditions that may trigger disorientation, such as the following:

- Recent illness such as the flu
- Difficulty with urinating
- Recent head injury
- Diabetes
- Lung disorder
- Medication errors, such as taking medications in the wrong combination or not as directed
- Exposure to other drugs or alcohol

The physical examination will include a thorough evaluation of the nervous system, including the brain. The doctor may also perform neurological cognitive tests, magnetic resonance imaging (MRI) of the head, blood and urine tests, and an electroencephalogram (EEG), depending on the signs and symptoms.

After the necessary tests, the doctor may be able to identify the cause of the disorientation and will determine if it is a symptom of a persistent illness such as chronic obstructive pulmonary disease; that of a permanent disorder (see Chapter 37, p. 861, and *Supporting Mrs. Thomas, Part I: Certain Illnesses Can Cause Dementia*, on the next page); or that of an acute condition such as delirium.

Ways to Minimize or Prevent Disorientation

Although some types of disorientation cannot be prevented, other types can be prevented through good health practices and lifestyle choices such as the following:

- Getting regular hours of sleep
- Eating a balanced diet that has plenty of vitamins and minerals
- Not drinking alcohol in excess
- Keeping careful control of blood sugar if diabetes is present
- Not smoking

DELIRIUM

Disorientation that occurs suddenly is called **delirium**—a condition of severe disorientation and

Supporting Mrs. Thomas, Part I: Certain Illnesses Can Cause Dementia

Eileen Thomas is a 68-year-old woman who lives with her husband in her own home. She was a chronic smoker for 40 years but quit 2 years ago, when she was diagnosed with chronic obstructive pulmonary disease (COPD). Mrs. Thomas's husband reports to their family doctor that recently she seems "confused": she has been leaving the stove on, forgetting to turn off the tap in the kitchen sink, and so on.

Mrs. Thomas's doctor tells the family that because of her long-term smoking (and other health issues), she has hardening of the arteries (atherosclerosis), which prevents oxygen from going to her brain in the normal manner. Although she is put on medication, her family is told that her condition cannot be cured and that she has dementia. As a support worker, you are to assist Mrs. Thomas with bathing and cooking meals, and her husband now buys the groceries for the family. You need to monitor her for unsafe behaviours and report your observations to your supervisor.

rapid changes in brain function. It is usually caused by a treatable physical or mental health disorder; it is often temporary and disappears once the illness has been treated. It can occur due to a reaction to medications, infection or other illness, poor nutrition, food poisoning, dehydration, or emotional trauma. Major life changes—such as the death of a loved one or a move into a facility—can also cause delirium.

Delirium should always be treated as an emergency. It often is the first or only sign of a physical disorder in older adults and in people with dementia. If you observe any sudden occurrence of signs and symptoms of delirium, inform your supervisor at once. ***The cause of the delirium needs to be determined, and the delirium needs to be treated immediately. In many cases (such as with stroke), the symptoms can become permanent or could progress and cause death.***

Signs and Symptoms of Delirium

Delirium involves a rapid alternation between mental states. For example, someone with delirium may become drowsy, then agitated, and then drowsy again. Other signs and symptoms include the following:

- Attention disturbance, such as an inability to maintain goal-directed, purposeful thinking or behaviour, or difficulty concentrating
- Incoherent speech and inability to stop speech patterns or behaviours
- Disorientation to time or place
- Changes in sensation and perception (which increases the disorientation)
- Sign of illusions or hallucinations
- Altered level of consciousness or awareness
- Altered sleep patterns; drowsiness
- Levels of alertness may vary—the client is usually more alert in the morning and less alert at night (drowsiness)
- Decrease in short-term memory and recall
- Changes in motor activities, movement
- Emotional or personality changes, such as anxiety, anger, **apathy** (appearance of indifference), depression, **euphoria** (exaggerated expression of well-being), or irritability

Diagnosis and Treatment of Delirium

The client with delirium should be seen as soon as possible by a physician, who will most likely order blood work (including blood and alcohol levels), EEG, computed tomography (CT) or MRI scanning of the clients' head, chest X-ray, or a lumbar puncture (spinal tap) to determine the cause of the delirium. The client is usually admitted to a hospital and treated as an inpatient. Acute disorders that cause delirium may coexist with chronic disorders that cause dementia.

The goal of treatment is to control or reverse the cause of the symptoms, and treatment depends on the specific condition causing delirium. Sometimes, treatment requires stopping medications (or alcohol consumption). Disorders that contributed to disorientation—for example, heart failure, decreased oxygen, or psychiatric conditions (such as depression)—will be treated. Successful early treatment for

It is more important to contain behaviors than to restrain behaviors

Supporting Mrs. Thomas, Part II: Recognizing Delirium and Acting Quickly

Mrs. Thomas has been your client for several months now, and although she has occasionally displayed unsafe behaviours—such as leaving the stove on—her condition has remained unchanged. On a particular day recently, Mrs. Thomas was acting completely differently. When you arrived, you found that she was very drowsy; then she woke up, became very tearful and agitated, threw some dishes on the floor, and finally fell asleep on the sofa.

As her support worker, you were understandably concerned, so you immediately notified your supervisor. Your supervisor advised you to call 9-1-1 and to accompany Mrs. Thomas to the hospital. The paramedics examined Mrs. Thomas and rushed her to the hospital by ambulance. At the hospital, it was found that the cause of this sudden, erratic behaviour was viral meningitis. The doctors expected that Mrs. Thomas would recover completely to her pre-meningitis state.

coexisting medical and psychiatric disorders often greatly improves mental functioning.

Some clients may require medications to control their aggressive, agitated behaviours or behaviours that are dangerous to themselves or to others. Medications are usually given in very low doses, with adjustments made as needed. For some clients, admission to a psychiatric facility may be necessary, especially if the dangerous behaviours continue. See the *Supporting Mrs. Thomas, Part II: Recognizing Delirium and Acting Quickly* box.

DEMENTIA

Dementia is a general term that describes the progressive loss of brain functions, including cognitive and social functions. It is not a single disease but a group of illnesses that involve memory, behaviour, learning, decision making, and communication. Dementia is ***not*** a normal part of aging. In fact, most older adults do not have dementia. While dementia can affect people in their 40s and 50s, it is more common after 65 years of age. Dementia affects a person's ability to perform complex as well as simple tasks. Usually, dementia starts slowly and progresses gradually to a worse state. Problems with complex tasks—such as driving, managing money, planning meals, and working—appear first. Over time, problems occur with simple tasks, such as bathing, dressing, eating, using the toilet, and walking; everyday skills are eventually lost.

When it is diagnosed, dementia is then categorized as either a mild or major neuro-cognitive disorder, depending on the extent of loss of cognitive and social functioning. A **neuro-cognitive disorder** is a disorder associated with dementia based on the extent of the client's decline in attention, functioning, learning, memory, language, deliberate motor movement, and social functioning.

There are many different forms and causes of dementia. Sometimes, dementia is caused by conditions that are treatable, in which case the dementia is usually reversed (cured) or slowed. See **BOX 36–2** for a detailed list of signs and symptoms of dementia.

Treatable (or Reversible) Forms of Dementia

Dementias that may be treated and sometimes reversed (usually referred to as *disorientation*) are caused by the following:

- ***Metabolic problems.*** An underactive thyroid gland can lead to disorientation or to delirium, both of which can be reversed when the thyroid condition is corrected. Low blood sugar (hypoglycemia) can cause disorientation or dementia if untreated. Abnormal sodium or calcium levels in the body can cause mental changes.
- ***Brain injury.*** Some brain injuries result in internal bleeding in the skull, which can cause a rapid onset of dementia symptoms. Without prompt detention and surgery to correct the bleeding, the client would most likely die or have permanent changes to cognitive function.
- ***Brain tumour.*** Delirium or dementia may result from a brain tumour, depending on the location,

BOX 36–2 Signs and Symptoms of Dementia

Early Warning Signs of Dementia

- Memory loss that affects daily activities (e.g., misplacing items or putting them in odd places)
- Disorientation (e.g., getting lost in familiar places or forgetting how to use simple, everyday items such as a microwave)
- Repeating words or sentences; problems finding the right words or following conversations
- Poor judgement (e.g., going outdoors in the snow without shoes)
- Problems with common tasks (e.g., dressing, cooking, driving)
- Changes in mood, behaviour, or personality (e.g., unfounded jealousy, suspiciousness, or poor social behaviour)
- Loss of interest in activities or hobbies (e.g., an avid gardener now letting weeds overrun the garden)

Signs of Progression of Dementia

- Forgetting recent events
- Forgetting simple directions
- Forgetting conversations
- Forgetting appointments
- Forgetting names (including those of family members)
- Forgetting the names of everyday things (e.g., clock, radio, TV, and so on)
- Forgetting words
- Substituting unusual words and names for forgotten ones
- Loss of train of thought
- Forgetting English (if it was a second language) and speaking only in the native language
- Cursing or swearing
- Misplacing items
- Putting things in odd places
- Having difficulty using debit cards, writing cheques, or balancing chequebooks
- Giving away large amounts of money
- Not recognizing or understanding numbers
- Having difficulty following conversations
- Having difficulty reading
- Having difficulty writing
- Becoming lost even in familiar settings
- Forgetting where they are
- Wandering from home
- Not knowing how to get back home
- Not being able to tell or understand time
- Not being able to tell or understand dates
- Not being able to handle everyday tasks (e.g., leaving the iron or stove burners on, leaving the food burning on the stove, and so on)
- Impairment of the skilled motor system, resulting in the loss of the ability to perform learned, purposeful movements, including activities of daily living (ADLs), such as bathing, brushing teeth, and so on. This motor system impairment is called **apraxia**.
- Distrusting others
- Being stubborn
- Withdrawing from society
- Being restless
- Becoming suspicious
- Becoming fearful
- Not wanting to do things
- Sleeping more than usual

size, and type of tumour. Surgery or chemotherapy may be used to treat the tumour.

- ***Alcohol.*** Long-term alcohol abuse can lead to dementia that may or may not be reversible.
- ***Nutritional deficiencies.*** Deficiencies in nutrients, such as vitamins B_1, B_3 or B_{12}, can contribute to dementia-like mental impairment.
- ***Infections.*** Many infections (e.g., UTI, an infected wound, or tuberculosis) can cause disorientation or delirium, which can be reversible if treated. However, in many cases, infections can go unreported because the client's disorientation is mistaken for an irreversible type of dementia.
- ***Poisoning.*** Environmental exposure and ingestion of lead and other heavy metals, or abuse of substances such as inhalants, may cause cognitive and behavioural changes, often mistaken for dementia.

Irreversible Forms of Dementia

Most forms of dementia cannot be reversed and have no prevention or cure. As a result, the client's brain function will decline over time. Some medications are now available to help delay brain function decline and have been helpful for some clients, but their effectiveness depends on the client's situation and the type of dementia. Irreversible dementia eventually interferes with all ADLs and will, unfortunately, contribute to the client's death. See the *Supporting Mrs. Thomas, Part III: The Impact of Dementia on a Family* box.

Supporting Mrs. Thomas, Part III: The Impact of Dementia on a Family

Mrs. Thomas has fully recovered and returned to her pre-meningitis state, but she is becoming increasingly forgetful. Last week, you noticed that she needed help with buttoning up her clothing while she was getting dressed. Mrs. Thomas herself mentioned to you that she "forgot" to undo her pants when she had to go to the washroom and soiled herself. On your last two visits, she did not recognize you but could read your name tag. Earlier this week, her husband told you that she did not recognize him when he was helping her undress for bedtime and started punching him, accusing him of trying to molest her. She also started to yell at her reflection in the mirror because she did not recognize herself.

Her husband took her to her doctor, and after numerous tests, the doctor told Mr. and Mrs. Thomas that her dementia was probably due to Alzheimer's disease. The doctor said that Mrs. Thomas's symptoms had progressed at a very rapid rate and her cognition would probably decline quickly. Mrs. Thomas's husband was very upset about the diagnosis; the couple had made plans to drive across Canada to visit their children and their grandchildren. Mr. Thomas told you that he was very grateful for your support in his wife's care.

PRIMARY DEMENTIAS

Dementias that are irreversible can be identified as either as **primary dementias**, which do not result from any other disease, or **secondary dementias**, which occur as a result of a physical disease or injury. The most common examples of primary dementias are discussed below.

Alzheimer's Disease and Related Dementias

The most common form of dementia, **Alzheimer's disease and related dementias (ADRD)**, account for over 64% of all dementias in Canadians.[1] ADRD are *primary* disorders of the brain; they are not caused by another illness or disease. Depending on its extent, it can be categorized as either a minor or major neuro-cognitive disorder.[2] Dr. Alois Alzheimer first identified Alzheimer's disease in 1906. The two distinguishing characteristics he found were (1) *plaques*, deposits in the brain that become toxic to brain cells at excessive levels, and (2) *tangles*, which interfere with vital processes and eventually choke off living cells.[3] The brain physically shrinks as these brain cells die, and ultimately how the brain functions is affected.[3] What happens in ADRD is that the nerve cells in the brain become sick and progressively less and less able to pass on messages to other nerve cells, and eventually these cells die. It is the loss of "connectivity" (the ability of one cell to communicate with another), which occurs long before the cells die, that is responsible for the symptoms of Alzheimer's disease.[4]

ADRD usually occurs after age 65 years and is often diagnosed after 80. However, it can also affect people in their 40s and 50s. Currently, ADRD has no cure, but there are some medications that can slow its progress. The cause of ADRD is unknown, but a family history of ADRD is a known risk factor.[3] The progression (i.e., the rate of decline of cognitive functioning) of ADRD varies from client to client and can span from 3 to 20 years. On average, people live with the disease between 8 and 12 years. The progression can be described as a series of stages; these stages (see p. 815) provide a guide to the pattern of the disease and help caregivers make care decisions.

Warning Signs of Alzheimer's Disease and Related Dementias

The Alzheimer Society of Canada has developed the following list of signs to look for when Alzheimer's disease is suspected. It is important for the person exhibiting these signs to be examined by a physician:[5]

1. Memory loss affecting day-to-day abilities—forgetting things often or struggling to retain new information
2. Difficulty performing familiar tasks—forgetting how to do something you have been doing your whole life, such as preparing a meal or getting dressed
3. Problems with language—forgetting words or substituting words that do not fit the context
4. Disorientation in time and space—not knowing what day of the week it is or getting lost in a familiar place
5. Impaired judgement—not recognizing a medical problem that needs attention or wearing light clothing on a cold day
6. Problems with abstract thinking—not understanding what numbers signify on a calculator, for example, or how they are used
7. Misplacing things—putting things in strange places, like an iron in the freezer or a wristwatch in the sugar bowl
8. Changes in mood and behaviour—for example, going from being easygoing to quick-tempered
9. Changes in personality—behaving out of character, such as feeling paranoid or threatened
10. Loss of initiative—losing interest in friends, family, and favourite activities

Vascular Dementia

Vascular dementia, sometimes known as *multi-infarct dementia,* is one of the most common forms of dementia, second only to Alzheimer's disease in older adults. Vascular dementia is caused by chronic, reduced blood flow to the brain—usually as the result of a stroke or series of strokes. In many cases, the strokes are so small that symptoms may not be noticeable. These strokes are known as "silent strokes" or *transient ischemic attacks* (*TIAs*). Over time, the damage adds up, leading to memory loss, disorientation, and other signs of dementia. Research has shown that there is a real connection between heart health and brain health, and heart problems such as dysrhythmia (problems with the heart's rhythm) have been shown to cause strokes.

Vascular dementia results in a subtle, progressive decline in memory and cognitive functioning. It is caused when the blood supply carrying oxygen and nutrients to the brain is interrupted by a blocked or diseased vascular system. If blood supply is blocked for longer than a few seconds, brain cells can die, causing damage to the cortex of the brain—the area associated with learning, memory, and language.

Depending on each client's health condition and the severity of the stroke or strokes, vascular dementia may come on gradually or suddenly. Currently, there is no known cure, but the good news is that making certain lifestyle changes and using practical strategies may help prevent strokes, compensate for cognitive losses, and slow the disease's development.

Vascular dementia affects different people in different ways, and the speed of progression varies from person to person. Some symptoms may be similar to those of other types of dementia and usually reflect increasing difficulty to perform everyday activities such as eating, dressing, or shopping.

Behavioural and physical symptoms can come on dramatically or very gradually, although it appears that a prolonged period of TIAs—the mini-strokes mentioned above—leads to a gradual decline in memory, whereas a bigger stroke can produce profound symptoms immediately. Regardless of the rate of appearance, vascular dementia typically progresses in a stepwise fashion, where lapses in memory and reasoning abilities are followed by periods of stability, only to give way to further decline.

Common mental and emotional signs and symptoms of vascular dementia include the following:

- Slowed thinking
- Memory problems; general forgetfulness
- Unusual mood changes (e.g., depression, irritability)
- Hallucinations and delusions
- Disorientation, which may get worse at night
- Personality changes and loss of social skills[6]

Dementia With Lewy Bodies

Dementia with Lewy bodies (DLB) is one of the most common types of progressive dementia. The central feature of DLB is progressive cognitive decline, combined with three additional defining features: (1) severe fluctuations in alertness and attention—for example, sleep disturbances, frequent drowsiness, lethargy, lengthy periods spent staring into space, or disorganized speech; (2) recurrent visual hallucinations; and (3) Parkinson's disease–like motor symptoms such as rigidity and the loss of spontaneous movement. People with DLB may also suffer from depression. The symptoms of DLB are caused by a buildup of Lewy bodies—accumulated bits of protein—inside the nuclei of neurons in areas of the brain that regulate particular aspects of memory and motor control.

The similarity of symptoms between DLB and Parkinson's disease and between DLB and Alzheimer's disease can often make coming up with a definitive diagnosis difficult for the physician. As well, Lewy bodies are often found in the brains of people with Parkinson's disease and in those with ADRD, a finding that suggests either that DLB is related to these other causes of dementia or that an individual can have both DLB and one of these other diseases at the same time. DLB usually occurs sporadically in people with no known family history of the disease. However, rare familial cases have occasionally been reported.

Fronto-Temporal Degeneration Dementia

Fronto-temporal dementia (FTD) is another type of dementia. It accounts for about 5% of all dementias and generally occurs between 40 and 60 years, with women slightly more affected than men.[7] FTD is characterized by dramatic changes in personality, behaviour, and thought processes. Changes in personal and social conduct occur in the early stages of the disease and include loss of inhibition, apathy, social withdrawal, mouthing of objects, and ritualistic compulsive behaviours. These symptoms may lead to misdiagnosis as a psychological or emotion-based problem, or, in older adults, these symptoms can be mistaken for withdrawal or eccentricity.

Many of the early symptoms of FTD are frontal lobe symptoms, which tend to mark out the differences between FTD and the other types of dementia such as ADRD. In ADRD, the initial symptoms tend to be memory impairment, but in FTD, since the frontal lobes of the brain are affected, the first symptoms occur in emotional and social functioning. The mood changes, often leaning toward euphoria, lack of inhibitions, and deterioration in social skills, are clearly noticeable.

A client with FTD may become excessively extroverted, withdrawn, rude, impatient, or aggressive and may make inappropriate remarks in public. The person may exhibit altered sexual behaviour, with a markedly increased interest in sex, which can be linked to loss of inhibition; it can be very disturbing and can get the client into trouble with the police.[7]

Pick's disease is one type of FTD. Pick's disease is marked by the presence of abnormalities in brain cells, called *Pick's bodies*, which are found in the affected areas as well as elsewhere in the brain. Behavioural changes can be very subtle at first; dementia is recognized when behaviour becomes more bizarre. Because of the type of brain damage, the disease also causes gluttony (gross overeating) and increased alcohol intake. Clients with Pick's disease may have a compulsion to put objects in their mouth.[7]

Problems with language can occur in the early stages of FTD but are not as striking as those in the early stages of ADRD. Difficulty finding words and naming objects occurs initially, and as the disease progresses, memory and apraxia become more marked.[7] Someone suffering from FTD will have difficulty maintaining a line of thought, be easily distracted, and have difficulty maintaining conversation for any length of time.[7]

Mixed dementia, which has characteristics of both Alzheimer's disease and vascular dementia, is now believed to be more common than previously thought.[8] This new information is important because scientists now realize that the combination of two diseases may have a greater impact on the brain than only one disease. The symptoms may be similar to Alzheimer's disease or vascular dementia or to both in combination.

SECONDARY DEMENTIAS

In many cases, a client's dementia results from the physical effects of a disease process, from ingestion of damaging substances, or from injury. This type of dementia is called a *secondary* dementia. This section examines some types of secondary dementias.

Parkinson's Disease Dementia

Parkinson's disease is a progressive illness that affects the brain's ability to control movement, resulting in tremors, stiffness, slowness, difficulty walking, and loss of balance. In the later stages of the disease, some people may also develop dementia. Common symptoms include memory loss; difficulty concentrating, thinking, or completing routine tasks; and navigating the environment. People with Parkinson's disease may also develop depression (see Chapter 35), hallucinations, and delusions. See Chapter 37 for a more detailed description of Parkinson's disease.

Creutzfeldt–Jakob Disease

First identified in the 1920s, Creutzfeldt–Jakob disease (CJD) is a very rare disease that causes dementia.[9] CJD appears to have a genetic link or susceptibility in 5% to 15% of cases and can be passed on through infected brain tissue. It is believed to be caused by what are called *proteinaceous prions*, which can live in the body for years before any signs of the disease become obvious. CJD occurs in people between the ages of 50 and 70 years and is a rapid, progressive neurological disease that can affect both humans and animals.

Early signs and symptoms of CJD include fatigue, difficulty sleeping and insomnia, excessive sleepiness, changes in personality, anorexia, progressive deterioration of memory, behaviour disturbances, and spasms of the body. Depression and psychosis are seen in 10% of cases, along with delusions and hallucinations.

CJD is usually rapidly fatal. In later stages, the client will have poor balance and pain, which will cause increasing problems with stability and walking. Dementia becomes obvious, and it eventually leads to a mute, rigid state. Once the signs of CJD become apparent, the progress of the disease is very rapid. There is no known cure for CJD; symptoms are treated to help alleviate distress and pain and to make the client as comfortable as possible. About 90% of patients with CJD die within 1 year of the first symptoms.

Normal Pressure Hydrocephalus

People who have had a history of brain hemorrhage or meningitis are at increased risk for this type of dementia. It is caused by poor reabsorption of cerebrospinal fluid and the resulting buildup of fluid in the brain. The symptoms include difficulty walking, memory loss, and inability to control urination. It can sometimes be corrected with surgical installation of a shunt in the brain to drain off the excess fluid.

Substance-Induced Persisting Dementias

A client whose dementia is a result of the persisting effects of an abused substance, medication, toxic substance exposure, or alcohol may be diagnosed with substance-induced persisting dementia. In this case, the client's cognitive decline may be caused by any of the following:

- Toxic effects of that substance on the brain cells
- Substance-related effects on internal organs, such as liver, heart, and kidneys
- Acquired brain injuries (ABI) related to falls sustained while impaired or disoriented.

It is important to note that any client who has a substance-related persisting dementia should be treated respectfully at all times and no differently from any other client. Support workers need to remember the DIPPS principles and to always act professionally.

Wernicke–Korsakoff Syndrome

Wernicke–Korsakoff syndrome (WKS) is a brain disorder that is caused by lack of thiamine (vitamin B_1); affects the nervous system, including the brain; and is usually associated with alcohol use disorder (heavy alcohol consumption) over a long period. WKS causes impairment of memory and intellectual or cognitive skills such as problem solving or learning, as well as symptoms of nerve damage, including damage to areas of the brain. The most distinguishing symptom is confabulation (fabrication)—the making up of detailed, believable stories about experiences or situations to cover the gaps in the memory.[10]

WKS may also occur in other conditions that involve severe malnutrition. Because of the following, thiamine deficiency is often seen in people who consume excessive amounts of alcohol:

- Many heavy drinkers have poor eating habits. Their nutrition is inadequate and does not contain essential vitamins.
- Alcohol can inflame the stomach lining and impede the body's ability to absorb the key vitamins it receives.

Treatment involves thiamine replacement therapy by intravenous (IV) or intramuscular (IM) injection, together with proper nutrition and hydration. However, the amnesia and brain damage caused by the disease do not always respond to thiamine replacement therapy. In some cases, drug therapy is recommended. If treatment is successful, improvement will become apparent within 2 years, although recovery is slow and often incomplete.[11]

Other Causes of Secondary Dementia

Many other health conditions (see Chapter 37) can also cause secondary dementia, including the following:

- Acquired immune deficiency syndrome (AIDS)
- Huntington's disease
- Multiple sclerosis
- Syphilis

DEPRESSION AND DEMENTIA[12]

Delirium and depression (see Chapter 35) can easily be mistaken for dementia, as they all share many of the same signs and symptoms. For this reason, depression is sometimes called **pseudo-dementia**, meaning false (*pseudo*) dementia. On the other hand, some people who have early ADRD may *seem* depressed but not be. Their symptoms are so similar to depression that their behaviours might be mistaken as simple depression. Symptoms that are common to both depression and dementia include the following:

- Lack of concern for surroundings
- Loss of interest in activities and hobbies
- Social withdrawal and isolation
- Trouble concentrating
- Impaired thinking

However, ***experts estimate that up to 40% of people with ADRD suffer from major depressive disorder as well.*** Depression in the older adult is always of great concern to health care providers, and an accurate diagnosis by a physician is very important. People who have dementia are less likely to tell others of their sadness, hopelessness, guilt, or other feelings associated with depression. It may also be difficult to diagnose depression in clients who have ADRD because their symptoms may differ from those of people who do not have ADRD. Symptom differences may include the following:

- Symptoms of depression may not last as long for people with ADRD.
- Symptoms of depression may come and go in people with ADRD.
- Symptoms of depression may be less severe in people with ADRD.
- People with ADRD may be less likely to talk about or attempt suicide.

Getting appropriate diagnosis and treatment for depression can significantly improve the quality of life of people with ADRD. Treatment includes a combination of medication, counselling, and encouraged socialization and activities.

Supporting a Client With Dementia Who Is Depressed

- Consider encouraging participation in a support group, which is especially helpful to clients in early stages.
- Schedule a predictable daily routine.
- Schedule high-energy activities such as bathing during the client's best time of the day.
- Make a list of activities, people, or places the client enjoys and schedule these things more frequently.
- Assist the client to exercise regularly, particularly in the morning.
- Acknowledge and validate the client's sadness and frustration.

- Frequently express hope that the client will feel better soon.
- Celebrate small successes and occasions.
- Reassure the client that she is loved, respected, and appreciated as part of the family.
- Offer favourite foods to the client.
- Reassure the client that he or she will not be abandoned.

STAGES OF DEMENTIA

One staging system explains three stages of dementia: (1) early, (2) middle, and (3) late. Most dementias are explained in these three stages, which generally apply to ADRD and most other forms of dementia. Another staging system, used by medical professionals, is called the Global Deterioration Scale (also called the Reisberg Scale), which divides the disease process into seven stages. More information about this scale is available on the Internet or from your local Alzheimer Society.

Whichever staging system is used, it is important to remember that ***dementia affects each client differently***. The client's symptoms and behaviours will vary depending on which area of the brain is affected. In the early stages, different dementias can present quite differently but tend to become similar as they progress. Signs and symptoms become more severe with each stage, although the rate of decline will vary from client to client. Eventually, the client will be confined to bed and become totally dependent on others for care. Death occurs when the brain shuts down all body systems.[13]

The order in which the symptoms appear, as well as the length of each stage, will vary from client to client. There is no clear line between the end of one stage and the beginning of another. In many clients, stages will overlap; some may experience many of the symptoms in each stage, and others may experience only a few. There may be fluctuations in a client from day to day, and the person may appear more disoriented one day and less so the next day.

Stage 1: Mild (Early Stage)

A client with dementia is usually cared for at home until symptoms become severe. Clients with dementia may live with family members or may live alone in their own homes and receive support from family, friends, volunteers, and home care workers. The primary caregiver may be the client's spouse, adult child, another family member, or friend. Other caregivers may periodically provide relief to the primary caregiver. Respite care through community day programs and home care may also provide temporary help.

Clients with dementia often need help getting organized, solving simple problems, and remembering appointments, occasions, and medications (TABLE 36–1). They need support and supervision—for example, if a client wants to bake cookies, you will need to make sure that the setting is safe for the activity and that the oven is turned off when the client is finished. Safety is an ongoing concern for the client with dementia, since the person may wander away, swallow a poisonous substance, or leave an appliance on. Ensure a safe setting, and supervise the client at all times. It is your responsibility to follow the client's care plan.

You may need to help a client start an activity or task and then provide only support and encouragement. Some clients with dementia will, however, have problems completing tasks and will need frequent cues, reminders, and repeating of facts and conversations. For example, a client wants to mail a letter but cannot remember the word *stamps* or where they are kept. You help this client remember the word and then help find the stamps. Follow the care plan, which may specify that you should focus on the client's enjoyment of an activity rather than on achievement.

A client in this stage will usually be aware of the diagnosis and will be able to participate in decisions affecting future care. Symptoms can include mild forgetfulness and communication difficulties, such as finding the right word and following a conversation. Some clients are able to stay involved in activities. Some others may become passive or withdrawn, or they may become depressed or anxious because they are frustrated by their changing abilities. It is important to monitor the emotional well-being of the client.

Stage 2: Moderate (Middle Stage)

Further decline occurs in the client's mental and physical abilities in the middle stage (TABLE 36–2).

TABLE 36–1 Typical Symptoms and Support Strategies for Early Stage of Dementia

Abilities Affected	Typical Symptoms of Early Stage of Dementia	Support Strategies for Support Workers, Families, and Caregivers*
Mental abilities	Mild forgetfulness; forgetting recent events Difficulty learning new things and following conversations Difficulty concentrating or limited attention span Difficulties with orientation, such as getting lost or not following directions Communication difficulties such as finding the right word Difficulty finding words, finishing thoughts, following directions, and remembering names Occasional disorientation to person, time, and place Difficulty performing everyday tasks Poor judgement; bad decisions (including when driving)	Use labels, notes, calendars, alarms, or timers to assist with memory cues. Pill dispensers and dosettes may assist with remembering when to take medications. Post emergency numbers by the telephone so they are easy to see. Break tasks into small steps. Keep group sizes small to reduce noise and overstimulation. Encourage the client to engage in conversation. Ask the client short questions. Ask questions frequently, if necessary. Encourage activities that are manageable. Follow routines as much as possible. Have someone escort the client to doctors' appointments so as to assist the client to relay concerns to the doctor. Register the client with the Alzheimer Society MedicAlert Safely Home registry. The family should discuss the client's driving with the family doctor; the support worker should discuss concerns with the supervisor. The family should discourage the client from driving and offer to drive the client to a destination if needed.

Continued

TABLE 36–1 Typical Symptoms and Support Strategies for Early Stage of Dementia—cont'd

Abilities Affected	Typical Symptoms of Early Stage of Dementia	Support Strategies for Support Workers, Families, and Caregivers*
Moods and emotions	Blaming others for mistakes, forgetfulness, and other issues Mood shifts Symptoms of depression, irritability, or defensiveness	Encourage nutritious foods. Allow the client to verbalize thoughts and feelings. Encourage meditation or stress-relieving activities. Seek medical assistance to see if medications can help the client.
Behaviours	Lack of spontaneity—less outgoing or less interested in things Passive Withdrawn from usual activities Restless	Encourage the client to stay physically fit. Encourage social connectedness with family and friends. Encourage the client to participate in activities that bring meaning and pleasure. Encourage participation in activities and events.
Physical abilities	Mild coordination problems	Have the client focus on activities that can be performed safely. Encourage the use of safety features such as handrails and grab bars. Remove tripping hazards from the home environment, such as scatter rugs and loose cords. Increase the lighting to improve visibility in areas around stairs, hallways, and entrances.

*Also refer to this chapter for more suggestions.
Source: Alzheimer Society of Canada. (2016). *Stages of Alzheimer's disease.* Retrieved from http://www.alzheimer.ca/en/About-dementia/Alzheimer-s-disease/Stages-of-Alzheimer-s-disease.

TABLE 36–2 Typical Symptoms and Support Strategies for Middle Stage of Dementia

Abilities Affected	Typical Symptoms of Middle Stage of Dementia	Support Strategies for Support Workers, Families, and Caregivers
Mental abilities	Memory loss increases—failure to recognize family and friends Forgetting personal history Disorientation to time and place Increasing restlessness during the evening hours (*sundowning*) Increased episodes of disorientation Development of sleep problems Dulled senses—inability to tell the difference between hot and cold and to recognize dangers Movement and gait problems—walking slowly; having a shuffling gait Communication problems—inability to follow directions; difficulty reading, writing, and math; speaking in short sentences or single words; statements not making sense	Use **cueing** to assist the client—use pictures, notes, signs, or seasonal objects. If the client is struggling to remember, offer information such as names in the conversation. Speak slowly and clearly. Use simple language, and repeat the message if necessary. Avoid abstract questions such as "What do you think about . . . ?" Ask concrete questions instead, such as "Do you think it is cold today?" Use physical gestures to reinforce your message. Limit choices to one or two.
Moods and emotions	Loss of impulse control—foul language, poor table manners, sexual aggression, rudeness Personality change Disorientation Anxiety or apprehension Suspiciousness Mood shifts Anger, hostile behaviours; violent behaviour Sadness or depression	Remember that the client is not intentionally being difficult. Try to identify and address the emotions behind the client's behaviours. Do not focus solely on the client's words. Encourage a healthy lifestyle, including healthy eating, physical activity, and familiar and meaningful activities. Reassure and comfort the client. Encourage the client to reminisce as a helpful strategy. Avoid disagreeing, arguing, or trying to convince the client that he is incorrect.

Continued

TABLE 36–2 Typical Symptoms and Support Strategies for Middle Stage of Dementia—cont'd

Abilities Affected	Typical Symptoms of Middle Stage of Dementia	Support Strategies for Support Workers, Families, and Caregivers
Behaviours	Declining ability to concentrate Restlessness (pacing, wandering) Repetition of movements and statements—moving things back and forth constantly Saying the same thing over and over again Delusions Aggression Uninhibited behaviours Passive behaviour	Remember that all behaviour has meaning. Try to identify the cause for that particular behaviour: Too much noise? Too many people? Hungry? In pain? Too hot? Cold? Uncomfortable? Irritated? Hungry? Need to toilet? Watch for behaviour changes that may result from a physical illness such as a UTI or the flu. Contact the Alzheimer Society to register the client in the MedicAlert Safely Home registry to help ensure the client's safety.
Physical abilities	Bowel and bladder incontinence Need for help with ADLs—bathing, feeding, and dressing self Fear of bathing; refusal to change clothes Disrupted sleep patterns Appetite fluctuations Language difficulties Visual–spatial problems	Know and maintain the client's preferred tastes and past routines. Keep style of clothing and hair simple and easy to maintain. Adjust schedules to make them as comfortable for the client as possible. Adapt activities to accommodate for lost abilities and make the most of the remaining abilities. Identify and prevent any potential hazards in the home (e.g., install grab bars). Have family or your supervisor consult an occupational therapist for advice on routines, activities, and ways to adapt the house to make it as safe and as accommodating as possible.

Source: Alzheimer Society of Canada. (2016). *Stages of Alzheimer's disease.* Retrieved from http://www.alzheimer.ca/en/About-dementia/Alzheimer-s-disease/Stages-of-Alzheimer-s-disease.

Memory will continue to deteriorate as the client forgets personal history and no longer recognizes family and friends. Some clients become restless and pace constantly or may wander off. Registering the client with the MedicAlert Safely Home program will provide peace of mind to the client's family, as the client can be easily located should she become lost.

A client may react in a number of ways to the loss of abilities. For example, the person may become less involved in activities or may repeat the same action or word over and over again. The local Alzheimer Society can provide education about the disease, resources, and support for clients and their families and can assist them to develop strategies to deal with difficult situations.

As the client's dementia progresses, the need for assistance increases. Usually, there comes a time when family and friends can no longer deal with the situation or meet all the client's needs. The client may be unable to tolerate wearing dentures or eyeglasses, which can increase the client's risk for injury. Such issues should be detailed in the client's care plan and noted by caregivers. Increased disorientation to time and place will also necessitate assistance with ADLs such as dressing, bathing, and using the toilet.

Community day programs, respite care, home care, and help from family members, friends, and volunteers are no longer enough at this stage. Long-term care is needed when at least one of the following occurs:

- Family members and friends are not able to meet the client's needs.
- Family members themselves have health problems.
- The client's behaviours present a danger to self or others.
- The client no longer recognizes the caregiver.

Many long-term care facilities have special care units (SCUs) for clients with dementia. The health care team ensures that their needs are met. Many facilities provide hospice care for those in the final stages of dementia.

When a client with dementia moves to a facility, the family or close friends usually continue to be involved in care, as they are an important part of the health care team. Some family members and friends may take part in facility activities, and, for many clients with dementia, they can provide comfort and support. Often, the client may be admitted to a locked SCU that will provide the safety and security the client needs. This type of unit will reduce the client's risk for injury if the client is prone to wandering.

Stage 3: Severe (Late Stage)

In this last stage, the client is incapable of remembering, communicating, or performing self-care (TABLE 36–3) and requires care 24 hours a day. Eventually, the client will become bedridden, have difficulty eating or swallowing, and lose control of bodily functions. This stage eventually ends with the client's death, often from secondary complications such as pneumonia.

SUPPORTING CLIENTS WITH DEMENTIA

Each client with dementia has unique care needs, depending on the form of dementia, the stage of the dementia, and the care setting. The *Think About Safety: The ABCDs of Managing Responsive or Challenging Behaviours* box on page 834 lists general guidelines for caring for clients with dementia. The care plan and your supervisor will give you specific instructions for each client.

Meeting Basic Client Needs

Many clients are able to remain in their own homes longer if their environment can be adapted to function effectively and safely. Over time, however, clients with dementia become dependent on others for all care—safety, hygiene, grooming, dressing, and elimination, as well as nutrition and fluids, exercise, health, comfort, and therapy. Follow the care plan. Other ways to assist the client to meet basic needs include the following:

- Meet food and fluid needs (see Chapter 28). Provide finger foods. Cut food into small bits and pour out liquids, as needed.
- Provide good skin care (see Chapters 24, 30, and 31). Keep skin free of urine and stool.

TABLE 36–3 Typical Symptoms and Support Strategies for Late Stage of Dementia

Abilities Affected	Typical Symptoms of Late Stage of Dementia	Support Strategies for Support Workers, Families, and Caregivers
Mental abilities	Loss of ability to remember, to communicate verbally, or to function independently Inability to process information Severe speaking difficulties Severe disorientation to time, place, and people Seizures (see Chapter 37) Constant state of disorientation—inability to recognize self, family members, or others Total dependence on others for all ADLs Total urinary and fecal incontinence	Use the senses to allow the client to connect: *Touch:* Hold the client's hand. Brush the hair. Give a gentle massage to the hands, legs, or feet. Have the client stroke a pet or a soft cloth. *Smell:* Olfactory (smell) memories can be very powerful! Introduce items such as perfumes, a flower, or food that the client once enjoyed. *Vision:* DVDs with quiet scenes of nature or calming sounds can be relaxing for a client. *Hearing:* Reading in a comforting tone can be soothing for the client, even if the person can no longer understand the words. *What* you say is not as important as *how* you say it!
Moods and emotions	Withdrawal from conversations	Fill a box with items that represent the person's interests, favourite activities, past work, and happy memories. Have photos and other memorabilia around for the client to see. Provide the client with the opportunity to hear, smell, taste, or see items that are associated with familiar rituals of spirituality that the client would remember.

Continued

TABLE 36–3 Typical Symptoms and Support Strategies for Late Stage of Dementia—cont'd

Abilities Affected	Typical Symptoms of Late Stage of Dementia	Support Strategies for Support Workers, Families, and Caregivers
Behaviours	Nonverbal communication (eye contact, crying, groaning) Inability to speak (groaning, grunting, or screaming)	Look closely at the client, and try to identify the source of the client's communication responses. Use cueing, whenever possible, to identify the causes of these behaviours.
Physical abilities	Increased sleep problems or sleeping longer and more often Confinement to bed—inability to sit or walk Loss of ability to speak Loss of control of bladder and bowels Difficulty eating and swallowing—increased risk for choking and aspiration Inability to dress or bathe Loss of weight Coma, death	Provide a safe, calming environment away from distractions. Ensure that the client is in a comfortable, upright position during and after meals. Allow plenty of time for the client to eat. Offer small, frequent meals and snacks rather than three big meals. Change the client's position every 2 hours, and provide proper skin care (see Chapters 25, 26, and 30). Set a toileting schedule (see Chapters 32 and 33). Provide adequate hydration during the day (see Chapter 28). Monitor bowel movements (see Chapter 33).

Source: Alzheimer Society of Canada. (2016). *Stages of Alzheimer's disease.* Retrieved from http://www.alzheimer.ca/en/About-dementia/Alzheimer-s-disease/Stages-of-Alzheimer-s-disease.

- Promote urinary and fecal elimination (see Chapters 32 and 33).
- Provide incontinence care as needed (see Chapters 32 and 33).
- Provide frequent toileting at regular intervals throughout the day and night.
- Promote exercise and activity during the day (see Chapter 26). Activity helps reduce wandering and sundowning behaviours (see p. 830). The client may also sleep better.
- Reduce intake of coffee, tea, and cola drinks, which contain caffeine. Caffeine is a stimulant that can increase restlessness, disorientation, and agitation.[14]
- Provide a quiet, restful setting (see Chapter 12). Soft music is better than loud TV programs.

- Play soft music during care activities such as bathing and during meals.
- Promote personal hygiene (see Chapter 30), but do not force the client into a shower or tub, as clients with dementia are often afraid of bathing. Try bathing the client when she is calm, using the client's preferred bathing method—tub bath, shower, bed bath, or towel bath. Follow the care plan. Provide privacy, and keep the client warm. Do not rush the client.
- Provide oral hygiene (see Chapter 30).
- Choose clothing options that are comfortable and easy to put on—for example, front-opening garments. Pullover tops are harder to put on, and the client may become frightened when the head is inside the pullover top.
- Clothing that closes with Velcro is easy to put on and take off. Buttons, zippers, snaps, and other closures that are hard to handle can frustrate the client.
- Offer simple clothing choices. Let the client choose between two shirts or blouses, two pants or slacks, and so on.
- Lay out clothing in the order it will be put on. Hand the client one clothing item at a time. Describe or show the client what to do, and do not rush him.
- Have equipment ready for any procedure to reduce the amount of time the client is involved in care measures.
- Observe for signs and symptoms of health problems (see Chapter 37).
- Prevent infection. Assist with handwashing when necessary (see Chapter 23).

Safety

Clients need a safe, quiet setting. They do not recognize safety hazards and are at risk for falls. If a client with dementia falls, he may not understand why it is unsafe to move after the fall. Because you should never use force or hold a client down, you may need to allow the client to move about. Talk to the client in a quiet and soothing voice until someone can assist you.

Clients may feel fearful even in a safe, quiet setting. They do not understand what is happening to them, so always explain calmly what you are going to do. Be prepared to repeat yourself since clients with dementia are often not able to retain information. Clients may be at increased risk for injury if they are combative or aggressive. Family members or caregivers (who are tired and weary) may be more likely to restrain or confine clients in their care so as to be able to manage them.

Ways to ensure client safety include the following:

- Remove harmful, sharp, and breakable objects—such as knives, scissors, glass, dishes, razors, and tools—from the area.
- Provide eating and drinking utensils that cannot be easily broken by the client so as to help prevent cuts and injuries.
- Place safety plugs in electrical outlets.
- Keep cords and electrical equipment out of reach.
- Remove electrical appliances—for example, hair dryers, curling or flat irons, makeup mirrors, and electric shavers—from the bathroom.
- Store personal care items—shampoo, deodorant, lotion, and so on—in a safe place.
- Use baby locks on doors to cabinets that contain medications or cleaning products.
- Store household cleaners and medications in locked storage areas.
- Store dangerous equipment and tools in a safe place.
- Supervise the client when the client smokes.
- Store cigarettes, cigars, pipes, matches, and other smoking materials in a safe place.
- Practise safety measures to prevent falls, burns, choking, poisoning, and fires (see Chapter 22).
- Keep all doors to kitchens, utility rooms, and housekeeping closets locked.

Hygiene, Grooming, and Dressing

Clients with moderate or severe dementia do not understand the need for personal hygiene and aseptic practices. They have to rely on the health care team to ensure good skin care (to prevent skin breakdown) and to help prevent the spread of infection. You assist them with handwashing at the following times:

- After they have urinated or defecated
- After they have coughed, sneezed, or blown the nose
- Before or after they have handled or eaten food
- Any time their hands become soiled

During personal care, look for signs or symptoms of conditions that may cause pain (e.g., skin lesions, rough pieces of clothing, or dental problems). It is important to know that these clients may resist your efforts to keep them clean and dry, as they do not understand what is happening or why. They may fear harm or danger when you get too close or touch them, so they may become agitated and combative (hitting or kicking); shout and cry out for help; or pull away during care. Sudden movements can cause skin tears. Refer to the section "Managing Challenging or Responsive Behaviours" on page 834.

Elimination Needs

Clients with moderate and severe dementia may urinate in the wrong places—for example, garbage cans, planters, and heating vents. Some may remove incontinence products and throw them on the floor or in the toilet. Some may soil themselves, the furniture, or the walls. Offer to assist with elimination needs frequently at regular times during both day and night. Provide perineal care after urinary and fecal elimination. Ask your supervisor for help if a client resists you. Never restrict fluid intake in an effort to control elimination.

Nutrition

Clients with dementia may become distracted during meals, or it may be hard for them to sit long enough to eat a meal. Some with later stage dementia forget how to use eating utensils, so finger foods can be offered to them instead. Some clients have problems swallowing (see Chapter 28), and some have to be fed. Some clients will resist your efforts to assist them with eating, and disoriented clients may throw or spit food. A quiet and calm environment in the dining area and special mealtimes are often helpful. Clients may be able to eat small amounts more frequently, rather than only three times a day.

Fluids

Clients with moderate and severe dementia are at risk for dehydration, as they do not recognize thirst. Encourage them to drink fluids regularly. Keep water and other fluids nearby, and offer fluids whenever you are around them. Remember that adequate fluids can reduce the risk for serious problems such as UTI or constipation.

Exercise

Inactivity and immobility are risk factors for pneumonia and pressure ulcers. Exercise is therefore important for clients with dementia, but they may resist it because they do not understand what is happening and may fear harm. They may become agitated and combative or cry out for help. Do not force a client to exercise or take part in activities. Stay calm. Ask your supervisor for help if needed. Follow the care plan.

Health Issues

Many clients with dementia have other health issues or injuries. However, they may not notice or recognize pain, fever, constipation, incontinence, or other signs and symptoms. Changes in usual behaviour may signal pain, discomfort, or delirium, which should be medically investigated immediately (see p. 807). A client who normally moans and groans all the time may become quiet and withdrawn; a client who is usually friendly and outgoing may become agitated and aggressive; a client who is nonverbal and quiet may become restless and cry easily. Loss of appetite may also signal pain. Report any changes in a client's usual behaviour to your supervisor.

The client must be kept free from abuse and neglect. Caring for clients with dementia is often very frustrating because some behaviours can be hard to deal with. Family caregivers and health care providers can become frustrated and short-tempered. Protect clients with dementia from abuse. Report any signs of abuse to your supervisor at once. If you are becoming frustrated with a client, talk to your supervisor. An assignment change may be needed.

Comfort

Comfort is important in the care of a client with dementia, so make sure that the client is physically comfortable. A quiet environment, talking in a calm voice, massage, soothing touch, music, and aromatherapy are all comforting and relaxing. Make sure that the client's clothing is also comfortable.

Sleep

- Dementia interferes with a person's ability to make decisions and to remember, so it is your responsibility to meet a disoriented client's physical and safety needs. Fatigue and visual changes, which are common with some dementias (e.g., Alzheimer's disease), can be stressful on the client. Ways to enhance the client's ability to fall asleep include the following:

- Follow bedtime rituals.
- Use night lights, which will help prevent accidents and disorientation.
- Limit caffeine intake during the day.
- Discourage naps during the day.
- Encourage exercise during the day.
- Reduce noises.

Socialization Therapy and Activities

Clients with dementia need to feel worthy and useful and to remain active in order to promote emotional and physical health. Clients should be encouraged to do what they can and what they enjoy. For example, a man who used to be a good dancer can take part in dancing activities. A woman who likes to draw can be encouraged to join a painting group. The social contact may be as important as the activity itself.

Adult day programs and long-term care facilities provide therapy and activities—such as music programs, art programs, fitness programs, and support groups—to meet the client's needs and cognitive abilities. Therapists may work with one client, a small group, or a large group.

In adult community settings, support workers often work with clients in the early stage of dementia. Many of these clients have care requirements but may be able to make some decisions for themselves. Your support enables these clients to remain in their homes.

Communication

Clients with dementia may develop communication problems. At first, they find it hard to find the right

Think About Safety

Supporting Clients With Disorientation or Dementia

- When visiting clients who have dementia, you should introduce yourself every time you see them, no matter how well they once knew you.
- Maintain the day–night cycle. Open curtains, shades, and drapes during the day. Close them at night. Use a night light at night. The client should wear regular clothes during the day—not sleepwear.
- To ensure the client's safety, try to keep the surroundings calm, quiet, and peaceful. Prevent loud noises, hurried movements, and congested hallways and rooms.
- Talk about current events and plans for the day. Keep discussions as short as possible. Allow time for the client to respond.
- Follow the client's established routine. Having a schedule for meals, bathing, exercise, TV, and other activities promotes a sense of order and of what to expect.
- When taking care of a client who is disoriented, frequently remind the person of her location.
- Break tasks into small steps when assisting the client.
- Do not rearrange furniture or the client's personal belongings.
- Encourage self-care.
- Be consistent.
- Place picture signs in rooms, bathrooms, dining rooms, and other areas (**FIGURE 36–1** on page 827). Follow your supervisor's directions.
- Keep personal items where the client can see them.
- Stay within sight to the extent possible. Do not leave the client unsupervised.
- Place memory aids (large clocks and calendars) where the client can see them.
- Keep noise levels low.
- Play music and show movies from the client's past.
- Provide frequent toileting at regular intervals.
- Select tasks and activities specific to the client's cognitive abilities and interests.
- Contact your local Alzheimer Society (or go online) for other suggestions on how to maintain client safety.

Providing Compassionate Care
The Client With Dementia

- ***Dignity.*** Clients with dementia do not choose to be forgetful, incontinent, agitated, angry, or rude. Nor do they choose to display other behaviours, signs, and symptoms of the disease. They cannot control what is happening to them; it is the disease that causes the behaviours. ***The dementia is responsible, not the client.***

  Treat all clients with dementia with dignity and respect. They have rights under human rights codes and long-term care legislation. In the advanced stages of dementia, they may not know or be able to exercise their rights, but they are still entitled to them. Be patient and calm when caring for clients with dementia. Always explain what you are going to do. Do not assume that the client cannot understand you.

  Take care never to make the client feel foolish about forgetting or misplacing something. Even in the later stages of dementia, clients can still feel embarrassment and shame. Protect the client's dignity when you are providing care. Only those involved in the client's care should be present for care procedures.
- ***Independence.*** The client has the right to autonomy. Clients with dementia should be encouraged to be independent for as long as safely possible. Encourage clients to do what they can for themselves.
- ***Preferences.*** Personal choice is important. Clients with early stage dementia can voice their preferences. Encourage clients with moderate stage dementia to make simple choices—for example, choosing one of two sweaters or watching or not watching TV. The family or substitute decision maker usually makes choices regarding bath times, menus, clothing, activities, and other care if the client is not able to.

  A client may choose to use a special pillow or blanket. The client may insist on wearing a particular sweater or cardigan because the item may have special meaning, or it may provide comfort and security. Eventually, the client may not know why the item is important or may not even recognize it. However, do not remove the item, as it is still important to the person.

  With Alzheimer's disease and most other dementias, clients continue to experience all forms of emotions well into the final stages. When a client can no longer use language, being able to recognize the client's emotional state can help you determine wishes, preferences, fears, likes, and dislikes.
- ***Privacy.*** The client has the right to privacy and confidentiality. Provide space and privacy for the client to visit with others. Protect confidentiality. Do not share information about the client with others. Do not relate stories about the client's behaviour to others.
- ***Safety.*** A safe, quiet, and calm setting promotes quality of life. Follow the safety measures in Chapter 22. All clients have the right to be free from restraints, which require a physician's order in any case and are used only if it is the best way to protect the client, ***not*** for the convenience of the health care team. Restraints can worsen disoriented and agitated behaviours. Your supervisor will tell you when to use restraints.

word. As the dementia progresses, clients speak in short sentences or in a few words, and often their speech is not understandable. Ways to enhance your communication include the following:

- Approach the client in a calm, quiet manner.
- Approach the client from the front. Do not approach from the side or back, as doing so can startle the client.
- Smile. Most clients instinctively respond favourably to a person smiling.
- Address the client by name every time you are in contact.
- State your name. Show your name tag.
- Use language and terms the client will understand, particularly if the client is used to speaking another language. Family members will often assist you with this.

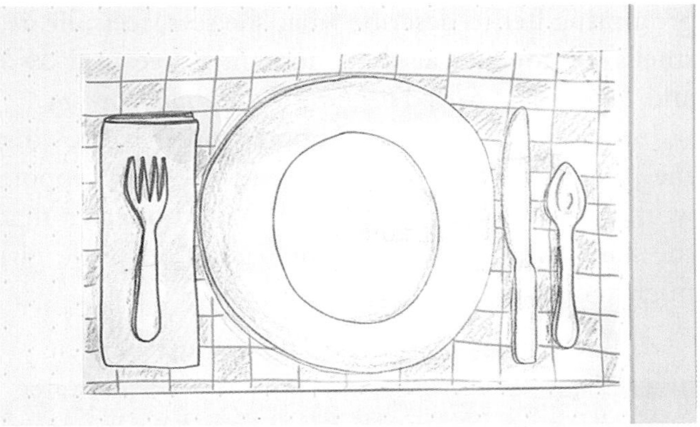

FIGURE 36–1 Signs provide cues to clients with dementia. This one is used to identify the dining room. (**Source:** Sorrentino, S.A., & Gorek, B. (2003). *Mosby's textbook for long-term care assistants* (4th ed., p. 670). St. Louis, MO: Mosby.)

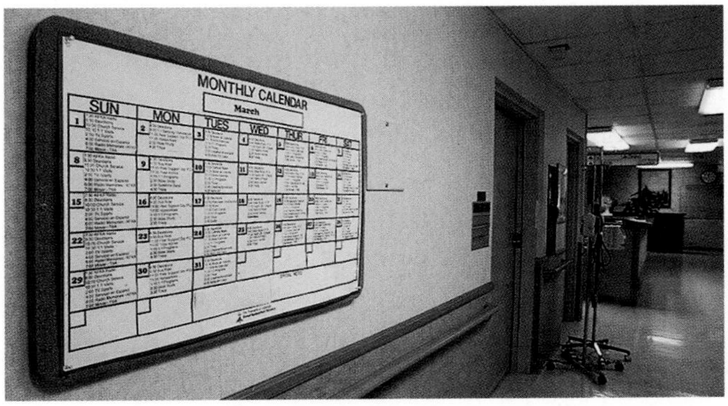

FIGURE 36–2 A large calendar listing the date and the day's events can be helpful to clients with disorientation or dementia.

- Give the date and time each morning. Repeat as needed during the day or evening.
- Explain what you are going to do and why.
- Give clear, simple directions and answers to questions.
- Ask clear and simple questions that require only simple answers. Give the client time to respond. Do not interrupt or rush her.
- Keep calendars and clocks with large numbers in the client's room and in other areas (FIGURE 36–2). Remind the client of holidays, birthdays, and special events.
- Have the client wear glasses and a hearing aid if the client uses them.
- Use touch to communicate (see Chapter 5).
- Place familiar objects and pictures within the client's view.
- Provide newspapers, magazines, TV, and radio. Read to the client if appropriate.
- Discuss current events with the client.
- Identify other people by their names. Avoid using pronouns (*he*, *she*, *they*, and so on).
- Practise measures to promote communication (see Chapter 5).
- Use gestures and cues. Pointing to objects may improve the client's understanding.
- Speak in a calm, gentle voice.
- Speak slowly. Use simple words and sentences.
- Do not criticize, correct, or argue with the client.
- Present one idea, question, or instruction at a time.
- Do not present the client with many choices.
- Provide simple explanations of all procedures and activities.
- Give consistent responses.
- Repeat information frequently. Usually, the client cannot remember new information.

MANAGING CHALLENGING OR RESPONSIVE BEHAVIOURS

Clients with dementia often display challenging behaviours, many of which may be disruptive to other clients or residents around them and may even challenge the abilities of the caregivers to provide compassionate care.

Challenging behaviours usually originate as a *response* to an illness, infection, or physical discomfort. They are, therefore, often referred to as *responsive* behaviours. It is important for you to remember that ***all behaviour has meaning. Clients who demonstrate behaviours that challenge caregivers are merely responding to something in their internal or external environment. It is the responsibility of all caregivers to try to understand these behaviours and to try to remedy the situation, following the DIPPS principles (dignity, independence, privacy, preferences, and safety).***

It is important to know that clients' responsive behaviours result from their dementia. Clients with dementia cannot control their actions, so you should never take their behaviours personally, become upset or angry with the clients, or blame yourself for their behaviours.

Clients with dementia may be unable to understand that they are cold or hungry because their brain may (1) no longer be able to sort out the vast number of messages received, (2) no longer send out the correct message to other parts of the brain, or (3) not be able to understand the meaning behind certain actions. As a result, the client with dementia may act out, become very resistant to staff, or even become very vocal or physically combative. Some clients with dementia may become aggressive toward other clients or toward the caregiving staff and may even spit, bite, or punch others. If a client is demonstrating aggressive behaviours, you need to ensure your own safety and that of others. You should also report unusual or increased instances of responsive behaviours. Your observations are very important in determining the causes of the person's behaviour (see the *Think About Safety: The ABCDs of Managing Responsive or Challenging Behaviours* box on p. 834).

As a support worker, you must learn how to safely and respectfully care for clients who can no longer communicate in the manner that they once did. You should try to determine what the client is trying to tell you. At all times, you should focus on the client's right to dignity, independence, privacy, preferences, and safety.

Validation Therapy

Validation therapy is a type of therapy for people with dementia that focuses on empathy and advocates accepting the affected person's perception of reality. Developed by Naomi Feil and practised throughout the world, validation therapy aims to make the client feel supported and respected. Rather than trying to bring the client with dementia back to our reality, this therapy suggests it is less stressful for the client if caregivers simply refrain from "challenging" or disagreeing with the client.[15]

For instance, if a person with dementia believes that she is waiting for her children, all now middle-aged, to return from school, family members and caregivers who use validation therapy would not argue the point or expect the person with dementia to have insight into her behaviour. They would not correct her beliefs but would simply allow the client to discuss *her perception of reality*.[15] The caregiver can focus on descriptive clues the client provides, prompting her to describe what she sees, feels, hears, smells, or touches at that moment.[15] See **BOX 36–3** and *Supporting Mrs. Yi: Using Validation Therapy*.

In this discussion, the support worker is allowing the client to lead the conversation. The support worker does not challenge Mrs. Yi, who states that she has a little girl, when, in reality, her little girl might be an older adult herself!

BOX 36–3 Principles of Validation Therapy

1. All people are unique and must be treated as individuals.
2. All people are valuable, no matter how disoriented they are.
3. There is a reason behind the behavior of disoriented old-old people.
4. Behavior in old-old age is not merely a function of anatomic changes in the brain, but reflects a combination of physical, social, and psychological changes that take place over the lifespan.
5. Old-old people cannot be forced to change their behaviors. Behaviors can be changed only if the person wants to change them.
6. Old-old people must be accepted nonjudgementally.
7. Particular life tasks are associated with each stage of life. Failure to complete a task at the appropriate stage of life may lead to psychological problems.
8. When more recent memory fails, older adults try to restore balance in their lives by retrieving earlier memories. When eyesight fails, they use the mind's eye to see. When hearing goes, they listen to sounds from the past.
9. Painful feelings that are expressed, acknowledged, and validated by a trusted listener will diminish. Painful feelings that are ignored or suppressed will gain strength.
10. Empathy builds trust, reduces anxiety, and restores dignity.

Source: Naomi Feil. (1993). *Validation therapy.* Retrieved from http://www.walking-in-their-shoes.com/validation-therapy.html.

Supporting Mrs. Yi: Using Validation Therapy

Mrs. Yi (who is 88 years old): I can't find my little girl.
Support worker: You are looking for your little girl? What is her name?
Mrs. Yi: Jia. Jia left the house this morning without a sweater, and it's cold outside!
Support worker: What did Jia wear this morning?
Mrs. Yi: It is so cold today. I know that Jia is cold.
Support worker: Yes, it is cold. Are you feeling cold?
Mrs. Yi: I am so cold.
Support worker: Let's get you a sweater to wear to keep you warm.
Mrs. Yi: I am so cold.

Gentle Persuasive Approaches

Across Canada and in some parts of the United States, many agencies have begun to use the **Gentle Persuasive Approaches (GPA)** program, designed to train health care workers in techniques used to handle and reduce responsive behaviours—for example, grabbing, biting, and hitting—that are associated with dementias such as Alzheimer's disease. Initially designed for long-term care home staff in 2004, GPA teaches workers to be self-protective, respectful, and nonviolent in vulnerable care situations and to prevent potential workplace injury.[16]

Preventing Wandering

Clients with dementia are not oriented to person, time, and place, so they may wander away and not be able to find their way back. They may wander off very quickly by foot, car, bicycle, or other means. They may be with you one moment and gone the next.

Judgement in these clients is poor. They cannot tell what is safe and what is dangerous, so they are at high risk for life-threatening accidents. They can walk into traffic or into a nearby lake, river, or forest.

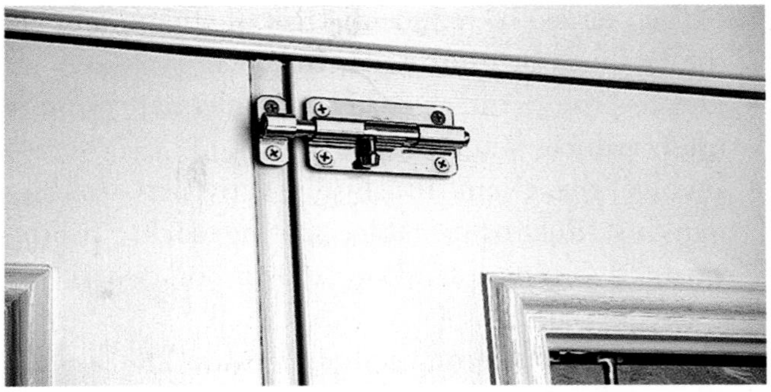

FIGURE 36–3 A slide lock is placed at the top of the door.

If not properly dressed, they are at risk for heat or cold exposure.

Wandering may have no cause or may have a legitimate cause that the client cannot articulate (tell you). For example, the client may be looking for something or someone—the bathroom, the bedroom, a child, or a partner. The client may also be experiencing pain, adverse effects of medications, stress, restlessness, or anxiety.

For clients living at home or in facilities, the Alzheimer Society of Canada provides, for a small fee, a nationwide service called MedicAlert Safely Home, which serves to identify and safely return people who wander off or become lost. A family member completes a form and provides a recent picture of the client. This information is entered into a national database, and the client is given an ID card and bracelet. Anyone finding a lost client can call the police, who then will call the family member or caregiver. Ways to prevent injury in clients who have a tendency to wander include the following:

- Follow facility policy for locking doors and windows. In community settings, locks are often placed at the tops and bottoms of doors (**FIGURE 36–3**), as the client is not likely to look for a lock in these places.
- Keep door alarms and electronic doors turned on. The alarm should be set to go off whenever the door is opened.
- Follow facility policy for fire exits. Everyone must be able to leave the building if a fire occurs.
- Make sure the client wears a facility ID bracelet or MedicAlert Safely Home registry ID at all times.
- Agencies may camouflage exits or hazardous equipment that cannot be put away (such as

oxygen tanks) to reduce the risk of clients' leaving the facilities or injuring themselves.
- Exercise the client, as ordered, as adequate exercise often reduces wandering.
- Involve the client in simple activities—folding napkins, dusting a table, sorting socks, rolling yarn, sweeping, sanding blocks of wood, or watering plants.
- Do not use restraints, as they tend to increase the client's disorientation and can make him agitated. Remember, too, that restraints require a physician's order.
- Do not argue with the client who wants to leave. The client does not understand what you are saying.
- Go with the client who insists on going outside. Make sure the client is properly dressed. Guide the client inside after a few minutes (**FIGURE 36–4**).

Secured Units

Some long-term care residents tend to wander throughout the facility or try to leave the building, which may put them at risk for injury. These residents may be moved to a secured unit—an area in the facility where entrances and exits are locked—which provides a safe setting for residents to move about but not wander away.

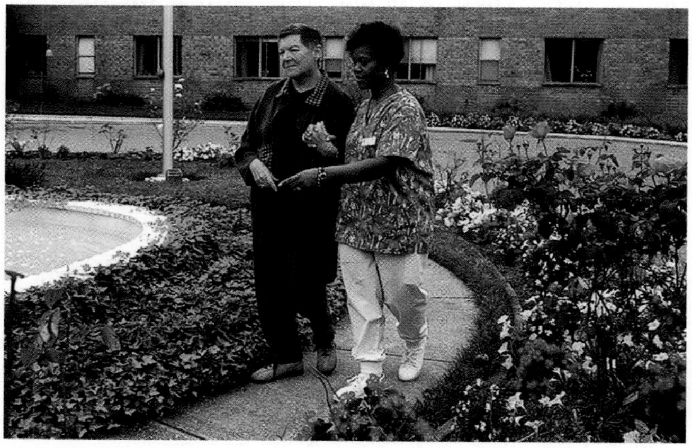

FIGURE 36–4 Walk with the client who wants to go outside, and then guide the client back inside after a few minutes. Note how this support worker is pointing out things for the client to look at. This action can sometimes help trigger the client's long-term memories. (**Source:** Sorrentino, S.A., & Gorek, B. (2003). *Mosby's textbook for long-term care assistants* (4th ed., p. 670). St. Louis, MO: Mosby.)

Secured units are considered a form of environmental restraint, so the facility must take care to use the least restrictive approach. A dementia diagnosis and a physician's order are needed to place a resident in a secured unit, and the health care team should regularly review the client's need to be in a secured unit, always taking care to protect the resident's rights.

As the dementia progresses to the advanced stage, a secured unit is no longer needed, as the client cannot sit or walk and is bedridden. Since wandering is not a risk anymore, the client is transferred to another unit.

Standards of care for special care units have been established by legislation. Staff must have special training in the care of people with dementia. The unit must have programs that promote clients' dignity, personal freedom, and safety.

Sundowning

Sundowning is a condition in which the signs, symptoms, and behaviours of dementia increase during the hours of darkness—in the late afternoon and evening hours. As daylight ends and darkness sets in, disorientation, restlessness, anxiety, agitation, and other symptoms increase. Behaviour worsens after the sun goes down and may deteriorate throughout the night. The client may be afraid of the dark or may see things that are not there because of poor lighting or shadows.

If the client tells you, for example, that there is a "strange person" in the room, you should never ignore the client's statement. Turn the light on, and reassure the client. Remove things that may be casting a shadow or disturbing the client, and provide the client with verbal reassurance. See the *Supporting Reverend Welikij: How Sundowning Can Upset Families* box, on page 833. Ways to reduce the likelihood of client injury or agitation due to sundowning include the following:

- Complete treatments early in the day if doing so will reduce the client's agitation.
- Provide a calm, quiet setting late in the day. Playing soft music may help.
- Ensure that the client is clean and dry and is in no danger of falling from the bed or chair.

- Do not restrain the client.
- Encourage exercise and activity early in the day.
- Hunger can increase restlessness. The client who is experiencing sundowning may be tired or hungry, may have to go to the washroom, or may not recognize the place.
- Promote regular elimination. The need to eliminate can increase restlessness.
- Do not try to reason with the client, as communication is impaired, and the person cannot think or speak clearly.
- Shadows can be disturbing for some clients. Keep the environment well lit.

Hallucinations and Delusions

A *hallucination* is seeing, hearing, or feeling something that is not real. Senses are dulled in affected people, who see animals, insects, or people who are not really present. Some may hear voices, feel bugs crawling on them, or feel that they are being touched by someone.

Delusions are false beliefs. A client with dementia may believe that a doll is a baby or that a spouse has been unfaithful. Some may believe that they are being held captive, killed, or attacked. A client may believe that the caregiver is someone else. Many other false beliefs that can cause intense fear or other emotions in the client can occur.

Ways to diminish the impact of hallucinations or delusions on the client with dementia include the following:

- Ensure the client wears eyeglasses and hearing aids, as prescribed. The problem can be made worse by impaired vision or hearing. Follow the care plan.
- Do not argue with the client.
- Reassure the client. Say that you will ensure protection from harm.
- Distract the client with some item or activity. Taking the client for a walk may be helpful.
- Use touch to calm and reassure the client (**FIGURE 36–5**).
- Eliminate noises that the client could misinterpret and that could be upsetting—for example, noises from the TV, radio, stereo, furnaces, air conditioners, appliances, and other sources.

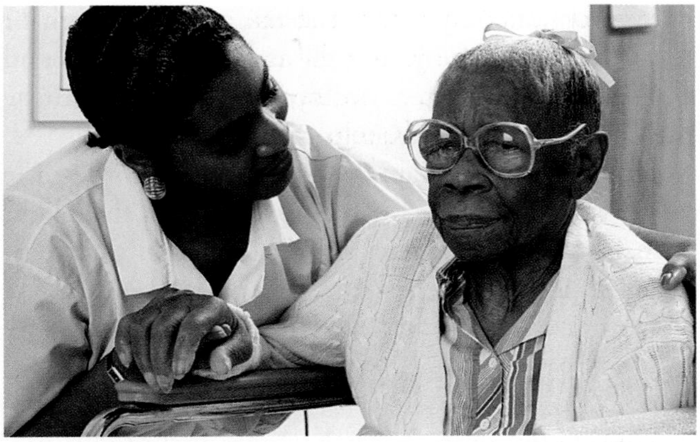

FIGURE 36–5 Use touch to calm the client with dementia. Note how this support worker is safely positioned to the side of the client, within the client's line of sight. (**Source:** Sorrentino, S.A., & Gorek, B. (2003). *Mosby's textbook for long-term care assistants* (4th ed., p. 670). St. Louis, MO: Mosby.)

- Check the lighting. Make sure there are no glares, shadows, or reflections.
- Cover or remove mirrors. The client could mistake the reflection for another person and become frightened.

Catastrophic Reactions

Catastrophic reactions are extreme responses to what the client perceives as extreme danger, disaster, or tragedy. The client may scream, cry, or be agitated or combative. These reactions are commonly caused by too much stimulation that can overwhelm the client—for example, being in a noisy dining room, hearing radio or TV noises, and being asked questions all at the same time.

Sometimes, clients have extreme reactions whenever anything out of the ordinary or unexpected happens. For example, a flickering light may be perceived as a fire, resulting in the client running away screaming. The client may even be frightened if someone approaches too quickly or stands too close.

Clients with dementia should never be "sneaked up on." Approach them from the side, in full view of them. Calmly address the client to get her attention, taking care not to startle her.

Agitation and Restlessness

The client may fidget, pace, hit, or yell and may resist care. Common causes of such behaviours are pain or discomfort, anxiety, lack of sleep, and too much or too little stimulation, as well as hunger, thirst, and the need to eliminate. A calm, quiet setting and the meeting of basic needs help calm the client.

Do not overstimulate the client. Use a calm, gentle voice when talking. Do not overwhelm the client with instructions or choices. Do not rush the client or be impatient.

Aggression and Combativeness

Aggressive or combative behaviours include hitting, pinching, grabbing, biting, or swearing. They may result from agitation and restlessness, pain, fatigue, too much stimulation, response to caregiver stress, and a feeling of being lost or abandoned. The behaviours often occur during care procedures that upset or frighten the client (e.g., bathing, dressing). See Chapter 5 for ways to deal with an angry client. It is your responsibility to always (1) follow the client's care plan regarding these procedures, (2) respect the DIPPS principles, and (3) ensure your safety and the safety of others.

Screaming

It is common for clients in the later stages of dementia who are very disoriented and have poor communication skills to scream to communicate. Clients may scream a word or a name or just make screaming sounds.

Possible reasons for screaming include hearing and vision problems, pain or discomfort, fear, and fatigue. Clients may have been overstimulated or understimulated. A disoriented client may react to a caregiver or family member by screaming.

Sometimes, the following measures are helpful:

- Providing a calm, quiet setting
- Playing soft music
- Having the client wear a hearing aid or eyeglasses, as prescribed
- Having a family member or favourite caregiver comfort and calm the client
- Using therapeutic touch (a noninvasive method of healing in which the caregiver places hands on the client in a gentle and nonthreatening manner) to calm the client

Abnormal Sexual Behaviours

Sexual behaviours can be labelled "abnormal" on the basis of how and when they occur. Clients with dementia are not oriented to person, place, or time. Abnormal sexual behaviours may involve the wrong person, the wrong place, and the wrong time.

Sometimes, clients with dementia are not able to control their behaviours. For example, some clients may touch and fondle their genitals for pleasure or masturbate in public. Masturbation in public is viewed as sexually aggressive behaviour, but some clients may not understand that their behaviour is socially offensive. Some clients with dementia may mistake someone for a sexual partner and may try to kiss, hug, or touch that person.

Some abnormal behaviours are not sexual in nature. Touching, scratching, and rubbing the genitals can signal infection, pain, or discomfort in the genitourinary system or some other underlying health problem that can cause soreness and itching (see *Supporting Reverend Welikij: How Sundowning Can Upset Families* on p. 833). Other causes can be poor hygiene or being wet or soiled by urine or stool. Clean the client quickly and thoroughly after elimination to ensure that the client is not wet or soiled.

Sexually aggressive behaviours have many causes, including the following:

- Disorientation
- Nervous system disorders
- Adverse effects from medications
- Fever
- Dementia
- Acquired brain injury

Report incidences of a client repeatedly touching the genitals. Try to determine the cause of the client's behaviour. Provide for privacy and safety. Tell your supervisor about the situation. A health care provider may assess the client for health issues or may encourage the client's sexual partner to show affection. Remember that normal practices such as hand holding, hugging, kissing, and touching are to be encouraged and may reduce the client's inappropriate behaviour. If you observe a client masturbating in public, lead the client to his room, and provide for privacy and safety.

Supporting Reverend Welikij: How Sundowning Can Upset Families

Reverend Welikij, 72, a retired clergyman, lived at home with his wife until several months ago. He was admitted to an extended care facility because of his dementia. Reverend Welikij was usually a quiet, soft-spoken man, but the staff at the facility had begun to notice that he was becoming increasingly agitated in the evenings. One night, he took his pants down and started pulling on his penis while his wife and daughter were visiting him in the lounge area. They were horrified and embarrassed and could not understand why he was behaving in such a way.

The support staff took him to his room to provide him with privacy, assisted him to the bathroom, and then to bed. They then reported this behaviour to the nurse in charge, who conveyed the information to his doctor. It was later found that Reverend Welikij had a UTI, and because he was unable to state that something was wrong, he acted out to show his discomfort.

His wife and daughter were very relieved when this information was relayed to them. They decided to visit him earlier in the evenings when he was "more like himself." This helped make Mrs. Welikij's visits with her husband less distressing.

Repetitive Behaviours

Repetitive means repeated over and over again. Clients with dementia sometimes repeat the same actions over and over. For example, a client may fold a napkin, may say the same words, or ask the same question again and again. Such behaviours are not hurtful to the client but can be annoying to caregivers and family members.

Harmless acts should be permitted, or the client could be distracted from the act with music, picture books, exercise, movies, or a walk.

Hoarding

Hoarding means collecting things and putting them away in a guarded manner. Clients who hoard items may hide them in drawers or under the beds. Some clients will hoard any and all items that they can find, and some will seek out specific items and hoard them. You should try to find out from the family why these items are significant to the client.

CAREGIVER NEEDS

Being a primary caregiver to a person with dementia can be extremely stressful physically, emotionally, socially, and financially. Many adult children in the "sandwich generation" have their energies divided between taking care of both their children and their parents, all of whom need attention. They not only care for two families but also often have full-time jobs outside their homes, which can add to their stress.

Caregivers can, therefore, suffer from anger, anxiety, sleeplessness, and depression. Some find it difficult to concentrate on anything and are always irritable. Abuse may occur in very stressful caregiving situations.

Because they are constantly under stress, caregivers are susceptible to health problems themselves, so they need to take care of their own health by ensuring a healthy diet, exercise, and plenty of rest. Caregivers must ask family and friends for help when their responsibilities become overwhelming.

Caregivers need much support and encouragement, so many of them join support groups sponsored by hospitals, long-term care facilities, and the Alzheimer Society of Canada, which has chapters in cities and towns across the country. People in similar situations voice their feelings, anger, frustration, guilt, and other emotions and share coping and caregiving strategies.

Caregivers, family members, and friends of a person with dementia often feel helpless. No matter what they do, the person only gets worse. Much time, money, energy, and emotion are needed to care for the person. Guilty feelings are common in these caregivers as well. Family and friends know that the person has not chosen to have dementia or to have its signs, symptoms, and behaviours. Nevertheless,

Think About Safety

The ABCDs of Managing Responsive or Challenging Behaviours

A = Activating Event

Remember that all behaviours have meaning.

Ask yourself:

- When and where did the behaviour occur?
- What was the client doing immediately before the behaviour occurred?
- What was happening around the client at the time?
- Assess environmental factors (in consultation with your supervisor or nurse):
- Noise (e.g., loud TV or music, staff change of shift, mealtime clatter)
- Clutter (e.g., furniture, people)
- Bright lights or glare on the floor
- Mirrors
- Room temperature (e.g., too hot or too cold)
- Recent changes in environment (e.g., renovations, staff or client changes)
- Does the environment provide a safe area for clients to wander around?
- Does the environment encourage independence, dignity, and mobility?
- Does the environment accept the client's cultural and lifestyle habits?
- Has there been a recent change in medication?

Determine whether the client has any of the following (in consultation with your supervisor or nurse):

- Impaired vision or hearing
- Acute illness (e.g., UTI, pneumonia)
- Chronic illness (e.g., angina, diabetes)
- Chronic pain (e.g., arthritis, ulcers, headaches)
- Dehydration
- Constipation
- Fatigue or physical discomfort

Observe for psychological factors (in consultation with your supervisor or nurse):

- Does the client have a history of psychiatric illness?
- Has the client experienced a recent loss or an accumulation of losses?
- Does the client appear sad (e.g., tearful or withdrawn)?
- Are past events influencing present behaviours (e.g., post-traumatic stress disorder [PTSD], abuse)?
- Does the client appear to be responding to hallucinations?

B = Behaviour

Determine whether the client has the following behavioural symptoms (in consultation with your supervisor or nurse):

- Physical aggression
- Screaming
- Restlessness
- Agitation
- Wandering
- Culturally inappropriate behaviours
- Lack of sexual inhibitions
- Hoarding
- Constant questioning
- Cursing
- Shadowing (i.e., following someone, often imitating their actions)

Psychological Symptoms

Determine whether other clients or relatives have described the client as having symptoms indicating the following (in consultation with your supervisor or nurse):

- Anxiety
- Depression
- Paranoia
- Hallucinations
- Delusions

C = Consequences

Ask yourself the following questions:

- What was the consequence of the behaviour for the client, for staff, and for other clients?
- Was the client told off, ignored, restrained, sedated, or guided back to where the client had been? The consequence of the behaviour is very much dependent on the staff's interpretation and reaction to the behaviour. At this stage,

Continued

Think About Safety—cont'd

communication is the main factor to influence the behaviour and its consequence.

- Remember the three parts of communication:
  - i. body language (55%)
  - ii. tone and pitch of voice (38%)
  - iii. words used (7%)

The attitude and manner of the care staff are extremely important. Clients with cognitive impairment are extremely sensitive to nonverbal cues and mirror the affective behaviour of those around them. A patient, calm, and gentle manner is contagious and has a positive effect. It is important to be aware that if your body language indicates that you feel tense, frustrated, or angry, it may contradict the words you are using.

D = *Decide* How to Support Clients; Help *Decrease* Their Challenging Behaviours; and *Debrief* Others

- Stop before you approach the client, think about what you are about to do, and consider the best way to do it. Plan your actions and explain who you are, what you want to do, and why you want to do it. Never assume the client will not understand you!
- Smile! Clients will take their cue from you and will mirror your relaxed and positive body language and tone of voice.
- Go slowly! You may have a lot to do and be in a hurry, but the client is not. How would you feel if someone came into your bedroom, pulled back your blankets, and started pulling you out of bed without giving you time to wake up properly?
- Go away when it is necessary! If the client is resistive or aggressive but is not causing harm to self or others, leave the person alone. Give the client time to settle down, and approach again later.
- Give them space! Any activity that involves invasion of personal space increases the risk for assault and aggression. Every time you provide care to a client, you are invading that person's space.
- Stand aside! Always provide care from the side of the client, not from the front, where you are an easy target to hit, kick, and so on.
- Distract them! Talk about the things that the client enjoyed in the past, and give the client a face towel or something to hold on to while you are providing care.
- Keep it quiet! Excess noise can disorient and agitate the client. Check the noise level, and if it is high, reduce it. Turn off the radio or TV if it is upsetting the client.
- Do not argue! Arguing will only disorient, irritate, and further agitate the client.
- Brainstorm and debrief! Discuss with the rest of the team how all of you can best meet the physical, environmental, and psychological needs of the clients in your care.
- Follow the care plan.
- Report and record what caused the behaviours, all behaviours observed, and what you did to support the client.

(See **FIGURE 36–6, *A* AND *B*.**)

Sources: Regional Dementia Management Strategy Document Library. (2001, Bendigo Health Care Group). Bendigo, Australia. Retrieved from www.dementiamanagementstrategy.com. Reprinted by permission of Bendigo Health's Collaborative Health Education and Research Centre.

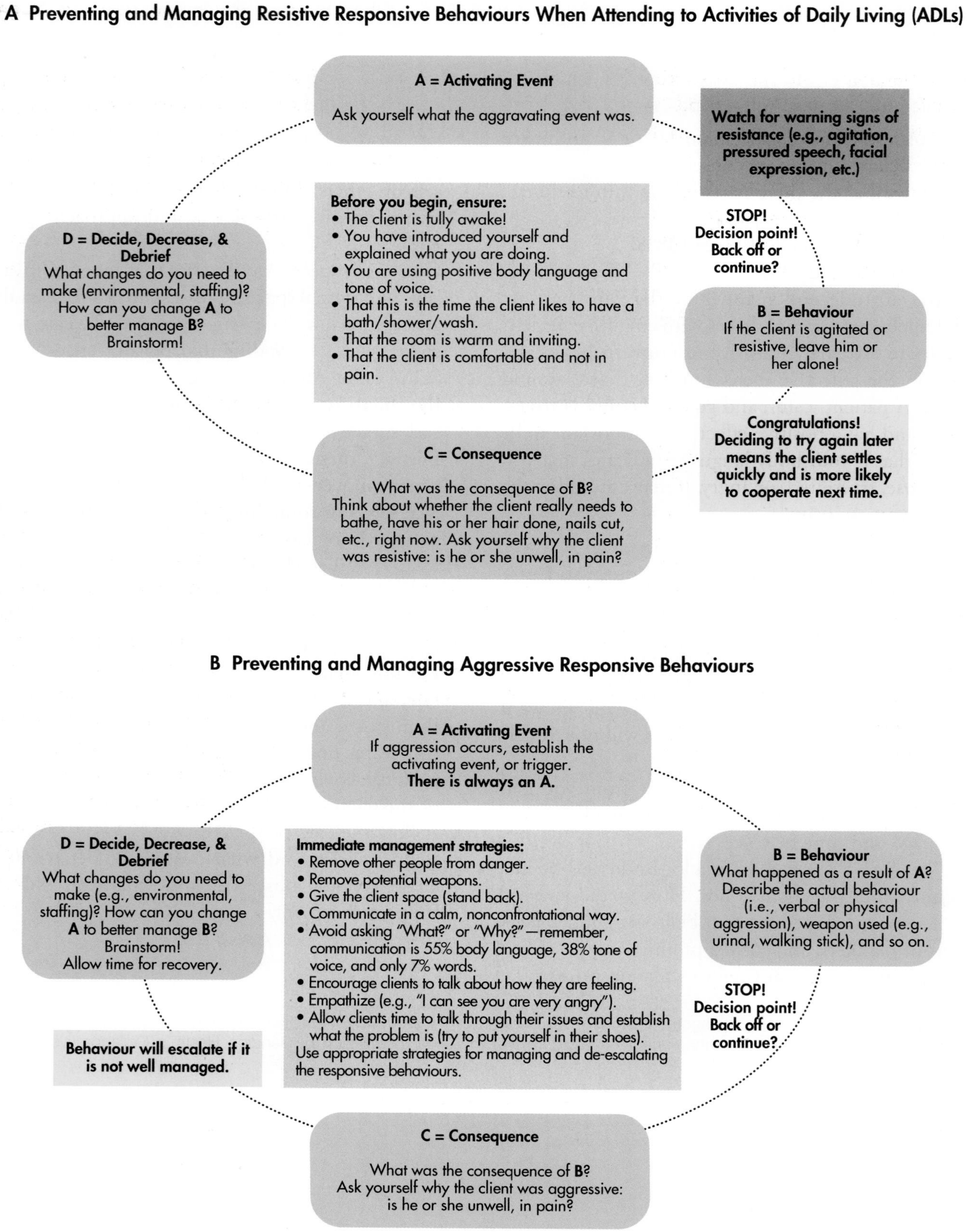

FIGURE 36–6 The cycle of challenging behaviours. **A,** Preventing and managing resistance when attending to activities of daily living (ADLs). **B,** Preventing and managing aggression. (**Source:** Regional Dementia Management Strategy Document Library. (2001). Bendigo Health Care Group. Bendigo, Australia. Retrieved from http://www.dementiamanagementstrategy.com/Pages/ABC_of_behaviour_management/Management_strategies.aspx. Reprinted by permission of the Centre for Rural Rehabilitation & Aged Care.)

sometimes, behaviours are frustrating, embarrassing, or threatening. Family and friends may be upset and angry that their loved one can no longer show love or affection.

As a support worker, you play a key role in caregiver relief. You may assist the primary caregiver or other caregivers, or you may care for the client to give the caregiver some time off from his responsibilities. Follow the care plan, and perform your tasks competently. The caregiver should have confidence in your skill and ability in order to relax and let go of control for some time. The care plan may ask you to encourage the caregiver to take care of personal needs and to leave the home to have a break while you are there. You may observe signs and symptoms of caregiver stress and signs of depression and abuse. Report these observations immediately to your supervisor (see the *Case Study: Supporting Caregivers of Clients With Dementia* box).

CASE STUDY Supporting Caregivers of Clients With Dementia

Mrs. Munroe, 70, has Alzheimer's disease. She has stage 2 (moderate) dementia. She lives at home with her husband, who is her primary caregiver. Leila is assigned to provide morning respite care. This is her fourth visit. Mrs. Munroe is incontinent; she also needs assistance with feeding, bathing, and dressing. She is frequently rude and aggressive and becomes angry if someone stands too near her or tries to make her do something. Quick, sudden movements and loud noises also upset her. The care plan calls for Mr. Munroe to take a break—preferably away from the house—while Leila takes care of Mrs. Munroe's needs. Mr. Munroe is reluctant to leave, since he is anxious about his wife.

Discussion

Leila's visit is scheduled for 3 hours. She knows that Mr. Munroe will not leave until he is satisfied that his wife is in competent hands. Leila starts her visit by sitting down with Mrs. Munroe at the kitchen table and talking quietly and gently. She explains that she is going to make breakfast and gives Mrs. Munroe two food choices. Leila makes breakfast while she continues talking with Mrs. Munroe in a quiet, reassuring voice. Mr. Munroe is anxiously watching everything from the living room. When Mrs. Munroe is settled, Leila suggests to Mr. Munroe that he go out for a coffee, and he reluctantly agrees to go. When he comes back 1 hour later, Mrs. Munroe has been bathed and dressed, and she is sitting quietly watching TV. Mr. Munroe feels better for having had a break, and now he feels confident in Leila's ability to care for his wife.

CHAPTER REVIEW

KEY POINTS

- Disorientation, delirium, and dementia are not a normal part of aging.
- Diseases that affect the brain can affect cognitive functioning, which involves the following functions of the brain: (1) memory, (2) thinking, (3) reasoning, (4) ability to understand, (5) judgement, and (6) behaviour.
- Disorientation is the inability of a person to think with the usual clarity. There are numerous causes of disorientation. Disorientation may be temporary or permanent. Permanent disorientation is caused by physical changes to the structure of the brain.
- Delirium is disorientation that occurs suddenly. It is usually caused by treatable physical or mental health disorders. Delirium should always be treated as an emergency requiring medical attention.
- *Dementia* is a general term that describes the progressive loss of functions, including cognitive and social functions. Dementia usually gets worse over time.
- Early warning signs of dementia include the following: (1) memory loss that affects daily functioning; (2) disorientation; (3) repeating words or sentences; having problems finding words or following conversations; (4) using poor judgement; (5) having difficulty completing common tasks; (6) changes in mood, behaviour, or personality; and (7) loss of interest in hobbies or activities.
- All caregivers should be aware of ways to support clients who have dementia. These clients face the following challenges: (1) environmental challenges, (2) communication challenges, (3) wandering, (4) sundowning, (5) hallucinations or delusions, (6) sleep disturbances, and (7) impaired ability to meet basic needs.
- Dementia usually progresses in three stages: (1) early, (2) moderate or middle, and (3) late. You should be aware of the typical symptoms of each stage and the care that you must provide accordingly.
- The ABCDs of managing challenging (*responsive*) behaviours are (A) *activating* event, (B) *behaviour*, (C) *consequences*, and (D) *deciding* how to support clients, *decreasing* their challenging behaviours, and *debriefing* others.
- When a client displays responsive behaviours, remember the DIPPS principles and ensure your safety and the safety of others.

CRITICAL THINKING IN PRACTICE

Mrs. Uma is 82 years old and lives in a long-term care facility. Today she seems irritable and does not recall your name. These issues are not normal for her. She says she is tired and does not want to eat breakfast. When should you report these changes? Why is it important to monitor for such changes in older adults?

REVIEW QUESTIONS

Answers to these questions are at the bottom of page 840.

Circle the BEST answer.

1. Cognitive function relates to:
   A. Memory loss and personality
   B. Thinking and reasoning
   C. Ability to toilet oneself
   D. How emotional a person can get
2. If a client is disoriented after moving to a long-term care facility, this disorientation is likely to be:
   A. Temporary due to medications
   B. Due to emotional stress caused by the move
   C. Due to an infection
   D. Due to brain injury
3. Which of the following statements about delirium is true? It:
   A. Is a permanent state of disorientation
   B. Is unavoidable and happens to most clients
   C. Is an emergency and can be a reaction to medications
   D. Should be ignored so as not to embarrass the client

4. Which of the following statements about dementia is true? Dementia:
   A. Can affect people in their 40s
   B. Is a normal part of aging
   C. Is less common in people over 65 years of age
   D. Can result in colour-blindness

5. Which of the following statements about secondary dementias is true?
   A. They occur only in older people.
   B. Diet and medications can cure the disease.
   C. Their cause is unknown.
   D. They result from physical disease, ingestion of damaging substances, or injury.

6. A common sign or symptom of dementia is:
   A. Headache
   B. Paralysis
   C. Dyspnea
   D. Poor judgement

7. People in the early stage of dementia:
   A. Usually remain in their homes with support
   B. Are totally dependent on others for care
   C. Are confined to bed
   D. Are usually placed in secured units

8. Joe Dunn has Alzheimer's disease (ADRD). Which statement is true?
   A. ADRD occurs only in older people.
   B. Diet and drugs can control the disease.
   C. ADRD and delirium are the same thing.
   D. There is no known cure for ADRD.

9. Mr. Dunn is screaming. You know that screaming is:
   A. An agitated reaction
   B. His style of singing
   C. A sign of heart disease
   D. A repetitive behaviour

10. Mr. Dunn is offered simple choices. This is because:
    A. He is not really a choosy person
    B. He is not very smart
    C. His wife makes all of his decisions
    D. More choices would only disorient and agitate him

11. Secured units:
    A. Prevent the disoriented client from wandering and getting lost
    B. Are rarely used because they are restrictive and inhumane
    C. Are necessary only when a client is in the severe or late stage of dementia
    D. Prevent a client's family from visiting

12. Mr. Dunn has moderate dementia and tends to wander. You should do the following:
    A. Tell him about safe areas for wandering
    B. Keep him in his pyjamas so he will not want to wander far
    C. Keep him on bed rest and give him comfort care
    D. Make sure the door alarms are turned on

13. *Sundowning* means that:
    A. The person becomes sleepy when the sun sets
    B. Behaviours become worse in the late afternoon and evening hours
    C. Behaviour improves at night
    D. The person is in the third stage of dementia

14. Which of the following safety points should you follow for Mr. Dunn?
    A. All safety hazards should be painted red.
    B. Mr. Dunn should wear a large sign that says he is a safety risk.
    C. Sharp and breakable objects should be removed from his environment.
    D. He can keep his smoking materials but should smoke only in designated areas.

15. Besides ensuring a quiet, calm environment, what else should you keep in mind when caring for Mr. Dunn in a facility?
    A. Introduce yourself every time you see him.
    B. Mr. Dunn no longer has rights, as he is too disoriented.
    C. Never touch Mr. Dunn as it could scare him.
    D. Clients should be encouraged to bathe each other, as it gives them a sense of purpose.

16. Support workers usually have much contact with family members in the following way:
   A. Offering advice to the family
   B. Telling the family that they are not helping out enough
   C. Providing support and relief to the family
   D. Telling the family about other clients

17. A type of dementia that is caused by a series of small strokes resulting in brain tissue death is called:
   A. Lewy body dementia
   B. Creutzfeldt–Jakob disease
   C. Fronto-temporal dementia
   D. Vascular dementia

Match each definition with a key term in the list below. Note there are more key terms than definitions.
   A. Agitation
   B. Catastrophic reactions
   C. Delusions
   D. Depression
   E. Hallucinations
   F. Hoarding
   G. Pacing
   H. Sundowning
   I. Wandering

18. Becoming restless and agitated in the late afternoon or night
19. Believing things that are not true
20. Seeing things that are not there
21. Walking back and forth in the same area
22. Becoming withdrawn and having no energy or interest in doing things
23. Being excited, restless, or troubled
24. Collecting and putting things away in a guarded manner
25. Moving from one area to another aimlessly

Answers: 1.B, 2.B, 3.C, 4.A, 5.D, 6.D, 7.A, 8.D, 9.A, 10.D, 11.A, 12.D, 13.B, 14.C, 15.A, 16.C, 17.D, 18.H, 19.C, 20.E, 21.G, 22.D, 23.A, 24.F, 25.I

Chapter opener image: Fotoluminate LLC/Shutterstock.com

CHAPTER 37

Common Diseases and Conditions

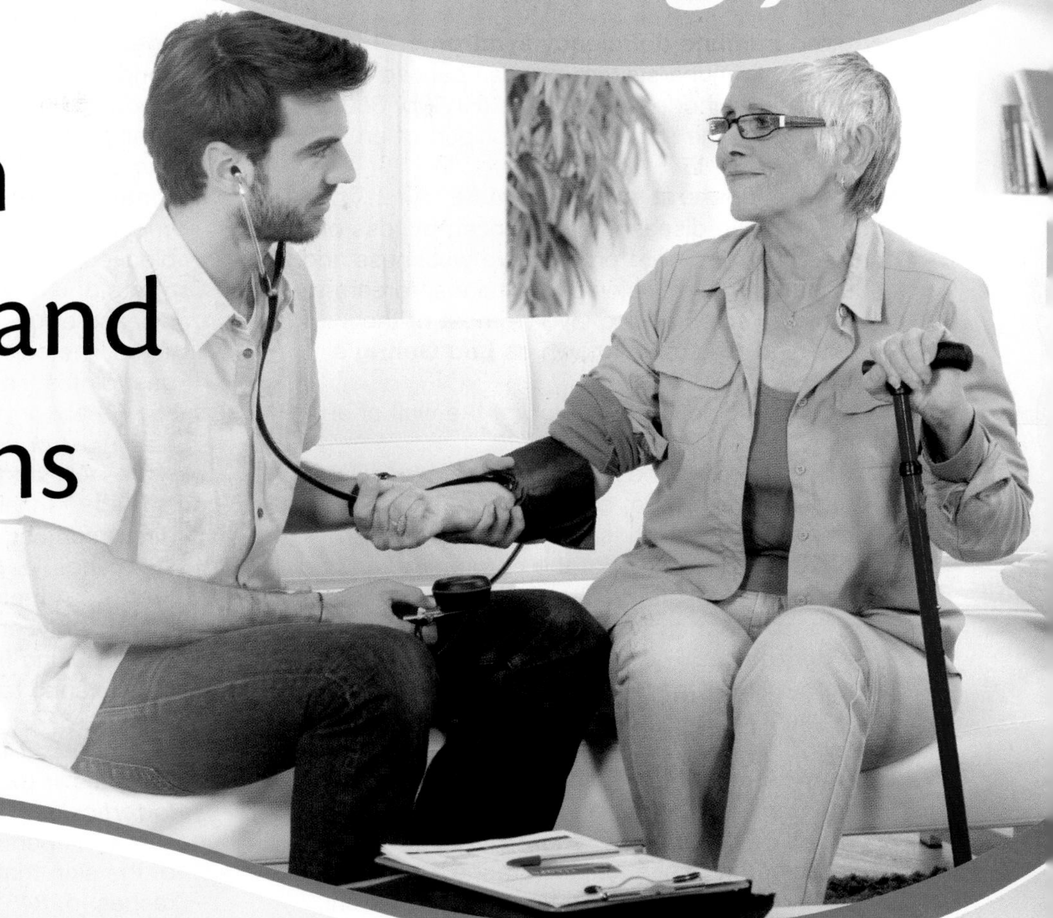

OBJECTIVES

After reading this chapter, the learner should be able to do the following:

- Describe the common disorders of the integumentary system and the care required.
- Describe the common musculo-skeletal disorders and the care required.
- Explain how to care for clients in casts and with fractures.
- Describe the effects of amputation.
- Describe the common neurological disorders and the care required.
- Identify the causes and effects of brain and spinal cord injuries and the care required.
- Describe the common cardiovascular disorders and the care required.
- Describe the common respiratory disorders and the care required.
- Describe the common digestive disorders and the care required.
- Describe the common urinary disorders and the care required.
- Describe the common endocrine disorders and the care required.
- Describe the common types of cancers and some of the treatments available.
- Describe the common communicable diseases and the care required.
- Describe the common immune system disorders and the care required.

KEY TERMS

acquired immune deficiency syndrome (AIDS) Immune system disease caused by human immunodeficiency virus (HIV). *p. 880*

amputation The removal of all or part of an extremity. *p. 854*

amyotrophic lateral sclerosis (ALS) A degenerative disease characterized by loss of the motor neurons, with progressive weakness and atrophy of the muscles of the hands, forearms, and legs, spreading to involve most of the body and face. Also known as **Lou Gehrig's disease**. *p. 862*

aneurysm A localized dilation of the wall of an artery or heart chamber. *p. 860*

angina pectoris Chest (*pectoris*) pain (*angina*) caused by ischemia, a lack of blood supply to the heart muscle, which is usually caused by an obstruction or spasm of the coronary arteries because of **coronary artery disease**. *p. 864*

arrhythmia Abnormal (*a*) heart rhythm (*rhythmia*). *p. 867*

arthritis Joint (*arthr*) inflammation (*itis*). *p. 855*

arthroplasty Surgical replacement (*plasty*) of a joint (*arthro*). *p. 855*

asthma A respiratory disorder characterized by recurring episodes of paroxysmal dyspnea (intermittent spasms of shortness of breath); wheezing on expiration, inspiration, or both, caused by constriction (narrowing) of bronchi; coughing; and thick bronchial secretions of mucous. *p. 867*

athlete's foot A highly contagious fungal skin infection that causes the affected foot to peel, burn, itch, and turn red. *p. 848*

benign Noncancerous. *p. 876*

benign prostatic hypertrophy (BPH) An enlarged prostate gland. *p. 873*

boil See **furuncle**. *p. 848*

cancer A group of diseases characterized by out-of-control cell division and growth, which can occur in many body systems. *p. 876*

cholecystitis Inflammation of the gallbladder. *p. 870*

chronic obstructive pulmonary disease (COPD) A persistent lung disorder that obstructs (blocks) the airways; refers to chronic bronchitis and emphysema. *p. 868*

cirrhosis Persistent liver disease characterized by normal liver cells being replaced by scar tissue. *p. 870*

colitis Inflammation of the colon. *p. 870*

congestive heart failure (CHF) An abnormal condition that occurs when the heart cannot pump blood normally. Blood backs up and causes an abnormal amount (congestion) of fluid in the tissues. Also known as *heart failure*. *p. 866*

coronary artery disease (CAD) A condition of impaired cardiac pumping due to narrowed or blocked arteries. *p. 863*

Crohn's disease A persistent inflammatory bowel disease of unknown origin, usually affecting the ileum, the colon, or another part of the gastrointestinal (GI) tract. *p. 870*

cyst An abnormal, closed sac, which may contain air, fluids, or semi-solid material. *p. 848*

cystitis A bladder infection. *p. 872*

dermatitis Inflammation of the skin caused by direct contact with an irritating or allergy-causing substance. *p. 845*

diabetes A metabolic disorder characterized by hyperglycemia (high blood sugar levels) and resulting from low levels of insulin or a resistance to insulin's effect at a cellular level. *p. 874*

diverticulosis The condition (*osis*) of having small pouches in the colon that bulge outward (*diverticulum*). *p. 871*

eczema A persistent inflammatory condition of the skin that can include recurring skin rashes. *p. 845*

epilepsy A group of neurological disorders characterized by recurrent episodes of convulsive seizures, sensory disturbances, abnormal behaviour, loss of consciousness, or some or all of the above. *p. 857*

fibromyalgia A condition associated with aching, stiffness, and fatigue in muscles, ligaments, and tendons. *p. 857*

fracture A broken bone. *p. 850*

furuncle A skin disorder caused by the infection of a hair follicle. Also called a **boil**. *p. 848*

gastro-esophageal reflux disease (GERD) A disorder of the digestive system that causes heartburn. *p. 869*

gout A disease caused by the accumulation of uric acid in the cartilage of a joint, especially in the tendons. Also called *metabolic arthritis*. *p. 857*

heart attack See **myocardial infarction**. *p. 865*

hemiplegia Paralysis (*plegia*) of one side (*hemi*) of the body; the arm and leg, body organs, vision, the tongue, and the swallowing mechanisms on the affected side can all be compromised. *p. 859*

hepatitis Inflammation (*itis*) of the liver (*hepat*) that may be caused by bacterial or viral infection, parasitic infestation, alcohol, drugs, toxins, or transfusion of incompatible (not matching) blood type. *p. 870*

hives See **urticaria**. *p. 845*

Huntington's disease An inherited neurological disorder that causes uncontrolled movements, emotional disturbances, and cognitive losses. *p. 861*

hyperthyroidism A condition caused by an overactive thyroid gland. *p. 876*

hypothyroidism A condition caused by an underactive thyroid gland. *p. 876*

impetigo A contagious skin disorder caused by bacteria. *p. 848*

irritable bowel syndrome (IBS) A disorder of the bowel characterized by abdominal pain and changes in bowel habits. *p. 870*

Lou Gehrig's disease See **amyotrophic lateral sclerosis**. *p. 862*

malignant Describes any condition in the body that, if untreated, may be a threat to health (e.g., malignant hypertension). Specifically, it describes a tumour that invades and destroys other cells or tissues. Also known as *cancerous*. *p. 876*

metastasis The spread of cancer to other parts of the body. *p. 876*

multiple sclerosis (MS) A persistent, slowly progressive disease, in which the body's immune system attacks the protective myelin sheaths that surround the nerve cells of the brain and spinal cord (a process called *demyelination*), resulting in damaged areas that are unable to transmit nerve impulses. *p. 861*

myocardial infarction (MI) Death (*infarction*) of heart tissue (*myocardium*) caused by lack of oxygen to the heart. Also known as **heart attack**. *p. 865*

osteoarthritis (OA) A type of arthritis that causes the cartilage that occupies the joints of the body to wear away, causing pain in and disfigurement to the joints. *p. 855*

osteomyelitis Inflammation or infection of the bone. *p. 852*

osteoporosis A bone disorder (*osteo*) in which the bone becomes porous and brittle (*poros*). *p. 855*

paralysis Complete or partial loss of ability to move a limb or muscle group. *p. 862*

paraplegia Paralysis (*plegia*) from the waist down. *p. 862*

Parkinson's disease Neurological disorder in which the cells in certain parts of the brain are gradually destroyed; causes tremors, muscle stiffness, slow movement, and poor balance. *p. 860*

phlebitis An inflammation of a vein. *p. 867*

pneumonia Infection of the lung tissue. *p. 867*

psoriasis A persistent skin disorder that affects the skin and joints. It commonly causes red scaly patches to appear on the skin. *p. 848*

pyelonephritis Inflammation of the kidney and renal pelvis because of bacterial infection. *p. 872*

quadriplegia Paralysis (*plegia*) of all four (*quad*) limbs and the trunk; paralysis from the neck down. *p. 862*

renal calculi Kidney (*renal*) stones (*calculi*). *p. 872*

scabies A highly contagious skin infection caused by a mite. *p. 845*

scleroderma A progressive autoimmune disease that involves the hardening (*sclero*) of the skin (*derma*) and connective tissue throughout the body. *p. 849*

seborrheic keratosis Noncancerous skin growth that is common in older adults. *p. 849*

sexually transmitted infections (STIs) Diseases that are spread through sexual contact. *p. 881*

shingles A viral infection causing a painful rash of raised blisters, which can appear anywhere on the body, usually on one side. It is caused by the same virus that causes chicken pox. *p. 845*

transient ischemic attack (TIA) A temporary interruption of blood flow to the brain. *p. 858*

tumour A new growth of abnormal cells that could be **malignant** or **benign**. *p. 876*

urinary tract infection (UTI) An infection in the urinary system. *p. 871*

urticaria A common skin condition characterized by raised, usually itchy **wheals**. It is commonly caused by an allergic reaction to food, food additives, or drugs. Also known as **hives**. *p. 845*

wheal A circular, red, spongy lesion that evolves (develops) and changes over minutes to hours. It is usually surrounded by an area of redness called a *flare*. *p. 845*

As a support worker, you will have a supervisor who will direct the care you give; however, understanding diseases and health conditions will help you better provide the care your clients need. This chapter gives basic information about common diseases and conditions. Some diseases and conditions are acute, others are chronic or persistent, and some others can even result in the death of clients. Many diseases and health conditions are progressive—that is, they gradually get worse over time. Others are disabling or life threatening.

While caring for clients, you must encourage them to be as independent as possible. Some clients with progressive, disabling, or life-threatening illnesses or health conditions become immobile and bedridden. See Chapter 26 for more information on caring for these clients. Portray a positive attitude and always remember the priorities of support work (see the *Providing Compassionate Care: Caring for Clients With Diseases or Conditions* box).

A review of Chapter 17 will be helpful when you study this chapter. See Chapters 35, 36, 39, and 40 for descriptions of health problems not discussed in this chapter.

INTEGUMENTARY DISORDERS

The integumentary system is made up of skin and its appendages, such as hair, nails, and sweat and oil glands. Many skin disorders cause discomfort to clients (also refer to Chapter 24). Treatments for skin disorders may seem very easy to do, and you may have done the treatment at home on your own family, but you cannot perform any treatment that is not

Providing Compassionate Care
Caring for Clients With Diseases or Conditions

- ***Dignity.*** The care you give affects the client's life. Although the physical support you provide is very important, clients also need emotional support, as it promotes the client's dignity. It shows that you care about the whole client, not just his physical needs. Remember, many clients dealing with serious health problems are coping with change, loss, and fear. Imagine what life must be like for the client.

  Whenever the client needs someone to talk to, your being there is important. You may not have to say anything. Just be a good listener, and use touch if appropriate. Do not avoid being near the client for fear of getting the disease. It is very important not to judge the client or assume that he "deserves" the disease, especially in caring for clients with communicable diseases. Many clients with health problems rely on their spiritual faith to cope with their conditions. Respect all expressions of spirituality. Report to your supervisor if the client asks to speak with a spiritual advisor.
- ***Independence.*** The more clients can do for themselves, the better off they are. Always encourage clients to do what they can for themselves—even clients in advanced stages of diseases.
- ***Preferences.*** Protect the client's right to personal choice. Always explain what you are going to do prior to doing it. The client's consent is necessary. Make sure to involve the client in deciding when to begin the care or procedures. Always ask clients about their preferences, and respect them. If their preferences conflict with the care plan, notify your supervisor.
- ***Privacy.*** Protect the client's right to privacy and confidentiality. Remember to close doors and privacy curtains before procedures. Expose only the body part involved in the procedure. Always keep your conversations private. Discuss the client's health problems only with your supervisor and the health team members involved in the client's care. Do not give information to families and visitors. Do not discuss clients with your family and friends.
- ***Safety.*** Clients with health problems are at high risk for falls, choking, and other accidents (see Chapter 22). Know the safety measures required for each client. Always remember to follow Standard Practices. They protect you and others.

within your scope of practice. FIGURE 37–1 shows some common skin disorders.

Urticaria

Urticaria (also known as **hives**) is a common skin condition characterized by raised, usually itchy wheals (FIGURE 37–1, *A*). It is commonly caused by an allergic reaction to food, food additives, or drugs. A **wheal** is a circular, red, spongy lesion that evolves and changes over minutes to hours. It is usually surrounded by an area of redness called a *flare*. Urticaria can vary in size from a few millimetres to wheals covering a whole extremity and causing severe itching. Urticaria can be caused by allergies to a number of things. Common allergic reactions are to foods such as shellfish or to drugs. If you observe signs of urticaria on your client, report it immediately to your supervisor. Treatments may include antihistamines as well as topical lotions or creams to relieve the itching. It is important to record what your client has ingested (eaten) and any substances she has been in contact with, such as powders or creams. Urticaria usually disappears in a matter of hours after ingestion.

Dermatitis

Dermatitis is an inflammation of the skin caused by direct contact with an irritating or allergy-causing substance (FIGURE 37–1, *B*). *Contact dermatitis* can be caused by exposure to a material that the client has become allergic to. Some other common allergens that can cause dermatitis are poison ivy, poison oak, latex, cosmetics, perfumes, and some plants. Symptoms can include itching, skin redness, skin tenderness, swelling, or warmth of the exposed area.

Irritant dermatitis can be caused by reaction to materials such as soaps, detergents, or chemicals and usually resembles a burn. Your role as the support worker will be to follow the care plan and ensure that further exposure to the irritant is prevented.

Eczema

Eczema is an inflammatory condition of the skin. Eczema may look different from person to person. In most cases, it is characterized by dry, red, and extremely itchy patches of skin (FIGURE 37–1, *C*). In other cases, it can involve *papular* (solid elevation of the skin) or vesicular (solid elevation of the skin containing fluid) lesions. Eczema occurs in both children and adults and often first appears in infancy. Areas of high perspiration and creases of the elbows and knees are often prone to skin breakdown from eczema. Treatment usually focuses on preventing scratching. The care plan will tell you what treatments are to be carried out. One of the most common treatments is to apply lotions or creams to keep the skin as moist as possible. Eczema is a persistent condition, and research is ongoing to find medications to control outbreaks.

Shingles

Shingles is a viral infection causing a painful rash of raised blisters, which can appear anywhere on the body, usually on one side (FIGURE 37–1, *D*). It is caused by the herpes varicella zoster virus, which is the same virus that causes chicken pox. The shingles rash can appear anywhere on the body, but the most common sites include the trunk, buttocks, or face. The blister outbreak lasts about two weeks. Shingles can cause extreme and sometimes debilitating pain, itching, or tingling along the affected nerve root, whether the rash is present or not. The pain may linger for weeks, months, or even years.

Once a person becomes infected with this virus, it never leaves that person's body, but it exists in a dormant (inactive) state. Stress, illness, and a weakened immune system can reactivate the virus in the form of shingles, usually travelling along one of the nerve pathways in the body. If the shingles rash appears on the face and spreads to the eye, it can lead to cornea scarring and chronic tearing in the affected eye. Shingles can be spread through skin contact to people who have not acquired immunity to herpes varicella zoster.

Scabies

Scabies is a highly contagious skin infection caused by a mite. The mite burrows under the skin to deposit its eggs, causing intense, itchy skin rashes (FIGURE 37–1, *E*). Scabies is transmitted by skin-to-skin contact between people. Since it takes approximately 4 to 6 weeks for symptoms to develop after the initial

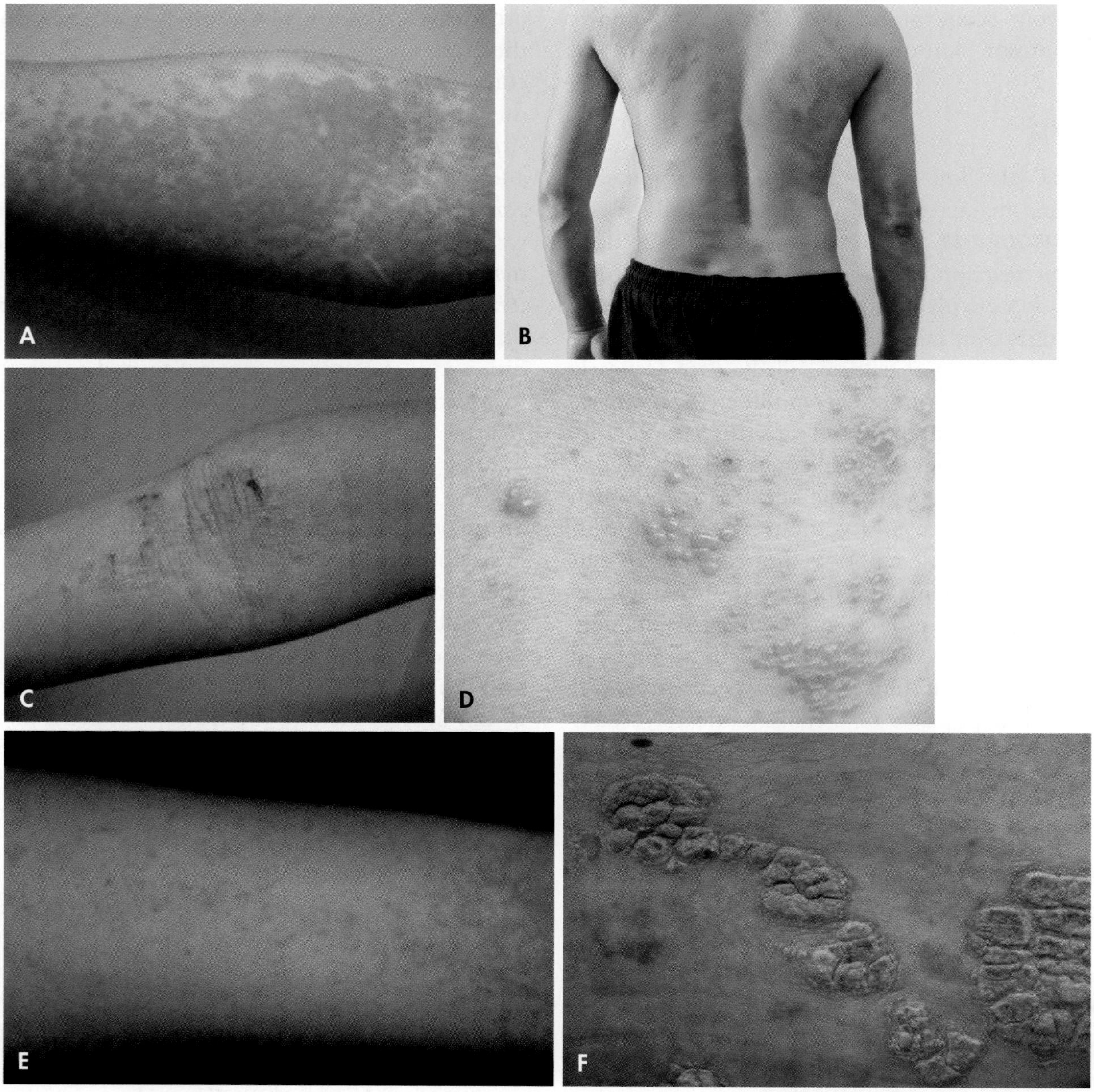

FIGURE 37–1 Common skin disorders. **A,** Urticaria. (**Source:** James Heilman, M.D. This file is licensed under the Creative Commons Attribution-Share Alike 3.0 Unported license: https://creativecommons.org/licenses/by-sa/3.0/deed.en.) **B,** Dermatitis. (**Source:** chaphot/Shutterstock.com) **C,** Eczema. (**Source:** James Heilman, M.D. This file is licensed under the Creative Commons Attribution-Share Alike 3.0 Unported license: https://creativecommons.org/licenses/by-sa/3.0/deed.en.) **D,** Shingles (herpes varicella zoster). (**Source:** komkrit Preechachanwate/Shutterstock.com) **E,** Scabies. (**Source:** Steschke. This file is licensed under the Creative Commons Attribution-Share Alike 3.0 Unported license: https://creativecommons.org/licenses/by-sa/3.0/deed.en.) **F,** Psoriasis. (**Source:** James Heilman, M.D. This file is licensed under the Creative Commons Attribution-Share Alike 3.0 Unported license: https://creativecommons.org/licenses/by-sa/3.0/deed.en)

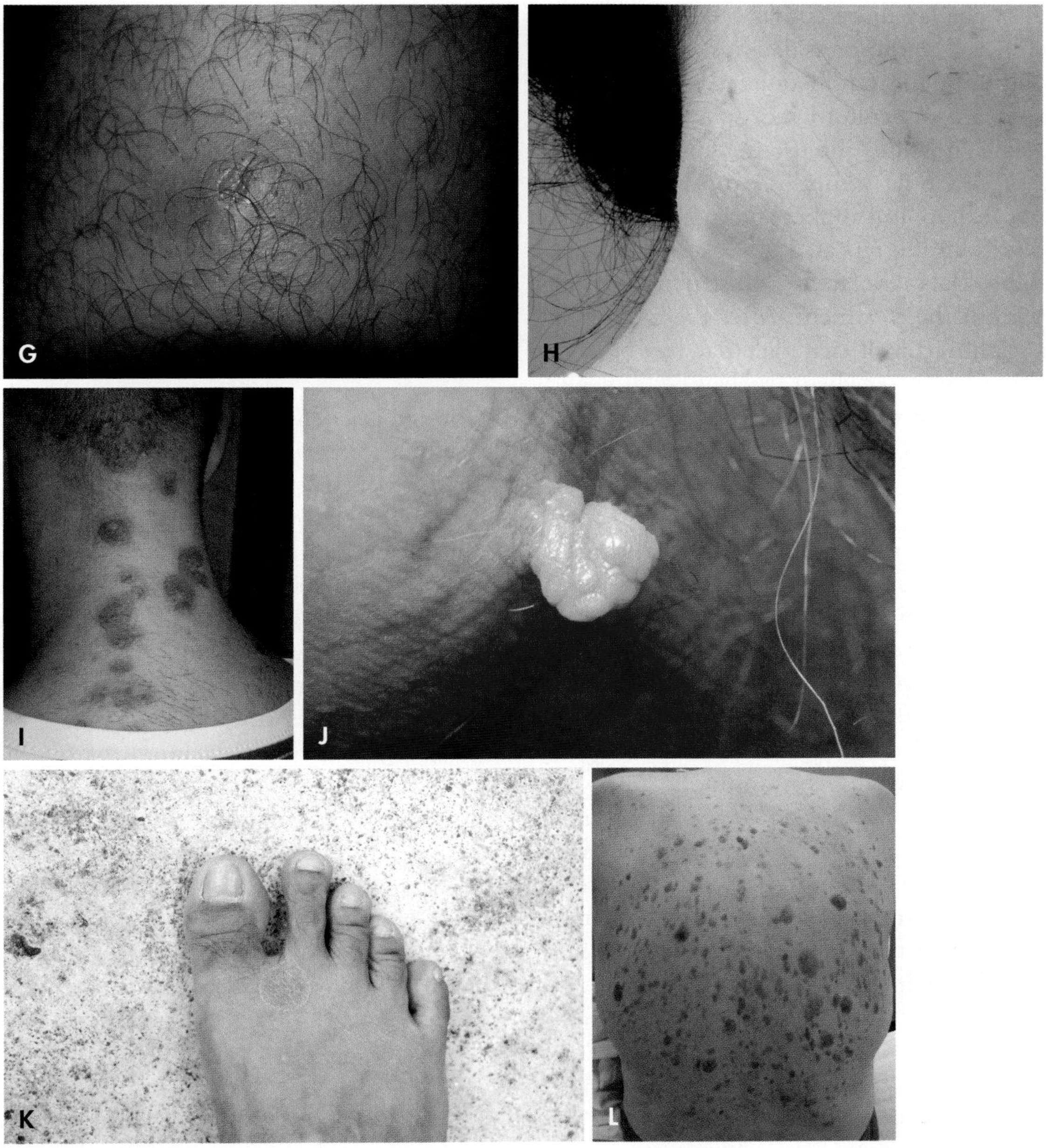

FIGURE 37–1, cont'd G, Boils (or furuncles). (**Source:** Mahdouch. This file is licensed under the Creative Commons Attribution 1.0 Generic license: https://creativecommons.org/licenses/by/1.0/deed.en.) **H,** Cyst. (**Source:** © BSIP SA/Alamy Stock Photo) **I,** Impetigo. (**Source:** Åsa Thörn. This file is licensed under the Creative Commons Attribution-Share Alike 3.0 Unported license: https://creativecommons.org/licenses/by-sa/3.0/deed.en.) **J,** Skin tag. (**Source:** ©/Alamy Stock Photo) **K,** Athlete's foot. (**Source:** witsanu deetuam/Shutterstock.com.) **L,** Seborrheic keratosis. (**Source:** James Heilman, M.D. This file is licensed under the Creative Commons Attribution-Share Alike 3.0 Unported license: https://creativecommons.org/licenses/by-sa/3.0/deed.en.)

infestation, a client can be contagious for at least a month before the condition is diagnosed. As a result, it can spread through a family or a facility. The mites and burrows are difficult to see, so scabies is frequently misdiagnosed as intense itching of the skin before the red papular eruptions form. Treatment usually involves a topical application to kill the mites. Some applications are repeated a week later. Ensure that you follow the manufacturer's instructions if you are carrying out the treatment. After the treatment, thorough washing of all material that has been in contact with the infected client (such as bedding and clothing) in the past 4 days is recommended.

Psoriasis

Psoriasis is a persistent skin disorder that causes red scaly plaques (patches) on the skin and can be found anywhere on the body (**FIGURE 37–1, *F***). These scaly patches are areas of excessive skin production that accumulate and become inflamed. As the skin deposit accumulates, it takes on a silvery-white appearance. The cause of psoriasis has not yet been identified, but stress and excessive alcohol consumption can aggravate the condition. A client with psoriasis can suffer from physical discomfort, itching, and poor self-image because of the appearance of the skin. Treatments available are numerous and will be different for each client. You need to follow the client's care plan for the treatment of the affected areas.

Boil

A **furuncle**, or **boil**, is a skin disorder caused by the infection of a hair follicle, usually by a type of bacterium (a disease-causing organism) called *Staphylococcus*. Boils appear as red, pus-filled lumps, which are painful (**FIGURE 37–1, *G***). The most common sites for boils are the back, underarms, shoulders, thighs, and buttocks. When the boil is ready to drain or discharge the pus, a yellow or white point will appear in its middle. The care plan may include applying warm compresses to the boil, a process referred to as "bringing it to a head." You cannot predict when the boil may break, so use Standard Practices when providing care to the area of the boil. Your supervisor will inform you of the nursing care required when the boil drains.

Cyst

A **cyst** is an abnormal, closed sac that can occur anywhere in the body. The sac, which may contain air, fluids, or semi-solid material, has a distinct membrane enclosing it (**FIGURE 37–1, *H***). Once the cyst has formed, it will remain in the tissue unless it is removed by surgery or by taking medication to dissolve the sac.

Impetigo

Impetigo is a contagious skin disorder that is caused by either *Streptococcus* or *Staphylococcus* bacteria. When a person scratches a cut or scratch that has become infected and touches another part of the body, the bacteria can spread. The infected area forms a crust, which then drains, thus also spreading the bacteria (**FIGURE 37–1, *I***). The usual treatment for small areas of infection is application of an antibiotic ointment. If the impetigo is widespread, an oral antibiotic may be prescribed.

Impetigo is commonly found on the hands and face of children. The most common way of getting impetigo is by coming into contact with an infected person. If you are caring for a client with impetigo, use Standard Practices when washing around the area. Encourage the client to perform frequent hand hygiene. Washing the client's linens and dishes separately from others' will help avoid spreading pathogens.

Skin Tag

A *skin tag* is a small flap of flesh-coloured skin that looks like a droplet or "tag" of skin (**FIGURE 37–1, *J***). Skin tags are not painful but, depending on where they appear, can get caught in jewellery, zippers, or even bra hooks. They are most common on women and on older adults.

Athlete's Foot

Athlete's foot is a highly contagious fungal skin infection that causes the affected foot to peel, burn, itch, and turn red (**FIGURE 37–1, *K***). It is easily spread through contact in moist areas, such as locker rooms or showers, or by exchanging footwear. It can be treated by drying the foot thoroughly, including between the toes, and by using over-the-counter (OTC) medications or, in severe cases, prescription medications.

Scleroderma

Scleroderma is a rare, progressive autoimmune disease that involves the hardening (*sclero*) of the skin (*derma*) and connective tissue throughout the body. There are two main types of scleroderma: (1) *Localized scleroderma* is less severe and usually affects the skin. Muscles and bones may be affected, but internal organs are not. The lesions on the skin can appear either as hard, oval, white lesions with a purple ring around them or as hard, reddish scales. (2) *Generalized scleroderma* affects both the skin and the internal organs, causing damage to the organs. There is no cure for scleroderma, and treatment usually involves medications to soften the skin and reduce inflammation. Clients may be self-conscious because of the appearance of their skin. As the support worker, you must treat them with respect. Treatment for the affected internal organs varies, depending on the damage.

Seborrheic Keratosis

Seborrheic keratosis is a noncancerous growth that is common in older adults. These growths can appear on many areas of the skin, either alone or in groups. They may be dark or multicoloured, and they usually have a grainy surface, though they can be smooth and waxy (**FIGURE 37–1, *L***). They may be mistaken for moles or skin cancer.

Skin Cancer

Skin cancer is a malignant growth on the skin that usually develops in the epidermis and so is easily visible (**FIGURE 37–2**). The two most common types of skin cancer are *basal cell carcinoma* and *squamous cell carcinoma*; both types are unlikely to spread to other parts of the body. The most dangerous type of

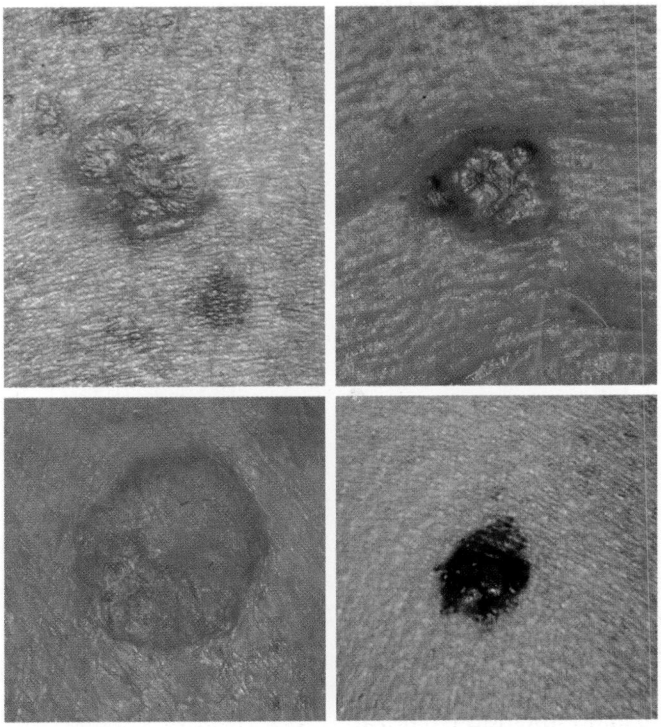

FIGURE 37–2 A and B, Two common presentations of basal cell carcinoma. **C,** Squamous cell carcinoma. **D,** Malignant melanoma. (**Source:** Seidel, H.M., Stewart, R.W., Ball, J.W., et al. (2003). *Mosby's guide to physical examination* (5th ed., p. 209). St. Louis, MO: Mosby.)

skin cancer is *malignant melanoma*, which can be fatal if not treated early.

Basal cell carcinoma is the most common type of skin cancer, accounting for 90% of all skin cancers. It usually presents as a raised, smooth, pearly bump and occurs on an area that has been exposed to the sun, such as the neck or shoulders. Small blood vessels may be seen in the tumour. Frequently, crusting and bleeding occur in the centre of the tumour, so it can be mistaken for a sore that does not heal.[1]

Squamous cell carcinoma is the second most common type of skin cancer. It starts in the epidermis as a red, scaly, thickened patch on sun-exposed skin, eventually penetrating the underlying tissue if not treated. Bleeding and ulceration can occur. It is easily treated when found early. In a small percentage of cases or if it is not treated, this cancer spreads (*metastasizes*) to other parts of the body.

Malignant melanoma is a less common but highly dangerous form of skin cancer. It is the eighth most common form of cancer in Canada.[2] It is caused by excessive exposure to ultraviolet (UV) light from either the sun or tanning beds and from repeated sunburns. Prevention measures include avoiding overexposure to the sun and using a broad-spectrum sunscreen with SPF 15 or greater throughout the year when outdoors.

All melanomas look different. Signs of a melanoma include the following mole traits:

- More than one colour (may be shades of black, brown, or blue or sometimes white, grey, red, or pink)
- Asymmetrical
- Irregular border or jagged edges
- More than 6 mm in diameter
- Itchy
- Changes in texture
- Oozing
- Bleeding

Early detection is critical. The appearance of a new mole during adulthood should be checked by a physician.

Treatment of skin cancer usually includes removal of the lesion, ensuring that the edges are free of cancer cells. The lesion may be removed by surgery, radiation therapy, or cryotherapy (freezing off the lesion).

MUSCULO-SKELETAL DISORDERS

Musculo-skeletal disorders affect bones, joints, muscles, and the ability to move. Some disorders are caused by injury, and others result from aging or disease.

Fractures

A **fracture** is a break in the bone. Along with the break, the tissues around the fracture, including muscles, blood vessels, nerves, and tendons, are usually injured. Fractures are open or closed (**FIGURE 37–3**). A *closed fracture* (*simple fracture*) means that the bone is broken but the skin is intact. An open fracture (*compound fracture*) means that the broken bone has come through the skin.

Fractures are usually caused by falls and other accidents but can also result when bones are weakened by diseases such as cancer, alcoholism, and osteoporosis. Signs and symptoms of a fracture include the following:

- Limb appearing bent or out of position
- Pain
- Swelling
- Limited movement of limb or loss of function

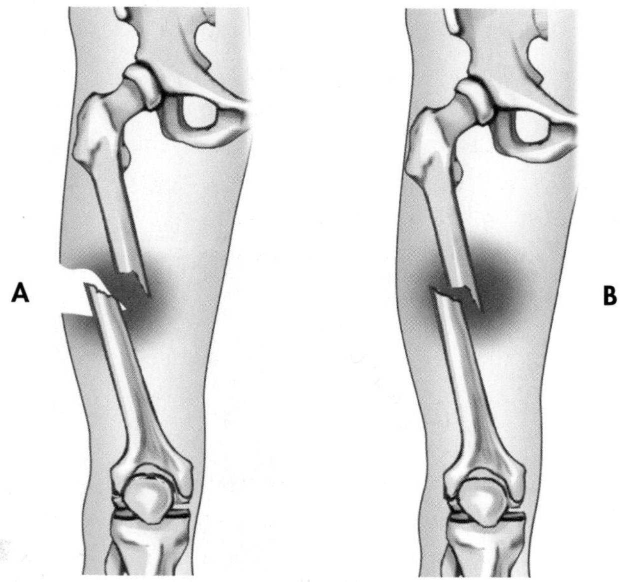

FIGURE 37–3 A, Open fracture. **B,** Closed fracture. (**Source:** Thibodeau, G.A., & Patton, K.T. (2010). *The human body in health and disease* (5th ed., p. 196). St. Louis, MO: Mosby.)

- Bruising and colour changes in the skin at the fracture site
- Bleeding (internal or external)

To help the broken bone heal, the bone ends are brought into normal position—called *reduction*. *Closed reduction* involves moving the bone back into place without opening the skin. *Open reduction* involves surgery to expose the bone and bring it back into alignment. Nails, rods, pins, screws, plates, or wires are sometimes used to keep the bone in place. After reduction, the site of the fracture is immobilized; that is, movement of the bone ends is prevented by using a cast or traction (see the *Focus on Children: Fractures* box). The location and the seriousness of the fracture will determine the type of immobilization used.

The goal in managing fractures is to ensure that the affected limb segment will achieve maximal possible function after it has healed.

Casting and Cast Care

Casts are applied to immobilize a fracture for an extended length of time in order for it to heal in its correct position. Casts that stay in place for the duration of the healing process are made of plaster, fibreglass, or plastic. Some casts, though, are of removable plastic material. Before applying a plaster or fibreglass cast, the injured part is covered with a stockinette, which protects the skin, and then a layer of padding. Plaster casting material, which comes in rolls, is moistened and wrapped around the padding. Fibreglass casts dry quickly, usually in 20 to 30 minutes. A plaster cast dries in 24 to 48 hours. It is odourless, white, and shiny when dry. When wet, it is grey and cool and has a musty smell. Any client complaints about increasing pain or numbness and tingling in the casted limb should be reported immediately to the supervisor.

Proper care of a cast is important. As a support worker, you may assist with care of the cast. All casts will generate heat when they are drying, so it is important not to cover the cast during this period so as to keep it cool and allow it to dry. The client's care plan may tell you to elevate the client's casted limb. Elevating the limb reduces swelling and pain in the injured area. Removable plastic casts can be inflatable to compress the injury or fracture. The benefits of this type of cast are that it can be removed for physiotherapy or hygiene and it can reduce ankle stiffness and muscle atrophy as well as decrease healing time (**BOX 37–1**).

> **FOCUS ON CHILDREN**
>
> **Fractures**
>
> Falls and accidents involving motor vehicles, bicycles, skateboards, scooters, and in-line skates are common causes of fractures in children. Fractures in infants and certain types of fractures, such as a spiral fracture (often caused from twisting the body part), may also be signs of child abuse.

Traction

Traction is rarely used anymore to treat fractures and bone dislocation. However, two main types of traction are still in use: skin traction and skeletal traction.

- ***Skin traction***[3]—temporary measure before a surgical repair to help prevent displacement between fractured bone pieces. Weights are suspended at the end of the bed and are counterbalanced by the client's own body weight. This traction is held in place either with wide strips of medical adhesive tapes attached to the skin of the limb segment below the fracture or with a foam boot that is securely fitted to the client's foot. Positioning in a slight Trendelenburg position (see Chapter 25) will keep the client from sliding to the foot of the bed. This type of traction can cause damage to the client's skin, so usually no more than 10% of the client's body weight (to a maximum of 5 kg) is recommended for the traction weights. If heavier weights are used, the superficial skin layers of the leg can be irritated or even pulled away from underlying layers, and the risk for friction injury in the client's coccyx region increases (see Chapter 24).
- ***Skeletal traction***[3]—most common for femur fractures. A surgical pin with weights attached to it is placed through a bone farthest from the fracture. An apparatus to facilitate traction is then applied to the client (**FIGURE 37–4**).

BOX 37–1 Guidelines for Cast Care

- Sometimes, with an open reduction, a window is cut in the cast so that the incision and healing process can be observed; as well, allowing oxygen to reach the incision can assist in the promotion of healing. Any blood loss under the cast may leave a faint outline on the cast. This outline should be marked on the cast and dated so as to see if the outline grows, which may indicate further blood loss.
- Keep a plaster cast dry. A wet cast loses its shape. For a cast that is near the perineal area, a nurse may apply a waterproof material around the perineal area once the cast has dried.
- Do not let the client insert anything into the cast. Itching under the cast will cause an intense desire to scratch. Items used for scratching (pencils, coat hangers, knitting needles, back scratchers, etc.) can open the skin, and an infection can develop. Items used for scratching can also wrinkle the stockinette or be lost in the cast, causing pressure and skin breakdown.
- Elevate the client's arm or leg in a cast on pillows. Elevation reduces swelling.
- Ensure you have adequate help and use proper body mechanics when turning and repositioning the client. Plaster casts can be heavy and awkward, and you could easily lose your balance.
- Position the client as directed by your supervisor and the care plan.
- Report these signs and symptoms immediately:
  - Pain—warns of a pressure ulcer, poor circulation, or nerve damage
  - Swelling and a tight cast, numbness, pale skin, or cyanosis (blue colour of the skin)—all signs of reduced blood flow to the area
  - Numbness or inability to move fingers or toes—a sign of pressure on a nerve
  - Temperature changes on the skin—cool skin means poor circulation; hot skin means inflammation
  - Chills, fever, nausea, vomiting, odour, or drainage on or under the cast—may signal an infection under the cast

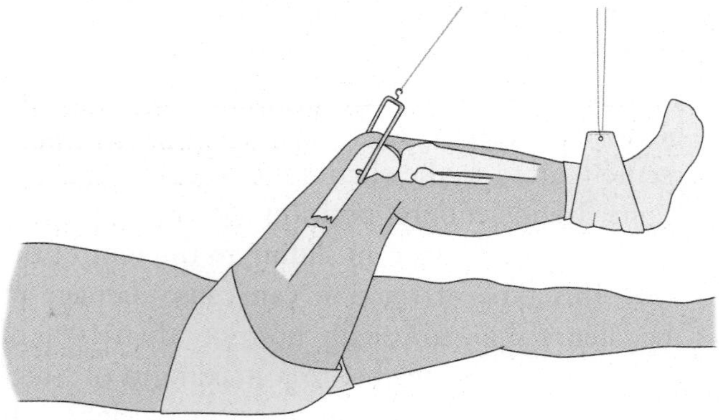

FIGURE 37–4 Skeletal traction for a femur fracture using a Steinmann surgical pin to stabilize the limb and promote healing. (**Source:** Monica Schroeder/Science Source)

Hip Fractures

Fractured hips are common in older adults, especially in older women. Two signs of a fractured hip are shortening of the leg and outward rotation of the leg. Fractured hips in older people are a serious concern because they heal more slowly. The person is also put at risk for life-threatening postoperative complications such as pneumonia, urinary tract infections, and thrombi in the leg veins, as well as for pressure ulcers, constipation, and confusion.

The fractured hip is fixed in position with a pin, nail, plate, screw, or artificial hip joint. The client needs preoperative and postoperative care (see Chapter 45), usually including rehabilitation after surgery. If home care is not possible, the client will need subacute or long-term care. Unless complications develop, most clients return home after successful rehabilitation (see the *Focus on Home Care: Clients Recovering From Hip Fractures* box). **BOX 37–2** describes the postoperative support care these clients require.

Osteomyelitis

Osteomyelitis is the inflammation or infection of the bone marrow, often caused by *Staphylococcus*

BOX 37–2 Caring for Clients With Hip Fractures

- If the client must remain in bed, follow the guidelines for bed care.
- Transfer, turn, and reposition the client, as directed. Turning and positioning depend on the type of fracture and the surgery performed. Usually, the client is not positioned on the operated side.
- Keep the operated leg abducted (away from the median plane) at all times—whether the client is supine, is being turned, or is in a side-lying position (**FIGURE 37–5, *A***). Use pillows or abductor splints, as directed (see **FIGURE 37–5, *B***).
- Prevent external rotation (turning outward) of the hip. Use trochanter rolls, pillows, sandbags, or abductor splints, as directed (see Chapter 24).
- Provide ROM exercises, as directed. Do not exercise the affected leg.
- Provide a straight-backed chair with armrests. The client will need a high, firm seat, so avoid placing the client in a low, soft chair.
- Position the chair on the client's unaffected side when transferring, as per the client's care plan.
- Do not let the client stand on the affected leg unless allowed by the physician.
- Support and elevate the affected leg, as directed, when the client is in a chair.
- Apply elastic stockings, as directed (see Chapter 30).
- Remind the client not to cross the legs while seated or lying in bed.

bacteria. It can be a complication of a bone fracture or of orthopedic surgery and often occurs in the femur and tibia. If not recognized early, it can be very difficult to cure and can lead to persistent pain, loss of function, constant drainage, and even death. Osteomyelitis occurs more frequently in males, possibly because they suffer a higher number of trauma injuries.

As a support worker caring for a client with a recent fracture, ***you must report any symptoms that might indicate osteomyelitis***: acute localized pain,

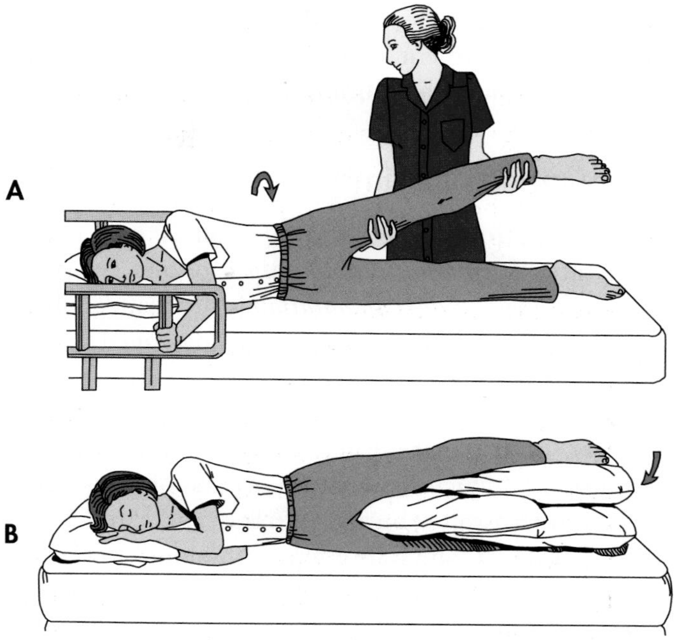

FIGURE 37–5 A, The hip is abducted when the client is turned. **B,** Pillows are used to maintain the hip in abduction. (**Source:** Phipps, W.J., Sands, J.K., & Marek, J.F. (1999). *Medical–surgical nursing: Concepts and clinical practice* (6th ed.). St. Louis, MO: Mosby.)

FOCUS ON HOME CARE

Clients Recovering From Hip Fractures

The artificial hip joint can dislocate (move out of place) with adduction, internal rotation (turning inward), or bending of the leg at the hip joint by more than 90 degrees. Lying on the affected side, sitting in low seats, sitting with the legs crossed, bending from the waist, and putting on shoes and socks or stockings would involve these movements and should be avoided for 6 to 8 weeks after surgery.

An occupational therapist helps the client learn to perform self-care activities, including using self-help devices for dressing (see Chapter 27). The client needs a raised toilet seat for elimination and a shower chair for bathing. When in bed, he or she uses a pillow or abductor splint between the legs. A physiotherapist helps the client learn muscle-strengthening exercises. A walker is usually needed for walking.

redness, drainage, fever, and malaise (tiredness) in the client. Treatment may include surgery to drain the area, followed by administration of antibiotics.

Amputation of a Limb

An **amputation** is the removal of all or part of an extremity. A *traumatic amputation* occurs by accident, whereas *surgical amputation* is performed when an extremity has been so severely damaged in an accident that it has to be removed, when amputation is necessary to treat or prevent disease (such as cancer), or if gangrene has occurred. *Gangrene*—a condition in which tissue death occurs—is caused by infection, frostbite, burns, injuries, and circulatory disorders, all of which interfere with blood flow, thus depriving tissue of oxygen and nutrients. Poisonous substances and waste products build up in tissue, and, as a result, the affected tissue dies and becomes black, cold, and shrivelled (**FIGURE 37–6**). If untreated, gangrene can spread through the body and cause death. The most common cause of amputation is complications from diabetes.

Amputation of all or part of an upper extremity—including fingers, hand, forearm, or entire arm—may be necessary. Similarly, all or part of the lower extremity—including toes, foot, lower leg below or above the knee, or entire leg—may be amputated. The client may experience *phantom limb pain*, which is the perception that the limb is still part of the body and that it is in pain. The client may also feel burning or tingling that seems to stem from the amputated limb. The dominant theory for the cause of this pain is the irritation of the nerve endings in the stump (the remaining part of the limb), which is a normal reaction that may last only for a short time after surgery or for many years.

The client who has undergone an amputation needs a lot of supportive care, since the amputation affects the client's whole life, including body image, daily activities, and work.

Prostheses

Most clients with amputations are fitted with *prostheses* (prosthetic devices; singular, *prosthesis*)—artificial replacements for missing body parts (**FIGURE 37–7**). A prosthesis can be made for any body part—for example, the hand, arm, leg, eye, or breast.

To fit an arm or leg prosthesis, the stump is first conditioned, which involves shrinking and shaping the stump into a cone shape using an elastic stocking or bandage (**FIGURE 37–8**). It is important to wash the

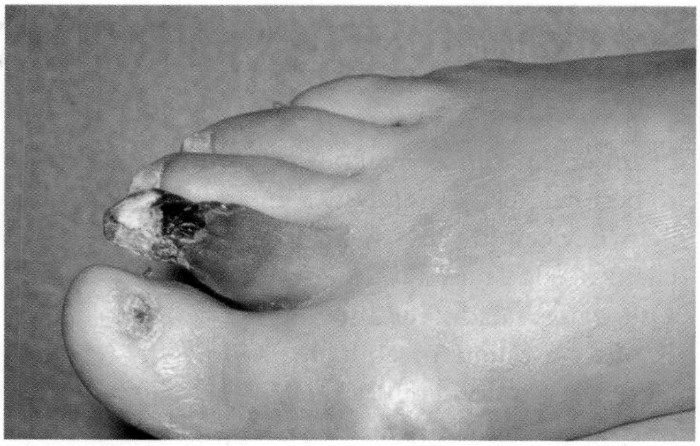

FIGURE 37–6 Gangrene. (**Source:** © Medical-on-Line/ Alamy Stock Photo.)

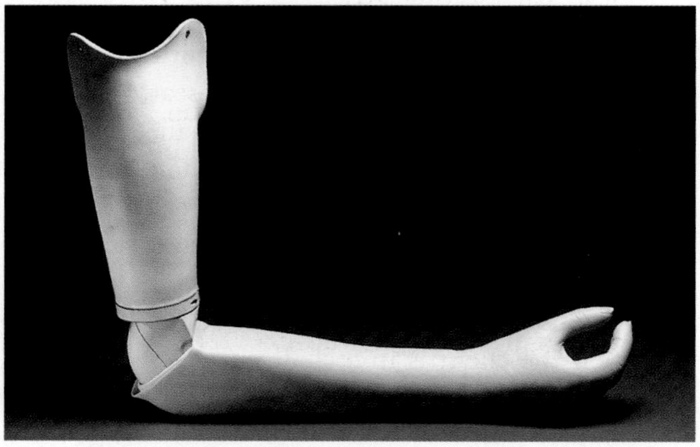

FIGURE 37–7 Arm prosthesis. (Courtesy: Motion Control, Inc., Division of Fillauer Companies, Inc., Salt Lake City, UT.)

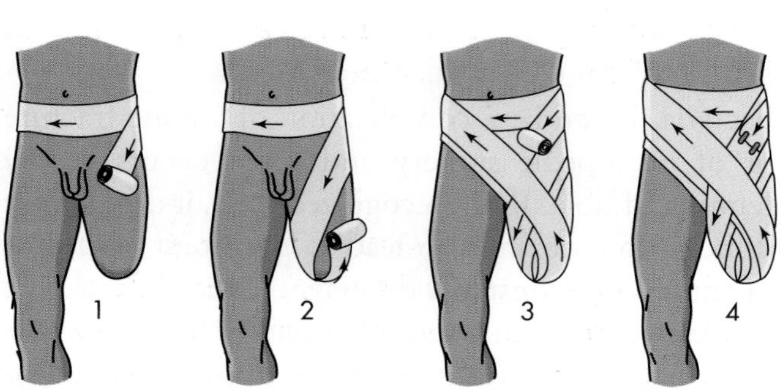

FIGURE 37–8 A mid-thigh amputation is bandaged to shrink and shape the stump. (**Source:** Monahan, F.D., Sands, J.K., Neighbors, M., et al. (2007). *Phipps' medical–surgical nursing: Health and illness perspectives* (8th ed., p. 880). St. Louis, MO: Mosby.)

elastic stocking, as normal moisture could accumulate and cause the stocking to break down, which, in turn, would increase the possibility of breakdown of the skin or healed incision. The client needs to exercise to strengthen the other limbs, and physiotherapists and occupational therapists help the client learn how to use the prosthesis. Research is being done on prosthetic devices that will enable more mobility for the client. Currently available prostheses allow for limited movement and can be cumbersome.

Prostheses and Skin Care

Proper skin care is important for clients with prostheses. For those with leg or arm prostheses, the stump is confined in the prosthesis. Since the skin in this area is not exposed to air, it may become hot and moist, which can cause irritation, blisters, and skin infections.

Follow the client's care plan. The skin at the prosthesis site requires daily care. Damp skin inside the prosthesis can become irritated, so the skin usually needs to be cleaned at the end of the day to keep it thoroughly dry. Wash the skin with warm water and soap—sometimes with medicated soap, depending on the client's needs. Rinse the skin thoroughly with warm water to remove any soap residue, and towel-dry gently. The client's care plan may call for skin lotion or cream to be applied to the entire stump area in order to keep the skin soft and prevent skin damage.

Notify your supervisor at once if the client complains of pain at the prosthesis site. Also, report any signs of redness, swelling, or drainage at the site.

Most prostheses are washed every day with warm soapy water, rinsed well, and towel-dried. Prostheses are very valuable, so do not handle them unless instructed to in the care plan. Keep the prosthesis in its box or container when not in use.

Osteoporosis

Osteoporosis is a bone (*osteo*) disorder in which the bone becomes porous and brittle (*porosis*), meaning it can break easily. Bones of the spine, hips, and wrists are affected most often. Osteoporosis is common in older adults and in postmenopausal women. After menopause, ovaries stop producing the hormone estrogen, resulting in bone changes. Lack of dietary calcium is also a major cause of osteoporosis.

Smoking, high alcohol intake, lack of exercise, prolonged bed rest, and immobility are risk factors for osteoporosis. For bone to form properly, it must continually bear weight. If not, calcium is not absorbed, and the bone becomes porous and brittle. Back pain, gradual loss of height, and a stooped posture occur. Fractures are a great risk if the client falls or has an accident. Sometimes, bones are so brittle that the slightest activity—for example, turning in bed or getting up from a chair—can cause a fracture. Always keep this risk in mind when moving your clients.

Because there is no cure for osteoporosis, prevention is important. The diet must contain enough calcium and vitamins. Estrogen is prescribed for some women after menopause but is not used as much as in the past. Other medications prescribed are bisphosphonates, selective estrogen receptor modulators (SERMs), calcium, and vitamin D, and more medications are being developed. Weight-bearing exercises—for example, strength training (lifting weights), walking, jogging, dancing, and stair climbing—may also prevent osteoporosis.

Some clients with osteoporosis wear a back brace or corset or use walking aids. While you provide support care to a client, protect the client from falls and accidents. Transfer, turn, and reposition the client gently.

Arthritis

Arthritis—which means joint (*arthr*) inflammation (*itis*)—is the most common joint disease. *Inflammation* means swelling, redness, heat, and pain. Pain and decreased mobility occur in the affected joints. Arthritis occurs in all ages. Clients with severe arthritis may require **arthroplasty**—surgical replacement (*plasty*) of a joint (*arthro*) to relieve pain and restore joint motion. Ankle, knee, hip, shoulder, wrist, finger, and toe joints can be removed and replaced with an artificial joint.

There are different types of arthritis. The two most common are osteoarthritis and rheumatoid arthritis.

Osteoarthritis

Osteoarthritis (OA) is the most common form of arthritis. It causes the cartilage that occupies the joints of the body to wear away, causing pain in and disfigurement to the joints. Obesity and a sedentary lifestyle are the main contributors to OA. It affects 13% of adults in Canada.[4] It tends to occur in people over 40 and becomes more common with increasing age. Approximately 80% of Canadians are affected by osteoarthritis by age 75.[5]

OA usually affects the weight-bearing joints—the hips, knees, ankles, and spine. However, joints in the fingers and thumbs can also be affected. In OA, cartilage (the material that cushions the ends of the bones) gradually breaks down, and, eventually, the involved bones rub together, causing pain, especially when the joint is moved. In OA, joints become swollen, stiff, and painful.

Pain is often less severe in the morning and worsens during the day. Pain occurs with weight-bearing and joint motion, and severe pain can interfere with rest and sleep. The joints become stiff after the client has not moved for a period, and cold weather and dampness can increase the symptoms.

Bones can also thicken and form growths called *spurs*, which change the shape of the bone and joint. Spurs called *Heberden's nodes* are common in the fingers (**FIGURE 37–9**).

OA has no cure. Treatment involves relieving pain and stiffness, and physicians often prescribe Tylenol or special arthritis medications as well as heat or cold applications. Treatment for obese clients often includes weight loss through a low-fat, low-calorie diet. During the advanced stage of OA, the client may need a cane or walker. Measures to prevent falls are important, and assistance with activities of daily living (ADLs) is given as needed. Elevated toilet seats are helpful for clients with limited range of motion (ROM) in the hips and knees.

Rheumatoid Arthritis

Rheumatoid arthritis (RA) is a persistent and progressive disease that affects 1 in 100 Canadians.[6] It usually occurs in people between the ages of 25 and 50. However, RA can affect people of all ages, from toddlers to older adults, and is found to be more common in women than in men (see the *Focus on Children: Arthritis* box).

RA affects connective tissue throughout the body. The immune system does not recognize the connective tissue as "normal" and attacks and destroys it. The disease can destroy connective tissues of the heart, lungs, eyes, kidneys, and skin, but it affects mainly the joints, which become painful, swollen, and stiff. RA usually occurs on both sides of the body, but not always. Pain and stiffness are usually worst when the client wakes in the morning but gradually decrease during the day. RA usually starts with the smaller joints in the fingers, hands, and feet and moves on to the larger joints (wrists, elbows, and shoulders; ankles, knees, and hips). Eventually, the normal tissue is replaced by scar tissue, and deformities in the joints can develop (**FIGURE 37–10**). In time, the organs in the body also become affected by RA. Fatigue and fever are common.

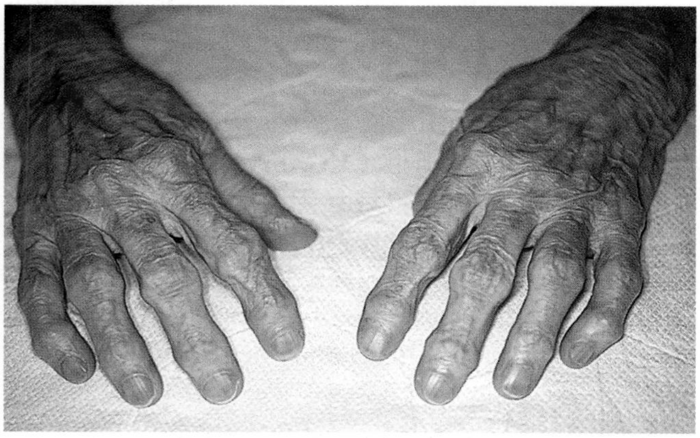

FIGURE 37–9 Spurs that occur in the end joints of fingers are called Heberden's nodes. (**Source:** Swartz, M.H. (2009). *Textbook of physical diagnosis* (6th ed., p. 626). Philadelphia, PA: Saunders.)

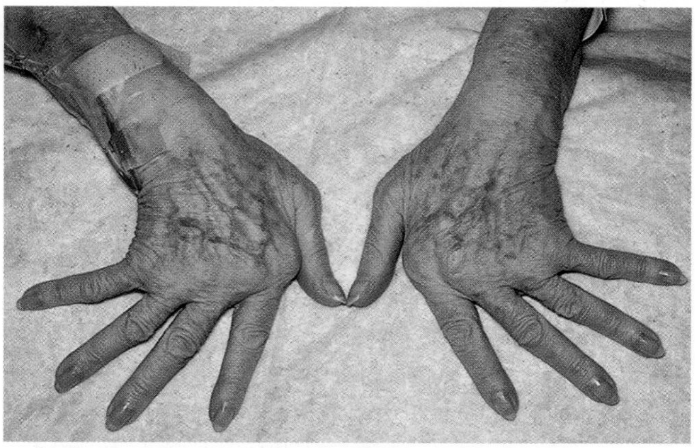

FIGURE 37–10 Deformities caused by rheumatoid arthritis. (**Source:** Swartz, M.H. (2009). *Textbook of physical diagnosis* (6th ed., p. 625). Philadelphia, PA: Saunders.)

> **FOCUS ON CHILDREN**
>
> **Arthritis**
>
> RA in children is called *juvenile rheumatoid arthritis (JRA).* JRA can affect the child's growth and development; as well, eye inflammation can be a complication.

Treatment goals are to maintain joint motion, control pain, and prevent deformities. Rest is balanced with exercise. Adequate sleep—8 to 10 hours—is necessary each night, along with morning and afternoon rest periods. Bed rest is needed if several joints are involved and if fever is present.

Clients with RA benefit greatly from ROM exercises, and some may need walking aids or splints. Taking safety measures to prevent falls is important. Physicians prescribe medications as well as heat or cold applications for relief of pain and inflammation. Some clients may need joint replacement surgery.

Gout

Gout, also called *metabolic arthritis,* is a disease caused by the accumulation of uric acid in the cartilage of a joint, especially in the tendons. It usually affects the big toe first but can affect other joints as well. The signs and symptoms of gout include severe and sudden pain, swelling, redness, warmth, and stiffness of the joint and possibly a low-grade fever. Even simply placing a blanket over the affected area may cause severe pain to the client with gout. Treatment involves pain medication and anti-inflammatory drugs. Applying ice packs may help relieve pain. Follow the care plan.

Fibromyalgia

Fibromyalgia is a condition associated with aching, stiffness, and fatigue in muscles, ligaments, and tendons and often affects the neck, shoulders, upper back, lower back, hips, legs, knees, and feet. Because of the pain and stiffness in the affected parts, the client commonly experiences fatigue and sleep disturbances. Persistent fatigue makes even simple tasks difficult. Clients diagnosed with fibromyalgia have usually gone through many tests to rule out other disorders. The process can be very frustrating for them because there are, as yet, no specific tests to identify this condition. As a support worker, you need to sympathize with your clients and encourage them to accept the treatments indicated on their care plans.

There is no cure for fibromyalgia. Heat and cold applications, massage, and regular stretching and ROM exercises are helpful. Occupational therapy may be required, along with prescribed medications to relieve pain, relax muscles, and promote sleep.

NERVOUS SYSTEM DISORDERS

The nervous system communicates signals between the brain and the body, so nervous system disorders affect physical and cognitive functions. *Physical functions* include tasks such as moving, touching, seeing, hearing, and controlling the bowel and bladder. *Cognitive functions* include tasks controlled by the mind (the word *cognitive* is related to knowledge), such as thinking, reasoning, understanding, remembering, learning, reading, and problem solving.

Epilepsy

Epilepsy is a group of neurological disorders characterized by recurrent episodes of convulsive seizures, sensory disturbances, abnormal behaviour, loss of consciousness, or some or all of the above. Temporary changes occur in the brain because of a burst of electrical energy, which results in a seizure, affecting awareness, movement, or sensations. A *seizure* (or *convulsion*), in some people, can be a violent and sudden contraction or tremor of muscle groups, uncontrolled movements, and loss of consciousness; in others, the seizure may be so subtle that it can go unnoticed. Seizures can involve the entire brain or just one part of the brain. Some clients have a warning of a seizure, or an *aura,* before it starts.

Some infants can have a single seizure caused by a very high fever. A single seizure does not mean epilepsy, however; in epilepsy, seizures recur. Known causes of epilepsy include the following:

- Brain injury before, during, or after birth
- Lack of oxygen before, during, or after birth

- Problems with brain development before birth
- An injury or infection during the mother's pregnancy
- Head trauma (accidents, gunshot wounds, sports injuries, falls, blows to the head)
- Chemical imbalance
- Poor nutrition
- Brain tumour
- Childhood fevers
- Poisons such as lead and alcohol
- Infections, such as meningitis and encephalitis
- Stroke

Children and young adults are commonly affected, but epilepsy can develop at any time during a person's life. It can occur because of any problem affecting the brain—for example, cerebral palsy, developmental disability, autism, and Alzheimer's disease.

There is no cure for epilepsy at this time, but it is normally controlled by medication. Surgery has been used for clients suffering from severe, uncontrolled seizures. When controlled, epilepsy usually does not affect learning and ability to perform ADLs. Activity limitations occur only in severe cases. For example, if a client is at risk of having a seizure at any time, her job choices and activities such as driving may be limited. Each province and territory has regulations regarding driver's licences for clients with epilepsy.

If a client experiences an epileptic seizure, your responsibility is to prevent self-injury. Stay with the client and call for assistance. Lower the client to the floor if possible, and move objects away from him. You should move the client away from sharp edges, place something soft under the head, and, if possible, move him onto his side to avoid asphyxiation (choking on vomit). If it is not possible to move the client onto his side during the seizure, gently try to move his head to the side, but do not force any movement of body parts. After the seizure is over, put the client in the recovery (three-quarter prone) position, and check the client for injury. If the seizure lasts longer than 5 minutes or if more seizures follow one after another, you should call emergency services immediately.

***Never* place anything in the client's mouth during a seizure.** Doing so can cause injury to you or your client. Clients will not swallow their tongues but may bite them during the seizure.

After a seizure, the client may be exhausted and confused and may not be aware that a seizure has occurred. Stay with the client until he returns to his normal condition. You may need to help the client wash and change clothes, as some clients may vomit, void, or soil themselves during or after a seizure. Some clients may fall into a deep sleep, and some may experience a headache after a seizure.

You should record your observations—duration of the seizure, parts of the body involved, any mannerisms noted, and your client's behaviour after the seizure has stopped.

Stroke

Stroke, or *cerebral vascular accident (CVA),* is the fourth leading cause of death in Canada and also the leading cause of nervous system disabilities in adults.

The Heart and Stroke Foundation of Canada defines *stroke* as a sudden loss of brain function. Stroke is caused by one of the following:

- An interruption of blood flow to the brain, often caused by a blood clot
- The rupture of a blood vessel in the brain

When a vessel to the brain is blocked or bursts, blood supply to a part of the brain is suddenly obstructed, and the brain cells in the affected area do not get oxygen and nutrients. A brain injury results, and the functions controlled by that part of the brain are lost or impaired.

Temporary interruption of blood flow to the brain is called a **transient ischemic attack (TIA)**. Even though a TIA results in no permanent brain injury, it is an important warning sign, as sometimes a TIA occurs before a stroke. So a client having a TIA needs immediate medical attention.

The risk for stroke increases with age—most strokes affect people aged 65 years or older. Men are at a slightly higher risk than women, but more women than men die from strokes. Risk factors other than gender include high blood pressure, smoking, diabetes, heart disease, high blood cholesterol, lack of exercise, and high alcohol intake.

Common warning signs of a stroke are listed in **BOX 37–3**. A stroke is a medical emergency, so the client needs immediate medical attention. Call emergency services.

If the client survives the stroke, some brain injury is likely. The injured area in the brain cannot send messages to control certain parts of the body, so normal function is affected, depending on the area of the brain injury (**FIGURE 37–11**). The effects of stroke include the following:

BOX 37–3 Warning Signs of a Stroke

- Weakness—sudden loss of strength or numbness in the face, arm or leg, even if temporary
- Trouble speaking—sudden difficulty speaking or understanding or sudden confusion, even if temporary
- Vision problems—sudden trouble with vision, even if temporary
- Headache—sudden severe and unusual headache
- Dizziness—sudden loss of balance, especially with any of the above signs

Source: Heart and Stroke Foundation of Canada. (2016). *Stroke signs.* Retrieved from http://www.heartandstroke.on.ca/site/c.pvI3IeNWJwE/b.3581689/k.780C/Stroke__Warning_Signs.htm.

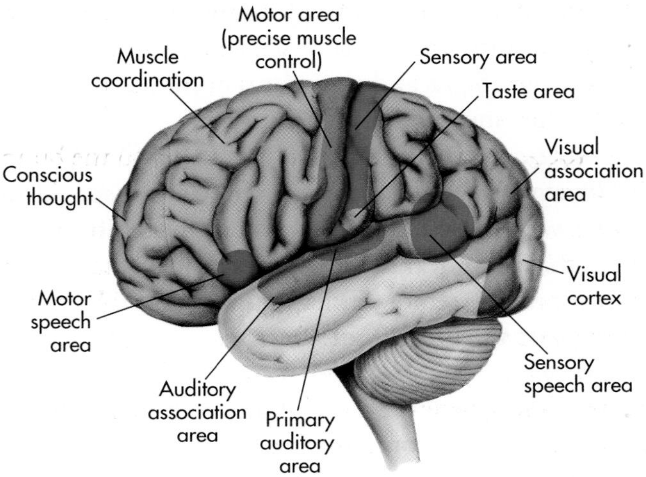

FIGURE 37–11 Functions lost because of a stroke depend on the area of brain injury. (**Source:** Thibodeau, G.A., & Patton, K.T. (2010). The human body in health and disease (5th ed., p. 251). St. Louis, MO: Mosby.)

- **Hemiplegia**—paralysis (*plegia*) of one side (*hemi*) of the body; the right arm and leg or the left arm and leg could be affected
- Weakness on one side of the body
- Loss of facial muscle control
- Changing emotions (the person may cry easily, sometimes for no apparent reason)
- Difficulty swallowing (*dysphagia*)
- Dimmed vision or loss of vision
- Loss of ability to speak or understand others; *aphasia* (see Chapter 39)
- Changes in sight, touch, movement, and thought
- Impaired memory
- Urinary frequency, urgency, or incontinence
- *Aphasia*—loss of speech

Following a stroke, the client's behaviour is affected. The client may forget about or ignore the weaker side because of loss of movement and feeling on that side. If vision is affected, the client may not see one side of the visual field. This impairment can cause the client to eat food from only one side of the plate or to read only one side of a page.

After a stroke, clients may no longer recognize familiar objects or know how to use them. Telling time may be hard for these clients, and they may not recognize people. Memory problems and difficulty learning and remembering new information are common. Clients may forget what to do or how to do it, or if they do know, their bodies may not be able to act, making it difficult for them to carry out ADLs (see Chapter 36).

Depression is a common after-effect of illness or disability. It is particularly common after a stroke as a result of the brain injury. As a support worker, encourage your clients to share their feelings during this difficult period. Sometimes, their emotional responses may seem exaggerated or inappropriate. Outbursts of anger, moaning, laughing, or crying for little or no reason often occur. Remember, these reactions are beyond clients' control, so be patient and kind with them. Report any changes in the client's behaviour or mood to your supervisor.

Rehabilitation usually starts immediately after a stroke, and many clients are able to improve or regain lost functions. Speech therapy, physiotherapy, and occupational therapy are usually ordered by the physician. In addition, a swallowing assessment may be

Facial drooping Arm weakness speech difficulties Time to call F.A.S.T done to provide guidelines within the care plan to reduce the risk for choking and aspiration problems. Self-help devices may be necessary (see Chapter 27), and the client may depend partially or totally on others for care. Most stroke survivors return home and require home care, but some may need subacute or long-term care, depending on their needs and conditions. Some clients require assistance with ADLs, but they are encouraged to do as much as possible for themselves. Clients who are immobile need skin care to prevent pressure ulcers, and they also may require a bladder or bowel control training program and ROM exercises. Communication methods are established for clients with language impairments (see Chapter 39).

Aneurysm

An **aneurysm** is a localized dilation (expansion, and thus weakness) of the wall of an artery or heart chamber. It may be caused by atherosclerosis (see p. 864) and hypertension (see p. 863) or, less frequently, by trauma, infection, or a congenital weakness in the vessel wall. Aneurysms are common in the aorta but can also occur in peripheral vessels. In older people, the popliteal artery is a common site for an aneurysm. The effect of an aneurysm will depend on the area damaged.

Clients with aneurysms are usually asymptomatic (without symptoms), which explains the occurrence of sudden death when an aneurysm ruptures. Most aneurysms are discovered on routine physical examination or with X-rays. Once diagnosed, the primary goal is to prevent a rupture. If an aneurysm ruptures, surgical repair is needed to stop the bleeding, but this surgery can be very complicated, especially if the aneurysm is in an abdominal, thoracic, or brain artery.

Acquired Brain Injuries

Acquired brain injury (ABI) is damage to brain tissue caused by a disease, a medical condition, an accident, or violence. When the head is subjected to violent forces, the brain is bashed against the skull, resulting in bleeding, swelling, and bruising of brain tissue. Brain injury can be permanent.

Most ABIs are caused by motor vehicle accidents (MVAs). Other common causes are falls, sports and recreational injuries, acts of violence, work-related accidents, and other nervous system injuries—for example, spinal cord injuries. As well, conditions during birth, near drowning, choking, suffocation, or stroke can cause ABIs. Brain injury can also occur without any outward signs of physical damage—for example, when babies are shaken violently (known as *shaken baby syndrome*). Some acquired brain injuries are caused by lack of oxygen to the brain because of accidents, diseases, and certain conditions. Lack of oxygen destroys brain cells and can cause permanent brain injury.

Signs and symptoms depend on the severity and location of the injury. See Chapter 35 for ways that ABIs can affect cognition and memory. Disorientation, poor coordination, personality changes, headache, dizziness, fatigue, problems with vision, sensitivity to noise or light, or problems with sleep may occur. Behavioural changes include moodiness, irritability, or an inability to sit still. Cognitive problems include difficulty making decisions, problems with attention or concentration, or problems recalling simple words. Severe brain injury can result in intellectual disability, speech problems, breathing difficulties, and loss of bowel and bladder control. Rehabilitation (see Chapter 27) is required for these clients. Care depends on their needs and abilities.

Parkinson's Disease

Parkinson's disease is a neurological disorder in which cells in certain parts of the brain are gradually destroyed. It is progressive, and as yet, there is no cure. The disease is usually seen in people over 50 years of age. Signs and symptoms become worse over time. They include the following:

- ***Tremors***—often start in one finger and spread to the whole arm; pill-rolling movements (rubbing of the thumb and index finger) may occur and progress to tremors in legs, jaws, and face
- ***Stiff muscles***—stiffness in arms, legs, neck, and trunk
- ***Masklike expression***—inability to blink or smile; a fixed stare is common
- ***Slow movement***—a slow, shuffling walk and inability to lift the feet
- ***Stooped posture and impaired balance***—inability to walk, with increased risk for falls

Other signs and symptoms that can develop over time include swallowing and chewing problems, constipation, and bowel and bladder problems. Sleep disturbances and depression as well as *dementia*—memory loss, slow thinking, and emotional changes (see Chapter 36)—can also occur. Speech changes include slurred speech, monotone, and soft speech. Some clients may talk too fast or repeat what they say. Allow your client the time required to communicate.

Medications specific for Parkinson's disease are prescribed, along with exercise and physiotherapy to help improve or maintain strength, posture, balance, and mobility. The client needs to have regular rest periods and avoid stress, as tiredness and stress can make the symptoms worse. The client may need help with ADLs. Measures to promote normal elimination are practised, and safety practices to prevent falls and choking are followed. As a support worker, treat the client with dignity and respect. Remember, the client's masklike facial expression does not show the person's true feelings.

Huntington's Disease

Huntington's disease is an inherited neurological disorder. It destroys brain cells and causes uncontrolled movements, emotional disturbances, and cognitive losses. Signs and symptoms may appear any time between the ages of 20 and 60 years. They begin with twitching, fidgeting, and clumsiness, and over time, the client's arms and legs constantly move, making walking impossible. The client may have difficulty eating and swallowing and is unable to perform many ADLs.

Clients with Huntington's disease also may have slurred speech, depression, irritability, and apathy. Cognitive losses include loss of intellectual speed, attention, and short-term memory. Concentration on intellectual tasks becomes increasingly difficult as the disease progresses. Currently, there is no cure, and there are no treatments to prevent or control the disease.

Support care depends on the client's needs. Safety practices should be followed to prevent falls, choking, and other accidents. Emotional support is necessary for all clients, but it is particularly important for these clients, as they are often relatively young and in long-term care facilities. Also, often, more than one member of the family has the disease.

Multiple Sclerosis

Multiple sclerosis (MS) is a persistent, slowly progressive disease in which the body's immune system attacks the protective myelin sheaths that surround the nerve cells of the brain and spinal cord (a process called *demyelination*), resulting in damaged areas that are unable to transmit nerve impulses.

Canada has one of the highest rates of MS in the world. Symptoms usually start between the ages of 15 and 40 years, with women being affected more often than men.[7] The onset is gradual, and symptoms vary greatly from client to client. A client can also have different symptoms at different times, with conditions improving during periods of remission.

The common symptoms of MS are as follows:

- Blurred vision, double vision, or blindness
- Extreme fatigue
- Loss of balance, dizziness, difficulty walking, and clumsiness
- Muscle weakness and stiffness
- Tingling, numbness, or a burning feeling in one area of the body
- Sensitivity to heat
- Difficulty speaking
- Difficulty swallowing
- Bladder and bowel issues
- Impotence or diminished sexual arousal
- Short-term memory loss
- Difficulties concentrating
- Impaired judgement or reasoning

There is no cure as yet for MS, but research is ongoing, and every day, more progress is being made. A number of drugs used to treat MS are keeping clients in remission for longer periods. Some clients are seeking alternative methods of treatment, some of which involve travel to another country for procedures not yet available in Canada. Support care depends on the client's needs and condition. At first, the client may need home care, especially help with housekeeping, to prevent fatigue. As mobility decreases, the client depends more on others, and measures have to be taken to prevent injury and to promote bowel and bladder elimination. Eventually, the client may require long-term care.

Amyotrophic Lateral Sclerosis

Amyotrophic lateral sclerosis (ALS), also known as **Lou Gehrig's disease**, is a degenerative disease characterized by loss of the motor neurons, with progressive weakness and atrophy of the muscles of the hands, forearms, and legs, eventually spreading to involve most of the body and face. In Canada, about 3 000 people are currently living with this disease, which occurs most commonly between the ages of 40 and 70 years.[8]

ALS is a progressive disease in which nerve cells in the brain and spinal cord are gradually destroyed. The rate of progress of the disease differs with each client. Usually, the first sign of the disease is difficulty using fingers and hands. The client may not be able to pick up a cup, lace shoes, pull up zippers, or do buttons. The client then has difficulty walking, so stumbling and falling are common. Eventually, all muscle control is lost, and the client is unable to speak, swallow, move, or breathe independently. Eventually death occurs.

Clients with ALS are alert and can think clearly through the course of the disease. Even if these clients cannot speak, remember that they can still understand what you and others say. The speech pathologist may recommend new communication methods. Follow the care plan. Emotional support is very important, as these clients are very aware of what is happening to their bodies, and the progression of the disease is quite distressing. They eventually become confined to bed and are usually placed in a side-lying position.

Spinal Cord Injuries

The spinal cord is a pathway that allows communication between the brain and the rest of the body, so when it is damaged, the nerves cannot send messages between the brain and the different parts of the body, and partial or total paralysis may occur. **Paralysis** is the complete or partial loss of ability to move a body part or muscle group. Spinal cord injuries, most of which are permanent, are often caused by MVAs.

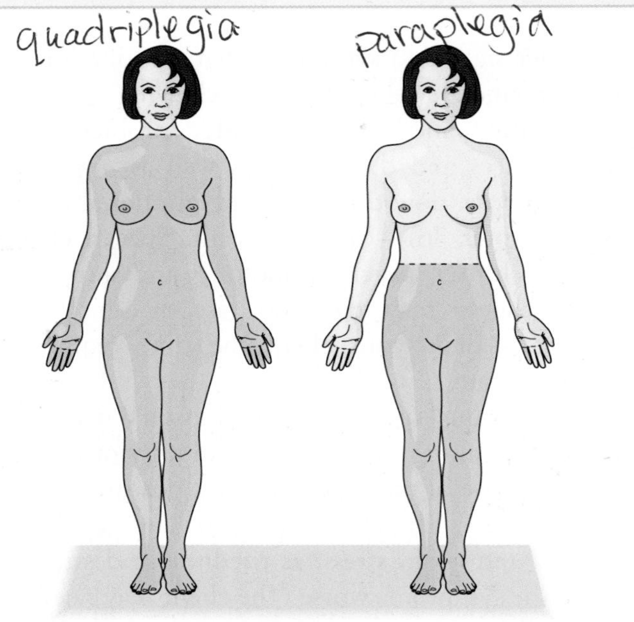

FIGURE 37–12 The shaded areas indicate the areas of paralysis.

Which parts of the body are paralyzed depends on where the spinal cord was injured. The higher up the spine the injury occurs, the greater the loss of function is (**FIGURE 37–12**). Spinal cord injuries at the thoracic level (chest area) or lower may cause **paraplegia**—paralysis (*plegia*) from the waist down. Injuries in the cervical region (neck) may cause **quadriplegia**—paralysis (*plegia*) of all four (*quad*) limbs and the trunk; the client is paralyzed from the neck down. These clients often need cervical traction and a special bed that keeps the spine straight at all times.

Clients who have had recent spinal cord injuries require rehabilitation (see Chapter 27), and the rehabilitation program depends on the client's needs and remaining abilities. **BOX 37–4** describes the care clients with paralysis usually need.

CARDIOVASCULAR DISORDERS

The cardiovascular system involves the heart and blood vessels. The heart pumps blood continuously through the vessels, and blood delivers oxygen, nutrients, and other substances to the body's cells and removes waste products. Cardiovascular disorders involve problems in the heart or in the blood vessels and are the leading causes of death in Canada.[9]

BOX 37–4 Care of Clients With Paralysis

- Assist with ADLs and home management tasks. Follow the care plan.
- Prevent falls. Follow the care plan for safety measures and the use of bed rails.
- Keep the call bell within reach (in facilities). Check the client often if she is not able to use the call bell. Encourage your client to call out for help if unable to use the call bell.
- Prevent burns by checking the temperature of bathwater, heat applications, and food.
- Turn and reposition the client at least every 2 hours. Follow the care plan.
- Maintain good alignment. Use supportive devices according to the care plan.
- Prevent pressure ulcers. Follow the care plan.
- Assist with transfers.
- Follow bowel and bladder training programs.
- Assist with ROM and other exercises, as ordered by the physician.
- Assist with food and fluids as needed. Provide self-help devices, as ordered. Feed the client if necessary.
- Follow the client's rehabilitation plan.
- Give emotional support.

BOX 37–5 Risk Factors for Hypertension

- ***Age.*** Blood pressure tends to rise with age, beginning at about age 35.
- ***Ethnicity.*** The incidence of hypertension is statistically higher among Canadians of South Asian, Indigenous, or African descent
- ***Family history.*** If a parent has hypertension, the adult child has a greater chance of also developing it. The risk increases if both parents have hypertension.
- ***Obesity.*** The risk increases if the excess weight is stored around the abdomen.
- ***Diabetes.*** People with diabetes are at increased risk for hypertension.
- ***Stress.*** Repeated exposure to stress may raise blood pressure levels.
- ***Alcohol.*** Excessive alcohol consumption increases blood pressure.
- ***Smoking.*** Cigarette smoking may contribute to hypertension in some people.

Hypertension

Hypertension is abnormally high blood pressure. The systolic pressure is 140 mm Hg or higher, or the diastolic pressure is 90 mm Hg or higher (see Chapter 15). Elevated measurements must occur on two consecutive occasions to consider a diagnosis of hypertension. The risk factors identified by the Heart and Stroke Foundation of Canada are listed in BOX 37–5.

Narrowed blood vessels are a common cause of hypertension because when vessels become narrowed, the heart has to pump with more force to move blood through the vessels. Other causes of hypertension include underlying medical issues such as kidney disorders, head injuries, complications of pregnancy, and tumours.

Hypertension can damage other body organs. The heart may enlarge so that it can pump with more force. Blood vessels in the brain may burst and cause a stroke, and blood vessels in the eyes, kidneys, and other organs may be damaged.

At first, hypertension may not cause signs or symptoms, so many people with hypertension do not even know they have it. Usually, it is discovered when blood pressure is measured during routine checkups. Signs and symptoms develop as the disorder progresses. Headache, blurred vision, and dizziness may be reported. Complications of hypertension include stroke, heart attack, kidney (renal) failure, and blindness.

Certain medications can lower blood pressure. The client with hypertension needs to quit smoking, exercise, and get enough rest. A sodium-restricted (low-salt) diet and, if the client is overweight, a low-calorie diet are ordered by the physician.

Coronary Artery Disease

Coronary arteries are located in the heart and supply the heart with oxygen-rich, nutrient-rich blood. **Coronary artery disease (CAD)** is a condition in which the coronary arteries are narrowed or blocked

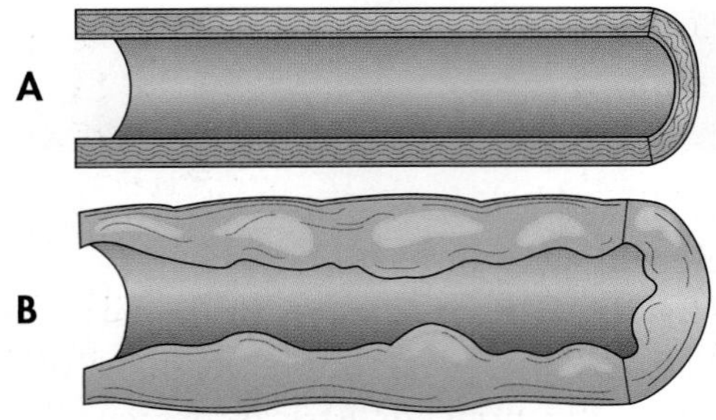

FIGURE 37–13 A, Normal artery. **B,** Fatty deposits on the walls of arteries with atherosclerosis. (Courtesy of the Heart and Stroke Foundation of Canada. (2015).)

by thickening and narrowing of the artery walls—called *atherosclerosis*. Atherosclerosis is caused by a buildup of cholesterol (a soft, waxy substance) and other fatty substances along the inside walls of the arteries (**FIGURE 37–13**). When coronary arteries become narrowed or blocked, blood flow to the heart is slowed or stopped. The heart muscle does not get enough oxygen and nutrients, so it cannot work properly, leading to chest pain and heart attack. Risk factors for CAD include the following:

- Hypertension
- High blood cholesterol
- Lifestyle factors (lack of exercise, obesity, smoking, excessive alcohol, stress)
- Uncontrolled diabetes
- Age (it is more common in older adults)
- Gender (it is more common in men)
- Family history of CAD

Treatment for CAD involves reducing the risk factors. Nothing can be done about the person's gender, age, and family history. However, efforts can be directed at weight loss, regular exercise, quitting smoking, and maintaining a healthy diet. Controlling blood pressure and diabetes also is important.

Some clients need coronary artery bypass grafting (CABG). This surgery creates a bypass (new path) around the diseased part of the artery and thus increases blood flow to the heart. Less invasive procedures such as *angioplasty* and *vascular stenting* are now available. There are pros and cons to each procedure. CABG involves general anaesthesia and a longer recovery time, but the beneficial effect of the surgery lasts longer as arteries remain patent (clear) longer. Stenting is done under local anaesthesia, is less invasive, and has a shorter recovery time, but the effect of the procedure may be more limited.

Angina Pectoris

Angina pectoris means chest (*pectoris*) pain (*angina*) caused by CAD. It occurs when the heart muscle does not get enough oxygen. Clients with angina are at risk for a heart attack. Physical exertion is the most common trigger for angina. Other triggers include emotional stress, extreme cold or heat, heavy meals, alcohol, and smoking.

The chest pain associated with angina has been described as a feeling of heaviness, tightness, or pressure. Usually, the pain occurs on the left side, and some clients feel severe pain that lasts 2 to 15 minutes. Pain may travel (radiate) to the jaw, neck, shoulders, back, and arms (**FIGURE 37–14**). Sometimes, angina is mistaken for indigestion or heartburn when felt in the upper abdominal area. Besides pain, the client may experience shortness of breath, nausea, sweating, dizziness or light-headedness, fatigue, or palpitations (quick heartbeats). Women, older adults, and people with diabetes may have symptoms that differ from these usual symptoms. The signs and symptoms the client experiences will cause the client to stop all activity and seek rest. Rest often relieves the symptoms in 3 to 15 minutes, as it reduces the heart's need for oxygen. Therefore, normal blood flow is achieved and heart damage is prevented.

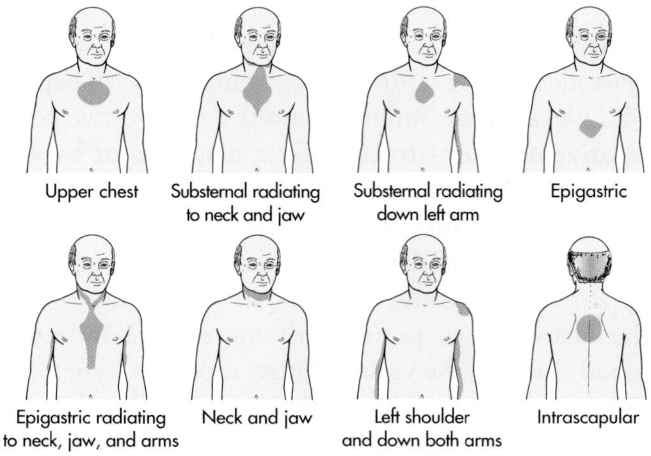

FIGURE 37–14 Shaded areas show where the pain of angina pectoris is located. (**Source:** Lewis, S.M., Heitkemper, M.M., & Dirksen, S.R. (2007). *Medical–surgical nursing: Assessment and management of clinical problems* (7th ed., p. 797). St. Louis, MO: Mosby.)

Besides resting and avoiding common triggers, clients are often prescribed nitroglycerin in tablet, ointment, patch, or spray form to relieve angina. The client carries the medication at all times and takes a dose whenever an angina attack occurs. If a client has taken the maximum amount of nitroglycerin and there is no pain relief, call emergency services and your supervisor.

Myocardial Infarction

Myocardial infarction (MI) means death (*infarction*) of heart tissue (*myocardium*) caused by lack of oxygen to the heart because of sudden interruption of blood flow to the heart. Atherosclerosis or a thrombus (blood clot) obstructs blood flow through an artery, and sudden cardiac death (*cardiac arrest*) can occur as a result. The area of damage may be small or large (**FIGURE 37–15**). Common terms for MI are **heart attack**, *coronary*, *coronary thrombosis*, and *coronary occlusion*. An estimated 1.6 million Canadians are living with heart disease or the effects of stroke, and 1.3 million Canadians are living with heart disease.[10] Defibrillation, when used with cardiopulmonary resuscitation (CPR), can improve cardiac arrest survival rates to more than 50% if delivered in the first few minutes. For every one minute delay in defibrillation, the survival rate decreases by 7% to 10%.

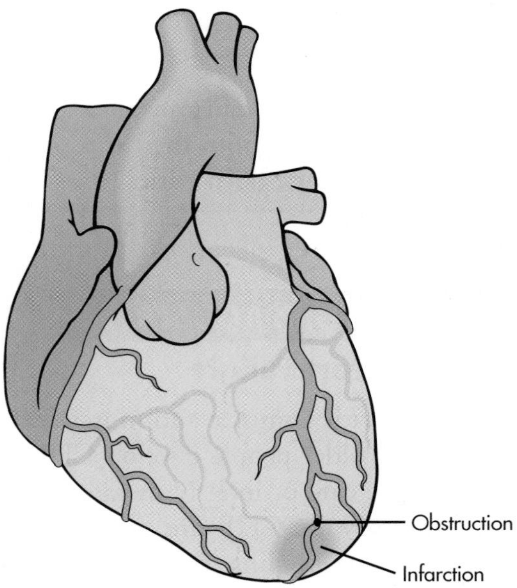

FIGURE 37–15 Myocardial infarction. (**Source:** Lewis, S.M., Heitkemper, M.M., & Dirksen, S.R. (2000). *Medical–surgical nursing: Assessment and management of clinical problems* (5th ed., p. 861). St. Louis, MO: Mosby.)

A client having an MI may have one or more of the signs and symptoms listed in **BOX 37–6**. Many clients deny that they are having an MI. The average client waits almost 5 hours before getting help; however, it must be remembered that an MI is an emergency. Research being conducted on atypical myocardial infarctions indicates that many women, especially older women, ignore the early warning signs that can occur at least a month before an MI. Unusual fatigue, sleep disturbances, shortness of breath, indigestion, and anxiety are signs often ignored by women. As a support worker, you need to report any of these symptoms in your client to your supervisor. Treatments are directed at relieving pain, stabilizing vital signs, giving oxygen, and calming the client; medications need to be given as well.

BOX 37–6 Signs and Symptoms of Myocardial Infarction

- Sudden, severe chest pain, usually on the left side
- Pain described as crushing, stabbing, or squeezing; most people complain of feelings of tightness, heaviness, pressure, fullness, or burning in the chest
- Pain that radiates to the neck and jaw, and down the arm or to other sites
- Pain that is more severe and lasts longer than with angina
- Pain that is not relieved by rest and nitroglycerine
- Indigestion
- Shortness of breath
- Nausea or vomiting
- Dizziness
- Perspiration
- Cyanosis (bluish lips and nail beds from lack of oxygen in the blood)
- Cold and clammy skin
- Low blood pressure
- Weak and irregular pulse
- Fear and anxiety; a feeling of doom (disaster)

The client is treated in a hospital coronary care unit (CCU), which has emergency equipment and medications needed to prevent life-threatening complications. The client is kept in the CCU for 2 to 3 days (depending on your area) and then transferred to another nursing unit once stable.

The client who has suffered an MI is allowed to increase his level of activity gradually. Medications and measures to prevent complications are continued. Rehabilitation, with the goal of preventing another heart attack, is begun in a hospital and continued when the client returns home. The rehabilitation includes an exercise program and teaching about medications, dietary changes, activity, and lifestyle modifications. Activities, including sexual activity, return to normal levels slowly, and the client can return to work when advised by the physician.

Congestive Heart Failure

Congestive heart failure (CHF), or simply *heart failure*, is an abnormal condition that occurs when the heart cannot pump blood normally. Blood backs up and causes an abnormal amount (congestion) of fluid in the tissues. CHF may affect the right side, left side, or both sides of the heart.

The right side of the heart receives blood from body tissues and pumps it into the lungs to get oxygen. With right-sided heart failure, blood backs up into the veins. Fluid collection in the body produces weight gain. *Pitting edema* (swelling due to excess fluid in the tissues—see Chapter 28) becomes evident in the feet and ankles, and the neck veins become enlarged. The liver becomes engorged, which impairs its function. Congestion in the abdomen may cause digestive problems, including loss of appetite, abdominal pain, and (eventually) weight loss.

The left side of the heart receives blood from the lungs and pumps it into the rest of the body. With left-sided heart failure, blood collects in lung tissue, resulting in difficulty breathing (*dyspnea*), increased sputum (mucus in the lungs), cough, and gurgling sounds in the lungs. Dyspnea is worse when the client is active or is lying down, so it disrupts sleep. The client may wake up with a feeling of suffocation. Fatigue and weakness in the limbs are common.

In advanced CHF, the brain may not get enough oxygen, causing confusion and behaviour changes. Poor blood flow to the kidneys results in impaired kidney function and low urine output.

CHF can be treated and controlled by medications that can strengthen the heart and reduce the amount of fluid in the body. Treatment also includes a sodium-restricted diet and administration of oxygen. Weight is measured daily to check for weight gain, an early sign of fluid buildup. Most clients with CHF prefer the semi-Fowler's or Fowler's position for ease of breathing. As a support worker, you may be involved in the following:

- Maintaining bed rest
- Measuring intake and output
- Measuring daily weight, ideally before eating and after voiding
- Restricting fluids, as ordered by the physician
- Assisting with transfers or ambulation
- Assisting with self-care activities
- Maintaining good positioning and body alignment according to the care plan
- Applying elastic stockings to reduce leg swelling

See the *Focus on Children: Congestive Heart Failure* and *Focus on Older Adults: Congestive Heart Failure* boxes.

FOCUS ON CHILDREN

Congestive Heart Failure

Congenital heart defects can cause CHF in children. (*Congenital* comes from the Latin word *congenitus*, meaning "to be born with.")

FOCUS ON OLDER ADULTS

Congestive Heart Failure

Because the heart is a muscle and muscles weaken with age, many older people develop CHF. Some may need home care or long-term care.

Older adults with CHF are at risk for skin breakdown. Tissue swelling, poor circulation, and fragile skin combine to increase the risk for pressure ulcers. Effective skin care and regular position changes are essential.

Arrhythmias

Arrhythmias are abnormal (*a*) heart rhythms (*rhythmias*). They happen when the heart's electrical system malfunctions. Sometimes, heartbeats are skipped, or extra beats occur. Usually, the client's health is not affected, but some arrhythmias are more serious. They can cause dizziness, shortness of breath, fainting, or death. Avoiding caffeine (coffee, tea, colas, and chocolate) and alcohol can sometimes prevent arrhythmias. Medications are needed for severe arrhythmias.

Pacemakers—medical devices that are implanted in the client's body to regulate the heartbeat—are used to treat some arrhythmias. They monitor heart rates, and when necessary, they give small electric shocks to stimulate heartbeats. Pacemakers can run on batteries for several years. Clients with pacemakers should avoid any areas or equipment that have strong electrical or magnetic fields, such as some microwaves, security systems, or therapeutic magnetic mattress pads. People who have pacemakers should also ask their doctor about being around cellphones and MP3 players, high-tension wires, metal detectors, industrial welders, electrical generators, and even some machines for medical procedures, such as magnetic resonance imaging (MRI).

Phlebitis

Phlebitis is inflammation of a vein. It occurs most often in the legs. Phlebitis can be caused by bacterial infection, chemical irritation, trauma, lupus, or a genetic condition. Signs and symptoms include redness and warmth in the area, pain, burning, and swelling. Provide supportive care according to the care plan.

Thrombus

A *thrombus* is a blood clot that forms in a blood vessel. If it occurs in a large blood vessel, it will decrease blood flow through the blood vessel. If it occurs in a small blood vessel, it may completely stop blood flow, which can result in the death of the tissue below the blockage. A thrombus can form as a result of a stroke, a heart attack, deficiencies in the blood's clotting ability, or extended periods of inactivity, such as following surgery (see Chapter 45). A thrombus or a part of it may dislodge and travel through the body until it lodges in another blood vessel. A travelling blood clot is called an *embolus*, which can eventually move to the lungs and cause severe respiratory problems and death.

To avoid the formation of blood clots, your clients should be encouraged to keep active. It is especially important to encourage leg exercises if your client is confined to bed. Follow the care plan.

RESPIRATORY DISORDERS

The respiratory system is made up of the lungs and their airways. The airways bring oxygen into the lungs and remove carbon dioxide from the body. Respiratory disorders interfere with this function and threaten life.

Asthma

Asthma is a respiratory disorder characterized by recurring episodes of *paroxysmal dyspnea* (intermittent spasms of shortness of breath); wheezing on expiration, inspiration, or both, caused by constriction (narrowing) of bronchi; coughing; and thick bronchial secretions of mucous. The client with asthma becomes short of breath and produces wheezing sounds, which may be frightening for her. The client may also experience a rapid pulse, perspiration, and cyanosis. Allergies; exercise; cold air; outdoor activity in hot, humid weather; smog; and emotional stress are common causes of asthma attacks.

Clients with asthma have medications to treat the disorder but, for severe attacks, may require emergency department treatment. You must call emergency services as soon as you see your client in distress. The client and family are taught how to prevent asthma attacks, as repeated attacks can damage the respiratory system.

Pneumonia

Pneumonia is an infection of lung tissue. Alveoli (tiny air sacs within the lungs) in the affected area fill with pus, mucus, and other liquid, and oxygen and carbon dioxide are not exchanged properly, causing insufficient oxygen in the blood.

Bacteria and viruses can cause pneumonia. Clients who are immobile are at higher risk for developing pneumonia. The onset can be gradual or sudden. Signs and symptoms include shaking, chills, severe chest pain, a cough that produces rust-coloured or greenish sputum (*phlegm*, or mucus), high temperature, rapid breathing and pulse rate, cyanosis (blue-tinged skin), and confusion.

While providing support care, follow Standard Practices. Transmission-Based Practices (see Chapter 23) may be ordered by the physician to prevent the spread to others, especially in facilities, where frail clients with compromised immune systems may be very vulnerable to pneumonia. It is important that the support worker be aware of what the precautions are and how to strictly adhere to isolation procedures. Immunizations for pneumonia for high-risk clients are now available.

Bronchitis

Acute *bronchitis* is inflammation of the bronchi (the large airway passages entering the lungs; singular, *bronchus*) caused by bacteria or viruses and can last for several days or weeks. Chronic bronchitis is not generally caused by a virus (see "Chronic Obstructive Pulmonary Disease," below).

A client with acute bronchitis usually has a cough that produces sputum. The colour of the sputum will indicate if the infection is viral or bacterial. Green-coloured mucus may indicate a bacterial infection, but only a lab test will confirm the type of infection and will determine the treatment the physician will prescribe. Fever, fatigue, shortness of breath, and chest pain may accompany the cough. Bacterial bronchitis is treated with antibiotics, and viral bronchitis will usually disappear on its own. While providing support care to a client, if you observe blood-tinged sputum, report it immediately to your supervisor.

Chronic Obstructive Pulmonary Disease

Chronic obstructive pulmonary disease (COPD) refers to chronic bronchitis and emphysema, which often occur together. It is the fourth leading cause of death worldwide and is expected to climb to third place by 2030, according to the World Health Organization.[11] For Canadian women, COPD causes more deaths than breast cancer does.[11] COPD is a persistent lung disorder that obstructs (blocks) the airways and makes breathing difficult. It is a progressive disease, gradually worsening over time.

Smoking is the most common cause of COPD. Long-time exposure to chemical fumes and to certain dusts is another cause.

COPD cannot be cured but can be controlled. The client must quit smoking and avoid second-hand smoke. Medications to open the airways are usually delivered by metered-dose inhalers (MDIs), or "puffers" (see Chapter 43). Breathing exercises and oxygen therapy may also be ordered. Fluid intake is encouraged to decrease the thickness of secretions, and efforts are made to prevent respiratory tract infections. If one occurs, prompt treatment is necessary.

Chronic Bronchitis

Chronic bronchitis is a persistent inflammation of the bronchi. Large amounts of mucus are produced in the bronchi, and the bronchial walls swell. The mucus is thick and difficult to cough up, so it cannot be cleared completely and thus obstructs the airways, making airflow into and out of the lungs difficult. Therefore, the body cannot get normal amounts of oxygen. The excess mucus also provides a place for the growth of microbes, so infection is a risk. Coughing is the first and most common symptom of chronic bronchitis. The client also has difficulty breathing and tires easily. Eventually, breathing becomes difficult even when the client is resting.

Emphysema

Emphysema occurs when the walls of the alveoli (small cavities; singular, *alveolus*) are damaged and become less elastic than normal. They do not expand and shrink as normal during inhalation and exhalation, and as a result, when the client breathes out, air is trapped in some of the alveoli and not exhaled. As the disease progresses, more alveoli become involved, and more air is trapped. The normal exchange of oxygen and carbon dioxide cannot occur in the affected alveoli. As more air is trapped in the lungs, the person develops a *barrel chest* (**FIGURE 37–16**).

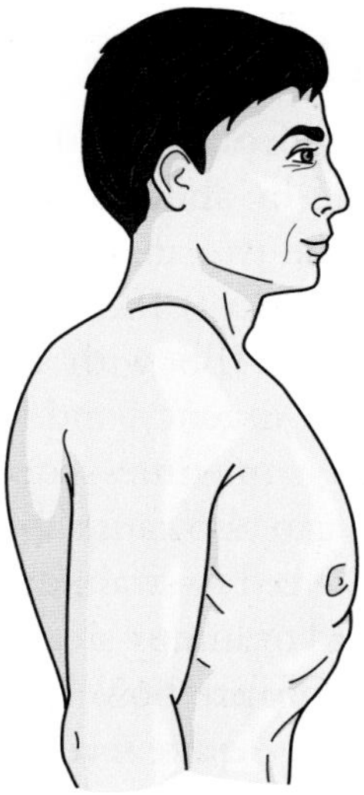

FIGURE 37–16 Barrel chest caused by emphysema.

Breathing is very difficult for people with emphysema. Sometimes, they lose weight because eating is difficult when they are out of breath. Clients with emphysema usually prefer to sit upright and slightly forward because breathing is easier in this position.

Treatments include the following:

- Antibiotics to fight infection
- Medications to ease chest pain, cough, and fever
- Proper diet
- Proper fluid and hydration
- Fowler's or semi-Fowler's position to make breathing easier
- Oxygen therapy

DIGESTIVE DISORDERS

The digestive system breaks down food for absorption by the body and also eliminates solid wastes. See Chapter 33 for a more detailed discussion on some digestive disorders—diarrhea, constipation, flatulence, and fecal incontinence.

Vomiting

Vomiting (*emesis*) is the act of expelling stomach contents through the mouth. It signals illness or injury that can be life threatening. *Vomitus* (material vomited) can be aspirated (inhaled into the lungs) and obstruct the airway. Vomiting large amounts of blood can lead to shock. Practise the following measures when a client vomits:

- Follow Standard Practices.
- Turn the client's head well to one side to prevent aspiration.
- Place a kidney basin or other container under the client's chin.
- Remove vomitus from the client's immediate environment.
- Provide oral hygiene to help remove the taste of vomitus.
- Eliminate odours.
- Change linens or client's clothing, as necessary.
- Observe vomitus for colour, odour, and undigested food. Vomitus that looks like coffee grounds may contain digested blood, which could indicate internal bleeding and must be reported immediately.
- Estimate the amount of vomitus. In the community, you may not have an accurate means of measuring the amount of vomitus. You could estimate a cupful or plateful or follow your agency's policy to determine small, medium, and large amounts. Some facilities will require you to measure and record the amount of vomitus according to their policy.
- Report immediately to your supervisor that the client has vomited, and report your observations. Some facilities may require you to keep the vomitus so that it can be observed or sent to a laboratory for analysis.

Gastro-Esophageal Reflux Disease

Gastro-esophageal reflux disease (GERD) is a common disorder of unknown cause. The muscle band at the end of the esophagus and the start of the stomach relaxes at inappropriate times, allowing the stomach acids to go up the esophagus. Clients refer to it as "heartburn," which is the most common symptom of GERD. Other symptoms include a sour taste in the mouth, bad breath, belching, and difficulty or pain when swallowing. Treatment usually involves medication and may include raising the head of an adjustable bed or putting blocks under the head of the bed to keep the top part of the body at a higher level than the stomach.

Gallbladder Disease

The *gallbladder* is a pear-shaped sac that stores bile (see Chapter 17). For reasons yet unknown, the components of bile often form stones in the gallbladder, which can cause inflammation, called **cholecystitis**. Stones can obstruct the flow of bile into the digestive system. Symptoms of cholecystitis include severe pain in the abdomen, nausea, vomiting, and, in some cases, jaundice. Treatment may include surgery and a low-fat diet.

Liver Disease

The liver plays an important part in carbohydrate and protein metabolism and produces bile. Two of the most common disorders of the liver are hepatitis and cirrhosis. Liver transplantations can successfully treat some liver diseases.

Hepatitis may be caused by a bacterial or viral infection (viruses can be hepatitis A to hepatitis G), a parasitic infection, alcohol, drugs, toxins, or a transfusion of incompatible blood. (See pp. 878–880 for a discussion on communicable hepatitis diseases.)

Cirrhosis occurs as a result of persistent liver disease. Liver tissue is gradually replaced by scar tissue, which affects liver function. It is most commonly caused by alcoholism and hepatitis C virus. There is no cure for cirrhosis, but treatment can halt further damage. Some signs and symptoms are weight loss, jaundice, enlarged liver, fatigue, and accumulation of fluid in the abdomen.

Celiac Disease

Celiac disease is an inborn metabolic disorder that results in the inability to tolerate gluten protein. Gluten is found in wheat, oats, and barley. The disease affects adults and young children and causes abdominal distension, vomiting, diarrhea, muscle wasting, and extreme lethargy. Diarrhea is usually large in volume, foul smelling, and pale in colour. The only effective treatment is a gluten-free diet. As the support worker, you must ensure that you follow the care plan regarding your client's diet. Since many foods can contain traces of gluten, accurate reporting of foods that cause symptoms can help identify foods the client should avoid.

Irritable Bowel Syndrome

Irritable bowel syndrome (IBS) is a disorder of the bowel characterized by abdominal pain and changes in bowel habits. The two main types of IBS are (1) IBS with diarrhea and (2) IBS with constipation. A client suffering from IBS with diarrhea often has abdominal bloating, urgency, and frequent loose and watery stools that sometimes contain mucus. IBS with constipation can also cause abdominal bloating. Clients frequently need to strain during bowel movement, produce hard or lumpy stools, and are left with the feeling of incomplete bowel emptying. Abdominal pain, which can be quite severe, is usually relieved after bowel movement.

The cause of IBS is not yet known, although stress is thought to trigger episodes. Treatment will vary, depending on which type of IBS the client is diagnosed with. Medication for IBS with diarrhea would consist of antidiarrheals, and medications for IBS with constipation would consist of stool softeners or laxatives. For some clients, avoiding nonsoluble fibrous foods can help control episodes.

Compassion is required when caring for a client with IBS since the condition can be quite stressful and embarrassing. You may be asked to record the dietary intake of your client to determine which foods trigger episodes.

Colitis

Colitis is inflammation of the colon. Signs and symptoms of colitis include fever, pain, abdominal tenderness, rectal bleeding, and ulcerations in the colon. Treatment may include antibiotics and anti-inflammatory drugs. A reduction in the intake of carbohydrates has helped some clients. Surgery may be required to remove the affected part of the colon.

Crohn's Disease

Crohn's disease is a persistent, inflammatory condition of the GI tract characterized by flare-ups and periods of remission. It can affect all age groups, and no exact cause has been identified for this disorder. The disease can affect any part of the GI system, but it most commonly affects the last part of the small intestine and the large intestine. Symptoms can vary, depending on the area affected. The most common symptoms are abdominal pain, diarrhea, and weight loss. Some clients have episodes of bloody diarrhea and can have as many as 20 bowel movements in a day. Bowel obstructions can occur because of the narrowing of the intestines from persistent inflammation and, if severe enough, can become life threatening.

Crohn's disease can also affect other body systems. Some complications include skin rashes, arthritis, eye inflammation, mouth ulcers, and anemia.

Treatment for a flare-up usually involves medications to reduce inflammation and infection, if present. During remission, the goal of treatment is to build up the client's physical and mental ability to cope with the next flare-up when it occurs. There is no cure for Crohn's disease, a fact that is difficult for many clients to accept.

Crohn's disease affects each client differently, depending on the areas of the bowel and other body systems affected. Your observations, recording, and reporting are very important to help your client during a flare-up. For example, a client vomiting or having a fever could mean a bowel obstruction; a client complaining of pain around the anus could indicate an inflammation or start of an abscess, and joint pain could be the start of arthritis associated with Crohn's disease.

It is very important to record the colour and approximate volume of each bowel movement and to describe if blood is visible. During flare-ups, clients can lose weight because of decreased food intake and malabsorption. They may hesitate to eat, being fearful of more bouts of diarrhea. Follow the care plan for dietary intake.

Diverticular Disease

Diverticular disease is very common in older adults. It is characterized by the development of small pouches that bulge outward through weak spots in the colon (**FIGURE 37–17**). Each pouch is called a *diverticulum* (*diverticulare* means "turn inside out"). The condition of having these pouches is called **diverticulosis** (*osis* means "condition of").

When feces enter the pouches, the pouches can become inflamed and infected—which is called *diverticulitis* (*itis* means "inflammation"). The client has abdominal pain and tenderness on the lower left side of the abdomen. Fever, nausea and vomiting, chills, cramping, and constipation are likely to be present. Bloating, rectal bleeding, frequent urination, and pain while urinating can also occur.

A ruptured pouch is a rare complication that results in feces spilling out into the abdomen, leading to a severe, life-threatening infection. A pouch also can cause a block in the intestine (intestinal obstruction) that feces and gas cannot move past. These conditions require surgery.

A low-fibre diet and constipation are risk factors for diverticular disease. To treat it, the physician orders dietary changes and, in some cases, antibiotics. Surgery to remove the diseased part of the bowel is needed for severe disease, obstruction, and ruptured pouches. Sometimes, a colostomy is necessary (see Chapter 33).

URINARY DISORDERS

The kidneys, ureters, bladder, and urethra are the major structures of the urinary system. Disorders can occur in one or more of these structures.

Urinary Tract Infections

Urinary tract infections (UTIs) are common, and infection in one area of the urinary system can

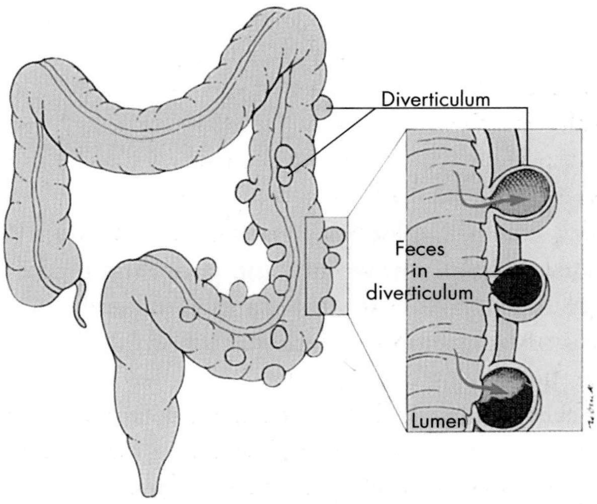

FIGURE 37–17 Diverticular disease.

lead to infection of the entire urinary system (see Chapter 32).

Normally, the urinary system is sterile, meaning it has no microbes. However, microbes can enter the system through the urethra. Catheterization, urological examinations, infections through sexual intercourse, poor perineal hygiene, incomplete bladder emptying, and poor fluid intake are common causes of UTIs. UTIs are frequently acquired in health care settings.

Women are at high risk because microbes can easily enter the short urethra. Prostate gland secretions help protect men from UTIs. However, an enlarged prostate increases the risk for a UTI, so older men are more likely than younger men to get one.

Cystitis means inflammation (*itis*) of the bladder (*cyst*). **Pyelonephritis** is an inflammation (*itis*) of the kidney (*nephr*) and renal pelvis (*pyelo*) due to bacterial infection. Signs and symptoms are as follows:

- Urinary frequency and urgency
- Oliguria—scant (*olig*) urine (*uria*)
- Dysuria—difficult or painful (*dys*) urination (*uria*)
- Pain or burning during urination
- Foul-smelling urine
- Hematuria—blood (*hemat*) in the urine (*uria*)
- Pyria—pus (*py*) in the urine (*uria*)
- Fever and chills
- Pain in the lower abdomen or back

In older adults, sudden confusion can indicate a possible urinary infection. Treatment includes antibiotics and increased fluid intake—usually 2 000 mL/day.

Renal Calculi

Renal calculi are kidney (*renal*) stones (*calculi*). Prolonged bed rest, immobility, and poor fluid intake are risk factors. Stones vary in size and in mineral content. Signs and symptoms include the following:

- Severe, cramping pain in the back and side, just below the ribs
- Pain in the abdomen, thigh, and urethra
- Nausea and vomiting
- Fever and chills
- Urinary frequency and urgency
- Oliguria—scant (*olig*) urine (*uria*)
- Dysuria—difficult or painful (*dys*) urination (*uria*)
- Hematuria—blood (*hemat*) in the urine (*uria*)
- Foul-smelling urine

Treatment involves medication for pain relief and increased intake of fluids—about 2 000 to 3 000 mL a day. Increased fluids cause stones to leave the body through the increased excretion of urine. All the client's urine must be strained to catch any stones that may be passed during urination (see Chapter 32). Sometimes, however, surgical removal of stones may be necessary. Dietary changes can help prevent further formation of stones, so dietitians are usually part of the health care team.

Renal Failure

Renal failure (kidney failure) occurs when the kidneys do not function or are severely impaired. When the kidneys fail, waste products are not removed from blood, and the body retains fluids. As fluids build up in the bloodstream, the client may have puffy and swollen face, hands, and feet. Hypertension and CHF can result. Renal failure can be acute or persistent.

Acute Renal Failure

Acute renal failure occurs suddenly after severely decreased blood flow to the kidneys caused by severe bleeding, heart attack, CHF, burns, infections, or severe allergic reactions. Acute renal failure is usually a temporary condition. With treatment, the condition may be reversed. However, it is a very serious condition, as it can result in death.

Acute renal failure occurs in phases. First, *oliguria* (scant amount of urine) occurs, when urine output is less than 400 mL in 24 hours. This phase lasts a few days to 2 weeks. Then *diuresis*—the process (*esis*) of passing (*di*) urine (*uria*)—occurs, and large amounts of urine are produced, about 1 000 to 5 000 mL/day. Kidney function improves and returns to normal during the recovery phase. The disease process can take from 1 month to 1 year. However, some people do not recover and develop chronic renal failure.

The physician orders medications, restricted fluids, and diet therapy. The care plan will likely include the following:

- Measuring and recording urine output every hour if your client has a catheter (an output of less than 30 mL per hour should be reported immediately)
- Measuring and recording intake and output of fluid
- Restricting fluid intake
- Daily weight measurements using the same scale
- Frequent oral hygiene
- Measures to take if the client is confined to bed
- Measures to prevent infection

Chronic Renal Failure

In *chronic renal failure*, the kidneys cannot meet the body's needs. The nephrons of the kidneys are destroyed over many years. Hypertension and diabetes are common causes; some others are infections, urinary tract obstructions, and tumours.

Signs and symptoms appear when 80% to 90% of kidney function has been lost. A few of the many signs and symptoms are yellow skin; dry, itchy, or brittle skin; inflammation of the mouth; bruises and bleeding; hypertension; and a burning sensation in the legs and feet.

Every body system is affected because waste products build up in the blood. There is no cure; in the early stages, however, diet therapy, fluid restriction, and medications may slow kidney damage. The general care required for clients in chronic renal failure is described in **BOX 37-7**.

Once the client has lost considerable kidney function, dialysis becomes necessary. *Dialysis* is the process of removing wastes and excess water from blood. Only specially trained nurses can perform this procedure. Initially, it is done in a dialysis unit, but, eventually, some clients may be able to have home dialysis, and you may be the caregiver. Your supervisor will ensure that you are aware of your responsibilities and scope of practice when giving care. Some clients may require kidney transplantation.

BOX 37-7 Care of Clients With Chronic Renal Failure

- Limit fluids.
- Measure the client's blood pressure with the client in the supine, sitting, and standing positions.
- Measure weight daily with the same scale and at the same time of day.
- Measure and record intake and output of fluids.
- Use bath oils, lotions, and creams on the skin to prevent itching. Follow the care plan.
- Provide frequent oral hygiene, as clients' mouths are often dry.
- Encourage rest.
- Prevent complications of bed rest if the client is confined to bed.

Benign Prostatic Hypertrophy (BPH)

Benign prostatic hypertrophy (BPH) is an enlarged prostate gland. The prostate gland surrounds the urethra, the tube that carries urine from the bladder out of the body. As the prostate enlarges, it may partially block the urethra. As a result, affected men may have problems urinating.[12]

BPH is very common in older men. In fact, about half of all men older than 75 have some symptoms of it. BPH is not a form of cancer, nor does it cause prostate cancer. It also does not cause erection difficulties or affect a man's ability to father children.[12]

BPH can cause urinary problems such as the following:[12]

- Difficulty stopping or starting urination
- Frequently feeling the need to urinate, which can interrupt sleep
- A weak or slow urine stream
- A feeling that the bladder is not empty even after urination
- Urinary dribbling (leaking)
- Blood in the urine, especially when trying to force a urinary stream

If your client cannot urinate without extreme difficulty, the bladder may be blocked, and your supervisor should be notified. This problem is rare but may cause backed-up urine (urinary retention), leading to bladder infections, bladder stones, or kidney damage.[12]

ENDOCRINE DISORDERS

The endocrine system is made up of glands that secrete chemical messengers called *hormones*. Hormones affect other organs and glands and are essential for body function. Endocrine disorders result in hormone levels that are either too high or too low. The most common endocrine disorder is diabetes.

Diabetes

Diabetes is a disorder in which the body cannot produce or use insulin properly. *Insulin* is a hormone secreted by the pancreas and needed for the proper use of sugar (*glucose*). It helps the sugar obtained from foods to get into cells. Without enough insulin in the body, sugar builds up in blood—referred to as *hyperglycemia*, which means high (*hyper*) sugar (*glyc*) in blood (*emia*). When cells do not have sugar for energy, they cannot perform their functions. Left untreated, mild hyperglycemia can lead to long-term complications. Severe hyperglycemia can be life threatening.

Today, more than nine million Canadians live with diabetes or pre-diabetes. Approximately 10% of people with diabetes have type 1 diabetes, and the number of people with type 2 diabetes is increasing dramatically. There are three types of diabetes:

- ***Type 1 diabetes***—occurs most often in children and young adults but can occur at any age. The pancreas does not produce insulin, leading to severe hyperglycemia. These clients develop symptoms early in the disease and need treatment of daily insulin injections. It is sometimes called *insulin-dependent diabetes mellitus* (*IDDM*).
- ***Type 2 diabetes***—usually develops in adulthood but can occur in children as well. Type 2 is the most common type of diabetes. Either the pancreas does not produce enough insulin, or the body does not effectively use the insulin that is produced. Obesity and family history are risk factors. Risk also increases after age 40 years. Almost 80% of Canadians come from populations that are at higher risk for type 2 diabetes (e.g., Indigenous, Hispanic, Asian, South Asian, or African descent).[13]

  The hyperglycemia is often mild enough that the client may not notice the symptoms. Treatment often consists of diet and exercise or oral medications. Insulin is sometimes required. Type 2 diabetes is sometimes referred to as *non–insulin-dependent diabetes mellitus (NIDDM),* although this name is misleading since some clients must take insulin.
- ***Gestational diabetes***—develops during pregnancy and usually disappears after the baby is born. However, the woman who experiences gestational diabetes is at risk for developing type 2 diabetes later in life.

Common signs and symptoms of type 2 diabetes are the following:

- Increased thirst
- Frequent urination
- Constant hunger
- Unusual weight loss
- Extreme fatigue
- Dry, itchy skin
- Blurred eyesight

It is important that diabetes be controlled. If left untreated or poorly managed (as often happens with type 2 diabetes), the high levels of blood sugar slowly damage both small and large blood vessels in the body, potentially causing numerous complications, including blindness, kidney disease, nerve damage, sexual dysfunction, and circulatory disorders. Circulatory disorders can lead to stroke, heart attack, and slow wound healing. Foot and leg wounds have very serious consequences for people with diabetes, as infection and gangrene can occur and sometimes lead to amputation.

There is no cure for diabetes, but the disease can be managed to reduce or prevent long-term complications. All clients with diabetes must follow a careful diet, and overweight clients need to lose weight. Exercise is included as part of the treatment plan, as regular exercise helps lower blood sugar levels, promotes weight loss, and reduces stress. Oral medications may also be necessary. Regular and proper foot and nail care provided by a professional is extremely important, as corns, blisters, and calluses on the feet can lead to infection and necessitate amputation. The client's feet should be inspected daily, and any cuts, lesions, or nonintact skin surface should be reported immediately to the supervisor.

When you are caring for a client with diabetes, your reports and observations are extremely important, as you could be the first one to observe changes in your client's condition.

Diabetes requires blood sugar monitoring—glucometers are now available to allow clients themselves to do finger-prick blood tests to determine the levels of sugar in blood and the amount of insulin needed. Clients with type 1 diabetes need to test their blood sugar level on an average of three to four times a day before each insulin dose, and those with type 2 diabetes usually need to monitor their levels once daily. Blood sugar monitoring is a delegated act that you may be trained to do as part of your role.

Clients with type 1 diabetes require insulin injections usually one to four times daily; some clients with type 2 diabetes also need insulin. Most clients administer their insulin themselves. The exact type and dose of insulin must be taken as ordered by the physician so as to prevent complications from insulin therapy. If too much insulin is taken, hypoglycemia occurs. *Hypoglycemia* means low (*hypo*) sugar (*glyc*) in blood (*emia*). If not corrected (by intake of sugar), hypoglycemia can lead to coma or death. Immediately report signs and symptoms of hyperglycemia or hypoglycemia to your supervisor.

As the support worker, you may prepare meals for adults and children with diabetes. Diet is a very important part of managing diabetes. Follow the client's diet plan carefully, and serve meals and snacks on time. You need to record the amount of food your client consumes at every meal and snack. Calories not consumed at a meal or snack need to be replaced in the course of that day, or your client may experience a reaction. Refer to the care plan. Signs and symptoms of hypoglycemia and hyperglycemia are described in TABLE 37–1. The care plan will tell you what to do if your client is having a reaction.

hypo - low hyper - high

TABLE 37–1 Hyperglycemia and Hypoglycemia

Causes	Warning Signs and Symptoms	
Hyperglycemia (High Blood Sugar)		
Undiagnosed diabetes Not enough insulin or diabetes medication Overeating, or eating the wrong kind of foods Too little exercise Stress—physical or emotional	Tiredness or fatigue Hunger Thirst Frequent urination Leg cramps Blurred vision Dry, itchy skin Flulike achiness Sweet breath odour	Headache Flushed face Rapid, weak pulse Low blood pressure Slow, deep, and laboured breathing Confusion Nausea and vomiting Convulsions Loss of consciousness
Hypoglycemia (Low Blood Sugar)		
Too much insulin or diabetes medication Omitting or delaying a meal or snack Eating too little food Too much exercise Vomiting	Hunger Weakness Trembling, shakiness Sweating Headache Dizziness Faintness Irritability, anxiety	Confusion, disorientation Rapid pulse Low blood pressure Rapid, shallow breathing Changes in vision Cold, clammy skin Unconsciousness Convulsions

Hyperthyroidism

Hyperthyroidism is caused by an overactive thyroid gland, which results in too much thyroid hormone being produced. All of the body's processes are regulated by thyroid hormone, so all of the body's functions speed up because of excess thyroid hormone. Since all body functions are affected, there can be different signs and symptoms, including weight loss, increased hunger, hyperactivity, palpitations, nausea, vomiting, irritability, and depression. Treatment may be the surgical removal of some or all of the thyroid gland, administration of one dose of radioactive iodine to destroy some of the thyroid cells, or medications that inhibit the production of thyroid hormone.

Hypothyroidism

Hypothyroidism is caused by an underactive thyroid gland. With decreased production of thyroid hormone, all of the body processes are slowed down. Signs and symptoms present are the opposite of the signs and symptoms of hyperthyroidism: weight gain, impaired memory, fatigue, sluggishness, irritability, constipation, and slower heart rate. Treatment consists of a thyroid supplement.

CANCER

Cells reproduce for tissue growth and repair and usually divide in an orderly and controlled way. **Cancer** is a group of diseases characterized by out-of-control cell division and growth leading to the development of a lump or mass of cells. This new growth of abnormal cells is called a **tumour**. Tumours can be **benign** (noncancerous) or **malignant** (cancerous). Benign tumours grow slowly and are contained in one area. They do not usually cause death. Malignant tumours grow rapidly and invade other tissues and affect several body systems (**FIGURE 37–18**).

Metastasis is the spread of cancer to other body parts (**FIGURE 37–19**). Cancer cells break off from the tumour and travel to other body parts, where new tumours grow. Death occurs if the cancer cannot be treated or controlled.

Cancer can occur in almost any body part. Common cancer sites are the lungs, breasts, prostate, colon and rectum, uterus, urinary tract, and skin. Cancer is the second leading cause of death in Canada and occurs in all age groups.[14] In Canada, one out of every four cancers diagnosed in women are breast cancers, and one out of every 30 women will die from it.[15] Prostate cancer is the most common cancer among Canadian men (excluding nonmelanoma

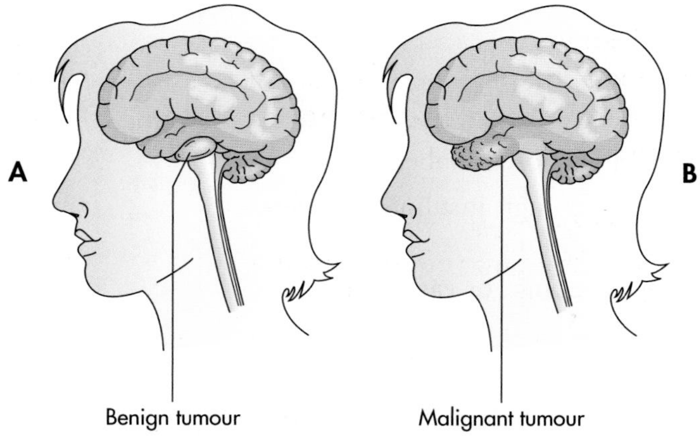

FIGURE 37–18 A, Benign tumours grow within a localized area. **B,** Malignant tumours invade other tissues.

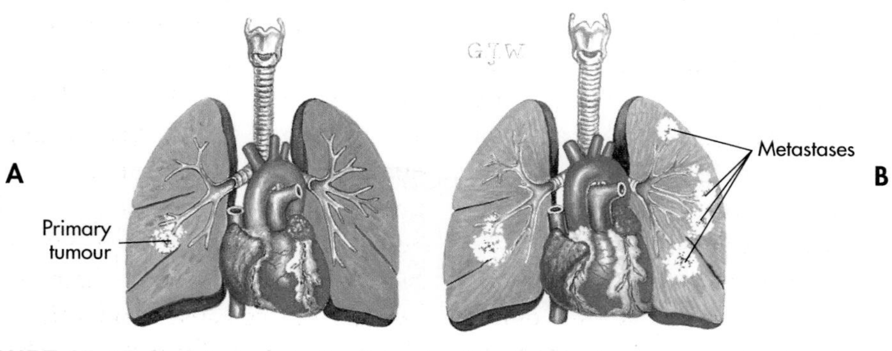

FIGURE 37–19 A, A tumour in the lung. **B,** The tumour has metastasized to the other lung. (**Source:** Belcher, A.E. (1992). *Cancer nursing*. St. Louis, MO: Mosby.)

skin cancer). It is the third leading cause of death from cancer in men in Canada.[16] One type of *leukemia* (acute lymphocytic leukemia, a type of blood cancer) is the most common cancer in children.[17]

The exact causes of cancer are unknown. However, certain factors contribute to its development, including the following:

- A family history of cancer
- Smoking
- Alcohol abuse
- High-fat, high-calorie, low-fibre diet
- Exposure to radiation (including sun exposure)
- Exposure to certain chemicals (carcinogenic, or cancer-causing, agents)
- Hormones
- Viruses

Treatment is most successful when the cancer is detected as early as possible. The warning signs identified by the Canadian Cancer Society are listed in **BOX 37–8**.

Treatment depends on the type of tumour, its location and size, and whether it has spread. One or many treatments may be used, with the following goals:

- Cure the cancer
- Keep the cancer from spreading
- Slow the cancer's growth
- Relieve symptoms caused by the cancer

The three most common cancer treatments are surgery, radiation therapy, and chemotherapy. Recently, stem cell transplantation has been used to treat some types of cancers, especially those affecting bone marrow. Surgery to remove tumours is localized (contained to one area) and involves the removal of malignant tissue as well as surrounding tissue and lymph nodes that might contain cancer cells. If the tumour has not spread to other areas, surgery has a greater chance of success.

Radiation therapy destroys living cells, and, like surgery, it is used for treating localized cancers. Radiation therapy uses high-energy rays directed at the tumour to destroy cancer cells. It can be used alone or in combination with surgery and chemotherapy. Treatment is usually given over a period of weeks. During treatment, normal cells can be destroyed along with cancer cells. Adverse effects of radiation therapy include discomfort, nausea and vomiting, fatigue (tiredness), anorexia (loss of appetite), and diarrhea. Skin breakdown can occur in the area being radiated, so the physician may order special skin care procedures. The markings drawn on the body to show where the radiation will be administered should not be washed off.

Chemotherapy involves powerful drugs that kill cancer cells. These drugs can be administered orally or intravenously. Like radiation, chemotherapy affects normal cells as well as cancer cells, so adverse effects can be severe. The digestive tract may be irritated, and nausea, vomiting, and diarrhea may result. Some other adverse effects are inflammation of the mouth (*stomatitis*) and hair loss (*alopecia*), and because of decreased production of blood cells, the client may tire easily and is at risk for bruising, bleeding, and infection.

BOX 37–8 Warning Signs of Cancer

- A new or unusual lump or swelling in the breast, testicles, or any other part of the body
- Any sore that does not heal anywhere on the body or in the mouth
- Obvious change in the shape, size, or colour of a mole or wart
- A nagging cough, hoarseness, or a croaky voice
- Difficulty swallowing
- Blood in the urine, stool, or phlegm
- Unusual bleeding or discharge of any sort from the nipple or vagina
- Change in bladder habits, such as pain or difficulty urinating
- Any change in bowel habits (constipation or diarrhea) that lasts more than a few weeks
- Persistent indigestion
- Unexplained weight loss, fever, or fatigue
- Unexplained aches and pains
- Any new growth on the skin, or patches of skin that bleed, itch, or become red

Source: Canadian Cancer Society. (n.d.). *Finding cancer early.* Retrieved from http://www.cancer.ca/en/prevention-and-screening/early-detection-and-screening/finding-cancer-early/?region=ns.

Stem cell transplantation involves infusion of healthy stem cells into the body. Stem cell transplantation may be necessary if bone marrow stops working and does not produce enough healthy stem cells. The procedure can help the body make enough healthy white blood cells, red blood cells, or platelets and reduce the risk of life-threatening infections, anemia, and bleeding. This procedure is also known as *bone marrow transplantation* or *umbilical cord blood transplantation*, depending on the source of the stem cells. Stem cell transplantation can use cells from the client's own body (*autologous stem cell transplantation*) or stem cells from donors (*allogenic stem cell transplantation*). The procedure is not widely available across the country, but certain cancer centres are undertaking trial cases.

Clients with cancer have certain needs, and their care often includes the following:

- Providing relief or control of the pain
- Ensuring adequate rest and exercise
- Providing fluids and good nutrition
- Preventing skin breakdown
- Preventing bowel elimination issues (constipation results from pain medications; diarrhea results from chemotherapy)
- Managing the adverse effects of radiation therapy and chemotherapy

The client with cancer has great emotional and social needs. Anger, fear, and depression are common in these clients. The appearance of the affected area following surgery may cause the client to feel unwhole, unattractive, or unclean. The client and family need much emotional support. Talk to the client. Do not avoid the client because you feel uncomfortable.

COMMUNICABLE DISEASES

A communicable disease is caused by microbes that spread easily, so the disease can be transmitted from one host to another. Communicable diseases are spread in different ways (see Chapter 23):

- *Direct contact*—with the infected person
- *Indirect contact*—with contaminated dressings, linens, or surfaces
- *Airborne transmission*—when the client sneezes or coughs
- *Vehicle transmission*—through blood transfusions or by ingesting contaminated food, fluids, or drugs
- *Vector transmission*—via animals, fleas, ticks, mites, and mosquitoes

While providing support care, you often cannot tell by looking at clients if they have a communicable disease. Sometimes, even the clients with communicable diseases may not know that they have one. Therefore, you must follow Standard Practices when working with all clients. Standard Practices prevent the spread of communicable diseases. You may also have to follow Transmission-Based Practices with certain clients, if so ordered by a physician (see Chapter 23). Follow the care plan.

TABLE 37–2 outlines common childhood communicable diseases; however, adults can also contract (get) these diseases. This section discusses hepatitis, acquired immune deficiency syndrome (AIDS), sexually transmitted infections (STIs), influenza (the flu), and tuberculosis.

Hepatitis

Hepatitis means inflammation (*itis*) of the liver (*hepat*). It is characterized by jaundice, anorexia, abdominal and gastric discomfort, abnormal liver function, clay-coloured stools, and tea-coloured urine. It can be caused by a bacterial, viral, or parasitic infection; by alcohol, drugs, or toxins; or through transfusion of incompatible blood. When the viral infection of the liver first occurs, it is called *acute hepatitis*, which may or may not cause recognizable symptoms, such as nausea, vomiting, and pain in the abdomen. Acute hepatitis often lasts less than 1 or 2 months. After about 2 weeks, dark urine and jaundice (a yellowish colour in the skin and whites of the eyes) develop in some, but not all, clients. Some clients with hepatitis have light-coloured stools, muscle pain, drowsiness, irritability, and itching, as well as diarrhea and general ache in the joints accompanied by redness and swelling.

For mild cases of acute viral hepatitis, no medication or other treatment is available or necessary. The disease runs its course and resolves by itself. The primary goals for managing acute viral hepatitis are

TABLE 37–2 Common Communicable Childhood Diseases

Disease	Transmission	Signs and Symptoms
Chicken pox (varicella)	Direct contact or airborne contact with respiratory secretions; direct contact with skin lesions	Fever, rash, and skin lesions
Measles (rubeola)	Direct or indirect contact with nasal secretions	Fever, cough, rash, inflammation of the mucous membranes of the nose, nasal discharge, bronchitis
Mumps	Direct contact with saliva droplets	Fever, headache, swollen salivary glands, earache
Pertussis (whooping cough)	Airborne or direct contact with droplets from the respiratory tract	Fever, sneezing, severe cough at night; coughs that are short and rapid followed by a "whoop" or crowing sound with inhalation
Rubella (German measles)	Airborne or direct contact with secretions from the nose and pharynx	Fever, headache, loss of appetite, nasal inflammation, sore throat, cough, rash
Scarlet fever	Airborne or direct contact with nasal and pharyngeal secretions	Fever, chills, headache, vomiting, abdominal pain, red and swollen tonsils and pharynx, rash

providing good nutrition, preventing additional damage to the liver, and preventing transmission to others.

Some cases of acute hepatitis do not resolve. If hepatitis lasts longer than 6 months, it is called *chronic hepatitis*. Chronic hepatitis causes liver damage over a long period. The normal cells of the liver are eventually replaced with scar tissue—a condition known as *cirrhosis*, which can cause complete liver failure. When the liver fails, the client will need life-saving liver transplantation.

There are three major viruses that cause hepatitis in Canada: hepatitis viruses A, B, and C. All can be passed from one person to another. Vaccines are now available for protection against hepatitis A and B, and a vaccine against hepatitis C is currently being developed.

- ***Hepatitis A virus*** is spread by the fecal–oral route; that is, the virus is transmitted when traces of feces are ingested. Food, water, and drinking and eating vessels (cups, bowls, and cutlery) can be contaminated with feces. The virus is ingested when contaminated food or water is consumed or when a person eats or drinks from a contaminated vessel. Risk factors include crowded living conditions and poor sanitation and hygiene.

  While providing support care, always wear gloves and follow Standard Practices when assisting with perineal care, cleaning incontinent clients, and handling bedpans and rectal thermometers. Clients with fecal incontinence, confusion, or dementia can cause contamination. Carefully look for contaminated items and areas. Practising hand hygiene is essential for everyone. Assist the client with hand hygiene if necessary. Hepatitis A does not cause chronic hepatitis (see the *Focus on Children: Hepatitis* box).
- ***Hepatitis B and C viruses*** are present in an infected person's blood and certain body fluids (semen and vaginal secretions) and can be spread through sexual intercourse or by sharing needles

FOCUS ON CHILDREN

Hepatitis

Hepatitis A is more common among preschool and school-aged children than among adults because the virus spreads easily among children. Poor hygiene practices after defecation lead to contamination of eating and drinking vessels, toys, and other surfaces. Also, young children often put their hands, toys, and other items in their mouths.

with an infected person. These viruses can be spread during blood transfusions and childbirth (from the mother to the child) and also by needle stick injuries and by direct contact between open skin and infected blood or body fluids (see Chapter 23). Therefore, follow Standard Practices when contact with blood or body fluids is likely. Transmission-Based Practices are ordered as necessary. Hepatitis B (in 10% to 15% of cases) and hepatitis C (in 70% to 85% of cases) can cause chronic hepatitis.

Acquired Immune Deficiency Syndrome

Acquired immune deficiency syndrome (AIDS) is a disease of the immune system caused by *human immunodeficiency virus (HIV)*. AIDS affects the person's ability to fight infections. Clients with AIDS may get infections such as pneumonia and tuberculosis (TB) and are also at increased risk for cancers. Sometimes, they experience central nervous system damage, which may cause memory loss, loss of coordination, paralysis, mental health disorders, and dementia.

A person may be infected with HIV but not have any signs or symptoms of AIDS. This person is a carrier and can transmit the virus to others. There is no cure for HIV infection; however, several medications have been developed recently that slow its progression to full-blown AIDS. With current treatment, people who are infected can remain AIDS-free for many years.

HIV is spread from an infected person to another person through an exchange of certain body fluids—blood, semen, vaginal secretions, or breast milk. HIV is transmitted mainly through the following means:

- Unprotected sexual intercourse with an infected person (*unprotected* means "without a condom"); the virus enters the bloodstream through small breaks in the mucous membranes of the rectum, vagina, penis, or mouth
- Needle-sharing among intravenous (IV) drug users
- HIV-infected mothers to their babies at birth or during breastfeeding
- ***Infected body fluids coming in direct contact with broken skin;*** needle stick injuries can thus spread HIV (see Chapter 23)

HIV is *not* spread through saliva, tears, urine, sweat, sneezing, coughing, and insects or through casual contact, including hugging, touching, or shaking hands with an infected person.

AIDS is the last stage of HIV. If HIV infection is not treated, AIDS develops about 10 years after the initial infection. The following are possible warning signs of AIDS:

- Rapid weight loss
- Dry cough
- Fever or night sweats
- Fatigue
- Swollen glands in the armpits, groin, or neck
- Diarrhea that lasts for more than a week
- White spots or unusual blemishes on the tongue, in the mouth, or in the throat
- Pneumonia
- Red, brown, pink, or purplish blotches on the skin or inside the mouth, nose, or eyelids
- Memory loss, confusion, or dementia

You may be providing support care to clients who have AIDS or who are HIV carriers. With some procedures, you may come in contact with the client's blood. Following Standard Practices is important to protect yourself and others from being infected by HIV. ***These precautions apply when you are caring for all clients.*** Remember, you may care for a client who has HIV infection but shows no symptoms, or you may care for a client who has undiagnosed HIV infection. As long as you strictly follow all Standard Practices, you need not fear working with clients with HIV infection or AIDS (see the *Focus on Older Adults: HIV and AIDS* box).

FOCUS ON OLDER ADULTS

HIV and AIDS

AIDS is often considered a young person's disease. Also, people often think that older adults are not sexually active and are therefore not at risk for AIDS. However, older adults can get and spread HIV in the same ways as younger adults, the exceptions being through childbirth and breastfeeding. Consider every client as potentially infectious. Follow Standard Practices with all clients.

Sexually Transmitted Infections

Sexually transmitted infections (STIs) are spread through sexual contact (TABLE 37–3). Some clients may not be aware that they are infected, and some others may know and still not seek treatment, commonly because of embarrassment.

STIs are usually associated with the genital area, but other areas such as the rectum, ears, mouth, nipples, throat, tongue, eyes, and nose may also be affected. Most STIs are spread only through sexual contact. The use of condoms helps prevent the spread of STIs and is also very important for preventing the spread of HIV infection and AIDS. Some STIs can be spread through a break in the skin, contact with infected body fluids (blood, semen, saliva), or contaminated blood or needles. Following Standard Practices is, therefore, necessary at all times.

Influenza

Influenza ("the flu") is a respiratory tract infection caused by a virus. In Canada, the flu season lasts from November or December through April or May. Millions of people suffer from the flu. Influenza is highly contagious and spreads when an infected person coughs or sneezes. It can also be spread by indirect contact—for example, by touching an object such as a doorknob or a telephone that was recently handled by an infected person.

Onset is usually sudden, with headache, chills, and cough, followed by fever, loss of appetite, muscle aches, and tiredness. Coldlike symptoms, including runny nose, sneezing, watery eyes, and throat irritation, occur, as well as nausea, vomiting, or diarrhea, especially in children. Recovery is usually complete in 1 to 2 weeks. However, some people develop serious and life-threatening complications—for example, pneumonia.

While providing supportive care, good hygiene and Standard Practices are essential to reduce the risk for infection. Washing your hands before and after client contact is crucial. The most effective method of prevention is the flu vaccine, which is necessary yearly for people at high risk. At-risk people include the following:

- People 65 years of age and older
- Residents of long-term care facilities
- People who have chronic diseases
- Caregivers and people who live with someone in a high-risk group

Your employer may request or require that you get a yearly flu vaccination, as it protects you and your clients.

Tuberculosis

Tuberculosis (TB) is a persistent bacterial infection generally transmitted by the inhalation or ingestion of infected droplets and usually affecting the lungs, although infection of multiple organ systems can occur.

TB was a major cause of death in the early 1900s. When TB medications were introduced in the 1940s, a dramatic decline in the number of TB cases resulted. However, TB still occurs and is a major health problem in many parts of the world. In the late 1980s, the number of cases of TB began to increase again.

The bacteria causing TB (*Mycobacterium tuberculosis*) are spread by airborne droplets (see Chapter 23) when the infected person coughs, sneezes, or speaks and others in the environment inhale the bacteria. Anyone who has close, frequent contact with an infected person is at risk. TB is more likely to occur in close, crowded areas, such as inner-city neighbourhoods. People with HIV infection are also at risk.

Sometimes, bacteria can reside in a person and not cause an infection until many years later. The person may not have symptoms at first, and the disease may be found during a routine chest X-ray or a TB skin test. Early signs and symptoms are tiredness, loss of appetite, weight loss, fever, and night sweats. Coughing occurs and becomes more frequent as the disease

TABLE 37–3 Sexually Transmitted Infections

Disease	Signs and Symptoms	Treatment
Genital herpes	Recurrent, painful, fluid-filled sores on or near the genitalia (FIGURE 37–20) The sores may have a watery discharge Itching, burning, and tingling in the genital area Fever Swollen glands	No known cure Medication can be given to control discomfort
Venereal warts	*Males*—Warts appear on the penis, anus, or genitalia *Females*—Warts appear near the vagina, cervix, and labia	Application of special ointment that causes the warts to dry up and fall off Surgical removal may be necessary if the ointment is not effective
Gonorrhea	Burning on urination Urinary frequency and urgency Vaginal discharge (females) Urethral discharge (males)	Antibiotic medications
Syphilis	*Primary syphilis*—appears 10 to 90 days after exposure: painless chancre (a type of sore) on the penis, in the vagina, or on genitalia; chancres may also be present elsewhere on the body *Secondary syphilis*—appears about 2 months after the chancre, lasting up to 1 year: rash, general fatigue, loss of appetite, nausea, fever, bone and joint pain, hair loss, lesions on the lips and genitalia *Tertiary syphilis*—appears 3 to 15 years after infection: damage to the cardiovascular system and central nervous system, blindness, dementia	Antibiotic medications

progresses; increased sputum production and chest pain also occur.

Clients with active TB may need to be treated in a hospital, and when they return home, they must continue taking TB medications daily for several months.

Clients with TB need to cover their noses and mouths with tissues when coughing or sneezing and then flush the tissues down the toilet. In health care facilities, tissues used by clients with TB are placed in a biohazard bag and disposed of according to facility policy. Standard Practices and Airborne Precautions must be practised during care of a client with TB (see Chapter 23).

IMMUNE SYSTEM DISORDERS

The immune system protects the body from microbes, cancer cells, and other harmful substances. It defends against threats inside and outside the body. Immune system disorders occur from problems with the immune response. The response may be inappropriate, too strong, or lacking. See discussion of the immune system in Chapter 17.

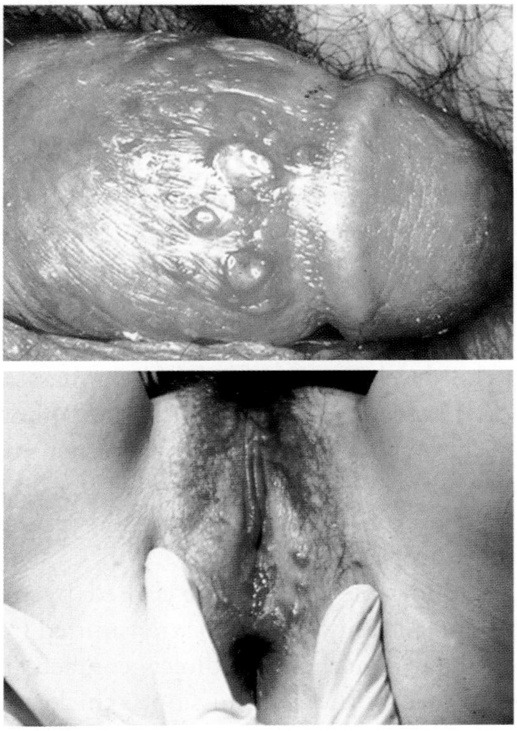

FIGURE 37–20 Genital herpes. **A,** Sores on the penis. **B,** Sores on the perineum. (Courtesy of USPHS, Washington, DC.)

HIV, which causes AIDS, is an example of an acquired viral infection that destroys important white blood cells and weakens the immune system.

Autoimmune Disorders

Autoimmune disorders occur when the immune system attacks the body's own (auto) healthy cells, tissues, or organs. They can affect any part of the body and often affect several parts of the body at the same time (FIGURE 37–21). Autoimmune disorders can change how organs function and can also cause an organ to grow abnormally. Some of the more common autoimmune disorders discussed earlier in this chapter include the following:

- Multiple sclerosis
- Rheumatoid arthritis
- Scleroderma
- Type 1 diabetes
- Celiac disease
- Inflammatory bowel disease (including Crohn's disease, colitis, and IBS).

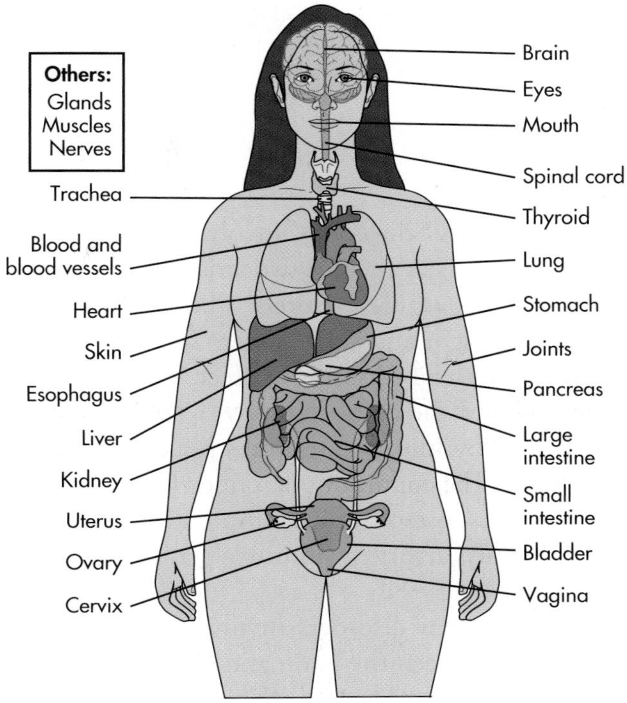

FIGURE 37–21 Body parts that can be affected by autoimmune disease

Other common autoimmune disorders include the following:

- ***Hashimoto's disease.*** Antibodies react against proteins in the thyroid gland, causing gradual destruction of the gland. Eventually, it will not produce enough thyroid hormone. The person has fatigue, weakness, weight gain, sensitivity to cold, muscle aches, stiff joints, facial swelling, and constipation.
- ***Graves' disease.*** Antibodies to a receptor on the thyroid gland can cause the gland to overproduce thyroid hormone, leading to a hyperthyroid condition. The person has anxiety, problems sleeping, rapid heart rate, weight loss, sweating, muscle weakness, shaky hands, and bulging eyes.
- ***Lupus.*** This inflammatory disease can damage the joints, skin, kidneys, heart, lungs, and other body parts. A "butterfly rash," across the nose and cheeks is common. Lupus can be difficult to diagnose as symptoms can vary and be mistaken for other illnesses. Clients with lupus may have periods of illness alternating with periods of remission. Some people with lupus are able to live normal lives, whereas others may be very sick. Follow the care plan carefully, as each client's treatment will be different.

CHAPTER REVIEW

KEY POINTS

- Integumentary disorders involve skin and its appendages. They include urticaria (hives), dermatitis, eczema, scabies, psoriasis, boils (furuncles), cysts, impetigo, and skin cancer.
- Musculo-skeletal disorders affect bones, joints, muscles, and the ability to move. Some disorders are caused by injury, and others result from aging or disease. The conditions described for this system are fractures, osteomyelitis, amputation of a limb, osteoporosis, arthritis, fibromyalgia, scleroderma, and gout.
- Nervous system disorders involve the disruption of signals between the brain and other parts of the body. These disorders can affect physical and cognitive functions. Conditions described include epilepsy, stroke, acquired brain injuries, Parkinson's disease, Huntington's disease, multiple sclerosis (MS), amyotrophic lateral sclerosis (ALS), and spinal cord injuries.
- Cardiovascular disorders involve the heart and blood vessels. Disorders described are phlebitis, thrombus, hypertension, coronary artery disease (CAD), congestive heart failure (CHF), and arrhythmias.
- Respiratory disorders involve the lungs and their airways. Disorders described are asthma, pneumonia, bronchitis, and chronic obstructive pulmonary disease (COPD).
- Digestive disorders impact the proper breaking down of food for absorption by the body and also the elimination of solid wastes. Disorders include gastro-esophageal reflux disease (GERD), gallbladder disease, liver disease, celiac disease, irritable bowel syndrome (IBS), colitis, Crohn's disease, and diverticular disease.
- Urinary disorders involve the kidneys, ureters, bladder, and urethra, which are the major structures of the urinary system. Disorders can include urinary tract infections (UTIs), renal calculi, and renal failure, which can be acute or persistent.
- Endocrine disorders involve the glands that secrete hormones. These disorders result in hormone levels that are too high or too low. The three most common endocrine disorders are diabetes, hyperthyroidism, and hypothyroidism.
- Cancer includes a group of diseases characterized by out-of-control cell division and growth leading to the development of a lump or mass of cells. When cancer cells break off from the tumour, they travel to other body parts, where new tumours grow. Cancer can occur in almost any body part. Common cancers are bowel, breast, prostate, and skin cancers.
- Communicable diseases are caused by microbes that spread easily and can be transmitted from one person to another by direct contact, indirect contact, airborne transmission, vehicle transmission, or vector transmission. There are a number of common communicable childhood diseases. Other communicable diseases more common in adults include hepatitis (types A, B, and C), acquired immune deficiency syndrome (AIDS), sexually transmitted infections (STIs)—which include genital herpes, venereal warts, gonorrhea, and syphilis—influenza, and tuberculosis.
- Immune system disorders occur from problems with the immune response. *Autoimmune disorders* occur when the immune system attacks the body's own (auto) healthy cells, tissues, or organs. Common autoimmune disorders include multiple sclerosis, rheumatoid arthritis, scleroderma, type 1 diabetes, celiac disease, inflammatory bowel disease (including Crohn's disease, colitis, and IBS), Hashimoto's disease, Graves' disease, and lupus.

CRITICAL THINKING IN PRACTICE

Kim Kris has severe pain on his left side over his kidney area. He does not want to eat and has had difficulty getting out of bed. The doctor has diagnosed him with shingles. Can a person have shingles without having any visible rash? What are your responsibilities when caring for someone who has shingles?

REVIEW QUESTIONS

Answers to these questions are at the bottom of the page.

Circle T if the answer is true, and F if the answer is false.

1. T F A sore that does not heal is a warning sign of cancer.
2. T F Stroke is a complication of hypertension.
3. T F A common treatment for hypertension is a high-sodium diet.
4. T F The pain of angina is relieved with rest and nitroglycerin.
5. T F *Myocardial infarction* means heart attack.
6. T F A pacemaker is a device used to treat renal failure.
7. T F Clients with congestive heart failure need to drink extra fluids.
8. T F Smoking is the most common cause of COPD.
9. T F The flu season in Canada is June through October.
10. T F Stroke often causes hemiplegia.
11. T F Clients with Parkinson's disease often have blank, expressionless faces.
12. T F Clients with Huntington's disease are not affected intellectually.
13. T F Canada has one of the lowest rates of MS in the world.
14. T F A client with advanced ALS cannot speak or move but can hear and understand.
15. T F Clients with brain or spinal cord injuries require amputations.
16. T F Arthritis usually affects bones and muscles.
17. T F Fibromyalgia is a respiratory disorder.
18. T F Clients with osteoporosis have an increased risk for fractures.
19. T F When lifting a cast, support it with your palms, not your fingertips.
20. T F After a hip pinning, the operated leg is abducted at all times.
21. T F Hyperglycemia means low sugar in the blood.
22. T F Diabetes can cause circulatory disorders.
23. T F Good foot care is especially important for people with diabetes.
24. T F Vomiting can cause aspiration.
25. T F Passing a kidney stone is called *cystitis.*
26. T F Clients with chronic renal failure need increased fluid intake.
27. T F Hepatitis B virus is spread by the fecal–oral route.
28. T F HIV is spread by infected urine.
29. T F HIV remains in the infected person's body for life.
30. T F STIs are usually spread by sexual contact.
31. T F Urticaria (hives) is caused by an allergic reaction.
32. T F Eczema is a skin infection caused by a mite.
33. T F Psoriasis is caused by the infection of a hair follicle.
34. T F A cyst can contain air, fluids, or semi-solid material.
35. T F Impetigo is not contagious.
36. T F There is no cure for scleroderma.
37. T F Gout usually affects the big toe.
38. T F Lupus is a persistent autoimmune disease.
39. T F If your client is having an epileptic seizure, you should put something between the teeth so that he will not swallow his tongue.
40. T F GERD occurs when stomach acids go up the esophagus.
41. T F Cholecystitis is inflammation of the gallbladder.
42. T F Celiac disease is a disorder of the large intestine.
43. T F A client with IBS can suffer from diarrhea or constipation.
44. T F Crohn's disease is a persistent inflammatory condition of the bowel.
45. T F Hyperthyroidism is caused by an underactive thyroid gland.

Answers: 1.T, 2.T, 3.F, 4.T, 5.T, 6.F, 7.F, 8.T, 9.F, 10.T, 11.T, 12.F, 13.F, 14.T, 15.F, 16.F, 17.F, 18.T, 19.T, 20.T, 21.F, 22.T, 23.T, 24.T, 25.F, 26.F, 27.F, 28.F, 29.T, 30.T, 31.T, 32.F, 33.F, 34.T, 35.F, 36.T, 37.T, 38.T, 39.F, 40.T, 41.T, 42.F, 43.T, 44.T, 45.F

Chapter opener image: Phovoir/Shutterstock.com

CHAPTER 38

Developmental Disorders and Disabilities

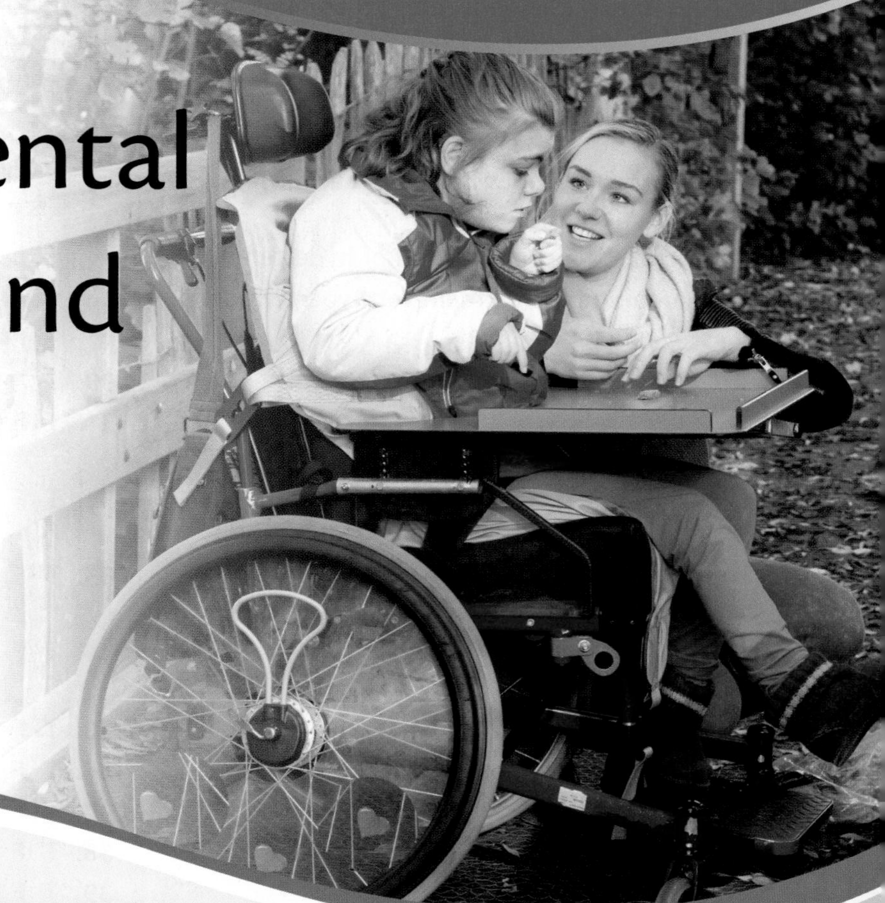

OBJECTIVES

After reading this chapter, the learner should be able to do the following:

- Explain the impact a developmental disorder or disability can have on a client's family.
- Identify common developmental disorders and disabilities and describe their causes.
- Discuss how common developmental disorders and disabilities affect functioning.
- Describe and understand how to care for clients with developmental disorders and disabilities.

KEY TERMS

attention-deficit/hyperactivity disorder (ADHD) A disorder that causes inappropriate levels of inattention as well as hyperactive and impulsive behaviour. *p. 896*

autism spectrum disorder (ASD) A neurodevelopmental disorder that impairs a person's ability to communicate and interact with others. It can include restricted repetitive behaviours, interests, and activities. *p. 897*

cerebral palsy (CP) A disorder affecting muscle control (*palsy*) caused by an injury or abnormality in the motor region of the brain (*cerebral*). *p. 892*

cognitive disability See **intellectual disability**. *p. 889*

developmental disability A permanent disability that a person is born with or that begins before 18 years of age. *p. 887*

diplegia Loss of ability to move (*plegia*) corresponding parts on both (*di*) sides of the body; both arms or both legs are affected. *p. 893*

Down syndrome (DS) A congenital disorder caused by an extra chromosome; DS results in varying degrees of intellectual disability. *p. 892*

fetal alcohol spectrum disorders (FASD) A group of physical and mental abnormalities that occur in children as a result of alcohol consumption by the mother during pregnancy. *p. 895*

fragile X syndrome The most common form of inherited developmental disorder. *p. 890*

intellectual disability Impaired ability to learn. Also known as **cognitive disability**. *p. 889*

seizure Brief disturbance in the brain's normal electrical function; affects awareness, movement, and sensation. *p. 894*

spastic Uncontrolled contractions of skeletal muscle and smooth muscle. *p. 893*

spina bifida A congenital disorder caused by improper closing of the spine before birth. *p. 894*

tonic–clonic seizure A seizure involving convulsions. *p. 894*

A *disability* is any loss of physical or mental function (see Chapter 4). Many disabilities begin in adulthood due to diseases, medical conditions, and injuries. A **developmental disability** is a permanent disability that a person is born with or that begins before 18 years of age. Developmental disabilities are caused by various conditions, illnesses, accidents (e.g., poisoning, trauma), diseases, or developmental (genetic) disorders (e.g., cerebral palsy, Down syndrome) that injure or affect the normal development of the brain or body before birth, during birth, or during childhood or adolescence.

Developmental disorders and disabilities can be mild, moderate, or severe. They can affect physical function, mental function, or both, limiting the person's ability to function in at least three of the following life activities:

- Self-care (e.g., eating, dressing, hygiene)
- Understanding and expressing speech and language
- Learning
- Mobility (i.e., getting around independently)
- Self-direction (e.g., solving problems, making choices and decisions)
- Independent living
- Economic self-sufficiency (i.e., earning enough income to support oneself financially)

This chapter will discuss the causes of the most common developmental disorders and disabilities and how they affect an individual's functioning. Most clients with developmental disorders and disabilities need lifelong assistance, support, and special services, which are provided by the health care team involved in the client's care.

THE IMPACT OF DEVELOPMENTAL DISORDERS AND DISABILITIES ON THE FAMILY

Families of children with developmental disorders and disabilities may face many challenges. As the support worker, be sensitive to the family's situation. Some family members you work with may be adjusting to a recent diagnosis of a disability in a child in their family. They may still be figuring out the new roles and routines for everyone in the family, so they may be under great stress. Other families may have already established their roles and routines. Remember, every family situation is different.

Most children with disabilities live with their families at home, and many attend regular schools with the help of teacher's aides. Being a primary caregiver for a child with a disability can be an all-consuming task, as it often takes great amounts of time, energy, and work. Many caregivers have to balance caregiving with other responsibilities, including full-time jobs and caring for other children. Parents of children with disabilities may not ever leave their child with others so as to spend time alone with each other because they do not want to impose on family or friends to care for the child. Also, they may not be able to spend as much time with their other children as they would like.

Some parental caregivers may feel that their child is considered "different" by society and worry about the stigma associated with their child's disorder or disability. They may encounter discrimination and other barriers. The constant stress and work of caregiving can lead to burnout (see Chapter 7)—the caregiver's becoming physically and emotionally exhausted. There can be economic and financial burdens as well, as special equipment and adaptive and assistive devices are expensive and may not be covered under the family health plan or the provincial or territorial plan.

Home care and other community agencies often provide needed support and services. The types of community agencies available vary by region. Families in large cities will more likely have easier access to support groups and agencies compared with families in small towns and rural communities. Many families may have to rely on the Internet for access to information and group support.

As a support worker, you will be working closely with the family caregivers. You may take on some household tasks so that the parents can spend more time with the child who has a disability and with their other children. You may provide respite care so that the parents can have a break from caregiving. You also may directly assist the child, according to the care plan. For example, you might help with the child's rehabilitation activities under the supervision of a physiotherapist or occupational therapist. You may accompany the child to and from school

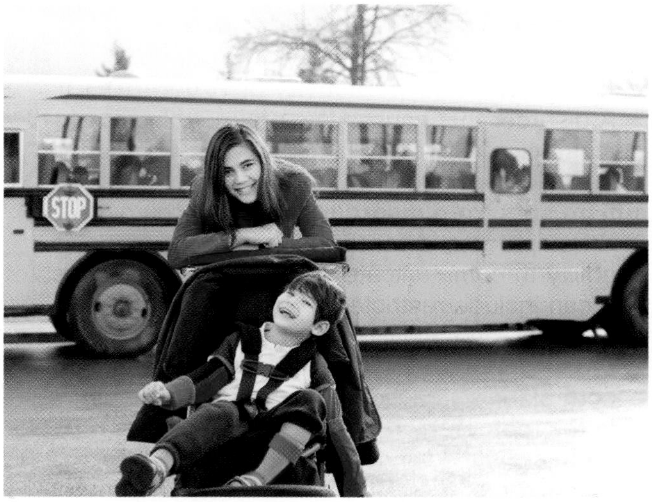

FIGURE 38–1 You may accompany a child with a disability to and from school. (**Source:** Jaren Jai Wicklund/Shutterstock.com)

(**FIGURE 38–1**) or work with children with disabilities in schools. Children with severe disabilities may need long-term care in special facilities.

As the child and parents grow older, caring for the adolescent or adult child often becomes physically difficult. Parents may not be able to lift or move the adolescent or adult child. Parents who are the caregivers may become ill, injured, or disabled, or may die. Through all these situations, the client with the developmental disorder or disability continues to need care.

Adolescents and adults with developmental disabilities live in community or residential settings, in their own homes, or in group homes. Some may live in specially licensed long-term care facilities. Support workers in these facilities require special training to meet the needs of clients with developmental disabilities. Often, the client's family continues to be involved in the care. Remember that family members have cared for the client for most of the person's life, so they understand the client's condition and needs very well. Include family members, whenever appropriate, when you provide care and services.

TYPES OF DEVELOPMENTAL DISORDERS AND DISABILITIES

Developmental disorders and disabilities include, but are not limited to, the following:

- Intellectual disabilities
- Down syndrome

- Cerebral palsy
- Epilepsy
- Spina bifida
- Fetal alcohol spectrum disorders
- Attention-deficit/hyperactivity disorders
- Autism spectrum disorder

A number of children and adults have more than one condition that causes a disability. TABLE 38–1 lists other conditions that cause developmental disabilities.

Intellectual Disabilities

An **intellectual disability** (**cognitive disability**) is an impaired ability to learn and results in below-average intelligence and limitations in the ability to function in certain areas of daily life. (*Intelligence* relates to learning, thinking, and reasoning.) The client can learn new skills but does so at a slower than normal rate. A client with an intellectual disability often has difficulties with communication, self-care, and social interaction. In the past, intellectual disability was called *mental retardation,* a term now considered unacceptable in Canada.

An intellectual disability can be caused by any genetic abnormality, injury, or disease that impairs the development of the brain. Some common causes of intellectual disabilities are listed in **BOX 38–1** on page 891. People with an intellectual disability often have other disabilities as well.

Intellectual disabilities range from mild to severe. Tests that measure intelligence are called IQ (intelligence quotient) tests. An average person without an intellectual disability has an IQ score of about 90 to 110. People with IQ scores between 70 and 55 are considered to have *mild intellectual disability.* They may be slow to learn but are able to attend regular schools. As adults, they can function in society with some support. They can work and live in the community and need only occasional support. People who have IQ scores below 55 are considered to have *moderate intellectual disability* and need daily support at home and at work. People with IQ scores below 25 are considered to have *severe intellectual disability* and need constant support in all areas.

The Canadian Association for Community Living is a national association dedicated to serving people with intellectual disabilities and their families. The association's goal is to ensure that people with intellectual disabilities have opportunities to live meaningful, dignified lives. The association's philosophy is that people with intellectual disabilities can and should be allowed to participate in all aspects of community living. Children should live in families, be integrated into regular schools whenever possible, and interact with other children with or without disabilities. Adults with intellectual disabilities have

TABLE 38–1 Some Conditions Leading to Developmental Disabilities

Acquired brain injury	*Damage to brain tissue caused by disease, medical condition, accident, drug overdose, or violence.* Some accidents and diseases reduce or cut off oxygen to the brain, thereby destroying brain cells and causing brain injury. For example, conditions during birth, near drowning, choking, suffocation, and stroke can all cause brain injury. Certain infections (meningitis, encephalitis) or chemicals (mercury and lead poisoning) also destroy brain tissue. Unfortunately, people who use street drugs risk ingesting toxic substances and overdosing. Blows to the head—for example, those received through motor vehicle accidents, falls, sports injuries, and child abuse (including shaking)—can batter the brain and cause brain injury. Acquired brain injuries can be permanent and severe, causing personality changes, vision problems, speech problems, muscle control problems, and intellectual disability.

Continued

TABLE 38–1 Some Conditions Leading to Developmental Disabilities—cont'd

Congenital heart disease	Congenital heart disease involves abnormalities in the structure or function of the heart that are present before birth. Affected babies who survive may tire easily or experience delayed growth. Most congenital heart conditions must be corrected by surgery.
Fragile X syndrome	The most common inherited cause of mental impairment and the most common known cause of autism spectrum disorder, **Fragile X syndrome** is a genetic condition caused by changes in the X chromosome that prevent the chromosome from making the protein that it normally does. Some individuals are carriers who have a small defect in the gene (called *permutation*) and show no symptoms. One in 259 women carry the fragile X gene, and there is a 50% chance of her passing it on to her children; about 1 in 800 men carry the fragile X gene and pass it on to all of their daughters but not to their sons. The fragile X gene can be passed down unnoticed through generations before a child is affected with full mutation. Boys and girls can both be affected, but boys are usually affected more severely. Most males with full mutation will have developmental disabilities. Only one third to one half of girls have significant intellectual impairment. There is ongoing research into the causes for males being more affected, but recent reports suggest that since girls have two X chromosomes, even if affected, they still have one strong X chromosome, whereas males have only the one X chromosome, which, if damaged, causes full mutation. Common symptoms of fragile X syndrome are the following: • Mental impairment, ranging from learning disabilities to developmental disabilities • Attention deficit and hyperactivity • Anxiety and unstable mood • Autistic behaviour • Long face, large ears, flat feet • Hyperextension of joints, especially fingers • Seizures (affecting about 25% of people with fragile X)
Hydrocephalus	Hydrocephalus is a condition in which fluid collects in the brain (*hydro* means water, and *cephalo* means head). Left untreated, it causes the head to become enlarged and increases pressure on the brain. If the child survives, intellectual disability and neurological damage may result. To treat hydrocephalus, a shunt (a long, flexible tube) is placed in the brain and connected to a body cavity, usually the abdomen or a heart chamber. The shunt is completely enclosed inside the body. Fluid drains from the brain through the tube into the body cavity. Shunts usually stay in place for the remainder of the person's life.

Continued

TABLE 38–1 Some Conditions Leading to Developmental Disabilities—cont'd

Phenylketonuria (PKU)	In this inherited condition, the body lacks an enzyme necessary to process a certain amino acid (phenylalanine). When this amino acid builds up in the blood, it injures brain tissue. Left untreated, PKU causes intellectual disability and neurological disorders. PKU can be detected with a blood test in the first few days of life. With proper treatment, brain injury can be avoided. Treatment involves maintaining a strict diet throughout life. In Canada, all newborns are routinely tested for PKU.
Shaken baby syndrome	This term refers to the physical and cognitive impairments caused by violently shaking a baby or young child. Babies and young children have weak neck muscles, and shaking them violently causes the head to swing back and forth with great force. As a result, the brain bangs against the skull wall, causing bleeding behind the eyes and in the brain. Permanent brain injury, seizures, partial or total blindness, paralysis, intellectual disability, or death can occur. Less violent but frequent shaking of a young child can also cause long-term effects, including attention deficits and learning disabilities.

BOX 38–1 Causes of Intellectual Disability

Genetic Conditions
- Abnormal genes inherited from one or both parents (e.g., fragile X syndrome and PKU)
- Missing or extra chromosomes (e.g., Down syndrome)

Problems During Pregnancy
- Alcohol or drug use
- Poor nutrition
- Exposure to certain environmental hazards, such as X-rays or certain chemicals
- Illnesses such as rubella (German measles) or syphilis
- Uncontrolled medical conditions such as diabetes mellitus or human immunodeficiency virus (HIV)

Problems at Birth
- Premature birth
- Low birth weight
- Lack of oxygen to the baby's brain during birth

Problems After Birth
- Childhood diseases such as whooping cough, chicken pox, and measles
- Infections such as meningitis and encephalitis
- Acquired brain injury caused by accidents, disease, or abuse
- Severe malnutrition or neglect

the right to control their lives to the fullest extent possible—that is, they should make choices and decisions about their care and how they live. They should have friends, work at jobs, enjoy adult activities, and contribute to their communities.

People with intellectual disabilities have sexual, emotional, and social needs and desires, just like everyone else. They have the right to privacy and to love and to be loved. Some adults with intellectual disabilities have life partners; some marry and have children.

Most people with intellectual disabilities are able to control their sexual urges, but a few are unable to. The nature of their sexual responses and where they display them may be inappropriate (see Chapter 16 for a discussion on how to deal with sexually aggressive clients). Children and adults with intellectual disabilities are vulnerable to sexual abuse. Report

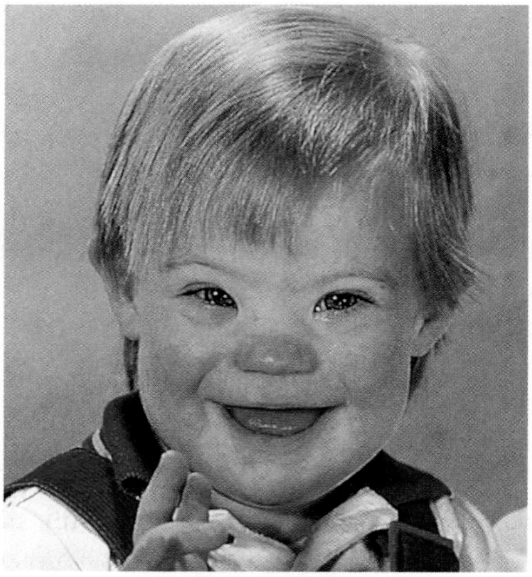

FIGURE 38–2 A child with Down syndrome. (**Source:** Thibodeau, G.A., & Patton, K.T. (2010). *The human body in health and disease* (5th ed., p. 676). St. Louis, MO: Mosby.)

signs of sexual abuse immediately (see Chapter 16). Children with intellectual disabilities need to be educated about sexual abuse, safe sex, and other issues related to sexuality.

Down Syndrome

Down syndrome (DS) is a disorder caused by an extra chromosome, so the affected person has 47 chromosomes. It occurs due to an error at fertilization and is a congenital (present at birth) condition. In Canada, DS is one of the most common congenital chromosomal disorders. For every 10 000 births, 14 babies are born with DS.[1]

DS causes varying degrees of intellectual disability—usually moderate to severe. The child also has distinguishing physical features caused by the extra chromosome (**FIGURE 38–2**):

- Small head
- Oval-shaped eyes that slant upward
- Flat face
- Short, wide neck
- Large tongue
- Wide, flat nose
- Small ears
- Short stature
- Short, wide hands with stubby fingers
- Weak muscle tone

Many children with DS have congenital heart defects and tend to have vision and hearing disorders as well. They are at risk for ear infections, respiratory infections, and thyroid gland problems. People with DS may start to show symptoms of dementia after age 35, and Alzheimer's disease is commonly diagnosed in their 40s. Genetic counsellors relate this prevalence to the effect of the extra chromosome.

Early intervention programs ideally begin soon after birth and will help identify the best methods for teaching each particular child. Clients with DS may need physiotherapy as well as speech-language and occupational therapies, training for self-care skills, and health and sex education. A tendency for weight gain and constipation are frequent problems in these clients, so they need a well-balanced diet and regular exercise. With good nutrition, adequate physical activity, and consistent mental stimulation, many people with DS live well into their 60s.

Cerebral Palsy

Cerebral palsy (CP), a disorder affecting muscle control (*palsy*), is caused by an injury or abnormality in the motor region of the brain (*cerebral*). Depending on which area(s) of the brain have been injured, one or more of the following may occur:

- Involuntary movements
- Poor coordination and posture
- Muscle weakness
- Difficulty or inability to walk
- Difficulty or inability to speak

CP may occur before, during, or shortly after birth. Lack of oxygen to the fetal or newborn brain is the usual cause. Infants at risk include the following:

- Those born prematurely
- Those with a low birth weight
- Those who do not cry in the first 5 minutes after birth
- Those who need mechanical ventilation
- Those who have bleeding in the brain
- Those with heart, kidney, or spinal cord abnormalities
- Those with blood problems
- Those who have seizures

Acquired brain injury in infancy and early childhood also can result in CP (see Chapter 35 and TABLE 38-1, on p. 889).

Certain body movements and body parts are affected by CP. The following types of CP are the most common:

- ***Spastic cerebral palsy.*** Spastic means uncontrolled contractions of skeletal muscles (*spastic* comes from the Greek *spastikos*, meaning "to draw in"). Muscles contract or shorten and remain stiff and unable to relax. One or both sides of the body may be involved, so posture and balance are affected, and movement is stiff and jerky. If the client's arms are affected, she may have difficulty eating, writing, dressing, and doing other activities of daily living (ADLs). If the client's legs are affected, she may have difficulty walking or moving. The spastic form is the most common type of CP (about 50% of all cases).
- ***Athetoid cerebral palsy.*** The client cannot control body movements (*athetoid* comes from the Greek *athetos*, meaning "not fixed"). The client has involuntary, constant, slow weaving or writhing motions that occur in the trunk, arms, hands, legs, and feet. The client might have difficulty reaching for and grasping objects and remaining upright for sitting or standing. Sometimes, the muscles of the tongue, face, and neck may be affected, causing the client to drool or grimace.
- ***Ataxic cerebral palsy.*** The client has weak muscle tone and difficulty coordinating movements (absence of [*a*] arrangement or order [*taxis*]), so the person appears very unsteady and shaky when walking and has trouble maintaining balance.

The following terms are used to describe the types of CP according to the body parts affected:

- ***Monoplegia***—*mono* means one. This type of CP is a paralysis of a single limb, usually an arm.
- ***Hemiplegia***—*hemi* means half; *plegia* means "complete or partial loss of ability to move." CP affects one side of the body—the right arm and leg or the left arm and leg. The other side functions normally. The client may be able to walk but might look a little awkward.
- ***Diplegia***—*di* means two. With diplegia, there is a loss of ability to move (*plegia*) corresponding parts on both (*di*) sides of the body. In most cases of diplegia caused by CP, both legs are affected—so the client has difficulty walking—but the upper body is not affected. (In extremely rare cases, both arms are affected, but not the legs.)
- ***Quadriplegia***—*quad* means four. CP affects all four limbs (both arms and both legs). The client cannot walk or use the arms. Usually, the client also has difficulty with movement of the facial muscles and the trunk. Talking and eating may be difficult, and the client needs a wheelchair to get around.

Some clients with CP are only mildly affected. Their movements are awkward, but they can walk independently, and they do not have intellectual disability. However, other clients with CP are severely affected and can have many other accompanying impairments and problems, including the following:

- Intellectual disability
- Learning disability
- Hearing impairment
- Speech impairment
- Vision impairment
- Difficulty swallowing
- Drooling because of difficulty swallowing saliva
- Bladder and bowel control problems
- Seizures
- Attention-deficit/hyperactivity disorder (short attention span, poor concentration, and increased activity)
- Breathing problems due to poor posture
- Pressure ulcers from immobility

Care depends on the severity of the CP and the needs of the client. The goal is for the client to be as independent as possible. Physiotherapy, occupational therapy, and speech therapy, the use of eyeglasses or hearing aids, and surgery and medications for muscle problems can all help. As a support worker, you may be required to assist the client with CP with range-of-motion (ROM) exercises and ADLs.

Epilepsy

Epilepsy is a condition characterized by recurrent (occurring repeatedly from time to time) seizures (*epilepsia* means seizure). A **seizure** is a brief disturbance in the brain's normal electrical function, which affects awareness, movement, and sensation.

Seizures that affect only one part of the brain are called *partial seizures*. Seizures that affect the whole brain are called *generalized seizures*. The area of the brain affected by the seizure temporarily loses its ability to function normally, so seizures may cause different reactions, depending on the part of the brain affected. For example, some seizures cause the person to briefly stare and appear unresponsive; others (as in **tonic–clonic seizures**) involve a violent and sudden contraction or tremor of muscle groups. The person loses consciousness and falls to the floor. All muscle groups contract and relax, causing jerking and twitching movements of the body. Urinary and bowel incontinence may occur. A tonic–clonic seizure usually lasts for 1 to 7 minutes. A single seizure does not mean that the person has epilepsy since a number of factors can cause a single seizure. For a diagnosis of epilepsy, the person has to have recurring seizures. The electrical system in the brain is permanently damaged, making it susceptible to seizures.

Children and young adults are commonly affected, but epilepsy can develop at any time during a person's life. Often, the cause of epilepsy in a particular person is not known. It can be caused by any problem affecting the brain—for example, CP, intellectual disability, autism spectrum disorder, Alzheimer's disease, stroke, tumours, and acquired brain injury (see TABLE 38-1, on p. 889).

There is no cure for epilepsy, but medications are prescribed by a physician to try to prevent seizures. These medications may control seizures in many people but may not work in others, so some may need brain surgery to reduce the frequency of seizures.

When controlled, epilepsy usually does not affect learning and the ability to perform ADLs. In severe cases, epilepsy may limit the activities of those affected. For example, a person who has frequent seizures may not be allowed to drive, which may limit job choices and opportunities. For these clients, safety measures are needed at home, in the workplace, and for transportation and recreation.

Clients with epilepsy have an increased risk for premature death. They have higher rates of suicide; sudden, unexplained death; and accidental death, especially drowning.

As a support worker, you must observe and report all activity before, during, and after a seizure.

Spina Bifida

Spina bifida is a congenital disorder caused by improper closing of the spine before birth (*spina* means backbone, and *bifida* means split in two parts). Spina bifida is a *neural tube defect* (NTD) that can range from mild to severe. With NTDs, the brain, spinal cord, and the protective coverings for these organs do not fully develop. These defects occur during the first months of pregnancy. Consuming sufficient folic acid before conception and during early pregnancy greatly reduces the risk of having a baby with neural tube defects (see Chapter 28).

Bones of the spinal column (vertebrae) protect the spinal cord. In the case of spina bifida, the vertebrae do not close properly, leaving the spinal cord unprotected. The spinal cord contains nerves that send messages to and from the brain, and because in spina bifida the spinal cord is unprotected, nerve damage occurs. Affected body parts do not function properly, and partial or complete paralysis and loss of bowel and bladder control may result. Infection of the exposed spinal cord is also a risk.

Spina bifida can occur anywhere in the spine. The lower back is the most common site. Types of spina bifida include the following:

- ***Spina bifida occulta***—(*occult* means hidden). This type is the mildest form of spina bifida. A slight deficiency occurs in the vertebral closure. However, the spinal cord and the membranes (*meninges*) that cover it remain in place. Skin usually covers the defect; in other words, the defect is hidden. The person may have a dimple or tuft of hair on the back (FIGURE 38–3); however, the spinal cord and nerves are normal. It rarely causes disability, and, often, there are no symptoms. Foot weakness as well as bowel and bladder disorders may occur.
- ***Spina bifida cystica***—(*cystica* means cyst or sac). Part of the spinal column is in a pouch or sac that protrudes from the opening in the spine. A membrane or a thin layer of skin covers the sac, which looks like a large blister. Because the pouch is

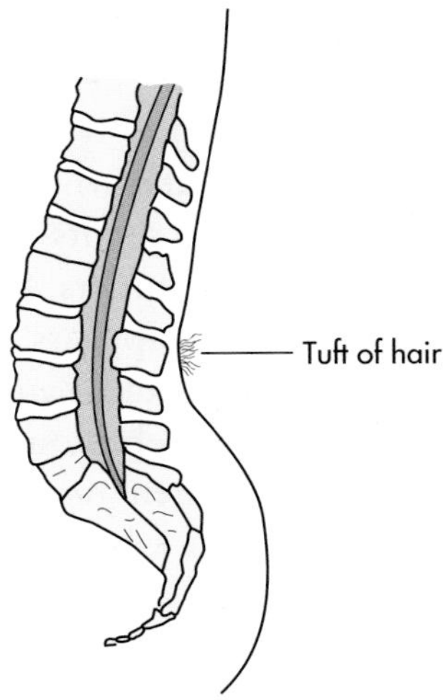

FIGURE 38–3 Spina bifida occulta.

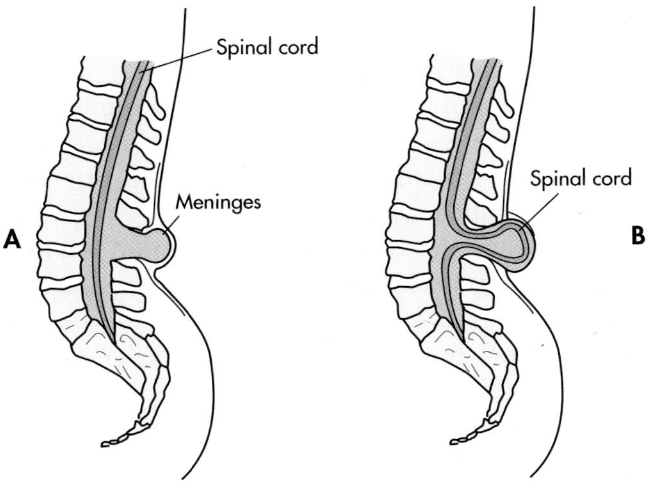

FIGURE 38–4 Spina bifida. **A,** Meningocele. **B,** Myelomeningocele.

easily injured, infection is a risk. There are two types of spina bifida cystica (**FIGURE 38–4**):

- *Meningocele*—(*meningo* comes from *meninx*, meaning membrane; *cele* means hernia or swelling). Meninges are the connective membranes that cover and protect the brain and spinal cord. The cerebrospinal fluid also protects the brain and the spinal cord. With this type of spina bifida, a sac containing meninges and cerebrospinal fluid protrudes from the spine (see **FIGURE 38–4, *A***). The sac does not contain nerve tissue, so the spinal cord and nerves are unaffected, and nerve damage usually does not occur. This defect can be corrected by surgery.
- *Myelomeningocele* (or *meningomyelocele*)—(*myelo* means spinal cord). With this type of spina bifida, a sac containing nerves, a part of the spinal cord, meninges, and cerebrospinal fluid protrudes from the spine (see **FIGURE 38–4, *B***). This type is the most common and most serious form of spina bifida, in which there is severe nerve damage. The spinal cord is damaged or not properly developed. Loss of function occurs below the level of damage. Leg paralysis, lack of sensation, and lack of bowel and bladder control are common. The baby's back is closed with surgery, usually soon after birth. Some children and adults with this form of spina bifida walk with braces or crutches, but some will need wheelchairs.

Clients with spina bifida may have other disorders or conditions—for example, those related to learning, attention, language, reading, and math. They are at risk for obesity, gastro-intestinal disorders, and mobility issues. Skin breakdown, depression, and social, emotional, and sexual issues are other risks. Hydrocephalus (see TABLE 38-1, on p. 889) often occurs with certain types of spina bifida.

Fetal Alcohol Spectrum Disorders (FASD)

Fetal alcohol spectrum disorders (FASD) are a group of physical and mental abnormalities that occur in a child as a result of alcohol consumption by the mother during pregnancy. In Canada, one child is born with FASD every day. It is the most common preventable developmental disorder.

Physical problems include low birth weight, weak muscle tone, and poor weight gain. Cardiac (heart) disorders, hearing loss, and abnormalities of the spine and joints may also occur. The client may have characteristic facial features, including an abnormally small head, small eye openings, a thin upper lip, and a small chin.

A child with FASD may have an intellectual disability and may have other behavioural, learning, and emotional disorders, including poor attention span, hyperactivity, poor motor skills, and slow language development. Older children and adults with FASD may often have memory problems, poor judgement, difficulties with ADLs, inability to manage anger, poor social skills, and mental health problems. Some adults with FASD work and live independently, but some will need support and help from family and community services. Women with FASD can have a normal baby as long as they do not consume alcohol during pregnancy.

Attention-Deficit/Hyperactivity Disorders (ADHD)

Attention-deficit/hyperactivity disorder (ADHD) causes inappropriate levels of inattention as well as hyperactive and impulsive behaviour. ADHD is one of the most common childhood disorders, along with attention-deficit disorder (ADD). The two disorders are grouped together within the same category because of the similarities between symptoms. Approximately 3% to 7% of school-aged children have ADHD, and some research indicates that larger cities may have rates as high as 10% to 15%.[2] The *Diagnostic and Statistical Manual of Mental Disorders*, fifth edition (*DSM-5*), states that ADHD is two times more common in boys than girls,[3] although some researchers suggest that girls with ADHD may be overlooked because they tend to be more inattentive than hyperactive. A child is more likely to develop ADHD if a close biological family member also has it. Children with learning or communication problems may also be more likely to have ADHD.[4]

ADHD has always been considered a children's disorder, but increasingly, in the past 25 years, adults, too, have been diagnosed and medicated for this problem. It is believed that an adult who is newly diagnosed with ADHD likely had the disorder in childhood but it went undiagnosed. Although symptoms can be caused by other events, such as a head injury, hyperthyroidism (see Chapter 37), or seizure disorders, true ADHD appears during early childhood and may be diagnosed even before age 7. It used to be thought that the majority of children ultimately grew out of ADHD before reaching adulthood. However, it is now known that these disorders often do not disappear as children mature.

ADHD symptoms exist over a long term, occur in more than one environment, and are severe enough to impair someone's everyday functioning. Hyperactive people often appear as if they *need* to move. Therefore, they are almost constantly moving and frequently make excessive noise. People who have chronic difficulties in maintaining focus or completing their work, who repeatedly engage in disruptive or antisocial behaviours such as lying and cheating, who have poor social skills, and who act impulsively (i.e., without thinking about results of actions) may have one or more of these disorders. Sometimes, the person with attention deficit appears to act without prior thought or intention and can be intrusive, rude, and dangerous. These behaviours can result in accidents. For example, children may not think about landing when they jump off a ledge to catch a ball. For adults, ADHD interferes with both work and family functioning. Symptoms of ADHD can include the following:

- Disorganization and difficulty with task completion
- Inability to sit still
- Trouble with follow-through on promises or commitments
- Difficulty structuring time and setting priorities (e.g., chronic lateness)
- A tendency to say what comes to mind without considering the timing or appropriateness of the remark
- A tendency toward addictive behaviours
- A craving for excitement and frequently searching for high stimulation
- Trouble focusing attention and easily distracted (e.g., tunes out or drifts away in the middle of a page or a conversation)
- Mood swings
- Easily flustered, tense
- Short temper, likely with a history of explosive episodes

Experts consider ADHD to be a chronic condition that has no cure, although a number of treatment options can help people successfully manage their ADHD. For example, encourage the client to keep a food diary in order to monitor if preservatives or other food additives can be contributing to the client's ADHD.[5] Treatment for people with this disorder may include medications as well as psychotherapy, depending on the client and the symptoms. It is important that the client get assistance from a health care provider as soon as possible after diagnosis.

Autism Spectrum Disorder

Autism spectrum disorder (ASD) is a neurodevelopmental disorder that impairs a person's ability to communicate and interact with others. *Autos* means self, and the client with ASD withdraws into the self. It may seem as if clients with ASD are in their own world and uninterested in others. For example, they may not notice when someone enters a room, and some children with ASD may prefer to play alone. Some avoid physical contact and become very upset when touched.

ASD begins in early childhood—between the ages of 18 months and 3 years. In Canada, about 1 child in 94 is diagnosed with ASD.[6] It is one of the most common brain disorders affecting children; boys are affected more often than girls.[7]

ASD is a number of related complex neurobiological conditions that can affect the normal function of the gastro-intestinal, immune, hepatic, endocrine, and nervous systems. It can impact normal brain development, leaving individuals with symptoms such as communication problems, decreased interest in various activities, reduced willingness to engage in activities, difficulty with typical social interactions, and a tendency to repeat specific patterns of behaviour. Both verbal and nonverbal communication are affected, and some individuals are unable to understand the facial expressions of others. This disorder may also affect the development of fine and gross motor ability in some clients.

ASD may range from mild (e.g., an individual with Asperger's syndrome who has difficulties with social function but who otherwise functions well intellectually and at work) to severe (e.g., a child with severe autism who is developmentally delayed and who is unable to function independently). The following symptoms are common:

- Develops language skills slowly, if at all
- Repeats words or phrases
- Cannot start or maintain conversations
- Repeats body movements (hand flapping, finger flicking, rocking)
- Has short attention span
- Avoids eye contact
- Spends time alone
- Shows little reaction to pain
- Dislikes cuddling
- Has frequent tantrums for no apparent reason
- Has strong attachment to a single item, idea, activity, or person
- Needs routines; dislikes change
- Lacks fear
- Does not respond to others
- Is too active or too quiet
- Displays aggressive or violent behaviour
- Tends to injure self

Since individuals on the autism spectrum may have varying degrees and combinations of symptoms, treatment needs to be specific to the individual. Every client is very different. However, as a support worker caring for children or adults with ASD, remember the following:

- Strict routines are usually important. The client may become very upset if the routine is disrupted. Follow the client's routine whenever possible. Warn the client if the routine must be changed.
- The client needs to develop social and work skills. Some adults with ASD work and live independently, but some need support and help from family and community services. Some may live in group homes or residential care facilities.
- Children with ASD require careful supervision. Some should never be left alone.

There is no cure for autism spectrum disorder, but with therapy, the client may learn to change or control behaviours. Behaviour modification—rewarding positive behaviours and correcting negative behaviours—is used to encourage social behaviours. Speech and language therapy is encouraged to assist the client in improving communication skills. Music, auditory, recreation, and sensory therapies may also assist the client.

SUPPORTING CLIENTS WITH DEVELOPMENTAL DISORDERS AND DISABILITIES

Clients with developmental disorders and disabilities often have complex care needs, especially if their disabilities are severe. You must be familiar with special equipment and self-help devices needed for each client. Follow the care plan, and consult with your supervisor if you have questions. For example, Gordon, 10, has severe cerebral palsy. He cannot walk and has limited use of his hands. He tends to slide down in his wheelchair, so a postural support is used to help keep him in good body alignment. He must be repositioned frequently to prevent pressure ulcers. Gordon also has a hearing impairment and a speech disorder; he wears hearing aids in both ears and uses a computer to communicate. Gordon has splints on his ankles to prevent contractures. He uses a special spoon strapped to his wrist to help him eat.

When working with children and adults with developmental disorders or disabilities, remember to consider the client before the disorder or disability. For example, Gordon is an intelligent, sensitive 10-year-old who enjoys reading, going on outings, and visiting with his support worker. He also happens to have severe CP and uses a wheelchair.

Clients with developmental disorders or disabilities have the same rights and needs as everyone else. Each client is unique. The effects of disabilities vary, depending on the client. Your supervisor and the care plan will tell you how to meet each client's needs in the best way. As always, your priority when caring for these clients is to promote their dignity, independence, preferences, privacy, and safety (see the *Think About Safety: Caring for Clients With Developmental Disorders and Disabilities* box and the *Providing Compassionate Care: Caring for Clients With Developmental Disorders and Disabilities* box.)

You can help a child with a developmental disorder or disability and the child's family in the following ways:

- Encourage the family to maintain a consistent daily schedule.
- Maintain a regular bedtime.
- Use lists, charts, or memory aides to remind the client about important duties, dates, and times.
- Encourage regular physical activity.
- Encourage structured social activities, such as sports or dancing. Such activities can also improve the child's social strengths and self-esteem.
- Suggest the client study in a quiet area, away from noisy distractions.
- Suggest counselling, which can assist the client and family to cope and help the client learn how to adapt to the world environment.
- Encourage the client to take medication at the same time every day and to report any adverse effects to the client's health care provider immediately.
- Encourage the client to eat a nutritionally balanced diet and to follow Canada's Food Guide for Healthy Eating.

Think About Safety

Caring for Clients With Developmental Disorders and Disabilities

- Follow the care plan for supervision for a client with autism. Some clients, especially children, will need constant supervision, as they are not aware of the dangerous situations in the home and can walk out of the home at any time and not be aware of any dangers on the streets; also, they may not know how to get home.
- Clients who have difficulty eating or swallowing should not eat or drink without supervision.
- When caring for a client with spina bifida cystica, be careful when working around the sac, as the tissue can be very fragile. Injury can lead to infection.
- If your client has a seizure, ensure that there is nothing within reach that could harm the client; do not hold the client down; keep track of the duration of the seizure and the parts of the body affected; if the seizure lasts longer than 5 minutes, call the emergency medical service in your area. After the seizure has stopped, place the client on the left side in case the client vomits; stay with the client until he or she recovers.

Providing Compassionate Care
Caring for Clients With Developmental Disorders and Disabilities

- ***Dignity.*** Adults and children with developmental disabilities deserve to be treated with respect and in a manner that promotes their dignity. Remember to consider the client before the disability. The words you use are an important way to show respect. For example, say, "clients with disabilities." Do not refer to them as "handicapped," "disabled," or "crippled." Also, do not identify the client by the disability. For example, it is correct to say, "Mr. Joshi has autism spectrum disorder." Do not say, "Mr. Joshi is autistic." Say, "Susan has an intellectual disability," not "Susan is retarded."

  Have empathy, not pity. Remember, empathy is understanding the experiences and feelings of others; pity is feeling sorry for others, which implies that you are superior to the person.

  Also, promote dignity through your actions. Extend the same courtesies and consideration that you show all clients. Be friendly, and talk with your clients. Be a good listener, and show interest in their lives. Children with disabilities are like all children; they need attention and love. They also need to play and have fun. Adults with disabilities are like all adults; they need support and encouragement. Treat them like adults. Shake hands when introduced. Offer to shake hands even if the client has an artificial limb, has limited function in the hand, or has to use the left hand. Speak directly to the client in a normal tone of voice. Address adults using their titles and last names, unless they tell you otherwise.
- ***Independence.*** The goal for clients with disabilities is for them to be as independent as possible. Do not make assumptions about what the client can and cannot do. Follow the care plan. Encourage the client to use self-help devices whenever possible. Be patient, and do not rush the client.
- ***Preferences.*** Clients have the right to personal choices. Provide opportunities for the client to make choices and decisions. Ask first if the client wants help and how you can provide help. All clients must consent to procedures before you start. If the client does not want you to continue, stop. Contact your supervisor. Also, adapt your work to allow for the family's choices and preferences (unless directed otherwise in the care plan).
- ***Privacy.*** Medical and personal information about the client is confidential. Talk about the client only with members of the health care team who need to know. Do not expose the client. Provide privacy when performing procedures. Drape the client so as not to expose the client's body. Remember that adults with disabilities have sexual needs. Many have partners or are married. Allow for privacy for sexual activity.
- ***Safety.*** Most developmental disorders or disabilities create safety hazards for the client. Check with your supervisor and the care plan to determine how to ensure the client's safety. Practise the safety measures described in Chapter 22. Also, be alert to signs of abuse. Report any suspected abuse to your supervisor immediately. Remember, you also must report child abuse directly to a public authority (see Chapter 16).

CHAPTER REVIEW

KEY POINTS

- Developmental disorders and disabilities can affect physical, mental, and intellectual functions.
- Developmental disorders and disabilities are always permanent and may be mild, moderate, or severe.
- There are various developmental conditions, and each condition can have a wide range of symptoms.
- A developmental disability can occur in the child because of the condition of the mother during pregnancy, or it can occur during birth, after birth, or during childhood or adolescence. The disability interferes with and impairs normal development in a child.
- The care plan for each client will differ, depending on the client's level of functioning, age, and symptoms.
- A developmental disorder or disability can affect the client and the family across the client's lifespan as the needs of the client change and the ability of family members to care for the client change as they age.
- The family and the client (depending on the client's age) should be included in planning care.

CRITICAL THINKING IN PRACTICE

A teenage client who has cerebral palsy has long fingernails that she likes to have filed and polished. Today, you notice that some of her fingernails are broken and have rough edges. You quietly try to file her nails before beginning her personal care, but as you begin, she resists. She swings her arms at you and yells. What *should* you have done prior to beginning nail care? Why is nail care important for this client? How might you provide care safely?

REVIEW QUESTIONS

Answers to these questions are at the bottom of the next page.

Circle the BEST answer.

1. All developmental disorders and disabilities are caused:
   A. During adulthood
   B. Due to trauma
   C. During pregnancy
   D. Before birth, at birth, or during childhood or adolescence
2. These statements are about developmental disorders and disabilities. Which one is true?
   A. Self-care, learning, and mobility are always affected.
   B. The disability is permanent.
   C. Physical and intellectual impairment always occur together.
   D. The person with a developmental disorder or disability cannot hold a job.
3. Down syndrome:
   A. Is a genetic disorder
   B. Is caused when the mother is stressed during pregnancy
   C. Can be transmitted through direct contact
   D. Is a form of depression
4. Cerebral palsy is usually caused by:
   A. An extra chromosome
   B. A high fever
   C. Lack of oxygen to the brain
   D. Infection during pregnancy
5. A person with the spastic type of cerebral palsy may have issues such as:
   A. Learning difficulty
   B. Drooling
   C. Difficulties with posture, balance, and movement
   D. Weaving motions of the trunk, arms, and legs

6. Which statement about attention-deficit/hyperactivity disorder (ADHD) is correct?
 A. It is never present in adults.
 B. Occurrence is more likely if a close biological family member has ADHD.
 C. It is more common in girls than in boys.
 D. People with ADHD have a reduced tendency toward addictive behaviours.

7. Symptoms of attention-deficit/hyperactivity disorder (ADHD) include:
 A. A short temper with explosive episodes
 B. Sitting still and playing for long periods of time
 C. Avoiding excitement and stimulation
 D. Ability to structure time and set priorities easily

8. Symptoms of autism spectrum disorder appear:
 A. At fertilization
 B. During pregnancy
 C. At birth
 D. In early childhood

9. A person with autism spectrum disorder has:
 A. Impaired movement
 B. Issues with relating to people
 C. Diplegia
 D. A buildup of an amino acid in the blood

10. A person with epilepsy always has:
 A. A chance of a seizure if the medication regime is not followed
 B. Diplegia
 C. Weak muscle tone
 D. Low IQ

11. Spina bifida involves:
 A. Improper closing of the spine
 B. Seizures
 C. Abnormalities in the structure of the heart
 D. Changes in the X chromosome

12. Fetal alcohol spectrum disorders are caused by:
 A. Acquired brain injury
 B. Shaking an infant
 C. The mother drinking alcohol during pregnancy
 D. Abnormal chromosomes

Answers: 1.D, 2.B, 3.A, 4.C, 5.C, 6.B, 7.A, 8.D, 9.B, 10.A, 11.A, 12.C

CHAPTER 39

Speech and Language Disorders

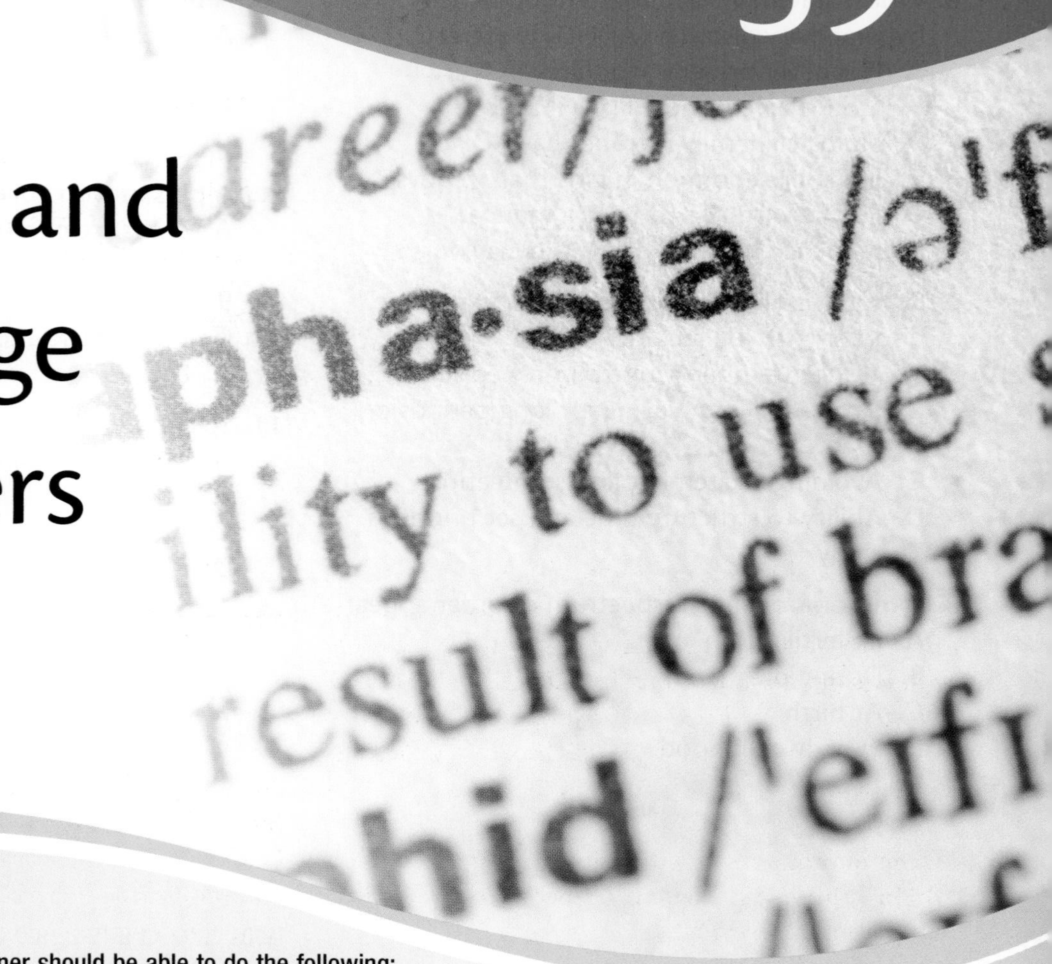

OBJECTIVES

After reading this chapter, the learner should be able to do the following:

- Describe types of aphasia.
- Describe apraxia of speech.
- Describe dysarthria.
- Describe how speech and language disorders are treated.
- Identify what communication aids are and how they assist the client.
- Describe how computers can assist clients with speech disorders.
- Describe the emotional effects of a language disorder.
- Describe how to communicate with clients with language disorders.
- Apply the procedures described in this chapter to clinical practice properly.

KEY TERMS

aphasia Partial or complete loss (*a*) of speech and language skills (*phasia*) caused by brain injury. *p. 903*

apraxia of speech Inability (*a*) to correctly move (*praxia*) the muscles used to speak. Apraxia is usually caused by a brain injury. *p. 904*

dysarthria Difficulty (*dys*) speaking clearly (*arthria*), caused by weakness or paralysis in the muscles used for speech. *p. 904*

expressive aphasia Difficulty speaking or writing. *p. 903*

expressive–receptive aphasia Difficulty speaking and understanding language. Also known as **global aphasia**. *p. 904*

global aphasia See **expressive–receptive aphasia**. *p. 904*

receptive aphasia Difficulty understanding language. *p. 903*

Imagine what life would be like if you were unable to speak or communicate! That is a daily reality for those with speech and language disorders. Speech and language disorders involve difficulty speaking, understanding, reading, or writing and, unfortunately, they can occur at any age. The causes include the following:

- Genetic problems or conditions present at birth
- Brain injury (e.g., caused by accident, infection, drug abuse, or stroke)
- Disease
- Hearing loss
- Brain tumours
- Problems with the body structures used for speech

Chapter 5 discussed effective communication between people who have no physical communication disorder. This chapter builds on the information presented in Chapter 5 and applies it to the process of communicating effectively with clients who have speech and language disorders. It should be noted that speech and language disorders are a result of injuries or decline in the brain's communication centre, as noted above. They should not be confused with the difficulty of people who speak another language to understand English.

Clients with speech or language disorders should always have a thorough health history taken, usually by a doctor or a nurse, as soon as possible before treatment begins. The client's history will provide details that can help the health care team better understand the health challenges the client has faced.

APHASIA

Aphasia is the partial or complete loss (*a*) of speech and language skills (*phasia*) caused by brain injury. Stroke (also called *cerebral vascular accident*, or *CVA*), head trauma, and brain tumours are the most common causes of aphasia. Some people with aphasia regain some or all of their language skills, but in some, aphasia is permanent. For example, people with dementia who develop aphasia do not typically regain verbal communication skills (see Chapter 36).

For communication to occur, a message must be sent, received, and interpreted. People with aphasia are unable to send messages, unable to understand the message received, or both.

Types of Aphasia

There are three basic types of aphasia:

1. **Receptive aphasia**—difficulty understanding language, including both spoken and written words. People with receptive aphasia cannot understand their own words or others', so their speech is mixed up or muddled. They also mix up sounds within words. A client trying to say "hospital," for example, may say "posital."
2. **Expressive aphasia**—difficulty speaking or writing. People with expressive aphasia can understand

spoken and written words, but their speech or written language is jumbled or slurred and difficult to understand. They think one thing but say or write another. For example, a client may want food but ask for a newspaper. People with expressive aphasia cannot think of the right words or put the right sounds together to form words and sentences. For example, a client trying to say, "Please give me a glass of water" may actually say "Come. Come. Come. Come." Some may leave out connecting words. Others can produce only meaningless sounds. Because people with expressive aphasia are very aware of their mistakes since *they* can understand what they are saying, they may become frustrated or depressed, leading them to cry or swear for no apparent reason.

3. **Expressive–receptive aphasia** (also known as **global aphasia**)—difficulty speaking and understanding written and spoken language. Some people with expressive–receptive aphasia can say only "yes" and "no" and make sounds such as "da da." Some others have lost all speech and language skills.

APRAXIA OF SPEECH

Apraxia of speech (*verbal apraxia*) is the inability (*a*) to correctly move (*praxia*) the muscles used to speak. People with this disorder are not able to control their lip, jaw, or tongue movements. As a result, they are not able to say the desired sounds and words. Apraxia of speech is caused by brain injury resulting from stroke, accident, brain tumour, or infection. Some babies are born with this disorder. Apraxia of speech can occur alone or with aphasia.

Understanding the speech of people with apraxia of speech is difficult, as they usually speak very slowly and may use words that sound similar to but not be exactly what they are trying to say. For example, a client may say "me" instead of "see." As well, the order of sounds within words may be mixed up. For example, a client may say "thootshub" instead of "toothbrush." Some people have problems putting words in the right order or finding the right words. Inconsistent speech is common—that is, a person may say something correctly one time and incorrectly another time.

DYSARTHRIA

Dysarthria is difficulty (*dys*) speaking clearly (*arthria*). It is caused by weakness or paralysis in the muscles used for speech. Common causes of dysarthria include cerebral palsy, multiple sclerosis, head injury, tumour, and infection.

People with dysarthria usually have slurred, slow, and soft speech and speak in flat, harsh, or nasal tones. They often have problems forming words, spacing their words, and breathing while speaking. Speech errors are usually consistent and predictable, so you may become familiar with a client's speech.

EMOTIONAL EFFECTS OF SPEECH AND LANGUAGE DISORDERS

How would you feel if you were not able to express your thoughts and feelings? How would you feel if you were not able to understand what others are saying? People with speech and language disorders experience emotions such as frustration, depression, and anger, as well as low self-esteem, shame, and guilt. **BOX 39–1** contains comments from people who have had aphasia.

Communication is important for functioning and for maintaining relationships with others. Being unable to communicate may cause a client to avoid social situations, or family and friends may avoid the client instead. Speech and language disorders can be very stressful for families, as the relations between all family members are usually affected.

Many of us often find sharing our thoughts and feelings with others difficult. It is even more difficult for someone who has a speech or language disorder since even everyday conversations require great effort. People with speech and language disorders may speak slowly, may struggle with words, or may mispronounce words frequently. These communication difficulties might be frustrating for both the affected person and the listener, who may have to struggle to understand. Family members may find themselves trying to correct the person or becoming irritated with the person if the same word or phrase is repeatedly mispronounced. The person who cannot speak clearly might be tempted to avoid speaking.

People with speech or language disorders may not be able to work, so they may suffer the added stress

BOX 39–1 Comments From People Who Have Had Aphasia

- "I wanted to speak, but no sounds came out of my mouth."
- "I felt … imprisoned in a tomb."
- "I noticed a change in me. I was another person, someone who was unable to express the little I knew. I was ashamed."
- "If you don't know words, you keep quiet … When it's noisy, you can't talk … People talk for us … Anyway, when we talk, it's not the way it used to be … you keep quiet."
- "Once I had to answer the intercom. I said 'Hello?' I heard the person speaking on the other end, but I couldn't understand him. So, to prove that it wasn't me who had the problem, I repeated, 'Hello! Hello! Hello!' as if to signal the line was bad. That's how I got out of that situation."
- "I feel useless … slightly distanced from the family because I can only understand things after some time. My world has shrunk."
- "I want to say something … just before I start saying it, she helps. Sometimes if she would stay back and let me finish, I would be all right."

Source: Joanette, Y., Lafond, D., & Lecours, A.R. (1993). The person with aphasia. In D. Lafond et al. (Eds.), *Living with aphasia: Psychosocial issues* (pp. 19–39). San Diego, CA: Singular Publishing Group.

of financial concerns. For some people, even routine tasks like shopping, cooking, paying bills, and doing household repairs may be impossible, so they are forced to depend on others to do what they used to be able to do themselves.

Emotional reactions vary from client to client and from family to family. Observe and listen to your clients and their families. Put yourself in their place. How would you feel and want to be treated in their position? Accept and understand displays of emotion.

TREATMENT FOR SPEECH AND LANGUAGE DISORDERS

A speech therapist (also called a *speech–language pathologist*) helps the client with a speech disorder learn to communicate and also helps family members learn new communication techniques. Methods used depend on the disorder, its cause, and its severity. Practice and exercises may help the client relearn speech and language skills. In the case of dysarthria, the client practises muscle-strengthening exercises and learns how to breathe while speaking.

People with speech and language disorders also learn how to improve existing skills. For example, a client learns to use body language and facial expressions to make communication more effective. Some people learn new skills such as sign language.

Those with severe speech and language problems may never regain their ability to speak and understand language. These clients may be helped by the following aids:

- ***Communication boards.*** These are boards with pictures or words that show functions or tasks (**FIGURE 39–1**). There are pictures or words related to activities of daily living, such as sleep, food, drink, medicine, and glasses. The client points to the things that are needed. The type of communication board depends on the client's needs. For those who can read, words rather than pictures are often used. For those with quadriplegia who are not able to speak or point, eye-gaze boards may be used. The client indicates needs by gazing at the picture or word on the board and either blinking or using another signal to accept it.
- ***Mechanical and electronic devices.*** These devices range in complexity and cost—from large computers that cannot be moved easily from place to place to handheld devices such as electronic talking aids (**FIGURES 39–2 AND 39–3**). The client touches a picture displayed on the screen, and the message

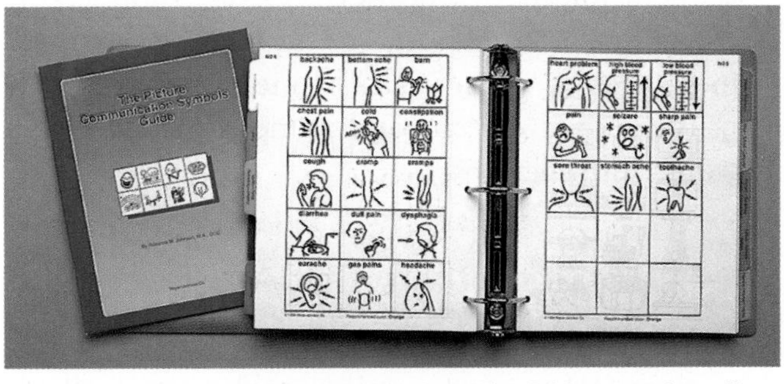

FIGURE 39–1 Communication board of images the client with aphasia can use to communicate with.

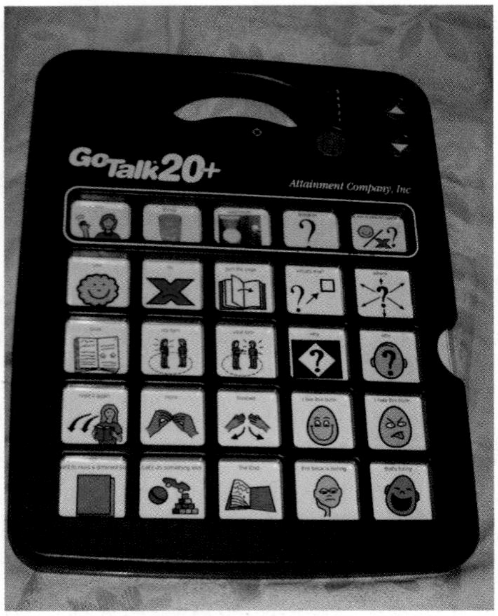

FIGURE 39–2 Electronic talking aid using symbols. (**Source:** Poule. This file is licensed under the Creative Commons Attribution-Share Alike 3.0 Unported license, https://creativecommons.org/licenses/by-sa/3.0/deed.en.)

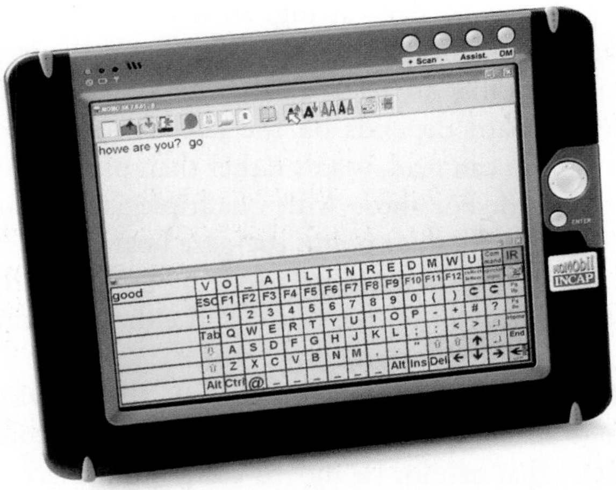

FIGURE 39–3 A computer that provides a speaking voice to its user. (**Source:** Courtesy SpecialNeedsComputers.ca, St. Catharines, ON.)

is then voiced by the device. For example, the client touches a picture of a sad face. A recorded message says, "I am sad." The message may also be printed on a screen, and some devices convert words into pictures.

The Use of Computers That Assist Clients With Speech and Language Challenges

A variety of communication tools are available to assist clients who have speech and language challenges to communicate more easily.[1] For example, people with verbal-expression communication disorders (such as dyslexia or verbal apraxia) often have difficulty reading or writing. Electronic devices that use a combination of screen reading, magnification systems, and alternate input provide computing access to people with such impairments. As well, electronic tablets that are small, easy to transport, and easy for most people to use can be customized with downloadable applications to assist the client (**FIGURE 39–4**).

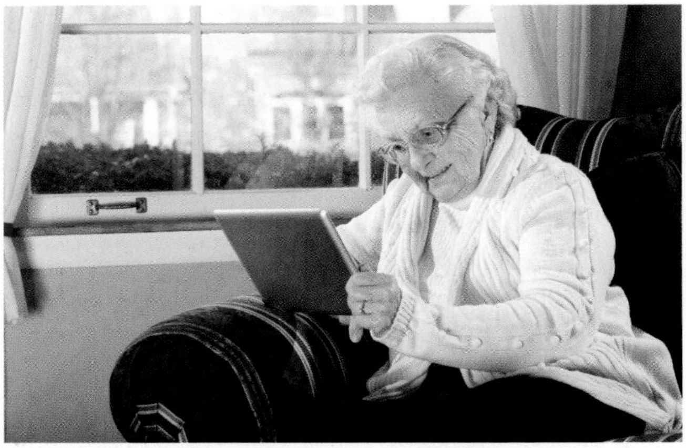

FIGURE 39–4 This tablet is simple, large enough to see any printed words or symbols, yet small enough for many clients with communication challenges to use. This client also uses the tablet to communicate electronically with her grandchildren who live in another province. (**Source:** Jim David/Shutterstock.com)

For clients who are unable to speak clearly but are able to type in the correct words or identify symbols that represent the words, there are systems available that can speak for them. Most of the software packages used for these applications can operate with a speech synthesizer. The speech that comes from the machine is electronically generated but can be adapted for a male or female voice. These computer-assisted electronic aids are expensive and may be difficult for some to carry around, but they have proven to be invaluable in improving the quality of life for those with speech and language challenges.

SUPPORTING AND COMMUNICATING WITH CLIENTS

As a support worker, to effectively communicate with your clients who have speech and language disorders, you must first know how you communicate in general. Do you speak clearly, or do you mumble? Do you use gestures? You may have to change the way you speak. Follow the care plan and your supervisor's instructions. Use the communication methods that are best for your client. While you are speaking, you should remember to be mindful of your facial expressions, as they can reflect any impatience or frustration you feel with the client.

The effort of understanding others and making oneself understood can be exhausting, especially to clients with speech and language disorders, so they often tire easily. Their other health problems may also cause fatigue. Be alert for signs of fatigue, such as drooping shoulders, irritability, lack of interest, and a decline in understanding. Reduce surrounding distractions (e.g., close doors and windows, turn down the volume of a television or radio), which can make concentrating difficult for the client. Some clients with speech and language disorders will appear withdrawn and uninterested. Spend extra time with these clients. Social interaction can promote self-esteem and recovery. Always include them in conversations, even if they cannot understand you.

Clients with speech and language disorders should be treated with respect and empathy. Remember DIPPS—the five principles of support work (see the *Providing Compassionate Care: Communicating With Clients With Speech and Language Disorders* box; also see the *Supporting Mr. Hamilton, Part 1: Communicating With Clients With Expressive Dysphasia* and *Supporting Mr. Hamilton, Part 2: Communicating With Clients With Expressive Dysphasia* boxes). Follow the guidelines in **BOX 39–2** on page 909.

Do NOT finish words for clients. Have patience.

Providing Compassionate Care
Communicating With Clients With Speech and Language Disorders

- ***Dignity.*** Showing respect, warmth, and compassion are important ways to promote dignity. Never talk about a client as if the person were not present. Address questions for and comments about the client to the client, not to others who are present. Some people with language disorders are embarrassed to speak in front of others, especially strangers, so do not force a client to talk in front of others (see the *Supporting Mr. Hamilton, Part 1: Communicating With Clients With Expressive Dysphasia* box).
- ***Independence.*** People with speech and language disorders must gain, regain, or maintain independence and control. Support, encouragement, and patience are important. Never show impatience, frustration, or worry when a client is having problems speaking or understanding. Do not talk down to the client. (The *Supporting Mr. Hamilton, Part 2: Communicating With Clients With Expressive Dysphasia* box describes a support worker patiently using body language and symbols to learn about a client's needs.) The care plan may list ways to encourage communication.
- ***Preferences.*** Limit the number of choices to help the client express preferences without difficulty. Be encouraging and supportive. A useful tip is to write down the available choices beforehand so that the client can pick one easily.
- ***Privacy.*** Keep information about your client confidential. Remember your role and relationship with the client at all times. Be professional in your communication. Learn to be comfortable with silence. Do not feel that you need to talk when the client is silent.
- ***Safety.*** Take extra time to explain procedures. Do not explain all the steps at once. Explain the step just before you do it. Avoid medical terms. Speak clearly and slowly. Be alert for signs the client has not understood you.

Supporting Mr. Hamilton, Part 1: Communicating With Clients With Expressive Dysphasia

Joshua Hamilton, 57, survived a cerebral vascular accident several months ago. In addition to a few other health challenges, he has expressive aphasia. Marta, his support worker, has been assigned to Mr. Hamilton to assist him with his basic care at home.

Mr. Hamilton frequently asks Marta questions that she does not understand. Here is an example of a recent conversation:

Mr. Hamilton: Wuld ples git bassen eaten?
Marta: Could you please repeat that, Mr. Hamilton?
Mr. Hamilton: (raises his voice) Plasin get eatin puck.
Marta: Would you like something to eat?
Mr. Hamilton: (looks puzzled and upset) Dat stan woo.
Marta: (pretends to eat) Would you like a snack?
Mr. Hamilton: (shakes his head but says nothing)
Marta: (pretends to drink) Something to drink?
Mr. Hamilton: (nods his head and looks relieved)
Marta: (gets a glass and cup)
Mr. Hamilton: (gestures toward the cup)
Marta: (gets a tea bag) Would you like a cup of tea?
Mr. Hamilton: (nods)

In this situation, Marta was not sure what exactly Mr. Hamilton wanted. She thought the words *eaten* and *eatin* suggested that Mr. Hamilton wanted something to eat. He was, in fact, trying to say "tea." Marta did not know this, but she knew from reading his care plan and speaking to his family that Mr. Hamilton liked tea. Using body language and symbols, Marta discovered what Mr. Hamilton wanted, and by being patient and persistent, she was able to meet Mr. Hamilton's needs.

Supporting Mr. Hamilton, Part 2: Communicating With Clients With Expressive Dysphasia

Marta has noticed that Mr. Hamilton sometimes repeatedly says unrelated words, such as "bun … bun … bun … bun" instead of using the correct words. According to Mr. Hamilton's care plan, this impediment (obstacle) is a result of his global aphasia and occurs most frequently when he is tired, hungry, overstimulated, or in need of toileting. Occasionally, he will repeat a word over and over again and seems to get into a pattern of repeating himself, even though he has used the words correctly since his stroke.

Following the suggestions in his care plan, Marta reminded Mr. Hamilton to use another word the next time he repeats the same word or phrase. Here is an example of how she did this during a meal:

Mr. Hamilton: (gestures toward his food) Gum … gum … gum … gum …
Marta: (pointing at one of the foods on his plate with the spoon) Not "gum" (spoken gently). Potatoes?
Mr. Hamilton: (shaking his head)
Marta: (pointing at another food on his plate) Meat?
Mr. Hamilton: (nodding his head) Gum … gum …
Marta: (putting the meat on his spoon) Not "gum" (spoken gently). Meat.

Marta made sure to speak clearly and gently, used short sentences, and faced Mr. Hamilton. She also remembered to smile so she would not appear annoyed or angry in any way, knowing that Mr. Hamilton may be very sensitive to signs of impatience or frustration in others.

Mr. Hamilton: (nodding his head) Meat.

Marta then proceeded to assist Mr. Hamilton with his food.

BOX 39–2 Guidelines for Communicating With Clients With Speech and Language Disorders

- ***Minimize distractions.*** Distractions make concentration difficult and can also upset the client. Reduce background noise and activity. Close doors and windows. Turn off the television and radio (if the client agrees), and keep cellphones on silent mode. Make sure there is nothing in your hands or on your lap.
- ***Adjust the lighting.*** Make sure the client can see your face clearly and that you can see the client's. Turn down lights and adjust window coverings to reduce glare. Do not position yourself between the client and a window. The client may not be able to see you in the glare.
- ***Give the client your full attention.*** Sit close by and face the client. Look directly into the client's eyes so that the client can look at your face. Get the client's attention before you speak. Show that you are listening by using gestures and facial expressions. Do not perform other tasks while you are talking to the client.
- ***In the beginning of your work relationship with the client, you can start by asking questions to which you know the answer.*** Doing so helps you become familiar with the client's speech.
- ***Determine the subject being discussed.*** Knowing the topic helps you understand the main points. Look for nonverbal clues. Do the client's gestures, eyes, and body language tell you anything? Does the client use words or partial words that might describe an item or concept?
- ***Follow the client's lead.*** Alter your communication method, as needed. For example, Mrs. Schmidt becomes frustrated when you ask her questions. You learn that she responds better when you use gestures to demonstrate your question. If Mrs. Schmidt seems tired or has lost interest, allow her to rest. Bring up the subject at a later time.
- ***Speak slowly, clearly, and in a normal tone of voice.*** Adjust your speech to suit the client's needs. Talk to adults in a mature, professional manner. Do not use slang or figures of speech. Some clients may not understand them.
- ***Give the client time to respond.*** Do not rush the client. Pause between sentences to allow the client time to think and respond. Do not answer questions, including your own questions and those from others, when they are addressed to the client.
- ***Use simple words and short sentences.*** Avoid long, complex sentences. Focus on key words—mostly action words and words for people, places, or things. For example, say "Let's go for lunch" instead of "It's time for me to transfer you to the dining room for lunch."
- ***Be patient.*** Repeat your words, as needed. Rephrase your sentences if the client does not understand you.
- ***Use positive statements.*** Positive statements are easier to understand than negative statements. For example, say, "Bend your arm" instead of "Don't straighten your arm."
- ***Use appropriate questioning and paraphrasing techniques.*** Ask questions that require only a short answer or a shake of the head. Paraphrase (summarize in your own words) what the client has said. Ask the client if you have understood correctly (see Chapter 5).
- ***Provide cues, as needed.*** Help clients express themselves by giving them cues about a word they cannot recall. If it is an object, ask: "What does it look like?" "What is it used for?" and "Where is it found?" Encourage the use of gestures and pointing. If you think you understand what the client says, verify your assumption by asking if *this* is what she means. If the client's gestures or words suggest you have misunderstood, encourage the client again to use gestures, pointing, or symbols. For example, Mrs. Lin points to her sweater. You get it for her, and she puts it on. You have understood her need.
- ***Try other communication methods.*** Some people may write better than they speak. Follow the care plan. Use writing and communication boards, as needed.
- ***Pay attention to your own facial expressions and nonverbal cues.*** Your facial expressions can reveal if you are frustrated or impatient, and your client could easily detect this.

CHAPTER REVIEW

KEY POINTS

- Aphasia is the partial or complete loss of speech and language skills. These skills may be slowly regained or may be lost permanently.
- The three types of aphasia are (1) receptive, (2) expressive, and (3) expressive–receptive (global) aphasia.
- Apraxia of speech is the inability to move the muscles used in speech.
- Dysarthria is difficulty speaking clearly.
- People with speech and language disorders experience many emotions, such as frustration, depression, and anger, which can be stressful to both the client and the family.
- As a support worker, you should be aware of communication aids and how to communicate with a person with a speech or language disorder.

CRITICAL THINKING IN PRACTICE

Mr. Avery had a stroke. He has hemiplegia, receptive aphasia, and dysphagia. Explain how you will plan to perform the care measures listed below from his care plan. Apply learning from this and other chapters.

- Transferring him from the bed to the wheelchair
- Communicating with him
- Dressing and undressing him
- Assisting him with food and fluids
- Performing a safety check of the room

REVIEW QUESTIONS

Answers to these questions are at the bottom of the next page.

Circle the BEST answer.

1. People with receptive aphasia have problems with:
   A. Speaking and writing
   B. Pronouncing vowels
   C. Understanding language
   D. Moving the mouth, tongue, and lips

2. People with expressive–receptive aphasia have problems with:
   A. Speaking and writing
   B. Understanding language
   C. Moving the mouth, tongue, and lips
   D. Speaking and understanding language

3. Apraxia of speech is caused by:
   A. Brain injury
   B. Laziness of the client
   C. Increased tone in the muscles used to speak
   D. Lack of coordination in the muscles used to walk

4. People with dysarthria:
   A. Cannot read or write
   B. Understand what is said
   C. Make unpredictable speech errors
   D. Can control the muscles used to speak

5. People with speech and language disorders:
   A. Are not affected emotionally
   B. Cannot improve their communication
   C. Often have problems relating to family and friends
   D. Are consistent in the way they react emotionally to their disorders

6. When communicating with clients who have speech and language disorders, you should:
A. Speak in a very loud voice
B. Leave them out of conversations
C. Ask others what they are trying to say
D. Provide cues about words they cannot recall

7. If you do not understand what a client has said, you should:
A. Use body language and symbols
B. Ask to be assigned to another client
C. Pretend that you did understand
D. Ignore the client to make the client stop talking

8. Why should instructions be stated using positive phrases ("Bend your leg") rather than negative phrases ("Do not straighten your leg")?
A. Using negative terms may be confusing for the client.
B. Positive terms are usually more direct.
C. Negative terms usually focus on what the client has already done.
D. All of the above.

Answers 1.C, 2.D, 3.A, 4.B, 5.C, 6.D, 7.A, 8.D

CHAPTER 40

Hearing and Vision Disorders

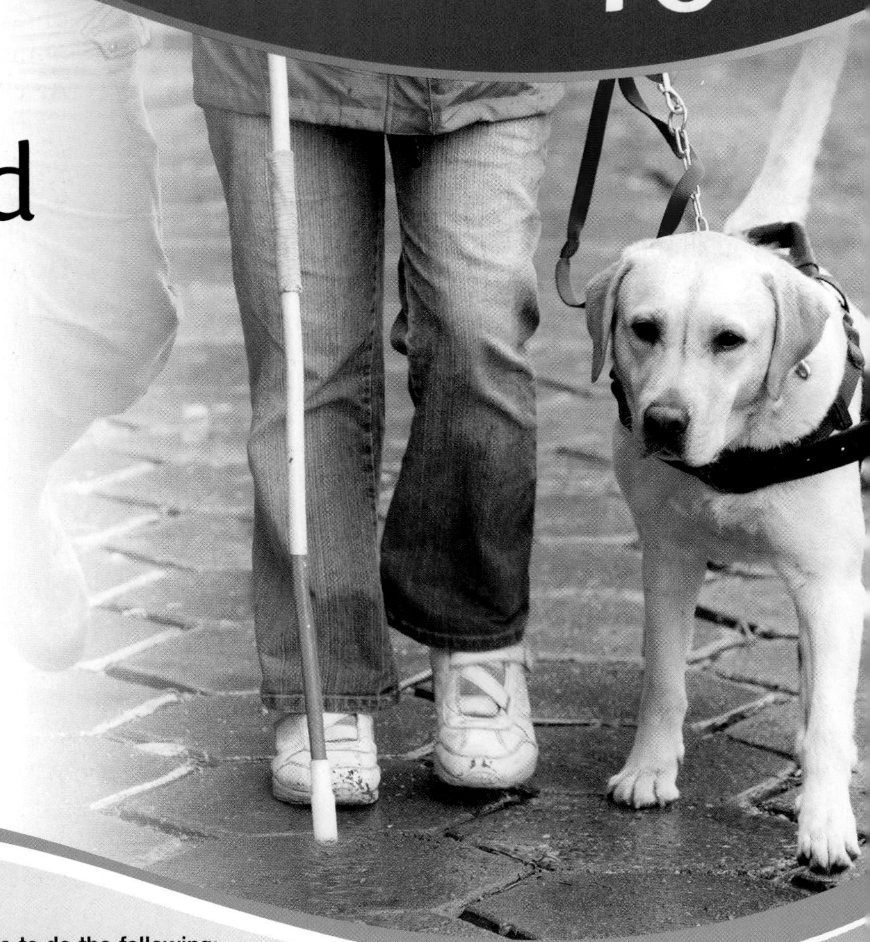

OBJECTIVES

After reading this chapter, the learner should be able to do the following:

- Describe the major ear disorders.
- Describe the effects of hearing problems.
- Describe aids for clients with problems.
- Explain how to care for clients with hearing loss.
- Describe the major eye disorders.
- Describe aids for clients with vision problems.
- Explain how to care for clients with vision loss.

KEY TERMS

age-related macular degeneration (AMD; ARMD) The breakdown (degeneration) of the macula (the light-sensitive part of the retina). AMD is a disease associated with aging that gradually destroys sharp, central vision. *p. 919*

Braille A writing system for the visually impaired that uses raised dots for each letter of the alphabet. *p. 922*

cataract Clouding of the eye's lens. *p. 921*

cerumen Ear wax *p. 914*

diabetic retinopathy A disorder (*pathy*) caused by diabetes, in which the blood vessels in the retina are damaged. *p. 920*

glaucoma An eye disease that causes pressure within the eye and vision loss. *p. 921*

Ménière's disease An inner ear disorder that can affect both hearing and balance. *p. 914*

otosclerosis A condition (*osis*) in which hardening (*sclero*) of the ossicles in the middle ear (*oto*) occurs, interfering with transmission of sound. *p. 914*

presbycusis The gradual hearing (*cusis*) loss associated with aging (*presby*). *p. 914*

presbyopia The gradual inability to focus (*opia*) on close objects; a condition associated with aging (*presby*). *p. 921*

retinal detachment The separation of the retina from its supporting tissue. *p. 920*

tinnitus Ringing in the ear. *p. 914*

vertigo Dizziness. *p. 914*

The senses of sight and hearing are important for communicating, learning, moving about, and performing activities of daily living (ADLs). They also help keep us safe by alerting us to danger.

Hearing and vision problems are common among all age groups, and common causes include conditions present at birth, diseases, and accidents. Some hearing and vision loss (and loss of other senses) is a natural part of aging.

As a support worker, you will care for many clients with hearing and vision disorders. Some clients may have minor disorders that can be corrected with hearing aids and glasses, whereas others may have severe losses (see the *Providing Compassionate Care: Clients With Severe Hearing or Vision Loss* box).

EAR DISORDERS

The ear is needed for hearing and balance. Ear disorders range from slight hearing impairments to complete deafness. Hearing impairments may occur suddenly, but they are usually gradual in onset. To prevent hearing loss, there needs to be more public awareness that ear protection should be used when using any loud machinery, even lawn mowers. Of greater concern are the consequences of children, teens, and young adults listening to music that is too loud—for example, blasting the music on car stereos or in their earphones—which can lead to future hearing problems. Hearing loss may affect one or both ears. See Chapter 17 for a review of the structure and function of the ear. Ear structures are shown in **FIGURE 17–17**.

Common causes of hearing impairment include the following:

- ***Otitis media***—infection (*itis*) of the middle (*media*) ear (*ot*)—is common in infants and children and may be acute or chronic. Normally, the ear's Eustachian tube (see Chapter 17) allows fresh air to enter the middle ear and fluids to drain from it. However, a cold or flu, large adenoids or tonsils, or an allergy such as hay fever can block the Eustachian tube, causing otitis media.[1]

  In very young children, the symptoms of *acute otitis media*—irritability, poor appetite, or ear pain—may be thought to be teething or a fever, which is a common effect of immunization. Therefore, it is very easy for otitis media to go undetected in infants and young children.[1]

  In *chronic otitis media*, the fluid in the middle ear builds up slowly and becomes thick and more difficult to drain. Chronic otitis media can damage the eardrum and the bones of the middle ear (the *ossicles*), which conduct sound to the inner ear and are essential for hearing. Permanent hearing loss can result from chronic otitis media.

- **Otosclerosis**—a condition (*osis*) in which there is an abnormal formation of new bone (*sclero*) in the middle ear that gradually immobilizes the stapes (stirrup bone) and prevents it from vibrating in response to sound, causing a progressive loss of hearing. Otosclerosis interferes with the transmission of sound. It is a hereditary condition that is a common cause of hearing loss and **tinnitus** (ringing in the ear) in adults. Surgery can often restore some hearing.
- **Ménière's disease**—an increase of fluid in the inner ear that causes pressure in the middle ear, resulting in **vertigo** (dizziness), tinnitus, and hearing loss. Clients experiencing dizziness must lie down to prevent a fall. Severe dizziness can cause nausea and vomiting. Usually, only one ear is affected.
- **Presbycusis**—the gradual hearing (*cusis*) loss associated with aging (*presby*). It usually occurs after age 50 years. There is no cure, but hearing aids and *speech reading* (lip reading) are helpful to those affected.
- ***Temporary hearing loss***—the blockage of the ear canal with **cerumen** (ear wax). Temporary hearing loss is common in older adults. A buildup of ear wax can lead to a client's gradual loss of balance. Both hearing and balance may be improved when the cerumen is removed by a physician or a nurse. Always encourage your client to allow wax to remove itself naturally rather than cleaning the auditory canal with cotton swabs, which can cause irritation, increase wax production unnecessarily, and cause the wax to impact and potentially perforate the eardrum.

HCAs Never Remove Ear wax

Providing Compassionate Care
Clients With Severe Hearing or Vision Loss

- ***Dignity.*** Clients with hearing loss or vision loss need patience and respect, not pity. Speak clearly in a normal tone of voice. Do not shout, and do not mumble or use slang terms. Do not talk to the client as you would to a child. Include the client in conversations with others. Never ask another person (such as a family member) to speak for the client. When speaking of a client's disability, always use the noun form of the disability, not the adjective form—for example, "Mrs. Kabir has a hearing loss," not "She is the deaf client." If a client uses sign language and has an interpreter, speak to the client, not to the interpreter.
- ***Independence.*** Remember, clients who are impaired in one area are not impaired in all areas. Do not make assumptions about their abilities or limitations. Clients with hearing loss or vision loss should be allowed to do as much for themselves as possible. Tell the client what you are doing step by step. Indicate when the procedure is over. When clients use self-care (assistive) devices to maintain independence, make sure they have access to these needed devices.
- ***Preferences.*** Follow your clients' choices and directions. Ask how you can help. Assist only if the client wants you to.
- ***Privacy.*** Respect your client's privacy. Always let the client know when you are in the room. If the client cannot hear you knock, make sure the client can see you entering the room. If the client cannot see you, announce your arrival clearly. Also, tell the client if others join you in the room.
- ***Safety.*** A safe setting is critical to clients with hearing loss or vision loss. Clients with hearing loss cannot hear sounds that signal danger, and those with vision loss cannot see obstacles in their path, so they are at great risk for falls. Follow the safety measures described in Chapter 22. Follow the care plan for safety measures specific to each client. In facilities, keep the call bell within easy reach.

Always tell your client when you are leaving the room. Remember your role and relationship with your clients at all times. Keep information about clients confidential. Communicate in a professional manner.

Effects of Hearing Impairment

Signs and symptoms of hearing impairment vary and are not always obvious. A person's behaviour or attitude may change because of a hearing impairment. For example, a person may not respond when others talk or ask questions and may become angry that others are not speaking loudly enough. Family and friends may not be aware of the issues, and they may become frustrated when communicating with the affected person and, therefore, may avoid talking with that person.

Some people deny that they have a hearing impairment, as they may not want to believe that they are any different from others or to admit to a sign of aging. Some people refuse to get or use a hearing aid.

The obvious signs of hearing impairment in adults and children include the following:

- Speaking too loudly
- Leaning forward to hear
- Turning and cupping the unaffected ear toward the speaker
- Responding inappropriately
- Asking for words to be repeated

Hearing impairment can affect all aspects of a person's health—physical, emotional, social, intellectual, and spiritual.

Additionally, hearing loss may cause speech problems. Not being able to hear one's own voice affects pronunciation and the volume of voice. Hearing loss may result in slurred speech and faulty pronunciation. Some people with severe hearing loss speak in a flat tone and drop word endings, and some cannot speak at all.

The Canadian Hearing Society is an excellent resource for clients, families, and support workers. It offers information and educational material on hearing impairment as well as aids for people who are hearing impaired.

Aids for People With Hearing Loss

A number of aids help people with a hearing impairment to communicate. These include hearing aids, special telephone systems, signalling devices, and hearing dogs.

Hearing Aids

A *hearing aid* is a device that fits inside the ear, behind the ear, or in the ear canal and makes sounds louder (**FIGURE 40–1**). It does not cure the hearing impairment, but it improves a client's hearing. Since both background noise and speech are made louder, you should help minimize background noise to enable your client to adjust to the hearing aid. Remember that the hearing aid makes speech *louder*—not clearer.

Hearing aids can cost up to $5000 per aid. Dropping a hearing aid can damage it and cause an added expense for your client or the family, so be very careful when handling them. Follow your supervisor's instructions regarding the appropriate care for a hearing aid, and report a missing or damaged hearing aid to your supervisor. Ensure that your client's name is on the device.

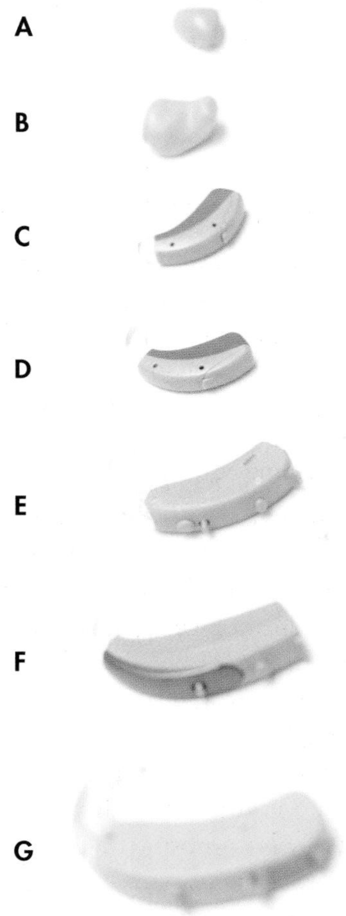

FIGURE 40–1 Hearing aids vary according to the client's needs. **A,** A completely-in-the-canal (CIC) hearing aid is molded to fit inside your ear canal. **B,** An in-the-canal (ITC) hearing aid is custom molded and fits partly in the ear canal. **C, D, E, F, G,** Behind-the-ear (BTE) hearing aids hook over the top of your ear and rest behind the ear. (**Source:** aerogondo2/Shutterstock.com)

Tips for troubleshooting common hearing aid problems are provided in **BOX 40–1**. Regular care of hearing aids should include the following:[2]

- Store hearing aids in a safe place that is dry and cool.
- Look for visual signs of damage such as cracks, broken parts, clogged openings, or moisture droplets.
- Check to make sure the battery is working by turning the hearing aid on, cupping it in your hand, and listening for a whistle. (Some hearing

BOX 40–1 Troubleshooting Common Hearing Aid Problems

Problem	Cause	Possible Remedy
Not working	Not turned on	Turn the "MTO" switch to *M*
	Battery weak or dead	Replace with fresh battery
	Battery polarity reversed	Make sure the battery is properly inserted
	Blocked ear mould	Clean ear mould
	Aid clogged with wax	Clean receiver opening
	Volume too low	Turn up the volume
Aid whistles	Improper seating in the ear	Insert correctly
	Volume up too high	Reduce volume
	Excessive wax in the ears	Have wax removed by a doctor or by a nurse on a doctor's order
	Ear mould loose	Get new ear mould—need appointment with hearing aid dispenser
	Internal feedback	Factory repair
Intermittent volume	Battery weak	Replace battery
	Poor battery contacts	Clean contacts
	"On" switch intermittent	Clean switch
	Moisture	Blow out moisture from the ear mould
	Damaged internal components	Factory repair
Not loud enough or sound distorted	Volume too low	Turn up the volume
	Battery weak	Replace battery
	Ear mould loose	Get new ear mould—need appointment with hearing aid dispenser
	Blocked ear mould	Clean ear mould
	Excessive wax in the ears	Have wax removed by doctor or by a nurse on a doctor's order
	Change in hearing	Appointment for hearing test

Source: The Canadian Hearing Society. (2002). Get Connected: Facts on Hearing Aids. Fact Sheet #7: Care of the hearing aids (p. 4). Toronto, ON. Retrieved October 20, 2011, from http://www.chs.ca/info/ha/7.html. Reprinted with permission.

aids turn on and off by opening up the battery chamber.)

- Check the hearing aid batteries so they do not suddenly run out of power. If batteries are dead, discard them in an appropriate manner. Switch the battery off if the aid is not being used. If the aid is not used for a long period of time, remove the battery. Clean battery contacts regularly with a cotton swab and check that the contacts are not bent.
- Wash the hearing aid if required. The type of hearing aid your client is using will determine the daily care you need to provide. The care plan will tell you what needs to be done and what tools to use. For example, some hearing aids must not be washed, but some need to be washed every time they are removed from the ear.
- Remove earwax from the hearing aid to prevent temporary malfunction or permanent damage. Change filters often so they do not collect wax or dirt.
- If you cannot clean the hearing aid completely, the supervisor or client may need to contact a hearing professional for help.
- Accumulated earwax may prevent sounds from travelling from the hearing aid into the middle ear. The client should never remove earwax from the ear since doing so can damage the ear. Instead, the client's doctor should be contacted to have the ear canals cleaned.
- Unless permitted by the manufacturer, the client should not wear the hearing aid when showering, swimming, or using a hair dryer. Avoid hair spray or other types of spray.

Technology for Hearing Assistance

Technology is advancing rapidly to provide assistance to clients with hearing impairment or complete hearing loss.

- ***Enhanced headphones.*** These headphones amplify the sound of people's voices. Some can be used for watching television or listening to music.
- ***Special telephone systems.*** *TTYs* (once called *telephone teletypes*) allow people with hearing loss to communicate through the telephone system. Users type messages back and forth to one another. *Amplified telephone handsets* make the caller's voice louder. *Extension bells* make the telephone ring more loudly.
- ***Signalling devices.*** These devices attach to such items as telephones, doorbells, and smoke alarms. When the device makes a sound, a light flashes to alert the person. Some devices include a vibrating option that can be felt.
- ***Emails.*** Text messaging through computers and cellphones has improved the ability of clients with hearing impairment to communicate with those who can hear. Speaking computer software programs are also available.
- ***Hearing dogs.*** Special dogs are now being trained to alert a person with a hearing impairment to different sounds, such as the ringing phone, the doorbell, an alarm, a baby's crying, and so on.
- ***Closed captioning.*** Since 1993, all TVs with screens larger than 13 inches have had built-in decoder circuitry that allows clients with a hearing impairment to enjoy the same programs as everyone else, using closed captioning.

Caring for Clients With Hearing Impairment

Some clients with hearing impairment wear hearing aids while others have hearing loss that cannot be improved by the use of hearing aids. Other clients prefer not to wear a hearing aid, or feel that they cannot afford the cost of a hearing aid. Some clients learn sign language (**FIGURE 40–2**), and some have hearing dogs that alert them to sounds. Other clients speech read by watching facial expressions, gestures, and body language. Follow the guidelines listed in **BOX 40–2** on page 919 when caring for clients with severe hearing loss.

Some clients who have experienced a gradual loss of hearing may not be fully aware that they no longer hear clearly. Unfortunately, this hearing loss can impact the client's ability to communicate comfortably in social situations, leading to feelings of frustration and embarrassment because of having to frequently ask people to repeat themselves. As a result, a client who has experienced gradual hearing loss may begin to avoid socialization with others, increasing isolation (see the *Supporting Mrs. Lopez: The Isolating Effects of Hearing Loss* box on page 919).

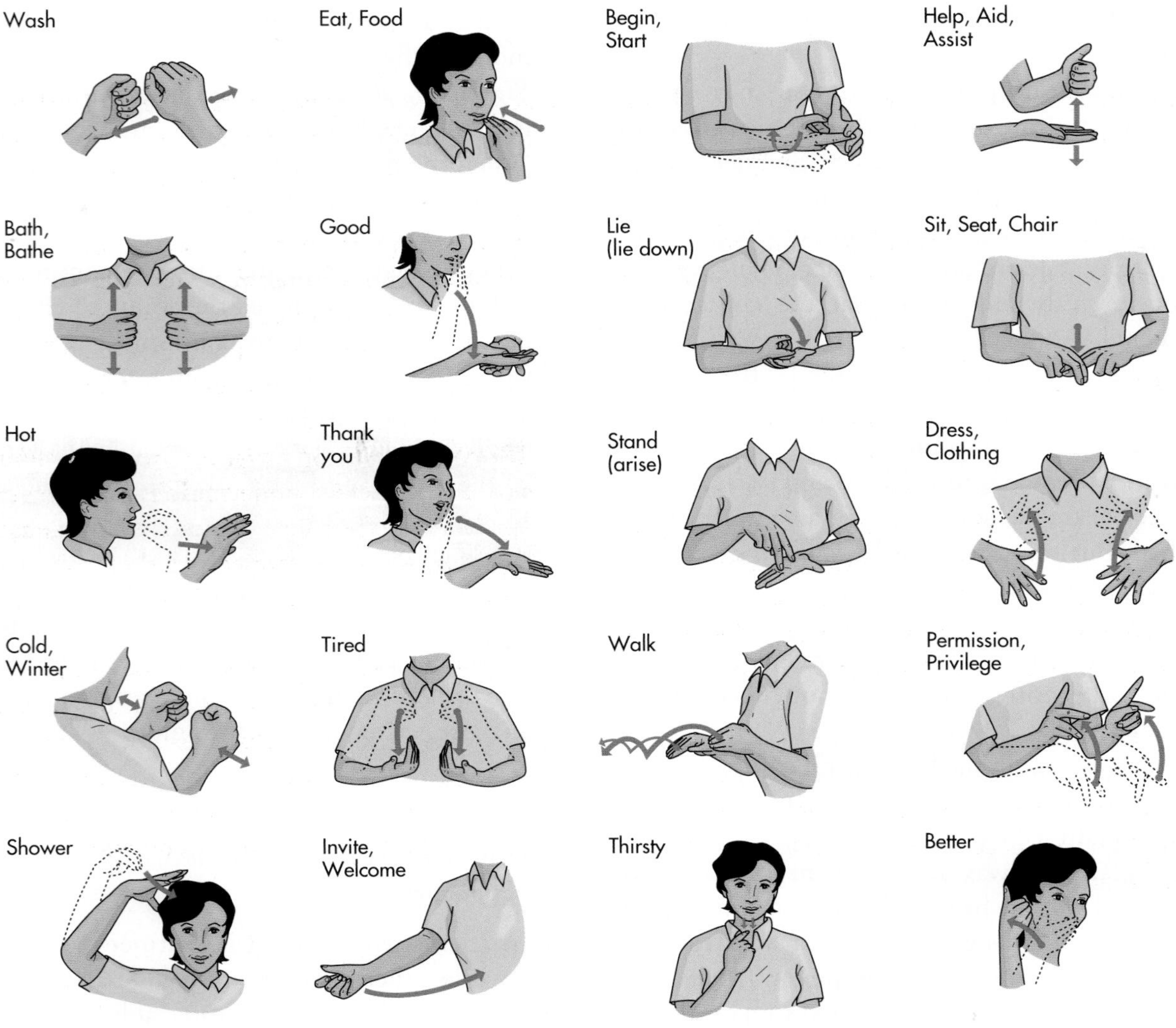

FIGURE 40–2 Sign language examples.

Clients with significant hearing loss are also at risk for injury if they cannot hear a smoke alarm or the kettle whistling (see Chapter 22). It is the responsibility of all health care team members to ensure the client remains safe at all times. Remember, some clients with hearing loss also have a speech or language disorder. Follow the guidelines listed in Chapter 39 for communicating with clients with speech or language disorders.

EYE DISORDERS AND VISION IMPAIRMENT

Eye disorders and vision impairment, ranging from very mild vision loss to complete vision loss, can occur at all ages. Health conditions, accidents, and eye diseases are among the causes of vision impairment. The level of vision impairment varies—some people cannot sense light at all and have no vision; others can sense some light but cannot see details; and still others have some vision but cannot see well. Someone who is *legally blind* is able to see objects at 6 m (20 ft.), whereas a person with normal vision (**FIGURE 40–3, *A*** on page 920) can see objects at 60 m (200 ft.). See Chapter 17 for a review of the structure and function of the eye. Eye structures are shown in **FIGURE 17–16** on page 285.

Vision impairment may occur suddenly or gradually, necessitating surgery, eyeglasses, or contact lenses. Common eye disorders and causes of vision impairment include the following:

- ***Conjunctivitis*** An inflammation of the clear membrane that covers the white part of the eye and lines the inner surface of the eyelids (see Chapter 23). The nonmedical term is *pink eye*.

BOX 40–2 Guidelines for Caring for Clients With Hearing Loss

- ***Alert the client to your presence.*** Get the client's attention. Raise an arm or hand, or lightly touch the client's arm. Do not startle or approach the client from behind.
- ***Adjust the lighting.*** Stand or sit in good light. Clients with hearing loss may need to see your face for speech reading. Shadows and glares affect their ability to see your face.
- ***Reduce background noise.*** Turn radios, televisions, air conditioners, and fans down or off if possible.
- ***Focus your attention on the client.*** Face the client. Stand or sit on the side of the unaffected ear. Do not turn or walk away, and do not do other tasks while talking to the client.
- ***Speak in a normal tone.*** Speak slowly and clearly. Do not shout. Do not cover your mouth when talking. Do NOT exaggerate your words.
- ***Check communication aids.*** Make sure the client is wearing any needed hearing aids, eyeglasses, or contact lenses. The client needs to see your face for speech reading. Help the client to put on aids if necessary.
- ***Adjust your language.*** State the topic of conversation clearly. Use simple words and short sentences. Focus on key words. Learn what works for the client. Try saying things in a different way if the client does not understand you.
- ***Use other communication methods.*** You may be unable to communicate using speech. Use nonverbal communication, including body language, to communicate messages (see Chapter 5), or write the key words on paper.
- ***Watch for signs of fatigue.*** Drooping shoulders and a decline in understanding are examples. Avoid tiring the client. If you are able to use sign language, it is recommended that you sign for only 30 minutes at a time to avoid tiring the client.
- ***Observe for and report environmental hazards.*** Devices that rely on sound notification (such as telephones, alarm clocks, doorbells, stove timers, or kettle whistles) may be now unsuitable for the client. Report this development to your supervisor and document your observations.

Supporting Mrs. Lopez: The Isolating Effects of Hearing Loss

Mrs. Lopez has experienced gradual but significant hearing loss and now avoids social situations because she feels left out of conversations. She is afraid of embarrassing herself by giving the wrong response, and straining to hear a conversation makes her tired. She no longer listens to the radio or watches TV. She has stopped going to church because she cannot hear the sermon. She is alone so much that she feels isolated and bored. As a support worker, how can you help her to adjust to her ongoing condition and decrease her boredom or isolation?

- **Age-related macular degeneration (AMD; ARMD)**—the breakdown (*degeneration*) of the macula, the central part of the retina. The retina is the inner layer of the eye that senses light and colour. The macula is a small spot in the retina where vision is keenest and where the highest concentration of cones for colour vision are. AMD is associated with aging and is the most common cause of vision impairment in people over 50. In fact, for adults over the age of 55, AMD is the leading cause of blindness in North America.[3] The condition starts with gradual or sudden partial loss of vision but is not painful. The central vision becomes fuzzy or shadowy, and over time, vision gets worse (see **FIGURE 40–3, *B***). AMD varies in severity—some people completely lose their sight; others may have some sight; and some may lose central vision but still have some *peripheral* vision (the sides, top, and bottom areas of vision). There is no cure for AMD. Macular degeneration can

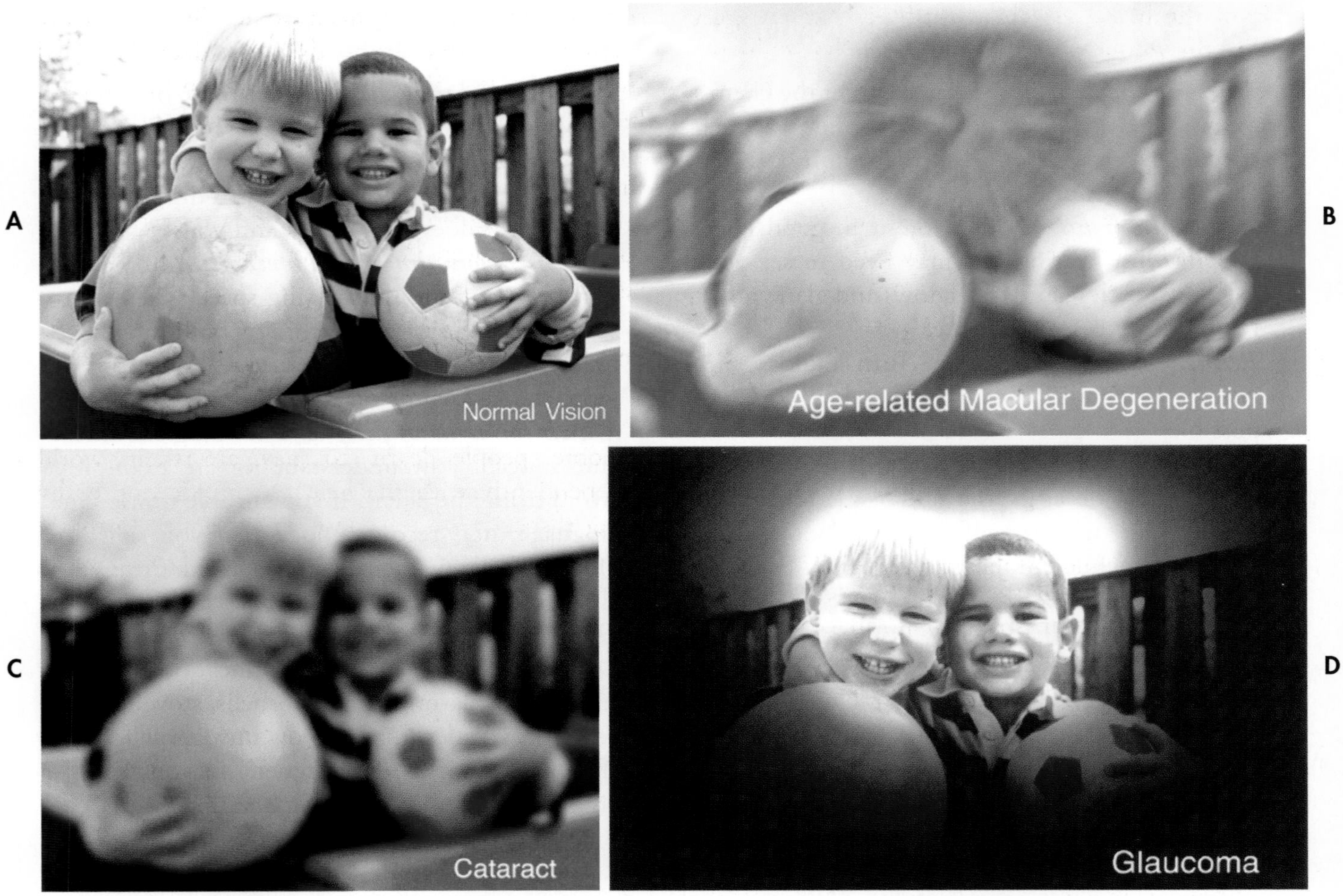

FIGURE 40–3 This is what a scene looks like to someone with **A,** normal vision. **B,** age-related macular degeneration. **C,** cataract. **D,** glaucoma. (**Source:** National Eye Institute, National Institute of Health.)

also affect younger adults and children. There are two types of AMD:

- *Wet AMD:* Blood vessels behind the retina start to grow under the macula. These blood vessels leak blood and fluid. Loss of central vision occurs quickly. An early symptom is straight lines appearing wavy. Wet AMD is considered advanced and more severe than dry AMD.
- *Dry AMD:* Light-sensitive cells in the macula slowly break down. Central vision in the affected eye gradually becomes blurry. As dry AMD gets worse, a blurred spot is seen in the centre of the eye. Central vision is gradually lost. Usually, both eyes are affected. Dry AMD is more common than wet AMD.

- **Retinal detachment**—the separation of the retina from its supporting tissue. The *vitreous* (the gel-like contents of the eyeball) thickens as the person ages. Shrinkage or contraction of the vitreous can tug on the retina, leading to a retinal tear. The retina cannot function when detached, and permanent vision loss in the affected eye can result. The causes of retinal detachment include eye injury, a head injury, a fall, eye disease, a condition such as diabetes, excessive nearsightedness, or a congenital thinning in the retina.[4] Symptoms may include flashing lights in the corner of the affected eye or the presence of "floaters." Vision may be saved by surgically reattaching the retina. It is important for the client to be assessed as soon as possible by an eye doctor.
- **Diabetic retinopathy**—a disorder (*pathy*) caused primarily by type 1 diabetes, in which the blood vessels in the retinas are damaged. Blood can leak

from the blood vessels. New blood vessels grow over the retina, creating scar tissue that pulls the retina away from the back of the eye. Retinal detachment and vision impairment may result. Routine visual exams are urged for all people with diabetes.

- **Cataract**—the clouding of the eye's lens, which prevents light from entering the eye (**FIGURE 40–3, *C***). The term *cataract* comes from the Greek word that means "waterfall." Cataracts are most common in older adults, although younger people are being diagnosed every day. A person with a cataract experiences gradual blurring, dimming of vision, and sensitivity to light and glares. Vision is eventually lost. A cataract can occur in one or both eyes. Surgery is the only treatment. A tiny incision is made into the eye, the cloudy lens is removed, and a plastic lens is implanted into the eye. Following surgery, vision returns to near-normal.
- **Glaucoma**—an eye disease that causes pressure within the eye, damaging the optic nerve. Blindness eventually results unless treated. Glaucoma is usually an age-related disease that may be gradual or sudden in onset. Signs and symptoms include *tunnel vision* (the field of vision being reduced until the person can see only straight ahead), blurred vision, and multicoloured halos around lights (**FIGURE 40–3, *D***). Treatment involves medications and possibly surgery, with the goal of preventing further damage to the optic nerve. Damage that has already occurred, however, cannot be reversed.
- **Presbyopia**—the gradual inability to focus (*opia*) on close objects. This condition is associated with aging (*presby*), with most people experiencing this normal decline in vision usually after age 40. Corrective and contact lenses, as well as good lighting, can be helpful.

Effects of Vision Impairment

Severe vision loss affects a client's physical, emotional, social, intellectual, and spiritual health. For example, Mr. Barak, 78, has AMD. He feels the loss of his independence and self-esteem, as even simple tasks such as dressing take much longer, and he is not able to read the newspaper. He does not go out alone because he is afraid of falling or getting lost, so he no longer attends his mosque. There are many resources available from the Canadian National Institute for the Blind (CNIB) that can help him—for example, talking books, many different types of aids to help with ADLs, technology advances, support for clients and families, devices for entertainment, and medical devices. Computers and computer software are also available for clients with vision loss.

Although the process is long and hard, many people with severe vision loss learn to lead independent lives. They learn to move about, perform ADLs, and read using a different method.

Some people learn to navigate their world independently with the help of a guide dog or by using a special white cane with a red tip. Both are recognized worldwide as signs that the person using them has vision loss. The guide dog serves as the eyes of the person with vision loss, recognizing danger and guiding the person through traffic. Clients are trained by a professional on the use of a white cane, and clients for whom a guide dog is appropriate will attend special training sessions.

Vision Aids and Corrective Measures

Eyeglasses

Eyeglasses correct vision impairment and are worn for reading or seeing objects at a distance or both. Some people wear them all the time while awake. Some people feel upset when they first realize they need glasses, but adjustment is usually rapid. Most accept the fact that glasses will be needed as they grow older.

Glasses are costly, so protect the client's glasses from damage. When not worn, they should be kept in their case. Glasses should be labelled with your client's name. Lenses are made of hardened glass or plastic to avoid breakage. Remove eyeglasses carefully.

Glass lenses are washed with warm water and dried with soft tissue. Plastic lenses are easily scratched, so special cleaning solutions, tissues, and cloths are used to clean and dry them.

Remove eyeglasses by holding the part of the frames sitting on both ears. Lift the frames off the ears, and bring the glasses down and away from the client's face.

Contact Lenses

Contact lenses (contacts)—hard or soft—fit directly on the eye. Many people prefer contacts because they cannot be seen, do not break easily, and can be worn even while playing sports. The disadvantage is that contacts can be easily lost. Depending on the type of lens, contacts can be worn continuously for 12 to 24 hours or even for 1 week. Contacts are usually removed for swimming and sleeping.

Remove and clean clients' contact lenses according to the manufacturer's instructions and your employer policy. Report any eye redness or drainage to your supervisor. Also, report complaints of eye pain or blurred vision. Ensure that you use gloves to decrease the risk of pathogen spread.

Laser Surgery for Vision Correction

Laser surgery is used to correct a number of different vision problems. Not all people are suited for laser vision correction, and suitability must be determined by the eye surgeon who specializes in this procedure.

Intra-Ocular Lens Implants

Cataract surgery, as mentioned, involves replacing the eye's natural lens with an artificial lens. The intra-ocular lens implant used in this surgery is a clear hard plastic, soft plastic, or silicone disc about the size of a small button that is usually implanted behind the iris. Because soft lenses can be inserted through a small incision, recovery time after the surgery is shortened. The artificial lens restores the focusing ability that the cataract took away from the client.[5]

After cataract surgery, clients are instructed to administer a special eye drop regimen and to wear special sunglasses that are more effective at blocking the sun's rays than regular sunglasses are. Some clients experience dry eyes temporarily, although this issue can be easily treated with drops. The importance of follow-up care and appointments must be stressed to the client.

Aids for Reading

Many people with vision impairment learn to read **Braille**—a writing system that uses raised dots in a certain pattern to represent each letter of the alphabet. The first 10 letters also represent numbers 0 to 9 (**FIGURE 40–4**). The person uses the fingers to feel the pattern of dots and determine the letter. Numerous books, magazines, newspapers, and computer keyboards are available in Braille. Braille is hard to learn, especially for older adults, so some people with vision loss never learn to read Braille.

Other reading aids include books with large print, audiobooks, and magnifiers (some with reading lamps attached to them).

Communication Aids

Examples of communication aids are calendars in Braille, large-print clocks that voice the time in hours or minutes, telephones with Braille keypads and extra-large numerals, and cheque- and envelope-writing guides. Computer software is continually being developed to assist people with visual impairment.

Devices for Entertainment

Examples of devices for entertainment are televisions with descriptive captions for movies and shows (usually available through the network provider), as well as playing cards and bingo cards with large numbers or in Braille.

Medical Devices

Examples of medical devices for people with visual impairment include pillboxes with the days or times written in Braille that let the person feel if the pill has been taken and "talking prescription devices" that provide voice messages describing how to take the medication.

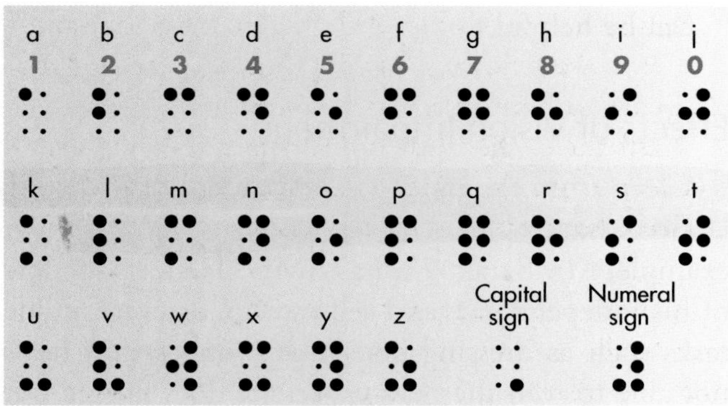

FIGURE 40–4 Braille.

Artificial Eyes

Surgical removal of an eye is sometimes necessary because of injury or disease. The person is then fitted with an *ocular prosthesis*, an artificial eye made of glass or plastic that matches the other eye in colour and shape. Prostheses may be permanent implants or removable. If the prosthesis is removable, the person is taught to remove, clean, and re-insert it and also to perform routine prosthesis care (**FIGURE 40–5**).

As a support worker, you may care for clients with artificial eyes, which are the client's property. As you would protect hearing aids, eyeglasses, and other valuable devices, protect the artificial eye from loss and damage. Provide care for the artificial eye in a safe place. For example, do not hold it over a sink because it can easily roll down the drain if dropped. You may assist your client in caring for the artificial eye and the eye socket where it is placed. Follow these measures when the artificial eye is removed and will not be re-inserted immediately:

- Wash the artificial eye with mild soap and warm water. Rinse it well.
- Line a container with a soft cloth or 4 × 4 gauze square to prevent damage.
- Fill the container with water or a saline (salt) solution.
- Place the artificial eye in the container. Close the container.
- Label the container with the client's name (if in a facility, include the room number).
- Place the container in the drawer in the bedside stand or in another safe place, as directed by the client.
- Wash the eye socket with warm water or saline. Use a washcloth or gauze square. Use a gauze square to remove excess moisture.
- Wash the eyelid with mild soap and warm water. Clean from the inner to the outer part of the eye (see Chapter 30). Dry the eyelid.

A client with an artificial eye has vision loss on the side of the artificial eye, but vision in the other eye may be normal or only slightly or moderately impaired.

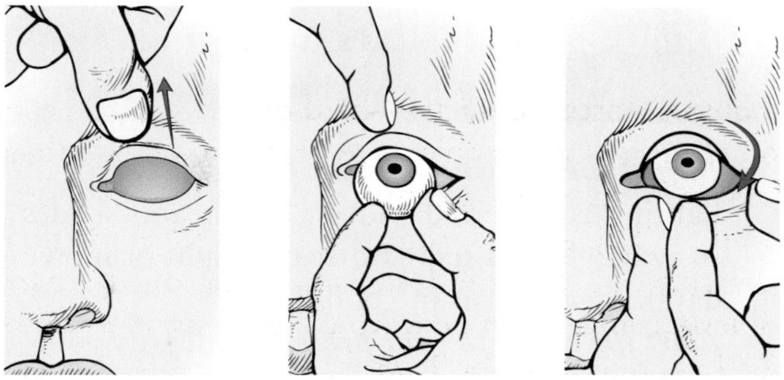

FIGURE 40–5 Inserting an artificial eye. (**Source:** Lewis, S.M., Heitkemper, M.M., & Dirksen, S.R. (2000). *Medical–surgical nursing: Assessment and management of clinical problems* (5th ed., p. 467). St. Louis, MO: Mosby.)

Caring for Clients With Vision Loss

People with vision loss often have highly developed senses of hearing, touch, smell, and taste. They are sensitive to the tone of a person's voice. When talking with clients with vision loss, pay attention to your voice, which needs to convey nonverbal cues you usually give with body language. Your voice should communicate warmth and respect. **BOX 40–3** contains guidelines for caring for clients with vision loss.

Think About Safety

Providing a Safe Setting for Clients With Vision Loss

- Outdoor walks and stairs must be clear of ice and snow. Tell your supervisor if they are not.
- Hallways and rooms must be free of clutter.
- If escorting a client who is blind, walk slightly ahead and allow him to rest his arm on you. Let the client hold you rather than holding the client (see **FIGURE 40–6**).
- Keep doors open or closed, never partially open, to avoid the client walking into the door.
- Remember that furniture and other items are arranged to suit the client's needs. Always replace items where you found them. Avoid rearranging furniture and other items.
- Orient the client to a new setting. Describe the layout, and identify the location and purpose of furniture or equipment. Let the client move about and touch and locate furniture if he can.
- In facilities, keep the call bell within the client's reach.

BOX 40–3 Guidelines for Caring for Clients With Vision Loss

- ***Adjust the lighting.*** Ask the client what type of lighting is preferred. Adjust blinds and shades to avoid glare (usually worse on bright or snowy days). Stand or sit in good light.
- ***Alert the client to your presence.*** Identify yourself when you enter the room. Give your name, title, and your reason for being there. Do not touch the client before indicating your presence. Address the client by name. Tell the client when you are leaving the room.
- ***Assist with walking.*** Walk slightly ahead of the client at a normal pace (FIGURE 40–6). Offer your right or left arm. Tell the client which arm you are offering, and the client can then take that arm. Never push, pull, or guide the client in front of you. Tell the client when approaching a curb or steps. Say if you will step up or down. Inform the client of doors, turns, furniture, and other obstructions. Give specific directions. For example, say "right behind you," "on your left," or "in front of you." Avoid phrases such as "over here" or "over there."
- ***Assist with eating.*** Read menus to the client. Avoid using table linens and china with patterns and designs. These items should be solid colours and provide contrast. For example, a white plate should be placed on a dark placemat. Explain the location of food and beverages on the tray. Use the face of a clock to describe their location (see Chapter 28), or guide the client's hand to each item on the tray. Cut meat into small bits, open containers, butter the bread, and perform other activities, as needed.

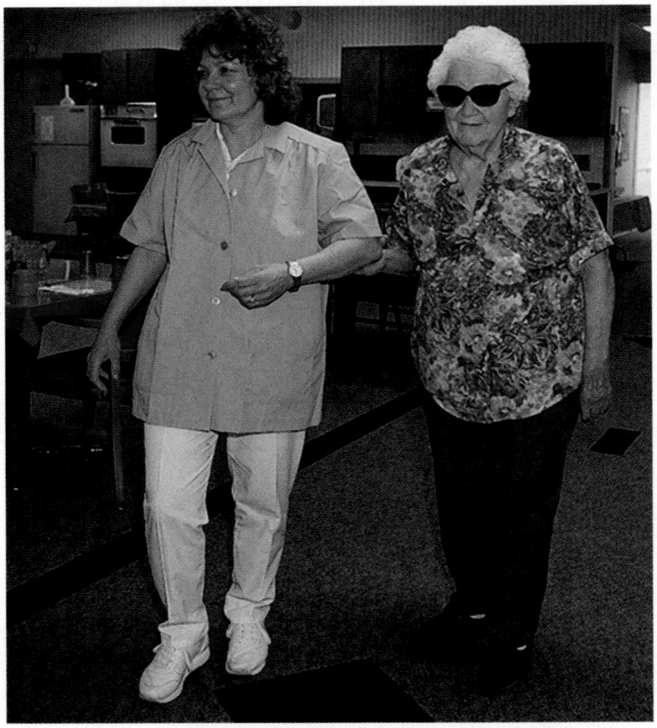

FIGURE 40–6 This client, who has vision loss, walks slightly behind the support worker, keeping her arm resting lightly on the support worker.

CHAPTER REVIEW

KEY POINTS

- Common causes of hearing impairment include otitis media, otosclerosis, Ménière's disease, dominant progressive hearing loss, presbycusis, and temporary hearing loss.
- The effects of hearing loss will vary from client to client. Some clients will blame others for not speaking clearly or loud enough for them to hear. Others may withdraw from embarrassment because they are not able to hear conversations.
- There are a number of aids to help people with a hearing impairment, including hearing aids, special telephone systems, signalling devices, text messaging, hearing dogs, and closed captioning on TVs.
- Guidelines to providing care to a client with hearing loss are as follows: (1) Alert the client to your presence; (2) adjust the lighting; (3) reduce background noise; (4) focus your attention on your client; (5) speak in a normal tone; (6) check communication aids; (7) adjust your language; (8) use other communication methods; and (9) watch for signs of fatigue in the client.
- Vision impairment can range from mild to complete blindness. Common causes are (1) age-related macular degeneration, (2) retinal detachment, (3) diabetic retinopathy, (4) glaucoma, (5) cataract, and (6) presbyopia.
- The effects of vision loss depend on the age of your client and when the symptoms start.
- The aids available for your client with vision loss include (1) eyeglasses, (2) Braille books, (3) books with large print, (4) audiobooks, (5) magnifiers, and (6) large-print clocks, and more aids are in development.
- When caring for clients with vision loss, (1) adjust the lighting; (2) alert the client to your presence; (3) assist with walking when required; and (4) assist with eating if required.

CRITICAL THINKING IN PRACTICE

Mr. Tyler is waiting in the dining room for lunch to be served. He asks for help deciding on which foods he would like that meal. Mr. Tyler is hard of hearing. You repeat the meal options several times. He struggles to hear you. What will you do? What can be done to promote better hearing and understanding of your message?

REVIEW QUESTIONS

Answers to these questions are at the bottom of the next page.

Circle the BEST answer.

1. Which effect of hearing problems is often not obvious to others?
   A. Loneliness and social isolation
   B. Speaking too loudly
   C. Asking to repeat things
   D. Answering questions inappropriately

2. Mr. Poulin has Ménière's disease. Which of the following is likely true?
   A. He has a middle ear infection.
   B. Vertigo is a major symptom.
   C. Hearing aids will correct the problem.
   D. He has vision problems because of it.

3. You are talking to Mr. Poulin. You should do the following:
   A. Speak clearly, distinctly, and slowly.
   B. Sit out of direct light.
   C. Shout.
   D. Sit on the side of his affected ear.

4. Mr. Poulin's hearing aid is not working. First, you should:
   A. See if it is turned on
   B. Wash the hearing aid with soap and water
   C. Have it repaired
   D. Change the batteries

5. Which is true of age-related macular degeneration?
- **A.** Surgery usually corrects the problem.
- **B.** There is no cure.
- **C.** Eyeglasses will improve vision.
- **D.** It is most common in young adults.

6. Glaucoma is:
- **A.** An ear disorder common among children
- **B.** Sign language for people with hearing loss
- **C.** A disease that damages the optic nerve
- **D.** A symptom of cataracts

7. When not worn, glasses should be:
- **A.** Left on the bed or chair within easy reach
- **B.** Left out of the case on the bedside table
- **C.** Kept in a cleaning solution
- **D.** Kept in their case

8. Braille involves:
- **A.** A white cane with a red tip for walking
- **B.** Raised dots arranged to represent letters of the alphabet
- **C.** An artificial eye
- **D.** Books on CD, audiotape, or MP3

9. Mrs. Ho has vision loss. You should do the following:
- **A.** Offer her your arm and walk slightly behind her
- **B.** Speak loudly to her
- **C.** Announce your presence when entering her room and let her know when you leave the room
- **D.** Leave the room quickly

10. Which of the following is unsafe for Mrs. Ho?
- **A.** Keeping doors open or closed
- **B.** Informing her of steps and curbs
- **C.** Turning lights on
- **D.** Rearranging furniture

Answers: 1.A, 2.B, 3.A, 4.A, 5.B, 6.C, 7.D, 8.B, 9.C, 10.D

Chapter opener image: Cylonphoto/Shutterstock.com

CHAPTER 41

Oxygen Needs

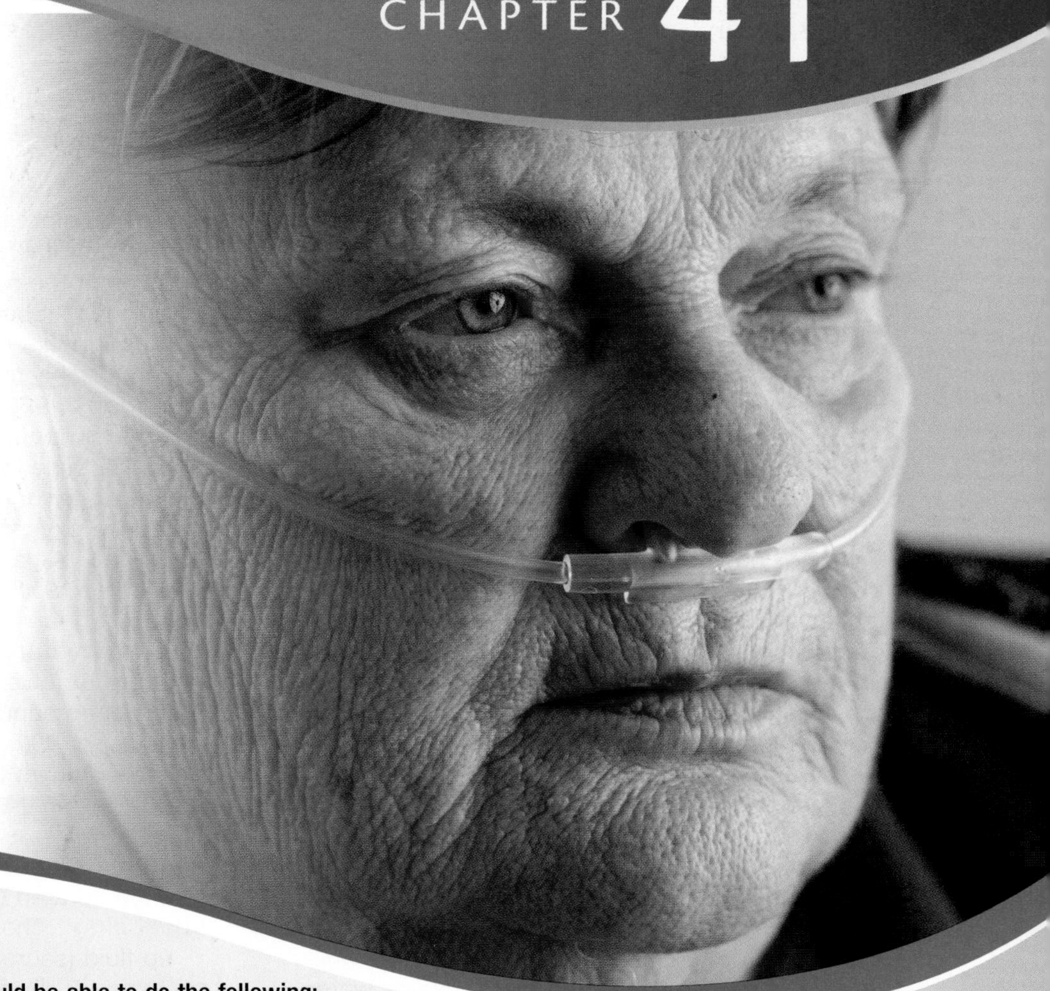

OBJECTIVES

After reading this chapter, the learner should be able to do the following:

- Describe factors that affect oxygen needs.
- Identify the signs and symptoms of hypoxia and altered respiratory function.
- Describe tests used to diagnose respiratory problems.
- Explain measures that promote oxygenation.
- Describe devices used to administer oxygen.
- Explain how to safely assist a client with oxygen therapy.
- Describe the safety measures for suctioning.
- Explain how to assist in the care of clients with artificial airways, on mechanical ventilation, and with chest tubes.
- Apply the procedures described in this chapter to clinical practice properly.

KEY TERMS

apnea The lack or absence (*a*) of breathing (*pnea*). *p. 932*
bradypnea Slow (*brady*) breathing (*pnea*); respirations are fewer than 12 per minute. *p. 932*
chest tube A hollow plastic tube surgically inserted into the chest cavity, which allows for the removal of trapped air (*pneumothorax*) and the drainage of blood or fluid (*hemothorax* or *pleural effusion*). *p. 956*
Cheyne–Stokes Respirations that gradually increase in rate and depth and then become shallow and slow; breathing may stop (*apnea*) for 10 to 20 seconds. *p. 932*
cyanosis An abnormal condition, evidenced by bluish colour in the skin, lips, mucous membranes, and nail beds caused by a lack of oxygenated blood in the visible tissues. *p. 933*
distilled water Sterile and pure water that has been boiled and allowed to cool and condense. *p. 943*
eupnea Normal breathing. *p. 931*
face mask A mask used to deliver oxygen that covers the client's nose and mouth. *p. 941*
flowmeter A device that regulates the flow of oxygen to the nasal cannula or face mask. *p. 940*
flow rate The volume of a substance, such as oxygen or fluids, administered over a prescribed period. *p. 942*
hemoptysis Bloody (*hemo*) sputum (*ptysis*, meaning "to spit"). *p. 931*
humidified oxygen Oxygen that contains water vapour. *p. 943*
hyperventilation Respirations that are more rapid (*hyper*) and deeper than normal. *p. 932*
hypoventilation Respirations that are slow (*hypo*), shallow, and sometimes irregular. *p. 932*
hypoxia A deficiency (*hypo*) of oxygen in the cells (*oxia*). *p. 932*
intubation The process of inserting an artificial airway. *p. 949*
Kussmaul respiration Deep, rapid respiration characteristic of diabetic acidosis or other conditions causing acidosis. *p. 932*
mechanical ventilation The use of a **ventilator** to move air into and out of the lungs. *p. 954*
nasal cannula A flexible tube inserted into the nares of the nose to deliver oxygen *p. 940*
orthopnea Shortness of breath (*dyspnea*) when lying in a flat or supine position; ability to breathe comfortably (*pnea*) only when sitting or standing (*ortho*). *p. 929*
orthopneic position Sitting up (*ortho*) and leaning over a table to breathe. *p. 933*
oxygen-conserving devices Devices that help reduce oxygen wastage. *p. 939*
pollutant A harmful chemical or substance in air or water. *p. 931*
respiratory arrest Stoppage of breathing. *p. 930*
respiratory depression Slow, weak respirations at a rate of fewer than 12 per minute; respirations are not deep enough to bring enough air into the lungs. *p. 930*
SOB Acronym for "short of breath." *p. 929*
SOBOE Acronym for "short of breath on exertion." *p. 929*
sputum Mucus from the respiratory system that is expectorated (expelled) through the mouth. *p. 946*
suctioning The process of withdrawing or sucking up fluid (secretions). *p. 952*
tachypnea Rapid (*tachy*) breathing (*pnea*); respirations are 24 or more per minute. *p. 932*
tracheostomy A surgically created opening (*ostomy*) through the neck into the trachea (*tracheo*). *p. 950*
ventilator A machine used to provide airflow into and out of the lungs. *p. 954*

Suctioning is a delegated task
Trach is a delegated task

Oxygen (O_2) is a gas that is part of the air we breathe. It has no taste, odour, or colour. Oxygen is the most important basic need for life, and without it, death will occur within minutes. Breathing is something that we take for granted until we experience difficulty breathing. People who have certain illnesses or are in stressful situations might experience difficulty breathing, which can affect the amount of oxygen in their blood cells.

As a support worker, you will often work with clients who have difficulty breathing or absorbing enough oxygen into their bodies. To survive, these

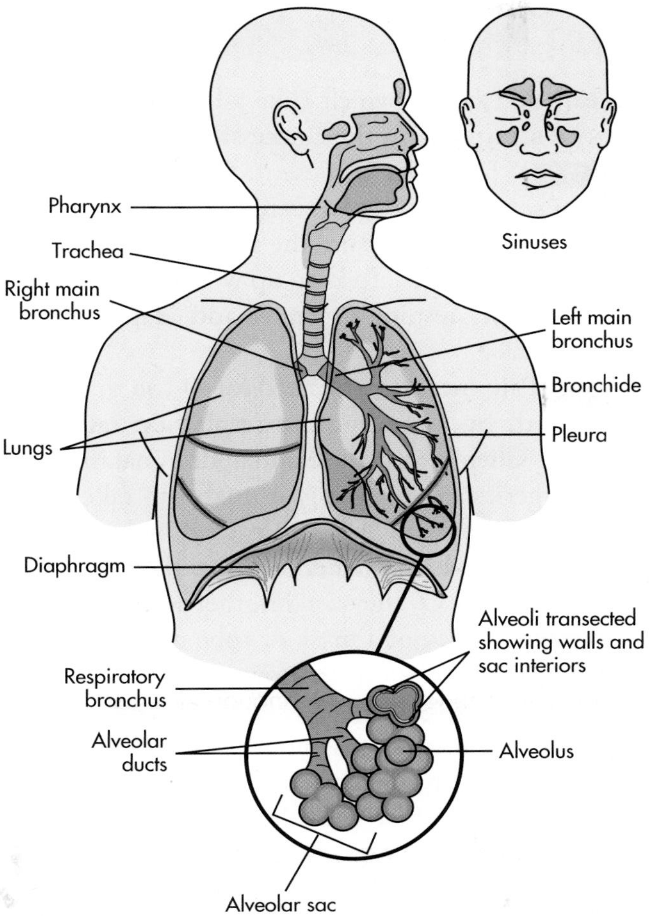

FIGURE 41–1 The respiratory system.

clients require oxygen, which is supplied to them through a nasal tube or mask. It is your responsibility to know how to provide safe and effective care to clients (**FIGURE 41–1**). See Chapter 17 for a description of the respiratory system.

Oxygen therapy is handled in the same way as any medication. The physician prescribes the amount of oxygen, the device to use, and the times for therapy. Some clients may need oxygen constantly, whereas others may need it for relief of symptoms such as chest pain (in those with heart disease) or shortness of breath (in clients with respiratory diseases who may have enough oxygen while at rest but become short of breath with mild activity).

As with any task, before giving or assisting with any care described in this chapter, you should make sure of the following:

- Your province or territory allows you to perform the task.
- The task is in your job description at your facility or agency.
- You have the necessary training.
- You know how to use the equipment.
- You have reviewed the task with a nurse.
- A nurse or respiratory technician will supervise you.

FACTORS AFFECTING OXYGEN NEEDS

For cells to get enough oxygen, the respiratory and cardiovascular systems must function properly. Any disease, injury, or surgery involving these systems can affect the body's ability to absorb oxygen from the air and deliver it to the cells. Body systems depend on each other, so altered function of any system (e.g., nervous, musculo-skeletal, urinary system) can affect oxygen absorption and delivery. Major factors affecting oxygen absorption and delivery are discussed in **BOX 41–1**.

ALTERED RESPIRATORY FUNCTION

The function of the respiratory system involves three processes that must work together. Respiratory function is altered if even one of these processes is affected:

1. Air moves into and out of the lungs.
2. O_2 and CO_2 are exchanged at the alveoli.
3. The blood transports O_2 to the cells and removes CO_2 from them.

The client who is short of breath (**SOB**) or who is short of breath on exertion (**SOBOE**) has altered respiratory function; that is, something is preventing the person from breathing easily. Altered respiratory function may be an acute or chronic problem. When unable to breathe easily, a client may panic or feel anxious. The client becomes uncomfortable, is usually visibly struggling to breathe, and often wants to sit up in the bed or in a chair since it may be more difficult to breathe when lying flat (**orthopnea**) (**BOX 41–2** on page 931).

Struggling to breathe is both exhausting and dangerous for the client, as usually more energy is used (and therefore more oxygen) doing so. Report your observations to your supervisor promptly and accurately so that quick action may be taken to correct

BOX 41–1 Factors Affecting Oxygen Needs

- ***Respiratory system function.*** The airway must be open (*patent*), and there must be an adequate number of alveoli (single-celled air sacs in the lungs) to effectively absorb oxygen and excrete carbon dioxide (CO_2), which is a waste product.
- ***Cardiovascular system function.*** Oxygen is required by all cells to produce energy to carry out their proper functions, and blood must flow normally to and from the heart to all bodily cells. When blood vessels are narrowed by disease or other causes, blood flow will be affected. Capillaries and cells must exchange O_2 and CO_2 efficiently.
- ***Red blood cell count.*** Blood must have enough red blood cells (RBCs), which are produced in bone marrow and contain hemoglobin. Hemoglobin contains iron, and it picks up oxygen in the lungs and carries it to the cells. Health challenges that reduce RBCs in the blood include chemotherapy, leukemia, iron-deficiency anemia, and blood loss.
- ***Nervous system function.*** Nervous system diseases and injuries can affect respiratory muscles, making breathing difficult or impossible. Brain injury as well as use of narcotics and depressant drugs can affect the respiratory rate, rhythm, and depth.
- ***Aging.*** Respiratory muscles weaken and lung tissue becomes less elastic with advancing age, making coughing more difficult. If the person cannot cough to remove secretions from the upper airway, pneumonia (infection of the lungs) can develop. For this reason, older adults are at risk for respiratory complications after surgery.
- ***Exercise.*** The body requires more O_2 when it is exercised, to supply energy needed by cells. The O_2 demand throughout the body is usually met by increasing the respiratory rate and depth (in the lungs).

  Clients with heart and respiratory disease may have enough O_2 while they are at rest, but with even a slight increase in activity, their bodies may not be able to bring in enough O_2 and deliver it to the cells for energy. This lack of O_2 stresses the heart and lungs, which (like all tissues) require oxygen to perform their necessary tasks.
- ***Fever.*** When fever is present, O_2 needs increase because the body is working hard to fight the infection that is causing the fever; the metabolic rate also increases. To keep up with the body's O_2 needs, the respiratory rate and depth must increase.
- ***Pain.*** Pain increases the need for O_2, so the body responds by increasing the respiration rate and depth. Clients with chest and abdominal injuries or surgeries are unwilling or unable to take deep breaths because of the pain caused by breathing in and out, which further increases their need for O_2. The extra O_2 they need is, therefore, supplied to them by way of a mask or tube until they can take deep breaths on their own.
- ***Drug (narcotic or barbiturate) overdose.*** Normally, when used as prescribed, the proper amount of a drug will control moderate to severe pain (narcotics) or provide sedation (barbiturates). When a narcotic, such as morphine or meperidine (Demerol), or a barbiturate is taken for "recreational" purposes; mixed with alcohol or other drugs that have not been prescribed; or taken beyond the safe dosage, the breathing centre in the hypothalamus of the brain is affected. The brain cannot tell the person to take deep breaths, so respirations are suppressed and become dangerously slowed or even stopped, possibly resulting in a loss of consciousness or death. Substance abusers are at risk for **respiratory depression** (breaths not deep enough to bring enough air into the lungs) and **respiratory arrest** (stoppage of breathing) from overdoses of these drugs.
- ***Smoking.*** Those who smoke inhale air that is mixed with harmful substances that can damage the lung tissue and have been proven to cause lung cancer and chronic obstructive pulmonary disease (COPD). Smoking is also a risk factor for coronary artery disease.
- ***Allergies.*** An *allergy* is a sensitivity to a substance—for example, pollen, dust, foods,

Continued

BOX 41–1 Factors Affecting Oxygen Needs—cont'd

drugs, or smoke—that causes the body to react with signs and symptoms such as a runny nose, wheezing, or congestion. As part of the allergic reaction, the upper airway mucous membranes may swell. With severe swelling, the airway can close, resulting in shock and death. More commonly, however, people with allergies are at risk for chronic bronchitis and asthma.

- ***Pollutant exposure.*** A **pollutant** is a harmful chemical or substance in air or water. Air pollutants—for example, dust, fumes, toxins, asbestos, coal dust, and sawdust—damage the lungs. Exposure to pollutants can occur at home, in the workplace, or in the community.
- ***Nutrition.*** Good nutrition that includes iron and vitamins (vitamin B_{12}, vitamin C, and folic acid) is necessary to produce RBCs, without which the body cannot transport O_2 to cells.
- ***Alcohol.*** Alcohol depresses the brain. Excessive amounts reduce the cough reflex and increase the risk for aspiration, which can cause obstructed airway and pneumonia.

BOX 41–2 Signs and Symptoms of Altered Respiratory Function

- Signs and symptoms of hypoxia (see BOX 41–3, on p. 933)
- Any abnormal breathing pattern
- Complaints of shortness of breath or being "winded" or "short-winded"
- Cough (note frequency and time of day)
  - Dry and hacking
  - Harsh and barking
  - Productive (produces sputum) or nonproductive
- Sputum (see p. 946)
  - Colour—clear, white, yellow, green, brown, or red
  - Odour—none or foul
  - Consistency—thick, watery, or frothy (with bubbles or foam)
  - **Hemoptysis**—bloody (*hemo*) sputum (*ptysis*, meaning "to spit"); note if the sputum is bright red, dark red, blood-tinged, or streaked with blood
- Noisy respirations
  - Wheezing
  - Wet-sounding respirations
  - Crowing sounds
- Chest pain
  - Location
  - Constant or intermittent (comes and goes)
  - Client's description (stabbing, knifelike, aching)
  - What makes it worse (movement, coughing, yawning, sneezing, sighing, deep breathing)
- Cyanosis
  - Skin
  - Mucous membranes
  - Lips
  - Nail beds
- Changes in vital signs
- Body position
  - Sitting upright
  - Leaning forward or hunched over a table

the problem and prevent it from getting worse. ***You should be aware, however, that if the client is uses an oxygen tank, you should never turn up the oxygen level if the client's care plan does not direct you to do so. In certain circumstances, turning up the oxygen could cause extreme harm to the client and can make the client even more short of breath!***

Abnormal Respiratory Patterns

The normal respiration rate for adults is 12 to 20 per minute. Infants and children have faster rates (see TABLE 15–3, on p. 240). Normal respirations are quiet, effortless, and regular, and both sides of the chest should rise and fall in a uniform manner. The medical term for normal respirations is **eupnea**.

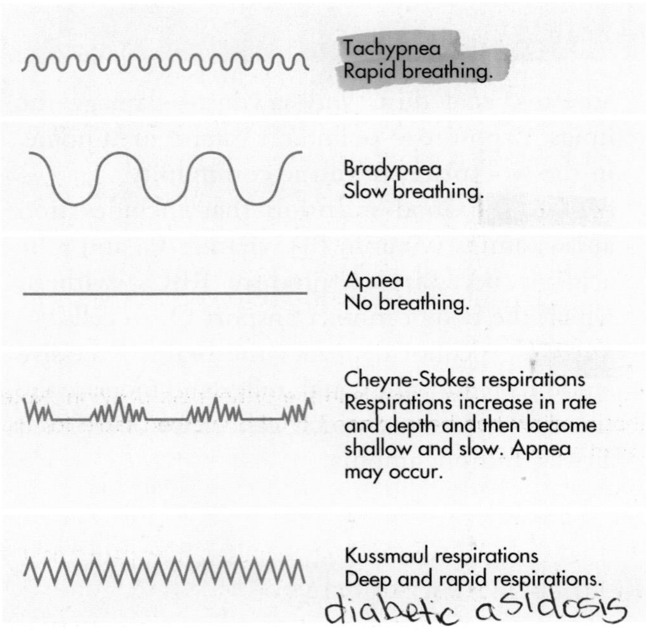

FIGURE 41–2 Some respiratory patterns. (Adapted from Phipps, W.J., Neighbors, M., Marek, J. et al. (2003). *Medical–surgical nursing: Health and illness perspectives* (7th ed.). St. Louis, MO: Mosby.)

The following respiratory patterns are abnormal (**FIGURE 41–2**):

- **Tachypnea**—rapid (*tachy*) breathing (*pnea*). Respirations are 24 or more per minute. Fever, exercise, pain, airway obstruction, and hypoxemia are common causes.
- **Bradypnea**—slow (*brady*) breathing (*pnea*). Respirations are fewer than 12 per minute. Drug overdoses and nervous system disorders are common causes.
- **Apnea**—the lack or absence (*a*) of breathing (*pnea*). It occurs in cardiac arrest and respiratory arrest. Sleep apnea and periodic apnea of newborns are other types of apnea.
- **Kussmaul respirations**—deep and rapid respirations characteristic of diabetic acidosis or other conditions causing acidosis.
- **Hypoventilation**—slow (*hypo*), shallow, and sometimes irregular respirations. Common causes include lung disorders (such as pneumonia) that affect the alveoli. Other causes include obesity, airway obstruction, side effects of drugs, and nervous system and musculo-skeletal disorders affecting the respiratory muscles.
- **Hyperventilation**—rapid (*hyper*) and deeper-than-normal respirations. Its many causes include asthma, emphysema, infection, fever, nervous system disorders, hypoxia, anxiety, pain, and some drugs.
- ***Dyspnea***—difficult, laboured, or painful (*dys*) breathing (*pnea*). Heart disease, exercise, and anxiety are common causes.
- **Cheyne–Stokes**—respirations that gradually increase in rate and depth and then become shallow and slow. Breathing may stop (*apnea*) for 10 to 20 seconds. Drug overdose, heart failure, renal failure, and brain disorders are common causes. Cheyne–Stokes respirations are common when death is near.
- ***Orthopnea***—shortness of breath (*dyspnea*) when lying in a flat or supine position and ability to breathe comfortably (*pnea*) only when sitting or standing (*ortho*). Common causes include emphysema, asthma, pneumonia, angina pectoris, and other heart and respiratory disorders.

Hypoxia

Hypoxia—a deficiency (*hypo*) of oxygen in the cells (*oxia*)—is one of the results of abnormal respiratory functioning, and it is caused by any illness, disease, injury, or surgery that affects respiratory function. Hypoxia is a life-threatening condition because without enough oxygen to function, cells will be damaged or die.

The brain is very sensitive to an inadequate supply of oxygen. Restlessness, dizziness, and disorientation are early signs of hypoxia. It is important that you report signs and symptoms of hypoxia (**BOX 41–3**) immediately. The sooner hypoxia is diagnosed, the sooner oxygen can be given and the cause of the hypoxia treated.

PROMOTING OXYGENATION

For the body to get enough oxygen, air must move deeply into the lungs and reach the alveoli, where O_2 and CO_2 are exchanged. Disease and injury can prevent air from reaching the alveoli. Pain, immobility, and narcotics interfere with deep breathing and with coughing up secretions. These factors allow the secretions to collect in the airway and lungs, interfering with air movement and lung function. Secretions

BOX 41–3 Signs and Symptoms of Hypoxia

- Restlessness
- Dizziness
- Disorientation
- Confusion
- Behaviour and personality changes
- Difficulty concentrating and difficulty following directions
- Apprehension
- Anxiety
- Fatigue
- Agitation
- Increased pulse rate
- Increased rate and depth of respirations
- Sitting position, often leaning forward
- **Cyanosis** (an abnormal condition evidenced in light-skinned clients by bluish colour in the skin, mucous membranes [lips, gums, and around the eyes], and nail beds; in darker-skinned clients, cyanosis may be easiest to see in the mucous membranes and nail beds)
- Dyspnea

also provide an environment for microbes to grow and multiply, with the possibility of leading to a life-threatening infection.

To completely meet the client's oxygen needs, the care plan will list measures to promote oxygenation. Some of the measures require the administration of O_2 or other activities that simply involve movement—for example, a short walk—to expand the client's lungs. Some other measures that are commonly listed in care plans are discussed below.

Positioning and Rest Periods

For clients confined to bed, breathing is usually easier in the semi-Fowler's or Fowler's position. Clients who experience orthopnea (shortness of breath when lying in a flat or supine position) often prefer to sit up and lean over a table (called the **orthopneic position**). You can increase the client's comfort by placing a pillow on the overbed table (**FIGURE 41–3**). Make sure that the client has sufficient rest periods

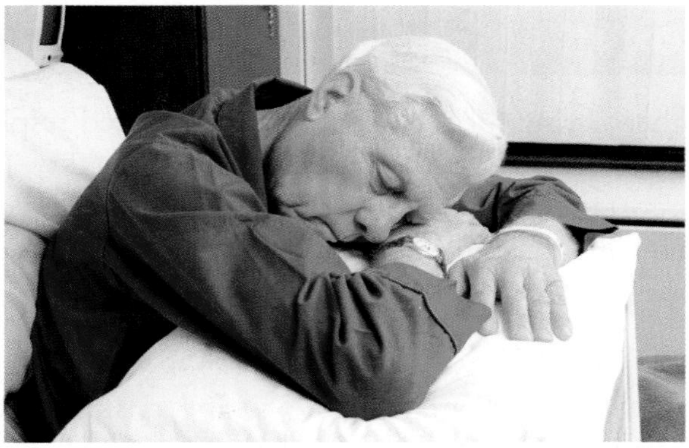

FIGURE 41–3 The client is in the orthopneic position. Note that a pillow has been placed on the overbed table for the client's comfort.

between activities so that she can breathe more easily without struggling for oxygen (**BOX 41–4**).

When a client is confined to bed for long periods, it is important that the person changes positions frequently, at least every 2 hours. If not, the lung cannot expand on one side, and secretions could pool (collect) at the bottom of the lung. Unless the physician has placed restrictions on positioning, the client should never lie on one side for a long time. You should always follow your client's care plan.

Coughing and Deep Breathing

Coughing removes mucus from the lungs, and deep breathing moves air into most parts of the lungs. Therefore, coughing and deep-breathing exercises help clients with respiratory disorders. These exercises are done after surgery and during bed rest; however, clients may be reluctant to do them as they may cause pain after injury or surgery, or the client may be afraid of opening an incision during coughing.

Coughing and deep breathing help prevent pneumonia and *atelectasis*. The walls of healthy lungs (lined in a sticky mucous membrane) expand with every deep breath and are thereby prevented from collapsing and sticking to each other. In atelectasis, a portion of the lung collapses after mucus collects in a section of the airway, preventing air from entering that part of the lung. Clients who do not perform deep-breathing and coughing exercises risk developing atelectasis because mucus is then allowed to collect in their lungs, increasing the chance of the sticky, mucus-lined lungs' not expanding. The mucus that collects in

BOX 41–4 Caring for a Client Who Has Altered Respiratory Function

When caring for the client who has altered respiratory function, whether at home or in a facility, it is important to provide care, such as the following, that will relax the client and reduce the client's need for more oxygen:

Positioning

- Assist the client into the sitting position—the semi-Fowler's or high Fowler's position whenever possible—as it makes breathing easier. Clients who are sitting up can expand their lungs much more easily than those who are lying down. Place several pillows behind the client's back or use a large foam wedge if the client has one.
- Use a reclining chair for the client's naps or sleeping. A reclining chair can allow the client to sleep in a partially upright position, which gives the lungs more room to breathe.
- If the client is in a hospital bed, mechanically elevate the head of the bed to reduce the client's need to move in bed without help.

Time Management

- Provide care at a time when the client is as well rested and comfortable as possible.
- Allow for frequent rest periods.
- Be organized. Arrange to do all of your care in the shortest, least strenuous way possible.

Client Care

- Assist the client with moving and turning to reduce oxygen need as much as possible.
- Never wear powders or apply powders on the client, as they can irritate the airway and cause the client to have difficulty breathing.
- Make sure the client is as comfortable as possible. Discomfort can cause a client to become anxious, and anxiety will increase the need for oxygen. Smooth out the sheets on the bed, and turn the pillow over to the smoother, cooler side. Make sure that the client does not have any restrictive clothing on.
- Encourage relaxation. Feelings of tension can contribute to breathlessness, and muscle tension can make the act of breathing harder. You can help reduce the client's tension level by promoting pleasant activities as well as relaxation exercises.
- Make sure that the bedside and the surrounding area are clean and dust-free. Wipe down all surfaces with a damp cloth (do not use disinfectants around the client as they can trigger an allergic reaction). Remove any clutter from the room as clutter can trap dust.
- If you must make the client's bed, make sure that the sheets are never shaken in the air (see Chapter 34).
- Open a window or use a fan to get air moving in the room; air movement will help the client to feel less short of breath.
- Make sure the client is well hydrated. Most clients who are short of breath tend to breathe through the mouth, which can dry the lips, oral mucous membranes, and the throat. Apply water-soluble jelly to the lips ***(never use oil or grease, as these substances are combustible and may create a risk for fire)***. Have the client drink fresh water frequently, at least once every hour. Avoid the use of straws, as drinking from a straw increases the breathing effort and requires more energy.
- In the winter, use a humidifier or place pans of water near radiators to moisten the room air that is breathed in. A humidifier can help loosen up thick phlegm (mucus) in the lungs so that it is coughed up easily, and it will also keep the throat and nasal passages from becoming too dry. Wash the humidifier or pans daily to prevent bacteria from colonizing in this warm, moist setting.
- If it is allowed on the client's care plan, offer throat lozenges or hard candy to help moisten a dry throat. Sucking on lozenges or candy increases

Continued

BOX 41–4 Caring for a Client Who Has Altered Respiratory Function—cont'd

the production of saliva, which moistens the throat as the lozenge or candy is swallowed.

Other Professional Responsibilities

- Avoid wearing perfumes that can trigger an allergic reaction, which would only make breathing more difficult for the client.
- Be friendly and professional at all times, but try not to engage the client too much in conversation. Ask the client questions that require short or one-word answers only.

Oxygen Therapy

- Oxygen supports combustion, so you must keep combustible items (e.g., clothing, towels, and sheets that are static-charged) away from the oxygen source to reduce the risk for a fire.

the lungs and the mucus on the walls are attracted to each other, causing that portion of the lung to collapse. The postsurgical period, bed rest, lung disease, and paralysis are risk factors for atelectasis.

The frequency of coughing and deep breathing varies among clients. For example, physicians may order the exercises every 1 to 2 hours or four times a day while the client is awake. Your supervisor and the care plan will tell you which clients are suitable candidates for the exercises and when the exercises should be done. You will also be told the required number of deep breaths and coughs for the client. Follow the care plan.

Report and record the following observations after assisting the client with coughing and deep breathing:

- The number of times the client coughed and took deep breaths
- How the client tolerated the procedure

Assisting With Coughing and Deep-Breathing Exercises

Advocate on behalf of the client's quality of life by promoting:

Dignity • Independence • Preferences • Privacy • Safety *(see BOX 1–4, on p. 17)*

PRE-PROCEDURE

1 Identify the client, according to employer policy. *This eliminates the possibility of mistaking one client for another.*
2 Explain the procedure to the client.
3 Practise proper hand hygiene.
4 Provide for privacy.

PROCEDURE

5 Help the client to a comfortable sitting position—dangling, semi-Fowler's, or Fowler's. *Lung expansion is easier and better if the client is placed in the sitting position than in the lying position.*
6 Have the client take deep breaths:
   a Have the client place the hands over the rib cage (**FIGURE 41–4**).
   b Ask the client to exhale. Explain that the ribs should move as far down as possible.
   c Have the client take a breath as deep as possible. Remind the client to inhale through the nose.
   d Ask the client to hold the breath for 3 seconds.
   e Ask the client to exhale slowly through pursed lips (**FIGURE 41–5**).

Breathing through pursed lips increases lung pressure and exercises the lungs when breathing out. The client should exhale until the ribs move as far down as possible.

Continued

Assisting With Coughing and Deep-Breathing Exercises—cont'd

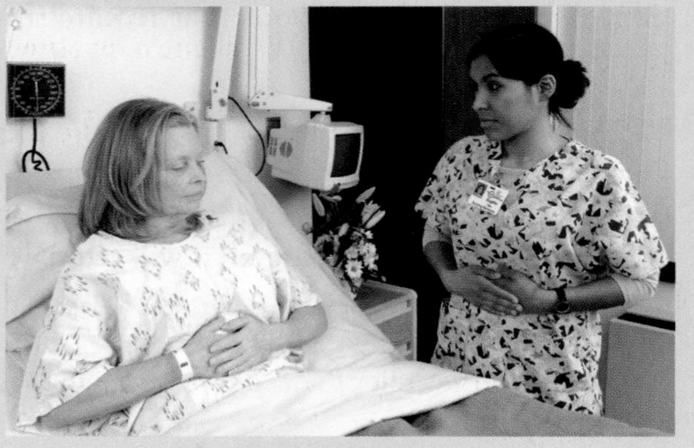

FIGURE 41–4

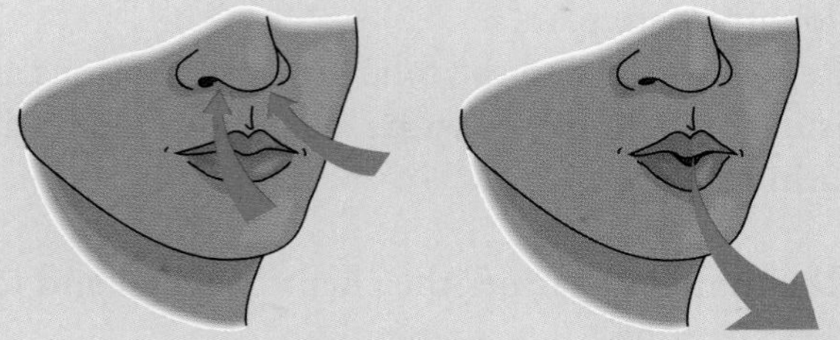

FIGURE 41–5

f Repeat steps *a* through *e* four more times.
This exercise encourages the client to take full breaths.

7 Ask the client to cough:
a Have the client interlace the fingers over the incision for support (FIGURE 41–6, *A*) or hold a pillow or folded towel over the incision for support (FIGURE 41–6, *B*).
Holding the abdomen can decrease abdominal discomfort when taking deep breaths and coughing.

A

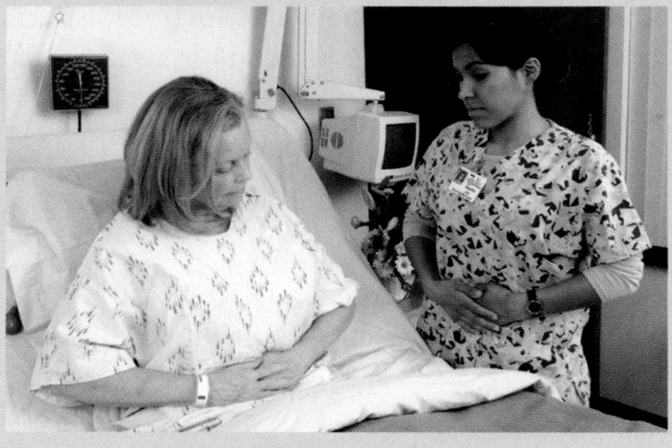

FIGURE 41–6 A

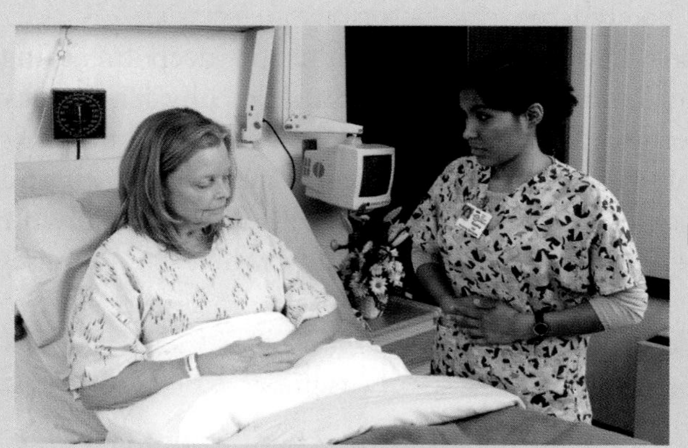

B

FIGURE 41–6 B

b Have the client take in a deep breath as in step 6.
c Ask the client to cough strongly twice with the mouth open.

POST-PROCEDURE

8 Provide for safety and comfort.
9 Place the call bell within reach.*
This provides an easy, safe way for the client to contact the staff if necessary.
10 Follow the care plan for bed rail use.*
This reduces the risk for client injury.
11 Remove privacy measures.
12 Practise proper hand hygiene.

Report and Record your actions and observations, according to employer policy.
This is done for legal reasons and to keep the rest of the health care team informed.

*Steps marked with an asterisk may not apply in community settings.

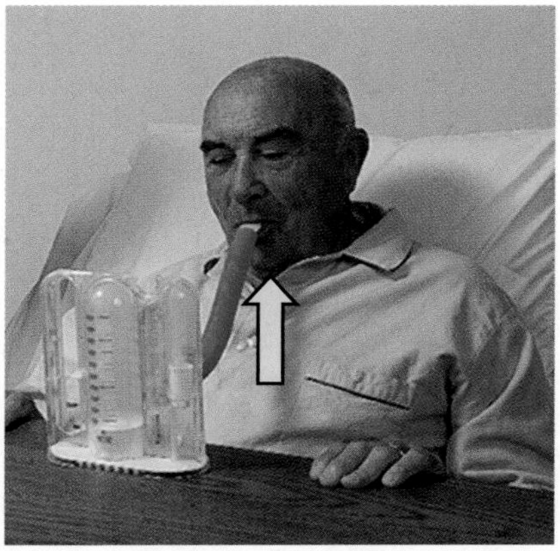

FIGURE 41–7 A client using a spirometer. The arrow shows direction of airflow.

Incentive Spirometry

An *incentive* provides encouragement. A *spirometer* is a machine that measures the amount (volume) of air inhaled. The client is encouraged to inhale until a preset volume of air is reached. The incentive spirometer is made up of a breathing tube, an air chamber, and an indicator (called a *piston*), which will rise with each inhalation. The piston allows the client to see air movement during inhalation (FIGURE 41–7). The piston is made from a flat disc, plastic balls, or bars. The client inhales as deeply as possible and holds that breath for a certain time, usually at least 3 seconds.

Incentive spirometry is also called *sustained maximal inspiration (SMI) (sustained* means "constant"; maximal means "the most or the greatest"; and *inspiration* means "breathing in").

The goal of using a spirometer is to improve lung function and prevent respiratory complications. A spirometer may be given to some clients to use at home and to those in hospital who have had surgeries, but they can be used by anybody the doctor thinks would benefit. By taking long, slow, and deep breaths, the client moves air deep into the lungs; secretions become loose; and O_2–CO_2 exchange occurs between the alveoli and capillaries.

The device is used as follows:

1. The spirometer is placed upright.
2. The client exhales normally.
3. The client seals the lips around the mouthpiece of the device.
4. The client takes a slow, deep breath until the balls in the spirometer rise to the desired height.
5. The client holds the breath for 3 to 6 seconds to keep the balls floating.
6. The client removes the mouth from the mouthpiece and exhales slowly. The client may cough at this time.
7. After taking some normal breaths, the client uses the device again.

Your supervisor and the care plan will tell you the following:

- How often the client needs to use incentive spirometry
- How many breaths the client needs to take
- The desired height that the floating balls should reach

Follow employer policy for cleaning and replacing the mouthpiece.

ASSISTING WITH OXYGEN THERAPY

Disease, injury, and surgery can all interfere with a client's ability to breathe easily, either directly (e.g., if the client has asthma) or indirectly (e.g., if the client has just had abdominal surgery and it hurts too much to take a deep breath). If the level of O_2 in the blood is lower than normal (*hypoxemia*), the physician orders oxygen therapy.

Your Role in Oxygen Therapy

As a support worker, ***you do not "give" oxygen***. In many provinces, support workers are trained to perform oral suctioning, to transfer oxygen from a liquid source tank to a portable tank (often called a *stroller unit*), and to ensure the client's oxygen unit is functioning well. The nurse and respiratory therapist, however, are responsible for starting and maintaining a client's oxygen therapy. You assist in providing safe care to clients receiving oxygen (see BOX 41–4 on p. 934 for a list of your duties and responsibilities).

Oxygen Sources

Whether the client is at home or in a continuing care facility, oxygen may be supplied by one of three main

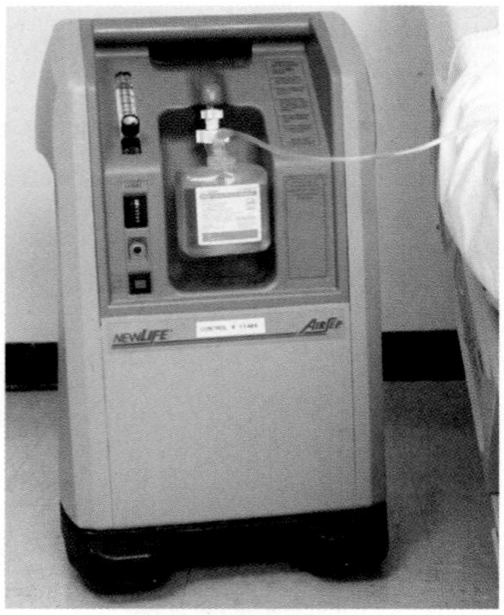

FIGURE 41–8 Oxygen concentrator.

delivery systems: oxygen concentrator, oxygen cylinder, and liquid oxygen system.

Oxygen Concentrator

This machine makes oxygen by taking in room air and filtering out the oxygen (FIGURE 41–8). It must be plugged into a grounded electrical outlet. Because the oxygen concentrator "makes" the oxygen, it does not need to be replaced or refilled regularly. Ambulatory clients may use portable oxygen cylinders along with their concentrators to help them to be mobile and also to be prepared for a power failure. Oxygen concentrators are used in facilities and community settings, while cylinders are used by the client while on outings from home. Some suppliers offer lightweight aluminum cylinders for easier handling.

Oxygen Cylinder

An oxygen cylinder is a tank of compressed oxygen. Large tanks are used inside the home, and small tanks are used for outings or travel. Some clients may be ambulatory but still need continuous oxygen therapy as they go about their daily lives, so they use portable oxygen cylinders (tanks) carried in a shoulder bag or wheeled in a cart (FIGURE 41–9). Large cylinders are often used for babies who need special breathing equipment.

The length of time a cylinder lasts will depend on the amount of oxygen the client uses. A gauge on the cylinder shows how much oxygen is left in it (FIGURE 41–10). Check the gauge often, and tell your supervisor if the oxygen in the cylinder is low.

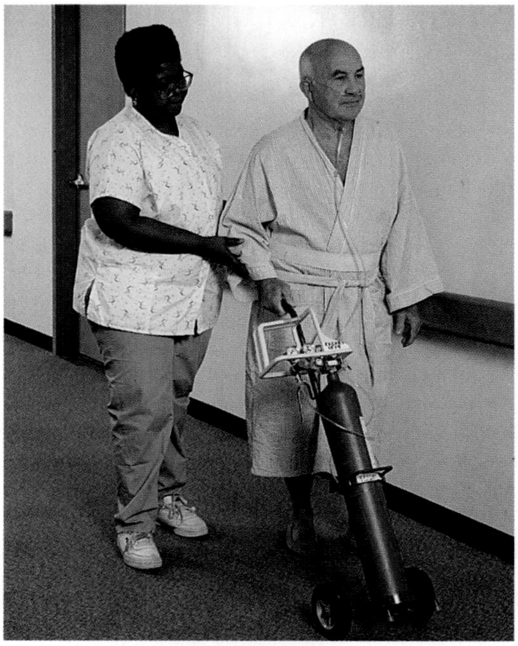

FIGURE 41–9 A client is using a portable oxygen tank while walking.

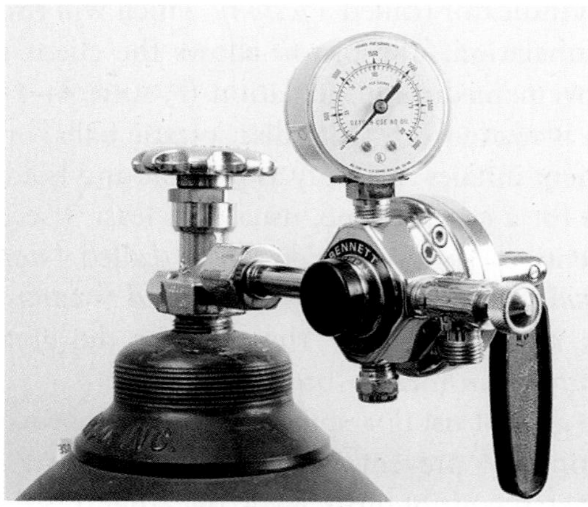

FIGURE 41–10 The gauge shows the amount of oxygen remaining in the tank.

Oxygen cylinders are used for clients in facility or community settings. In hospitals and some continuing care facilities, oxygen is piped directly to each client's unit by way of a *wall oxygen outlet* (FIGURE 41–11) from a centrally located oxygen supply.

Liquid Oxygen System

The liquid oxygen system stores oxygen in its liquid form. The liquid is kept in large stationary containers called *reservoirs*. A portable unit that can be worn over the shoulder is filled from a stationary unit

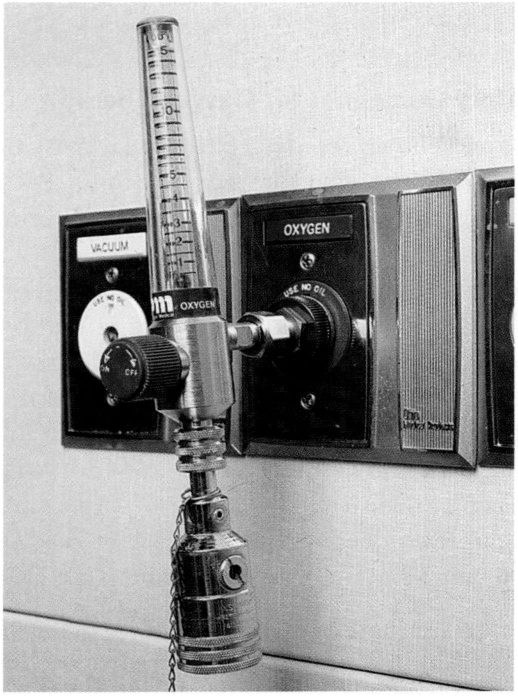

FIGURE 41–11 Wall oxygen outlet.

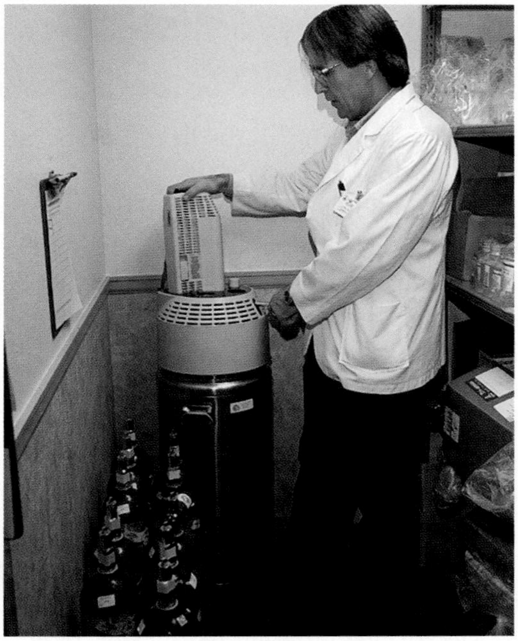

FIGURE 41–12 Liquid oxygen system.

(**FIGURE 41–12**) and has enough oxygen for about 8 hours of use. The liquid turns into gas before it leaves the container and is breathed in by the client.

A gauge shows the amount of oxygen in the unit. Tell your supervisor if the amount is low. Liquid oxygen is very cold and, if touched, can freeze the skin. Follow employer procedures and the manufacturer's instructions when working with liquid oxygen. Liquid oxygen systems are used for clients in facility or community settings.

With the oxygen systems described above, oxygen is delivered continuously while the client inhales and exhales. However, a lot of the oxygen is wasted when the client exhales. **Oxygen-conserving devices** help reduce this wastage so that the client's oxygen supply lasts longer, and the client can thus go for longer outings. Conserving devices also cut down on the number of oxygen cylinders that have to be delivered to the client.

Oxygen Therapy and Safety

Remember, you ***assist*** with oxygen therapy; you do ***not*** administer oxygen. However, it is your responsibility to provide safe care to clients receiving oxygen. Follow the safety guidelines in the *Think About Safety: Safety Guidelines for Oxygen Therapy* box, as well as the fire safety guidelines in **BOX 41–5**.

Oxygen and Fire Safety

Oxygen is the chemical necessary for combustion to take place. With higher-pressurized oxygen—such as with compressed oxygen cylinders—the risk for combustion increases when in the presence of both a source of ignition and a combustible material. For example, if a client had compressed oxygen nearby and was close to a source of ignition (e.g., a lit cigarette), the client's clothing would ignite more easily and burn hotter and faster than it would if surrounded only by room air. Fires caused by an accident with oxygen devices can cause significant damage to property and even loss of life. It is very important to keep an oxygen source away from heat and open flame. Follow employer policies and the fire safety guidelines in **BOX 41–5**.

The physician, nurse, or respiratory therapist is responsible for teaching the client and family members about oxygen safety. However, people sometimes forget or disregard safety rules (see the *Supporting Mr. Kaluwa: Oxygen Safety at Home* box on page 941). You may observe a client, visitor, or family member creating a safety hazard—for example, a home care client attempting to light a gas stove

BOX 41–5 Oxygen and Fire Safety Guidelines

- Place "No Smoking" signs in the room and on the room door.
- Remove smoking materials from the room (e.g., cigarettes, cigars, pipes, matches, lighters).
- Remove materials from the room that ignite easily (e.g., alcohol, nail polish remover, oils, petroleum jelly, greases).
- Keep the oxygen source and tubing away from heat sources and open flames (e.g., direct sunlight, lit cigarettes, candles, lamps, stoves, heating ducts, radiators, heating pipes, space heaters, kerosene heaters).
- Turn off electrical items before unplugging them.
- Use electrical equipment (e.g., razor, radio, TV) only if it is in good repair.
- Use only electrical equipment that has a three-prong plug whenever possible.
- Do not use materials that cause static electricity (wool and synthetic fabrics).
- Know the location of fire extinguishers and how to use them (see Chapter 22).
- If a fire occurs, turn off the oxygen. Then move the client to safety.
- Remind the client about oxygen safety. Report safety hazards immediately.

while using oxygen or a family member wanting to smoke while the oxygen device is on. Such situations are very dangerous, so warn the individuals of the dangers and the safety hazards. Also, call your supervisor immediately and report the situation.

Think About Safety

Safety Guidelines for Oxygen Therapy

- Never remove the device (cannula, mask) used to administer oxygen.
- Report to your supervisor if the client removes the device.
- Make sure the device is secure but not tight.
- Check for signs of skin irritation caused by the device. Check behind the ears, under the nose (cannula), and around the face (mask). Also check the cheekbones.
- Keep the client's face clean and dry when a mask is used.
- Never shut off oxygen flow.
- Do not adjust the flow rate unless allowed by your scope of practice limitations and your employer's policy.
- Tell your supervisor immediately if the flow rate is too high or too low.
- Tell your supervisor immediately if the humidifier is not bubbling.
- Secure connecting tubing in place. Tape or pin it to the client's garment, according to employer policy.
- Make sure there are no kinks in the tubing.
- Make sure the client does not lie on any part of the tubing.
- Report signs and symptoms of hypoxia, respiratory distress, or abnormal breathing patterns to your supervisor immediately (see **FIGURE 41–2** on p. 932, **BOX 41–2** on p. 931, and **BOX 41–3** on p. 933).
- Provide oral hygiene, as directed. Follow the care plan.
- Make sure the device is clean and free of mucus.
- Maintain an adequate water level in the humidifier.

Oxygen Administration Devices

The physician orders the device used to administer oxygen. The devices that are commonly ordered are described below.

Nasal Cannula

The **nasal cannula** (**FIGURE 41–13**) is used at home or in a hospital setting to deliver O_2 to a client in need of extra oxygen. It consists of a set of two prongs that are placed in the client's nostrils and a plastic tube that fits behind the ears. The prongs from which oxygen flows curve downward to prevent drying of the sinuses.

The nasal cannula is connected to an oxygen tank, to a portable oxygen generator, or to a wall connection in a hospital through a **flowmeter**, which regulates the

Supporting Mr. Kaluwa: Oxygen Safety at Home

Joe Kaluwa, 88, is a retired farmer who lives in his home with his wife, Lily. Mr. Kaluwa started smoking at the age of 13, and now, after a lifetime of smoking, he has advanced emphysema and COPD. Mr. Kaluwa has been repeatedly instructed to quit smoking, but he continues to smoke a pack of cigarettes a day. Mrs. Kaluwa has forbidden smoking inside the house, so he goes outside to smoke—in the backyard during summer and in the garage in winter.

Mr. Kaluwa was hospitalized recently for his COPD and was discharged yesterday. He was sent home with a nasal cannula through which oxygen is administered to him, and he was instructed to use it all 24 hours of the day. While in the hospital, he had been warned not to allow anyone to smoke around his oxygen because of the risk for combustion.

A respiratory therapist set up his oxygen tank and tubing at his home. You have been assigned to provide support care and to ensure that he maintains his oxygen therapy. Today, upon your arrival for your first visit to Mr. Kaluwa, you find him sitting in his backyard, calmly smoking a cigarette. He is still connected to his oxygen tubing, with the nasal cannula in place in his nose and around his ears and the portable tank next to him. You take a quick look at his oxygen meter and find that the device is on. Mr. Kaluwa notices that you look surprised, and he tells you that he "turned down his oxygen" to be able to smoke safely. What should you do?

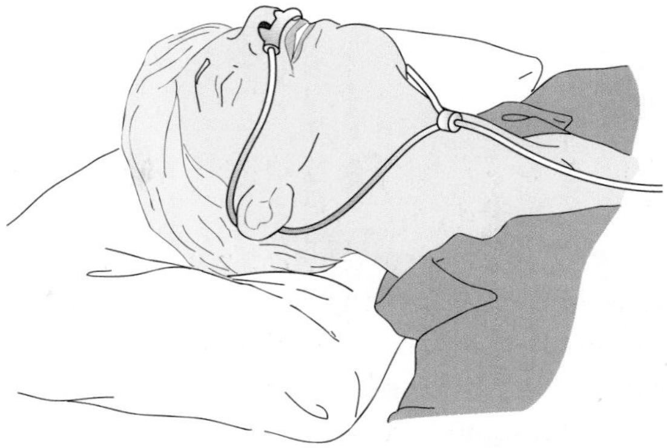

FIGURE 41–13 Nasal cannula.

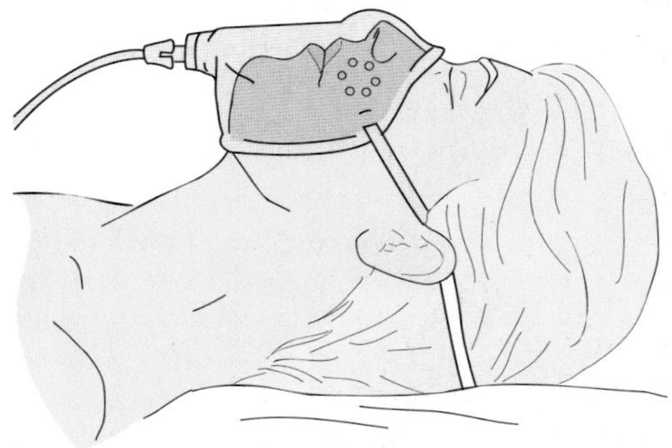

FIGURE 41–14 Simple face mask.

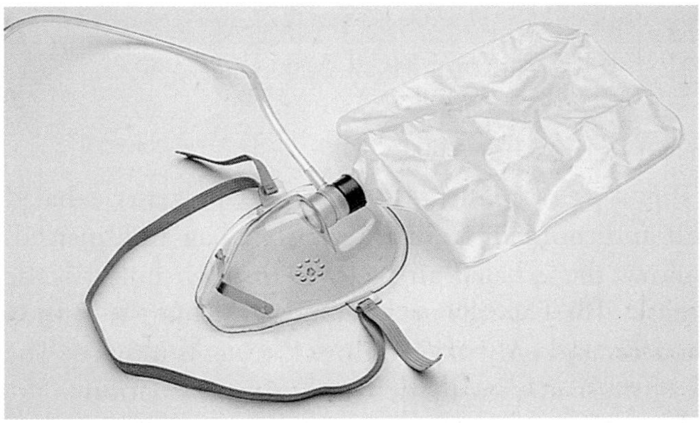

FIGURE 41–15 Partial-rebreather mask.

flow of oxygen. The client can eat and talk with the cannula in place. If the prongs are placed too tightly, nasal irritation or pressure on the ears and cheekbones may occur. You should always report signs or complaints of skin irritation or soreness.

Simple Face Mask

The simple **face mask** (**FIGURE 41–14**) covers the nose and mouth and is connected to an oxygen source. The mask has small holes on the sides through which room air enters during inhalation and CO_2 escapes during exhalation.

Partial-Rebreather Mask

With the partial-rebreather mask (**FIGURE 41–15**), a bag is added to the simple face mask to collect exhaled air. When breathing in, the client inhales O_2 as well as some exhaled air and some room air. The bag should not totally deflate during inhalation.

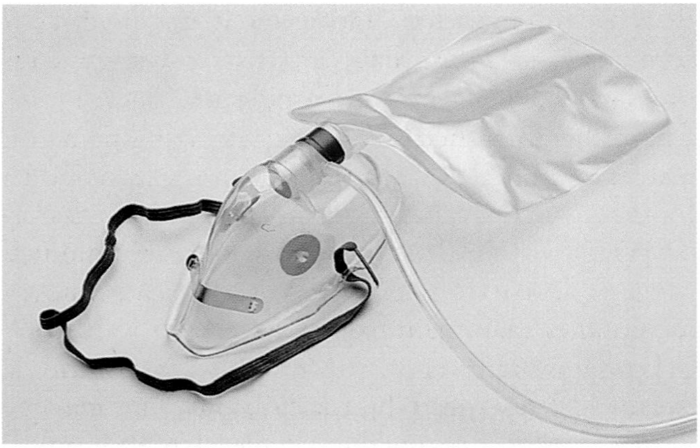

FIGURE 41–16 Non-rebreather mask.

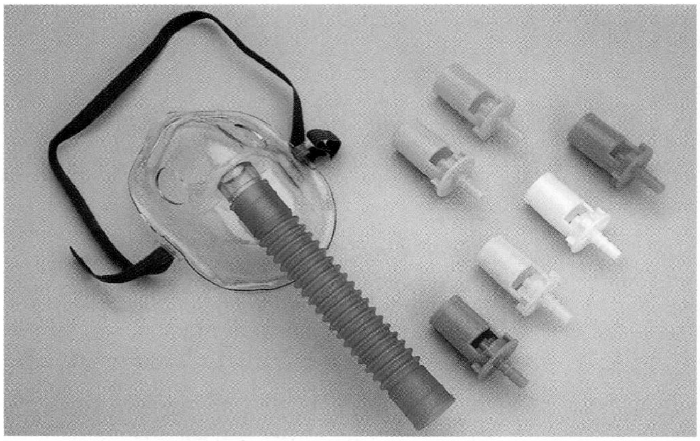

FIGURE 41–17 Venturi mask.

Non-Rebreather Mask

This type of mask (FIGURE 41–16) prevents exhaled air and room air from entering the bag and, instead, allows the exhaled air to leave through holes in the mask. The bag fills up with oxygen from the oxygen source, and only oxygen from the bag is inhaled. The bag must not totally deflate during exhalation.

Venturi Mask

The venturi mask (FIGURE 41–17) allows precise amounts of oxygen to be given. Special colour-coded plastic adaptors that fit into the mask are connected to the source of oxygen. Each colour is coded to show what amount of oxygen the mask delivers.

Special care is needed when masks are used. Masks make talking difficult, so listen carefully when the client is trying to say something. Moisture can build up under the mask. Keep the client's face clean and dry to help prevent irritation from the mask. Report any signs of skin irritation. Masks are removed for eating, and usually O_2 is administered via a nasal cannula during that time.

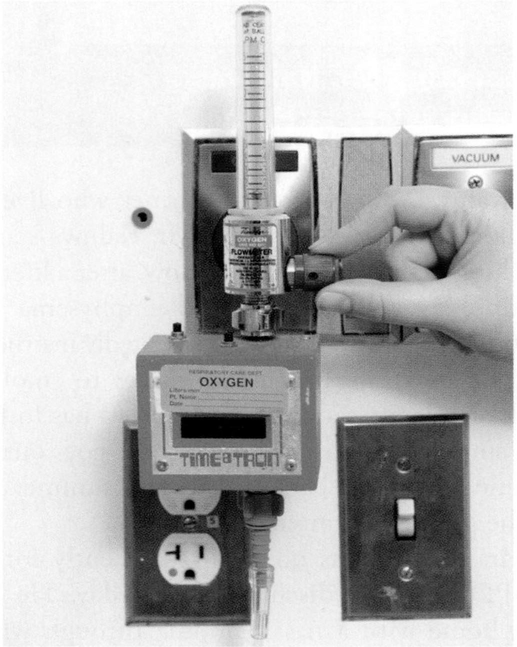

FIGURE 41–18 The flowmeter is used to set the oxygen flow rate.

Oxygen Flow Rates

The amount of oxygen ordered by the physician and administered to the client is called the **flow rate**. The flow rate is measured in litres per minute (L/min), and the oxygen flow rate can range from 2 to 15 L/min. A nurse or respiratory therapist sets the flow rate (FIGURE 41–18).

Your supervisor and the care plan will specify the client's flow rate. While giving care to your clients who are receiving oxygen, always check the flow rate. Tell your supervisor immediately if the flow rate is too high or too low. A nurse or respiratory therapist will then adjust the flow rate. Some employers may allow support workers to adjust oxygen flow rates. If you are allowed to adjust the flow rate, follow employer policies and procedures.

Preparing for Oxygen Administration

Humidified Oxygen

Oxygen is a dry gas. If it is not humidified (made moist), it can dry the mucous membranes of the

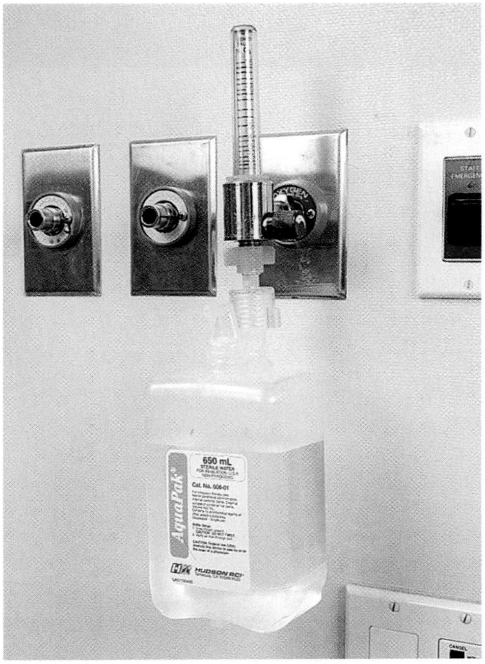

FIGURE 41–19 Oxygen administration system with humidifier.

airways. A *humidifier* (**FIGURE 41–19**) is a system by which oxygen is forced through distilled water, allowing it to bubble up and be collected in the tubing for the client to breathe. **Distilled water** is pure, sterile water that has been boiled and allowed to cool and condense. Tap water is not used, as it contains impurities that can irritate the mucous membranes and damage the equipment. The humidifier is then attached to the oxygen administration system (wall outlet, oxygen tank, or oxygen concentrator). It then produces **humidified oxygen**; that is, oxygen that contains water vapour. Humidified oxygen is less drying and irritating to delicate mucous membranes than plain oxygen is.

Low flow rates (1 to 2 L/min) by nasal cannula usually do not need humidification. You may be responsible for checking the water level in the humidifier and cleaning and refilling it. Follow employer procedures and your supervisor's directions.

You do not administer oxygen, but your supervisor may ask you to set up the oxygen administration system. You are told the following:

- The client's name and room and bed number (in facilities)
- The oxygen administration device ordered
- Whether humidification was ordered

Tell your supervisor when you finish setting up the oxygen administration system. A nurse will turn the oxygen on, set the flow rate, and apply the administration device.

Setting Up for Oxygen Administration 123

Advocate on behalf of the client's quality of life by promoting:

Dignity • Independence • Preferences • Privacy • Safety *(see BOX 1–4, on p. 17)*

PRE-PROCEDURE

1 Identify the client, according to employer policy. *This eliminates the possibility of mistaking one client for another.*
2 Explain the procedure to the client.
3 Practise proper hand hygiene.
4 Collect the following supplies:
 - ☐ **Oxygen administration device with connecting tubing**
 - ☐ **Flowmeter**
 - ☐ **Humidifier (if ordered)**
 - ☐ **Distilled water (if using a humidifier)**

 By collecting all of the necessary equipment beforehand, you will not have to leave your client's side and can eliminate wasting time and energy in obtaining the forgotten equipment.

Continued

Setting Up for Oxygen Administration—cont'd

PROCEDURE

5 Make sure the flowmeter is in the "Off" position.
It may spark if in the "On" position!
6 Attach the flowmeter to the wall outlet or to the tank.
7 Fill the humidifier with distilled water.
Distilled water does not contain the bacteria and impurities that are found in tap water.
8 Attach the humidifier to the bottom of the flowmeter.
Humidified oxygen keeps delicate mucous membranes moist, preventing them from drying out.
9 Attach the oxygen administration device and connecting tubing to the humidifier.
Do not set the flowmeter. Do not apply the oxygen administration device on the client.
These tasks are not within your scope of practice.

POST-PROCEDURE

10 Provide for safety and comfort.
11 Place the call bell within reach.*
This provides an easy, safe way for the client to contact the staff if necessary.
12 Discard packaging in the appropriate container(s).
This keeps the unit clean and tidy for others.
13 Make sure the cap on the distilled water bottle is secure. Store it according to employer policy.
This makes it easier to find the next time it is needed.
14 Practise proper hand hygiene.
15 Tell your supervisor when you are finished. A nurse will:
- ☐ Turn on the oxygen and set the flow rate
- ☐ Apply the oxygen administration device

Report and Record your actions and observations, according to employer policy.
This is done for legal reasons and to keep the rest of the health care team informed.

*Steps marked with an asterisk may not apply in community settings.

ASSISTING WITH ASSESSMENT AND DIAGNOSTIC TESTING

The physician orders tests to determine the cause of a breathing problem. Numerous respiratory tests are available (**BOX 41–6**). Most of these tests are done at hospitals or clinics, and some are done in continuing care facilities. They are done by a physician or a specially trained nurse, respiratory therapist, or laboratory technician. You may assist the client before and after a test, as directed by your supervisor, the care plan, and the assignment sheet.

You are likely to assist with pulse oximetry and to collect sputum specimens (see p. 948). Both procedures may provide the physician with information about the state of the client's respiratory system.

Pulse Oximetry

A *pulse oximeter* is a device used to measure (*meter*) oxygen (*oxi*) concentration in arterial blood as well as to measure pulse rate. *Oxygen concentration* is the amount (percent) of hemoglobin that contains oxygen. The normal range is 95% to 100%. For example, if 97% of all the hemoglobin carries O_2, tissues get enough oxygen. If only 90% of the hemoglobin contains O_2, tissues do not get enough oxygen to function. The pulse oximeter can detect low

BOX 41–6 Common Respiratory Tests

- ***Chest X-ray (CXR)***—an X-ray of the chest; taken to evaluate changes in the lungs.
- ***Lung scan***—performed to see which areas are not getting air or blood. The client inhales radioactive (*radioactive* means "giving off radiation") gas and is injected with a radioisotope (a *radioisotope* is a substance that gives off radiation). Lung tissue getting air and blood "takes up" the radioactive substances, and a scanner then senses the areas with radioactive substances.
- ***Bronchoscopy***—a scope (*scopy*) passed into the trachea and bronchi (*broncho*). Airway structures are checked for bleeding and tumours. Tissue samples (biopsy) are taken, or mucous plugs and foreign objects are removed. After the procedure, the client is NPO (receives nothing by mouth) and watched carefully until the gag and swallow reflexes return, usually in about 2 hours.
- ***Thoracentesis***—the pleura (*thora*) is punctured, and air or fluid is removed (*centesis*) from it. The physician inserts a needle through the chest wall into the pleural sac when injury or disease causes it to fill with air, blood, or fluid, and respiratory function is affected.

  Sometimes fluid is removed for laboratory study, and sometimes anticancer medications are injected into the pleural sac. After the procedure, which takes only a few minutes, the client is checked frequently for shortness of breath, dyspnea, cough, sputum (see p. 946), chest pain, cyanosis, vital sign changes, and other respiratory signs and symptoms.
- ***Pulmonary function tests***—tests that measure the amount of air moving into and out of the lungs (volume) and how much air the lungs can hold (capacity). The client takes as deep a breath as possible and, using a mouthpiece, blows into a machine. The tests are used to evaluate clients at risk for lung diseases or postoperative lung complications and to measure the progress of lung disease and its treatment.
- ***Arterial blood gases (ABGs)***—the puncturing of a radial or femoral artery to obtain arterial blood and measure the amount of oxygen in it. Hemorrhage from the artery must be prevented, so pressure is applied to the artery for at least 5 minutes after the procedure and longer if the client has blood clotting problems.

oxygen levels before any signs or symptoms appear, and the measurements are used to prevent and treat hypoxia.

A pulse oximeter, which consists of a computerized monitor and a sensor (probe), is a very delicate and expensive piece of equipment that should always be handled gently. ***Never drop or handle a pulse oximeter roughly, as doing so can affect the delicate sensors within it.*** Most employers now consider pulse oximetry a regular part of taking a client's vital signs, so the support worker should be aware of the correct method of attaching the pulse oximeter and reading it (see the procedure *Measuring the Pulse and Oxygen Concentration Using a Pulse Oximeter* in Chapter 15).

The sensor is attached to the client's finger, toe, nose, earlobe, or forehead (**FIGURE 41–20**). Two light beams on one side of the sensor pass through the tissues. A detector on the other side measures the amount of light passing through the tissues. Using this information, the oximeter measures O_2 concentration, and the value and pulse rate are displayed on the monitor. Oximeters have alarms, which sound if O_2 concentration is low, if the pulse is too fast or too slow, or if other measurable problems occur.

Small, handheld oximeter units are available for home use. Usually, the client's oxygen concentration and vital signs are measured simultaneously. Because the device is portable and used for many clients, you must test its accuracy: After applying the sensor, check the client's radial pulse and compare it with the displayed pulse. The pulse rates should be the same.

Selecting the ideal sensor site on the client is important. Your supervisor or the care plan will tell you which site to use based on the client's condition. Swollen sites and sites with skin breaks should be

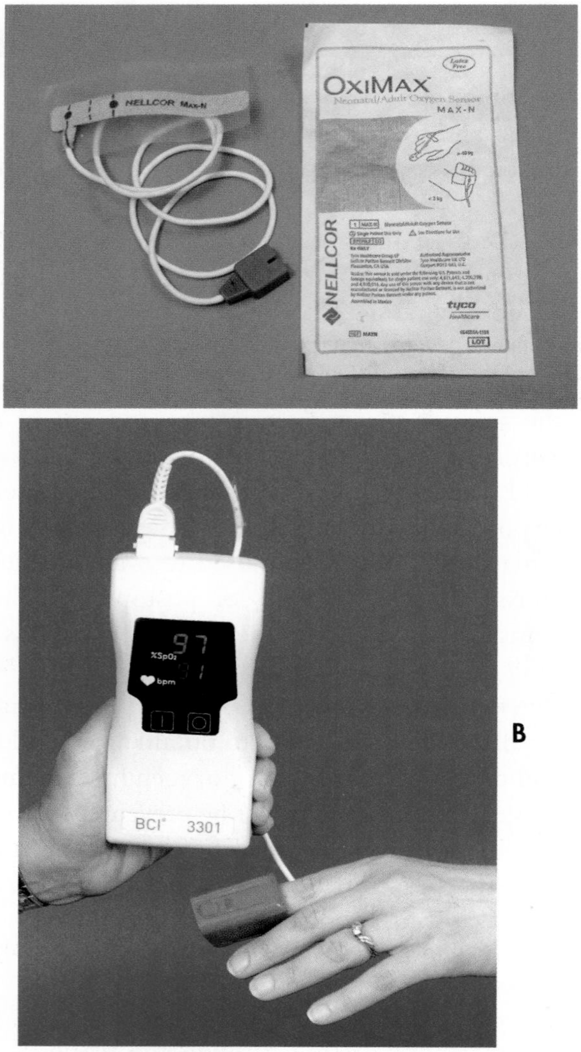

FIGURE 41–20 **A,** The sensor tubing is supplied in individual packages. One end of the tubing is attached to the pulse oximeter, and the other end is then clipped over the client's nail bed. **B,** A pulse oximeter sensor attached to a finger.

avoided. Because aging and vascular disease often cause poor circulation, blood flow to the fingers or toes is sometimes poor. In such a case, the earlobe, nose, or forehead site is used.

Bright light, nail polish, artificial nails, and movements can affect measurement accuracy. To prevent inaccurate readings, place a towel over the sensor to block out bright light; remove the client's nail polish or use another site; and do not use a finger site if the client wears artificial nails. Movements from shivering, seizures, or tremors affect finger sensors. The earlobe is a better site if a client has these problems. Blood pressure cuffs affect blood flow, so if using a finger site, do not measure blood pressure on that side.

Report and record measurements accurately. Use the abbreviation SpO_2 (S = saturation, p = pulse, O_2 = oxygen) when recording the oxygen saturation value. Also, report and record the following:

- The date and time
- What the client was doing at the time of measurement
- Oxygen flow rate and the device used
- Reason for the measurement (routine or change in the client's condition)
- Other observations, such as the client's cooperation with wearing the pulse oximeter

Pulse oximetry does not replace good observations. The client's condition can change rapidly. Observe for signs and symptoms of hypoxia—such as a change in the client's behaviour or ability to comprehend instructions—which can signal a drop in the client's SpO_2 level.

Collecting Sputum Specimens

Respiratory disorders cause the lungs, bronchi, and trachea to secrete mucus. Mucus from the respiratory system is called **sputum** when expectorated (expelled) through the mouth. Note that sputum is *not* saliva (spit), which is a thin, clear liquid produced by the salivary glands in the mouth.

Sputum specimens can be collected from clients in the community, in continuing care facilities, and in the hospital. Sputum specimens are studied for blood, microbes, and abnormal cells. For this test, the client must cough up sputum from the bronchi and trachea (not saliva from the mouth!); doing so can often be painful and hard to do. Specimens should be collected in the morning because secretions are more easily coughed up upon awakening.

The client should rinse the mouth only with water to decrease saliva and remove food particles. Instruct the client ***not*** to use mouthwash before the procedure because it can destroy some of the microbes in the mouth and give a false reading.

Ensure that the client has privacy for this procedure. The procedure can be embarrassing for the client,

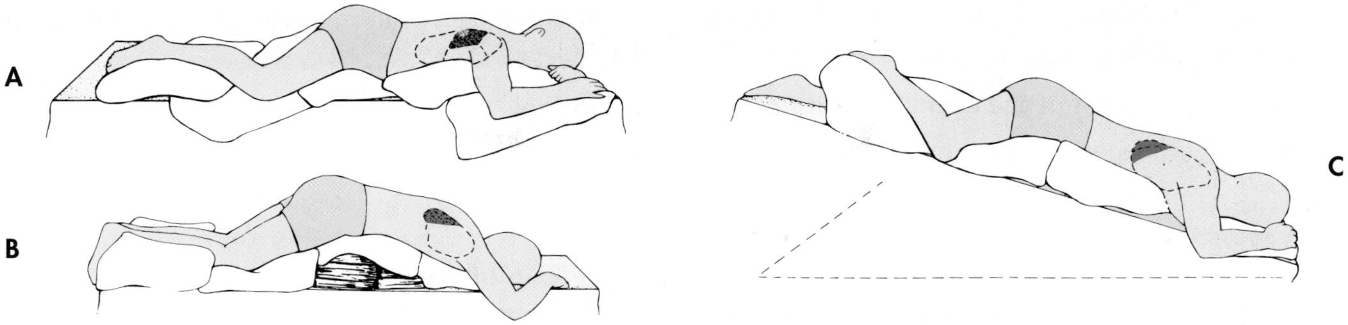

FIGURE 41–21 Some positions used for postural drainage. (*Note:* A nurse or respiratory therapist is responsible for postural drainage. ***Do not place the client in these positions without supervision.***) **A,** Draining the right upper lobe. **B,** Draining the right middle lobe. **C,** Draining the right lower lobe. (**Source:** Potter, P.A., Perry, A.G., Ross-Kerr, J.C., et al. (2014). *Canadian fundamentals of nursing: Concepts, process, and practice* (5th ed.). Toronto, ON: Elsevier.)

as the sputum is unpleasant to look at, and the coughing and expectorating sounds may disturb others nearby. If possible, collect the specimen when the roommate or family members are out of the room. Cover the specimen container, and place it in a bag in order to keep the contents out of sight. Always follow Standard Practices (see Chapter 23) when collecting a sputum specimen.

Postural Drainage

Some clients do not have the strength to cough up sputum, so the nurse or respiratory therapist places them in a certain position to allow secretions to drain by gravity (gravity causes fluids to flow downward). Coughing is then made easier for them after postural drainage. The client is positioned in such a way that a lung part is at a higher level than the airway (**FIGURE 41–21**). Positioning depends on the lung part that needs draining.

If it is within your scope of practice for your province or your agency, you may have to assist with postural drainage. Do not attempt to position the client without supervision (see the *Focus on Children: Assisting With Treatments* box).

Report and record the following observations after collecting a sputum specimen:

- The time the specimen was collected
- The amount of sputum collected
- How easily the client coughed up the sputum
- The consistency of the sputum

ARTIFICIAL AIRWAYS

Artificial airways keep the airway patent (open) and are used in the following circumstances:

- The airway is obstructed from disease, injury, secretions, or aspiration.
- The client is semi-conscious or unconscious.
- The client is recovering from anaesthesia.
- The client needs mechanical ventilation.

FOCUS ON CHILDREN

Assisting With Treatments

Breathing treatments and suctioning are often needed to obtain sputum specimens from infants and small children. The nurse or respiratory therapist gives the breathing treatment, and the nurse suctions the trachea for the sputum specimen. The infant or child is likely to be uncooperative during suctioning. You can assist by comforting the child. You might be asked to hold the child's head and arms still.

Collecting a Sputum Specimen

123

Advocate on behalf of the client's quality of life by promoting:

Dignity • Independence • Preferences • Privacy • Safety

(see BOX 1–4, on p. 17)

PRE-PROCEDURE

1 Identify the client, according to employer policy.
This eliminates the possibility of mistaking one client for another.

2 Explain the procedure to the client.

3 Practise proper hand hygiene.

4 Collect the following supplies:

- ☐ **Sputum specimen container and label**
- ☐ **Laboratory requisition**
- ☐ **Disposable bag**
- ☐ **Gloves**
- ☐ **Mask (if needed)**
- ☐ **Tissues**
- ☐ **Cup of water**
- ☐ **Kidney basin**

By collecting all the necessary equipment beforehand, you will not have to leave your client's side and can eliminate wasting time and energy in obtaining the forgotten equipment.

5 Label the specimen container.
It is easier and cleaner to do this before the container is used.

6 Provide for privacy. If able, the client can go into the bathroom for the procedure.

PROCEDURE

7 Put on gloves. Put on a mask.
This decreases the risk for pathogen spread.

8 Ask the client to rinse the mouth with clear water. If the client is in bed, offer a glass of water and allow the client to spit into the kidney basin.
This removes food particles or medications that may be present in the client's mouth.

9 Have the client hold the container. Only the outside can be touched.
The inside of the container is sterile. Touching it will contaminate it.

10 Ask the client to cover the mouth and nose with tissues when coughing.
This decreases the risk for pathogen spread.

11 Ask the client to take two or three deep breaths and cough up the sputum.
Taking two or three breaths first will fill the lungs with enough oxygen to initiate a deep cough.

12 Have the client expectorate directly into the specimen container (see FIGURE 41–22). Sputum should not touch the outside.
This decreases the risk for pathogen spread.

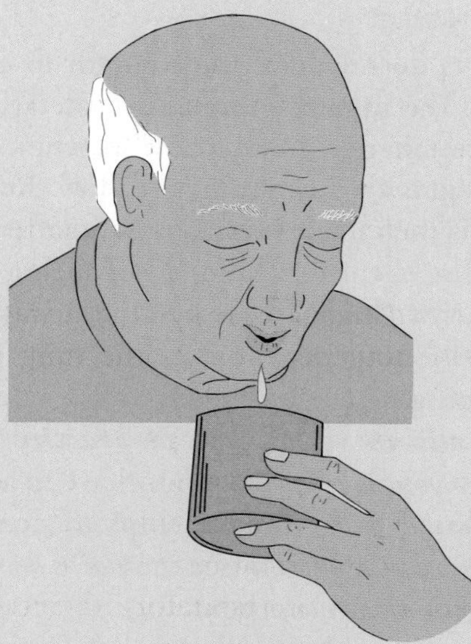

FIGURE 41–22

Continued

Collecting a Sputum Specimen—cont'd

13 Collect 15 to 30 millilitres (mL) (1 to 2 tablespoons) of sputum unless you have been told to collect more.
This is the required amount for a sputum test.

14 Put the lid on the container. Do not touch the inside of the lid.
This traps the contents and keeps them intact.

15 Place the container in the bag. Attach the requisition to the bag.
This ensures the correct lab test will be applied to the sample.

16 Remove your gloves. Remove your mask. Dispose of them in the appropriate container.

17 Practise proper hand hygiene.

POST-PROCEDURE

18 Provide for safety and comfort.

19 Place the call bell within reach.*
This provides an easy, safe way for the client to contact the staff if necessary.

20 Remove privacy measures.

21 Practise proper hand hygiene.

22 Take the bag to the appropriate area.
This is to ensure proper follow-up of the sample.

23 Practise proper hand hygiene.

Report and Record your actions and observations, according to employer policy.
This is done for legal reasons and to keep the rest of the health care team informed.

*Steps marked with an asterisk may not apply in community settings.

Types of Artificial Airways

Intubation is the process of inserting an artificial airway. Artificial airways are usually plastic and disposable and come in adult, pediatric, and infant sizes. The following airways are commonly used:

- ***Oro-pharyngeal airway***—inserted through the mouth and into the pharynx (**FIGURE 41–23, A**). A nurse, paramedic, or respiratory therapist inserts the airway, usually in a hospital or, in an emergency situation, on the way to a hospital.
- ***Naso-pharyngeal airway***—inserted through a nostril and into the pharynx (**FIGURE 41–23, B**). A nurse, paramedic, or respiratory therapist inserts the airway, usually in a hospital or, in an emergency situation, on the way to a hospital.
- ***Endo-tracheal (ET) tube***—inserted through the mouth or nose and into the trachea (**FIGURE 41–23, C**). A physician, a nurse with special training, or a paramedic with special training inserts it using a lighted scope. A balloon (called a *cuff*) at the end of the tube is inflated to keep the airway in place.
- ***Tracheostomy tube***—inserted through a surgical incision (*ostomy*) into the trachea (*tracheo*) (**FIGURE 41–23, *D***). Some tubes have cuffs; the cuff is inflated to keep the tube in place. Tracheostomies are done by a physician in both emergency and nonemergency situations; they can be either temporary or permanent.

Care of a Client With an Artificial Airway

Clients with an artificial airway are normally cared for in a hospital setting until they are able to be at home, and, as the support worker, you are given directions by a nurse. The client's vital signs need to be checked often, and the client must be observed for hypoxia and other respiratory signs and symptoms. The client needs frequent oral hygiene, as the

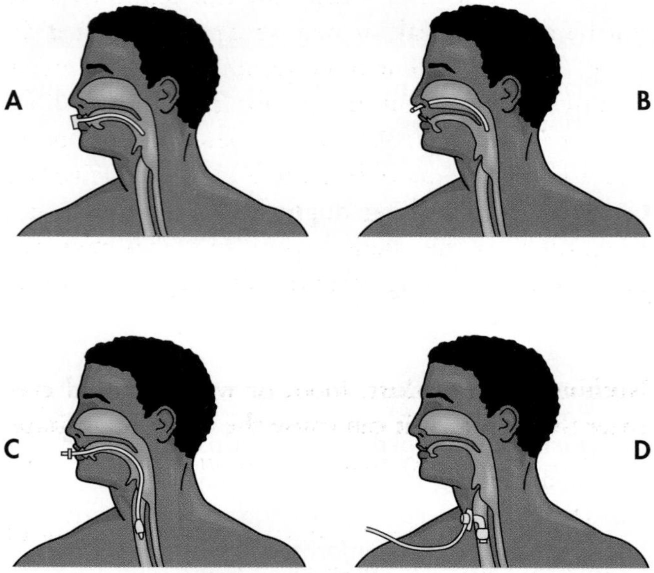

FIGURE 41–23 Artificial airways. **A,** Oro-pharyngeal airway. **B,** Naso-pharyngeal airway. **C,** Endo-tracheal tube. **D,** Tracheostomy tube.

oral mucous membranes may become dried and cracked. Your supervisor and the care plan will tell you when and how to perform oral hygiene. If an airway comes out or is dislodged, you need to tell your supervisor immediately.

Talking is hard with oro-pharyngeal and naso-pharyngeal airways. Clients with ET tubes cannot speak, but some tracheostomy tubes allow clients to speak. Paper and pencils, magic slates, communication boards, and hand signals can all be used to communicate. Follow the care plan.

Gagging and choking sensations are common with artificial airways. Comfort and reassure the client. Remind the client that the airway helps breathing. Use touch to show you care.

Tracheostomies

A **tracheostomy** is a surgically created opening (*ostomy*) through the neck into the trachea (*tracheo*). A tracheostomy tube is usually inserted through this opening, and the client breathes through the tracheostomy tube. A humidifier attachment may be needed for about 1 month after tracheostomy surgery because the trachea is now exposed to drier air.

FOCUS ON CHILDREN

Congenital Conditions

Some children are born with congenital (*congenital* means "present at birth") conditions, and some of these conditions affecting the neck and airway require tracheostomies. Some infections and foreign body aspiration cause airway structures to swell or be blocked and obstruct airflow, which necessitates emergency tracheostomies.

Types of Tracheostomies

Tracheostomies can be temporary or permanent, depending on the client's circumstances. In temporary situations, tracheostomies may have been inserted because of a severe breathing crisis or blockage. In permanent cases, airway structures have been surgically removed, along with the client's larynx and epiglottis. Clients who have head and neck cancers, severe airway trauma, or brain injury may require permanent tracheostomies. Generally, a surgeon will consider a tracheostomy only when there is no other option (see the *Focus on Children: Congenital Conditions* box). Certain groups—for example, babies, smokers, and older adults—are more vulnerable to complications following a tracheostomy.

The long-term care of clients depends on whether the tracheostomy tube is temporary or permanent. If it is temporary, it will be removed when no longer needed, and the incision will be allowed to heal closed, leaving a small scar in the neck area. If the tracheostomy is permanent, the hole (*stoma*) will stay open. However, the opening tends to narrow with time, and further surgery may be needed to widen it. The outer tracheostomy tube needs to be changed every few months, and the site is inspected at each change. The client may be referred to a speech pathologist for alternative means of communication.

Supporting the Client With a Tracheostomy

A tracheostomy tube is made of plastic or metal and has three parts (**FIGURE 41–24**):

- ***Obturator***—used to insert the outer cannula and then is removed; it has a round end. (The

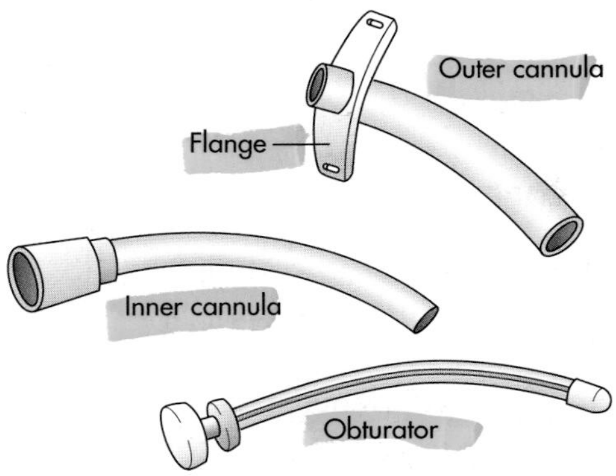

FIGURE 41–24 Parts of a tracheostomy tube.

obturator is placed within easy reach in case the tracheostomy tube falls out and needs to be re-inserted. It is taped to the wall or to the bedside stand.)

- ***Inner cannula***—an inner tube; it requires cleaning whenever it gets blocked with secretions, once to several times every day. It is removed for cleaning and mucus removal and then re-inserted and locked in place. The inner cannula maintains the hygiene of the airway because it can be removed, cleaned, and then replaced. Some plastic tracheostomy tubes do not have inner cannulas.
- ***Outer cannula***—secured in place with ties around the neck or a Velcro collar. The outer cannula is not removed.

The cuffed tracheostomy tube provides a seal between the cannula and the trachea (see **FIGURE 41–23, *D***). This type is used with mechanical ventilation. The cuff prevents air from leaking around the tube and also prevents aspiration. A nurse or respiratory therapist inflates and deflates the cuff.

If the tube is not secured properly, it could come out with coughing or if pulled on (extubation). Damage to the airway is possible if the tube is loose and moves up and down in the trachea. ***Call your supervisor if the outer cannula comes out or is loose.***

The tube must remain patent at all times to enable the client to breathe. Some clients can cough secretions up and out of the tracheostomy; some clients may require suctioning. ***Call your supervisor if the client shows signs and symptoms of hypoxia or respiratory distress.***

The client with a permanent tracheostomy may not be able to speak or may speak with great difficulty. Assist the client to communicate with you by writing or using a communication board (see **FIGURE 39–1** on page 905). When the client tries to speak, you must remember to be patient and supportive (see Chapter 39). Speaking might be very difficult and frustrating for the client, especially if you have difficulty understanding what he is trying to tell you.

Safety Measures

Nothing (such as dust, food, or water) should ever enter the stoma, as it can cause the client to aspirate. The following safety measures are important:

- Dressings should never have loose gauze or lint or anything that the client can inhale.
- The stoma or tube should always be covered when the client goes outside. The client should cover the stoma with a scarf or shirt or blouse that buttons at the neck to prevent dust, insects, and other small particles from entering the stoma.
- The stoma should never be covered with plastic, leather, or similar materials. These materials prevent air from entering the stoma, making it difficult for the client to breathe.
- The client should take tub baths, instead of showers. If showers are taken, a shower guard should be worn, and the client should hold a handheld nozzle to direct water away from the stoma.
- Assist the client with shampooing. Remember that water should never enter the stoma.
- The stoma should be covered when the client has a shave.
- The client must not be allowed to swim, as water will enter the tube or stoma.
- MedicAlert jewellery should always be worn, and clients should also carry a MedicAlert ID card whenever they leave their homes.

Tracheostomy Care

Clients require care to their tracheostomy site when there are excessive secretions, when the ties or collar holding their tracheostomy in place become soiled, or when the dressing around their tracheostomy becomes soiled or moist. Such care is usually provided every 8 to 12 hours, or according to the client's care plan. Remember to follow Standard Practices

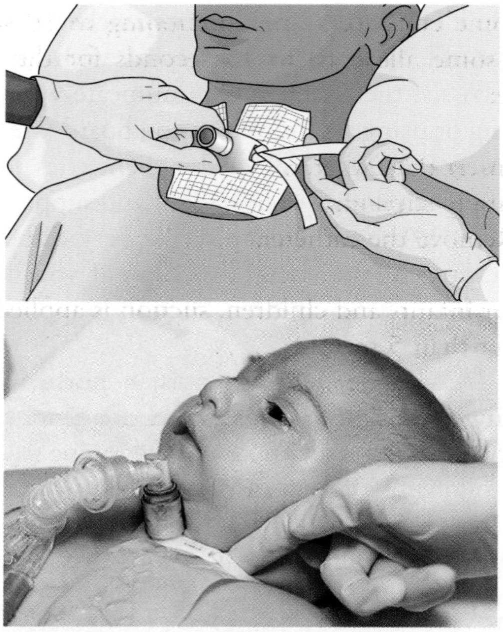

FIGURE 41–25 **A,** A finger is inserted under the ties. **B,** For children, only a fingertip is inserted under the ties. (**Source** (for *B*): Hockenberry, M.J., & Wilson, D. (2007). *Wong's nursing care of infants and children* (8th ed.). St. Louis, MO: Mosby.)

(see Chapter 23) when assisting with tracheostomy care. Tracheostomy care involves the following:

- ***Cleaning the inner cannula***—removes mucus and keeps the airway patent. Cleaning is not necessary with inner cannulas that are disposable.
- ***Cleaning the stoma***—prevents infection and skin breakdown.
- ***Applying clean ties or a Velcro collar***—prevents infection. Remember when the ties are removed, you need to hold the outer cannula in place. The ties or collar must be secure but not tight, and you should be able to slide a finger under the ties or collar (**FIGURE 41–25,** ***A***). (See the *Focus on Children: Tracheostomy Care* box).

SUCTIONING AN AIRWAY

Injury and illness often cause secretions to collect in the upper airway, resulting in the following problems:

- They obstruct airflow in and out of the airway.
- They provide an environment for microbes.
- They interfere with O_2–CO_2 exchange.
- Hypoxia can occur.

Usually, coughing removes secretions, but some clients are unable to cough, or the cough is too weak to remove secretions. Some clients cannot expectorate or swallow secretions after coughing. These clients need suctioning to remove secretions.

Suctioning is the process of withdrawing or sucking up fluid (secretions). A tube connects to a suction source (wall outlet or suction machine) at one end and to a suction catheter at the other end. The catheter is inserted into the airway, and secretions are withdrawn through the catheter.

Suctioning Sites

The upper airway (nose, mouth, and pharynx) and the lower airway (trachea and bronchi) are suctioned.

- ***Oro-pharyngeal route***—the mouth (*oro*) and pharynx (*pharyngeal*) are suctioned. A suction catheter is passed through the mouth and into the pharynx.
- ***Naso-pharyngeal route***—the nose (*naso*) and pharynx (*pharyngeal*) are suctioned. The suction catheter is passed through the nose and into the pharynx.
- ***Lower airway suctioning***—done through an ET tube or through a tracheostomy tube.

> **FOCUS ON CHILDREN**
> **Tracheostomy Care**
>
> As with adults, in children the ties must be secure but not tight. You should be able to slide only a fingertip under the ties (**FIGURE 41–25,** ***B***). Ties are too loose if you can slide your whole finger under them. When assisting with tracheostomy care, you must hold the child still. Position the child's head so that the neck is slightly extended.

Safety Measures Related to Suctioning

If not done correctly, suctioning can cause serious harm to the client. As suctioning removes oxygen from the airway, the client may be unable to breathe during suctioning, and hypoxia and life-threatening complications can arise. The respiratory, cardiovascular, and nervous systems can be affected, and cardiac arrest, infection, and airway injury are possible. ***It is your responsibility to ensure that suctioning is within your scope of practice for your province or territory and within your agency.***

The client's lungs are hyperventilated—given extra (*hyper*) breaths (*ventilate*)—before suctioning from an ET tube or tracheostomy. An Ambu bag (**FIGURE 41–26**) is attached to an oxygen source; then the oxygen delivery device is removed from the ET or tracheostomy tube, and the Ambu bag is attached to the ET or tracheostomy tube. To give a breath, the bag is squeezed with both hands. A nurse or respiratory therapist gives three to five breaths. Remember, oxygen is considered a medication, and you do ***not*** administer medications. Therefore, you may operate an Ambu bag attached to an oxygen source only if it is within your scope of practice.

Some employers limit suctioning to 10 seconds, and some allow 10 to 15 seconds for the suction cycle:

1. Insert the catheter.
2. Apply suction.
3. Remove the catheter.

For infants and children, suction is applied for no longer than 5 seconds.

You might be asked to assist a nurse with suctioning. You need to understand the principles and safety measures involved in safe suctioning (**BOX 41–7**).

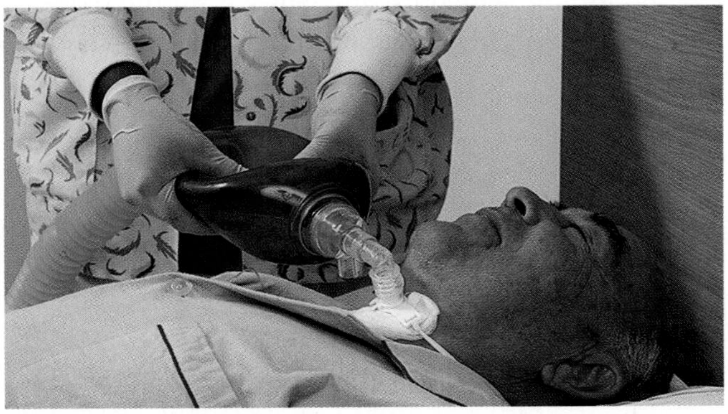

FIGURE 41–26 The Ambu bag. A nurse compresses it with two hands.

BOX 41–7 Principles and Safety Measures for Suctioning

- If suctioning is within the support worker's scope of practice in your province or territory and at your agency, you should be taught the correct way to do it by a nurse or a respiratory technologist.
- Review the procedure with your supervisor (a nurse). Know what is expected of you.
- Suctioning is done as needed (prn). Coughing and signs and symptoms of respiratory distress signal the need for suctioning. Your supervisor will tell you what signs to look for.
- Standard Practices should be followed. Secretions can contain blood and are potentially infectious.
- In some circumstances, sterile technique must be used (see Chapter 23).
- Your supervisor will tell you the size and type of catheter to collect (**FIGURE 41–27**). Airway injury can occur if the catheter is too large.
- Needed suction equipment and supplies should be kept at the bedside so that they are readily available when the client needs suctioning.
- When suction is applied, air is sucked out of the airway, so suction should not be applied while inserting the catheter.
- The catheter is cleaned with water or saline after removal.

Continued

BOX 41–7 Principles and Safety Measures for Suctioning—cont'd

- The catheter should be inserted smoothly to prevent injury to the mucous membranes.
- The suction catheter should be passed (inserted) no more than three times. The risk for injury increases each time the catheter is passed.
- When suctioning, ***you should not suction any deeper than the client's oral cavity. This means that the catheter should not go past the back of the client's teeth (or the gum area).*** Suctioning near the client's epiglottis can trigger a strong gag reaction. Suctioning that far back is allowed in deep suctioning, which usually falls within the scope of practice only of nurses or respiratory technicians.
- Check the client's pulse, respirations, and pulse oximeter readings before, during, and after the procedure. Also observe the level of consciousness. Tell your supervisor immediately if any of the following occur:
  - A drop in pulse rate, or a pulse rate less than 60 beats per minute
  - Irregular cardiac rhythms
  - A drop or rise in blood pressure
  - Respiratory distress
  - A drop in the SpO_2 (see p. 946)

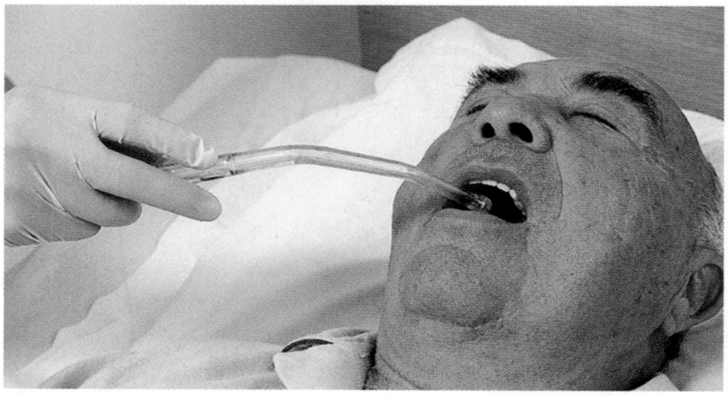

FIGURE 41–27 The Yankauer suction catheter (also called a *tonsil suction*) is often used when there are large amounts of thick secretions.

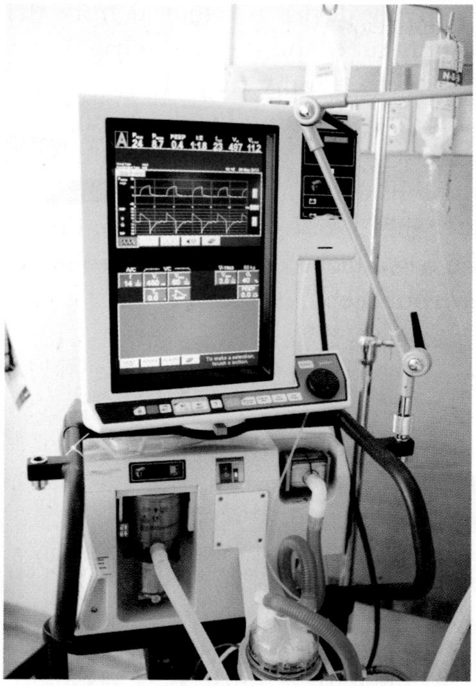

FIGURE 41–28 A mechanical ventilator. (**Source:** Happy Together/Shutterstock.com)

MECHANICAL VENTILATION

In the case of some severe problems, a client may not be able to breathe, or normal blood oxygen levels are not maintained. These problems include (1) hypoxia caused by weak muscle effort, airway obstruction, and damaged lung tissue; (2) nervous system diseases and injuries that can affect the respiratory centre, interfering with messages between the lungs and the brain; and (3) drug overdoses that can depress the brain's hypothalamus or the breathing control centre. In these situations, mechanical ventilation may be needed to save the client's life. **Mechanical ventilation** is the use of a machine to move air into and out of the lungs (**FIGURE 41–28**), allowing O_2 to enter the lungs and CO_2 to leave them. ***It is your responsibility to ensure that assisting with mechanical ventilation is within your scope of practice for your province or territory and your agency.***

Mechanical ventilation is always initiated in a hospital. Some people need it for a few hours or days, while others need it for longer. Clients requiring mechanical ventilation will have a **ventilator** attached to some form of artificial airway, such as an ET tube or a tracheostomy tube.

BOX 41–8 Guidelines for Caring for Clients Receiving Mechanical Ventilation

- Keep the call bell within reach (in facilities).
- Make sure hoses and connecting tubing have slack. They must not pull on the artificial airway.
- Answer call bells promptly. The client is in a situation in which she must depend on others for basic needs.
- Explain who you are and what you are going to do whenever you enter the room.
- Give the day, date, and time every time you give care.
- Report signs of respiratory distress or discomfort at once.
- Do not change settings on the machine or reset alarms.
- Follow the care plan for communication. Since the client cannot talk, use agreed-upon hand or eye signals for "yes" and "no." All health care team members must use the same signals, or confusion, not communication, may occur. Some clients may be able to use paper and pencil, magic slates, communication boards, or hand signals to communicate. Follow the care plan.
- Ask questions that have simple answers. It may be hard for the client to write long responses.
- Watch what you say and do, whether you are near or away from the client and family. They pay close attention to your verbal and nonverbal communication. Do not say anything that could upset them.
- Provide comfort and reassurance by talking to the client. It is also comforting when you talk about seemingly "light" topics such as the weather, pleasant news events, gifts, and cards.
- Meet the client's basic needs. Follow the care plan.
- Use touch to reassure and comfort the client.
- Tell the client when you are leaving the room and when you will return.

Clients needing mechanical ventilation are very ill or have other problems and injuries. Some are confused or disoriented or cannot think clearly. Many are frightened by the machine and by thoughts of dying. Some feel relieved to get enough oxygen. Many fear the prospect of needing the machine for life. Mechanical ventilation can be painful for those who have chest injuries or have had chest surgery. Tubes and hoses restrict movement and can cause more discomfort.

Follow the guidelines in **BOX 41–8** if you are providing care for a client on mechanical ventilation. In such a situation, your supervisor (usually a nurse) would have to show you how to connect the ET or tracheostomy tube to the ventilator in case of an emergency. Ventilators have alarms that sound when something is wrong—for example, the client gets disconnected from the ventilator. When any alarm sounds, ***first check to see if the client's tube is attached to the ventilator. If it is not, attach it to the ventilator. The client can die if not connected to the ventilator.*** Then tell your supervisor at once about the alarm. ***You should never reset alarms.***

FOCUS ON HOME CARE

Mechanical Ventilation

Home care is often arranged for clients receiving mechanical ventilation. Portable ventilators are used in home care. A nurse will teach you how to care for each client. Family members are also taught how to assist with the client's care. Always make sure that a nurse is available by phone when you are in the client's home.

Often, clients need to be weaned from the ventilator. That is, clients gradually need to breathe without the ventilator. Weaning can take many weeks. A physician, respiratory therapist, and nurse plan the weaning process. (See the *Focus on Home Care: Mechanical Ventilation* box.)

CHEST TUBES

Air, blood, or fluid can collect in the pleural space (sac or cavity) when the chest has been penetrated because of injury or surgery. A **chest tube** is a hollow plastic tube surgically inserted into the chest cavity, which allows for the removal of trapped air (*pneumothorax*) and the drainage of blood or fluid (*hemothorax* or *pleural effusion*).

- ***Pneumothorax*** is air (*pneumo*) in the pleural space (*thorax*).
- ***Hemothorax*** is blood (*hemo*) in the pleural space (*thorax*).
- ***Pleural effusion*** is the escape and collection of fluid (*effusion*) in the pleural space (*pleural*).

Air, blood, or fluid collecting in the pleural sac causes pressure, which makes the lungs collapse. Therefore, air does not reach affected alveoli, and O_2 and CO_2 are not exchanged, resulting in respiratory distress and hypoxia. Sometimes, the accumulated pressure is great enough to threaten the heart's ability to pump blood, and the situation becomes life threatening. Hospital care is required in these cases. A physician inserts the chest tube to remove the air, fluid, or blood (**FIGURE 41–29**). After the client's condition has been stabilized, the client may need rehabilitation or subacute care.

Chest tubes attach to connecting tubing, which, in turn, attaches to a tube in a drainage container (**FIGURE 41–30**). This drainage system must be airtight to prevent air from entering the pleural space. Sometimes suction is applied to the drainage system. You may be asked to assist a nurse with the client's care. Follow the guidelines in **BOX 41–9**.

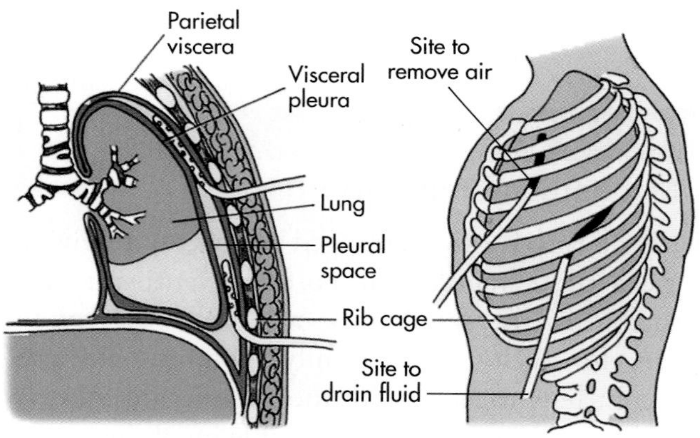

FIGURE 41–29 Chest tubes inserted into the pleural space. (**Source:** Perry, A.G., Potter, P.A., & Ostendorf, W.R. (2014). *Clinical nursing skills & techniques* (8th ed., p. 657). St. Louis, MO: Mosby.)

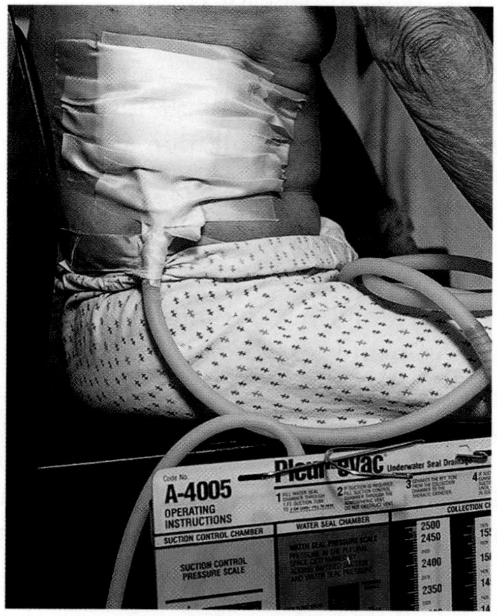

FIGURE 41–30 Chest tubes attached to a disposable water-seal drainage system. (**Source:** Perry, A.G., Potter, P.A., & Ostendorf, W.R. (2014). *Clinical nursing skills & techniques* (8th ed., p. 656). St. Louis, MO: Mosby.)

BOX 41–9 Guidelines for Caring for Clients With Chest Tubes

- Keep the drainage system below the level of the client's chest.
- Check vital signs, as directed. Report vital sign changes at once.
- Report signs and symptoms of hypoxia, complaints of pain, difficulty breathing, and respiratory distress at once.
- Keep connecting tubing coiled on the bed. Allow enough slack so the chest tubes are not dislodged when the client moves. If tubing hangs in loops, drainage collects in the loop.
- Prevent tubing kinks, which can obstruct the chest tube, causing air, blood, or fluid to collect in the pleural space.
- Observe chest drainage. Report any change in chest drainage at once, including increases in drainage or the appearance of bright red drainage.
- Record chest drainage according to employer policy.
- Turn and reposition the client, as directed. Be careful and gentle to prevent chest tubes from dislodging.
- Assist the client with coughing and deep-breathing exercises, as directed.
- Assist with incentive spirometry, as directed.
- Note any bubbling in the drainage system. Tell your supervisor at once if bubbling increases, decreases, or stops.
- Tell your supervisor at once if any part of the system is loose or disconnected.
- Keep sterile petrolatum gauze at the bedside. It is needed if a chest tube comes out.
- Call for help at once if a chest tube comes out. Cover the insertion site with sterile petrolatum gauze. Stay with the client. Then follow the nurse's directions.

CHAPTER REVIEW

KEY POINTS

- Oxygen is a basic necessity of life. Death occurs within minutes if breathing stops, and serious illnesses can occur without enough oxygen.
- Factors affecting oxygen needs include (1) respiratory system status, (2) cardiovascular system status, (3) red blood cell count, (4) nervous system function, (5) aging, (6) exercise, (7) fever, (8) pain, (9) drug (narcotic or barbiturate) overdose, (10) smoking, (11) allergies, (12) pollutant exposure, (13) nutrition, and (14) alcohol.
- Normal adults take 12 to 20 breaths per minute on average. Tachypnea is rapid breathing (24 breaths or more per minute), and bradypnea is slow breathing (12 or fewer breaths per minute).
- All health care workers should be familiar with the signs and symptoms of hypoxia and must know to report them to the supervisor.
- You can promote oxygenation through (1) proper positioning and frequent rest periods and (2) encouraging coughing and deep breathing.
- As a support worker, you must be familiar with oxygen therapy and aware of the scope of practice for support workers in your province or territory.
- You may be responsible for *assisting with* oxygenation assessment (such as pulse oximetry) and diagnostic testing (such as collecting sputum samples).
- If it is within your scope of practice in your province or territory, you may be asked to support a client who (1) has a tracheostomy, (2) may need suctioning, (3) is mechanically ventilated, or (4) has a chest tube.

CRITICAL THINKING IN PRACTICE

You are a student training in the clinical setting. You are helping a support worker transfer a resident to a wheelchair. The support worker asks you to connect the person's nasal cannula to the portable O_2 tank and turn it on to 2 L/min. Support workers in your agency are not allowed to adjust O_2 flow rates. How will you respond? What will you do if the support worker adjusts the flow rate?

REVIEW QUESTIONS

Answers to these questions are at the bottom of page 960.

Circle the BEST answer.

1. Alcohol and narcotics affect oxygen needs because they:
   A. Depress the breathing centre in the brain
   B. Are pollutants
   C. Cause allergies
   D. Cause a pneumothorax
2. Hypoxia is:
   A. The lack of oxygen
   B. Not enough oxygen in the cells
   C. Not enough oxygen in the blood
   D. The amount of hemoglobin that contains oxygen
3. An early sign of hypoxia is:
   A. Dysphasia
   B. Cyanosis
   C. Restlessness
   D. Decreased pulse and respiratory rates
4. A client can breathe deeply and comfortably only while sitting. This state is called:
   A. Bradypnea
   B. Orthopnea
   C. Biot's respirations
   D. Kussmaul's respirations
5. Which of the following is a sign of altered respiratory function?
   A. Joint pain
   B. Nausea and vomiting
   C. Severe abdominal pain
   D. Wheezing or crowing sounds
6. A client's SpO_2 is 98%. Which of the following is true?
   A. The client needs suctioning.
   B. The pulse oximeter is wrong.
   C. The client's pulse is 98 beats per minute.
   D. The measurement is within normal range.

7. Which of the following is a common site for a pulse oximetry sensor?
   A. Wrist
   B. Index finger
   C. Upper arm
   D. Second toe

8. The best time to collect sputum is:
   A. On awakening
   B. After meals
   C. At bedtime
   D. After suctioning

9. A sputum specimen is needed. You should ask the client to:
   A. Use mouthwash
   B. Brush the teeth
   C. Apply lubricant to the lips
   D. Rinse the mouth with clear water

10. You are assisting a client with coughing and deep breathing. Which of the following is true?
    A. The client exhales through pursed lips.
    B. The client should do this just after eating.
    C. The client exhales deeply through the nose.
    D. The client needs to be in a comfortable lying position.

11. Which of the following is useful for deep breathing?
    A. Chest tubes
    B. Pulse oximeter
    C. Incentive spirometer
    D. Partial-rebreather mask

12. You are assisting with oxygen therapy. You can:
    A. Start the oxygen
    B. Decide what device to use
    C. Turn the oxygen on and off
    D. Keep the connecting tubing secure and free of kinks

13. A client has a tracheostomy. Which of the following is true?
    A. The outer cannula is removed for cleaning
    B. The obturator is inserted after the outer cannula
    C. The outer cannula must be secured in place
    D. The client is rarely at risk for aspiration

14. A client who has a tracheostomy can do the following:
    A. Sing
    B. Shave
    C. Shower
    D. Swim

15. A client has a tracheostomy. For the client's safety, the old ties are removed after:
    A. The stoma is cleaned
    B. The dressing is removed
    C. The inner cannula is removed
    D. The outer cannula is held in place

16. These statements are about suctioning. Which one is true?
    A. You can perform the procedure without wearing gloves.
    B. Suctioning is done every 2 hours.
    C. Suction is applied while inserting the catheter.
    D. A suction cycle is no more than 10 to 15 seconds.

17. Chest tubes:
    A. Insert air into the lungs
    B. Remove trapped air from the chest cavity
    C. Are artificial airways
    D. Provide mechanical ventilation for the client

18. Which of the following is used to hyperventilate the lungs?
    A. Ambu bag
    B. Pulse oximeter
    C. Incentive spirometer
    D. Partial-rebreather mask

19. Mr. Long requires mechanical ventilation. Which of the following is true?
    A. He cannot move.
    B. His call bell is useless right now.
    C. You can reset alarms on the ventilator.
    D. He has an endo-tracheal (ET) tube or a tracheostomy tube.

20. An alarm sounds on Mr. Long's ventilator. What should you do first?
A. Reset the alarm
B. Ask him what is wrong
C. Call your supervisor immediately
D. Check to see if his airway is attached to the ventilator

21. A client has a pneumothorax, which is the collection of:
A. Air in the pleural space
B. Blood in the pleural space
C. Fluid in the pleural space
D. Respiratory secretions in the pleural space

22. Chest tubes are attached to a disposable water-seal drainage system. You should do the following:
A. Encourage the client to stay in bed
B. Hang the tubing in as straight a line as possible
C. Keep the drainage system below the client's chest
D. Re-insert the tubing if it is accidentally disconnected

Answers: 1.A, 2.B, 3.C, 4.B, 5.D, 6.D, 7.B, 8.A, 9.D, 10.A, 11.C, 12.D, 13.C, 14.B, 15.D, 16.D, 17.B, 18.A, 19.D, 20.D, 21.A, 22.C

CHAPTER 42

Home Management

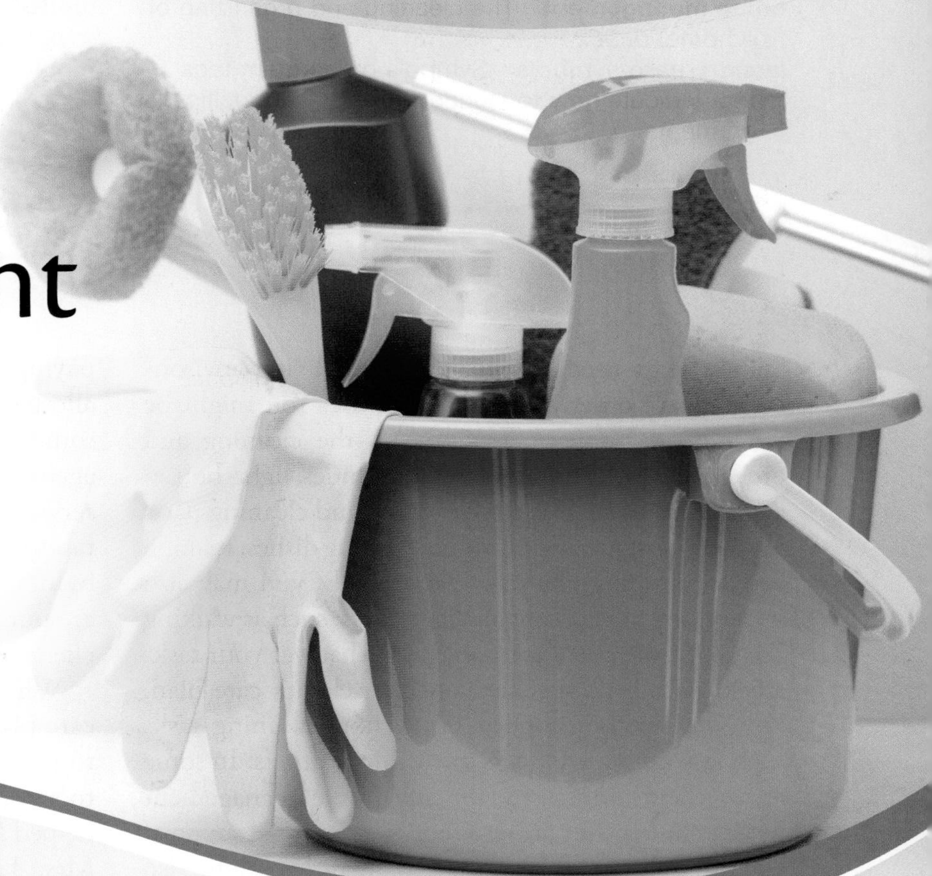

OBJECTIVES

After reading this chapter, the learner should be able to do the following:

- Describe why home management is important.
- Explain the support worker's role in home management.
- Describe the support worker's role in handling clients' money.
- Explain how to use cleaning supplies safely.
- Describe how to clean bedrooms, living rooms, bathrooms, and kitchens.
- Describe how to do laundry properly.
- Differentiate between the various laundry care symbols.

KEY TERMS

home management The cleaning and organizing of a home. *p. 962*
laundry care symbols Symbols on garment tags that indicate how to launder or care for specific garments. *p. 974*
mildew The black discoloration caused by mould. *p. 972*
mould A microscopic fungal parasite. *p. 972*

Some clients need help keeping their living environment clean, orderly, healthy, and safe. You might be assigned to **home management**—the cleaning and organizing of a home—which includes light housekeeping tasks, such as straightening and cleaning parts of rooms, vacuuming, dusting, washing dishes, making beds, and doing laundry. Occasionally, you may also be required to take care of clients' pets, such as walking the dog if the client is unable to. Whatever your tasks are, they will be specified on each client's care plan. You will not be assigned heavy housecleaning tasks such as washing windows or cleaning carpets. In some areas, clients must pay for any home management services unless they are also receiving personal support.

Hospitals and long-term care facilities might also have support workers do basic housekeeping tasks. However, most facilities have a housekeeping staff. This chapter focuses on home management in community care settings.

YOUR ROLE IN HOME MANAGEMENT

A clean and orderly setting is important for health and safety. Dust, dirt, and damp areas promote the growth of microbes, and clutter can cause falls and serious injury. People who have illnesses or disabilities, those recovering from surgery or injuries, new parents, caregivers tending to sick family members, and older adults may not be able to do regular housekeeping.

Who Pays for What Services?

The client, family, and case manager decide what household tasks need to be done and list them in the client's care plan. Clients are usually responsible for paying for these services out of the money they are allotted for home care. In some circumstances and in some provinces and territories, however, the funding agency is billed directly by the agency providing the services, without the client's involvement. Whereas tasks such as regular cleaning and laundry are funded by home care services, some tasks, such as pet care, are not funded and so are paid for separately by the client or family.

While you must complete the tasks listed in the care plan, there will be occasions that you will have to prioritize tasks. For example, one of your tasks is to straighten and clean the bathroom after you have helped Mrs. Jacob with personal care. However, since Mrs. Jacob is incontinent of urine, you need to provide skin care and help her change into clean clothes. The client's immediate personal care needs take priority.

Whatever the household task, remember the principles of compassionate care (see the *Providing Compassionate Care: Home Management* box).

Assisting the Client With Tasks Involving Their Money

As a support worker, you may occasionally be required to accompany your client to do personal banking, buy groceries, or pay bills. When assisting your client with these tasks, you should keep the following points in mind:

- This duty must be clearly written in the client's care plan and must follow the policies of your employing agency. The care plan should specify *exactly* what your responsibilities are. Some clients with severe arthritis, for example, may just need

Providing Compassionate Care
Home Management

- ***Dignity*** is the state of feeling worthy, valued, and respected. All people deserve a neat, clean, peaceful setting, but illness, disability, surgery, or injury may limit a person's ability to clean. Helping with home management promotes comfort, emotional well-being, and dignity. Treat your client's home and belongings with respect and care.
- ***Independence*** is the state of not depending on others for control or authority. For some clients, accepting help means a loss of control. Respect your client's wishes for independence and control. As they recover, some clients gradually assume responsibility for home management. Occupational therapists help some clients learn new ways to perform household tasks. For example, Mr. Ho, who had an arm amputated, is trying to make his bed using techniques he learned in occupational therapy, but his progress is slow. Do not make the bed for him. Be patient, and praise him for trying and for the amount of work he has done.
- ***Preferences*** are the rights to select or the act of selecting someone or something over another or others. Follow your client's preferred methods for household tasks, which will be listed in the care plan. Respect that all people have different preferences and standards. For example, Mrs. Neal may not show any interest in having a neat bedroom, but she may not tolerate even a tiny stain on her blouse. Use the client's preferred cleaning products—for example, a client may use vinegar and water instead of a commercial floor cleaning product.
- ***Privacy*** is the state of being free from unsanctioned intrusion, as well as the degree to which an individual can determine which personal information is to be shared with whom and for what purpose. It is one of the most important and comprehensive of all human rights, and yet it is one of the hardest to protect.

  Some clients or families may view your presence as an intrusion. Find out if there are any areas of the home that the client considers private or "off limits" to you. If there are rooms, parts of rooms, or items that a client does not want touched or cleaned, respect these wishes. Never judge or criticize a client's housekeeping standards. Never talk to others about the cleanliness of a client's house. Doing so would be unprofessional and unethical.
- ***Safety*** is the state of being free from actual, threatened, or imagined danger, risk, or injury. Some cleaning solutions have WHMIS labels (see Chapter 22). Read these and other product labels carefully. Follow all use and storage instructions. Do not let people walk on mopped floors, which may be slippery and cause a fall. Put away buckets and cleaning solutions when you are finished with them. Store cleaning solutions out of reach of children and adults with dementia. Clear away clutter. If the client's safety is at risk, talk to your supervisor.

assistance with handling their money because they cannot hold it without dropping it. Others may need you to pick up some groceries and provide an account of the purchases.

- Your supervisor should be able to answer any questions that you might have about your agency's policies regarding financial responsibilities.
- You should not agree to anything that is not specified on your client's care plan. If you have any concerns or questions, consult your supervisor.
- All money that you handle should be recorded in the appropriate manner. Some agencies, for example, record all transactions on a page to which the support worker is required to attach receipts. When you are given money to purchase an item, you will be responsible to record how much cash was given to you and the amount of change that you are returning. You should be aware of your particular responsibilities in this matter.
- Always provide receipts for any transaction that you did on your client's behalf. If your agency's policy is to notify your supervisor before and after banking, you should do so promptly.

- Remember that the client's personal identification number (PIN) and bank account numbers are private, and you should NOT have access to them. If the client has difficulty typing in the numbers, for example, a banking associate should be asked to do so. You should step far enough away that you do not hear the numbers.
- Many agencies do not allow support workers to assist the client in doing personal banking and, instead, request that family members (or a court-appointed representative) take on this responsibility. This policy protects support workers from being accused in the case of any money being lost. However, if you are self-employed and are asked to assist the client with personal banking or shopping, you will not have a supervisor to contact if a situation arises. It is important that you have a clear understanding of what your expected duties are and that you keep very accurate records of what you have done and where the client has put her money.

Supporting Mrs. Yeung: Conflicting Home Management Demands

Rosa's client, Mrs. Yeung, 67, is recovering from heart surgery. Mrs. Yeung asks Rosa to wash the bathroom floor. Rosa explains that the care plan does not specify washing the floor, but Mrs. Yeung is upset because she wants the floor washed.

Mrs. Yeung tells Rosa that she feels too ill to clean her house and wants Rosa to do it for her. Rosa explains that she must be on time for her next appointment and suggests that Mrs. Yeung voice this need to the case manager. Rosa shows that she cares by listening and offering a means to a solution to Mrs. Yeung, who regains her composure. Rosa reports the matter to her supervisor.

Dealing With Conflicting Demands

Many people have set routines and want things done in certain ways. However, because of time constraints or for health and safety reasons, it may not be possible for you to follow the set procedure. Or you may have to deal with conflicting demands if the care plan says one thing but the client wants something different (see the *Supporting Mrs. Yeung: Conflicting Home Management Demands* and *Supporting Mrs. Washington: Part 1: Using the Client's Home Equipment Safely* boxes). Listen to your client, but if a conflict arises between the client's preferences and the care plan, discuss the conflict with your supervisor. Also, discuss with your supervisor any complaints the client may have.

GETTING ORGANIZED

Usually, home management tasks are assigned in addition to personal care and other tasks. The key to completing home management tasks as well as your other duties is to use your time wisely. Review the time management skills described in Chapter 7. Follow the guidelines in **BOX 42–1** and these general points:

- ***Set priorities.*** Follow the care plan. Do the most important tasks first.
- ***Set a routine.*** Discuss the routine with your client. Agreeing on the routine will help you manage your time.
- ***Gather all supplies beforehand.*** By doing so, you will avoid wasting time and energy.
- ***Use your time well.*** Start with tasks that have waiting periods or that run automatically. For example, if laundry and personal care activities are on your list, start the laundry first. Leave soiled linens to soak while you help your client with the bath.
- ***Finish tasks, and put items away.*** Finish tasks that you have started. After finishing, put all items away in their proper places.
- ***Set time limits for each task.*** Having a time limit helps you stay organized and finish on time.
- ***Focus on the task.*** Do not let your mind wander. For example, do not carelessly wipe a counter while talking to your client. Focus on the person first. Then clean the counter properly.
- ***Put the client's needs first.*** Remember your first priority is to promote the client's comfort, well-being, and safety. Follow the care plan.

Supporting Mrs. Washington: Part 1: Using the Client's Home Equipment Safely

Ida Washington is an 82-year-old woman who lives alone in her own home. Last month, Mrs. Washington fell down her front steps and broke her hip. She requires weekly support worker assistance with her bath, grocery shopping, laundry, and light housework, as she does not have anybody else who can help her. You are the support worker who was assigned to Mrs. Washington.

Mrs. Washington is very happy to have assistance with bathing, shopping, and housecleaning, but she is very particular about how her laundry is done. She uses a very old washing machine to wash her clothes, and she hangs her wet laundry outside to dry on a clothesline. She does have an electric clothes dryer, but she uses it only in the wintertime.

On your first day, Mrs. Washington explains that she wants her clothing separated by colour and washed in her washing machine. She gives you instructions on how to wash her clothing, and you notice that her instructions differ from those on the care labels on some items. As well, you are unfamiliar with her brand of washing machine and are nervous about operating it safely. What should you do?

BOX 42–1 Cleaning Guidelines

- ***Clear away clutter.*** Put items in their proper places. Nothing should be on the floor or counter unless it belongs there. Do not leave items on stairs or in high-traffic areas. Ask the client where things belong. If the client does not know, place items neatly out of the way, and tell the client where you put them. Check with the client before throwing anything away, as even a scrap of paper may be important.
- ***Work from higher to lower.*** Begin in higher areas and work your way to the bottom. Dust and dirt from higher surfaces fall on lower surfaces. For example, when vacuuming stairs, start at the top of the stairs and work down to the bottom.
- ***Work from far to near.*** For example, when wiping a kitchen counter, make brisk strokes from the back to the front. When washing a floor, start at the far end of the room and work toward the door.
- ***Work from dry to wet.*** Begin with rooms and areas without sinks, tubs, showers, and toilets, and then clean bathrooms and kitchens. Sweep the floors before washing them.
- ***Work from cleanest to dirtiest.*** This helps avoid contaminating clean areas with microbes from a dirtier area. For example, wipe the cleanest part of the counter first. Clean the area used for food preparation last.
- ***Change cleaning cloths and water frequently.*** Do not wait for these to become visibly dirty before changing them. Use fresh cloths for each task. For example, use one cloth for dusting and another for wiping counters.
- ***Use a damp cloth for dusting.*** The moisture in a damp cloth picks up dust, whereas a dry cloth simply stirs the dust around.
- ***Rinse and dry washed surfaces.*** Rinsing removes soapy residue and drying removes dampness.
- ***Avoid soiling a clean area.*** For example, do not walk on a washed floor until it is dry.

EQUIPMENT AND SUPPLIES

Many cleaning agencies will bring their own cleaning equipment and supplies. However, it is the policy of many home care support agencies that, when cleaning is required, the support worker will use the client's equipment and supplies. Some homes have appropriate cleaning equipment and supplies, but not all. The following items are needed for cleaning. Clean and store items after use.

Equipment

- ***Clean rags, sponges, cloths, or paper towels.*** After use, wash rags, sponges, and cloths in hot, soapy water. Hang them to air-dry, or dry them in a dryer.
- ***Broom, dustpan, and brush.*** After use, shake the broom and brush into a large, moistened bag. Wipe the dustpan with a damp cloth.
- ***Microfibre dusting, mopping, and sweeping tools.*** Microfibre tools are highly effective, and many clients (and cleaning agencies) prefer them to the more traditional cleaning tools. These products are sold under a number of trade names, including Swiffer.
- ***Mop and bucket.*** Wash and rinse both after use.
- ***Toilet brush.*** Rinse in a bucket of cold water. Flush the water down the toilet.
- ***Utility gloves.*** Wash in hot, soapy water, and hang to dry.
- ***Vacuum cleaner.*** Use the right attachments to clean carpets and upholstery. Follow manufacturer's instructions. Replace filter bags as needed. Make sure the cord and plug are in good repair.
- ***Dishwashing materials.*** After use, clean all the cloths, sponges, scouring pads, and brushes.

Supplies

- ***Detergents***—for laundry and dishwashing
- ***All-purpose cleaners***—for counters, floors, and other surfaces
- ***Glass cleaners***—for mirrors
- ***Special cleaners***—for bathrooms, toilets, mirrors, ovens, and so on
- ***Cleansers and scouring powders***—for scrubbing
- ***Disinfectants***—to destroy pathogens. (There are many disinfectants available for home surface use. Bleach can be used as a laundry disinfectant but must be used ***with caution*** because it can damage fabrics.)
- ***Baking soda***—to eliminate refrigerator odours, counter stains, and so on
- ***White vinegar***—can be used to clean mirrors (Mix one part white vinegar to three parts water.)

If supplies and equipment are lacking, you may have to clean with what the client has on hand. Use your problem-solving skills (see the *Supporting Mrs. Washington: Part 2: Finding Safe Cleaning Product Alternatives* box).

USING CLEANING PRODUCTS SAFELY

Cleaning products can cause harm if not used and stored properly. Remember the following points:

- ***Read all labels carefully.*** Follow manufacturers' instructions. Be familiar with the WHMIS hazard labels (see Chapter 22).
- ***Never mix cleaning products.*** Some products contain chemicals that create poisonous fumes when mixed. Mixing anything containing bleach and ammonia, for example, produces a deadly gas called chlorine. Remember to read product labels and to follow the instructions on the container.
- ***Choose cleaning products that are safest to use.*** Many people have sensitivities or allergies to scents or to the products themselves, so avoid highly scented products or harsh chemicals.
- ***Wear utility gloves when using cleaning products.*** Do not use disposable gloves. They are too thin and can easily puncture; therefore, they would not protect you from harsh chemicals.
- ***Use caution when using cleaning products and chemicals to avoid splashing.*** If any chemical does splash and land on your skin (or in your eye), you should know how to treat it; therefore, you should always read the label *before* you use the product. ***Report any splashes to your supervisor.***
- ***Never use products in unlabelled containers.***
- ***Store products in their original containers.***
- ***Keep cleaning products away from food.***
- ***Keep cleaning products out of reach of children and away from adults with dementia.***

Supporting Mrs. Washington: Part 2: Finding Safe Cleaning Product Alternatives

You arrive at Mrs. Washington's house, ready to assist with her bathing and to clean her bathroom afterward. While gathering the necessary equipment, you notice that Mrs. Washington has cloths and paper towels but no cleaners. She also does not have a floor mop. At most agencies (including your new agency), the policy is to try to find cleaning substitutes before calling the office.

You are able to locate a bottle of white vinegar in the kitchen and make a cleaning solution with water and vinegar in a bucket. You use this mixture to clean the bathroom. You decide that because Mrs. Washington's bathroom is small, you can wash her floor using a cloth and the vinegar-and-water solution. Later, you report your actions to your supervisor, and you identify what supplies are needed at Mrs. Washington's house. Your supervisor tells you that she is pleased that you were resourceful in finding alternative cleaning solutions and did not skip cleaning Mrs. Washington's bathroom just because she did not have name-brand cleansers. Your supervisor then asks if you can think of a way to make your own "mop" in case of a similar situation in the future.

- ***Use products only for their intended purpose.*** Some products can harm the surfaces you are trying to clean!
- ***Keep aerosol cans away from heat sources.***
- ***Ask the client before using a strong cleaner on a surface.***
- ***Rinse strong, abrasive cleaners immediately after use.***
- ***Do not scrub vigorously.*** You could damage a delicate surface.

CLEANING BEDROOMS, LIVING ROOMS, KITCHENS, AND BATHROOMS

Clients' living habits vary. Some use their living rooms infrequently, while others may eat and sleep in the living room. Some clients spend all their time in bed and even eat their meals in the bedroom. Whatever the situation, all rooms should be kept clean and orderly. Important tasks and supplies for cleaning bedrooms are detailed in **BOX 42–2**. **BOX 42–3** lists the key steps to follow when cleaning bedrooms and living rooms.

Cleaning Kitchens

A clean kitchen is critical to preventing the spread of foodborne illnesses (see Chapter 28). **BOX 42–4** details how to clean the kitchen thoroughly. When cleaning kitchens, remember the following:

- Do not pour dirty or contaminated liquids down the kitchen sink. Flush them down the toilet.
- Use one cloth for counters, another for wiping floors, and another for dishes.
- Use paper towels to dry your hands. Do not dry your hands on a towel used for dishes.
- Change cloths daily or as needed. Wash in bleach (or alternative) and hot water.
- Use paper towels when possible.
- Clean the microwave after every use.
- Do not dispose of soiled diapers in the kitchen garbage.

Cleaning Bathrooms

Bathrooms need special attention because microbes easily grow and spread in damp places, so family members must keep bathrooms clean. Because bathroom surfaces are so low, it is important to practise proper body mechanics (see Chapter 25) at all times when cleaning them. Toilets must be cleaned thoroughly with a disinfectant or toilet bowl cleaner. Wear utility gloves for cleaning toilets. Brushes or sponges used to clean the toilet must not be used for cleaning other areas in the house. **BOX 42–5** lists all the tasks and supplies required for cleaning a bathroom thoroughly.

Since some cleaners can scratch porcelain surfaces, use special cleaners for the bathroom. If they are not

Text continued on page 972

BOX 42–2 Cleaning Bedrooms

Task	Supplies and Equipment	Process
Make the bed or straighten linens		See Chapter 34.
Change the linens	Sheets Pillowcases Protective sheets or pads Blankets Comforter or bedspread	See Chapter 34.
Straighten the room		Straighten items on bedside table. Remove old magazines and newspapers, used tissues, drinking glasses, and so on (with permission from the client). Place reading material and glasses within reach. Put away clothing, shoes, and other items (with permission from the client). Look for items under and behind the bed. Empty the wastebasket.
Replenish supplies	Pitcher and glass Tissues and toilet paper Other supplies, as necessary	Discard stale water; wash pitcher and glass; and refill pitcher and glass. Replenish other supplies as needed.
Wipe surfaces	Two cloths Hot, soapy water	Wipe doors, doorknobs, and light switches. Dry with dry cloth.
Dust	Damp cloth	Dust all surfaces, including dressers, bookshelves, windowsills, bedside tables, and lamps.
Clean commodes	Toilet bowl cleaner or disinfectant Bucket of hot water Utility gloves Toilet brush or sponge Fresh cloths or paper towels	Wear gloves. Flush contents in the toilet; do not splash. Clean the commode bowl, under the bowl, and under and behind the seat. Clean and dry commode surfaces with fresh cloths or paper towels.
Clean floors	*Depending on floor surface:* Vacuum Broom, dustpan, and brush Mop and bucket of hot, soapy water Damp mop	Vacuum carpet. Sweep and damp-mop the floor. Use dry mop for hardwood floors. Shake area rugs outside and vacuum them.

BOX 42–3 Cleaning Living Rooms

Task	Supplies and Equipment	Process
Straighten the room		Remove clutter and items that could cause falls (with permission from the client). Open windows (if possible) while you are cleaning to rid the room of stale air and odours. Keep windows open while using cleaning supplies in the house. Close windows after you have finished cleaning. Remove dirty dishes and ashtrays. Look under cushions and under furniture arms for food particles and other items. Bundle up old newspapers and place them in the recycling box (or the appropriate place). Sweep or vacuum crumbs off furniture. Plump up cushions.
Replenish supplies	Tissues Other supplies	Provide fresh water, tissues, reading materials, and other supplies.
Wipe surfaces	Two cloths Hot, soapy water	Wipe doors, doorknobs, and light switches. Dry with dry cloth.
Dust	Damp cloth	Dust all furniture, including the television and other electronic equipment.
Clean floors	*Depending on floor surface:* Vacuum cleaner Broom, dustpan, and brush Mop and bucket of hot, soapy water Dry mop	Vacuum the carpet. Sweep and damp-mop the floor. Use dry mop for hardwood floors. Shake area rugs outside and vacuum them.

BOX 42–4 Cleaning Kitchens

Task	Supplies and Equipment	Process
Clean surfaces (counters, stovetop, table)	Hot, soapy water Boiling water Disinfectant Baking soda Cloth or sponge Second cloth or paper towel to dry counter	Wipe surfaces with cloth and hot, soapy water; rinse and dry. Scrub with disinfectant, and rinse with boiling water if the surfaces were in contact with raw poultry, meat, fish, or eggs; dry thoroughly with paper towels. Use baking soda to remove stubborn counter stains. Wipe table (and mats) with cloth and hot soapy water.

Continued

BOX 42–4 Cleaning Kitchens—cont'd

Task	Supplies and Equipment	Process
Clean toasters or toaster ovens		Unplug the toaster, turn it upside down, and shake it gently to remove crumbs. Wipe up the crumbs. Remove crumb tray and wash, if necessary, in warm, soapy water. Dry carefully, and replace in toaster.
Clean microwave oven	Hot, soapy water or diluted vinegar solution on clean cloth or paper towel	Soften grease splatters inside the microwave by placing a cup of water into the microwave and microwaving it on High for 90 seconds. Wash the interior thoroughly, and dry it with a clean cloth or paper towel. (When cooking food in the microwave, remember always to cover the food with a dish or paper towel to prevent splatters.)
Clean cutting boards	Hot, soapy water Boiling water Disinfectant Cloth and dishwashing brush	Wash with hot, soapy water; rinse and pat dry with paper towels. Scrub with disinfectant and rinse with boiling water if the surfaces were in contact with raw poultry, meat, fish, or eggs; dry thoroughly with paper towels.
Wash dishes	Liquid detergent and hot water Dishcloth, scouring pads, or dishwashing brush	Scrape food remnants from dishes. Wash glassware and cups first, then utensils, plates, bowls, pots, and pans. Soak pots and pans in hot water if food is stuck on them. Rinse items well in hot water. Place items in a drainer to dry; air-drying is cleaner than towel-drying.
Use automatic dishwasher	Dishwasher detergent	Read instructions or ask family member to demonstrate use. Scrape large food particles and rinse dishes before loading (**FIGURE 42–1**). Place glasses and cups in washer upside down. Do not stack items on top of one another, as they will not be cleaned properly. Do not put the following in a dishwasher: electrical appliances, delicate glasses, fine china, sharp knives, cast iron, wood, or most plastics. Check with the client before putting pots and pans in the dishwasher. Use only dishwasher detergent; other soaps or detergents will damage the machine.

Continued

BOX 42–4 Cleaning Kitchens—cont'd

Task	Supplies and Equipment	Process
Clean kitchen sinks	Hot, soapy water Scouring powder Boiling water Disinfectant Paper towels	Clean with hot, soapy water and scouring powder. Clean with disinfectant and paper towels if the sink has been used for the preparation of poultry, raw meat, fish, or eggs; pour boiling water down sink after the sink has been cleaned; dry with paper towel. Wipe taps with hot, soapy water; dry with paper towel.
Clean refrigerator	Hot, soapy water Baking soda Cloth or paper towels	Open all containers; discard food items that have expired, do not look fresh, or are more than 2 days old (check with client). (See the *Supporting Mrs. Washington: Part 3: Respecting the Client's Wishes When Cleaning* box.) Remove items from shelves, one shelf at a time; remove shelves and wash with cloth and hot, soapy water; dry with paper towels or a clean cloth; replace items when shelf has been cleaned and dried. Clean the drawers and inside of door. Clean the interior (all surfaces) of the refrigerator. Place a small bowl of baking soda in the refrigerator to absorb odours. Wipe the door of the refrigerator and the handle.
Dispose of waste	Garbage bags Utility gloves Paper towels Hot, soapy water	Wear gloves. Remove and discard garbage; place in garage or throw down apartment chute. Whenever possible, place recyclable items in the proper container. Wash garbage can using paper towels and hot, soapy water. Place a fresh bag in the container. Check with the client on recycling of newspapers, cans, and glass.
Clean kitchen floors	Broom, dustpan, and brush Damp mop Hot, soapy water	Sweep the kitchen floor. Damp-mop the kitchen floor.

Supporting Mrs. Washington: Part 3: Respecting the Client's Wishes When Cleaning

It is now time to clean Mrs. Washington's kitchen. You perform all of the steps in BOX 42–4. While you are cleaning Mrs. Washington's refrigerator, you notice that many of the items in her fridge, such as her processed salad dressings, barbecue sauce, and margarine, are past their expiry dates by several months, and some had even expired the previous year. Before you throw them out, however, you check with Mrs. Washington.

Mrs. Washington seems to be annoyed at your suggestion to throw away some of her food and instructs you to put the items back in her refrigerator. You comply with her instruction and proceed with your duties in a pleasant manner. She does not mention the occurrence again.

You report your concern about the expired foods to your supervisor, and your supervisor, who does not seem shocked by the client's reaction, asks why you think Mrs. Washington is reluctant to throw away the outdated items from her fridge.

available, use laundry detergent (or a small amount of dish soap) or even a vinegar-and-water solution.

The bathrooms of clients who are at high risk for infection—for example, clients recovering from surgery and those undergoing chemotherapy—must be kept very clean. The care plan lists extra measures needed for these clients, such as the following:

- Clean the tub, shower, and sink with the appropriate disinfectant before and after use.
- Use paper towels for drying hands.

Mould and Mildew

Mould is a microscopic fungal parasite, and **mildew** is the black discoloration caused by mould that can cause a foul odour. Surfaces in all rooms should always be dried well to prevent growth of mould and mildew. Surface mould, or small to moderate amounts of mould, can be cleaned with water and dish detergent. Do not use bleach to remove mould. You should wear protective equipment, including waterproof utility gloves, eye protection and a mask when removing mould. If there is a lot of mould present, your supervisor may discuss with the client the need to address the underlying cause. Professional mould abatement specialists may be required to remove extensive mould growth. Sensitive individuals should not be in the same room and may choose to leave the house until the mould is removed.[1]

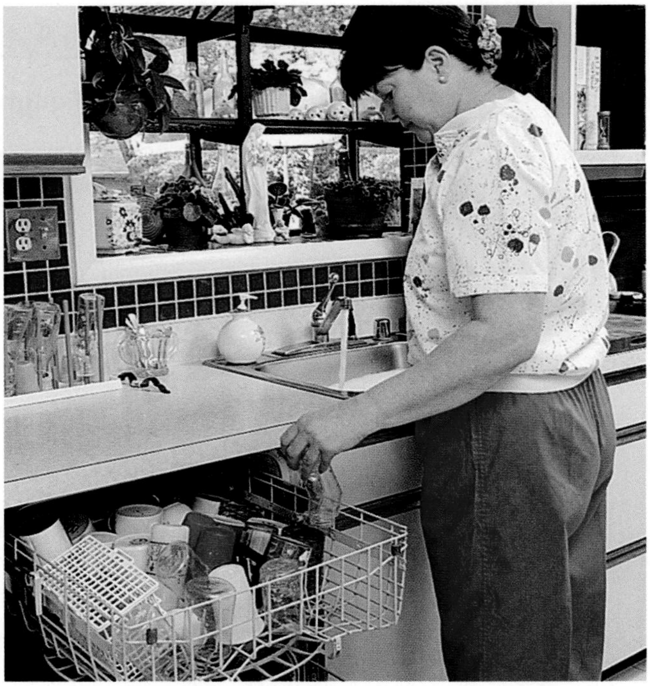

FIGURE 42–1 Some dishwashers require that dishes be rinsed before they are loaded. For all dishwashers, large food chunks and dried food should always be removed before loading.

DOING LAUNDRY

When you are doing laundry, your goal is to clean clothing items without damaging them. Many clients' houses and apartments will have laundry facilities. If not, a laundromat has to be used, and you will need the right amount of change to operate the washing machines and dryers. Find out if the client keeps change for this purpose.

Ask your client (or family member) which detergent, bleach, and fabric softener to use. Also, find

BOX 42–5 Cleaning Bathrooms

Task	Supplies and Equipment	Process
General guidelines and hygiene measures		Rinse and dry bar soaps after use. Flush the toilet with the seat down to prevent splashing and the spread of microbes. Rinse the sink after it has been used for washing, shaving, or oral hygiene. Remove and dispose of hair from the sink, tub, or shower. Hang damp towels and bath mats out to dry, or place them in a hamper. Wash bath mats, the wastebasket, and the laundry hamper every week. Put out clean towels. Wipe up water spills. Wipe out the bathtub or shower immediately after use. Provide enough toilet paper and tissue. Open shower doors to prevent mildew from developing inside the shower. Do not pour dirty or contaminated liquids in the sink. Flush them down the toilet.
Clean sinks	Cloths or sponge Utility gloves Hot, soapy water Disinfectant	Wipe the sink with hot, soapy water and disinfectant. Rinse, and dry with a dry cloth. Wipe and dry taps.
Clean bathtubs, showers, and shower curtains	Cloths or sponge Utility gloves Hot, soapy water Disinfectant	Wipe with hot, soapy water, and disinfect showers and shower curtains. Rinse, and dry with a dry cloth. Wipe and dry taps.
Replenish supplies	Toilet paper Tissues Soap and shampoo Toothpaste Other supplies, as needed	Check and replenish supplies.
Clean surfaces	Cloths or sponge Utility gloves Hot, soapy water Disinfectant	Wipe windowsills, bathroom tiles, soap holders, and door handles with hot, soapy water and disinfectant. Rinse and dry all surfaces.
Clean mirrors	Glass cleaner or white vinegar and water Paper towels	Wipe with paper towels and cleaner. Dry with paper towels.

Continued

BOX 42–5 Cleaning Bathrooms—cont'd

Task	Supplies and Equipment	Process
Clean toilets	Toilet bowl cleaner or disinfectant NEVER use bleach in the toilet bowl, as it could cause a toxic gas to be released Bucket of hot water Utility gloves Toilet brush or sponge Fresh cloths or paper towels	Wear gloves. Clean the toilet tank. Clean the toilet bowl, outside and inside; clean under the bowl and under and behind the seat. Clean and dry the toilet seat, toilet handle, and outer surfaces with fresh cloths or paper towels (FIGURE 42–2).
Clean floors	Bucket of hot, soapy water Disinfectant Utility gloves Mop, cloths, sponge, or vacuum	Clean the floor last. Dry the floor to prevent falls. Vacuum carpeted floors.

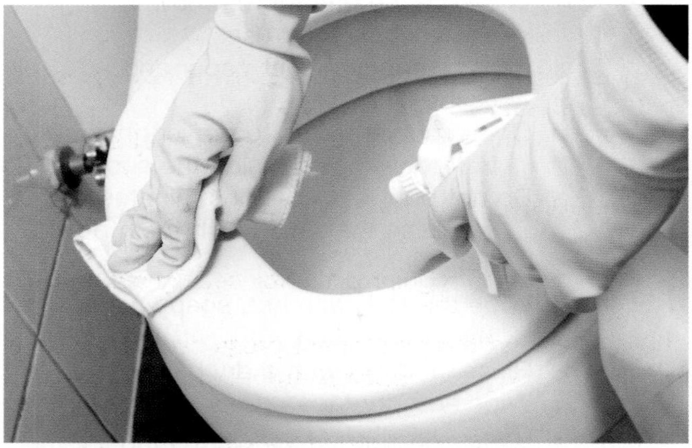

FIGURE 42–2 Preparing to clean the bathroom. Note the use of sturdy utility gloves when using household cleaners. Kneeling on a towel (which will later be washed) will help to prevent transfer of pathogens from the floor to the support worker's clothing. Cleaning items and clean paper towels should also be pulled from the roll and placed within reach before the gloves are contaminated. (**Source:** © Tifonimages | Dreamstime.com.)

out if there are any special laundry instructions. For instance, are garments air-dried or dried in a dryer? Follow your client's preferences. BOX 42–6 describes how to do laundry properly.

Laundry Care Symbols

Most garments have **laundry care symbols** on inside labels that indicate how to care for the garment (FIGURE 42–3). The standard symbols used in Canada since 2003 are consistent with American and international care symbols.[2]

The five basic black-and-white symbols inform consumers of washing, bleaching, drying, ironing, and professional cleaning instructions, with additional information provided using numbers (representing degrees Celsius), dots, and dashes. Other care symbols include those for dry cleaning, washing by hand, and drying naturally.

The five basic symbols are as follows:[2]

- ***The washtub symbol***—tells how to wash or not wash the garment. The water temperature is given in centigrade. The horizontal bars under the washtub symbol show how vigorous a wash cycle can be used—two bars mean use a gentle cycle; one bar means use a permanent press cycle; no bars mean use a normal cycle.
- ***The triangle symbol***—tells if bleach can be used. A blank triangle means any type of bleach can be used. Two diagonal lines in the triangle warn against using chlorine bleach.
- ***The square symbol***—tells how to dry items. A circle inside the square permits the item to go in the dryer. Other lines within the square provide instructions for natural drying (e.g., lay flat, hang to dry).
- ***The iron symbol***—tells if the garment can be ironed and at what temperature.
- ***The circle symbol***—tells if the garment needs to be dry cleaned.

BOX 42–6 Doing Laundry

Task	Process
Gather laundry	Walk through the house and gather items that require washing from hampers or areas specified by the client (for example, the towels on the floor in the bathroom).
Read manufacturer's instructions	Read the instructions on the washer, dryer, and laundry products. Read the garment's care label.
Sort items to be washed	Separate by fabric type. Separate heavily soiled or stained items. Separate any garments that require special care (such as washing by hand or dry cleaning). If unsure about washing or dry cleaning, ask the client. Sort by colour: whites, darks, and coloured fabrics. Close zippers, hooks, and buttons. Check pockets for tissue, change, and other items.
Presoak	Presoak heavily soiled and stained items. Use the hottest water safe for the fabric. Soak in bleach or borax for 30 minutes. See BOX 42–7 for information about removing blood, urine, and fecal stains.
Prewash	Prewash heavily soiled items in a washing machine if it has a prewash cycle or in a bucket, laundry tub, or bathtub if not. Scrub the soiled area by rubbing it together in your hands, and wring out before placing into the washer. Use the recommended amount of detergent. Use the hottest water safe for the fabric.
Select the water temperature and the cycle	Use hot water (54–65°C or 130–150°F) and the regular cycle for heavily soiled clothes, cloth diapers, and whites. Use warm water (38–43°C or 100–110°F) and the permanent press cycle for moderately soiled clothes and permanent press fabrics—for example, nylon, polyester, and acrylic. Use cold water (26–38°C or 80–100°F) for bright colours, fabrics with colours that may run, fragile fabrics, and lightly soiled garments. Use the gentle cycle when the label recommends it. Wash garments with colours that may run (e.g., black or bright reds) separately.
Load the machine	If the machine requires you to select the water level, judge the appropriate level for load size. For example, use a high water level for a full machine. Do not overload the washer. Wash bulky items separately. Use a measuring cup for the detergent (and fabric softener, if client uses liquid softener); follow the directions on the package. If the client has a front-loading washing machine, clean out the rubber gasket to prevent the accumulation of hair and lint. Front-loading washers must be wiped down and the door kept open between loads to prevent mildew accumulation, which would cause foul-smelling clothing.

Continued

BOX 42–6 Doing Laundry—cont'd

Task	Process
Load clothes into the dryer	To avoid the risk for fire, ***remove lint from the filter after each load*** unless using a commercial laundromat. Do not overload the dryer. Determine temperature as per instructions on garment labels. Do not put woollen sweaters or garments that may shrink (see labels) in the dryer; lay these items flat to dry on a towel or clothes rack. Use a sheet of fabric softener (as per client's preferences). Remove garments soon after dryer stops to prevent wrinkling. Remove lint from the filter.
Hang clothes on a clothesline	Check with the client before using clothespins on any article of laundry. Some articles are too delicate and need to be laid flat to dry on a clean towel or clothes rack. Wipe the clothesline down first with a clean, wet cloth to remove accumulated dirt. Clothing dries fastest when it is able to receive direct sunlight, so choose the area of the clothesline that receives sun instead of shade. Shake out each piece of clothing to remove wrinkles prior to hanging it on the line. Place clothespins on the edges of the article to be dried. Do not apply clothespins to the centre of a piece of clothing. Ensure the clothespin is firmly positioned. When the clothing is dry, fold each article as it is removed from the clothesline. Place the article of laundry in a clothes basket. Check garment labels before ironing.
Iron	Use a steam iron for heavily wrinkled clothing. Make sure the iron is hot before using it. After you have finished ironing, be sure to turn off the iron and unplug it. Many older irons do not have an automatic shut-off. Ensure that the hot iron is not in a place where people or pets can accidentally burn themselves.

When doing laundry, remember the following:

- Do not leave wet items in the washer. Moisture can cause mildew.
- If possible, dry items in a dryer rather than hanging them to dry. Quick drying helps eliminate microbes.
- Avoid leaving items in the dryer; doing so can wrinkle or damage the fabric.
- Use the hottest water and the longest wash cycle allowed for the item (see **FIGURE 42–3**).

Laundry Soiled With Body Substances

Soiling from blood, body fluids, secretions, or excretions is an ***infection control issue***. You should always follow employer policy and Standard Practices (see Chapter 23) when handling, transporting, or processing laundry soiled with these substances. Do the following when handling laundry soiled with body substances:

- Practise hand hygiene frequently.
- Wear gloves at all times when handling the soiled laundry. Remove the gloves properly (see Chapter 23) and discard them in the appropriate container.
- Place soiled laundry in leak-proof plastic bags. Secure bags to prevent spillage.
- Keep soiled laundry away from other laundry.
- Double-bag laundry if the outside of the first bag becomes contaminated with body substances.

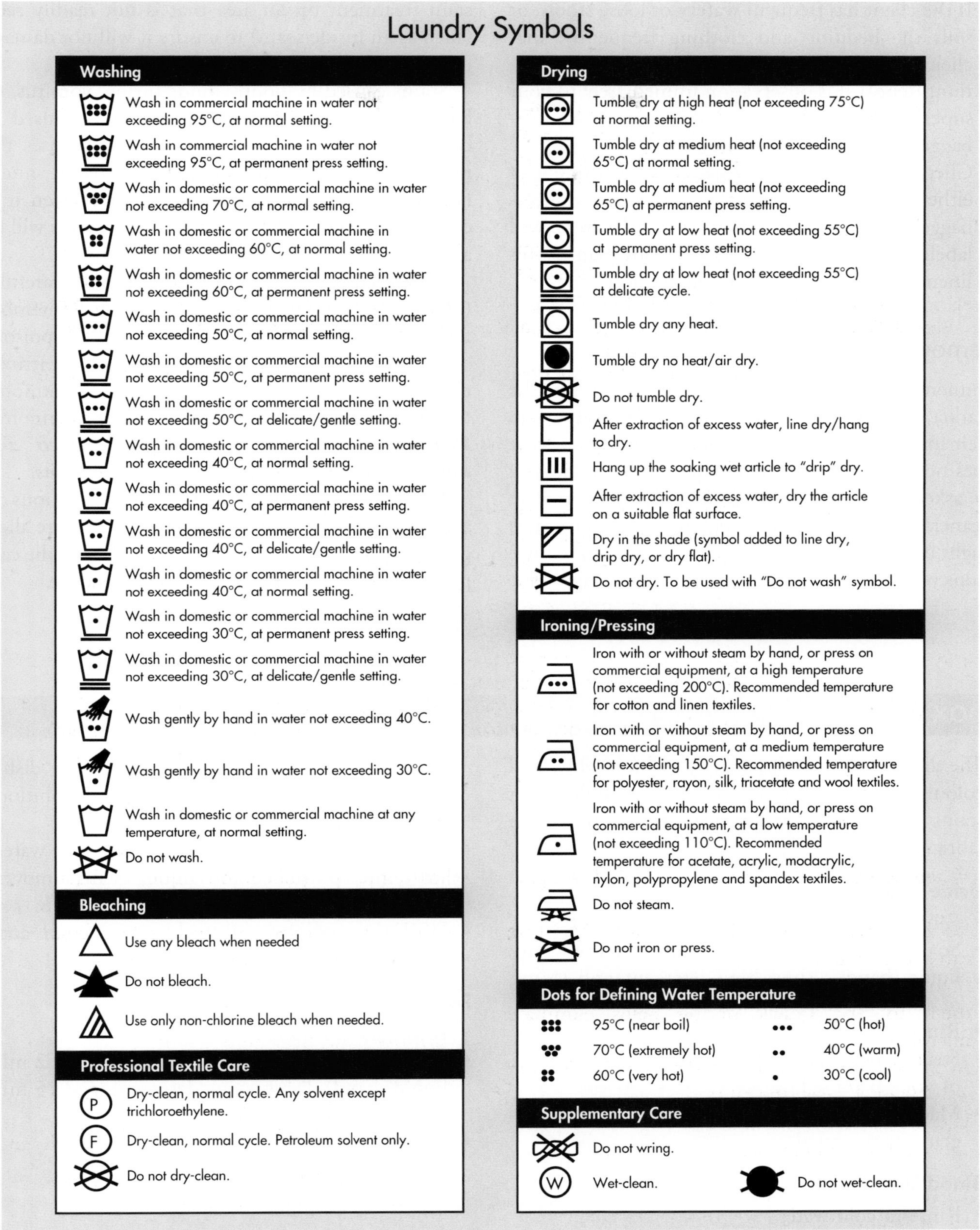

FIGURE 42–3 Laundry symbols. (**Source:** Innovation, Science and Economic Development's Office of Consumer Affairs. (n.d.) *Guide to apparel and textile care symbols.* Retrieved from https://www.ic.gc.ca/eic/site/oca-bc.nsf/eng/ca02009.html.)

- If the client has frequent watery or loose stools, or soils the bedding and clothing frequently, that client may be ill and may require medical attention. Report this observation immediately to your supervisor! Soiled linens should always be double-bagged and labelled as a biohazard.
- Clients on chemotherapy who are incontinent of either urine or feces must have their linens double-bagged separately from all other laundry items and labelled as a biohazard. Check the care plan, as this linen may have special care instructions.

Removing Stains

Numerous stain treatment products are on the market, and most do remove stains effectively when their instructions are followed carefully. If the client does not have any stain-removing products and you are asked to remove stains from clothing, alternative cleaners (such as a paste of baking soda and water) might be useful. You should never attempt to remove stains without the client's permission. Also, apply the stain treatment on an area that is not readily seen (such as an inside seam) to ensure it will not damage that article of clothing.

Stains caused by bodily fluids (urine, vomitus, or blood) or solids (stool) should always be rinsed in cold water. Rinsing them in hot water causes the protein in the bodily fluid or solid to change, much like how an egg changes its appearance when it is cooked. Without soaking in cold water, stains will be almost impossible to remove in the future.

When removing stains, handle chemicals carefully (BOX 42–7). Follow the label instructions. Remember that both chlorine bleach and ammonia are poisonous. Each of them, by themselves, can burn or irritate the eyes and skin. Take care not to inhale ammonia fumes; open a window when using ammonia. ***Remember never to mix chlorine bleach and ammonia because doing so creates a toxic gas.***

Before using bleach, check the care instructions on a garment. Also, be aware that some people are allergic to chemicals in cleaning products. Check the care plan. If you are not sure, ask your supervisor.

BOX 42–7 Removing Stains

The directions in this box apply to both white and colour-fast clothes and linens. If possible, treat stains immediately, before they become set in the fabric.

Urine Stains

- Rinse in cold water.
- Soak in a solution of 1 L of warm water, 2 mL liquid (hand) dishwashing detergent, and 15 mL of ammonia for 30 minutes.
- Rinse in cool water.
- Soak in a solution of 1 L warm water and 15 mL of vinegar for 1 hour.
- Machine-wash with chlorine bleach and detergent; dry as usual.

Blood Stains

- Rinse in cold water.
- Rub with a paste of powdered detergent and water or 5 mL of liquid commercial stain-remover detergent, 2 mL liquid (hand) dishwashing detergent, or a bar of soap. Let solution sit on the stained area for 15 minutes.
- Soak another 15 minutes in 1 L of cold water with the powdered or liquid stain-remover detergent.
- Wash in machine using chlorine bleach and detergent; dry as usual.

Fecal Stains

- Rinse in cold water.
- Soak in a solution of 1 L warm water, 2 mL liquid (hand) dishwashing detergent, and 15 mL ammonia for 30 minutes.
- Wash in machine using chlorine bleach and detergent; dry as usual.

RECYCLING ITEMS AND COMPOSTING

Most municipalities in Canada encourage residents to recycle their waste cardboard and paper, cans, jars, and other items. You should be aware of the items that are allowed to be recycled in the client's area, as each municipality has its own rules and specifics regarding recycling.

Some areas specify that certain types of waste must be disposed of in a container of a specific colour. For example, one municipality may insist that paper and cardboard be placed in a red container, cans and jars in a blue container, and wet waste that can be composted in a green container. If the client lives in an apartment building, you may be responsible for taking the recycling items to the assigned disposal area and putting them into their appropriate bins (**FIGURE 42–4**).

Recycling and composting reduces the amount of waste that would eventually fill our dumpsites and landfills and is an environmentally responsible action all of us can participate in.

PERFORMING TASKS NOT INCLUDED ON THE CLIENT'S CARE PLAN

Occasionally, you might be asked to perform a task not included on the client's care plan. Some of the tasks might seem easy to do, but others might not. For example, one client may ask you to make a sandwich, even though meal preparation is not on that client's care plan. Another client may ask you to wash the windows so that the client can clearly see the birds coming to the birdfeeder.

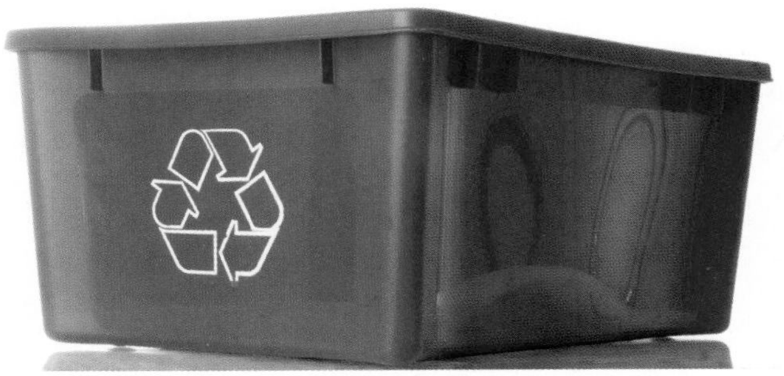

FIGURE 42–4 Recycling bin. (**Source:** © Can Stock Photo Inc./Colecanstock.)

You should remember that you will not be paid for performing any tasks that are not on the client's care plan. Some employers frown on the support worker providing "free" services (i.e., services that the client would normally have to pay your agency for you to perform). Some agencies' insurance companies will not compensate you if you are injured while performing a task that is not on your client's care plan. You should also be aware that if you provide "free" services, the client will probably expect the same services from other support workers in the future!

Some clients (or their friends or family) will see you as a source of free services (see the *Supporting Mrs. Washington: Part 4: Adhering to the Task List* box). You should know how to respond to the client or others when you are asked to perform a task that is not on the care plan. Remember that you should always be professional, calm, and respectful if you must refuse someone's request for unpaid services.

Consult With Your Supervisor

Before performing a task that is not on the client's care plan, it is always a good idea to consult your supervisor. Your supervisor is aware of your agency's policies regarding such situations. Occasionally, your supervisor will say that it is "up to you," especially if the request is not time-consuming or does not require special skills. For example, your client may ask you to feed the bird while you are near the canary's cage. This task is neither complicated nor time-consuming, so your supervisor might very well allow you to do it. Other favours, however, can be time-consuming and may put you behind in your schedule if you have other clients to see that day.

Some "favours" asked may be beyond your scope of practice, and you should ***never be persuaded to perform them***. For example, since Mrs. Patel's arthritis is acting up and she cannot handle her insulin syringe, she asks you to help her with it. In this situation, it is important that you call your supervisor immediately and consult with him, as there is considerable risk of harming the client. Your supervisor may go to the client's house to perform the task or send a nurse over instead.

Supporting Mrs. Washington: Part 4: Adhering to the Task List

Mrs. Washington finally agrees to your supervisor's suggestion that she allow you to wash her laundry at her next-door neighbour's home because you are reluctant to use her very old washing machine. Mrs. Washington's neighbour, Sue Black, is a very pleasant 30-year-old woman. Sue has been very nice to Mrs. Washington since her fall. She took care of her mail while she was in the hospital, and she recently suggested to Mrs. Washington that you could do her laundry at her house and she talked to your supervisor about it.

Because Sue is usually at work, she has given Mrs. Washington her house key so that you can use her washer and dryer while she is away. Today, Sue is home with a cold. She greets you at her door to let you into her house and asks that you do her a favour—that you fold the load of her clothing that is in her dryer and then do another load of her clothes before you leave Mrs. Washington's house for the day. Doing so would put you behind in seeing your next client. It would also be against your agency's policies, which say you cannot do work for people other than your list of clients. What should you do?

CHAPTER REVIEW

KEY POINTS

- The support worker may be required to assist in home management services—tidying and cleaning rooms, vacuuming, dusting, washing dishes, making beds, doing laundry—to enhance the health and well-being of a client. Support workers are not assigned heavy housecleaning tasks such as washing windows or cleaning carpets.
- The support worker's tasks will be specified on each client's care plan.
- Cleaning products should be used safely and stored properly. Remember the following points: (1) read all labels carefully, (2) never mix cleaning products, (3) wear utility gloves when using cleaning products, (4) never store products in unlabelled containers, (5) store products in their original containers, (6) keep cleaning products away from food, (7) be careful never to splash bleach or other chemicals, (8) keep cleaning products out of the reach of children, (9) use products only for their intended purpose, (10) keep aerosol cans away from heat sources, (11) ask the client for permission before using a strong cleaner on any surface, (12) rinse off harsh or strong cleaners after using, and (13) do not scrub vigorously.
- Specific guidelines for home management and cleaning include (1) clearing away clutter, (2) working from higher to lower, (3) working from far to near, (4) working from dry to wet, (5) working from cleanest to dirtiest, (6) changing cleaning cloths and water frequently, (7) using a damp cloth for dusting, (8) rinsing and drying washed surfaces, and (9) avoiding soiling a clean floor.
- Dry all surfaces well to prevent growth of mould and mildew. Surface mould can be cleaned with water and dish detergent. Do not use bleach to remove mould.
- You should be aware of specific stain-removing guidelines when doing laundry.
- You should be aware of the recycling guidelines in the client's residential area.

CRITICAL THINKING IN PRACTICE

Working for a home care agency, you have been assigned to assist with bathing and dressing for Mrs. Soto, a new client. She was recently sent home from a rehabilitation hospital after falling and breaking her hip. You notice that Mrs. Soto's family did not obtain the shower chair that was recommended. You do not know how to safely get her in and out of the tub without this chair, and she does not seem very steady on her feet. What should you do? What are your responsibilities in this situation?

REVIEW QUESTIONS

Answers to these questions are at the bottom of page 982.

Circle the BEST answer.

1. Home management duties include:
   A. Personal care and hygiene tasks
   B. Organizing the garage
   C. Light housekeeping tasks
   D. Cleaning the attic

2. Which of the following is a true statement?
   A. The client, family, and case manager decide on the required housekeeping tasks.
   B. Housekeeping tasks are never on the care plan.
   C. In consultation with the client, you can change the care plan tasks at any time.
   D. The care plan is only a suggestion for what you should be doing.

3. When cleaning a surface, you should:
   A. Work from the bottom to the top
   B. Work from near to far
   C. Work from cleanest to dirtiest
   D. Work from wet to dry

4. You need to do laundry, dust surfaces, and mop the floor. In which order should you do these tasks?
   A. Do laundry, dust, and mop
   B. Dust, mop, do laundry
   C. Mop, do laundry, dust
   D. Do laundry, mop, dust

5. When clearing clutter, you must:
   A. Use your judgement about important and unimportant items
   B. Throw away all stray pieces of paper
   C. Gather things in one place so the client can put them away later
   D. Ask the client before throwing anything away

6. You are not familiar with the client's cleaning products. You should:
   A. Contact your supervisor
   B. Follow the label directions
   C. Ask the client to buy new products
   D. Replace them with your favourite brand of products

7. When are utility gloves necessary?
   A. When loading the dishwasher
   B. When folding clean linens
   C. When cleaning the toilet
   D. When putting cleaning products away

8. When working in a kitchen, you should:
   A. Dry the dishes with a tea towel rather than let them air-dry
   B. Use paper towels to dry your hands
   C. Use one cloth to wash surfaces, dishes, and floors
   D. Pour contaminated liquid down the kitchen sink

9. When doing laundry, the hot-water cycle is used for:
   A. Diapers
   B. Lightly soiled clothes
   C. White lingerie
   D. Delicate fabrics

10. Which of the following should you do when handling linens soiled with body substances?
    A. Wash them with other garments in hot water
    B. Throw them away
    C. Ask the client to help you
    D. Follow Standard Practices

11. Why should you never mix bleach with anything containing ammonia (including urine)?
    A. The urine stains will become permanent.
    B. When mixed, they will form a poisonous gas.
    C. The bleach will not be as effective.
    D. Nothing will happen.

12. Why are fecal stains always rinsed in cold water?
    A. It is too wasteful to use hot water to rinse them out.
    B. Cold water is cheaper for the client.
    C. Using hot water will cause the item to shrink.
    D. Hot water can cause the protein in the fecal material to thicken.

Answers: 1.C, 2.A, 3.C, 4.A, 5.D, 6.B, 7.C, 8.B, 9.A, 10.D, 11.B, 12.D

Chapter opener image: Chutima Chaochaiya/Shutterstock.com

CHAPTER 43

Assisting With Medications

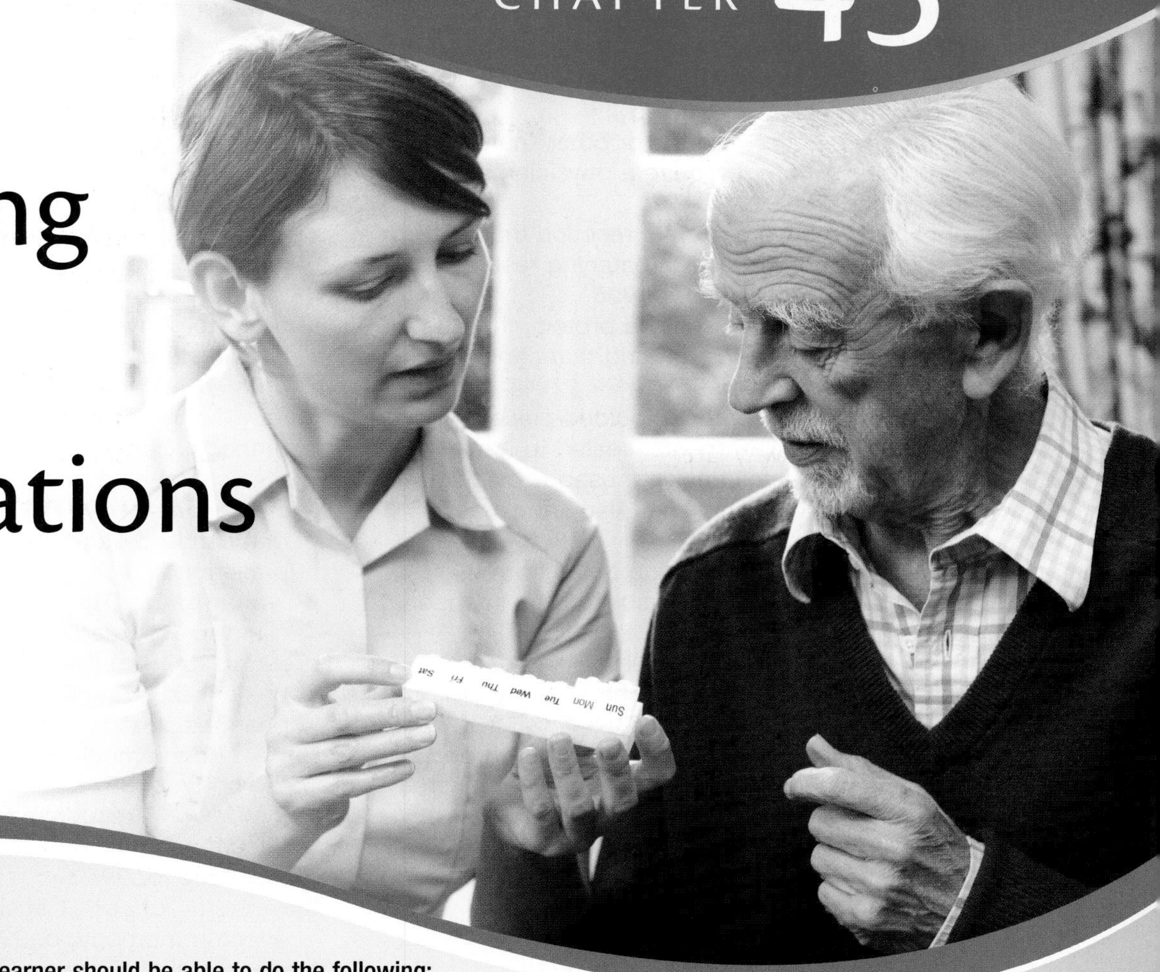

OBJECTIVES

After reading this chapter, the learner should be able to do the following:

- Identify the support worker's role in assisting with medications.
- Summarize how drugs work in the body.
- List the factors that affect drug action.
- List the different forms of medications.
- Differentiate between *assisting* with medications and *administering* medications.
- Identify guidelines to follow when assisting with medications.
- List the "rights" of assisting with medications.
- Summarize what to do if a medication error is made.
- Outline the support worker's main responsibilities when assisting with medications.
- Apply the procedures described in this chapter.

KEY TERMS

adverse effect A dangerous or unwanted side effect of a medication. *p. 995*

alternative remedies Herbal or other "natural" products that do not require a physician's prescription. *p. 991*

anaphylaxis A severe allergic reaction that occurs rapidly and causes a life-threatening response involving the whole body. *p. 996*

antigen A substance, usually a protein, that the body recognizes as foreign and that can evoke an immune response. *p. 995*

blister pack A transparent moulded piece of plastic with multiple compartments, sealed to a sheet of cardboard with a foil backing, used to package individual-dose medications. Also known as a *bubble pack*. *p. 986*

distribution The path the drug takes from the bloodstream to the body tissues of the intended site of action. *p. 987*

dosette Container that stores medications in separate compartments arranged by day or hour. Also known as *pillbox*. *p. 986*

drug antagonism An unusually weak drug effect that occurs when two or more drugs are taken at the same time. *p. 987*

drug interaction The combined action that a medication and another substance (such as another drug, alcohol, or food) has on the body. *p. 987*

drug synergism An unusually strong drug effect that occurs when taking two or more drugs at the same time. *p. 987*

excretion Exiting from the body, especially through the stool, urine, lungs, or skin. *p. 987*

generic name of a drug The name given to a drug approved by Health Canada. It is also known as the "official name" of a drug. *p. 992*

medication A drug or other substance used to prevent or treat disease or illness. *p. 987*

metabolization Chemical reactions that take place to convert a drug from smaller molecules into waste products before it can exit the body. *p. 987*

metered dose inhaler (MDI) A pressurized canister of medication that releases a single dose of medication as a mist. *p. 989*

over-the-counter (OTC) medication A medication that can be bought without a physician's prescription. *p. 990*

polypharmacy The use of more medications by a client than is medically required. *p. 990*

prescription (Rx) medication A medication that is prescribed by a physician and dispensed by a pharmacist. *p. 991*

route How a medication enters and is absorbed by the body. *p. 987*

side effect A response to a medication that occurs in addition to the intended or main response. *p. 995*

therapeutic effect Causing a desired, positive effect in the body. *p. 995*

trade name of a drug The name given to a drug by the manufacturer. Also known as *proprietary name*. *p. 992*

Medications are drugs and other substances used to prevent or treat diseases or illnesses. Many clients living in community settings engage in *self-directed medication management*, meaning that they take their medications independently.

As a support worker, however, you may be responsible for assisting a client with taking medications (see the *Supporting Mr. Whitehill: Assisting a Client With Taking Medications* box). Clients in a variety of situations and settings may need help for different reasons. For example, some clients need assistance with taking medications because they are not able to reach the medicines or open the containers; others may not be able to read the containers or may have

This chapter is adapted from Birchenall, J., & Streight, E. (2003). Mosby's textbook for the home care aide *(2nd ed., p. 345). St. Louis, MO: Mosby; and Lilley, L. L., Harrington, S., Snyder, J. S., et al. (2007).* Pharmacology and the nursing process in Canada. *Toronto, ON: Mosby Elsevier. The authors gratefully acknowledge the contributions of the authors of these textbooks.*

Supporting Mr. Whitehill: Assisting a Client With Taking Medications

Mr. Whitehill is an 86-year-old man who was recently referred to your agency while his wife is in hospital after having suffered a stroke. Mr. Whitehill has recently been diagnosed with dementia, and although he can dress and shower himself, he needs to be reminded when to do these things as well as when to take his medications. As a support worker, you have been hired to care for him 1 hour a day to help him with his morning care and with taking his medications. According to his care plan, he will take the pills out of his blister pack himself if you remind him to do so.

It is your first day, and you have observed that Mr. Whitehill has had no problem with showering, dressing, or feeding himself. It is now time for him to take his medications, so you have reminded him, but he does not seem to know how to take the pills out of the blister pack or which pills to take. He turns to you and asks for your help. What should you do? Do you know the scope of practice for support workers in your province?

BOX 43–1 *Assisting With* Versus *Administering* Medications

Assisting with medications and *administering* medications are two very different functions. *Assist* means "to help"; *administer* means "to give."

Assisting with medications involves helping clients to self-administer medications. For example, you hand them their medications, or you open the bottles or packages for them. Such tasks are strictly a *mechanical* function; that is, you perform the functions clients would normally perform with their own hands and feet to obtain the medication.

Administering medications involves measuring medications or getting them into the person's body, and it requires special judgement and knowledge. Clients and residents in facilities usually have medications administered to them, and some home care clients also need health care providers to administer their medications. However, administering medications is beyond your scope of practice. In some provinces and territories, ***in some special circumstances***, you may be asked by your supervisor to perform a controlled act, such as giving an insulin injection or administering some forms of medication to certain clients. ***You must never just assume this responsibility, as it is beyond your usual scope of practice. If you are asked to administer medication, it is your employer's responsibility to ensure that you are formally trained, supervised, and monitored by a registered staff member. It is then your responsibility to ask questions for clarification and to safely follow the instructions given. This function must be in your job description, as part of your employment agreement. Remember that you are ultimately responsible for any medications that you assist the client with!***

A small mistake when assisting with or administering medications can cause serious harm. Follow employer policies and provincial or territorial laws to protect your clients, your employer, and yourself. When assisting with medications, follow the "rights" of assisting with medications (p. 997). Check the care plan to see how much assistance the client requires.

shaky hands. Support workers working in a retirement home or group home may assist with medications as one of their duties.

Remember that assisting with medications must be specifically part of your job description and within your scope of practice in your province. Also remember that, depending on your province, a registered nurse, a licensed or registered practical nurse, or a registered psychiatric nurse must teach you how to do this task for each client. (See **BOX 43–1**.)

SCOPE OF PRACTICE: YOUR ROLE

Your role in assisting with medications depends on your provincial or territorial legislation, your employer's policy, and your training and education. (Refer to Chapter 9 for more information about the laws that govern support workers across Canada.) Ensure that you are clear about what your duties include and that you have been taught how to perform each of the tasks that you are expected to do. In many areas, for example, oxygen therapy is considered to be a medication, since there is great potential risk for harm to a client. Check with your employer or supervisor should you have any questions.

Your role may involve *one or more* of the following:

- Reminding the client to take a medication
- Bringing medication containers to the client
- Bringing prepoured medications, prefilled syringes, blister packs, or dosettes (pillboxes) to the client
- Reading the prescription label to the client
- Loosening or removing container lids or opening blister packs
- Checking the dosage on the medication label with the client's medication administration record (MAR)
- Providing water or other fluids, as needed
- Supervising the client as the client places the medication into the hand, measuring spoon, or cup
- Steadying the client's hand while the client places medications or administers eye drops, nasal sprays, and so on
- Documenting in the client's MAR the medications given, according to your agency's policy

You are *not* responsible for monitoring the outcome of the drug therapy. The physician, nurse, or case manager owns this responsibility. ***However, you must observe for and report any changes in the client's condition or behaviour.***

The nurse or pharmacist teaches the client about the medications that have been prescribed. Clients then should be able to take medications accurately and know the medications' desired effects, when and how to take the medications, any adverse effects to watch for, and foods or other medications to avoid. If your client does not have this information, notify your supervisor.

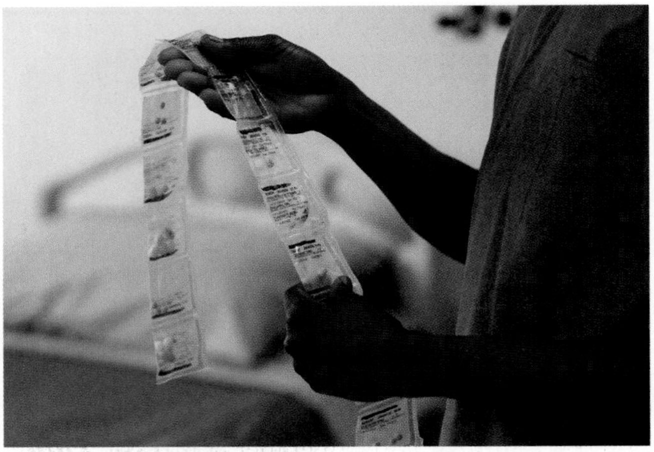

FIGURE 43–1 Blister (bubble) packs are supplied by the client's pharmacy and contain the medications the client has to take at that time. (**Source:** Brian Hillier.)

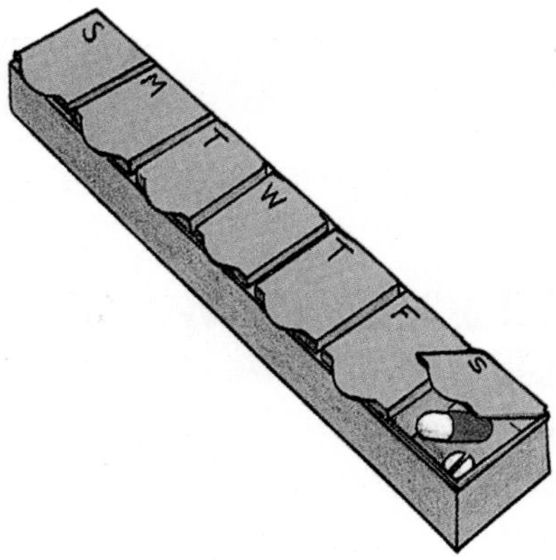

FIGURE 43–2 Dosettes are pillboxes that help clients keep track of their daily medications. (**Source:** Birchenall, J., & Streight, E. (2003). *Mosby's textbook for the home care aide* (2nd ed., p. 348). St. Louis, MO: Mosby.)

Many clients receive their medications in a **blister pack**, or bubble pack (**FIGURE 43–1**). Blister packs are supplied by the client's pharmacy with the client's medications for that day or time grouped together and plastic heat-sealed to a cardboard card. Clients open the appropriate blister pack (or direct you to do it for them) and take their medications.

Clients may store medications in a **dosette**, which is also known as a *pillbox* (**FIGURE 43–2**). Dosettes have compartments that organize the medications by day or by hour. They help clients remember what they have taken and what medications remain to be

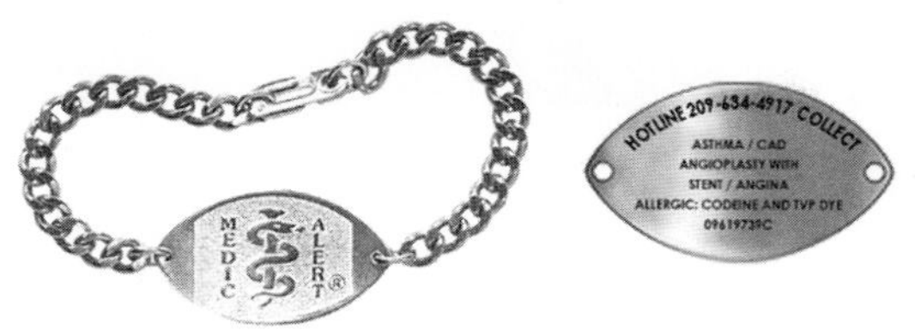

FIGURE 43–3 A MedicAlert bracelet contains the client's emergency medical information, including drug allergies, engraved on the back. (**Source:** Potter, P.A., Perry, A.G., Ross-Kerr, J.C., et al. (2006). *Canadian fundamentals of nursing* (3rd ed., p. 839). Toronto, ON: Elsevier Canada.)

taken each day. If the client is unable to fill the dosette, a nurse or family member may do so. ***Filling a dosette is not your responsibility.***

Before assisting with a medication, always check the MAR, which should list any medications the client is allergic to. Some clients may wear MedicAlert bracelets that indicate any drug allergies (**FIGURE 43–3**). Medication errors can occur easily, but they are always avoidable! See the *Think About Safety: Guidelines for Assisting Clients With Medications* box.

HOW MEDICATIONS WORK IN THE BODY

A **medication** (drug) is a chemical substance that causes a specific effect on the body and is prescribed for and taken by people to obtain various desired results in the body. Some medications might *treat illness* or pain—for example, ibuprofen to reduce the pain of a headache. Other medications *promote health*—for example, a stool softener to help reduce discomfort during bowel movement. And some medications *prevent illness*—for example, an antibiotic to prevent an infection after surgery.

Drug Action

Medications enter the body in a variety of ways. *How* the medication enters the body (so that it can start working) is known as the **route**. TABLE 43–1 lists some types of medications and their routes. Medication such as injections and intravenous medications are not included in the table because you will not be responsible for assisting with or administering them.

Depending on the route, the body must absorb and distribute the drug so that the drug can work. Absorption and distribution are also necessary to *metabolize* the drug so that the body can rid itself of the remaining materials (molecules of the drug the body no longer needs)—that is, *excrete* them from the body. For example, the blood pressure pill that a client swallows must enter the stomach, be broken down into small molecules, enter the bloodstream (*absorption*), and travel throughout the body to reach its intended tissues (**distribution**) so that it can cause the intended effect. After the drug has done what it was intended to do in the body, it must then be broken down into smaller waste particles and sometimes converted into other substances the body can use (i.e., **metabolization**, which usually takes place in the liver), and then be removed from the body, usually in the stool or in the urine (**excretion**).

Drug Interactions

The way that medications interact with other drugs or substances in the body (e.g., alcohol) is also important, as mixing these substances may cause an undesirable effect on the client, known as a **drug interaction**. For example, a client might take an over-the-counter (OTC) medication, herbal supplement, or vitamin, and, depending on its nature, it might interact with the prescription medication that the client's doctor prescribed.

The combined effect of two drugs being greater than the effect of either drug given alone is known as **drug synergism**. This combined effect can cause the client to become extremely drowsy, hyperactive, or nauseated. When combined, some medications can even affect that client's heart function or blood pressure. For example, taking an antihistamine when a narcotic is active in the person's system will make a person much more drowsy than if only one of the medications was taken.

Conversely, some medications will counteract the actions of other drugs when combined, called **drug antagonism**. For example, an antacid might prevent an antibiotic or birth control pill from being absorbed in the stomach.

Clients on prescribed medications should never drink alcohol or take OTC medications without first consulting a doctor, pharmacist, or nurse, as serious harm may result from combining medications and other drugs or alcohol.

TABLE 43–1 Types of Medications and Their Routes

Route	Form	Description	
Oral (taken by mouth and swallowed): Solids or semi-solids	Capsules	Small gelatin containers that hold medications	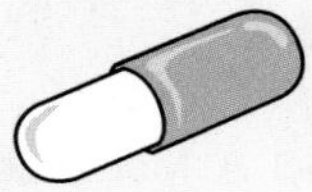
	Lozenges	Flat discs containing medication in a flavoured base; lozenges are held in the mouth, where they dissolve and slowly release medication	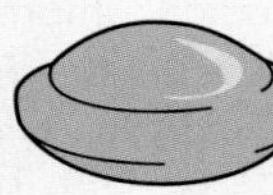
	Tablets	Dry, powdered medications that have been formed into hard discs or cylinders; *sublingual* medications are placed under the tongue and dissolved or absorbed into the body	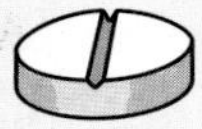
Oral: Liquids	Elixirs	Medication dissolved in liquid containing alcohol or water and flavourings	
	Suspensions	Medication suspended in a liquid that should be shaken or stirred before use	
	Syrups	Medication dissolved in a concentrated sugar solution	
Topical (applied to the skin or mucous membranes)	Ointments or creams	Semi-solid material containing medication; contained within the area where they are applied	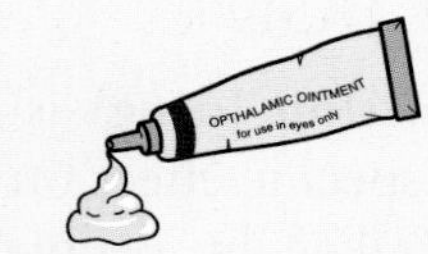
	Transdermal discs or patches	Medication on a small disc or patch that is applied to unbroken skin; absorbed into the bloodstream through the skin over a 24-hour period	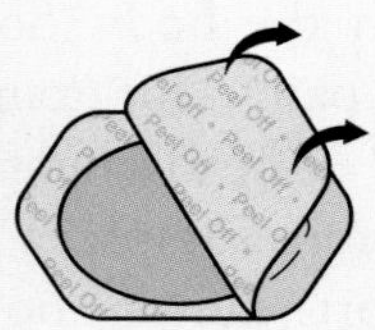
	Suppositories—rectal or vaginal	Solid form of medication for insertion into the rectum or vagina; body temperature causes the suppository to dissolve, and the medication is released and absorbed by the mucous membranes	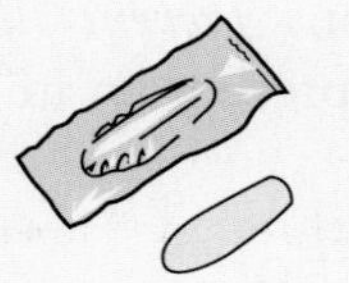
Eye/Ear/Nose	Drops	Liquid form of medication in a special container that allows one drop at a time to be administered; usually eye drops, ear drops, and nose drops	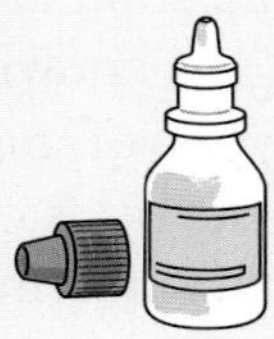

Continued

TABLE 43–1 Types of Medications and Their Routes—cont'd

Route	Form	Description
Parenteral (injected)	Liquid for injection	Liquid form of medication that is injected using a *syringe* (a device consisting of a plastic tube filled with medication, a plunger, and an attached needle); may be injected into muscle (*intramuscular*), a vein (*intravenous*), or under the skin (*subcutaneous*) 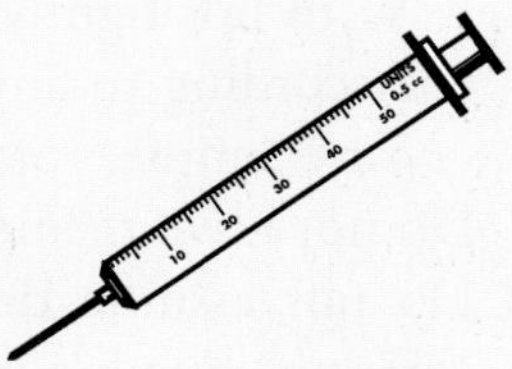
Inhalation (breathed in through the mouth or nose)	Aerosols	Medication particles suspended in air or gas that are inhaled into the lungs; administered through a **metered dose inhaler (MDI)**—often called a "puffer" or "inhaler"—which is a small cylinder used with a special delivery system (Many people use the MDI with holding chambers, especially people who are very young, old, or frail. The client uses it to inhale the medication through the mouth in specifically measured (metered) doses. The use of a holding chamber is preferred as it prevents the medication in the MDI from landing on the client's tongue, preventing tongue irritation or taste changes from the medication.) 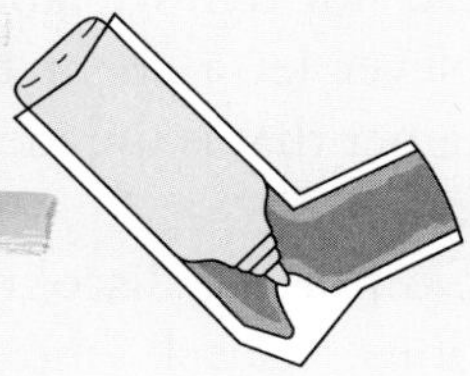

Adapted from Birchenall, J., & Streight, E. (2003). *Mosby's textbook for the home care aide* (2nd ed., p. 345). St. Louis, MO: Mosby.

Think About Safety

Guidelines for Assisting Clients With Medications

- Always follow employer policy.
- Always wash your hands, and work in a well-lit environment, away from avoidable distractions.
- Review the care plan with your supervisor before assisting the client with medications. Follow the "rights" of assisting with medications (see p. 997).
- Bring the right medication containers to the client. Read the labels carefully. Compare container labels with the care plan and the MAR.
- Know the correct dose of each medication. Check the care plan and the MAR.
- Give a glass of water (or other liquid) with oral medications, as ordered.
- Store medications:
  - In a special place just for the client's medications (separately from others' medications)
  - In a cool but dry place (not in the bathroom medicine cabinet)
  - Out of reach of children and of adults with dementia

Continued

Think About Safety—cont'd

- In the original labelled container
- With lids tightly closed
- According to any special storage directions—for example, "Store in the refrigerator"

- Do not leave medications at the client's bedside. Do not assume that the client will take them correctly. Remain with the client until the medication has been taken.
- Do not remove labels from the containers.
- Never let a client take medication from a container that is unlabelled or that has an unreadable label.
- Do not use discoloured or deteriorated medications. Check the expiry date on the labels before giving medications to the client. Notify your supervisor of expired or deteriorated medications.
- If you notice that the medications are running low, tell the client or family and your supervisor.
- Check with your supervisor before discarding any unused medications.
- Listen to the client. If the client questions something about a medication, STOP—do not assist with self-administration. Call your supervisor immediately.
- Report the following to your supervisor:
  - The client does not take medications correctly.
  - The client does not understand why the medication should be taken and does not know the dosage or the schedule.
  - The client refuses to take the medication or forgets or omits a dose; the client should not take a double dose if one has been omitted.
  - The client shows any adverse effects (for example, vomiting, rash, breathing difficulty, itching, or diarrhea).
  - The client wants to take medications (including OTC medications or alternative remedies) that are not listed on the MAR and care plan.
  - The client wants to take medications other than those in the dosette, such as outdated medication or medication that has been prescribed for someone else.
  - The client takes any other medications, recreational drugs, or alcohol. Mixing prescription medications with these substances may cause a drug interaction. A drug interaction may cause the medication's effects to be increased (*drug synergism*) or decreased (*drug antagonism*) or may even produce a new effect that neither would produce if taken alone.
  - The client complains that the medication is no longer working or producing the desired effect in the body. This may be a sign of *drug tolerance* and should be reported. The client's medication dose may need to be increased, or another medication may have to be substituted.
  - Never discard medications down the toilet, as the medication will eventually enter your municipality's water system, killing fish and wildlife. ***If medication drops (or is found) on the floor, you must discard it according to your agency's policies***, which may include having a witness and completing an incident report (see Chapter 22). You must also report and record this medication wastage according to your agency's policies.
- Record your actions, according to employer policy. When applicable, the client records both which medication was taken and the time it was taken on the MAR. Assist the client, as directed.
- Report and record if a medication has not been taken or has been omitted. Explain why.

Taking more than the prescribed dosage of medication or taking too many medications is called **polypharmacy** and can cause serious health problems. Suspected polypharmacy should always be reported to your supervisor. See the *Supporting Mrs. Lefcoe: The Effect of Polypharmacy on a Client* box.

TYPES OF MEDICATIONS

Medications come in many forms (see TABLE 43–1). Clients may take:

- **Over-the-counter (OTC) medications**—medications that can be bought without a physician's

Supporting Mrs. Lefcoe: The Effect of Polypharmacy on a Client

You live next door to Mrs. Lefcoe, who is a 79-year-old widow living alone since her husband died 5 years ago. She has three married children and numerous grandchildren, but they live in distant cities. You try to check on Mrs. Lefcoe weekly, and she has occasionally asked you to drive her to the grocery store during the winter months. Mrs. Lefcoe has a family doctor whom she likes because he is very pleasant. Since he has such a busy medical practice, she can see him only once a month. She gets her prescriptions filled at the pharmacy next to her doctor's office, always takes her prescribed medications on time, and follows instructions well.

Mrs. Lefcoe has never told her doctor that she also sees another family doctor on a monthly basis because she does not want "to hurt his feelings and make him stop having me as a patient." Her other family doctor used to treat her husband. After each appointment with this doctor, she gets any prescriptions filled at the pharmacy next to this doctor's office. She also takes these medications on time and as prescribed. Mrs. Lefcoe assumes that since she takes only *prescribed* medications and takes them as ordered, she is even "healthier." Mrs. Lefcoe also likes the attention she receives from her two doctors.

Last night, while walking to the bathroom, Mrs. Lefcoe became dizzy and collapsed. She remained on the floor all night, too weak to move. Fortunately, you spotted her through the front door when you stopped by to check on her the next day. She was rushed to hospital and was treated for medication overdose and dehydration. The doctors eventually diagnosed her with *polypharmacy* once they discovered that she was taking double doses of some medications and interacting doses of other medications. As a result, Mrs. Lefcoe became very ill, requiring hospitalization and then home care assistance after she was discharged home.

prescription—for example, acetaminophen (Tylenol) and cough syrup.

- **Alternative remedies**—herbal or other "natural" products that do not require a physician's prescription—for example, ginseng and shark cartilage. Alternative remedies are usually not considered part of conventional medicine.
- **Prescription (Rx) medications**—medications that require a physician's prescription and are dispensed by a pharmacist—for example, antibiotics and blood pressure medications.

You assist *only* with medications that are listed in the care plan. If a client requests your help with medications that are not in the care plan (including OTC medications and alternative remedies), notify your supervisor.

Clients might ask support workers to purchase or obtain OTC medications or alternative remedies for them. Refuse respectfully but firmly. Inform your supervisor of the client's request.

Drug Effects and Classifications

Medications can have *topical*, *local*, or *systemic* effects, according to *where* in the body the medication works. A cream that you rub on your skin might have a *topical* effect—that is, the cream works only on the skin surface. An eye drop medication might cause a *localized* effect—that is, it works only in the eye in which you put it. The pill that you take for your headache might have a *systemic* effect—that is, it might also help relieve pain elsewhere in your body.

Drugs are classified according to how they work—for example, an antibiotic works by eliminating or reducing harmful bacteria in the body. Generally speaking, most antibiotics share some common adverse effects, so there will be common observations or responsibilities for you to keep in mind when assisting a client with taking them. You should know that, in some clients, most drugs might cause nausea or vomiting.

TABLE 43–2 lists common responsibilities for you when assisting with medications under certain classifications and provides an example of a common drug (both its generic and trade names) in each classification. The **generic name of a drug** refers to its chemical name, while the **trade name of a drug** refers to its trademarked, packaged name given by the manufacturer. ***Although this list includes many of the main drug classifications and the observations or responsibilities that you might encounter in your support work, it does NOT address more complex issues such as drug interactions and does not discuss ALL of the necessary observations or responsibilities for each classification of drugs. These are only general guidelines. You MUST check with your supervisor to find out if there are any specific observations that must be made for a particular client.***

Factors Affecting Drug Action

Drugs should be stored in a dry, safe place so that they do not undergo any chemical change. Most drugs should never be stored in direct sunlight, and some drugs need to be stored in the refrigerator for them to remain chemically stable. You must read the label on the drug container and follow the instructions carefully.

TABLE 43–2 Drug Classifications and Your Responsibilities

Drug Classification	Drug Action	Example (Generic and Trade Names)	Observations and Responsibilities
Alzheimer's disease medications	Treat mild to moderate symptoms of Alzheimer's disease	donepezil hydrochloride (Aricept)	Report any nausea, diarrhea, vomiting, and muscle cramps; client may be fatigued easily
Analgesics (non-narcotic)	Relieve mild to moderate pain	acetaminophen (Tylenol)	Might cause stomach ache, so is often instructed to be taken with food
Analgesics (narcotic)	Relieve severe pain	acetaminophen 325 mg; caffeine and codeine 30 mg (Tylenol #3)	Report excessive drowsiness, constipation
Antacids	Relieve heartburn	calcium carbonate (Tums)	Should not be taken within 2 hours of another medicine as it might interfere with that drug's absorption
Anti-anginals	Relieve anginal chest pain	nitroglycerin (Nitrostat)	May cause dizziness in client; wear gloves while handling some of these drugs to avoid a bad headache
Anti-anxiety medications	Reduce anxiety	lorazepam (Ativan)	Might cause drowsiness and sleepiness; client should be careful when driving

Continued

TABLE 43–2 Drug Classifications and Your Responsibilities—cont'd

Drug Classification	Drug Action	Example (Generic and Trade Names)	Observations and Responsibilities
Antibiotics	Eliminate or reduce harmful bacteria	ampicillin (Novo-Ampicillin)	Check for diarrhea, vomiting; some clients may experience a bitter aftertaste Ensure clients finish the entire course prescribed, unless told not to by the doctor or pharmacist
Anticoagulants	Reduce blood clotting	warfarin (Coumadin)	May make clients more prone to bruising and bleeding; they must use care when brushing teeth or shaving Report bruises on body, blood in urine
Anticonvulsants	Reduce seizures	phenytoin sodium (Dilantin)	Make sure that mouth care is done often; thickening of the gingiva (gums) may cause tenderness when brushing teeth
Anti-emetics	Reduce nausea, motion sickness	scopolamine (Transderm-V)	Make sure the client has good mouth care to eliminate mouth sores and bad taste in mouth
Antihypertensives	Reduce blood pressure	ramipril (Altace)	Client should get up slowly to avoid dizziness or light-headedness
Antiparkinsonian agents	Reduce symptoms of Parkinson's disease	levodopa-carbidopa (Sinemet)	Report dizziness, pain, drowsiness, or irritability
Antipsychotics	Reduce psychosis, severe agitation, severe vomiting, or hiccups	haloperidol (Haldol)	Watch for hand tremors and dizziness; notify the nurse if you see any grimacing
Antitussives	Liquefy phlegm, making it easier to cough	dextromethorphan (Robitussin DM)	Should be taken after taking other drugs; clients must not drink fluids for 10 to 15 minutes to give chance for drug to be absorbed into throat tissues

Continued

TABLE 43–2 Drug Classifications and Your Responsibilities—cont'd

Drug Classification	Drug Action	Example (Generic and Trade Names)	Observations and Responsibilities
Antivirals	Reduce virus reproduction	acyclovir (Zovirax)	Report headache and nausea
Broncho-dilators	Reduce spasm in breathing passages	salbutamol (Ventolin)	Watch for dry mouth. May cause shakiness and tremors in hands and increased heart rate
Decongestants	Reduce nasal congestion	pseudoephedrine (Sudafed)	May cause dry mucous membranes and rebound congestion (congestion gets worse after drug wears off)
Diuretics	Lower blood pressure and body swelling by increasing urinary output	furosemide (Lasix)	Depending on the drug, some clients must eat more potassium-rich foods (bananas, baked white potatoes); more frequent urination may occur
Hypoglycemic agents	Improve insulin production in body	glyburide (Diabeta)	Report any nausea, vomiting, diarrhea, dizziness, or weakness
Insulin	Makes up for lack of natural insulin	insulin regular, human biosynthetic (Humulin R)	Report any blurred vision, dry mouth, extreme hunger, or chest palpitations
Laxatives	Help with bowel movements	bisacodyl (Dulcolax)	May cause diarrhea; encourage plenty of fluids and high-fibre diet to reduce need for laxatives
Nonsteroidal anti-inflammatory drugs (NSAIDs)	Reduce pain that comes with swelling	ibuprofen (Motrin)	May cause upset stomach, so should never be taken on an empty stomach
Thyroid replacements	Make up for lack of natural thyroid	levothyroxine sodium (Eltroxin)	Report menstrual irregularities, nausea, or vomiting

TABLE 43–3 Factors Affecting Drug Actions in the Body

Factor Affecting Drug Action in the Body	Description
Age	Young children and older adults may absorb, distribute, metabolize, and excrete drugs very differently from the way young adults do because their digestive organs may not be efficient enough.
Body size	A dose of medication that would have a **therapeutic effect** in a large, overweight adult might be an overdose in a small, thin adult of the same age because the drug level would be more concentrated in the small person. Note that some drugs are stored in the adipose tissue, which could lead to a buildup of that drug in the body over time.
Sex	Drugs affect men and women differently, depending on their body sizes, hormones, and other factors such as muscle mass.
Genetic factors	Some people have an inherited tendency to react to certain medications—for example, if Mr. Jones had a very unusual reaction to an anaesthetic, doctors may choose not to give the same anaesthetic to his daughter.
Emotional state	A severe emotional state will usually cause a person's heart rate and blood pressure to change, and these changes may, in turn, change the way a drug is absorbed, metabolized, and excreted.
Physical condition	Certain diseases will affect how well a drug is absorbed, distributed, metabolized, or excreted—for example, clients with kidney disease may not be able to excrete certain drugs through their urine as a person with healthy kidneys can.

The same drug can affect two people very differently because one person's body cells differ from those of another person, according to age, body size, gender, genetic factors, emotional state, and physical condition. TABLE 43–3 briefly describes how each of these factors affects drug actions.

Adverse Effects

Most medications have possible side effects. A **side effect** is another response to a medication that occurs along with the intended response. For example, some blood pressure pills will cause a client's heart rate to slow down, or a person taking pain medication may experience pain relief as well as drowsiness, nausea, and constipation. A medication may be ordered because of it's side effect. For example, one medication's side effect is to decrease saliva production in the mouth. A client may be given that medication prior to surgery to decrease sputum production and reduce the need for suctioning during surgery. Many side effects are predictable and harmless, but some can be so serious or harmful that the physician may order the medication to be stopped. A dangerous or unwanted side effect is an **adverse effect**.

Drug Allergy

A drug allergy is an abnormal response to a drug caused by the body fighting or attacking the drug (which is called an **antigen** when such a response occurs) by releasing chemicals called *antibodies*. Antibodies attack the antigen and can cause symptoms ranging from mild (skin rashes, swelling, puffiness, nasal drainage, itchy eyes) to moderate (fever, wheezing, extreme weakness, nausea, and vomiting) to severe (anaphylactic shock, severe low blood pressure, cardiac arrest).

Anaphylaxis—from the Greek *ana* (without) and *phylaxis* (protection)—is a severe sensitivity to an antigen (allergic reaction) that occurs rapidly and causes a life-threatening response involving the whole body. This reaction can lead to difficulty breathing and shock and can ultimately lead to death. In severe cases, anaphylactic shock can occur within seconds. Signs and symptoms include the following:

- Severe restlessness
- Increased anxiety
- Possible combativeness (from struggling to breathe)
- Sweating
- Shortness of breath
- Low blood pressure
- Irregular pulse
- Respiratory congestion
- Swelling of the larynx (laryngeal edema)
- Hoarseness
- Dyspnea

Anaphylactic shock is an emergency, and the emergency medical service (EMS) system must be activated immediately. The client needs special medications such as an epinephrine auto-injector to reverse the allergic reaction. Until emergency help arrives, keep the client lying down, ensuring that the airways are open. If cardiac arrest occurs, you must initiate cardiopulmonary resuscitation (CPR) at once.

BOX 43–2 Simple Medication Math Examples

(See Chapter 13 for a refresher on abbreviations.)

1. What is ordered: "Acetaminophen 500 mg tablets i to ii po q4h prn."
   Q: How many milligrams are in two tablets?
2. The side of the bottle of acetaminophen 500 mg tablets says, "Do not take more than 4 grams a day."
   Q. If the client takes one pill per dose, how many pills are allowed that day?
3. What is ordered: "Cough-Be-Gone cough syrup 15 mL po TID prn."
   Q: If 1 teaspoon equals 5 mL, how many teaspoons should this person take?
4. What is ordered: "Amoxicillin suspension 500 mg po QID." The bottle came with a dropper that says "250 mg per 5 mL."
   Q: a. How many millilitres should you give the client with each dose?
   b. How many times should you fill the dropper with each dose?

Answers:

1. Two tablets would contain a total of 1 000 mg.
2. The client should have no more than eight pills in one day.
3. The client should take three teaspoons of cough syrup for each dose.
4. a. You should give 10 mL of the amoxicillin for each dose.
   b. You would fill the dropper two times for each dose.

PERFORMING SIMPLE MEDICATION MATH

It is the role of the nurse to perform complex drug calculations, such as calculating how much insulin to give a client, which is ordered on a *sliding scale* (that is, the amount of insulin to give is based on the client's blood sugar results).

In areas throughout Canada where support workers may assist with medications, there are occasionally times when the support worker must perform simple calculations. Those instances usually involve *prn* medication (medication that is taken only when needed). In any case, the support worker should verify the dosage with the supervisor to ensure that the math calculation is correct. See **BOX 43–2** for examples of simple medication math.

DOCUMENTATION

The client's medication needs and your responsibilities are detailed in the care plan as well as on the client's MAR, which also serves as a record for actions taken. The exact form of the MAR varies by setting and employer. It always contains at least the following:

- The client's name
- The name, dose, and administration instructions for each medication
- A place to sign or initial after administering the medication

The MAR may also contain extra information, such as the client's allergies, expected adverse effects, and special instructions (see **FIGURE 43–4**).

In facilities, a nurse is responsible for signing or initialling the MAR, and in some, the MAR for each client is printed out daily.

In community settings, the MAR is kept only when it is necessary to track specific medications and dosages. Clients who administer their own medications may not need the MAR, but when one is required, it is kept in the client's home. If a nurse administers the medications, the nurse signs the MAR. If the client self-administers medications, the client signs the MAR as taught by the nurse. Observe as the client records the information on the MAR after the medication has been taken. Some clients may not be able to write because of physical disability or vision disorders, and you may then need to do the recording for these clients.

Follow your employer's policies and procedures for recording. Ask your supervisor for help if needed.

Understanding Abbreviations

An abbreviation is a shortened form of a word or phrase. The list on page 192 in Chapter 13 gives the more common abbreviations used in health care settings. Physicians, nurses, and pharmacists use many abbreviations when ordering and managing medications. The care plan and MAR should present information as clearly as possible. However, sometimes, abbreviations are used in these documents. Check with your supervisor about abbreviations used by your employer, especially when you are unsure about their meaning. Never guess about the meaning of an abbreviation, as doing so can cause serious harm to the client.

THE "RIGHTS" OF ASSISTING WITH MEDICATIONS

To help clients take medications accurately and safely, know and follow the "rights" of assisting with medications:

1. ***The right medication.*** Be sure you are assisting the client to take the right medication. The name of the medication is printed on the prescription label on the medication container (**FIGURE 43–5**). Read the label carefully, and make sure it is the same medication listed in the care plan and on the MAR. Check twice.
2. ***The right person.*** Be sure the medication is for your client. Check the prescription label on the medication container, and make sure it has the client's name (both first and last names). In some homes and facilities, two clients may have the same name. Make sure you are assisting the right client. Identify the client according to employer policy.
3. ***The right dose.*** The dose is listed on the prescription label, the care plan, and the MAR—for example, "Take one tablet daily" or "Apply ointment to left elbow twice a day." The correct amount of medication must be taken. For example, if Mrs. Jong removes two tablets from the container, and the prescription label and her care plan say that she has to take only one tablet at a time, you must point that out to her. When the medication is in liquid form, the dose measurements may be in imperial (ounces), household (teaspoons or tablespoons), or metric (millilitres) units. Be sure the client does not measure in teaspoons when the prescription calls for millilitres. Make sure the client uses measuring spoons and measuring cups—not household spoons or cups—to measure doses.
4. ***The right route.*** The prescription label, care plan, and MAR list the route (see TABLE 43–1).
5. ***The right time.*** For medications to work properly, they must be taken at the correct time. Medications may have to be taken once a day or two, three, or four times a day, as stated on the prescription label. For example, Mrs. Jong's prescription label states that the medication must be taken three times a day. The care plan and MAR

MEDICATION ADMINISTRATION RECORD

Name: Delbert Sullivan   Allergies: None known   Doctor's Name: J. Smith

Day		SUN	MON	TUE	WED	THUR	FRI	SAT
Date		7/11	7/12	7/13	7/14	7/15	7/16	7/17
Drug Name	Lasix (water pill)							
Dose	1 tablet							
Action	Increases urination							
Time	One (1) daily	0800	0800	0800	0800	0800	0800	0800
		JKS						

Special Instructions	Daily weight at 0800
	Drink plenty of fluids.
	Watch for and report any weight gain or swelling.
	Do not omit or increase dosage.
	Call doctor if unable to take medication.
Immediately Report	

Day		SUN	MON	TUE	WED	THUR	FRI	SAT
Date		7/11	7/12	7/13	7/14	7/15	7/16	7/17
Drug Name	Ferrous Sulfate (iron pill)							
Dose	1 tablet							
Action	Replaces iron in blood							
Time	Three (3) times daily	0900	0900	0900	0900	0900	0900	0900
		1300	1300	1300	1300	1300	1300	1300
		1700	1700	1700	1700	1700	1700	1700
		JKS						
		JKS						
		JKS						

Special Instructions	Take between meals.
	Take with full glass of water.
	Do not take with milk or antacids.
	Will change colour of stool to black.
	Do not crush tablet.
	May cause constipation.
Immediately Report	Nausea, vomiting, and diarrhea
	Abdominal pain

FIGURE 43–4 A sample medication administration record (MAR). (Adapted from Birchenall, J., & Streight, E. (2003). *Mosby's textbook for the home care aide* (2nd ed., p. 347). St. Louis, MO: Mosby.)

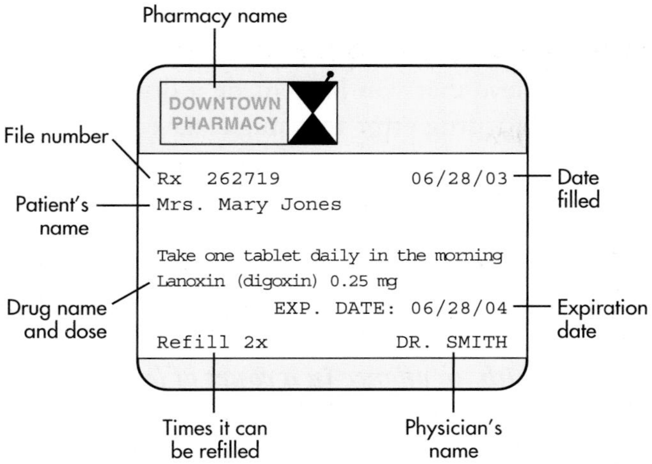

FIGURE 43–5 Read the prescription label before the client takes any medications. (**Source:** Birchenall, J., & Streight, E. (2003). *Mosby's textbook for the home care aide* (2nd ed., p. 349). St. Louis, MO: Mosby.)

state the exact times that the client needs to take the medication: 0600 hours, 1400 hours, and 2200 hours. Ensure that medications are given at the specified times. Taking medications at the wrong time of the day or taking them too close to or too far from meals and other medications can reduce their effectiveness and can even cause serious adverse effects.

Some medications have to be taken when the stomach is empty—that is, 1 hour before or 2 hours after a meal. Other medications need to be taken at mealtimes to reduce stomach irritation and promote absorption. The prescription warning labels for these medications will say "Take on empty stomach" or "Take with food or milk." Sometimes, clients must avoid certain foods or beverages when taking medications. Often, it is strongly recommended that alcohol and tobacco be avoided. Follow the warning labels on the prescription containers and the care plan.

Some medications (such as cough medicines or sublingual tablets) must be taken after all other oral medications are taken. It is important to know the *order* for taking several medications at one time. If you are uncertain about the order that medications should be taken, you should clarify it with your supervisor.

Clients may be confused about when to take their medications. For example, a client may say, "I can never remember. Do I take two tablets at 3 o'clock, or three tablets at 2 o'clock?" Tell your supervisor if there is evidence of confusion. The client may need a "refresher course" on taking medications properly.

Assist the client to take all medications at the right time. If you go on an outing with the client, bring along the medications that must be taken during that time.

6. ***The right day.*** Not all medications are taken daily; some are taken every second or third day. You need to check the MAR to ensure that the medication the client is taking is meant for that day.
7. ***The right reason.*** Medications should be taken for the right reason. A client saying, for example, "I took an extra pain pill to help me go to sleep" may indicate that the client is unaware of the risks associated with taking medication incorrectly. This situation should be reported to the supervisor.
8. ***The right expiry date.*** Just like foods, medications have expiry dates and should never be taken beyond their expiry date. In time, some medications either lose their potency (strength) or change chemically and become toxic for the client. If you have doubts about the expiry date, you should always check with your supervisor *before* assisting with that medication.
9. ***The right documentation.*** Any medication that is given must be documented properly, according to your agency policy. Medications are usually documented in the MAR. It is your responsibility to document any medication that you have assisted the client to take. If you have any questions about documenting, you need to ask your supervisor (who should be a nurse) to clarify it for you.

MEDICATION LABELLING REQUIREMENTS

In order to prevent medication errors, people must be able to understand the labels on the medications. In 2015, Health Canada released new regulations to improve drug safety by making product information easier for consumers to understand (see **BOX 43–3**).

BOX 43–3 New Canadian Labelling Requirements for Medications

In June 2015, new plain-language labelling regulations took effect for prescription drugs. In June 2017, the regulations will also apply to nonprescription drugs.

The regulations state that the information required on the label must be (1) prominently displayed, (2) easy for the purchaser to understand, and (3) expressed in plain language. Additionally, the text and graphics on the label cannot impede the comprehensibility (clarity) of the information on the label.

The regulations are not retroactive, but existing products are expected to conform to the new regulations as packaging is updated.

Another measure included in the regulations for consumer safety is a brand name assessment, which aims to ensure a new drug product would not be confused with another medication sold under a similar name.

Source: Health Canada. (2016), Guidance Document, *Questions and Answers: Plain Language Labelling Regulations,* Retrieved from http://www.hc-sc.gc.ca/dhp-mps/prodpharma/applic-demande/guide-ld/pll_qa_fin_qr_elc-eng.php

REPORTING MEDICATION ERRORS

If you believe that you have made a drug error (or you notice a drug error that might have been made by someone else), you need to report it to your supervisor immediately! It is the supervisor's responsibility to assess the situation and to determine the next course of action. ***Deliberate failure to report a medication error is possible grounds for immediate dismissal (losing your job) or civil action (being charged with an offence in a court of law).*** You are required to report the error even if you think it might get you into trouble! ***You can be in more trouble for failing to report the error than for making the error itself!***

Errors are caused by problems in technique (such as dropping a pill down the sink by accident), by omission (such as forgetting to give a medication), by incorrectly documenting a medication, or by failing to follow one or more of the "rights." ***A drug error can cause severe harm to the client, so errors must always be reported!***

Usually, an incident report must be filled out by you and your supervisor and a copy kept with the client's chart. Incident report statistics can also identify if there is a problem that is something beyond your control (such as how the medication is labelled by the pharmacy), so it is important to include as many details as possible in the incident report. See **FIGURE 22–29** on page 412 for a sample incident report.

Assisting With Oral Medications 123

Advocate on behalf of the client's quality of life by promoting:

Dignity • Independence • Preferences • Privacy • Safety *(see BOX 1–4, on p. 17)*

PRE-PROCEDURE

1 Identify the client, according to employer policy. *This eliminates the possibility of mistaking one client for another.*
2 Explain the procedure to the client.
3 Practise hand hygiene.
4 Assist the client with handwashing.
5 Collect the following supplies:
- ☐ **Oral medications**
- ☐ **Standard measuring spoon, cup, or other measuring device**

Continued

Assisting With Oral Medications—cont'd

- ☐ **Glass of water or other cool liquid**
- ☐ **Straw (optional)**

By collecting all the necessary equipment beforehand, you will not have to leave your client's side and can eliminate wasting time and energy in obtaining the forgotten equipment.

6 Provide for privacy.

PROCEDURE

For medications from a prescription container:

7 Check the label on each container and review the "rights" for this particular medication (see FIGURE 43–5 on p. 999) or on each prepoured medication: right medication, right person, right dose (e.g., be certain the strength of the solution/ointment in the container is correct), right route (e.g., be certain about which ear or both ears), right time, right day, right reason, and the right expiry date. Compare the label with the MAR and the care plan.
This reduces the risk for client injury.

8 Loosen lid(s) on container(s) if the client cannot do so. Tell the client the name of each medication (read from the label).

9 Place the container where the client can reach it, or hand the container to the client. Let the client read the name of the medication to you. Be sure the client wears eyeglasses if needed.

For medications from a blister pack:

10 Check the blister pack label and check for right medication, right person, right dose, right route, right time, right day, right reason, and right expiry date. Compare the label with the MAR and the care plan.
This reduces the risk for client injury.

11 Instruct the client to open the blister pack by pushing the soft plastic bubble and pushing the pills into a dish or saucer.
Having a dish or saucer handy beneath the blister pack will reduce the risk of dropping the pills as they exit the blister pack.

12 If the client cannot manually push open the blister pack, you can do so for the client.

For all medications:

13 Help the client pour the correct amount of liquid or count the correct number of pills.
This is a quick way to double-check that the client has all the medication needed.

Assist the client:

a *If the medication is to be swallowed:*

i Check the care plan to see if there is a specific order in which medications must be taken.
Certain medications, such as cough syrups, are meant to slowly coat the throat so should be taken last, for example, after water has been taken to assist the client to swallow pills.

ii Give a sip of water.
Providing a sip of water moistens the mouth and prevents pills from sticking to the client's tongue.

iii Support the client's hand, as necessary, to pour the medication.

iv Give a full glass of water or other cool liquid after the client puts the medication in the mouth (see exceptions in **i**, above).

v Remind the client to lower the chin while swallowing.
Lowering the chin will assist in the swallowing process and reduce the risk of aspirating the pills.

b *If the medication is to dissolve under the person's tongue:*

i Ask the client to put the medication under the tongue.

ii Ask the client to close the mouth and let the medication dissolve.

iii Remind the client not to chew or swallow the medication.
Chewing or swallowing these medications will prevent the medication from being absorbed properly under the tongue as it was designed to be.

iv Do not give food or fluids while the medication is dissolving.
Eating foods (or fluids) will prevent the medication from being absorbed under the tongue.

14 Close the container(s) after use.
This prevents accidentally spilling the medication.

Continued

Assisting With Oral Medications—cont'd

POST-PROCEDURE

15 Have the client record the medications taken correctly if applicable, or record this information for the client if specified in the care plan.
Medication self-administration should be recorded for legal reasons and to keep the rest of the health care team informed.
16 Store materials in their proper locations.
This makes them easier to find the next time they are needed.
17 Remove privacy measures.
18 Practise hand hygiene.

Report and Record your actions and observations, according to employer policy.
This is done for legal reasons and to keep the rest of the health care team informed.

Assisting With Rectal Suppositories or Enemas

123

Advocate on behalf of the client's quality of life by promoting:
Dignity • Independence • Preferences • Privacy • Safety *(see BOX 1–4, on p. 17)*

PRE-PROCEDURE

1 Identify the client, according to employer policy.
This eliminates the possibility of mistaking one client for another.
2 Explain the procedure to the client.
3 Practise hand hygiene.
4 Assist the client with handwashing.
5 Collect the following supplies:
- ☐ **Suppository**
- ☐ **Water-soluble lubricant**
- ☐ **Disposable gloves**
- ☐ **Toilet tissue**

By collecting all the necessary equipment beforehand, you will not have to leave your client's side and can eliminate wasting time and energy in obtaining the forgotten equipment.
6 Provide for privacy.

PROCEDURE

For suppositories:
7 Check the label on the suppository for right medication, right person, right dose, right route, right time, right day, right reason, and the right expiry date. Compare the label with the MAR and the care plan.
This reduces the risk for client injury.
8 Assist the client into bed and into the Sims' position on the left side.
*The descending colon lies on the left side of the body (see **FIGURE 17–24** on p. 293), so in this position, gravity will allow the suppository's medication to enter it from the anus and rectum.*
9 Help the client to lower or remove clothing to expose the anal area.
10 Unwrap the suppository.
11 Apply water-soluble lubricant to the suppository. Do not use petroleum jelly.
Petroleum jelly is not water soluble.
12 Give a glove to the client and see that it is put on.
13 Hand to the client the suppository to be inserted into the rectum. If necessary, don a glove and guide the client's hand.
14 Observe as the client inserts the suppository and wipes the anus with toilet tissue.

Continued

Assisting With Rectal Suppositories or Enemas—cont'd

15 Have the client remove and discard the glove into the waste container.

16 Remind the client to remain on the side for 15 to 20 minutes.
Remaining in this position will allow the suppository to dissolve and the medication to be absorbed.

For enemas:

This should be performed only if it is within your scope of practice for your province and you have been properly taught the correct procedure by a nurse.
Inserting any foreign object (such as an enema tip) into a client's anus and rectum can cause injury to the client. Proper training in performing this procedure will reduce the risk for client injury.

17 If it is within your scope of practice, perform steps 7 to 9 as above. Remove enema device from its packaging, and remove the cap covering the insertion tip.

18 Lubricate the insertion tip with water-soluble jelly.
This makes the tip easier to insert into the client's anus and rectum.

19 Insert the tip into the client's rectum, up to the end of the tip. (Remember to follow the manufacturer's instructions.)

20 Gently squeeze the contents of the enema into the client. Ask the client to take slow, deep breaths during this part of the process.
Squeezing gently will decrease the risk for abdominal cramping.

21 Frequently check on the client's level of comfort throughout the procedure. If the client develops cramping, ***stop immediately***, and consult your supervisor.
Abdominal cramping may be a sign of rectal injury or another serious medical problem and should be investigated before proceeding.

22 Remove the enema, and wipe the client's rectal area with toilet tissue. Discard the tissue into a garbage container.
This is to reduce the risk for pathogen spread.

23 If the enema was intended to assist in bowel evacuation, assist the client onto the toilet, a commode chair, or a bedpan, according to the client's level of mobility. Ensure that the client is sitting as upright as possible. Provide toilet tissue.
The upright position ensures better bowel evacuation than the lying position.

POST-PROCEDURE

24 Discard used materials in a waste container.
This decreases the risk for pathogen spread.

25 Assist the client with handwashing.

26 Provide the appropriate amount of privacy, and allow the client to defecate.

27 Have the client record medications taken if applicable. If specified in the care plan, record for the client.

28 Store materials in their proper location.
This makes them easier to find the next time they are needed.

29 Remove privacy measures.

30 Practise hand hygiene.

Report and Record your actions and observations, according to employer policy.
This is done for legal reasons and to keep the rest of the health care team informed.

Assisting With Eye Medications or Ointments

123

Advocate on behalf of the client's quality of life by promoting:

Dignity • Independence • Preferences • Privacy • Safety *(see BOX 1–4, on p. 17)*

PRE-PROCEDURE

1 Identify the client, according to employer policy.
This eliminates the possibility of mistaking one client for another.

2 Explain the procedure to the client.

3 Practise hand hygiene.

4 Assist the client with handwashing.

5 Collect the following supplies:
- ☐ **Eye medication or ointment**
- ☐ **Tissues or clean makeup remover pads**
- ☐ **Small hand mirror**
- ☐ **Disposable gloves (if necessary)**

By collecting all the necessary equipment beforehand, you will not have to leave your client's side and can eliminate wasting time and energy in obtaining the forgotten equipment.

6 Provide for privacy.

PROCEDURE

7 Check the label on the prescription container for right medication (e.g., be certain the preparation is for use in the eyes), right person, right dose (e.g., be certain the strength of the solution/ointment in the container is correct), right route (e.g., be certain about which eye or both eyes), right time, right day, right reason, and the right expiry date. Compare the label with the MAR and the care plan.
This reduces the risk for client injury.

8 Loosen lid on container if the client cannot do so.

9 Place the container within the client's reach, or hand it to the client. Be sure the client is wearing eyeglasses as needed.

10 Hold a mirror to help the client self-administer the eye medication.

11 Remove the client's eyeglasses, if worn.

12 Assist the client with:

a Eye medication (FIGURE 43–6):
- i Guide the client's hand to grasp the lower eyelid.
- ii Observe whether the client looks up and releases drops into the lower lid.
- iii Make sure that the dropper does not touch the client's eye.

Touching the eye with the dropper may injure the client's eye and would contaminate the dropper.
- iv Observe whether the client closes the eye to distribute the medication.

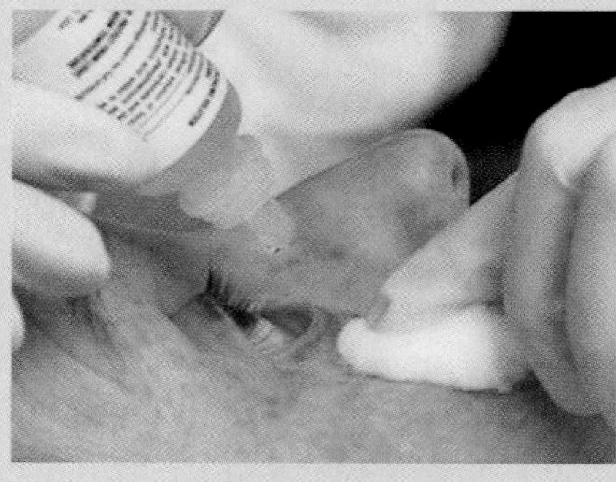

FIGURE 43–6 Insert the eye drop into the inside lower eyelid by holding it open with your gloved hand. (**Source:** Lilley, L.L., Harrington, S., & Snyder, J.S. (2005). *Pharmacology and the nursing process* (4th ed., p. 128). St. Louis, MO: Mosby.)

b Ointment (FIGURE 43–7):
- i Guide the client's hand to grasp the lower eyelid.
- ii Observe whether the client looks up and squeezes a small ribbon of ointment into the lower lid from the inner corner of the eye to the outer corner of the eye (FIGURE 43–8).
- iii Make sure that the tip of the tube does not touch the eye surface.
- iv Observe that the client closes the eye to allow the medication to dissolve and be distributed, and discard tissue.

Continued

Assisting With Eye Medications or Ointments—cont'd

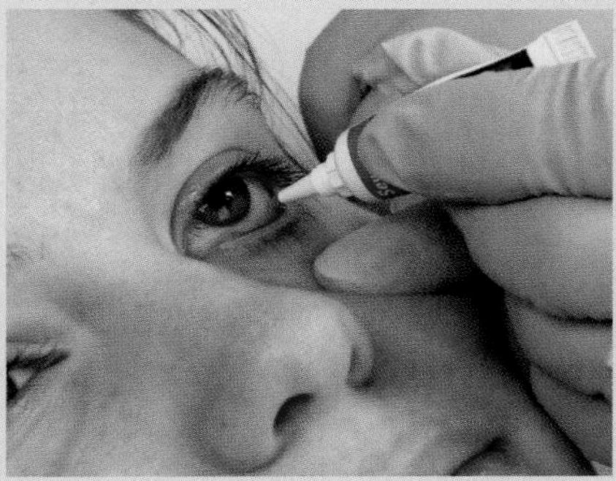

FIGURE 43–7 Applying eye ointment. (**Source:** Lilley, L.L., Harrington, S., & Snyder, J.S. (2005). *Pharmacology and the nursing process* (4th ed., p. 129). St. Louis, MO: Mosby.)

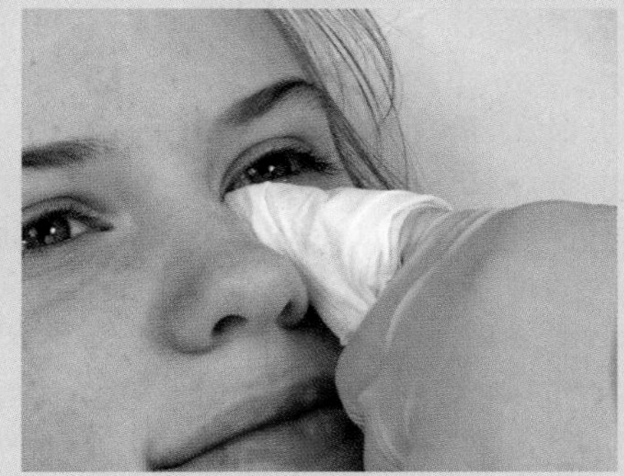

FIGURE 43–8 Apply gentle pressure to the inner corner of the eye for a few seconds after giving eye medications to ensure that they have time to be absorbed. (**Source:** Lilley, L.L., Harrington, S., & Snyder, J.S. (2005). *Pharmacology and the nursing process* (4th ed., p. 129). St. Louis, MO: Mosby.)

POST-PROCEDURE

13 Reseal the container.
This reduces the risk of contaminating the tip of the container.
14 Assist the client with hand hygiene.
15 Have the client record medications taken if applicable, or record for the client if specified in the care plan.
16 Store materials in their proper location.
This makes them easier to find the next time they are needed.
17 Remove privacy measures.
18 Practise hand hygiene.

Report and Record your actions and observations, according to employer policy.
This is done for legal reasons and to keep the rest of the health care team informed.

Assisting With Ear Drops

123

Advocate on behalf of the client's quality of life by promoting:

Dignity • **I**ndependence • **P**references • **P**rivacy • **S**afety

(see BOX 1–4, on p. 17)

PRE-PROCEDURE

1 Identify the client, according to employer policy.
This eliminates the possibility of mistaking one client for another.
2 Explain the procedure to the client.
3 Practise hand hygiene.
4 Assist the client with handwashing.
5 Collect the following supplies:
- ☐ **Ear drop medication**
- ☐ **Tissues or cotton balls**
- ☐ **Small hand mirror**
- ☐ **Disposable gloves (if necessary)**

By collecting all the necessary equipment beforehand, you will not have to leave your client's side and can eliminate wasting time and energy in obtaining the forgotten equipment.

6 Provide for privacy.

Continued

Assisting With Ear Drops—cont'd

PROCEDURE

7 Check the label on the prescription container and review the "rights": right medication (e.g., be certain the preparation is for use in the ears), right person, right dose (e.g., be certain the strength of the solution/ointment in the container is correct), right route (e.g., be certain about which ear or both ears), right time, right day, right reason, and the right expiry date. Compare the label with the MAR and the care plan.
This reduces the risk for client injury.

8 Loosen the lid on the container if the client cannot do so.

9 Place the container within the client's reach or hand it to the client. Be sure the client wears eyeglasses if needed.

10 Assist the client to lie on the side exposing the ear that is to receive the drop.
By positioning the client on the side, you help the ear drops to enter the middle ear using gravity.

11 Hold the mirror so the client can self-administer the ear medication. If the client cannot manoeuvre the ear dropper, you should assist, with permission (**FIGURE 43–9**). Ensure the tip of the dropper does not touch the ear.
Touching the tip of the dropper will contaminate it. It needs to remain sterile.

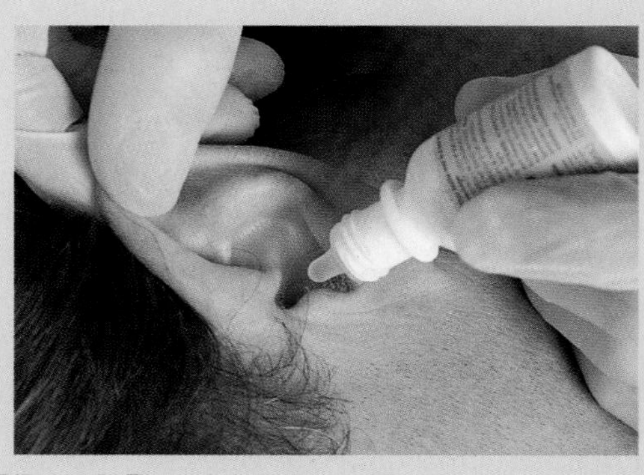

FIGURE 43–9 For adults, the external ear should be gently pulled upward and outward. If the client is an infant or child under 3 years of age, pull the external ear down and back. (**Source:** Potter, P.A., & Perry, A.G. (2005). *Fundamentals of nursing* (6th ed., p. 863). St. Louis, MO: Mosby.)

12 Ensure the drop or drops go into the ear canal. Gently massage the outside of the ear (the tragus), and then temporarily place a piece of cotton ball in the ear. The cotton ball can be removed after several minutes.
Gently massaging the ear tragus allows the medication to go as far into the ear canal as possible. The cotton ball holds the medication in place and prevents it from leaking out.

13 Repeat steps 10 to 12 to assist the client with inserting drop(s) into the other ear if necessary.

POST-PROCEDURE

14 Reseal the container.
This reduces the risk of contaminating the tip or the contents of the container.

15 Assist the client with hand hygiene.

16 Have the client record medications taken if applicable, or record for the client if specified in the care plan.

17 Store materials in their proper location.
This makes them easier to find the next time they are needed.

18 Remove privacy measures.

19 Wash your hands.

Report and Record your actions and observations, according to employer policy.
This is done for legal reasons and to keep the rest of the health care team informed.

Assisting With Transdermal Discs

123

Advocate on behalf of the client's quality of life by promoting:

Dignity • Independence • Preferences • Privacy • Safety (see BOX 1–4, on p. 17)

PRE-PROCEDURE

1 Identify the client, according to employer policy.
This eliminates the possibility of mistaking one client for another.
2 Explain the procedure to the client.
3 Practise hand hygiene.
4 Assist the client with hand hygiene.
5 Collect the following supplies:
- ☐ **Medicated transdermal disc**
- ☐ **Disposable gloves**
- ☐ **Small garbage bag**
- ☐ **Pen with nonsmear ink** (for labelling the patch)

By collecting all the necessary equipment beforehand, you will not have to leave your client's side and can eliminate wasting time and energy in obtaining the forgotten equipment.
6 Provide for privacy.

PROCEDURE

7 Check the label on the disc container for right medication, right person, right dose, right route, right time, right day, right reason, and the right expiry date. Compare the label with the MAR and the care plan.
This reduces the risk for client injury.
8 Put on gloves. Give the client a glove to put on.
9 Have the client remove, fold, and discard the old disc into a waste container. Wash the skin that had been covered by the old disc.
Washing the skin removes traces of medication or adhesive, which can irritate the skin.
10 Ask the client to select a new site for the new disc (any area without hair). Usually, the chest or upper arm area is used.
Hairy areas interfere with the adhesive and will prevent the patch from forming a good seal. Without a good seal, the client will not get the correct dosage of medication.
11 Observe or help the client to apply the new disc to the skin surface. Be sure that the medicated surface of the disc is not touched by ungloved fingers (FIGURE 43–10).
If you touch the disc with an ungloved hand, your skin may absorb some of the drug.

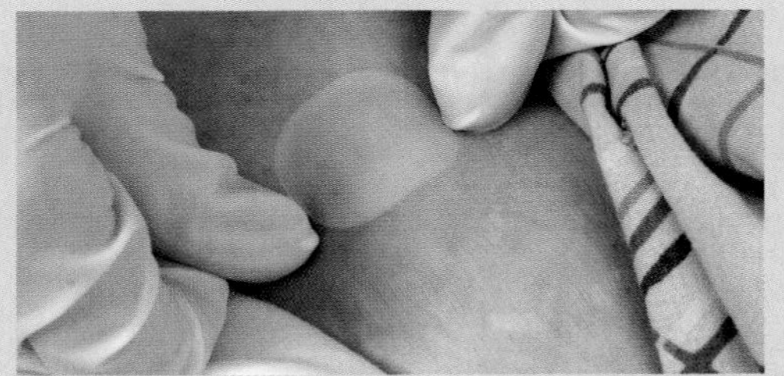

FIGURE 43–10 Ensure that the edges of the transdermal disc are secure after it has been applied on the client. (**Source:** Lilley, L.L., Harrington, S., & Snyder, J.S. (2005). *Pharmacology and the nursing process* (4th ed., p. 139). St. Louis, MO: Mosby.)

12 Write the date and time on the disc, making sure that your writing does not smudge.
Writing the date and time will ensure that the other health care team members know when the patch was applied. ***(Note: Some agencies require that you write on the disc before it is applied on the client; others prefer it done after applying the disc. As with all steps, ensure that you follow your agency's policies.)***

Continued

Assisting With Transdermal Discs—cont'd

POST-PROCEDURE

13 Discard the disc wrapper and other used materials into a garbage bag, and tie the bag. Dispose of the bag into a lidded garbage container.
Disposing of the patch in this way will ensure that the patch is not accidentally chewed by pets or children. There is enough medication in most patches to harm a child or a pet.
14 Remove gloves. Practise hand hygiene.
15 Have the client remove the glove, and discard it as well. Assist with hand hygiene.
16 Have the client record medications taken if applicable, or record for the person if specified in the care plan.
17 Store materials in their proper location.
This makes them easier to find the next time they are needed.
18 Remove privacy measures.
19 Practise hand hygiene.

Report and Record your actions and observations, according to employer policy.
This is done for legal reasons and to keep the rest of the health care team informed.

Assisting With Metered Dose Inhalers

123

Advocate on behalf of the client's quality of life by promoting:
Dignity • Independence • Preferences • Privacy • Safety (see BOX 1–4, on p. 17)

PRE-PROCEDURE

1 Identify the client, according to employer policy.
This eliminates the possibility of mistaking one client for another.
2 Explain the procedure to the client.
3 Practise hand hygiene.
4 Help the client with handwashing.
5 Collect the following supplies:
- ☐ **MDI container of prescription medication**
- ☐ **Disposable gloves** (if necessary)

It is important to plan thoroughly before starting any procedure. By collecting all the necessary equipment beforehand, you will not have to leave your client's side and can eliminate wasting time and energy in obtaining the forgotten equipment.
6 Provide for privacy.

PROCEDURE

7 a If the client is taking two asthma medications, always double-check, with either the client or your supervisor, which MDI the client should take first.
The order of these medications is very important because one medication helps to open the client's airway, which allows the other medication to then enter the client's lungs so that it can work more effectively.
b Check the label on the container for right medication, right person, right dose, right route, right time, right day, right reason, and the right expiry date. Compare the label with the MAR and the care plan.
8 Assist the client to shake the inhaler container vigorously.
Shaking the inhaler vigorously will activate the medication inside it, allowing it to work properly.

Continued

Assisting With Metered Dose Inhalers—cont'd

9 a Hand the MDI to the client, who then uses it to inhale the medication.(FIGURE 43–11).
b If two puffs are ordered, wait ***at least 1 minute*** between puffs of the first medication.
c If switching to another medication, wait ***at least 5 minutes*** before switching to the other medication.
This allows enough time for the first medication to work before switching to the other medication.

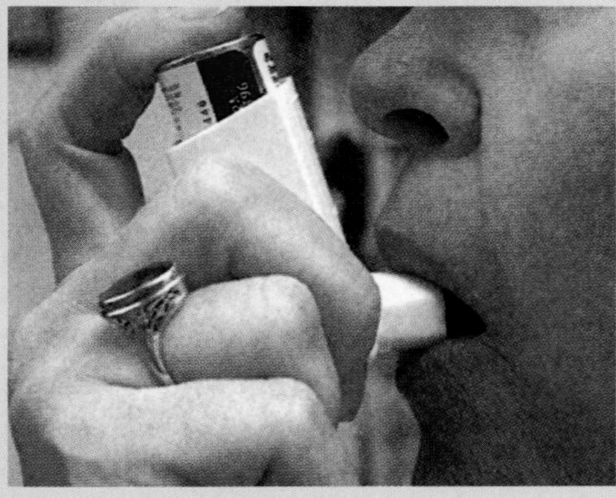

FIGURE 43–11 (**Source:** Birchenall, J., & Streight, E. (2003). *Mosby's textbook for the home care aide* (2nd ed., p. 354). St. Louis, MO: Mosby.)

POST-PROCEDURE

10 Have the client record medications taken if applicable, or record for the client if specified in the care plan.
Keeping track of medications used is a good habit for all clients so they can eliminate repeating doses or missing doses by accident.
11 Clean the MDI, according to the manufacturer's instructions, and store it in its proper location.
This makes it easier to find the next time it is needed.
12 Remove privacy measures.
13 Practise hand hygiene.

Report and Record your actions and observations, according to employer policy.
This is done for legal reasons and to keep the rest of the health care team informed.

Assisting With Metered Dose Inhalers With a Holding Chamber

123

Advocate on behalf of the client's quality of life by promoting:
Dignity • Independence • Preferences • Privacy • Safety (see BOX 1–4, on p. 17)

PRE-PROCEDURE

1 Identify the client, according to employer policy.
This eliminates the possibility of mistaking one client for another.
2 Explain the procedure to the client.
3 Practise hand hygiene.
4 Help the client with handwashing.
5 Collect the following supplies:
- ☐ **MDI container(s) of prescription medication**
- ☐ **Holding chamber**
- ☐ **Disposable gloves** (if necessary)

By collecting all the necessary equipment beforehand, you will not have to leave your client's side and can eliminate wasting time and energy in obtaining the forgotten equipment.
6 Provide for privacy.

Continued

Assisting With Metered Dose Inhalers With a Holding Chamber—cont'd

PROCEDURE

7 a If the client is taking two asthma medications, always double-check, with either the client or your supervisor, which MDI the client should take first.

The order of these medications is very important because one medication helps to open the client's airway, which allows the other medication to then enter the client's lungs so that it can work more effectively.

b Check the label on the container for right medication, right person, right dose, right route, right time, right day, the right reason, and the right expiry date. Compare the label with the MAR and the care plan.

This reduces the risk for client injury.

8 Assist the client to shake the inhaler container vigorously.

The inhaler must be shaken vigorously to activate the medication inside it.

9 Assist the client to remove the cap from the MDI container and insert it into the holding chamber.

The holding chamber helps medication to be inhaled into the client's lungs as intended and greatly reduces the amount of medication that would otherwise land on the clients tongue.

10 a Hand the MDI and the attached holding chamber to the client, who then uses it to inhale the medication (**FIGURE 43–12**).

The holding chamber is designed to prevent the medication from dropping onto the client's tongue.

The client should breathe normally for at least six breaths.

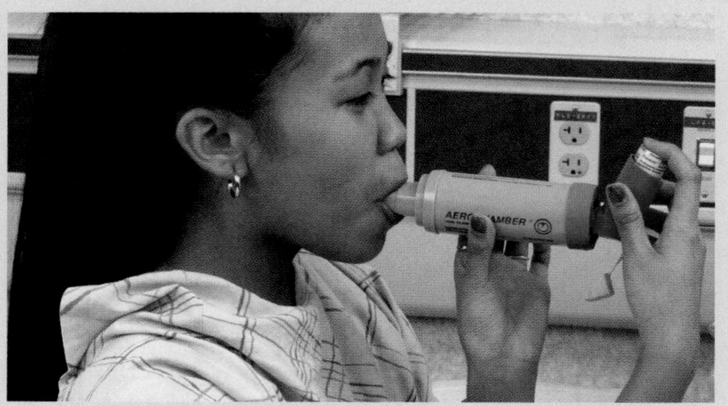

FIGURE 43–12 A holding chamber is often used when the client is unable to breathe deeply, although many doctors believe holding chambers should be used for all clients. With the holding chamber, the client can inhale the medication while breathing normally. (**Source:** Lilley, L. L., Harrington, S., & Snyder, J. S. (2005). *Pharmacology and the nursing process* (4th ed., p. 135). St. Louis, MO: Mosby.)

b If two puffs of one medication are ordered, wait ***at least 1 minute*** between puffs.

c If switching to another medication, wait ***at least 5 minutes*** before switching to the other medication.

This allows enough time for the first medication to work before switching to the other medication.

11 Repeat steps 8 to 10 with the second MDI if necessary.

12 Have the client rinse the mouth with water and spit out. Instruct the client ***not*** to swallow the water.

The water holds traces of medication, which may cause problems if left on the oral or digestive mucous membranes.

POST-PROCEDURE

13 Have the client record medications taken if applicable, or record for the client if specified in the care plan.

14 Clean the MDI, according to the manufacturer's instructions. Store the MDI in its proper location.

This makes it easier to find the next time it is needed.

15 Remove privacy measures.

16 Practise hand hygiene.

Report and Record your actions and observations, according to employer policy.

This is done for legal reasons and to keep the rest of the health care team informed.

CHAPTER REVIEW

KEY POINTS

- Assisting with and administering medications are different functions. *Assist* means "to help"; *administer* means "to give."
- A small mistake when assisting with or administering medications can cause serious harm.
- Assisting with medications involves helping clients to self-administer medications. It is strictly a *mechanical* function. As a support worker, you do what clients would do themselves if they could to obtain the medication.
- Administering medications is usually done in facilities and for some home care clients, but it is beyond your scope of practice. It involves measuring medications or getting them into the person's body.
- In some provinces and territories, ***in some special circumstances***, your supervisor may authorize and train you to perform a controlled act (e.g., giving an insulin injection). ***Never assume this responsibility, as it is beyond your usual scope of practice.***
- Medications are chemical substances that cause a specific effect on the body. Medications are taken or prescribed to (1) treat an illness, (2) promote health, or (3) prevent illness.
- All health care workers involved with administering or assisting with medications should be aware of drugs' effects and their classifications and the responsibilities associated with medications.
- Medication routes include (1) oral (solid, semi-solid, or liquids), (2) topical, (3) optic (eye), (4) otic (ear), (5) parenteral, (6) inhalation, and (7) suppository.
- The rights of clients related to medication administration by support workers include: the right medication, right person, right dose, right route, right time, right day, right reason, right expiry date, and right documentation.
- It is important for support workers to know the correct procedure for assisting with medications if doing so is within their scope of practice.

CRITICAL THINKING IN PRACTICE

You are a support worker working for a home care agency. You are allowed to assist with medications only if the client cannot physically open the medication packaging or has difficulty holding the pills. Today, one of your clients tells you she has a headache. You assist her to take her OTC medication. How would you do so in a safe and hygienic manner? What rules must you follow when reporting and recording this procedure in the client's chart? If you made a mistake with the medication, how do you correct the error?

REVIEW QUESTIONS

Answers to these questions are at the bottom of the next page.

Circle T if the answer is true, and circle F if the answer is false.

1. T F Support workers routinely administer medications.
2. T F A lozenge is a type of medication.
3. T F Over-the-counter (OTC) medications require a prescription.
4. T F You can purchase OTC medications for a client.
5. T F The physician, nurse, and case manager are responsible for monitoring the outcome of the drug therapy.
6. T F Adverse effects do not need to be reported.
7. T F You are responsible for filling pillboxes.
8. T F Any person administering or assisting with medications must record on the MAR according to the employer's policy.
9. T F Medications can be taken at any time, as long as the correct dose is given.
10. T F When assisting with medications, you must check that the client is taking the right medication.
11. T F All medications should be stored in the kitchen cabinet above the stove.

Circle the BEST answer.

12. Mrs. Stein has sore, swollen joints in her hands. You assist with her medications. Which of the following is *your* responsibility?
A. Loosening and removing container lids
B. Phoning the pharmacy to order more medication
C. Pouring the medication for her and administering it to her
D. Changing the times to take her medication

13. Which of the following is not one of the "rights" related to assisting with medications?
A. The right medication
B. The right colour
C. The right person
D. The right time

14. Mrs. Smith is asking for a headache pill that is not listed on her MAR. What should you do?
A. Phone her family doctor
B. Give it to her
C. Ask her daughter to give it to her
D. Check with your supervisor

15. A medication should be kept:
A. At the bedside, with the container open
B. In a warm, humid area
C. Along with other family members' or residents' medications
D. In its original labelled container

16. Which of the following should be reported to your supervisor? The client:
A. Refuses to take the medication
B. Needs to use a metered dose inhaler as specified on the MAR
C. Says that she does not like the taste of her medication but takes it anyway
D. Knows what to ask her doctor about her pills on her next appointment

Answers: 1.F, 2.T, 3.F, 4.F, 5.T, 6.F, 7.F, 8.T, 9.F, 10.T, 11.F, 12.A, 13.B, 14.D, 15.D, 16.A

CHAPTER 44

Heat and Cold Applications

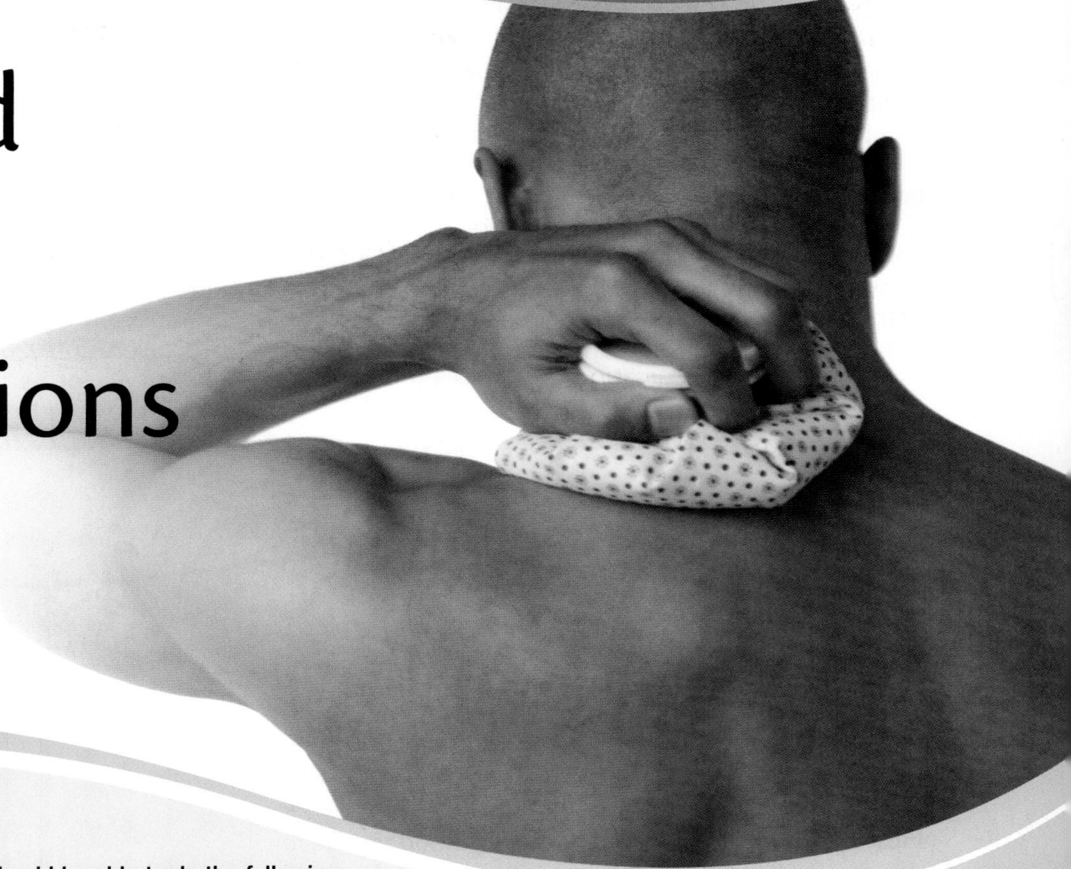

OBJECTIVES

After reading this chapter, the learner should be able to do the following:

- Identify the purposes, effects, and complications of heat and cold applications.
- List clients at risk for complications from heat and cold applications.
- List the guidelines for application of heat and cold.
- Perform the procedures described in this chapter in a safe manner.

KEY TERMS

aquathermia pad A waterproof plastic or rubber pad that can be applied to areas of muscle sprain, edema, or mild inflammation in the place of a heating pad or cold pack. *p. 1022*

blanket warmers Warming cabinets designed to heat bed linens. *p. 1014*

cold pack A commercial or homemade cold application; may be moist or dry. *p. 1027*

compress A soft pad that is moistened and applied over a body area. *p. 1017*

compression bandage A bandage designed to provide pressure to a particular area. Also known as a *tensor bandage*. *p. 1026*

constrict To squeeze or make narrow. *p. 1026*

dilate To expand or open wider. *p. 1016*

frostbite A medical condition in which skin and other tissues are damaged by extreme cold. *p. 1026*

gel pack A commercially produced hot-and-cold pack designed to keep its temperature over a period. *p. 1022*

RICE An acronym for "**R**est, **I**ce, **C**ompression, and **E**levate" as a method of treating recent injuries. *p. 1026*

sitz bath A shallow plastic bathtub, filled with warm water, designed to keep the buttocks and hips immersed while the person is in the sitting position. *p. 1020*

wheat bag (or beanbag) A type of heating bag that provides dry heat and is heated in a microwave. *p. 1018*

Physicians, nurses, and physiotherapists use heat and cold applications to reduce tissue swelling and promote healing and comfort. Heat and cold have opposite effects on body functions (**FIGURE 44–1**). Heat increases blood flow by *dilating* blood vessels in the area being heated (**FIGURE 44–1, *B***). Cold slows blood flow by *constricting* blood vessels in the area being cooled (**FIGURE 44–1, *C***). Both effects can be helpful, but there are risks associated with heat and cold applications, such as severe injuries and a decrease in the ability of that body part to function well. ***Because of these risks, a support worker should never use heat and cold applications unless they are in the client's care plan, and then only if this duty has been delegated by a nurse.***

Any client receiving a heat or cold application should be checked frequently for any signs of problems related to their use (TABLE 44–1). ***Inspect the skin beneath the application frequently, according to the care plan. It is advisable to check the skin every 5 minutes for the first two checks, and at least every 15 minutes after that. Because not every client will report discomfort, you should be particularly aware of signs of discomfort, such as restlessness, agitation, or other changes in behaviour.***

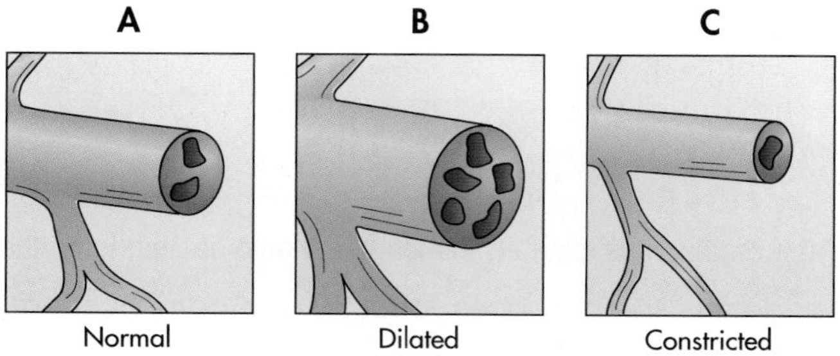

FIGURE 44–1 **A,** Blood vessel under normal conditions. **B,** Dilated blood vessel. **C,** Constricted blood vessel.

HEAT APPLICATIONS

Heat applications can be applied to almost any body part. They are often used for musculo-skeletal injuries or problems—for example, strains, low back pain, and arthritis (see TABLE 44–1). Heat applications in hospitals and clinics include the use of **blanket warmers**, which are warming cabinets designed to heat bed linens for chilled clients who are recovering from anaesthetic, receiving chemotherapy, or are too ill or frail to raise their own body temperature. Like all heat applications, it is important to ensure the linens are not so hot as to cause burns by adjusting the cabinet heating temperature and testing the

TABLE 44–1 Comparison Between Heat and Cold Applications

	Heat	Cold
Purposes	*For persistent (chronic) pain:* • Reduces pain of muscle cramps • Reduces pain related to arthritis • Promotes healing • Reduces joint stiffness	*For recent injury:* • Reduces swelling • Reduces pain • Slows bruising • Reduces itching from insect bites
How it works	Expands blood vessels and assists in increasing circulation to the area	Constricts blood vessels to reduce swelling and pain in the area
Examples	*Moist:* • Hot/warm compress • Hot/warm soak • Sitz bath *Dry:* • Wheat bags (or beanbags) • Heating pads • Heat rubs	*Moist:* • Cold/cool water compress • Cold/cool water soak *Dry:* • Cold pack, gel pack • Ice packs, bags, and collars • Cold rubs
Length of time for application*	Do not apply longer than 15 minutes at a time Check the client's skin every 5 minutes	Do not apply longer than 15 minutes at a time Check the client's skin every 5 minutes Cold applications are usually applied in 15-minute intervals (i.e., 15 minutes on followed by 15 minutes off)
Signs of problems: Stop application and report at once	Excessive skin redness in the area Excessive facial redness Blisters Complaints of discomfort, pain, or burning (or changes in the client's behaviour) Signs of skin irritation (such as redness, rash, itching, or burning)	Pale, white, or grey skin Cyanosis (bluish skin colour) Shivering Complaints of discomfort, pain, numbness, or burning (or changes in the client's behaviour) Signs of skin irritation (such as redness, rash, itching, or burning)
Complications from misuse	Burns Tissue death Circulatory shock	Frostbite Tissue death Circulatory shock

*These times were suggested by the Fowler–Kennedy Sports Medicine Clinic of Western University. Your supervisor may have more specific times as they pertain to each individual client. You should always follow the client's care plan and the policies of your employing agency.

Source: Fowler–Kennedy Sports Medicine Clinic, Western University, London, ON.

> **Think About Safety**
>
> **Heat and Cold Applications**
>
> Both heat and cold applications can be either moist or dry. You must thoroughly understand the purposes, effects, and complications of both heat and cold applications. ***Because of the risks involved, some employers allow only nurses to do heat and cold applications, while some others may permit support workers to do them as well. As always, you must be certain that the procedure is within your scope of practice.***
>
> Before you perform these procedures, it is ***your responsibility*** to make sure of the following:
>
> - Your provincial or territorial laws and employer's policies allow you to perform the procedure.
> - The procedure is in your job description.
> - You have the necessary training.
> - You are familiar with the equipment.
> - You have reviewed the procedure with a nurse.
> - A nurse is available to answer questions and to supervise you.

linens by placing a corner of them against the inner aspect of your wrist.

When heat is applied to skin, blood vessels in the area **dilate** (i.e., they expand or open wider) (see **FIGURE 44–1, *B***), allowing more blood to flow through them. This extra blood brings more oxygen and nutrients to the tissues for healing and removes excess fluid and wastes from the area faster. The extra blood causes the overlying skin to become red and warm to the touch. When heat is used correctly, muscles in that area relax, and painful swelling is reduced.

Complications

Burns result when heat is applied either for too long or at too high a temperature. Pain, excessive redness, and blisters are danger signs of burns. If you observe any of these signs, you should remove the application and report your observations immediately. If not treated right away, burns can lead to serious, life-threatening problems.

Some clients are at greater risk than others for burns and other complications from heat applications (see the *Think About Safety: Clients at High Risk for Complications From Heat or Cold Applications* box). It is your responsibility to observe these clients closely and to protect them from injury. Follow the guidelines listed in **BOX 44–1** when performing heat and cold applications.

> **Think About Safety**
>
> **Clients at High Risk for Complications From Heat or Cold Applications**
>
> - ***Clients with thin, delicate, or fragile skin.*** These clients include infants, young children, older adults, and fair-skinned people.
> - ***Clients who have decreased sensation (singular).*** Clients who have difficulty sensing heat, cold, or pain may not realize if the application is too hot or too cold and are at risk for skin damage. Examples of situations that may reduce a person's ability to feel pain include:
>   - Loss of consciousness
>   - Scarring of the skin
>   - Use of some medications
>   - Spinal cord injuries
>   - Stroke
>   - Diabetes
>   - Aging, which can cause decreased sensation due to changes in body function
> - ***Clients with dementia or confusion.*** These clients may not recognize pain, or they may not be able to communicate that they are in pain. You need to look for changes in the client's behaviour, which can signal discomfort.
> - ***Clients with metal implants.*** Metal conducts heat and cold, so deep tissues can be burned. Pacemakers and joint replacements are made of metal. ***Do not apply heat in the area of the implant.***

Moist and Dry Heat Applications

Moist heat application involves water coming in contact with the skin. Moist heat has certain advantages, including the following:

- Water conducts heat, so moist heat has a greater and faster effect than dry heat.

BOX 44–1 General Guidelines for Applying Heat or Cold

- Apply only when (1) ordered by a professional, (2) allowed by your employer, and (3) you are assigned to do so.
- Know how to use the equipment.
- Before applying moist applications, measure the temperature, according to your employer policy.
- Follow employer policies for safe temperature ranges (see TABLE 44–2).
- Do not apply hot applications above 41.1°C (106°F) because tissue damage can occur. ***Only a nurse can apply a very hot application.***
- Ask your supervisor what the temperature of the application should be for each client (see the *Think About Safety: Clients at High Risk for Complications From Heat or Cold Applications* box, on p. 1016).
  - Heat—cooler temperatures are used for clients at risk.
  - Cold—warmer temperatures are used for clients at risk.
- Know the precise site of the application. Ask your supervisor to show you the site.
- Before applying a dry heat or cold application, cover it with a flannel or terry-cloth cover, towel, or pillowcase, according to your employer policy.
- Do not leave clients at risk unattended.
- Observe the client's skin at least every 5 minutes for signs of complications (see TABLE 44–1, on p. 1015).
- Observe for changes in the client's behaviour, which may indicate pain.
- Remind the client not to change the temperature of the application.
- Prevent chills. When moist heat is applied, the increased blood flow to the affected area may cause reduced blood flow to other body parts, and the client may feel chilled. Cover the client with a blanket or robe. Eliminate room drafts. Offering the client socks to wear will help ensure warmth.
- Ask your supervisor how long to leave the application in place. Carefully watch the time. Heat and cold are applied for no longer than 15-minute periods.
- Provide for privacy. Properly drape and screen the client. Expose only the body part on which you will apply heat or cold.
- If it is safe to leave, place the call bell within the client's reach or remain within easy hearing distance.
- Follow Standard Practices. Wear gloves if you or the client has nonintact skin.

- Heat penetrates deeper with moist applications, so they have lower (cooler) temperature settings than dry heat applications and, thereby, help prevent injury to the client.

In *dry heat applications*, water does not come in contact with skin. The advantages of dry heat are as follows:

- The application stays at the desired temperature longer.
- Dry heat does not penetrate as deeply as moist heat, so this type of application may be chosen if the client is very thin or has a medical condition in which a penetrating heat application would be harmful to underlying tissues (such as having a bone screw or plate). However, it should be noted that because water is not used, dry heat needs higher (hotter) temperatures to achieve the desired effect.

With both types of applications, the client is at risk for burns. It is very important, therefore, to continually check on the client and inspect the skin under the application every 5 minutes. As mentioned, the application should never be left on the skin longer than 15 minutes (see the *Focus on Home Care: Dry Heat Applications* box).

Warm Compresses

Warm compresses are moist heat applications. A **compress** is a soft pad that is moistened and applied over a body area. Compresses can be hot or cold. A

TABLE 44–2 Heat and Cold Temperature Ranges

Temperature	Centigrade Range	Fahrenheit Range
Very hot	41.1°C to 46.1°C	106°F to 115°F
Hot	36.6°C to 41.1°C	98°F to 106°F
Warm	33.8°C to 36.6°C	93°F to 98°F
Tepid	26.6°C to 33.8°C	80°F to 93°F
Cool	18.3°C to 26.6°C	65°F to 80°F
Cold	10.0°C to 18.3°C	50°F to 65°F

compress is usually made of cloth—for example, a washcloth, small towel, or gauze dressing.

Your supervisor will tell you how long to leave the application in place (never more than 15 minutes). As with all heat applications, before applying the compress, test to see if it is too hot by placing a small corner of it on the inner aspect of your wrist. Check the skin every 5 minutes. To maintain the temperature, change the compress frequently. A layer of plastic wrap and a dry towel can be used to cover the compress and retain the heat.

Sometimes the care plan may order commercial compresses, which are premoistened and packaged in foil. Before you unwrap them, they are heated under an infrared lamp, as instructed by the manufacturer. Then they are unwrapped and applied in the same manner as "homemade" hot compresses. Commercial compresses are used once and then discarded.

FOCUS ON HOME CARE

Dry Heat Applications

Wheat or Bean Bags

The use of **wheat bags** (or **beanbags**) has become very popular because they are easy to use and inexpensive. They can even be made at home. These bags are warmed in the microwave, but the length of warming time depends on size, components, and the heating power of the client's microwave. If the client's care plan instructs you to apply them, you should ***always do the following:***

- Heat the bag in the microwave ***only for the length of time specified in the client's care plan.***
- ***Never leave the bean bag unattended while it is heating in the microwave.*** The contents can spark or even catch on fire (similar to microwave popcorn)! Always remove the bag immediately if you begin to smell something burning.
- After heating, ***shake the bag in order to mix the beans inside***, as they usually heat unevenly.
- ***Never place these bags directly on skin.*** They should always be wrapped in a pad or towel to avoid injuring the client. Check with your supervisor if you are unsure of the type of cover you should use.

Heating Pads, Electric Blankets, and Hot-Water Bottles

Some of your home care clients may have electric heating pads or hot-water bottles that apply dry heat. These items create serious fire and burn risks, ***so support workers are usually not permitted to apply electric heating pads or hot-water bottles.*** If a client asks you to apply an electric heating pad or hot-water bottle, explain that your employer's policy does not allow you to do this. Find another way to provide warmth to the client—such as giving a blanket or a sweater—and tell your supervisor about the client's request. If the client insists on using a heating pad or hot-water bottle while you are on duty, the client may need to sign a legal waiver (sometimes called a "Negotiated Risk Agreement") with your supervisor before you can apply it.

Applying Warm Compresses 123

Advocate on behalf of the client's quality of life by promoting:

Dignity • Independence • Preferences • Privacy • Safety *(see BOX 1–4, on p. 17)*

PRE-PROCEDURE

1 Identify the client, according to employer policy.
This eliminates the possibility of mistaking one client for another.

2 Explain the procedure to the client.

3 Practise proper hand hygiene.

4 Collect the following supplies:
- ☐ **Basin**
- ☐ **Bath thermometer**
- ☐ **Small towel, washcloth, or gauze squares**
- ☐ **Ties, tape, or rolled gauze**
- ☐ **Bath towel, large towel, or clean sheet**
- ☐ **Waterproof pad**

By collecting all the necessary equipment beforehand, you will not have to leave your client's side and can eliminate wasting time and energy in obtaining the forgotten equipment.

5 Provide for privacy.

6 Place the waterproof pad under the body part to be treated.
This keeps the bedding dry.

7 Fill the basin one half to two thirds full with hot water, as directed by your supervisor. Measure the water temperature.
Water can easily spill from an overfilled basin if it is carried.

8 Place the compress in the water.

9 Wring out the compress.
The compress should be wet enough to be effective, but not dripping.

10 Apply the compress to the area. Note the time.
It is important to time all heat and cold treatments to avoid thermal injuries in the client.

11 Ask the client if the compress feels comfortable. If the client is comfortable, cover the compress quickly with plastic wrap. Cover the plastic wrap with a bath towel (FIGURE 44–2).

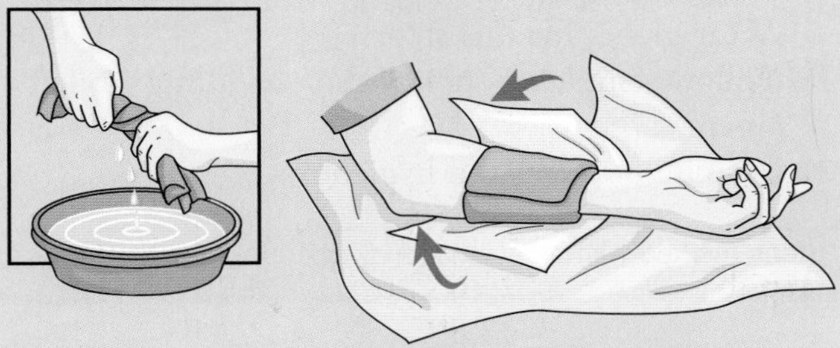

FIGURE 44–2 Cover a warm compress with plastic and a bath towel to prevent the compress from cooling down too quickly.

Secure the towel in place with ties, tape, or rolled gauze.
The plastic wrap prevents the towel from absorbing the moisture. The towel maintains the warmth of the compress as long as possible.

12 Place the call bell within reach. Follow the care plan for bed rail use.*
This provides an easy, safe way for the client to contact the staff if necessary.

13 Check the area every 5 minutes. The compress should never be applied longer than 15 minutes. Check for redness and complaints of pain, discomfort, or numbness. Remove the compress if any of these signs occur, and tell your supervisor immediately.
These are signs of thermal injuries and should be acted on quickly to avoid client injury!

14 Change the compress if it cools down.
The compress is effective as long as it is warm.

15 Remove the compress after 15 minutes or sooner, as directed by your supervisor. Pat the area dry with a towel.
Drying the skin with a patting motion is gentler than rubbing it with the towel.

Continued

Applying Warm Compresses—cont'd

POST-PROCEDURE

16 Provide for safety and comfort.
17 Remove privacy measures.
18 Clean the equipment. Discard disposable items. Wear gloves for this step.
19 Follow employer policy for handling soiled linen.
20 Practise proper hand hygiene.

Report and Record your actions and observations, according to employer policy.
This is done for legal reasons and to keep the rest of the health care team informed.

*Steps marked with an asterisk may not apply in community settings.

Warm Soaks

A warm soak is a warm, moist application that involves immersing a body part into heated water to promote circulation and muscle relaxation. Warm soaks are usually used for smaller body parts, such as a hand, lower arm, foot, or lower leg (**FIGURE 44–3**). A tub is used to soak larger parts (arm, leg, or torso). The soak lasts 15 minutes. Maintain the client's comfort and body alignment during the warm soak.

Remember to check the water temperature before soaking the body part. If the water is too hot, the skin can be burned as soon as it touches the water. If a water thermometer is not available, test the water by dipping your inner wrist in the water. If the water feels too warm, add some cold water and mix it in well.

Change the water, as necessary, to correct the temperature. Never add hot water while the body part is in the basin because you can burn the client. Instead, have the client remove the body part from the basin, assisting as necessary. Then you can safely add more hot water. Test the temperature again before assisting the client to put the body part back into the soak.

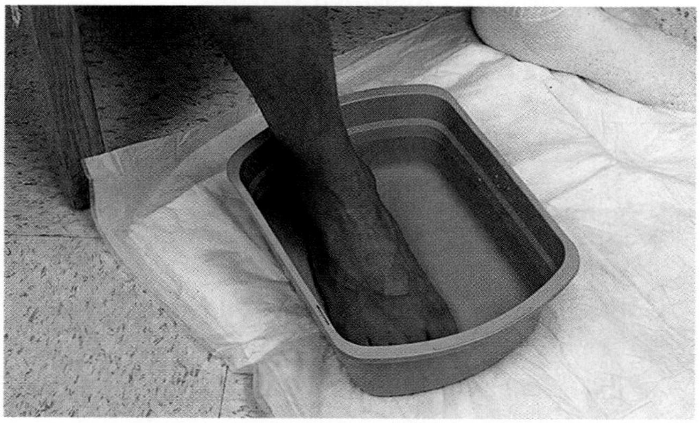

FIGURE 44–3 The warm soak.

The Sitz Bath

The **sitz bath**—also considered to be a warm, moist application—involves immersing the perineal and rectal areas in warm or hot water (*sitz* in German means "seat"). Some agencies use bidets instead of sitz baths. With bidets, the perineal and rectal areas are not immersed, but warm water gently flows over the area. Bidets have many of the beneficial effects of sitz baths. Sitz baths, usually lasting for about 15 minutes, are used after rectal surgery, female pelvic surgery, childbirth, and as treatment for hemorrhoids. They are used for the following purposes:

- To clean perineal or anal wounds
- To promote healing
- To relieve pain and soreness
- To increase circulation
- To stimulate voiding

The disposable plastic sitz bath fits onto the toilet seat (**FIGURE 44–4**). Plastic tubing runs from the bowl

The Warm Soak

123

Advocate on behalf of the client's quality of life by promoting:

Dignity • Independence • Preferences • Privacy • Safety (see BOX 1–4, on p. 17)

PRE-PROCEDURE

1 Identify the client according to employer policy.
This eliminates the possibility of mistaking one client for another.

2 Explain the procedure to the client.

3 Practise proper hand hygiene.

4 Collect the following supplies:
- ☐ **Water basin or an arm or foot bath**
- ☐ **Bath thermometer**
- ☐ **Bath blanket, large towel, or clean sheet**
- ☐ **Waterproof pad**

By collecting all the necessary equipment beforehand, you will not have to leave your client's side and can eliminate wasting time and energy in obtaining the forgotten equipment.

5 Provide for privacy.

PROCEDURE

6 Position the client for treatment.
The client will be more likely to participate if comfortable.

7 Place the call bell within reach.*
This provides an easy, safe way for the client to contact the staff if necessary.

8 Place a waterproof pad under the area to be treated.
This keeps the bedding dry.

9 Fill the water basin half full with warm water, as directed by your supervisor. Measure the water temperature. If a water thermometer is not available, test the water by dipping your inner wrist in the water. If the water feels too warm, add some cold water and mix it in well.
It is important to ensure that the water is not too hot so as to avoid causing thermal injuries to the client.

10 Place the client's body part into the water. Pad the edge of the basin with a towel. Note the time.
It is important to time all heat and cold treatments to avoid thermal injuries to the client.

11 Cover the client with a bath blanket, large towel, or clean sheet for extra warmth.
This ensures client warmth and privacy.

12 Check the area every 5 minutes. Check for redness and complaints of pain, discomfort, or numbness. Discontinue the soak if any of these signs are noticed. Wrap the body part in a towel, and inform your supervisor at once.
This reduces the risk for client injury.

13 Check water temperature every 5 minutes. Change the water, as necessary.
Wrap the body part in a towel while changing the water.
This prevents chilling of the client.

14 Remove the body part from the water after 15 minutes. Pat dry.
Drying the skin with a patting motion is gentler than rubbing it with the towel.

POST-PROCEDURE

15 Follow steps 16 through 20 in the procedure *Applying Warm Compresses*, on page 1019.

Report and Record your actions and observations, according to employer policy.
This is done for legal reasons and to keep the rest of the health care team informed.

*Steps marked with an asterisk may not apply in community settings.

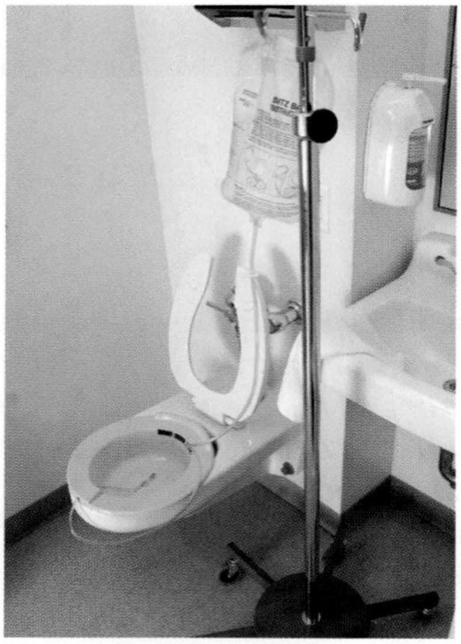

FIGURE 44–4 A disposable sitz bath with water bag, tubing, and clamp.

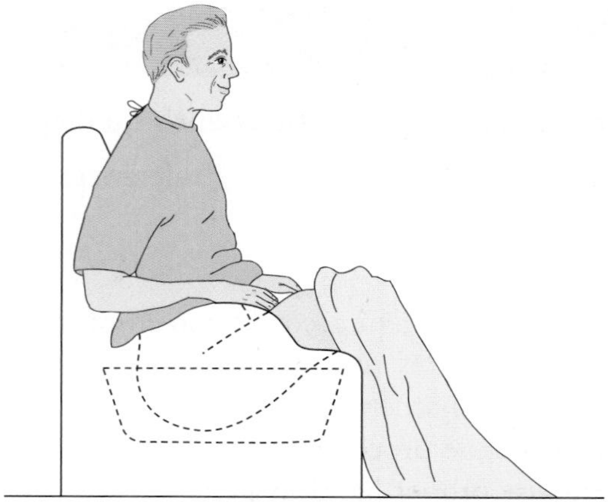

FIGURE 44–5 The built-in sitz tub. A blanket covers the client's legs to keep him warm and to respect his need for privacy.

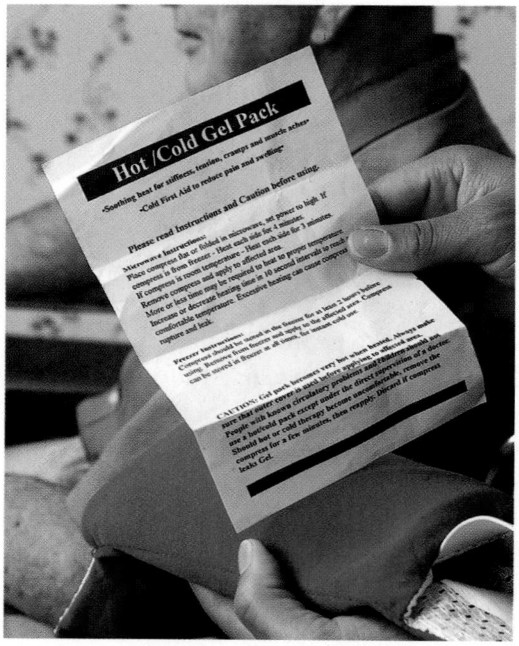

FIGURE 44–6 Commercial gel pack. The manufacturer's instructions explain how to activate the heat.

of the sitz bath to a water bag, and a plastic clamp closes the tubing. The sitz bath is filled with water at an appropriate temperature. (Check with your supervisor to determine a safe temperature.) The water bag is filled with warmer water. As the water in the sitz bath cools, the tubing is unclamped to allow the warmer water from the bag to flow into the sitz bath.

A *sitz tub* is a built-in fixture with a deep seat. The client sits in a seat filled with water (FIGURE 44–5), with the feet resting flat on the floor. Do not use an ordinary bathtub for a sitz bath. Immersing the legs and feet decreases the effectiveness of the procedure.

When a person uses a sitz bath, blood flow to the perineal and rectal areas increases. As blood flow to other body parts is reduced, the client may feel chilled. Cover the client's shoulders and knees for warmth. Reduced blood flow may also make the client feel faint, dizzy, weak, or drowsy. Check the client every 5 minutes for these signs. Stay in the room if it is not safe to leave the client alone. Allow as much privacy as possible. If it is safe to leave, place the call bell within the client's reach, or remain within easy hearing distance.

Warm Packs

A *pack* is a treatment that involves wrapping a body part with a wet or dry application. The application can be either warm or cold. Single-use (disposable) or reusable commercial packs are available (FIGURE 44–6). Some, such as some commercial **gel packs**, can be used alternately for heat and cold. The manufacturer's instructions will tell you how to activate the heat or cold.

An **aquathermia pad** is a waterproof plastic or rubber pad that can be applied to areas of muscle sprain, edema, or mild inflammation in the place of a heating pad or cold pack (FIGURE 44–7). The pad contains channels through which heated or cooled water flows. The device is connected by hoses to a

Assisting the Client to Take a Sitz Bath 123

Advocate on behalf of the client's quality of life by promoting:

Dignity • Independence • Preferences • Privacy • Safety (see BOX 1–4, on p. 17)

PRE-PROCEDURE

1 Identify the client, according to employer policy.
This eliminates the possibility of mistaking one client for another.
2 Explain the procedure to the client.
3 Practise proper hand hygiene.
4 Collect the following supplies:
- ☐ **Bath thermometer**
- ☐ **Large water container**
- ☐ **Two bath blankets, sheets, or large towels and clean garments**
- ☐ **Footstool, if the client is short**
- ☐ **Disinfectant solution**
- ☐ **Utility gloves**
- ☐ **Disposable sitz bath, if used.**
- ☐ **Wheelchair, if a built-in sitz tub is used**

By collecting all the necessary equipment beforehand, you will not have to leave your client's side and can eliminate wasting time and energy in obtaining the forgotten equipment.
5 Provide for privacy.

PROCEDURE

6 Assist the client to the bathroom or commode. Encourage the client to eliminate before the procedure.
Sitting in a sitz bath can give some clients the urge to void. This urge is reduced by having them eliminate prior to the sitz bath.
7 *If using a disposable sitz bath:*
- a Place the disposable sitz bath on the toilet seat.
- b Fill the sitz bath two thirds full with water. Measure the water temperature. (Your supervisor will tell you what water temperature to use.) If a water thermometer is not available, test the water by dipping your inner wrist in the water. If the water feels too warm, add some cold water and mix it in well.
- c Close the clamp on the tubing.
- d Fill the water bag with warmer water than that in the bowl. Your supervisor will tell you what water temperature to use. Measure the water temperature.
- e Hang the bag on a towel bar or from the top of the toilet tank. The bag must be at a higher level than the toilet seat.

It is important to ensure that the water is not too hot so as to avoid causing thermal injuries to the client.
8 *If using a built-in sitz tub:*
- a Transport the client by wheelchair to the room with the sitz bath.
- b Fill the sitz bath two thirds full with water. Your supervisor will tell you what water temperature to use. Measure the water temperature with a thermometer or your inner wrist.
- c Use towels to pad the metal part of the sitz tub that may be in contact with the client.

This will provide comfort for the client, as metal parts can feel hotter (or colder) to the client than the rest of the sitz bath.
9 Assist the client to remove or lower clothing below the waist, or raise the client's gown above the waist.
This will prevent clothing from getting wet.
10 Assist the client to sit in the sitz bath.
Providing assistance reduces the risk for client injury.
11 Place a bath blanket, sheet, or large towel around the client's shoulders. Place another over the legs for warmth.
This ensures client warmth and privacy.
12 Provide a footstool if the edge of the sitz bath causes pressure under the knees.
This reduces the risk for client injury.

Continued

Assisting the Client to Take a Sitz Bath—cont'd

13 Show the client how to open the clamp (of a disposable sitz bath) to let warmer water from the bag flow into the sitz bath. Assist as necessary.
14 Place the call bell within reach.*
This provides an easy, safe way for the client to contact the staff if necessary.
15 Stay with a client who is weak or unsteady.
This reduces the risk for client injury.
16 Check the client every 5 minutes for complaints or signs of weakness, faintness, and drowsiness. Check for a rapid pulse. If any signs occur, get assistance to help the client back to bed.
These are signs of thermal shock or fainting and should be acted on quickly to avoid client injury!
17 Assist the client out of the sitz bath after 15 minutes or as directed by your supervisor.
It is important to time all heat and cold treatments to avoid thermal injuries in the client.
18 Assist the client with drying off and dressing.
This ensures client safety.
19 Assist the client back to the hospital room or bedroom.

POST-PROCEDURE

20 Provide for safety and comfort.
21 Remove privacy measures.
22 Clean the sitz bath with disinfectant solution. Wear utility gloves.
23 Clean and return reusable items to their proper places.
This makes them easier to find the next time they are needed.
24 Follow employer policy for handling soiled linen. Wear gloves for this step.
25 Practise proper hand hygiene.

Report and Record your actions and observations, according to employer policy.
This is done for legal reasons and to keep the rest of the health care team informed.

*Steps marked with an asterisk may not apply in community settings.

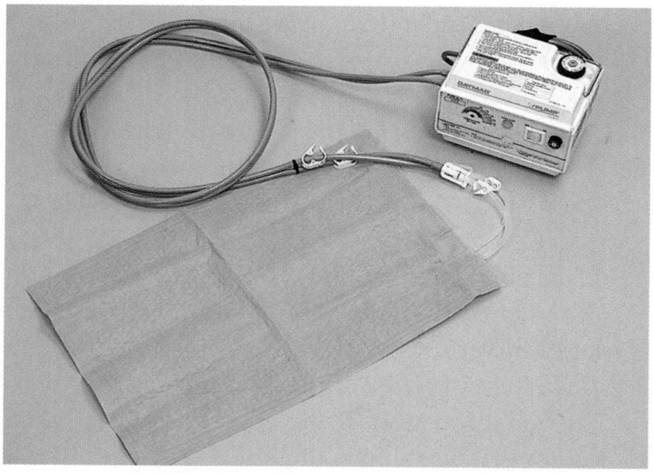

FIGURE 44–7 An aquathermia pad. (**Source:** Potter, P.A., & Perry, A.G. (2005). *Fundamentals of nursing* (6th ed., p. 1559). St. Louis, MO: Mosby.)

bedside control unit that contains a temperature regulator, a motor for circulating the water, and a reservoir of distilled water.

Some warm packs are put in boiling water for a few minutes or warmed in a microwave oven. Other types of packs require kneading or squeezing in order to activate them to heat up. Some packs can be either warmed in hot water (to heat) or placed in the freezer (to cool). Always read warning labels, and follow the manufacturer's safety instructions.

Reusable packs should never be placed directly on skin but should be covered with a clean, dry cloth, such as a dishcloth or towel. Follow employer policy and the manufacturer's instructions regarding how to cover the packs for use and how to clean them after use—typically by wiping with alcohol or washing with soap and water.

Applying a Warm Pack

123

Advocate on behalf of the client's quality of life by promoting:

Dignity • Independence • Preferences • Privacy • Safety (see BOX 1–4, on p. 17)

PRE-PROCEDURE

1 Identify the client, according to employer policy.
This eliminates the possibility of mistaking one client for another.

2 Explain the procedure to the client.

3 Practise proper hand hygiene.

4 Collect the following supplies:
- ☐ **Commercial pack or aquathermia pad**
- ☐ **Towel**
- ☐ **Pack cover**
- ☐ **Ties, tape, or rolled gauze (if needed)**
- ☐ **Waterproof pad**

By collecting all the necessary equipment beforehand, you will not have to leave your client's side and can eliminate wasting time and energy in obtaining the forgotten equipment.

5 Heat the pack. Follow the manufacturer's instructions.
The manufacturer's instructions should always be followed to prevent thermal injuries.

6 Put the pack in the cover.
This reduces the risk of the client getting burned.

7 Provide for privacy.

PROCEDURE

8 Place the pad under the body part.

9 Apply the pack quickly. Note the time.
It is important to time all heat and cold treatments to avoid thermal injuries in the client.

10 Secure the pack in place with ties, tape, or rolled gauze. Some packs are secured with Velcro straps (**FIGURE 44–8**).

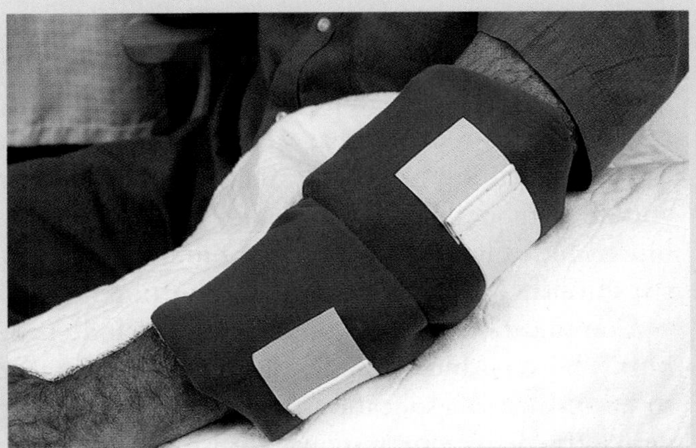

FIGURE 44–8 Warm pack secured with Velcro.

Securing the pad prevents it from slipping and keeps the heat contained.

11 Place the call bell within reach. Follow the care plan for bed rail use.*
This provides an easy, safe way for the client to contact the staff if necessary.

12 Check the area every 5 minutes for redness and check for complaints of pain, discomfort, or numbness. Remove the pack if any occur. Tell your supervisor at once.
These are signs of thermal injuries and should be acted on quickly to avoid client injury!

13 Change the pack if it cools down.
The pack loses its effectiveness after it cools down.

14 Remove the pack after 15 minutes or sooner, as directed by your supervisor. Pat the area dry with the towel.
It is important to time all heat and cold treatments to avoid thermal injuries to the client.

Continued

Applying a Warm Pack—cont'd

POST-PROCEDURE

15 Follow steps 16 through 20 in the procedure *Applying Warm Compresses* on page 1020.

16 If the pack is reusable, clean it according to employer policy and the manufacturer's instructions. Return the pack to its proper location.
This makes it easier to find the next time it is needed.

Report and Record your actions and observations, according to employer policy.
This is done for legal reasons and to keep the rest of the health care team informed.

*Steps marked with an asterisk may not apply in community settings.

COLD APPLICATIONS

Cold applications are often used to treat sprains, fractures, and fever (see **BOX 44–2**). They reduce pain, prevent swelling, and decrease circulation and bleeding. Cold applications also cool the body when fever is present.

BOX 44–2 Focus on First Aid

Remember "**RICE**" for recent injuries.

If someone you know or are caring for has suffered a recent injury, you should remember the acronym that you probably learned in your first-aid class: "RICE."

R: ***Rest*** the limb. Do not try to use it.

I: ***Ice.*** Apply ice packs to reduce swelling and decrease pain.

C: ***Compression.*** Wrap a **compression bandage**, designed to provide pressure to a particular area (also known as a *tensor bandage*), around the affected part, ensuring that it is not too tight. Signs that it is too tight include tingling and numbness, followed by increased pain and poor circulation (loss of colour) of the skin in the extremities of the affected body part.

E: ***Elevate*** the limb to reduce possible swelling.

Remember that the client should be assessed by a health care provider as soon as possible to determine if a fracture has occurred!

Cold has the opposite effect of heat on body functions. When cold is applied to the skin, blood vessels **constrict** (see **FIGURE 44–1, *C***, on p. 1014), resulting in decreased blood flow to the area and less oxygen and fewer nutrients being carried to the tissues. Cold applications are useful immediately after an injury. The decreased circulation reduces the amount of bleeding, bruising, and swelling, and cold has a numbing effect on the skin, which helps reduce or relieve pain in the affected part.

Complications

Cold applications should never be used on old injuries, as they can actually cause tissue damage, since the tissue over the old injury may be less sensitive to the cold. This tissue damage is called **frostbite**—a medical condition in which damage is caused to skin and other tissues due to extreme cold. Signs of frostbite include blisters; pale, white, or grey skin; cyanosis; shivering; numbness; pain; and burning.

Complications of cold applications include pain, burns, blisters, and cyanosis. Burns and blisters tend to occur due to applications being in direct contact with skin. It is your responsibility to check clients every 5 minutes, or more frequently for those who are at high risk for complications (see the *Think About Safety: Clients at High Risk From Heat or Cold Applications* box, on p. 1016), and to follow the guidelines listed in **BOX 44–1** on page 1017 in order to prevent injuries from cold applications. Be sure to peek under the application to inspect the skin.

In general, cold applications should be applied and removed in 15-minute intervals (15 minutes on and 15 minutes off). Timely removal of the cold application helps prevent tissue damage resulting from overconstricted blood vessels.

Moist and Dry Cold Applications

Cold applications can be moist or dry:

- Dry cold—ice bag, ice collar, or ice glove
- Moist cold—cold compress
- Moist or dry—cold packs

Moist cold applications penetrate deeper than dry ones, so the temperatures of moist applications should not be as low as those of dry applications. You should check the skin frequently (at least every 5 minutes, or more often, as directed by your supervisor).

Ice Bags, Ice Collars, Ice Gloves, and Dry Cold Packs

Ice bags, ice collars, and ice gloves are dry cold applications. The devices are filled with crushed ice.

Both reusable and single-use (disposable) **cold packs** are available commercially. To activate the cold, follow the manufacturer's instructions. You may need to strike, knead, or squeeze the pack. After use, reusable cold packs are cleaned and then kept in the freezer.

Devices with an outer covering can be placed directly on skin. Devices that come without a cover should be wrapped in a towel, pillowcase, or dishcloth. When the covering becomes moist, remove it and apply a dry one (see *Focus on Home Care: Ice Packs*).

Cold Compresses

A cold compress is a moist application that should not be left in place longer than 15 minutes. As with all heat and cold applications, the skin under the cold compress should be checked every 5 minutes for signs of blistering, increased pain, or frostbite.

FOCUS ON HOME CARE

Ice Packs

Disposable ice packs are commonly used in home settings. They are kept in the freezer until needed. A bag of frozen vegetables can be used as a makeshift ice pack. However, ***make sure the vegetables are not eaten later.*** Alternatively, plastic bags can be filled with ice; closed securely to prevent leaks; wrapped in a clean towel, dishcloth, or pillowcase; and used as ice packs. ***Remember to apply an ice pack only if your supervisor assigns this task to you, if you are familiar with your responsibilities, and if it is within your scope of practice in your province or territory!***

Applying an Ice Bag, Ice Collar, or Dry Cold Pack 123

Advocate on behalf of the client's quality of life by promoting:

Dignity • Independence • Preferences • Privacy • Safety *(see BOX 1–4, on p. 17)*

PRE-PROCEDURE

1 Identify the client, according to employer policy.
This eliminates the possibility of mistaking one client for another.

2 Explain the procedure to the client.

3 Practise proper hand hygiene.

4 Collect a cold pack with cover *or* the following supplies:
- ☐ **Ice bag, collar, or glove**
- ☐ **Crushed ice**

Continued

Applying an Ice Bag, Ice Collar, or Dry Cold Pack—cont'd

- ☐ **Cover, dishcloth, towel, or pillowcase**
- ☐ **Paper towels**

By collecting all the necessary equipment beforehand, you will not have to leave your client's side and can eliminate wasting time and energy in obtaining the forgotten equipment.

5 *Applying an ice bag, collar, or glove:*
- a Fill it with water and place the stopper. Turn the device upside down to check for leaks.
- b Empty the device.
- c Fill the device one half to two thirds full with crushed ice or ice chips (FIGURE 44–9).
- d Remove excess air by bending, twisting, or squeezing the device, or pressing it against a firm surface.

Excess air in the ice bag will reduce its effectiveness by creating an air barrier between the ice and the client's skin.
- e Place the cap or stopper on securely.
- f Dry the device with the paper towels.
- g Place the device in the cover.

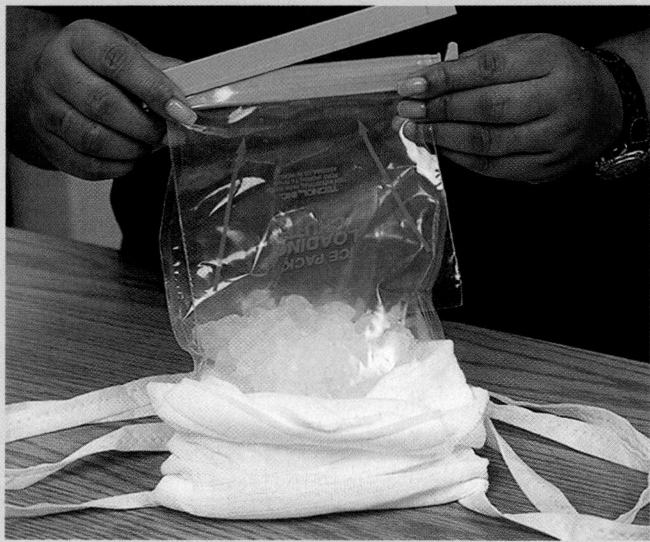

FIGURE 44–9

6 *Applying a cold pack:*
- a Squeeze, knead, or strike the disposable cold pack, as directed by the manufacturer.

This activates a chemical reaction to produce cold.
- b Place the device in the cover.

7 Provide for privacy.

PROCEDURE

8 Apply the device to the appropriate body part, as stated in the client's care plan. Secure it in place with ties, tape, or rolled gauze. Note the time.
It is important to time all heat and cold treatments to avoid thermal injuries in the client.

9 Place the call bell within reach. Follow the care plan for bed rail use.*
The call bell is a safe and easy way for the client to contact the staff if necessary.

10 Check the skin every 5 minutes. Check for signs of frostbite, including blisters; pale, white, or grey skin; cyanosis; shivering; numbness; pain; and burning. Remove the device if any of these signs occur. Tell your supervisor at once.
These are signs of thermal injuries and should be acted on quickly to avoid client injury!

11 Remove the device after 15 minutes or as directed by your supervisor.
It is important to time all heat and cold treatments to avoid thermal injuries in the client.

12 Provide for safety and comfort.

13 Remove privacy measures.

14 Clean equipment and the reusable cold pack (if used), according to employer policy and manufacturer's instructions. Discard disposable items, including the disposable ice pack (if used). Wear gloves for this step, and practise proper hand hygiene after removing and discarding the gloves. Return the pack to its proper location.
This makes it easier to find the next time it is needed.

Applying an Ice Bag, Ice Collar, or Dry Cold Pack—cont'd

15 Follow employer policy for disposing of soiled linen.
16 Practise proper hand hygiene.

Report and Record your actions and observations, according to employer policy.
This is done for legal reasons and to keep the rest of the health care team informed.

*Steps marked with an asterisk may not apply in community settings.

Applying Cold Compresses

123

Advocate on behalf of the client's quality of life by promoting:
Dignity • Independence • Preferences • Privacy • Safety *(see BOX 1–4, on p. 17)*

PRE-PROCEDURE

1 Identify the client, according to employer policy.
This eliminates the possibility of mistaking one client for another.
2 Explain the procedure to the client.
3 Practise proper hand hygiene.
4 Collect the following supplies:
- ☐ **Large basin with ice**
- ☐ **Small basin with cold water**
- ☐ **Gauze squares, washcloths, or small towels**
- ☐ **Waterproof pad**
- ☐ **Bath towel**

By collecting all the necessary equipment beforehand, you will not have to leave your client's side and can eliminate wasting time and energy in obtaining the forgotten equipment.
5 Provide for privacy.

PROCEDURE

6 Place the small basin with cold water into the large basin with ice.
The ice will keep the water in the small basin cold but will keep the ice separate, making it easier to wring out the compresses.
7 Place the compresses into the cold water.
8 Place the waterproof pad under the body part.
This keeps the furniture or bedding under the body part dry.
9 Wring out a compress. The compress should be wet but not dripping.
10 Apply the compress to the part. Note the time.
It is important to time all heat and cold treatments to avoid thermal injuries to the client.
11 Place the call bell within reach. Follow the care plan for bed rail use.*
This provides an easy, safe way for the client to contact the staff if necessary.
12 Check the area every 5 minutes. Check for signs of frostbite: blisters; pale, white, or grey skin; cyanosis; shivering; numbness; pain; and burning. Remove the compress if any signs occur. Tell your supervisor at once.
This reduces the risk for client injury.
13 Change the compress when it warms up. Usually, compresses need to be changed every 5 minutes.
Cold compresses lose effectiveness when they warm up.
14 Remove the compress after 15 minutes or sooner, as directed by your supervisor.
It is important to time all heat and cold treatments to avoid thermal injuries in the client.
15 Pat the area dry.
Drying the skin with a patting motion is gentler than rubbing it with the towel.

Continued

Applying Cold Compresses—cont'd

POST-PROCEDURE

16 Follow steps 12 through 16 in *Applying an Ice Bag, Ice Collar, or Dry Cold Pack* on page 1028–1029.

Report and Record your actions and observations, according to employer policy.
This is done for legal reasons and to keep the rest of the health care team informed.

*Steps marked with an asterisk may not apply in community settings.

CHAPTER REVIEW

KEY POINTS

- Before you perform these procedures, it is ***your responsibility*** to make sure of the following: (1) your provincial or territorial laws and employer's policies allow you to perform the procedure, (2) the procedure is in your job description, (3) you have the necessary training, (4) you are familiar with the equipment, and (5) you have reviewed the procedure with a nurse.
- Heat and cold have opposite effects on body functions. Whereas heat increases blood flow by *dilating* blood vessels in the area, cold slows blood flow by *constricting* blood vessels. You must thoroughly understand the purposes, effects, and complications of both heat and cold applications.
- Heat and cold applications can cause severe injuries, including a decrease in the ability of that body part to function well.
- Because of the risks, heat and cold applications should be used only if they are in the client's care plan. Support workers must not apply heat or cold unless delegated to do so by a nurse.
- Inspect the skin beneath the application every 5 minutes or according to the care plan. Heat or cold applications are not applied for longer than 15 minutes at a time.
- Not every client will report discomfort, so watch for signs of discomfort, such as restlessness, agitation, or other changes in behaviour.
- Both heat and cold applications can be either moist or dry. Water conducts heat and cold, so moist therapies have a greater and faster effect than dry therapies.
- Clients at greatest risk for complications from heat or cold applications include (1) clients with thin, delicate, or fragile skin; (2) clients who have decreased sensation; (3) clients with dementia or confusion; and (4) clients with metal implants.

CRITICAL THINKING IN PRACTICE

You have been instructed to remove Mr. Velez's hot pack. He says: "My knee feels much better with that on it. Can I leave it on longer?" What do you do? Is it safe, or are there risks to leaving the application in place? Explain. Are you allowed to apply or remove heat or cold applications in all settings? Explain why or why not.

REVIEW QUESTIONS

Answers to these questions are at the bottom of the next page.

Circle the BEST answer.

1. Which of the following is true about heat application?
   A. It will decrease the blood flow.
   B. It will cause an increase in muscle spasm.
   C. It will treat recent sprains.
   D. It can reduce joint stiffness.
2. Which of the following is the greatest threat from heat applications?
   A. Infection
   B. Burns
   C. Chilling
   D. Pressure ulcers
3. Who has the greatest risk for complications from a heat application?
   A. A 10-year-old boy
   B. A teenager
   C. A 40-year-old woman
   D. An older adult with diabetes
4. When checking the skin under a heat application, which of the following should you report?
   A. Rash
   B. Warm skin
   C. Relaxed muscles
   D. Client sleeping

5. The temperature of a hot application is usually between:
A. 26.6°C and 33.8°C
B. 33.8°C and 36.6°C
C. 36.6°C and 41.1°C
D. 41.1°C and 46.1°C

6. Which of these statements about moist heat applications is true?
A. Water is never in contact with the skin
B. Moist heat has a greater and faster effect than dry heat
C. Dry heat penetrates deeper than moist heat
D. Moist heat applications are more dangerous than moist cold applications

7. A client has a warm compress. Which of the following is true?
A. The warm compress is a dry heat application.
B. The compress is applied no longer than 5 minutes.
C. The area is checked every 5 minutes.
D. The compress should never be covered.

8. Which of these statements about sitz baths is true?
A. The foot and leg areas are immersed in warm or hot water for 15 to 20 minutes.
B. Weakness and fainting can occur.
C. Sitz baths should never be used on men.
D. The sitz bath lasts 1 to 2 hours.

9. Cold applications:
A. Reduce pain, prevent swelling, and decrease circulation
B. Dilate blood vessels
C. Prevent the spread of microbes
D. Are warmed in a microwave oven

10. Which of the following is a complication of a cold application?
A. Fever
B. Excessive thirst
C. Infection
D. Frostbite

11. Before applying an ice bag:
A. Prepare the bag by running it under hot water
B. Measure the temperature of the bag
C. Place the bag in a cover
D. Ask the client to void

12. Moist cold compresses are left in place no longer than:
A. 15 minutes
B. 30 minutes
C. 45 minutes
D. 60 minutes

Answers: 1.D, 2.B, 3.D, 4.A, 5.C, 6.B, 7.C, 8.B, 9.A, 10.D, 11.C, 12.A

Chapter opener image: Dan Kosmayer/Shutterstock.com

CHAPTER 45

Working in Acute Care

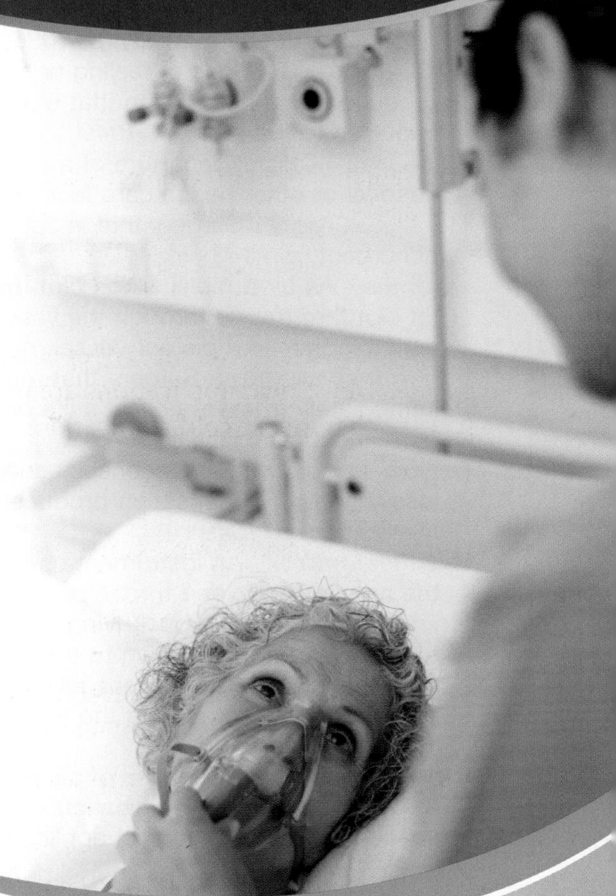

OBJECTIVES

After reading this chapter, the learner should be able to do the following:

- Describe how to promote well-being during the admission, transfer, and discharge procedures.
- Explain what to do before, during, and after a physical examination.
- Identify the equipment used during a physical examination.
- Describe how to prepare a client for an examination.
- Describe the possible examination positions and how to drape the client for each of these positions.
- Explain guidelines for assisting with a physical examination.
- Describe the common fears and concerns of surgical clients.
- Explain how clients are physically and psychologically prepared for surgery.
- Describe how to prepare a room for the postoperative client.
- List the postoperative signs and symptoms to report to the nurse.
- Explain how circulation is stimulated after surgery.
- Describe how to meet the client's hygiene, nutrition, fluid, and elimination needs after surgery.
- Perform the procedures described in this chapter.

KEY TERMS

admission Official entry of a client into a hospital or other health care facility. *p. 1036*
anaesthesia The loss of feeling or sensation, produced by a medication that blocks pain impulses to the brain. *p. 1049*
discharge Official departure of a client from a hospital or other health care facility. *p. 1038*
elective surgery Surgery that is scheduled but nonurgent. *p. 1043*
embolus An air bubble, blood clot (**thrombus**), or fat clot that travels through the vascular system until it lodges in a distant vessel. *p. 1051*
emergency surgery Surgery that must be done immediately to save a client's life or prevent permanent disability. *p. 1043*
general anaesthesia Unconsciousness and the loss of feeling or sensation produced by a medication. *p. 1049*
laryngeal mirror An instrument used to examine the mouth, teeth, and throat. *p. 1039*
lithotomy position A back-lying position in which the hips are brought down to the edge of the examination table, the knees are flexed, the hips are externally rotated, and the feet are supported in stirrups. *p. 1040*
local anaesthesia The loss of sensation in a small area, produced by a medication injected at the specific site or by a topical application. *p. 1049*
nasal speculum An instrument used to examine the inside of the nose. *p. 1039*
ophthalmoscope A lighted instrument used to examine the internal structures of the eye. *p. 1039*
otoscope A lighted instrument used to examine the external ear and the eardrum (tympanic membrane). *p. 1039*
percussion hammer An instrument used to tap body parts to test reflexes. Also known as **reflex hammer**. *p. 1039*
postoperative After surgery. *p. 1049*
preoperative Before surgery. *p. 1045*
reflex hammer See **percussion hammer**. *p. 1039*
regional anaesthesia The loss of sensation or feeling in a large area of the body, produced by the injection of a medication. *p. 1049*
thrombus A blood clot that forms in a blood vessel, which has the potential to become an **embolus**. *p. 1050*
tuning fork An instrument used to test hearing. *p. 1039*
urgent surgery Surgery that must be done soon to prevent further damage, disability, or disease. *p. 1043*
vaginal speculum An instrument used to open the vagina so that it and the cervix can be examined. *p. 1039*

In the past and in many municipalities, support workers did not play an active role in the everyday care of acute-care clients. However, this situation is certainly changing throughout the country, with more and more hospitals employing support workers to provide basic bedside care to clients and to assist the health care team. This chapter focuses on supporting the client during transitions, assisting with physical examinations, and supporting the client having surgery. In some provinces and territories, hospitalized people are called "patients," while in other provinces, they are referred to as "clients." For consistency, we have used the term *clients*.

The role that support workers play and their scope of practice when caring for clients in an acute-care setting (such as a hospital) differ somewhat from their roles and scope of practice in other settings (see Chapter 3). For example, there may be a need for more tasks to be delegated in an acute-care setting. ***Also, because acute-care clients (such as those who are undergoing investigative procedures or having surgery) can develop life-threatening health challenges quickly, it is important to observe for and immediately report changes in the client's condition to the nursing staff. As always, it is also important to stay within your scope of practice and not attempt anything that you have not been delegated or taught to do.***

SUPPORTING THE CLIENT DURING TRANSITIONS

Clients often need to move from one environment to another—for example, into a facility (*admission*) or out of a facility (*discharge*) or from one room or unit in a facility to another (*transfer*).

Transitions are difficult for most people. Do you remember how you felt the last time you moved? You might have felt sad if you had to leave friends and family behind, you might have felt strange and disoriented (out of place) in your new environment, or you might have experienced both feelings.

Clients should feel safe, comfortable, and relaxed in their environment, which may be any of the settings described in Chapter 3, including private homes, assisted-living dwellings, apartments, units in long-term care facilities, and hospital rooms. Consider the following examples:

- Mr. Kremer, 88, moves from his home to a long-term care facility, but he feels like a stranger there. Each time you approach him, you introduce yourself to him, explain your role, and what you will be doing. You make his room feel more like home by helping arrange the possessions he has brought with him. You introduce him to other staff and clients. He begins to feel more secure and comfortable.
- Jose Cruz, 17, is admitted to hospital following a car accident. He has some pain and is also anxious and fearful. A nurse gives him medication to control his pain. She explains what to expect during surgery and afterward. He feels better knowing what will happen next.

For clients who are unwell, moving from one environment to another can be very difficult. Many clients feel anxious, unsettled, and alone. Moving can even cause or increase signs of confusion or disorientation in some clients, especially older adults. You can promote clients' emotional well-being during transitions when you help them with the admission, transfer, and discharge processes.

The Hospital Unit

Hospital units have similarities to and differences from long-term care facilities. Each unit consists of client rooms and a nursing station. The nursing station is where change-of-shift reports take place and where the unit receptionist sits to answer phone calls. In many hospitals, it is also where client records are stored and the medication room is located. Each hospital unit has many other rooms within it as well: a *clean utility room*, where clean supplies are stored; a *soiled* (or *dirty*) *utility room*, where garbage and contaminated objects are kept; and a pantry (or kitchenette), with a refrigerator for storing client snacks, a microwave oven to heat (or reheat) client food, and storage for disposable eating utensils.

A hospital volunteer or staff member usually escorts newly admitted clients who are ambulatory to their assigned unit and notifies the nursing station of the new arrival. The nurse assigned to the client usually greets the client and begins the admission process. If the client is not in pain or distress, a support worker may be asked to greet the client and assist with the initial admission procedures. If you have been instructed to begin admission for a client, you should introduce yourself by name and title to the client and family (**FIGURE 45–1**). Call the client by name in the proper manner and lead the way to the client's room. Remember that the client and family may be feeling anxious, so be friendly and gentle, and do not rush them. See *Providing Compassionate Care: Welcoming a Newly Admitted Client,* on page 1037.

In a hospital that is *decentralized*, each client room will contain the client's records and any medications that were ordered. The medications are kept in locked cupboards on the wall that is shared with the hallway, and they have doors on either side to allow for access from inside the client's room and from the

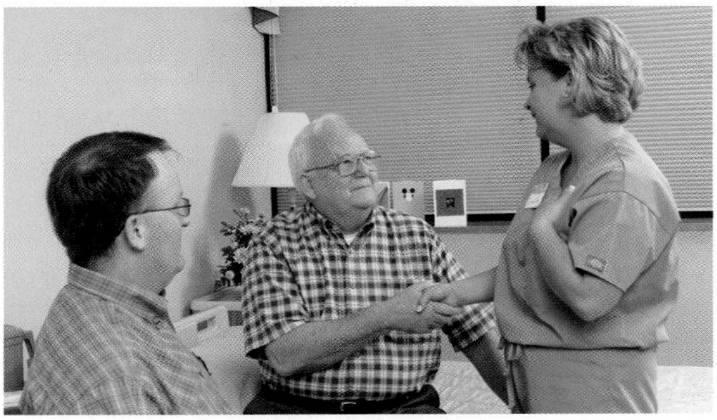

FIGURE 45–1 A support worker introduces herself to a new client and family member.

hallway for restocking. They are restocked by the appropriate person on a daily basis. Some decentralized hospitals also have small desks and computers, and some may have medication carts in the halls outside clients' rooms instead of medication cupboards if the rooms are too small to hold these items within them.

Most hospital rooms have medical apparatuses (such as blood pressure equipment) mounted on the wall near each client's bed for easy access when needed. Other equipment may also be present in clients' rooms according to their needs. For example, an intravenous (IV) pole (*IV standard*) is used to hang an IV infusion bag or feeding bag. Some hospital beds have an IV pole stored in the bed frame, or the IV pole may be a separate piece of equipment that is brought to the bedside when needed. (See Chapter 31 for instructions on how to dress and undress a client with an IV.)

Hospital rooms also have wall outlets for oxygen and suction (**FIGURE 45–2**) that are ready for use when required. Oxygen tanks, oxygen concentrators, and portable suction equipment, all of which are also common in long-term care and home care settings, may also be present. Because medical equipment is expensive and easily broken, only medically necessary equipment (except that mounted on the wall) is kept in the client's room. Equipment that is not required by the clients in the room should be properly cleaned and returned to the storage unit.

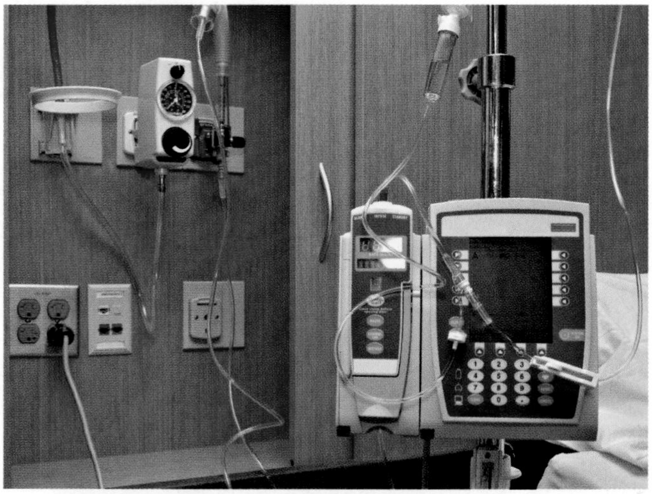

FIGURE 45–2 This hospital room has blood pressure equipment, an IV pole, and oxygen and suction outlets. (**Source:** Julio Yeste/Shutterstock.com)

Admitting a Client to an Acute-Care Facility

Admission is the official entry of a client into any health care facility where the client will be staying for any period of time, from overnight to indefinitely. The focuses of admission to any acute-care setting are diagnosis of the client's symptoms, treatment of or surgery for the client's illness, and improvement in the client's quality of life by providing pain and symptom relief, as well as rehabilitation and therapy if required.

Clients are admitted to hospital by a physician or a health care team, under the physician's admission *privileges* (rights). In many instances, clients are admitted to a specific hospital simply because it is the hospital where the client's doctor or team of doctors have admission privileges. In most hospitals, clients are usually assigned to an available room on a unit according to the client's main diagnosis. For example, clients who require heart monitoring will be admitted to a unit in which heart monitoring and treatment are the main focus.

The admission process can cause uncertainty, anxiety, and fear. Clients often worry about medical tests, treatment, and surgery. They may fear pain and serious health problems. Similarly, clients who face an uncertain length of time in the hospital often feel sad about leaving home. The facility is strange and unfamiliar—they do not know what to expect and where to go for things or who to approach if they have questions. They worry about getting meals, finding the bathroom, and getting help.

Except in emergencies, the hospital admission process starts in the admissions office. A member of the admitting staff gives the new client an ID number and a bracelet. The client signs a consent-for-treatment form, and the nursing unit is notified that a client is being admitted. As a support worker, you may be asked to prepare the room for the client. A porter, hospital volunteer, support worker, or an admissions office staff member brings the client to the nursing unit, sometimes by wheelchair or stretcher.

Providing Compassionate Care
Welcoming a Newly Admitted Client

- ***Dignity.*** Treat the new client and his belongings with respect. Introduce yourself by name and title to the client and family, and ask the client what name the staff should use. Do not rush into admission procedures. Treat the client and family as if they are guests in your home. Listen to their concerns or questions, and do not overload them with information. Explain details about routines and other matters only if the new client seems eager to hear them. Reassure clients that they do not need to remember everything. Remind them that they can ask questions and talk to the staff at any time.
- ***Independence.*** Show clients to their assigned rooms, and show them where to store their clothing and where the bathroom is. Explain how to use the various equipment in the room. Make sure clients can reach the phone, TV remote, and light controls.
- ***Preferences.*** Explain when visiting hours are and how to fill out the client's menu. Take note and promptly report if the client has food allergies or menu preferences because of religious or lifestyle reasons. Some clients request to have a family member present when the doctor visits, especially if the client has cognitive, language, or communication challenges. Such issues should also be reported to the nurse assigned to the client.
- ***Privacy.*** Show the new clients how to draw the privacy curtains (see **FIGURE 45–3**). Explain that the health care team respects all clients' right to privacy. Explain how you maintain privacy during personal care and other procedures.
- ***Safety.*** Explain how to use the call bell (see Chapter 22), and ensure that it is within easy reach. Clients (especially older adults) may become disoriented by being in unfamiliar surroundings, by changes in their sleep or eating habits, or by an increase in medications for pain or anxiety. Show the client around the bathroom, and point out safety features, such as grab bars (see **FIGURE 45–4**). Review safety and emergency procedures according to facility policy, and apply safety measures such as bed rails according to the client's care plan.

Admission procedures include the following:

- Weighing and measuring the client (see Chapter 15)
- Orienting the client to the room, nursing unit, and hospital
- Obtaining a urine specimen if ordered (see Chapter 32)

Transfers

A *transfer* occurs when a client is moved from one room or nursing unit to another or even to another facility. Transfers usually occur when a client's condition changes or when a room change is requested because roommates do not get along. Some clients are transferred for rehabilitation. A client may or may not welcome a transfer. The client's physician, nurse, or social worker usually explains the reason for the transfer.

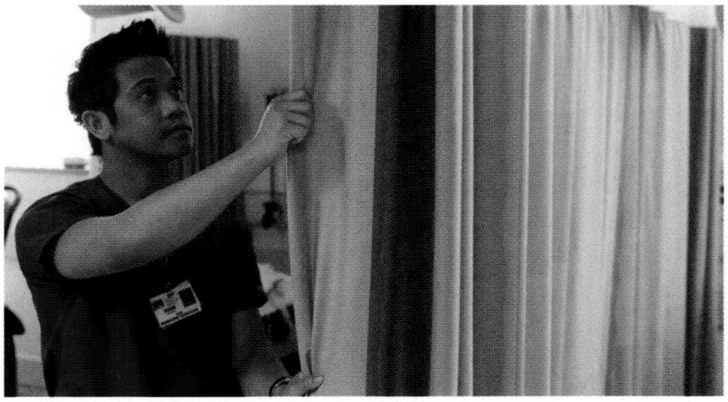

FIGURE 45–3 Curtains around the bed provide privacy in hospitals and long-term care facilities.

You may assist with the transfer or carry out the entire procedure. Clients are usually transported by wheelchair or stretcher or on their beds. Be sensitive and compassionate as you carry out the transfer procedure, as clients need support and reassurance. The client does not know the staff on the new unit, so

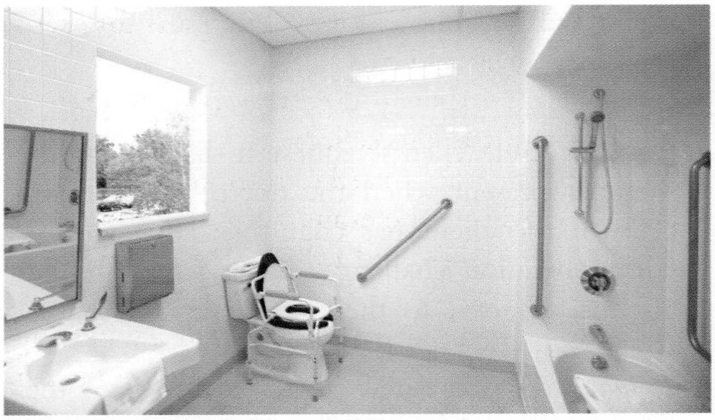

FIGURE 45–4 A facility bathroom. Note that there are several grab bars that can be used to assist the client. (**Source:** Brian Hillier.)

introduce the client to the staff and to the new roommate. Wish the client well as you leave.

Discharges

Discharge is the official departure of a client from a hospital or other health care facility. Discharged clients may have recovered enough to go home, and may need home care. Others are discharged to another hospital, to a long-term care facility, or to a hospice. The physician, nurse, dietitian, social worker, and other health care team members plan the client's discharge. If the client is going home, they teach the client and family about diet, exercise, medications, treatments, and dressing changes. The case manager arranges for home care, rehabilitation, special therapy, and equipment, if required.

You may help clients pack their belongings and get ready to leave and then transport them out of the facility. In a hospital, the physician must write a discharge order before a client is allowed to leave. In a long-term care facility, permission must be obtained from the nurse. In some facilities, the chart contains instructions as to when the client may leave and with whom.

Always use good communication skills when assisting with a client's discharge. Wish the client and family well as they leave the facility.

Sometimes, a client may want to leave without permission. If clients tell you that they want or intend to leave, notify the nurse immediately.

ASSISTING WITH PHYSICAL EXAMINATIONS

Physicians and nurses routinely perform physical examinations (exams) in a variety of settings for many reasons: (1) Routine health examinations are usually done in a physician's office to promote health. (2) Pre-employment physicals may take place in a physician's office or clinic and are done to determine fitness for work. (3) Physical examinations are used to diagnose and treat diseases and may be performed in a clinic, a physician's office, or a hospital emergency room. (4) Many long-term care facilities require new clients to have a physical exam when they arrive; some require clients to have physical exams at least once a year. (5) In some instances, clients may be referred to a specialist they have never met. Depending on the circumstances of the client's illness or injury, the specialist may wish to perform a thorough diagnostic exam on the client in a clinic, in her office, or in the hospital.

Clients who have been admitted to any acute-care facility will usually require one or more physical examinations during their hospital stay. In some provinces and territories, support workers in a facility may be asked to assist the physician or the nurse with a physical exam, and support workers in the community may assist physicians or nurses with some aspects of a physical exam.

Your Responsibilities Regarding Physical Examinations

Your responsibilities depend on your employer's policies and procedures, your scope of practice in your province or territory, the examiner's preferences, the setting you are working in, and the type of examination. You may do some or all of the following:

- Collect linens for draping the client for the procedure
- Collect examination equipment
- Prepare the room for the examination
- Transport the client to and from the exam room if your facility has an examination room
- Assist with lighting
- Measure vital signs, height, and weight
- Position and drape the client

- Hand equipment and instruments to the examiner
- Stay with the client before or during the exam to provide emotional support and to prevent falls
- Label specimen containers
- Dispose of soiled linen and discard used supplies according to the facility policy
- Clean equipment

Equipment

Instruments needed for a physical examination may include, but are not limited to, the following (**FIGURE 45–5**):

- **Ophthalmoscope**—a lighted instrument used to examine the internal structures of the eye.
- **Otoscope**—a lighted instrument used to examine the external ear and the eardrum (tympanic membrane). Some scopes are combination ophthalmoscopes and otoscopes, with parts for examining both eyes and ears.
- **Percussion hammer**—used to tap body parts to test reflexes. It is also called a **reflex hammer**.
- **Vaginal speculum**—used to open the vagina so it and the cervix can be examined.
- **Nasal speculum**—used to examine the inside of the nose.
- **Tuning fork**—an instrument used to test hearing.
- **Laryngeal mirror**—used to examine the mouth, teeth, and throat.

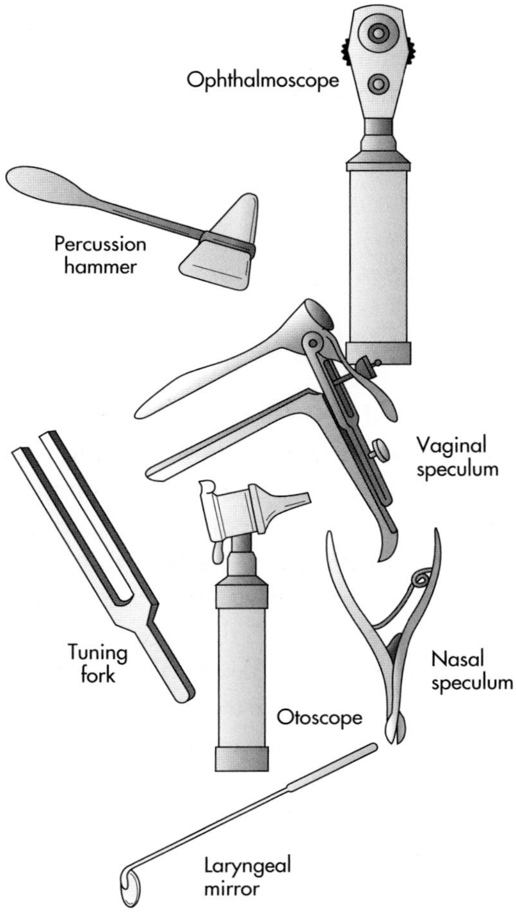

FIGURE 45–5 Some of the many instruments used for a physical examination.

Many facilities have examination trays in the supply department. If one is not available, collect the items ***listed in your facility's or agency's procedure manual or requested by the examiner***, and arrange them on a tray or table.

PREPARING THE CLIENT FOR A PHYSICAL EXAM

Many clients worry about having a physical examination because of possible findings or because of confusion or fear about what the examiner will do. Feeling discomfort and embarrassment, fearing exposure, and not knowing what the procedure involves all cause anxiety. As a support worker, you need to be sensitive to the client's feelings and concerns and prepare the client physically and psychologically for the examination.

The client has the right to know who will do the exam, the reason for the exam, when it will be done, and what the procedure involves. This information is given to the client by the physician or nurse. If a client asks you questions about an examination, reply that your supervisor will provide the necessary answers.

The exam is done only if the client gives consent. The client may want a different examiner or may want a family member to be present at the exam. Some clients want to have family members with them when exam results are explained to them. In the event that a client is not able to make an informed decision about an examination, the examiner must obtain permission from the appointed decision maker.

The client's right to privacy must be protected. In a facility, the examining area is screened and the room door closed. Depending on your employer's

FOCUS ON CHILDREN

Promoting Privacy and Comfort During a Physical Exam

Toddlers, preschool children, and school-aged children keep their underpants on for an examination. The underpants may be lowered or removed, as necessary, during the procedure.

The examination of an infant or a child is similar to an adult examination. However, a parent or other adult caregiver is required to be present. The parent or caregiver may need to hold the infant or child still for parts of the procedure if the child is uncooperative. Some parents or caregivers may be frightened by the child's reaction or by the examination itself. The child or infant may also have separation anxiety or fear of physical harm during the examination. Your calm, comforting attitude will help not only the child but also the parent or caregiver, who may be feeling anxious, too.

Most of the equipment is the same as for the adult examination; however, with children, toys are sometimes used to assess development, and vaginal speculums are never used.

policy, the client may have to remove all clothes for a complete examination and be asked to wear a hospital gown, which can reduce the feeling of nakedness and the fear of exposure. The client is also covered with a paper drape, bath blanket, or sheet. Explain to the client that only the body part being examined is exposed and that only minimum exposure will occur (see the *Focus on Children: Promoting Privacy* box). In a community setting, as well, you should cover the client with a sheet to ensure that only the areas being examined are exposed.

Clients are asked to void before the examination, as an empty bladder allows the examiner to feel the abdominal organs easily. A full bladder can change the normal position and shape of organs and can also cause discomfort, especially when the examiner is palpating (feeling) the abdominal organs. If a urine specimen is needed, ask the client to collect it when voiding before the exam. Explain how to collect the specimen (see Chapter 32), and when the client hands it to you, label the container.

Maintaining the client's warmth during the examination is important, so ensure that the client—especially one with an illness, an older client, or a child—is protected from chilling. Keep an extra blanket at hand, and take measures to prevent drafts.

The examiner may want height, weight, and vital signs measured, so obtain these before the examination starts and record the information on the examination form. The client is then positioned and draped for the examination. Take care to protect the client from falls and injury. Do not leave the client unattended.

Positioning and Draping the Client

For some examinations, special positions may be needed, and some of them may be uncomfortable and embarrassing for the client. The examiner will tell you how to position the client. Before helping the client assume and maintain the position, explain the following:

- Why the position is needed
- How to assume the position
- How the body is draped for warmth and privacy
- How long the client can expect to stay in the position

The *supine position* (*dorsal recumbent position* or *horizontal position*) is used to examine the abdomen, anterior chest, and breasts. The client lies flat on the back, keeping the legs together. If the perineal area is to be examined, the knees are flexed and the hips externally rotated (**FIGURE 45–6, *A***). The drape is extended over the client's body from the shoulders to the feet.

The **lithotomy position** (**FIGURE 45–6, *B***) is used to examine the vagina. The client lies on her back, and her hips are brought to the edge of the examination table. The knees are flexed, the hips externally rotated, and the feet supported in stirrups. The client is draped as for perineal care (see **FIGURE 30–26**, on p. 644). Some facilities provide socks to cover the client's feet and calves. If a client finds it difficult to assume this position, the examiner will tell you how to position the client.

The *knee–chest position* (**FIGURE 45–6, *C***) is used to examine the rectum and sometimes the vagina. The

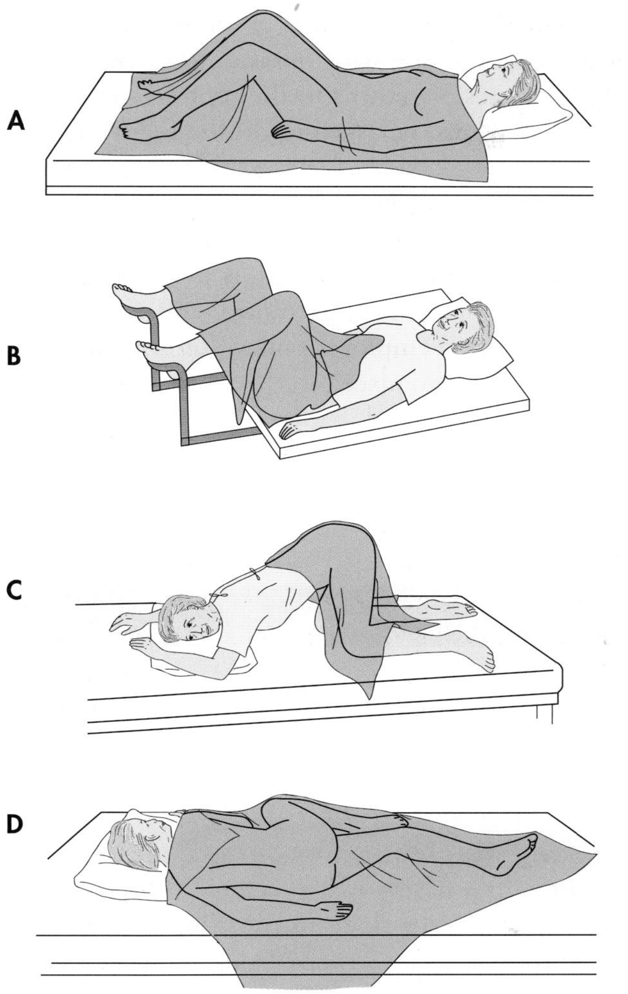

FIGURE 45–6 Positioning and draping for the physical examination. **A,** Supine position. **B,** Lithotomy position. **C,** Knee–chest position. **D,** Sims' position.

client kneels and rests the chest on the knees, with the head turned to one side. The arms are kept above the head or flexed at the elbows. The back is kept straight, and the body is flexed about 90 degrees at the hips. The client wears a gown and sometimes socks, and the drape is applied in a diamond shape to cover the back, buttocks, and thighs. This position is rarely used for older adults, who usually assume the side-lying position for rectal exams.

Sims' position (**FIGURE 45–6, *D***) is sometimes used to examine the rectum or the vagina. The client lies on the left side. The right leg is sharply flexed so that it is not on the left leg. The left arm is positioned along the client's back. The drape is applied over the client in a diamond shape. The corner near the examiner is folded back to expose the rectum or the vagina.

BOX 45–1 Guidelines for Assisting With a Physical Examination

- Perform hand hygiene before and after the examination.
- Provide for privacy by screening, closing doors, and draping. Expose only the body part being examined.
- Assist with positioning, as directed by the examiner.
- Place instruments and equipment near the examiner.
- If you are female, stay in the room when a female client is examined. When a male examiner examines a female client, another female must be present in the room for the legal protection of both the client and the examiner. The presence of a female attendant also provides psychological comfort to the client. Similarly, a female examiner may want a male attendant present when she examines a male client, again for the legal protection of both parties.
- Anticipate the examiner's need for equipment and supplies. When passing instruments during the physical exam, you should hand the instruments to the examiner with the handles toward the examiner. To keep the instrument sterile (if appropriate) or as clean as possible, you should handle the instrument only by holding it in the middle.
- Place a paper sheet or paper towel on the floor if the client is asked to stand (in a facility).
- Practise medical asepsis, and follow Standard Practices.

Assisting With the Examination

Depending on your province or territory and your facility's policies, you may be asked to prepare, position, and drape the client and also to assist the physician or the nurse during the exam. As a support worker, you will provide valuable help to the examiner and will provide comfort care to your client. When assisting with an examination, follow the guidelines in **BOX 45–1** (also see the *Focus on Children: Providing Privacy and Comfort During a Physical Exam* box).

Clients with dementia, serious injury, or an illness that can affect cognition may resist the examiner and may be agitated and physically aggressive because of confusion and fear. The client who refuses or actively resists an examination must not be restrained or forced to have the procedure. The client may react better at another time or with a family member present. The client's rights should always be respected.

Assisting After the Examination

After the examination has been completed, the client dresses and returns to the room if in a facility. Assist as needed. If a lubricant has been used for vaginal or rectal examination, wipe or clean the area before the client dresses or returns to the room.

You may also be asked to do the following:

- Discard disposable items.
- Replenish supplies for the next exam.
- Clean reusable items (such as otoscope and ophthalmoscope tips, speculum, and stethoscope), according to employer policy. Return them to the tray or storage place.
- Remove the used paper from the examination table. Cover the examination table with clean paper.

Preparing the Client for an Examination

123

Advocate on behalf of the client's quality of life by promoting:

Dignity • Independence • Preferences • Privacy • Safety *(see BOX 1–4, on p. 17)*

PROCEDURE

1 Identify the client, according to employer policy.
This eliminates the possibility of mistaking one client for another.

2 Explain the procedure to the client.

3 Perform hand hygiene.

4 Collect instruments and supplies, as listed in your facility's procedure manual or as requested by the examiner.
The type of examination and the condition of your client will determine the instruments and supplies needed for the examination.

5 Provide for privacy. In a facility, there will be curtains to provide privacy. In a community setting, you need to close the door to your client's room for privacy.

6 Ask the client to void. Offer the bedpan, commode, or urinal if necessary. Provide for privacy.
A full bladder can interfere with palpation of the abdomen and be very uncomfortable for the client.

7 Weigh and measure the client (see Chapter 15) if so instructed by your supervisor or examiner.

8 Help the client get on the examination table. Provide a footstool if necessary. (Omit this step if the exam is done in the client's room or in the client's home.)

9 For an examination done in the client's room, raise the bed to its highest level. Raise the far bed rail if used.

10 Position the client, as directed.
This helps provide a comfortable position for your client and ensure that your client is in the correct position for the examination.

11 Drape the client.
This provides privacy and some warmth for the client.

12 Place a bed protector under the client's buttocks.
This protects bed linens.

13 Raise the bed rail near you if used.

14 Ensure adequate lighting.
This ensures that the examiner has a clear line of vision.

15 Press the call bell for the nurse or examiner. Do not leave the client unattended.
This ensures the safety of your client.

- Label specimens. Take them to the designated area, according to employer policy.
- Clean and tidy up the client's unit or examination room. Follow employer policy for disposing of soiled linens.

Remember the client's right to privacy. The results of the examination are confidential. Only members of the health care team involved in the client's care need to know the reason for the exam and its results. If the client consents, the physician may provide the result to family members. The client may want to share the information with others. You should never disclose the results of the examination to the family, to co-workers, or to anyone else.

SUPPORTING THE CLIENT HAVING SURGERY

In hospitals, as a support worker, you will come in contact with clients before and after surgery. In long-term care facilities, you may care for many clients who are recovering from surgery. In the community, you may provide postoperative care to clients in their homes. Surgery is performed on clients for many reasons, including removal of a diseased organ or body part, removal of a tumour, or repair of injured tissue. Surgery may also be done to diagnose a disease, improve appearance, or relieve symptoms. A specially trained physician, called a *surgeon*, performs the surgery. The client is prepared by nurses and physicians for what happens before, during, and after surgery. Clients need both physical and psychological preparation before surgery.

A large number of surgeries—for example, repair of a hip fracture—require hospital stays; the client is admitted to the hospital before the surgery and stays for a few or several days after the surgery. However, outpatient surgery (also called *ambulatory surgery*, *day surgery*, or *same-day surgery*), which does not require an overnight hospital stay, is also done frequently. Clients undergoing these procedures are in the hospital for less than 24 hours.

Many outpatient surgeries are done in clinics or surgical centres that are part of hospitals or physicians' offices. For example, cataract surgery would be an outpatient procedure. As a support worker, you may be involved in caring for a client after the client returns home from surgery. Your employer will give you instructions regarding the care you need to provide to your client.

Some outpatient procedures will require *home preparation*. For example, to prepare for a colonoscopy, the client must take medication, as prescribed by the doctor, the day before the procedure to clear the colon of all fecal matter.

Surgeries may be elective, urgent, or emergency:

- **Elective surgery**—surgery that is scheduled but nonurgent (e.g., hip replacement surgery). Delaying the surgery does not result in permanent damage, disability, or death. The surgery may be scheduled 1 day before to months in advance. Often, clients are placed on waiting lists for elective surgery.
- **Urgent surgery**—surgery that must be done soon to prevent further damage, disability, or disease (e.g., cancer surgery and coronary artery surgery).
- **Emergency surgery**—surgery that must be done immediately to save a client's life or prevent disability. Clients who have been in accidents often require emergency surgery.

The reasons a client requires surgery will vary and may influence the client's mood prior to surgery. For example, if the client is facing diagnostic surgery to see if he has cancer, he may be tense, agitated, or even irritable. It is important to be empathetic and nonjudgemental of the client's actions at all times.

Purposes of surgical procedures include the following:

- ***Diagnostic***—investigative surgery to determine the cause of a client's symptoms or the extent to which an illness has affected the body. For example, a client who has been unable to conceive a child may require diagnostic surgery to explore why.
- ***Reconstructive***—surgery performed to restore the function or appearance of a body part or organ. For example, a client who has lost several fingers in a farming accident may require skin grafts and digit replacement to regain partial (or full) use of his hand.
- ***Palliative***—surgery performed to enhance the quality of the dying client's life, not to cure the

client. For example, a client with a large esophageal tumour may need to have the tumour removed or reduced to help her be able to eat.
- ***Curative***—surgery aimed at repairing (or removing) an injured or diseased body part in order to cure the disease. A client who has sustained abdominal injuries in a car accident would undergo surgery to repair any damaged areas.
- ***Transplant***—a surgical procedure in which a donor's tissue or organs(s) is implanted into a recipient's body in order to restore function and save the life of the recipient. Examples of transplanted tissues include skin, eyes (or parts of eyes), organs, bones, and bone marrow.

Psychological Care

Imagine you were in an accident, and when you woke up hours later, you were told that your right leg had been surgically amputated. How would you feel? Or if you were told you needed surgery the very next day, would you have fear of pain or death? Would you worry about who would care for your children and your home and who would earn money for your family while you were in the hospital?

Psychological preparation before surgery is very important. Illness or injury causes many fears and concerns (**BOX 45–2**), and if surgery is needed, these concerns increase. For example, clients may be afraid of the pain that they may experience after surgery. The entire health care team must communicate warmth, sensitivity, and caring to the client. Clients may express their fears to you, and as a support worker, you must respect these fears and concerns and the client's need to talk about them.

Feelings are influenced by past experiences. Some clients may have had surgery before, and some may not have had that experience at all. Family and friends may share experiences of their own surgeries with the client, which also can affect the client. Clients may have heard tragic stories related to surgeries—surgery on the wrong client, surgery on the wrong body part, instruments left in the body, death during surgery, and so on. Before surgery, some clients may not talk about their fears and concerns but just cry or be quiet and withdrawn; some may constantly talk about other things; some may pace restlessly; and some may act overly cheerful.

BOX 45–2 Common Fears and Concerns of Surgical Clients

Fears

Disfigurement and scarring
Disability
Pain during and after surgery
Dying during surgery
Anaesthesia and its effects
Exposure
Severe pain or discomfort after surgery
Tubes, needles, and other equipment used for care
Complications
Prolonged recovery
More surgery or treatments
Separation from family and friends
Nausea and vomiting

Concerns

Caring for children and other family members
Taking care of pets, the house, lawn, and garden
Payment of monthly bills, loans, mortgage, or rent
Insurance coverage for loss of earnings
Loss of control
Restrictions on lifestyle

Client Information

The physician explains to the client and family the need for surgery and the surgical procedure, risks, and possible complications. Options other than surgery as well as the risks of not having surgery are also explained. The physician or nurse gives information about when the surgery is scheduled, who will perform it, and how long it will take. The physician also answers all the questions and addresses any doubts the client and family may have about the surgery and what to expect and gives instructions about pre- and postoperative care. Consent for surgery must be given by the client or a substitute decision maker. In most provinces and territories, support workers cannot witness consent for surgery, as doing so is not within their scope of practice. If your client and the family request more information about the surgery, refer them to your supervisor.

Often, the health care team knows the results of the surgery before the client does. The physician informs the client and the family about the outcome of the surgery, deciding what and when to tell them. Clients and families are usually anxious to know the results and may ask you, nurses, and other health care workers for information. They may ask, for example, if reports are back from the laboratory or what the reports say. You should know what exactly the client is told, but you must take care not to reveal any information about the surgery or test results. If the client asks you for information, explain that you cannot give it and that you will get your supervisor to provide that information. Ensure that you report to your supervisor your client's concerns and questions so that the supervisor can answer the questions or direct the client to the doctor, who can address these issues. Your supervisor will tell you what the client and the family were told and when it was told. This information is confidential, so do not repeat it to anyone.

Your Role

As a support worker, you can assist in the psychological care of the surgical client. Do the following if you are involved in preoperative and postoperative care:

- Listen to the client when the client voices fears or concerns about surgery.
- Refer any questions about the surgery or its results to the nurse.
- Explain to the client the procedures that *you* will perform and the reasons for them.
- Communicate effectively. Use verbal and nonverbal communication (see Chapter 5).
- Report to your supervisor verbal and nonverbal signs of pain, fear, or anxiety that you have observed in the client.
- Report to your supervisor a client's request to see a spiritual advisor.

The Preoperative Period

The **preoperative** (before surgery) period may be many days or just a few minutes. If time permits, the client is prepared psychologically and physically for the effects of anaesthesia and surgery (see the *Focus on Children: Preparing for Surgery* box). Good preoperative preparation prevents complications after surgery.

Different kinds of medication are prescribed for preoperative preparation, and your supervisor will tell you the procedure to follow when assisting a client with these medications. Some medications may cause diarrhea and, therefore, dehydration in the client. You need to ensure that the client drinks lots of fluids. Instructions from the doctor will include what types of fluids are allowed. The client will need to stay close to a bathroom and may experience some cramping. The area around the anus can become quite sore with frequent defecation. You can assist the client with the use of adult unscented wet wipes, a water spray, or a barrier cream.

Home preparation before surgery can be tiring for older clients. It is important to ensure safety in the home if they become weak.

Preoperative Teaching

A nurse does the preoperative teaching and explains to the client what to expect before and after surgery. Teaching includes the following:

- ***Preoperative activities***—teaching about tests and their purposes, skin preparation, personal care, and the purposes and effects of medications.
- ***Deep-breathing, coughing, and leg exercises***—teaching and practising exercises that are to be done after the surgery. These are taught by either a nurse or a physiotherapist.
- ***The postanaesthesia care unit***—where the client wakes up from anaesthesia (**FIGURE 45–7**). Care that will be provided in the recovery room is explained.
- ***Food and fluids***—preoperative clients are NPO (nothing by mouth) for several hours. Some clients receive an intravenous (IV) infusion after surgery. The physician orders food and oral fluids once the client's condition is stable.
- ***Turning and repositioning***—the client usually is turned and repositioned every 2 hours after surgery. The client is taught what to expect.
- ***Early ambulation***—usually the client is encouraged to walk as soon as possible after surgery.

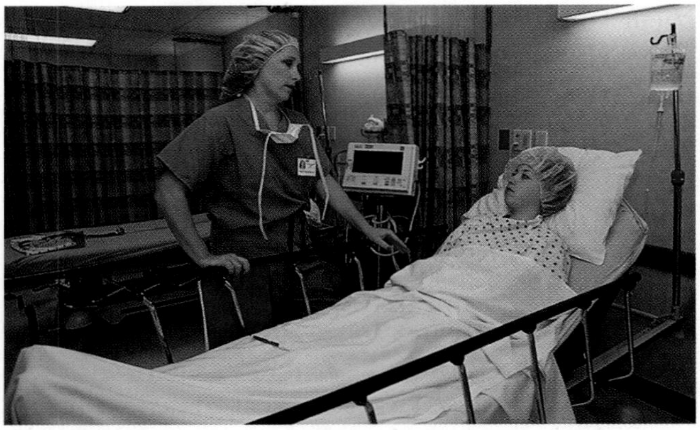

FIGURE 45–7 Postanaesthesia care unit (PACU) or recovery room.

FOCUS ON CHILDREN

Preparing for Surgery

The child who will be operated on, as well as the parents or caregivers, is psychologically prepared before the surgery if it is a scheduled surgery. Often, play is used to help the child understand what will happen. For example, dolls are used to show the anatomical site of surgery. The child and parents or caregivers are introduced to the members of the health care team who will be caring for the child. A tour of the operating room and the recovery room also is common.

- ***Pain***—the client is told about the type and amount of pain to expect and about medications for pain relief.
- ***Needed treatments and equipment***—the client may need a urinary catheter, nasogastric (NG) tube, oxygen, wound suction, a cast, traction, or wound dressings. Any treatment or equipment anticipated to be needed is explained to the client.
- ***Position restrictions***—the client is told if a certain position is required to be maintained after surgery—for example, after hip replacement surgery, the hip is abducted.

Special Tests

Before surgery, the physician orders tests to evaluate the client's circulatory, respiratory, and urinary systems. These tests include a chest X-ray, a complete blood count (CBC), and urinalysis. An electrocardiogram (ECG) detects any cardiac (heart) problems. In preparation for any needed transfusions to correct anticipated blood loss, the patient's blood is tested to determine blood type (type and cross-match). Other tests are done, depending on the client's condition and the requirements of the surgery. The client is prepared for the tests, as needed, and results are on the client's chart by the time of surgery.

Nutrition and Fluids

The client is usually allowed to have a light meal the day before the surgery and then is NPO for 6 to 8 hours before the surgery. These measures reduce the risk of vomiting and aspiration during general anaesthesia and after surgery. An NPO sign is placed in the client's room. Some clients may be required to take medications on the morning of surgery—for example, insulin or blood pressure medication. It is important that any such medication need is a doctor's order and that it is clearly written. Remember to remove the water pitcher and drinking glasses from the room when a patient is ordered NPO. If the time of surgery is delayed or cancelled, your client will need nutrition during the waiting period. Check with your supervisor about the type of diet and fluids allowed.

Elimination

Abdominal surgeries usually require a preoperative enema. Cleansing enemas are common before intestinal surgeries and are ordered to clear the colon of feces so that feces do not spill into the abdominal cavity when the intestine is opened.

Enemas are also given when straining or when a bowel movement could cause postoperative problems such as pain, severe bleeding (hemorrhage), or stress on the operated area. The physician specifies what enema to give and when, and usually a nurse administers the enema.

Some surgeries will necessitate urinary catheterization. For pelvic and abdominal surgeries, the bladder must be empty, as a full bladder is easily injured during surgery. Catheters also allow accurate urinary output measurements during and after surgery.

Personal Care

Personal care before surgery usually involves the following:

- ***Giving a complete bed bath, shower, or tub bath.*** A special soap or cleanser may be ordered. A bath and a shampoo help reduce the number of microbes on the body at the time of surgery.
- ***Removing makeup and nail polish.*** The skin, lips, and nail beds need to be observed for colour and circulation during and after surgery.
- ***Caring for hair.*** All hairpins, clips, combs, and similar items as well as wigs and hairpieces are removed. Some hospitals have both male and female clients wear surgical caps to keep hair out of the face and the operative area.
- ***Giving oral hygiene to promote comfort.*** Being NPO causes thirst and a dry mouth. Ensure that the client does not swallow any water during oral hygiene (see the *Focus on Children: Preoperative Oral Hygiene* box).
- ***Removing dentures.*** Before preoperative medications are given, dentures are removed, cleaned, and kept in a denture cup in a safe place. Some clients do not like being seen without their dentures, in which case allow them to wear their dentures as long as possible. This measure promotes the client's sense of dignity and self-esteem.
- ***Removing all jewellery.*** If body-piercing jewellery cannot be removed, it should be taped down.

Valuables

Valuables such as dentures, glasses, contact lenses, hearing aids, and jewellery are removed from clients for safekeeping. Artificial eyes and limbs also are removed, as these items are easily lost or broken during surgery. A note is made on the client's chart about the valuables removed and where they are kept. The client may not want to remove a wedding band or religious medal. In this case, the item is secured in place with gauze or tape, according to hospital policy.

FOCUS ON CHILDREN

Preoperative Oral Hygiene

A loose tooth can fall out during anaesthesia, and the child can aspirate the tooth. Therefore, during preoperative care, check for loose teeth when giving oral hygiene, and report any that you observe to the nurse. The nurse will note your observations on the preoperative checklist and inform the operating room (OR) staff.

Skin Preparation

The skin and hair shafts contain microbes that could enter the body through the surgical incision, and a serious infection could result. The skin cannot be sterilized, but skin *prep* can help reduce the number of microbes.

Hospital policy and the surgeon's preferences determine the area to be prepared for a specific surgery and the type of preparation to be done.

The Preoperative Checklist

A preoperative checklist (**FIGURE 45–8**) is placed at the top of the client's chart. The nurse makes sure that all items on the checklist have been completed because only when the list has been completed is the client considered to be ready for surgery. The nurse may ask you to do some things on the list, and when you complete each task, promptly report it to the nurse along with any observations. Except for positioning of bed rails, the entire checklist should be completed before preoperative medications are given.

Preoperative Medication

About 45 minutes to 1 hour before surgery, the preoperative medications are given by a physician or a nurse. One medication helps the patient relax and feel drowsy, and another dries up respiratory secretions to prevent aspiration. Drowsiness, lightheadedness, thirst, and dry mouth are normal and expected (see the *Focus on Children: Preoperative Medications* box on page 1049).

After the medications are given, safety measures are taken to prevent falls. Bed rails are raised, and the patient is not allowed out of bed from this point forward, so the client must void before the medications are given. If the client needs to void after the medications are given, a bedpan or urinal is used.

The bed is kept in the lowest position or raised to the highest position, according to hospital policy.

CREDIT • VALLEY
THE CREDIT VALLEY HOSPITAL
PRE-OPERATIVE CHECKLIST

Procedure: ______ **Date:** ______

Surgeon: ______ ☐ SDA ☐ SDC

SDC - Ride available? ☐ Yes ☐ No ☐ ICU/CCU

Allergies: ______

Allergy Bracelet: ☐ Yes

Infectious Disease Risk: ☐ Yes ☐ No ☐ Unknown

Yes: ______

Initial in box	YES	N/A	OR RN
Addressograph Plate			
Identification Bracelet			
Consent to Surgery			
Blood Consent			
History & Physical			
Surgical Consultation			
Pre Anaesthetic Questionnaire			
Pre-op Teaching			
Old Chart to OR			
Dentures Removed			
Capped/loose teeth/braces			
Retainers/Palate Expanders			
Contact Lenses Removed			
Hearing Aid Removed			
Prosthesis Removed			
Jewellery / Body PiercingRemoved/Taped			
Nail Polish Removed			
Undergarments removed			
Other:			
Operative Side ☐ Bil. ☐ R ☐ L ☐ N/A			
Operative Site Marked by MD			

Last void time: ______ / ______

NPO since: ______ / ______

VITAL SIGNS - Time

Temp ______ Pulse ______

Resp. ______ BP ______

Weight ______ kg SpO2 ______

Other Patient Information

Pre-operative

RN Signature/Init. ______ / ______

Date. ______

Physical & Emotional Assessment

☐ Oriented ☐ Confused
☐ Semi-Conscious ☐ Anxious
☐ Unconscious ☐ Language Barrier

Language Spoken at Home ______

	IMPLANTS		INIT.
AV Fistula	☐ R - ARM	☐ L - ARM	______
Total Hip	☐ R	☐ L	______
Total Knee	☐ R	☐ L	______
Pacemaker	☐ Yes		______

Location: ______

Other: ______ ______

LAB RESULTS/REPORTS

☐ Hemoglobin ☐ Sickle Cell
☐ Urinalysis ☐ Cap Blood Glucose: Result: ______
☐ Sickle Cell
☐ Electrolytes ☐ Urea ☐ Creat
☐ Glucose ☐ LFTs
☐ INR/PT / PTT ☐ ECG
☐ Gr & Reserve/OB Mom ☐ CXR
☐ Crossmatch ______ units ☐ Other:
☐ Autologous ______ units

Abnormal Results:

Medication Administration	**Initial**
	/
	/
	/
	/
	/
	/

IV Solution ☐ No

IV site/cath. size

RN Signature:

Operating Room

RN Signature/Init. ______ / ______

Date. ______

5322 D HR (Sept/2005)

PRE-OPERATIVE CHECKLIST

FIGURE 45–8 Preoperative checklist. (Courtesy of Credit Valley Hospital, Mississauga, ON.)

> **FOCUS ON CHILDREN**
>
> **Preoperative Medications**
>
> Some hospitals allow a parent or caregiver to stay with the child in the OR while anaesthesia is given. The person can stay until the child loses consciousness.

Move furniture out of the way to make room for the stretcher. Also, clear the overbed table and the bedside stand to prevent damage to equipment and valuables. Raise the bed to the highest position for transferring the client from the bed to the stretcher.

Transport to the Operating Room

A nurse or an attendant brings a stretcher to the client's room, and the client is transferred onto the stretcher and covered with a bath blanket or sheet to provide warmth and prevent exposure. The safety straps are secured and the side rails are raised to prevent falling. An orthopedic patient may be transferred to the OR in an orthopedic bed. A small pillow is sometimes placed under the client's head for comfort. Assist with all these tasks as required.

After identification checks have been made, the client's chart is given to the OR staff member.

The nurse responsible for preoperative care may go with the client to the OR entrance. Often, family members also are allowed to accompany the client to this point.

Anaesthesia

Anaesthesia is the loss of feeling or sensation produced by a medication. Anaesthetics are given by specially trained physicians called *anaesthetists*. There are three types of anaesthesia:

1. **General anaesthesia**—unconsciousness and the loss of feeling or sensation, produced by a medication that is given intravenously or that is inhaled (i.e., a gas).
2. **Regional anaesthesia**—loss of sensation or feeling in a large area of the body, produced by the injection of a medication. The client does not lose consciousness.
3. **Local anaesthesia**—loss of sensation in a small area, produced by a medication that is injected at the specific site.

The Postoperative Period

During the **postoperative** (after surgery) period, the client is taken to the postanaesthesia care unit (PACU) or, as it is called in some regions, the recovery room. In the PACU, which is near the OR, the client recovers from anaesthesia after the surgery. Recovery can take 1 to 2 hours, during which time the client is watched very closely. Some clients may suffer from nausea and vomiting. Vital signs are taken and observations are made frequently. The client leaves the recovery room when the following states are reached:

- Vital signs are stable.
- The respiratory function is good.
- The client can respond and is able to call for help if needed.

The physician gives the transfer order when appropriate or discharge order if the procedure was a day surgery.

Preparing the Client's Room

If you are employed in an acute-care setting, you will need to prepare the room for an inpatient client's return from the PACU. The room is prepared right after the client has been taken to the OR. The nurse tells you if special measures and equipment are needed. Preparations include the following:

- Making an open bed (see Chapter 34)
- Placing equipment and supplies in the room:
  - Thermometer
  - Stethoscope
  - Sphygmomanometer
  - Kidney basin
  - Tissues
  - Waterproof bed protector
  - Vital signs flow sheet
  - Intake and output (I&O) record
  - IV pole
  - Wound dressings
  - Other items, as directed by the nurse

- Raising the bed to its highest position
- Lowering bed rails
- Moving furniture to make room for the stretcher

Return From the Recovery Room

A PACU or recovery room nurse will call the client's unit to let that staff know when the client is ready for transfer. In many instances, the client's assigned nurse will assist the PACU porters in transporting the client from the PACU to the client's room. Staff from the nursing unit will then assist the PACU porters and assigned nurse to transfer the client from the stretcher to the bed and to position the client properly.

It is important to have an extra blanket ready for the client, as clients often feel cold after surgery because PACU units are often cold. Heated blankets are used in some facilities to warm clients after surgery.

Vital signs are taken by a nurse after the client has been positioned in bed. Vital signs are usually measured in the following frequencies:

- Every 15 minutes the first hour
- Every 30 minutes for 1 to 2 hours
- Every hour for 4 hours
- Every 4 hours

Depending on what surgery the client had, the client may be connected to a number of drains, pumps, or other equipment when she returns from surgery. It is important to ask the nurse before moving any of the devices. It is the nurse's responsibility to ensure that each device is working correctly. The nurse also observes the client and checks dressings for bleeding. Catheters, IV infusions, and other tube placements and functions are checked, and necessary care and treatments are given. Bed rails are raised, and the call bell is placed within the client's reach. The length of time before the family is allowed to see the client varies with each hospital.

Observations

The client requires careful monitoring during the postoperative period. After the client is stable, you may be asked to check the client frequently. The nurse tells you how often to check the client. Depending on the type of surgical procedure the client had, the client is at great risk for developing potentially life-threatening complications, especially in the first few hours following surgery. ***You must always be alert for the signs and symptoms*** listed in **BOX 45–3**, ***and report them to the nurse immediately.***

Positioning

Proper positioning after surgery promotes comfort and prevents complications. The type of surgery determines positioning and, possibly, position restrictions. The client is usually positioned for easy and comfortable breathing and to prevent stress on the incision. When the client is in the supine position, the head of the bed is usually raised slightly, and the client's head may be turned to the side, which will help prevent aspiration if vomiting occurs.

Repositioning every 1 to 2 hours helps prevent respiratory and circulatory complications. Turning may be painful for the client, so provide support, and turn the client with smooth, gentle motions. Pillows and other positioning devices are often used (see Chapters 25 and 26).

The nurse tells you when to reposition the client and the positions allowed. Usually, you assist the nurse, but sometimes, you will turn and reposition the client yourself once the client's condition is stable and the client is in a community setting or at home (see the *Focus on Older Adults: Postoperative Positioning* box on page 1052).

Coughing and Deep Breathing

Respiratory complications in the postsurgical period must be prevented. There are two major complications: (1) *pneumonia*, an inflammation and infection in the lung; and (2) *atelectasis*, the collapse of a portion of the lung. Coughing and deep-breathing exercises and incentive spirometry help prevent these complications (see Chapter 41) and are done every 1 to 2 hours when the client is awake. For comfort, the client should be instructed to splint the incision (hold his hands tightly over the incision) if possible (see the *Focus on Older Adults: Respiratory Complications After Surgery* box on page 1052).

Stimulating Circulation

After surgery, circulation must be stimulated, especially for blood flow in the legs. If blood flow is sluggish, a blood clot (**thrombus**) can form in the

BOX 45–3 Postoperative Observations That Must Be Reported Immediately

- Choking
- A drop or rise in blood pressure
- Bright red blood from the incision, drainage tubes, or suction tubes
- A pulse rate of more than 100 or less than 60 beats per minute
- A weak or irregular pulse
- A rise or drop in body temperature
- Hypoxia (see Chapter 41)
- The need for upper airway suctioning, signalled by any of the following:
  - Tachypnea (rapid breathing)
  - Dyspnea (difficult, laboured, or painful breathing)
  - Moist-sounding respirations
  - Gurgling or gasping
  - Restlessness
  - Cyanosis (bluish colour of the skin, lips, and nails)
- Shallow, slow breathing
- Weak cough
- Complaints of thirst
- Cold, moist, clammy, or pale skin
- Increased drainage on or under dressings or on bed linens (including turning pads, bottom sheets, and pillowcases)
- Complaints of pain or nausea
- Vomiting
- Confusion or disorientation
- Other measurements and observations, as directed by a nurse:
  - The amount, character, and time of the first voiding after surgery
  - Intake and output
  - Blood in the IV tubing
  - Redness or swelling around the IV insertion site
  - The appearance of drainage from a urinary catheter, NG tube, or wound suction
  - Any other observation that can indicate a change in the client's condition

deep leg veins (**FIGURE 45–9, *A***). An **embolus** is an air bubble, blood clot (thrombus), or fat clot that travels through the vascular system until it lodges in a distant vessel. An embolus can eventually lodge as far away as in the lungs (pulmonary embolus); once there, it can cause severe respiratory problems and even death (see **FIGURE 45–9, *B***).

Leg Exercises

Leg exercises help increase venous blood flow and thus prevent the formation of a thrombus. Leg exercises are easy to do; however, provide assistance if the client is weak. If the client has had leg surgery, a physician's order is needed for the exercises. Your supervisor will tell you when the client should do the exercises. The exercises are done at least every 1 or 2 hours while the client is awake. Have the client assume the supine position and do each of the following exercises five times (see Chapter 26):

- Make circles with the toes (ankle-rotating exercises).

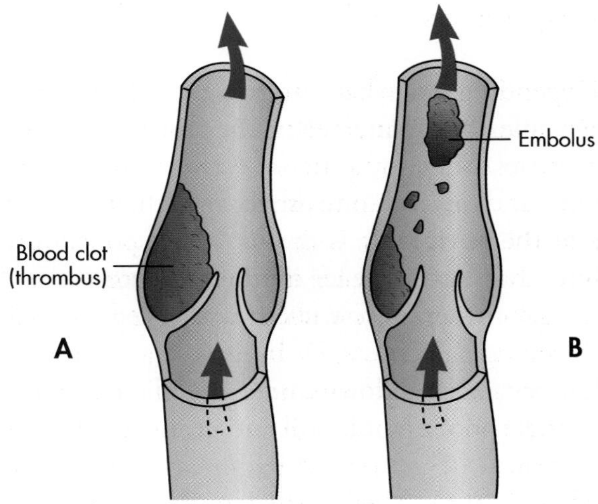

FIGURE 45–9 **A,** A thrombus (blood clot) is attached to the wall of a vein. The arrows show the direction of blood flow. **B,** Part of the thrombus has broken off and become an embolus. The embolus will travel in the bloodstream until it lodges in a distant vessel.

FOCUS ON OLDER ADULTS

Postoperative Positioning

Many older adults have stiff and painful joints even before surgery, and further soreness of muscles, bones, and joints often occurs from positioning on the operating room table. Take care to turn and reposition older adults slowly and gently.

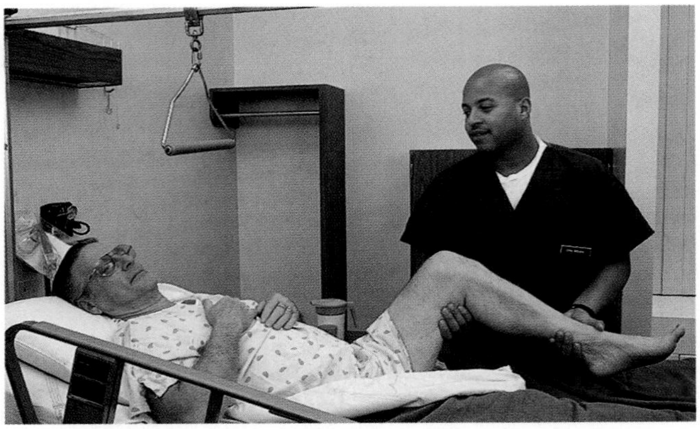

FIGURE 45–10 The client flexes and then extends the knee during postoperative leg exercises.

FOCUS ON OLDER ADULTS

Respiratory Complications After Surgery

Age-related changes increase the older adult's risk for respiratory complications following surgery. Since the respiratory muscles are weaker and lung tissue is less elastic, the client has less strength for coughing. Coughing, deep breathing, and incentive spirometry are, however, very important, and the client must be encouraged to do these exercises to prevent respiratory complications.

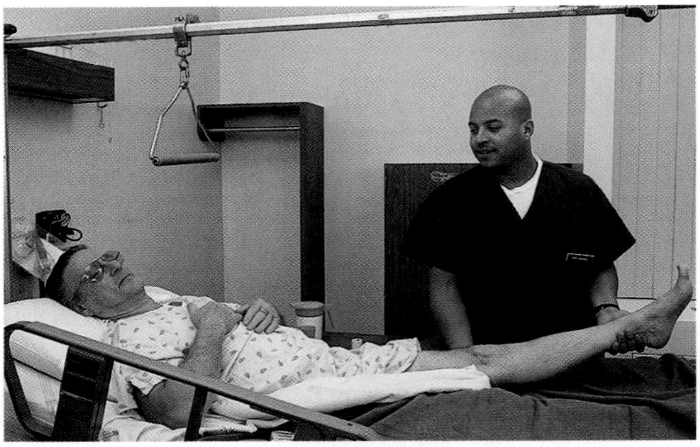

FIGURE 45–11 Assist the client with raising and lowering the leg.

- Dorsiflex and plantar flex the feet (calf-pumping exercises).
- Flex and extend one knee and then the other (**FIGURE 45–10**).
- Raise and lower one leg off the bed (**FIGURE 45–11**). Repeat this exercise with the other leg.

Do not place pillows under the client's calf as it may cause pooling of blood and create a risk for clot formation.

Elastic Stockings and Bandages

Elastic stockings and bandages are often used to help prevent the formation of a thrombus. The elastic exerts pressure on the veins, promoting venous blood flow to the heart. Elastic stockings or bandages are often ordered for postoperative clients and for regular use in those with heart disease and circulatory disorders.

Both elastic stockings and bandages could harm the client if applied improperly. Therefore, most hospitals allow only nurses to apply them to acute-care clients. If you are assigned this task, make sure that it is in your scope of practice and that employer policy allows you to do it. Also, ensure that you have been properly trained and are closely supervised (see Chapter 31 for a discussion on the application of elastic stockings and bandages).

Early Ambulation

Early ambulation prevents postoperative circulatory complications such as thrombus formation, pneumonia, atelectasis, constipation, and urinary tract infections. The client is usually encouraged to ambulate even on the day of surgery. The client first sits up with the legs over the edge of the bed (see "Helping the Client to Sit on the Side of the Bed (Dangle the Legs)" in Chapter 25). If blood pressure and pulse are stable, the client is assisted out of bed. Usually the client does not walk very far, just a few feet in the room. Walking distance is increased as the client gains strength.

The nurse will tell you when to help the client ambulate. Usually, you assist the nurse the first time the client ambulates.

Wound Healing

The surgical incision needs protection, so measures are taken to promote healing and prevent infection. Sterile dressing changes are done by a physician or a nurse. Some hospitals allow support workers to perform simple dressing care if the client is stable (see Chapter 24 for a discussion on wound healing).

Nutrition and Fluids

The client has an IV infusion upon her return from the OR. Continuation of the IV therapy depends on the type of surgery and the client's condition—for example, whether nausea and vomiting have resulted from the general anaesthesia. The client's diet progresses from NPO to clear liquids to full liquids to a light diet to a regular diet that is ordered by the physician. Frequent oral hygiene is important when the patient is NPO.

Some clients have NG tubes (see Chapter 29) after surgery. The NG tube is attached to suction equipment to keep the stomach empty. The patient remains NPO and receives IV therapy.

Elimination

Anaesthesia, the surgery, and being NPO can all affect normal fecal and urinary elimination, and medications for pain relief can cause constipation. You will be asked to take measures to promote elimination, as directed by the nurse (see Chapters 32 and 33).

Fluid intake and output (I&O) are measured during the postoperative period. It is important that the client urinates within 8 hours after surgery. Report the time and amount of the client's first voiding. If the client does not void within 8 hours, a catheterization is usually ordered. Some clients have catheters inserted routinely after surgery—for example, after bladder surgery (see Chapter 32 for care of the client with a catheter).

Adequate fluid intake and return to a regular diet are needed for normal bowel movement. Suppositories or enemas may be ordered if the client is constipated, and rectal tubes may be ordered for relief of flatulence (see Chapter 33).

Comfort and Rest

Pain is common after surgery. The degree of pain depends on the extent of surgery, the size and location of the incision site, and the presence of drainage tubes, casts, or other devices. In addition, as mentioned above, the client was placed in one position during surgery, often resulting in severe muscle strains and discomfort, usually in the chest, back, and arms, postoperatively. The physician orders medications for pain relief, and the nurse will tell you how to promote comfort and rest (see Chapter 12 for guidelines) listed as part of the client's care plan.

Some surgeries (such as *scopes*) involve inserting gas to inflate the dermis (skin) to allow the surgeon to have better visualization of the desired site. This gas is harmless to the body, but it can cause discomfort that resembles severe muscle cramping. Many clients also experience sore throats from being *intubated* (having a tube inserted into the throat for introduction of gas anaesthesia and for assistance with breathing).

Remember that people experience pain differently, and many factors, such as anxiety or fear, may enhance the pain the client is experiencing. Pain can also be a ***sign of an impending complication that is developing***, so it is important to always be empathetic to the client and to report any complaints of pain to the nurse.

Personal Hygiene

Personal hygiene is important for the client's physical and mental well-being. Wound drainage and skin prep solutions can irritate the skin and cause discomfort, and being NPO can cause dry mouth and breath odours. Moist, clammy skin from blood pressure changes or elevated body temperatures also cause discomfort. Frequent oral hygiene, hair care, and a complete bed bath the day after the surgery help refresh and renew the client's physical and psychological well-being. The gown should be changed whenever it becomes wet or soiled (see Chapter 30).

Think About Safety

Safety Precautions for Clients Having Surgery

- If your client is having a day surgery (e.g., colonoscopy), medications may be prescribed to be taken before the procedure, and these drugs can cause diarrhea. You must ensure that your client has access to the bathroom and that you can provide fluid replacement as prescribed by the physician.
- If you are employed in an acute-care facility and your client is having surgery, ensure that the side bed rails are raised once any preoperative medications have been administered so that your client does not roll out of bed. Your supervisor will tell you when you can lower the bed rails after the operation.
- Your supervisor will give you instructions regarding when your client will be NPO before surgery and after surgery. Follow the instructions, as giving a client something to drink before surgery could result in vomiting or aspiration. The physician will order fluid and food intake for your client after surgery.
- Depending on your agency's policy, you may be delegated by a nurse or physiotherapist to provide deep-breathing, coughing, and leg exercises.
- Ensure that you report your client's I&O to your supervisor, as required.
- If your client has received pain medications, you must be aware of the possibility of falls, so ensure that you are with your client at any time when he is out of bed.

CHAPTER REVIEW

KEY POINTS

- It is important to remember that acute-care clients can develop life-threatening health challenges quickly. Look for and report changes in the client's condition immediately to the proper person.
- You can promote clients' emotional well-being during transitions when you help them with the admission, transfer, and discharge processes.
- Physicians and nurses perform physical examinations to promote health and to diagnose and treat diseases. Some long-term care facilities require physical examinations of new admissions and yearly checkups thereafter.
- As a support worker, you may assist with exams. Your responsibilities depend on your employer's policies and procedures, as well as the examiner's preferences.
- You need to be sensitive to your client's feelings and concerns and help prepare the client physically and psychologically for the examination.
- Maintaining warmth and privacy during the examination is very important.
- A parent or another adult must be present when toddlers, preschool children, and school-aged children are being examined.
- If your client is having elective or emergency surgery, you may be required to provide preoperative care, postoperative care, or both. Your supervisor will give you directions for care. Your duties will depend on your employer's policies, the policies of the province or territory where you are employed, and the legislation in your area.
- A nurse or a physician will do the preoperative and postoperative teaching and will explain to the client and the family what to expect before and after surgery.
- Your client may share with you concerns and fears about the upcoming surgery, and you need to report these concerns to your supervisor.
- In a client's postoperative period, you must be vigilant in watching for any signs or symptoms of respiratory, circulatory, or skin conditions and report and record any concerns immediately to your supervisor.

CRITICAL THINKING IN PRACTICE

1. During an exam, you must leave the room several times for supplies. What problems does leaving the room cause? How could your need to do so have been prevented?
2. You are measuring a postoperative patient's vital signs. The person is restless. The vital signs are similar to previous measurements. What do you do? Is there anything you need to report? If so, when?

REVIEW QUESTIONS

Answers to these questions are at the bottom of the next page.

Circle T if the answer is true, and circle F if the answer is false.

1. T F A client is greeted by name when being admitted to a nursing unit in a hospital or long-term care facility.
2. T F Transfers are usually related to changes in a client's condition.
3. T F A nurse discharges the client before the client can leave a hospital.
4. T F The client's hair is kept out of the face for surgery by using pins, clips, or combs.
5. T F Nail polish and makeup can be kept on for surgery.
6. T F A drop in a patient's blood pressure should be reported to the nurse immediately.
7. T F The client is usually ambulated for the first time the day after the surgery.
8. T F Intake and output are measured after surgery.
9. T F A surgical client should void within 8 hours after surgery.

Circle the BEST answer.

10. The otoscope is used to:
- A. Examine the internal structures of the eye
- B. Examine the external ear and the eardrum
- C. Test reflexes
- D. Open the vagina

11. You are preparing Mrs. Janz for an exam. You should do the following:
- A. Do not tell her any details of the exam, as it is not part of your role
- B. Ask her to undress
- C. Take her vital signs
- D. Leave her alone while you go to tell the nurse that Mrs. Janz is ready

12. Mrs. Janz is lying on her back. Her hips are flexed and externally rotated. Her feet are supported in stirrups. She is in the:
- A. Supine position
- B. Lithotomy position
- C. Knee–chest position
- D. Sims' position

13. You will be assisting with Mrs. Janz's exam. Which of the following is true?
- A. Hand hygiene is done before and after the examination.
- B. Draping is not necessary if the door is closed.
- C. You leave the room while Mrs. Janz is examined.
- D. The examiner will position the client.

14. Which of the following statements is true?
- A. You cannot explain the reason for the exam to the client.
- B. You must keep the client safe from injury during the exam.
- C. You can tell the family the results of the exam.
- D. You explain what the examiner will do.

15. Which of the following is true of elective surgery?
- A. The surgery is done immediately.
- B. The need for surgery is sudden and unexpected.
- C. Surgery is scheduled for a later date.
- D. General anaesthesia is always used.

16. You can assist with a client's psychological preparation by explaining:
- A. The reason for the surgery
- B. The procedures you will be doing
- C. The risks and possible complications of surgery
- D. What to expect during the preoperative and postoperative periods

17. Preoperatively, Mr. Long is NPO. What does this mean?
- A. Nothing my mouth
- B. Allowed only water
- C. Given a regular breakfast
- D. Given a tube feeding

18. Mr. Long's preoperative medication has been given to him. He:
- A. Must remain in bed
- B. Is allowed to walk within his room
- C. Can use the commode to void
- D. Is allowed only sips of water

19. Mr. Long must do coughing and deep-breathing exercises after surgery to prevent:
- A. Bleeding
- B. A pulmonary embolus
- C. Respiratory complications
- D. Pain and discomfort

20. Postoperatively, Mr. Long's position is changed:
- A. Every 2 hours
- B. Every 3 hours
- C. Every 4 hours
- D. Every shift

Answers: 1.T, 2.T, 3.F, 4.F, 5.F, 6.T, 7.T, 8.T, 9.T, 10.B, 11.B, 12.B, 13.A, 14.B, 15.C, 16.D, 17.A, 18.A, 19.C, 20.A

CHAPTER 46

End-of-Life Care

OBJECTIVES

After reading this chapter, the learner should be able to do the following:

- Explain how culture, religion, and age influence attitudes toward death.
- Explain the importance of an advance directive.
- Describe the impact that grief can have on people.
- Describe the stages, phases, or tasks clients, families, and caregivers may encounter when dealing with grief.
- Explain how to help meet a dying client's needs.
- Describe the needs of the family of a dying client.
- Describe palliative care.
- Identify the signs of approaching death and the signs of death.
- Describe how to assist in giving postmortem care.
- Demonstrate the procedures described in this chapter.

KEY TERMS

grief The process of moving from deep sorrow caused by loss toward healing and recovery. *p. 1061*

grief counselling A support for people coping with the difficulties associated with the loss of a loved one. *p. 1061*

postmortem care Care of the body after *(post)* death *(mortem)*. *p. 1070*

rigor mortis The stiffness or rigidity *(rigor)* of skeletal muscles that occurs after death *(mortis)*. *p. 1071*

As a support worker, you will be required to help meet the physical, social, emotional, intellectual, and spiritual needs of clients who are dying, whether in a facility or in clients' homes. Your role may also involve providing support to a client's family and loved ones. Some family members may be very involved in care, whereas others may not be available because of distance or personal choice.

End-of-life care can be emotionally draining not only to the loved ones of the dying client but also to the client's caregivers. Witnessing and providing end-of-life care may remind caregivers of their own eventual death or of the deaths of their own loved ones. For some, having a dying client may cause feelings of helplessness since they are unable to "make the client better." Some health care team members may be unsure of their feelings about death or may be uncomfortable with dying clients or the subject of death being mentioned in conversation with the client.

Your feelings and beliefs about death and dying may affect the care you give when caring for a dying client, so you need to understand both the dying process and your own attitudes toward death and dying. This understanding will help you provide compassionate care. Before reading on, reflect on the following:

- What has been your experience with death?
- What are your feelings and beliefs about death and dying?
- How have your experiences and culture shaped your beliefs?

LIFE-THREATENING ILLNESS

Many life-threatening illnesses have no cure, and some injuries are so serious that the body cannot function. In these cases, recovery is not expected, and the illness or injury inevitably ends in death.

Health care providers cannot predict the exact time of death. A client may have days, months, weeks, or years to live. Some clients who are expected to live for a short time live for many years, whereas others who are expected to live longer die much sooner than predicted. Some clients die sooner than expected because they lose the will to live. No one can predict the length of time a client may have, as each client is unique.

The time spent knowing that death is approaching is often difficult for the client as well as the client's family, friends, and loved ones. The approach of death may be when people who are dying resolve existing interpersonal issues, put financial affairs in order, and decide on the extent of medical care they would like as they near their life's end. The loved ones of the dying client must begin to realize that they will not always have this person in their lives, and they may start to grieve the loss of their partner, friend, or family member.

ATTITUDES TOWARD DEATH

Personal beliefs, culture, religion, age, and experience influence attitudes toward death. Many people fear death; others believe they will regain health; and some accept and even look forward to death. A person's attitude toward death often changes with age and experience.

Until the beginning of the twentieth century, most Canadians died in their own homes, and families cared for loved ones who were dying. Death was considered a natural part of life. Today, however, most Canadians die in facilities. Many people have never seen a dying person or a dead body, so death can be a frightening experience for them.

Personal Beliefs, Culture, and Religion

Practices and attitudes about death differ among individuals, cultures, and religions (see the *Respecting Diversity: Death and Dying Rituals* box). Some people believe that there is no suffering and hardship, that they will be reunited with loved ones in the afterlife, and that sins and misdeeds will be punished then, too. Other people believe there is no afterlife. Many clients experience a strengthening of their religious beliefs when they face death, and such faith often provides comfort to the dying person and the family. Alternatively, clients may instead experience a loss of religious faith.

A client's personal, cultural, and religious beliefs also influence choices about end-of-life care and treatment of the body after death.

Dying With Dignity, the Right to Die, and Assisted Suicide

Many issues must be dealt with and discussed when a client is faced with a long (and sometime difficult) battle with a terminal illness. Most people fear pain and suffering. The goal of all palliative care is to reduce pain and suffering as much as possible for that person using pain medications and soothing comfort measures.

However, some people believe that "dying with dignity" should include removing breathing machines, feeding tubes, and other medical devices that only prolong life but do not cure the client. There are other people who believe that a terminal illness that brings pain and suffering is not life at all, and the client should have the right to choose when they will die. These people support *assisted suicide* (suicide that is aided by providing the client with the means to do it or the information on how to end his or her own life) or *euthanasia* (the act of putting another person painlessly to death).

The assisted suicide debate has been argued at every level in the Canadian legal system. In 2015, after many legal challenges of the federal law that criminalized assisted suicide, the Supreme Court of Canada legally reversed the position of Canada's Criminal Code, and, on June 6, 2016, assisted suicide became legal for any adult who is legally capable of making such a choice rationally as long as (1) the person clearly consents to the termination of his or her life, and (2) the person has an irreversible illness, disease, or disability that is causing intolerable pain or suffering and that cannot be reversed or acceptably reduced. This hotly debated law will have a wide-reaching impact on many Canadian lives and business industries, including medical tourism, health care, and law. At the time of this writing, physician, law, and health care worker groups are examining its legal implications.

Treatment of the Body After Death

People have various beliefs about the body's form after death. Some believe that the body keeps its physical form, whereas others believe that only the spirit, or soul, is present in the afterlife. Some believe in the concept of *reincarnation*, which is the belief that the spirit or soul is reborn in another human body or in another life form. These beliefs can influence the following:

- The client's (or family's) choice to be buried or cremated
- Whether an autopsy should be performed
- Whether or not organs should be donated for transplant
- Whether the body may be donated to science

Age and Experience

People's attitudes and responses to dying are highly individual. Age and stage of life are some of the major influences on people's feelings and reactions in regard to death.

Infants and toddlers have no concept of death. Between the ages of 3 and 5 years, children are curious and have some ideas about death because they know when family members or pets die, and

Respecting Diversity

Death and Dying Rituals

The following chart is intended to give a few examples of some cultural and religious beliefs and practices surrounding death and dying. ***Remember, individuals may not follow every belief and practice of their culture and religion.*** Each client is unique. Do not judge the client by your own standards. It is very important to talk to your client and the family to find out their wishes.

Hinduism	The dying person may be laid on the floor. A priest ties around the neck or wrist a thread that is not to be removed. After the client's death, a priest pours water in the client's mouth. Family members wash the body before cremation.
Sikhism	The body of the deceased person must wear or have the five Ks: *Kesh*, uncut hair; *Kangra*, wooden comb; *Kara*, wrist band; *Kirpan*, sword; *Kach*, shorts.
Buddhism	A monk is called in before a person's death, and he performs the last rites and chants at the dying person's bedside. Burial and cremation are both acceptable.
Shinto	Jewellery is removed from the body, and the body is then washed and dressed in a white kimono and straw shoes.
Islam	The dying person confesses sins. After death, the body is washed and wrapped in white cloth; the head is turned toward the right shoulder, facing east, toward Mecca.
Judaism	The body is washed by the burial society, and someone remains with the body (Orthodox and Conservative Jews) all the time. Whenever possible, burial is to take place within 24 hours after death.
Christianity	Rituals vary greatly among groups. Many give last rites or communion to the dying person. Many groups prefer burial to cremation.
Christian Science	A female client who dies should be handled only by a female staff member. Unless required by law, postmortems are not allowed.
Indigenous groups	The Inuit generally follow Christian practices. Funeral and mourning practices vary among different Métis, First Nations, and individual families. The large majority of First Nations people who are Christian usually prefer the funeral and burial practices particular to their church. Some follow Native spiritual traditions or incorporate aspects of these in Christian funerals.

Source: Potter, P.A., Perry, A.G., Ross-Kerr, J.C., et al. (2001). *Canadian fundamentals of nursing* (2nd ed., p. 600). Toronto, ON: Elsevier Canada.

they notice dead birds and insects. However, they may think that death is only a temporary state. Not answering their questions about death accurately and properly can cause fear and confusion. For example, children who are told "He is sleeping" may be afraid to go to sleep. Children between ages 5 and 7 know that death is final, though they may not think it will happen to them.

Adults often have more fears about death than children do. Adults may fear pain and suffering, dying alone, separation from loved ones, and loss of dignity. They may worry about the care and support of those left behind. Some people have regrets about missed opportunities, failed relationships, or unfulfilled hopes and dreams. People may feel that their lives did not have any meaning or, alternatively, that their lives did make a difference.

Older adults often have fewer fears about death, as they expect to die, and many have experienced the deaths of friends and loved ones. Some older adults welcome death as freedom from pain, suffering, and disability. As a support worker, you will have clients who may want to discuss their wishes about what should happen in the event of their death. Report their wishes to your supervisor, who will forward them to the family. Like younger adults, older adults often fear dying alone.

Although age and stage of life influence a person's response to dying, you cannot predict what a particular individual's response will be.

GRIEF

Loss is one of life's most stressful events. After the loss of a loved one (whatever the circumstance), it may take time for the person to heal emotionally. As each circumstance is different, each person responds to grief in his or her own way. Some people may need the support of family or friends to help them cope with grief, while others seek the assistance of trained professionals when struggling to cope with the changes in their lives.

What Is Grief?[1]

Grief (also called *bereavement*) is the emotional response to a loss or a death. Every client and family member will grieve differently based on past experiences, coping strategies, cultural beliefs, and spiritual beliefs. Coping with grief involves the processes of mourning and of adapting to the loss. A person will move back and forth through a series of stages and tasks many times over several years before the grieving process is complete.

Although no one really "gets over" a loss, the individual can heal and adapt to the loss. Many people associate grief with the death of an important person or pet. However, people experience grief after any important loss that affects their life, such as the loss of a job or relationship. Grief after diagnosis of an illness or other health problem is also common.

Grief is complicated and is different for everybody (See **BOX 46–1**). Feelings, thoughts, reactions, and challenges related to grief are very personal. Some people have thoughts or feelings that seem to be at odds with each other. For example, someone may feel very depressed about the loss but accept the loss at the same time.

In most cases, people navigate through grief with help from loved ones and other supporters and, in time, go back to their daily life. People may feel shocked, sad, angry, scared, anxious, or even numb, having a hard time feeling any emotions at all. Many people even feel relief or peace after a loss. The intensity of grief changes a lot over time. Holidays can often bring up strong feelings, for example. People work through grief in their own time and on their own path.

Some people need help from a mental health professional. Grief can be more complicated when the loss is sudden or unexpected, frightening, the result of an accident or disaster, or the result of a crime. Other factors also play a role: a person's experience of mental illness, lack of personal and social supports, and difficult personal relationships. A type of counselling called **grief counselling** supports people coping with the difficulties associated with the loss of a loved one.

Members of the health care team also experience the stages of grief. Caring for a dying client is a moving and emotional experience, and supporting a grieving family can be very difficult. As a support worker, you will grieve the loss of the client you have cared for. Do not turn away from these feelings, and try to develop your own support system that includes your supervisor and co-workers. Many facilities have support groups to help team members share their grief (see the *Case Study: Support Worker Grief* box).

Theories of Grief

There are several theories about the stages of the grieving process. Some are discussed below and in TABLE 46–1 on page 1063.

BOX 46–1 Supporting the Grieving Person

- Advise the person to connect with caring and supportive people, such as loved ones, neighbours, and co-workers and possibly a bereavement support group or community organization.
- Let the person know that it might take time to accept the loss. Everyone reacts differently to a loss, and there is no normal grieving period.
- Advise the person to allow herself to feel sadness, anger, or whatever she needs to feel and to find healthy ways to share her feelings and express herself, such as talking with friends or writing in a journal.
- Advise the grieving person to recognize that his life has changed. He may feel less engaged with work or relationships for some time. This disinterest is a natural part of loss and grief.
- Suggest reaching out for help. Inform the person that loved ones may want to give them privacy or may not feel comfortable asking him how he is doing. Tell him not to be afraid to ask for support.
- Holidays and other important days can be very hard. Advise the client that it may be helpful to plan ahead and think about new traditions or celebrations that support healing.
- Advise the person to take care of her own physical health. She should be aware of any physical signs of stress or illness and speak with her doctor if she feels that grief is affecting her health.
- The person may find comfort by offering support to other loved ones who are grieving. Reaching out to others may be helpful in the person's own journey.
- Advise the person to be honest with young people and children about what has happened and about how he feels. In return, the grieving person can encourage others to share their feelings.
- Encourage the grieving person to work through difficult feelings like bitterness and blame. These feelings can make it harder to move forward.
- Suggest the grieving person make a new beginning. As the feelings of grief become less intense, suggest she returns to interests and activities she may have dropped. In addition, suggest she think about trying something new.
- Suggest that the grieving person wait before making major life decisions. The person may feel differently as his feelings of grief lose their intensity. Sudden changes may also add to his stress.

Source: Adapted from Canadian Mental Health Association. (2015). *Grieving*. Retrieved from https://www.cmha.ca/mental-health/your-mental-health/grief/Grieving.

CASE STUDY Support Worker Grief

Indira works in a long-term care facility. She relates the following experience about her grief following the death of a resident:

"I cared for Mrs. Giovanni on and off for 5 years. We always talked while I gave care, and I got to know her quite well. She used to tell me about her early life in Italy before she came to Canada and show me photographs of her family.

"I was with her the day before she died. She wanted me to stay with her, and I did. I didn't know her end was so near. When I heard the next day that she had died, I was really upset. I hadn't been this sad when other residents had died. I felt sad for several weeks afterward.

"I shared my feelings with the nurse on my unit and with a co-worker. It helped to talk about it. Gradually, I accepted that my feelings were a natural reaction to loss and death. Looking back, I'm glad I got to know Mrs. Giovanni so well and made time for her the day before she died."

TABLE 46–1 Theories of the Grief Process

Kübler-Ross's Five Stages of Grief	Bowlby's Four Phases of Mourning	Worden's Four Tasks of Mourning
Denial	Numbing	Accepting the reality of loss
Anger	Yearning and searching	Working through the pain of grief
Bargaining	Disorganization and despair	Adjusting to the environment without the deceased
Depression	Reorganization	Emotionally relocating the deceased and moving on with life
Acceptance		

Source: Potter, P.A., & Perry, A.G. (2009). *Fundamentals of nursing* (rev. 7th ed., p. 464). St Louis, MO: Mosby.

Kübler-Ross's Stages of Grief

Kübler-Ross's theory identifies five stages that the client and family may undergo while grieving. These stages can be relevant when experiencing other types of grief, such as the loss felt in a marital breakup. *Not everyone who is grieving will go through every stage or experience them in any specific order.* Examples of behaviours during these stages are as follows:

- During *denial*, they refuse to believe that anything is wrong.
- In the *anger* stage, they may strike at anything or anybody.
- During the *bargaining* stage, they try to postpone the loss and hope the loss can be prevented.
- In *depression*, they may feel overwhelmed and lonely and may withdraw from others.
- With *acceptance*, they move forward with their lives and appreciate their memories of the person.

Bowlby's Phases of Mourning

Bowlby's attachment theory is the foundation for his theory on mourning. He describes four phases of mourning:

- The *numbing* phase may last for a few hours or longer. Mourners may describe it as feeling stunned.
- The *yearning and searching* phase arouses emotional outbursts and acute distress in most people. Trying to suppress these emotions will increase the amount of time needed to move through this phase.
- During the *disorganization and despair* phase, they try to examine how and why the loss occurred. They may try to blame someone for the loss.
- The final phase is *reorganization*. During this stage, people take on new roles, form new relationships, and acquire new skills.

Worden's Four Tasks of Mourning

Worden's four tasks of mourning imply that people who mourn can help themselves and be helped by people around them. Working through these tasks usually takes at least 1 year.

- ***Task 1***—to accept the reality of the loss. Even when death is expected, there is a period of disbelief.
- ***Task 2***—to work through the period of grief. There is emotional pain. For those who try to suppress the pain, this phase will last longer.
- ***Task 3***—to adjust to the environment in which the deceased is missing. As time passes, friends and family make less frequent contact, and the person starts to feel the full impact of the loss.
- ***Task 4***—to emotionally relocate the deceased and move on with life. The deceased will not be forgotten but will take a less prominent place in the person's life.

PALLIATIVE CARE

The World Health Organization (WHO) defines *palliative care* as "an approach that improves the quality of life of patients and their families facing the problem associated with life-threatening illness, through the prevention and relief of suffering by means of early identification and impeccable assessment and treatment of pain and other problems, physical, psychosocial and spiritual."[2] The focus of palliative care is on controlling symptoms and providing support to the client and family when there is no response to treatment.

The idea of hospice care began with giving a place of comfort to weary travellers in Europe during the Middle Ages. Centuries later, in 1967, Dr. Cecily Saunders opened the first free-standing research and teaching hospice in London, England. In 1976, pilot projects for palliative care were started at St. Boniface Hospital in Winnipeg and the Royal Victoria Hospital in Montreal. Soon after, hospice services in Canada proliferated both in the community and in hospital settings.

Depending on your location, the term *palliative* usually refers to the care given, and the term *hospice* refers to the place the care is given. In other areas, the terms *palliative care* and *hospice care* are used to mean the same thing—the compassionate care of dying persons directed at comfort and pain management, whether in a facility or the client's home. However, in some provinces and territories, *palliative care* is used more frequently to describe this care provided by health care teams within a specialized unit in a health care facility. The most common facility setting is the palliative care unit within a hospital. Long-term care facilities also provide palliative care.

A hospice program provides compassionate care to dying persons. Some cities and towns have community hospice organizations, which are usually nonprofit organizations run by volunteers and which sometimes work closely with home care programs.

Separate facilities called *hospices* also provide palliative care. Many hospices provide care in houses that once were private homes and that are often located in quiet neighbourhoods in parklike settings. The goal is to provide a comfortable, peaceful setting and to ensure comfort measures are provided to the client. Some hospices provide palliative care to specific client groups, such as those dying of acquired immune deficiency syndrome (AIDS) or cancer.

Hospice or palliative care is not intended to prolong life but to provide the best quality of life during the final days before death. The three main goals of hospice or palliative care are as follows:

1. ***To assist in controlling the pain and symptoms of illness.*** Most terminally ill clients fear pain more than death itself. Some of a dying client's fears and anxieties can be alleviated by providing good pain control.
2. ***To ensure that death is a natural process.*** The goal of care is not to prolong life but to provide the best quality of life during the final days before death. As a result, medical interventions such as respirators and tube feedings are not used to keep clients alive.
3. ***To provide compassionate care.*** A team of professionals, nonprofessionals, and volunteers with a special interest in the field of palliative care work with sensitivity to meet the needs of the dying client and the family. The right to die with dignity is strongly upheld.

Because palliative care is demanding and complex, it requires the expertise of more than one health care provider and, therefore, a team approach. The common goal or purpose behind all activities is to assist the dying client and his family in the best way possible. Team members vary, depending on the situation (**BOX 46–2**). Some clients may choose to include in the team a close friend as well as family members, all of whom can provide much emotional and physical care. Even in facility settings, family members and close friends are encouraged to help with the care of clients, and clients themselves can be active participants in their own care.

Although members of the team have one or more areas of expertise, their roles often overlap. For example, a support worker may provide assistance with personal care to a client in the community, but the hospice care nurse plays a similar role by bathing the client and monitoring skin condition. Or the nurse who assists with personal care may also provide counselling or physical therapy. Because roles overlap, it is important to ensure that the dying client receives the best care possible. Mutual respect between team

BOX 46–2 Palliative or Hospice Care Team Members in the Home

Care Provider	General Responsibilities
Client	• Participates in the decision-making process • Is included in all discussions about care, whenever possible
Caregivers	• May be family or friends • Participate in the decision-making process • Are included in all discussions about care, whenever possible
Home care coordinator	Assesses client needs and coordinates services in the home
Support worker	• Assists the dying client with personal care and household tasks • Monitors client's situation and reports significant observations • Provides emotional support to dying client and caregivers
Hospice volunteer	Provides emotional support and information about services available to a dying client and caregivers
Spiritual advisor	Provides spiritual and emotional support to the dying client and caregivers
Occupational therapist	• Teaches caregivers and the dying client to complete activities of daily living (ADLs) • Provides emotional support to the dying client and caregivers
Physician	• Monitors the dying client's health status • Prescribes and monitors medications for pain and symptom management • Educates and provides emotional support to the dying client and caregivers
Physiotherapist	Teaches physical exercise and recommends assistive devices to keep the client as independent as possible
Social worker	Provides supportive counselling
Nurse	• Monitors medications and assists with pain and symptom management • Assists with personal care • Educates and provides emotional support to the dying client and caregivers

Other individuals may also assist the client and family—for example, a nutritionist; a complementary therapist providing relaxation, massage, aromatherapy, acupuncture, therapeutic or healing touch, reflexology, music/art; and, of course, extended family and friends.

members as well as communication, accurate charting, and information sharing are all essential to ensuring the best care.

Caring for a Client Who Is Dying

The health care team helps meet the dying client's emotional, social, spiritual, intellectual, and physical needs, and every effort is made to promote physical and emotional comfort, whether the client is at home, in a hospice setting, or in a facility of any kind. The client's right to die in peace and with dignity is always kept in the forefront of these efforts (see **BOX 46–3** and the *Providing Compassionate Care: The Dying Client* box on page 1068).

Emotional, Social, Intellectual, and Spiritual Needs

Clients who are dying need accurate information to make informed decisions. They may want to talk about their fears, worries, and anxieties. Some may

BOX 46–3 The Dying Person's Bill of Rights

- I have the right to be treated as a living human being until I die.
- I have the right to maintain a sense of hopefulness, however changing its focus may be.
- I have the right to be cared for by those who can maintain a sense of hopefulness, however changing its focus might be.
- I have the right to express my feelings and emotions about my approaching death in my own way.
- I have the right to participate in decisions concerning my care.
- I have the right to expect continuing medical and nursing attention even though "cure" goals must be changed to "comfort" goals.
- I have the right not to die alone.
- I have the right to be free from pain.
- I have the right to have my questions answered honestly.
- I have the right not to be deceived.
- I have the right to have help from and for my family in accepting my death.
- I have the right to die in peace and with dignity.
- I have the right to retain my individuality and not to be judged for my decisions, which may be contrary to the beliefs of others.
- I have the right to discuss and enlarge my religious and spiritual experiences, regardless of what they may mean to others.
- I have the right to expect that the sanctity of the human body will be respected after death.
- I have the right to be cared for by caring, sensitive, knowledgeable people who will attempt to understand my needs and will be able to gain some satisfaction in helping me face my death.

Adapted from Barbus, A.J. (1975). The dying person's bill of rights. *American Journal of Nursing, 75*(1): 99.

want family and friends present, and some may want to be alone. Others may want someone from the health care team to stay with them. Often, clients prefer to talk at night, either because things are quiet and there are few distractions or because their fears and anxieties are worse at night. The following are ways you can meet a client's needs:

- ***Listening.*** If the client needs to share worries and concerns with you, let the client talk. You do not need to talk or worry about saying the wrong thing or finding comforting words. Sometimes, the client does not want to talk but just needs you around. Just being there and listening can be very helpful. If the client requests medical information, spiritual guidance, or counselling, immediately tell your supervisor. Remember, it is not your role to give clients information about their medical conditions.
- ***Touch.*** Touch conveys caring and support when words cannot. Touch, along with silence, is a powerful and compassionate way to communicate. However, always keep in mind that some clients may not like to be touched (see Chapter 10).
- ***Respect.*** The client may share thoughts about her religious or spiritual beliefs with you. Be respectful as you listen to the client.

Physical Needs

Dying may take minutes, hours, days, or weeks. Body processes slow down, the client grows weak, and changes occur in consciousness. The health care team encourages the client to do as much as possible independently during this period. As the client weakens, more help is provided with personal care. Eventually, the client may need to depend on others for all basic needs and ADLs.

- ***Pain relief and comfort.*** Some clients experience severe pain. Health care providers administer medications to relieve pain; as well, the care plan may call for other pain-relieving measures such as back massages, imagery, soft music, and relaxation techniques. Skin care, personal hygiene, and good alignment promote comfort. Follow the care plan.
- ***Comfort and positioning.*** Frequent position changes and supportive devices also promote comfort. You may need the help of another worker to turn the client slowly and gently. Semi-Fowler's position (Fowler's position with the knees slightly bent) is usually best for easing breathing

problems. Ask the client what position is most comfortable.

- ***Vision and eye care.*** At the end of life, vision blurs and gradually fails, so the client may find a darkened room frightening. The room should, therefore, be well lit (if the client wishes), but bright lights and glares should be avoided. Since the client's vision may be failing, explain what you are doing. Secretions may collect in the corners of the client's eyes. Ease the client's discomfort by providing eye care. Follow the care plan. It may call for applying protective ointment and moist pads to the client's eyes.
- ***Hearing.*** Hearing is one of the last functions to be lost. Many clients, even unconscious ones, are able to hear until the moment of death. Always assume that the client can hear, and continue to introduce yourself and give explanations and reassurance about the care you are giving, even when the client is unconscious. Speak in a normal voice, offer words of comfort, and avoid topics that could upset the client.
- ***Speech.*** The client may have difficulty speaking, so it may be hard to understand what she says. Some clients cannot speak at all. Anticipate clients' needs. Ask "yes" or "no" questions, and avoid asking questions that require long answers. Do not tire the client with questions, but do talk to the client.
- ***Mouth care.*** The client's mouth may feel dry, uncomfortable, or sore, and swallowing may be difficult and uncomfortable. Oral hygiene promotes comfort. Routine mouth care is given if the client can eat and drink. Frequent oral care is given as death nears and when the client has difficulty taking oral fluids. Provide good mouth care, as it is comforting to the client (see Chapters 12 and 30). Mucous membranes can become very dry, and sores can develop in the mouth. Oral hygiene is needed if mucus collects in the mouth and the client cannot swallow. Offer ice chips or small sips of fluids if the client has a dry mouth. Apply moisturizer to relieve dry, chapped lips. Follow the care plan.
- ***Nostril care.*** The client's nostrils may become crusted and irritated, usually by nasal secretions, oxygen cannulas, or nasogastric tubes. Clean the nose carefully. Apply lubricant, as directed by the care plan.
- ***Skin care.*** Circulation to the arms and legs slows as death approaches. Hands and feet may feel especially cold to the touch. Skin colour may change, and skin may appear pale or mottled (blotchy) and feel cold to the touch, but the client is usually not aware of feeling cold. The upper parts of the body may sweat as circulation to the peripheral parts fails. The body temperature may rise, and blankets may make the client feel too warm and cause restlessness, so only light bed coverings should be applied. Skin care, bathing, frequent position changes, and fresh garments and linens help keep the client comfortable. Measures must be taken to prevent pressure ulcers.
- ***Elimination.*** The dying client may have urinary or fecal incontinence. Follow the care plan for the use of incontinence products or bed protectors. Keep the client dry and clean. Give perineal care, as needed. Constipation and urinary retention are common, and the care plan may call for the use of enemas and catheter care, which may be delegated to you. Remember to follow Standard Practices.
- ***Nutrition.*** Nutritional needs decrease as the body can no longer deal with digesting food, so amounts of food should be reduced, and easily digestible types of food offered often.

Comforting the Family

The approaching death of a loved one is a stressful time for family members, who may be very tired, sad, and tearful. Watching a loved one die and dealing with the eventual loss of that person can be very painful. If the family wants a spiritual advisor to be present with them, let your supervisor know immediately.

Finding comforting words may be very hard. Show your feelings by being respectful, empathetic, and supportive. You may need to listen to a family member who wants to talk. However, do not feel that you have to talk. Use touch to show your concern. In a home care setting, you can show your support in many ways. You might help by taking on household tasks while the family cares for the dying client, or you might provide respite care to give the caregivers a break. Follow the care plan.

In facilities, family members are allowed to stay 24 hours a day if death is imminent. Palliative care

Providing Compassionate Care
The Dying Client

- ***Dignity.*** Treat the dying client with respect, dignity, warmth, and empathy. Be sensitive to the client's wishes. Listen when the client wants to talk. Respect the client's need for quiet and silence. Do not avoid the client if you feel uncomfortable or sad. Try to understand how your client is feeling.

  Whether a client is dying at home or in a facility, the environment should be comfortable and pleasant, quiet, well lit, and well ventilated. Try to keep equipment and supplies out of view, as some clients may find equipment such as suction machines and drainage containers upsetting to look at. Display expressions of concern (such as flowers and cards) in clear view, as some clients may find these comforting.

  Be sensitive to the client's needs. Provide comfort through care and touch if culturally appropriate for the client.

  Respect the client's religious views and practices. Do not impose your views on the client. Treat religious items and other personal possessions with care and respect.
- ***Independence.*** Encourage the client to do things without help if possible. Offer to assist before actually doing something for the client. The client has the right to autonomy.
- ***Preferences.*** The client has the right to make choices about the care, treatment, and environment, so respect these choices. Ask before providing care. Respect a client's decision to refuse treatment and not prolong life. In all health care settings, the client and family should be free to arrange the room as they wish to reflect the client's choices. Allowing such changes shows respect and helps the client feel cared for.
- ***Privacy.*** The dying client has the right to privacy. Remember, do not expose the client unnecessarily during care. The client has the right not to have the body seen by others, so follow proper screening and privacy procedures. Provide privacy during prayer and spiritual moments. The client and family have the right to have visits in private. In facilities, privacy may need to be arranged; for example, a roommate may have to leave while the family visits. Some clients may ask to see a spiritual advisor. The client also has the right to confidentiality; protect this right before and after death. Share information about diagnosis, health, and treatment only with those involved in the client's care. Maintain confidentiality about the client's final moments and cause of death as well as statements and reactions of the family.
- ***Safety.*** Clients who are dying are at high risk for falls, choking, and other accidents. Know the safety measures that must be taken for each client. The dying client has the right to be free from abuse, mistreatment, and neglect. It must be ensured that neither family members nor health care team members abuse or mistreat the client. Follow the safety measures described in Chapter 22.

rooms are available so that family members and the client can be together. The health care team helps make them as comfortable as possible.

- No matter what the setting, you need to respect the family's right to privacy while taking care not to neglect care because the family is present. Most facilities allow family members to give care. When they do, you may help them take beverage or meal breaks. Family members often hesitate to leave because they do not want their loved one to be alone. Offering to remain with the client can be a great relief for the family and make them feel better about taking a much-needed break.

LEGAL ISSUES

A person's right to die is a much-debated issue at present. Some clients do not want machines or other measures keeping them alive, so the client's informed consent is legally required by all provinces and territories for any such lack of treatment (see Chapter 9). Clients may give or withhold consent and make their own decisions about care. Some clients, however, may be unable to do so due to confusion, dementia, or other impairments, so a substitute decision maker often makes decisions for these clients.

Advance Directive

An *advance directive* (or *living will*) is a legal document in which a person states specific wishes about future health care, treatment, and personal care. Health care includes all medical treatment: diagnostic, therapeutic, preventive, and palliative. Personal care includes shelter, hygiene, nutrition, clothing, and safety.

An advance directive is used when the person can no longer make decisions or express personal wishes. Advance directives allow people to control their future health care. Without an advance directive, family members sometimes have to make difficult decisions on behalf of a loved one, and such decisions can result in conflict in the family.

Every province and territory has legislation about advance directives. Most advance directives have a dual function:

1. They allow a person to appoint a representative (proxy) to make medical care, treatment, and personal care decisions.
2. They give written instructions about medical care and treatment and personal care.

People often use advance directives to forbid certain types of treatment and care when there is no hope of recovery. For example, some people do not want life-sustaining measures that support or maintain life (e.g., tube feedings, ventilators, and cardiopulmonary resuscitation [CPR]). These measures and other machines keep a person alive when death is likely. An advance directive may instruct physicians not to start measures that prolong dying or to remove measures that prolong dying.

Advance directives are known by different names and have different powers, depending on provincial or territorial legislation—in Alberta, advance directives are called *personal directives*; in Manitoba, they are called *health care directives*; and in Ontario, these documents are called *powers of attorney for personal care* (in which a substitute decision maker is chosen). It is important to note that the word *attorney* in this use has a different meaning in Ontario or in your province or territory from in the United States. A person who is appointed an *attorney for personal care* does not have to be a lawyer.

Most people appoint a family member or friend to be their representative or proxy. In some cases, a lawyer may be named. The advance directive comes into effect *only* when a client can no longer make decisions about health care and personal care. At this point, the proxy, who has been given the legal right to make decisions for the client, steps in to make decisions on the client's behalf.

In most provinces and territories, residents name a proxy to make decisions about personal care as well as medical care and treatment. However, in some parts of the country, a proxy can be used only for decisions about medical care and treatment.

Not all clients name a proxy. When no proxy is named, family members, in consultation with the physician, decide for the client. Some provinces, however, require a court application before any decision can be made on behalf of an incapable person.

"Do Not Resuscitate" Orders

When sudden and unexpected death is possible, every effort is made to save the client's life. An emergency response system is activated, and CPR is started. In facilities, nurses, physicians, and emergency staff immediately get to the client's bedside, and in the community, ambulances and paramedics rush to the scene, bringing emergency and life-saving equipment with them. CPR and other life-support measures are continued until the client is resuscitated or until a physician declares the client dead. Clients and new staff need to clearly understand the policies and procedures of these facilities regarding resuscitation protocols.

Physicians often write "do not resuscitate" (DNR) or "no code" orders for clients who are not expected to recover. Such orders mean that the client will not be resuscitated and is allowed to die in peace and with dignity. The orders are written after consulting with the client and the family. The family or the proxy, in consultation with the physician, makes the decision about the DNR order if the client is not mentally able. Some people prepare an advance directive that contains DNR orders.

You may not agree with care and resuscitation decisions. However, you must follow the client's (or proxy's) wishes and the physician's orders, even if they are against your personal, religious, or cultural beliefs. If you are not comfortable with care and resuscitation decisions, discuss the matter with your supervisor.

> **FOCUS ON HOME CARE**
>
> **When Death Occurs**
>
> Some clients die at home, and you may be present at the time of death. Know your employer's policies and procedures. Call your supervisor, and follow the directions. Be supportive of the family. Respect the client's and the family's cultural values.

Signs of Death

Signs that death is near may occur rapidly or slowly. These include the following:

- ***Loss of movement, muscle tone, and sensation***—usually begins in the feet and legs and eventually spreads to other parts. When a client's mouth muscles relax, the jaw drops, and the mouth may stay open. The client's face often looks peaceful.
- ***Slowing of peristalsis and other digestive functions***—abdominal distension; fecal incontinence, urinary incontinence, or both; fecal impaction; nausea; and vomiting are common. The client usually refuses to eat or drink.
- ***Failure of circulation***—the pulse is fast, weak, and irregular. Blood pressure begins to fall. Skin may have a mottled appearance.
- ***Failure of the respiratory system***—presence of Cheyne–Stokes respirations. These respirations gradually increase in rate and depth, and then become shallow and slow, and then they stop for up to 30 seconds. Mucus collects in the airway and causes a wet, gurgling sound as the client breathes, known as the *death rattle*.
- ***Excessive fatigue and sleep***—as the client's metabolism slows down, the client may begin to sleep for prolonged periods throughout the day and night. The client may even become difficult to awaken or may lose consciousness. However, some clients do remain conscious until the moment of death.
- ***Changes in eating***—the client may not be interested in eating food once loved or may have cravings for odd food.
- ***Social withdrawal***—as the client's circulation decreases and organs begin to fail, the client's body is beginning to shut down. The client may gradually seem to lose interest in his surroundings; he may stop talking, may seem disinterested in activities (or people) and turn away visitors.
- ***Coolness in the tips of the fingers and toes***—the client's blood circulation slows and shifts away from the extremities in order to help the client's major organs. As a results, a noticeable cooling, development of a bluish tint to the client's skin, and cyanosis of the nail beds occur.

The physiological signs of death include absence of pulse, respirations, or blood pressure and fixed, dilated pupils. A physician determines that death has occurred and pronounces the person dead. In some parts of Canada, nurses are allowed to pronounce death when death is expected (see the *Focus on Home Care: When Death Occurs* box).

CARE OF THE BODY AFTER DEATH

Care of the body after *(post)* death *(mortem)* is called **postmortem care**, which begins after the client is pronounced dead and when no *autopsy* (an examination of the body to determine the cause of death) is required. You may be asked to assist with postmortem care, and during this process, you may have contact with blood or body fluids. Follow Standard Practices.

Postmortem care is done to maintain the body's appearance by helping prevent discoloration and skin damage. Remember, the right to privacy and the right to be treated with dignity and respect should be preserved even after a client's death. Remember to respect cultural diversity for this care.

Within 2 to 3 hours after death, rigor mortis develops. **Rigor mortis** is the stiffness or rigidity *(rigor)* of skeletal muscles that occurs after death *(mortis)*.

Postmortem care involves positioning the body in normal alignment before rigor mortis sets in. The family may want to see the body before it is taken to the morgue or funeral home. The body should be placed in a natural position for this viewing.

In some cases, the body is prepared initially only for viewing. Postmortem care is completed later at the funeral home. If the client dies at home, the funeral home usually provides postmortem care.

Postmortem care may involve repositioning the body to clean soiled areas and to put the body in good alignment. Movement of the body can cause sounds to come from the body as air is expelled. Do not be frightened by these sounds; they are normal and expected.

As a support worker, you will not have full responsibility for postmortem care, but you may assist in the procedure.

FUNERAL PLANNING

It can be difficult for clients and the family to discuss funeral arrangements. Some clients or families may have already made arrangements for the funeral. If prior arrangements have not been made, funeral directors will guide the family through the process and provide counselling sessions after the funeral to provide the necessary paperwork and information to settle the estate.

Assisting With Postmortem Care

123

Your client's and the family's cultural values and your employer's policies will determine this procedure.

Advocate on behalf of the client and family by promoting:

Dignity • Independence • Preferences • Privacy • Safety *(see BOX 1–4, on p. 17)*

PRE-PROCEDURE

1 Perform hand hygiene.
2 Collect the following supplies, depending on your facility's policies:
   - ☐ **Postmortem kit (body bag, identity [ID] tags, gauze squares)**
   - ☐ **Bed protectors**
   - ☐ **Wash basin**
   - ☐ **Bath towels and washcloths**
   - ☐ **Tape**
   - ☐ **Dressings**
   - ☐ **Gloves**
   - ☐ **Cotton balls**
   - ☐ **Gown or clean garments**
3 Provide for privacy.
4 Raise the bed to a comfortable working height.
   This helps prevent back strain.
   Make sure the bed is flat.*
   This is the "natural" sleeping position that is least distressing to the family.

PROCEDURE

5 Put on gloves.
6 Bathe soiled areas with plain water. Dry thoroughly.
   Clean the skin to reduce any odour from incontinence.
7 Place the body in the supine position. Straighten the arms and legs. Place a pillow under the head and shoulders (FIGURE 46–1).
   This keeps the body in alignment before rigor mortis sets in.

Continued

Assisting With Postmortem Care—cont'd

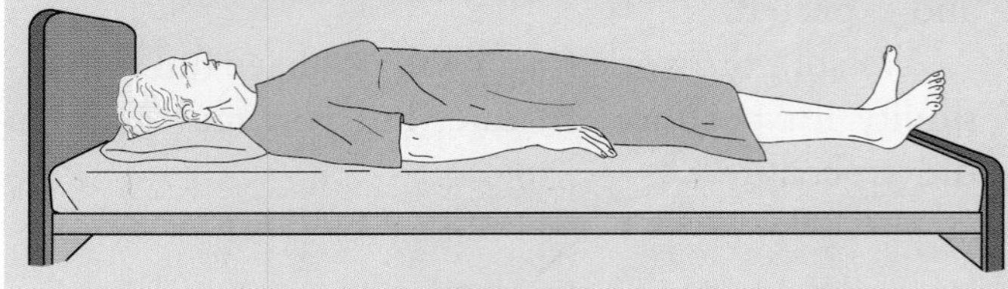

FIGURE 46–1

8 Close the eyes by gently pulling the eyelids over the eyes. According to employer policies, apply moist cotton balls gently over the eyelids if the eyes will not stay closed.
It may be upsetting for the family to view their relative with the eyes still open after death.

9 Insert the dentures if it is employer policy. If not, put them in a labelled denture container.

10 Close the mouth. It may be necessary (and subject to employer policy) to place a rolled towel under the chin to keep the mouth closed.
This keeps the mouth in alignment and shut before rigor mortis sets in.

11 Follow employer policies about valuables, including jewellery. In many facilities, the support worker and the nurse together make a list of valuables, and both sign a statement that the valuables have been placed in a sealed envelope.

12 Tape the wedding ring, if any, in place if doing so is your employer's policy.
Family members will decide how they want valuable items dealt with.

13 Follow employer policy and instructions in regard to drainage containers, tubes, and catheters.

14 Place a bed protector under the buttocks.
This prevents soiling of the bedding below if the client's sphincters release urine or stool.

15 Remove soiled dressings and apply clean ones.

16 Brush and comb the hair if necessary if it is culturally accepted.

17 Cover the body to the chin with a sheet if the family will view the body.

18 Put the client's belongings in a bag labelled with the client's name.*

19 Remove supplies, equipment, and linen. Tidy up the room. Provide soft lighting.*
Soft lighting is less likely to show the deceased client's skin colour mottling, which may be upsetting to the family.

20 Remove gloves. Perform hand hygiene.

21 When the family is viewing the body, leave the room, and return after the family leaves.

22 Perform hand hygiene. Put on gloves.

23 If required in your facility, fill out the ID tags. Tie one to an ankle or to the right big toe.*

24 Place the body in the body bag, or cover it with a sheet.*

25 Attach the second ID tag to the body bag if it is your employer's policy.*

26 Leave the denture cup with the body.

27 Provide for privacy.

28 Remove gloves.

29 Strip the bed after the body has been removed. Wear gloves.*

30 Remove gloves. Perform hand hygiene.

Report and Record your actions and observations, according to employer policy.
This is done for legal reasons and to keep the rest of the health care team informed.

- ☐ Report to your supervisor the time the body was taken by the funeral director.
- ☐ Document how personal property of your client was stored or whether it was sent with the funeral director. OR given to the family
Family members will be looking for these valuables, and they need to know how to recover the property.
- ☐ It is important also to document the location of your client's dentures.
It can be very upsetting to the family if their loved one's appearance is changed for funeral viewings by the absence of dentures.

*Steps marked with an asterisk may not apply in community settings.

KEY POINTS

- As a support worker, you will be required to help meet the physical, social, emotional, intellectual, and spiritual needs of clients who are dying and to support their families through the process.
- Personality, culture, religion, age, and experience influence people's attitudes toward death.
- As a support worker, you need to be aware of the cultural beliefs of your client and respect the death and dying rituals of the client and the family.
- The stages or phases of grief the client, the family, and you experience will vary in each case.
- Palliative and hospice care may be available in your community. The goal of care is to provide comfort and support to a dying client in the client's home or in a facility.
- As a support worker, you need to know your employer's policies and your legal obligations regarding advance directives and "do not resuscitate" orders.
- Care of the body after death will depend on the cultural beliefs of your client. Follow your employer's policy.
- Funeral directors are trained to assist families through the necessary processes and paperwork. They can also refer families to other support services.

CRITICAL THINKING IN PRACTICE

Mr. Wills was admitted to a hospital, where he was diagnosed with terminal cancer. Within a week, he has appeared to lose consciousness, and he now is receiving end-of-life comfort care. Mrs. Wills, his wife of 67 years, is always at his side and does not seem to think he is dying. She talks about the next time they visit the grandchildren, and how they like to garden. Is it normal for family members to behave in this manner? As a bedside caregiver for Mr. Wills, what should you say when Mrs. Wills talks about their future plans?

REVIEW QUESTIONS

Answers to these questions are at the bottom of page 1074.

Circle the BEST answer.

1. Which is true?
   A. Death from a terminal illness is sudden and unexpected.
   B. Doctors know when death will occur.
   C. An illness is terminal when there is no reasonable hope of recovery.
   D. All severe injuries end in death.
2. Adults of all ages often fear:
   A. Dying alone
   B. Reincarnation
   C. The five stages of grief
   D. Advance directives
3. People in the stage of denial:
   A. Are angry
   B. Make "deals" with God
   C. Are sad or quiet
   D. Refuse to believe they are dying
4. Palliative care is:
   A. Treatment that prolongs life
   B. Physical therapy for people with severe back pain
   C. Massage therapy and relaxation techniques to relieve pain
   D. Services for people with progressive and life-threatening illnesses that relieve or reduce uncomfortable symptoms
5. When caring for a dying person, you should:
   A. Listen and use touch when appropriate
   B. Do most of the talking
   C. Keep the room darkened
   D. Speak in a loud voice

6. As death approaches, the last sense to be lost is:
A. Sight
B. Taste
C. Smell
D. Hearing

7. Care of the dying person includes the following:
A. Forcing fluids
B. Low sodium diet
C. Active range-of-motion exercises
D. Position changes

8. The dying person is placed in:
A. The supine position
B. Fowler's position
C. A position comfortable for the client
D. The dorsal recumbent position

9. A woman is no longer able to make decisions about her own health care. Through an advance directive, she has appointed her sister as her proxy. Decisions about her health care are made by:
A. Her son
B. Her physician
C. Her sister
D. Her lawyer

10. A "do not resuscitate" order has been written for a client. This means:
A. Cardiopulmonary resuscitation (CPR) will not be done
B. The person has a living will
C. Life-prolonging measures will be carried out
D. The person will be kept alive as long as possible

11. Which of the following are signs of approaching death?
A. Decreased body temperature and rapid pulse
B. Increased movement and muscle tone
C. Increased pain and blood pressure
D. Cheyne–Stokes respirations

12. Postmortem care is done:
A. After rigor mortis sets in
B. After the person is pronounced dead
C. When the funeral director arrives for the body
D. After the family has viewed the body

Answers: 1.C, 2.A, 3.D, 4.D, 5.A, 6.D, 7.D, 8.C, 9.C, 10.A, 11.D, 12.B

Chapter opener image: Photographee.eu/Shutterstock.com

CHAPTER 47

Starting Your Career

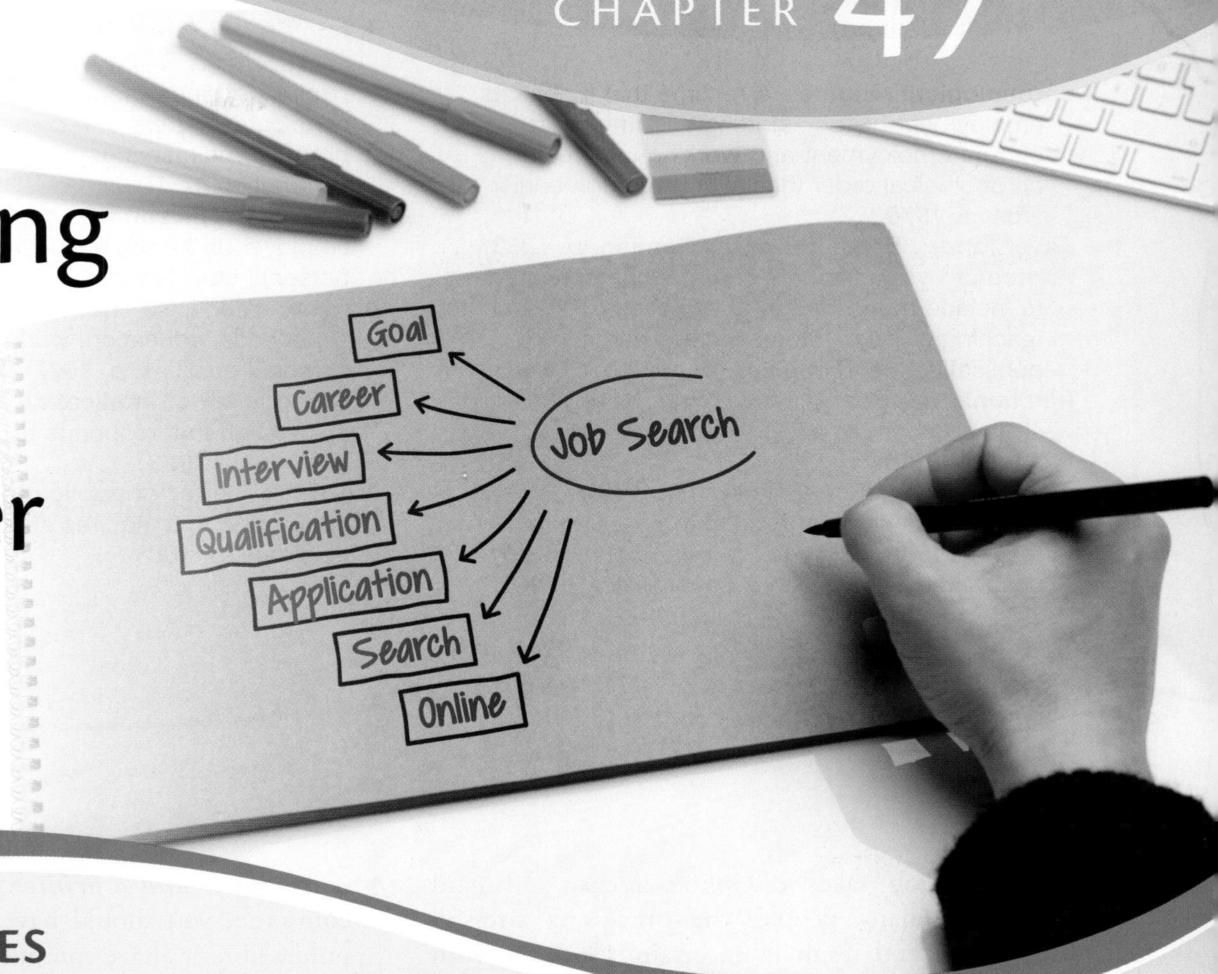

OBJECTIVES

After reading this chapter, the learner should be able to do the following:

- List the tools needed to prepare for your job search.
- Differentiate between a chronological resumé and a functional resumé.
- List three sources of advertised positions.
- Identify methods for finding out about unadvertised positions.
- List the details that are important in a letter of application.
- Summarize why one should take time completing application forms.
- List what interviewers are trying to determine during an interview.
- Summarize why the interview is a key element in the job search.
- Summarize why it is important to practise and plan before an interview.
- Name the ways to make a good impression at an interview.
- Summarize why it is important to write a thank-you note following an interview.
- Apply the techniques described in this chapter to the job application experience.

KEY TERMS

chronological resumé A resumé that highlights employment history, starting with the most current employment and working in reverse chronological order (backward) through earlier jobs. *p. 1078*

cover letter See **letter of application**. *p. 1083*

curriculum vitae (CV) A resumé that is lengthened to include a description of achievements, such as teaching experience, research, awards, publications, and degrees. *p. 1077*

functional resumé A resumé that highlights skills or functions and briefly lists positions held. *p. 1080*

letter of application A letter that is included with a resumé that summarizes the job applied for and reasons for applying for it; it can be solicited or unsolicited. Also called a **cover letter**. *p. 1083*

portfolio A binder containing the applicant's certificates, letters of recommendation, awards, proof of volunteering, or other pertinent information. *p. 1082*

reference A person who can speak to a potential employer about the applicant's skills, abilities, and personal qualities. *p. 1083*

resumé A concise one- to two-page summary of experience, education, work-related skills, and personal qualities. *p. 1077*

solicited letter of application A letter of application that responds to an advertised position. *p. 1083*

unsolicited letter of application A letter of application that inquires about potential openings. *p. 1083*

Finding a job takes discipline, focus, and hard work. For many people, the process is stressful because the end result is uncertain. However, with good preparation and a sound plan, the job search can be exciting and rewarding, as it gives you the opportunity to learn about yourself and to meet new people.

Today, support workers have a number of options to choose from when deciding the type of environment they would like to work in and who they wish to work for. While most beginning support workers seek employment at an agency or facility, others may choose to be self-employed to have greater flexibility in working around their personal responsibilities. Some support workers may find personal satisfaction being self-employed *and* employed at an agency, splitting time between both.

GETTING ORGANIZED

Your job search will be more successful if you get organized before you start. Choose a place in your home where you will work, and then make sure that you have the following tools in your workspace:

- ***A computer and a printer.*** If you do not own a computer, you should have access to one. Most public libraries have computers and printers available to the public. Most employers today post job openings on the Internet and request that resumés be sent by email, through a special section of the company's website, or through a third-party employment website.
- ***A telephone or cellphone with voice mail.*** Prospective employers should be able to reach you by telephone. If you have a cellphone, remember to set up your voice mail. The message on your voice mail should sound professional.
- ***Office supplies.*** Make sure that you have a supply of good-quality paper, a stapler (in case an employer requests a hard copy of your resumé), and pens.
- ***Resources.*** Many excellent books available at the library as well as Internet websites can provide needed information to help you with your job search. Look for books and websites that can show you how to prepare a resumé and cover letter. Your college library or local public library should have extensive resources on the job search (also, see **BOX 47–1**).

BOX 47–1 Useful Resources for Your Job Search

Resource	Description
What Color Is Your Parachute?	Well-known guide on job hunting
www.jobhuntersbible.com	Website for *What Color Is Your Parachute?*
http://www.youth.gc.ca/eng/topics/jobs/lmi.shtml	A Canadian government website with links to detailed labour market information on jobs and careers, as well as provincial, territorial, and local labour market information
www.careerbookstore.ca	Website with a comprehensive catalogue of books on all aspects of the job search
www.resumeedge.com	Free sample resumés and cover letters
http://www.youth.gc.ca/eng/topics/jobs/resume.shtml	A Government of Canada site with tips on resumé writing
www.job-interview.net	Sample interview questions
www.workopolis.com	Comprehensive website on all aspects of the job search that also posts health care positions and allows you to post your resumé for employers to view
Type keywords into your search engine (e.g., Google), such as "Support worker jobs in [your city or town]"	Using specific keywords will result in more focused search results
Many larger agencies have their own employer websites	These sites may post any job openings and provide links for applying to them

SETTING PRIORITIES AND GOALS

Before creating your resumé, think about your priorities and goals. Determine the following:

- What type of support work do you want to pursue?
- Would you prefer to work in a facility or a community setting?
- Do you want to be self-employed?
- Do you want full-time or part-time work?

As discussed in Chapter 3, there are different kinds of support work settings. If you were unsure during your program about where you would like to work, your clinical placements may have helped you make the decision. If you are still undecided, you may want to apply for work in a variety of settings.

PREPARING YOUR RESUMÉ AND PROFESSIONAL PORTFOLIO

Regardless of where you are applying to work, it is a good idea to prepare both resumés, which would be individualized for each position applied for, and a professional portfolio, which you could bring to show interviewers or potential clients.

Resumé

A **resumé** is a concise, one- to two-page summary of your experience, education, work-related skills, and personal qualities and is the first step toward a job interview. A resumé introduces you to possible employers, so it must look and sound professional. Employers use resumés to decide which job applicants to interview, and even small errors such as spelling mistakes may negatively influence the employer's decision. Some employers may ask for a **curriculum vitae**, or *CV*, which is a resumé that is lengthened to include a description of achievements, such as teaching experience, research, awards, publications, and degrees.

It is best to prepare your resumé well before you begin your job search. This gives you time to do it properly without rushing. As you prepare your resumé, keep the needs of prospective employers in mind. Consider what most employers look for in support workers (see Chapter 1). Remember, however, that each job is unique, so make adjustments to your resumé to fit the needs of each employer and setting. ***Remember to update your resumé frequently to reflect any new courses that you have taken or work experience that you have had since the last time you updated it.*** If you also store your resumé on a flash drive (memory stick), you have the advantage of portability when you need to print off copies and are away from home.

Keep a copy of the resumé on your hard drive as well as on a flash drive (memory stick) or external drive. Many employers require that you apply over the Internet, and you may be required to "copy and paste" sections of a prepared resumé onto their application sites. Since more employers expect resumés to be submitted electronically instead of in a printed form, you should always keep an updated resumé on your computer.

Elements of a Resumé

All resumés include information on the following:

- ***Experience.*** Employers want to know what you have done that qualifies you for the position. Experience does not have to be paid work. It can come from volunteer work, field placements, special projects, and recreational activities. Stress your skills and accomplishments rather than your duties and responsibilities.
- ***Education.*** Employers want to know if you have the educational qualifications required for the position. Your resumé should include the exact name of your certificate, the name of your educational institution, and the year you graduated. Also include additional training and any awards or honours you received.

The following elements are optional:

- ***Objective.*** An objective on a resumé states your immediate career goal and briefly lists relevant skills, abilities, and personal qualities. It appears at the top of the first page of your resumé, right after your name and address.
- ***Profile.*** A career profile summarizes your qualifications, highlighting particular skills and experience in one brief paragraph. It usually appears on the first page of your resumé, right after your name and address. Most people include either an objective or a profile but rarely both.
- ***Interests.*** Most career consultants advise against including a separate section on interests because it takes up valuable space. Instead, they suggest incorporating accomplishments in sports or hobbies into other sections of the resumé and doing so only if it is relevant to the job. For example, you may want to mention your skills in curling to show you are an experienced team player.

Getting Started on Your Resumé

Think of the resumé as an advertisement for those of your experiences, skills, and qualities that an employer might be seeking. Start by making a list of the skills and qualities an employer would want in a support worker; then make a list of your own skills and qualities and the experiences that helped you to develop those qualities.

If you are not able to identify your skills and qualities, start by thinking about your experiences. Ask yourself what you learned from each experience and how your experiences have influenced you.

Organizing Your Resumé

There are two basic resumé styles: (1) the chronological resumé and (2) the functional resumé.

Chronological Resumé

A **chronological resumé** highlights employment history, starting with your most current employment and working in reverse chronological order (backward) through earlier jobs (**FIGURE 47–1**). Because of its emphasis on work history, this style of resumé is best for those with the following:

- ***A steady history of employment in their chosen field***
- At least 2 years' employment with one employer
- Few gaps between jobs

SEAN TOOTOOSIS

16 Uptown Street, Apt. 4, Edmonton, AB T9Q 2PI, (403) 765-4321, stootoosis@elsewhere.net

---

PROFILE

- Experienced support worker who has cared for clients with diverse needs
- Skilled at motivating clients to regain their independence
- Dedicated to creating a caring, compassionate environment
- Discreet, hard-working, and loyal

EXPERIENCE

Support Worker, Hummingbird Agency, Edmonton, AB, August 2011–Present
- Provide personal care and support to diverse client population
- Skilled at caring for clients with quadriplegia and severe physical disabilities
- Selected to assist in training new staff and writing procedures for manual
- Praised for my calm, composed, empathetic manner with clients
- Demonstrated ability to work independently under minimal supervision

Support Worker, Primrose Group Home, Edmonton, AB, June 2008–July 2011
- Assisted developmentally disabled adolescents with activities of daily living
- Developed good listening and other interpersonal skills
- Demonstrated flexibility in meeting multiple needs and finishing tasks on time
- Commended by supervisor for initiative and problem-solving skills
- Served as leader of four-person team to redesign the home's living space

Lamantia Brickworks and Patios, Edmonton, AB, March 2003–May 2008
- Demonstrated leadership skills while supervising team of four bricklayers.

EDUCATION AND TRAINING

- Certificate in Personal Support Work, Western Canadian College, Edmonton, AB, 2008
- St. John's Ambulance First Aid and CPR Level C Certification, Edmonton, AB, yearly 2008–2015

OTHER

- Spoken languages: English and Cree

FIGURE 47–1 Chronological resumé.

Functional Resumé

A **functional resumé** highlights skills or functions and briefly lists positions held (**FIGURE 47–2**). Because it emphasizes skills and abilities, rather than specific jobs, a functional resumé is best for those with the following:

- Little work experience in their chosen field
- ***Long periods during which they were not in the workforce***
- Frequent job changes

A functional resumé should include your employment history with dates. A resumé that excludes this information might suggest that you have something to hide.

Creating Your Resumé

You will probably need to prepare several drafts of your resumé before you are satisfied. As you prepare your drafts, ask yourself the following questions:

- ***Is the information relevant?*** You have limited space to make an impression. Mention only those experiences that say something about how well you would perform on the job.
- ***Have I been completely honest?*** Emphasize your strengths, but do not misrepresent yourself. ***It is unethical to lie.*** Do not change your qualifications, job titles, education, or dates of employment. Do not exaggerate your limited accomplishments if you lack experience. Remember that some employers prefer to hire inexperienced workers because they may be more motivated, more flexible, and easier to train than those with experience.
- ***Have I expressed myself clearly?*** Be concise, and avoid using long words. Revise your draft to make sure it is clear. Avoid giving information in paragraphs; use bullet points instead. Sentences should be short and direct. Start them with action words, and avoid the use of the word "I." Remember, your resumé should be only one or two pages in length.
- ***Is my resumé consistent?*** Set up the page, headings, and sentences in a consistent format. Use bullets, bold type, italic type, or underlining in the same style throughout the document. Do not spell the same word two different ways (e.g., *honours* and *honors*). Use the same grammatical form for each point.
- ***Have I accounted for all my time?*** Do not leave blocks of time that are unaccounted for.
- ***Is my resumé correct?*** Read over the final document several times slowly and carefully. Do not trust your word processor's spell-check feature to catch all spelling errors (e.g., *their*, *they're*, and *there* are not always caught if misused). Some people have problems proofreading their own work because they read what they think they have written rather than what is actually on the page.

Begin by reading every word out loud. Make sure that what you have written makes sense as you hear it. If you find that you cannot judge your own work impartially and objectively, ask someone to read it aloud for you. Many employers use your resumé as a predictor for the type of support worker you will be. If there are errors, they may assume that you do not pay attention to your work, and you will not be called for an interview.

Follow this step by reading your document backward, starting at the end of the resumé and reading each sentence backward. You are more likely to catch typos and spelling mistakes when you read this way. Do not depend on computer spell-checks to find errors. When you are satisfied with your resumé, ask at least two reliable people to proofread it.

Formatting and Printing

To make a good impression, your resumé must look neat and professional:

- Choose a simple, professional-looking font (typeface) such as Times New Roman or Arial. Do not choose fancy or script-type fonts.
- Do not use more than one font.
- Keep the use of graphic devices such as **bold** or *italicized* type to a minimum.
- Do not crowd too much material on a page.

KAYLEE SAUVÉ

105 Pine Avenue, Hamilton, ON L4W 5Y3, (905) 725-9589, ksauve@link.com

---

OBJECTIVE

To provide support to clients in their homes and to deliver compassionate personal care.

SKILLS AND ABILITIES

- Listening skills: composed, respectful, and empathetic
- Speaking skills: won public speaking award in secondary school
- Language skills: speak English and French fluently
- Organizational skills: ability to complete work while meeting multiple demands
- Leadership skills: strong ability to motivate others; captain of winning basketball team
- Meal preparation skills: experienced; sound knowledge of food safety and nutrition
- Mature and responsible: child care worker for two families for six years
- Flexible: able to work in a variety of settings and adapt to different situations
- Self-reliant: confident working under minimal supervision
- Physically strong: unloaded trucks and lifted boxes at local food bank

EDUCATION

- Certificate in Personal Support Work, Ontario Institute for Applied Health Sciences, Hamilton, ON, 2011
- St. John's Ambulance First Aid and CPR Level C, Certification, Hamilton, ON, 2016
- Food Safety course, River College, Toronto, ON, 2015

EXPERIENCE

Sunset Nursing Home, Field Placement, Hamilton, ON, February 2015–April 2015
- Prepared and delivered meals for 35 residents

Ricky's Restaurant, Waitress, Hamilton, ON, Summers, May 2011–August 2015
- Greeted customers, served meals, prepared salads

Children's Caregiver, Hamilton, ON, Part-time, 2008–2014
- Cared for children ages 4 months through 9 years

Volunteer, Daily Food Bank, Hamilton, ON, January 2011–March 2014
- Unloaded trucks, stocked shelves, helped customers

FIGURE 47–2 Functional resumé.

Most computer programs have preset resumé designs that you can use to format your resumé. Many books and websites also present a variety of designs you can use. Some websites offer services such as formatting your resumé and posting it on the Internet. Because resumé formats change constantly, it may be worth securing the services of a professional resumé writer. Check the Internet for names in your area. Your school or college may also provide this service through the career centre.

If submitting your resumé in person or by mail, print it on good-quality white or ivory bond $8\frac{1}{2}'' \times 11''$ paper. ***Never*** use designed or patterned paper. If your resumé runs to two pages, staple the pages together. ***Never*** fold the corners down together. Paper clips can be used to hold your pages together, but many employers prefer staples.

The Professional Portfolio

Many interviewers or clients appreciate or even expect to see a portfolio when interviewing an applicant for the first time. A **portfolio** is a binder containing the applicant's certificates, letters of recommendation, awards, proof of volunteering, or other pertinent information. Its purpose is to easily reveal information about the applicant to the interviewer.

Each item within the portfolio should be placed in a plastic page protector and inserted into the binder in an organized manner. It is easiest when the items are sorted according to categories and labelled page dividers separate each section. Items should be in order of when they were obtained, with the most recent first, the second most recent after that, and so on. This way, the interviewer does not have to sift through the contents of the portfolio.

Your completed portfolio should contain the following:

- Copy of your resumé and cover letter, individualized for each specific employer
- List of references (with complete contact information) that you are prepared to leave with the interviewer
- Certificates that you have achieved
- Letters of recommendation and awards
- Workshops that you attended, along with the dates that you attended them
- Proof of volunteering
- Immunization record
- Police check (or vulnerable sector screen)
- Letters of reference from previous employers or clients
- Any other pertinent information

The interviewer or potential client may wish to make photocopies of some of the pages contained in your portfolio.

FINDING AND FOLLOWING LEADS

The main sources for advertised positions are online job sites, local newspapers, and college career services.

- ***Employment advertisements.*** Check national, local, and community newspapers daily for advertisements.
- ***The Internet.*** Many health care facilities post job openings on their websites. To search the Internet, use a search engine and type in search words such as "Health Care," "Home Health Care," "Home Care," "Home Health Services," "Community Health Care," "Retirement Homes," "Nursing Homes," "Nursing Services," "Not-For-Profit Jobs/Careers," and so on. General job search websites such as Monster, Indeed, and Workopolis (see **BOX 47–1**, on p. 1077) also post health care positions.
- ***College career services.*** Some colleges offer career counselling and placement services to students and members of the community. Employers post job openings on the bulletin boards at the college or on the college website.

Some positions are not advertised. To find out about unadvertised positions, try the following:

- ***Contact people you know.*** Friends, acquaintances, and professional contacts may help you to find work and advance your career. Make a list of people you know in the health care field, including course instructors and employers you worked for in your program placement. Ask these people if any positions are available at their workplace. They may be aware of jobs posted on bulletin boards or jobs that may become available.

- ***Check with your district home care program.*** The websites of your health district may list agencies that are used to deliver home care in the community as well as list contact information of local long-term care and retirement home agencies.
- ***Look in the Yellow Pages (www.yellowpages.ca).*** Look under the headings "Home Health Care," "Home Care," "Home Health Services," "Community Health Care," "Retirement Homes," "Nurses and Nurses Registries," "Nursing Homes," and "Nursing Services."
- ***Check your local library.*** Libraries often have lists of health care facilities and agencies.
- ***Attend job fairs.*** Job fairs are often held at community colleges or elsewhere in the community and may be advertised in the local newspapers, on local cable channels, or at your college.
- ***Check with your Canada Employment Centre.*** These centres often have information about local area employers and about specific job openings.

Selecting References

A **reference** is a person who can speak to a potential employer about your skills, abilities, and personal qualities. Determine who you want as references early in the job search. Do not use family members or friends as references. Previous employers are usually the best people to use as references. Other possibilities are people in positions of authority, such as teachers and camp directors. Here are some basic tips about references:

- ***Ask for the reference.*** Do not use someone as a reference without asking the person. Explain the type of work you are looking for. Do not assume the person will speak positively about you. Ask what the person would say your strengths and weaknesses are. Be reasonably certain the person will speak positively about you before listing that person as a reference. If you are applying for more than one position, be sure to ask if the person would give you a reference for each position.
- ***Make sure contact information is correct.*** Make sure you have accurate phone numbers or email addresses for your references to give prospective employers.
- ***Keep your references informed.*** Let your references know when you are going for a job interview so that they can be prepared for a phone call from your prospective employer. A reference who is prepared is more likely to give you a good reference.
- ***Follow up.*** Keep your references informed about your job search. If you got the job, thank them for their help. If you did not get the job, let them know.

PREPARING A LETTER OF APPLICATION

A **letter of application**, also called a **cover letter**, is included with a résumé. There are two kinds of letters of application:

1. A **solicited letter of application** responds to an advertised position (**FIGURE 47–3**).
2. An **unsolicited letter of application** inquires about potential job openings (**FIGURE 47–4**).

A letter of application should not simply summarize the information in your resumé. It should focus on what you can *offer* by summarizing how your skills and experiences are relevant to the job you are seeking. A good letter of application is persuasive, professional, and personalized. Try to find out the specific person who is responsible for hiring for the position, and direct your correspondence to that person. Most administrators do not like to receive applications or resumés from job seekers when there is a designated individual and department to deal with recruitment and hiring.

Determining the Employer's Needs

If a letter of application is solicited, study the advertisement carefully to determine what exactly the employer is looking for. Describe your experiences and skills that match what the employer wants. Consider if you have skills and qualities that are not listed in the advertisement but that could contribute to the position advertised. Even if you are new to support work, your course should have provided you with information about those qualities.

ADVERTISEMENT

Ferndale Lodge has two positions available for support workers. Reporting to the Director of Nursing Services, the successful candidates will provide personal care to residents. They must have excellent communication, problem-solving, and organizational skills. They must be able to cope with the demands of personal care service and remain calm and courteous with clients and their families at all times. They must be available to work days, evenings, nights, and weekends. Experience preferred but not required.

Reply in confidence to: Derek Sykes, Human Resources Director, Ferndale Lodge, Box 101, Littletown, BC V6X 2Z1.

453 Lower Town Road
Littletown, BC V6N 4N3

September 5, 2016

Mr. Derek Sykes
Human Resources Director
Ferndale Lodge
Box 101
Littletown, BC V6X 2Z1

Dear Mr. Sykes:

I am writing to apply for one of the support worker positions that were advertised in the September 4 issue of *The Star Daily*.

You specified that Ferndale Lodge is seeking qualified support workers with excellent communications, problem-solving, and organizational skills. I attended the support worker program at Central Vancouver College, where I developed strong organizational skills and finished in the top third of the class. Before enrolling in the support worker program, I worked as a full-time cashier while raising three children. In my position as a cashier for *Fresh Food,* I interacted with the public and treated all customers with respect, tact, and courtesy. I was promoted to the customer service desk, where I learned how to solve customers' problems efficiently and diplomatically.

I am a mature, hard-working person who enjoys working with people. I am also assertive, persuasive, and adaptable to new situations. Because I am highly motivated to begin a new career in support work, I would be a productive and enthusiastic employee. I am available to work all the times that you listed in your advertisement, including weekends.

Enclosed you will find a resumé that details my skills and experience. At your convenience, I would like to meet to discuss how I can contribute to Ferndale Lodge.

Sincerely,

Belinda Lau
(604) 345-6789
bflau@internet.ca

Enclosure

FIGURE 47–3 A sample advertisement and a solicited letter of application.

105 Pine Avenue
Hamilton, ON L4W 5Y3

Include return address

October 15, 2016

Include today's date

Ms. Katherine Ferrero
Director of Personnel
Mapleview Health Care Agency
1572 Maple Road
Hamilton, ON L9P 8B2

Identify the name and title of contact, and address of prospective employer

Dear Ms. Ferrero:

Include a greeting

I read in *The Sun Daily* on October 14 that Mapleview Health Care Agency is expanding its home care services. I am writing to ask you to consider me if you need support workers.

Identify the position

The article in *The Sun Daily* indicated that Mapleview Health Care Agency offers a wide range of services to people in their homes, including personal care, meal preparation, and housekeeping. While completing a support worker course at Ontario Institute for Applied Health Sciences, I acquired skills in all those areas. For my six-week field placement, I provided personal care to clients with dementia. In this position, I learned how to balance multiple demands by providing safe, dependable care in a timely manner to vulnerable people. Because many of them could not speak for themselves, I also had the opportunity to act as an advocate on their behalf at times.

Indicate your knowledge of the facility or agency

Indicate your qualifications

Link your skills to the job requirements; explain what you have learned from experience

I am a mature, responsible person who works well independently and as part of a team. Because I enjoy helping people, I know you would find me a competent and enthusiastic support worker.

Highlight personal qualities and other skills relevant to the job

Please find enclosed my resumé, which outlines my skills and experience in detail. I hope to have the opportunity to meet you to discuss how I can contribute to Mapleview Health Care Agency. Next week I will call you to discuss the possibility of an interview.

Indicate that your resumé is enclosed

Ask for an interview

Sincerely,

Kaylee Sauvē

Include a signature block

Kaylee Sauvé
(905) 725-9589
ksauve@link.com

Enclosure

FIGURE 47–4 An unsolicited letter of application.

If you write an unsolicited letter, find out as much as you can about the employer first. As mentioned earlier in this chapter, many agencies and facilities have websites that contain information about their health care goals and practices. For example, a facility's website might emphasize respect, compassion, and innovation as important goals. In your letter, you could indicate experiences in which you have demonstrated these qualities.

Organizing a Letter of Application (Cover Letter)

Use a standard letter format to organize your letter.

Front Matter

- ***Return address.*** Put your mailing address at the top left-hand corner of the page.
- ***Today's date.*** Include today's date on the left-hand side of the letter beneath your return address.
- ***Name, title, and address of prospective employer.*** Include the contact person's name, title, and address aligned with the left-hand margin. Ensure that this information is correct. You may have to call the facility or agency to confirm it. If you are unable to find out the person's name, you may have to exclude this information.
- ***Greeting.*** Greet the person you are writing to in a professional manner. If you do not know the name, write "Dear Sir or Madam."

Body

- ***Paragraph one.*** Identify the job, indicate how you learned about it, and explain your purpose for writing. In unsolicited letters, use this opening paragraph to ask about potential opportunities.
- ***Paragraph two.*** Explain how your qualifications, experience, and skills relate to the position you are seeking.
- ***Paragraph three.*** Describe personal qualities or additional skills that make you a suitable candidate.

Closing

- ***Paragraph four.*** Use the concluding paragraph to ask for an interview. If the letter is unsolicited, say that you will contact the reader at a future date. Refer the reader to the enclosed resumé.
- ***Signature block.*** End the letter in a professional manner by writing "Sincerely" or "Yours truly." Leave some space, and type your name at the end of the letter. Sign in ink above the typed name. Add your phone number and email address after your name. Type "Enclosure" at the bottom of the page to indicate that your resumé is enclosed.

Writing Your Letter of Application

You will probably have to write several drafts to create a convincing letter. First, concentrate on putting down your main points on an outline. As you revise the content of the letter, ask yourself the following questions:

- ***Have I emphasized relevant skills and qualities?*** Mention experiences that demonstrate the skills, qualities, and attitudes necessary to support work. For example, if you have worked as a sales clerk, emphasize your positive interactions with clients.
- ***Have I emphasized accomplishments and skills?*** Rather than simply listing the tasks performed, explain what your experience has taught you. You might say "Working as a sales clerk taught me how to interact with the public in a warm, courteous, and respectful manner."
- ***Have I used an appropriate tone?*** Your letter should be written in a respectful, capable, and professional tone. Be persuasive without being boastful. Minimize the use of the word "I" to sound more modest. If you lack experience, avoid an apologetic tone.
- ***Is my letter concise?*** Your letter should not be more than one page long. If it is longer, edit out some of the details.
- ***Does my letter sound and look professional?*** Proofread your letter carefully and have at least two reliable people also read it. Sometimes, it helps to read your letter out loud, trying to listen for grammar and sentence structure errors. Create it on a computer. Use a standard business letter format, and print out the letter on high-quality paper (if submitting a paper copy). Double-check that your contact information is correct. You should be completely sure that a prospective employer can reach you.

BOX 47–2 Sample of an Email to an Employer When Submitting a Resumé

Subject: Job Application and Resumé

Dear Sir or Madam:

I am applying for the position of Personal Support Worker that you advertised in the *London Free Press* on July 4, 2016, and have attached a cover letter with my resumé. As you can see, I am available for hire immediately.

Sincerely,

Mariane Blankette

Delivering Your Letter of Application and Resumé

Some employers request that the applicant deliver the resumé by mail or in person. Hand-deliver your letter of application and resumé whenever possible to make sure it arrives on time. Another method of delivery is courier. Make sure that it is directed to the correct department or room, especially if you are applying to a large agency such as a hospital. Follow up with a telephone call to find out if the letter reached the appropriate person. If you respond to an advertisement, send out your letter and resumé as soon as possible. Sometimes the earliest applicants get more attention simply because their applications arrived first.

Many employers request that letters and resumés be submitted by email (**BOX 47–2**). Because software programs vary, your resumé could lose its formatting, or the prospective employer could have difficulty opening your attachment. This issue can be avoided by sending your resumé in PDF format. Some employers refuse to accept electronic attachments, which can be infected with a virus, so you may be asked to copy and paste your letter into the body of your email. If you send your letter and resumé by email, send a hard copy as well. (However, if the employer asks the applicant not to submit a hard copy, you need to abide by this request.)

Tips on Conveying Professionalism Electronically

Since many employers post job opportunities on the Internet, and many applicants apply electronically, here are a few tips to ensure that you get the best attention:

- Your email background should be electronically neutral. Do not have a patterned or designed background.
- Ensure that your email address is a professional one. ***Never create a childish or offensive email address.***
- Never use abbreviations that are used on social media sites, known as "cyber-speak" (short forms for words or phrases, such as "LOL" or "CU later"). ***In any communication for professional purposes, whether on paper or online, you should use full sentences, appropriate punctuation, and correct and appropriate spelling and grammar.***
- Ensure that your resumé is in the correct file format (e.g., Microsoft Word or Adobe Acrobat). If you are unsure, contact the agency to find out or send the resumé in both formats.
- Do not have attachments or postscripts that open automatically (that indicate that you listen to a particular radio station, for example).

COMPLETING A JOB APPLICATION FORM

For some positions, you are expected to complete a preset job application form when employers need to find out specific information about their applicants. Institutions may use forms as a way to test applicants' reading, comprehension, and writing skills. It is a good idea to attach your resumé to the job application form, even when one is not required.

Most application forms ask for information about the following:

- Your legal eligibility to work in Canada
- Your education
- Your work-related skills
- Your employment history
- Names and phone numbers of employers
- Reasons for leaving previous jobs
- The names and phone numbers of three references

Remember that the completed application form says something about you. It should be professional looking and have no spelling or grammar mistakes or unfilled columns. Do a thorough job of filling out the form. If possible, take two copies of the form home with you. Use one as a rough copy and the other as your final copy. Ask someone reliable to read and check the final copy. If you make an error on the final copy, use correction fluid or tape to make the correction.

Application forms often require detailed information, such as the reason for leaving a job. You must answer every question truthfully. If you have been fired, or if you have an inconsistent work history, consider attaching a note of explanation.

Some employers require you to submit an online application form. Be just as careful with an online application as you would be with a hard copy. Ask someone reliable to read it over before you send it.

Using Social Networking Sites

The use of Internet social networking sites to apply for jobs or to post work availability has been increasing sharply. However, there are some important points to remember when posting information electronically:

- Manage your identity. You wish employers to be able to contact you, but some identifying information such as a personal address may be misused by some people.
- Control your privacy settings. You can restrict the information that is distributed.
- Pay attention to the professionalism of your social media page or personal website since employers will read it. Pictures of you and your friends drinking at a party, for example, will convince some employers not to contact you.
- Avoid errors in spelling and grammar and the use of slang terms, which may be interpreted as unprofessional by some potential employers![1]

THE INTERVIEW

You will not be hired as a support worker unless someone first interviews you and decides you are the right person for the job. During the interview, a prospective employer or client is trying to determine the following:

- Do you have the educational qualifications for the job?
- Do you have the skills necessary to do the job, or can you learn those skills?
- Will clients and co-workers respond well to you?
- Will you be a reliable, responsible, and motivated employee?

The interview is a key factor in any job search. From the interview, prospective employers decide if you have essential personal qualities such as compassion, respect, and enthusiasm. They can also judge if you are a good listener, if you speak clearly, and if you are at ease with others.

Interviewers may ask questions to find out the following:

- Can you handle the stress of working with seriously ill people?
- Can you deal with interpersonal conflict?
- Would you respond calmly and responsibly to an emergency?
- Are you capable of being firm and assertive with clients?
- Are you flexible enough to adapt to a variety of situations?
- Can you handle multiple demands and conflicts?
- Can you work under minimal supervision?
- Do you have initiative?
- Are you an effective team player?
- Can you handle routine problems on your own?
- Are you discreet?
- Do you respect individual differences?
- Are you a quick learner?
- Are you effective at managing your time?

Many interviewers ask situational questions, which are questions that are designed to find out what you would do in certain situations. You may be asked a question about an imaginary situation, or you may be asked to describe what you did in a particular situation you have encountered in the past.

Always be well prepared for an interview. When you are nervous, it can be difficult to think and speak clearly. If you have thought about possible questions and answers, you are more likely to be at ease. To prepare for an interview, think about the following:

- ***The position.*** Make sure you understand the nature of the position. Learn about the employer's services, clients, and philosophy. Read information about the employer that is available to the general public—for example, on its website and in brochures. Talk to friends, instructors, and acquaintances who know the agency or facility. Review the skills and qualities that are essential to support work.
- ***Your qualities, skills, and experience.*** Develop a clear understanding of yourself: your values, skills, qualities, interests, goals, strengths, and weaknesses. Write these down, along with specific experiences that illustrate each.
- ***Your portfolio.*** Review your personal portfolio and decide what you should highlight at each individual interview. What will impress each employer most? Bring your portfolio with you to your interview in case the interviewer wants photocopies of any of the pages.
- ***Your reference list.*** Most employers will require you to provide at least three references. Print off a list of references and a hard copy of your resumé, and attach them together. Your reference list should always be in the same font as the rest of your resumé.
- ***The interviewer.*** Put yourself in the interviewer's place. Review your letter of application and resumé. Why do you think you were selected for an interview? What concerns might the interviewer have about you? For example, if you are young and inexperienced, the interviewer may be concerned about your maturity level. If you have never remained in a job for more than a year, the interviewer may be concerned about your commitment. Be prepared to address these issues.

The Group Interview

More Than One Applicant

Occasionally, an agency may want to fill several positions, especially if it is short-staffed. In order to save time and trouble for the people who are doing the interviewing, the agency may group two or more applicants together in a room and ask each applicant specific questions. After one applicant has answered the question, the other applicants are invited to respond. Following this group interview, the applicants may then be interviewed individually.

The benefit for you of this interview type is that you might feel less nervous to know that "you are not alone." However, it can be intimidating to think that your answers are being compared with the answers of the other applicants in the room. Remember that, in this respect, it is no different from an individual interview because responses of various applicants will always be compared.

It is important to watch your body language and your responses during this type of interview. Try to watch each of the applicants as that person answers questions. You want to appear friendly and polite. Do not ever cut someone off while that person is speaking. This type of interviewing is a good technique for interviewers to identify a "team player" who has effective communication skills (see Chapter 5).

More Than One Interviewer

For some interviews, there is only one applicant but two or more interviewers, who will take turns asking the applicant questions. The interviewers usually read from a written list of prepared questions. Occasionally, the interviewers may ask the applicant an unscripted question for clarification of something the applicant has said.

This type of interview is usually very thorough, and the applicant may leave the room feeling overwhelmed. You should be aware that the interviewers are trying to determine if you can handle questions well and if you can answer them in an honest and sincere manner. They may ask you questions that test your ability to solve problems. These questions typically begin with "What would you do if . . ." The interviewers want to know how well you can apply what you have learned in your support worker education to the scenarios that they present to you. These responses can be easily practised with a friend or a classmate.

It is important to make eye contact with the interviewer who is speaking as a question is being asked (see Chapter 5). Remember, too, to use words and body language that show that you are friendly and approachable.

BOX 47–3 Common Interview Questions

- Tell me a little about yourself.
- What are your strengths?
- What are your weaknesses?
- Tell me about your last job.
- What did you like best or least about your last job?
- Why did you leave your last job?
- Why do you want to be a support worker?
- What do you think are the three most important qualities in a support worker?
- What do you think you can bring to support work?
- What do you think is the biggest challenge in support work?
- What do you like best or least about support work?
- Describe a situation in which you have met several demands.
- Describe a typical day in your last job.
- How did you manage your time in your last job?
- What did you learn from your last job?
- Give me an example of how you have worked as part of a team.
- Tell me about a time you showed initiative on the job.
- Tell me about a problem you had in your last job. How did you handle it?
- Tell me about a conflict you had with a client or co-worker. How did you handle it?
- What would your former supervisor tell me about your strengths and weaknesses?
- I am going to give you a made-up situation. Tell me how you would handle it.

Some employers may present a scenario that involves witnessing some kind of abuse by a co-worker. The employer may ask you how you would deal with this type of situation, both at the time of witnessing it and later.

Practising for Your Job Interview

Practice will give you confidence. When practising, focus on making eye contact with the interviewer, as well as on your listening skills, relaxation techniques, and responses to questions you think might be asked. Sit down only when invited to sit. Sit up comfortably straight without slouching. Try to remember your interviewer's name.

Developing Listening Skills

The ability to listen is an important skill for interviews. If you fail to listen, you will not make a good impression. Since listening is essential in support work, an employer is unlikely to hire a poor listener as a support worker. Be a good listener during the interview by avoiding the following:

- Failing to concentrate on what the interviewer is saying
- Failing to ask for clarification if the question is unclear
- Talking too much
- Responding to questions too quickly without thinking first about the answer

Practising Relaxation Techniques

You will probably listen more attentively if you feel relaxed in the interview. Deep-breathing exercises and other relaxation techniques can help you relax (see Chapter 7).

Practising Your Responses

Most interviewers ask similar questions. See **BOX 47–3** for a list of commonly asked questions. Practise your responses to these questions in front of a mirror or with a friend.

Planning

Plan ahead so that things go smoothly on the interview day.

- Decide what you are going to wear and make sure that the clothing is clean and pressed. Get a haircut if you need one.
- If the route to the venue of the interview is unfamiliar, do a "practice run" so that you will not get lost on the interview day. Leave yourself at least

30 minutes to spare in case of traffic delays on the way to the interview.
- In addition to your portfolio, bring notepaper and a pen that works.
- Do some research about the facility or agency by checking available websites. Doing so shows initiative and interest in working there.
- Plan a few informed questions to ask during your interview (see p. 1092).

Making a Good Impression

In an interview, first impressions are crucial. Poor impressions can be difficult to change, no matter how well you do later in the interview. From the moment you meet a prospective employer, you need to present a calm and professional image. This advice applies even when you stop by to pick up an application form. Pay attention to your grooming, your clothing, and your conduct.

Grooming

- Make sure your hair is clean, neat, and away from your face.
- Brush and floss your teeth. If you are a heavy coffee drinker or a smoker, bring breath mints with you (but do not have them in your mouth during the interview).
- Be careful not to wear too much makeup.
- Wear minimal jewellery. Avoid large bracelets, rings, and earrings.
- Remove body ornaments such as nose rings and eyebrow studs; cover any tattoos.
- Do not wear any perfume, cologne, or heavily scented lotions.
- Make sure your nails are trimmed. If you wear nail polish, use a neutral colour.
- Keep any facial hair trimmed and well groomed.
- If possible, wash and thoroughly dry your hands before you shake hands with the interviewer, especially if your palms perspire when you are nervous.

Clothing

- Men should wear clothing that is professional in appearance and businesslike, such as a shirt and dress pants. Women should wear a dress, blouse or sweater with either a skirt or tailored pants. Do not wear jeans, T-shirts, or shorts. Your outfit should fit properly, be in good repair, and be wrinkle-free.
- Wear clothing that fully covers undergarments such as panties, bras, or boxer shorts. Ensure these cannot be seen through the clothing.
- Avoid clothing that is tight fitting or revealing.
- Try clothing on at home and practise sitting and walking in the clothing in front of a mirror, if possible. Doing so is a good way to see if your clothing looks professional and feels comfortable when sitting. If you have access to one, inspect yourself in front of a full-length mirror.
- If wearing pantyhose or tights, make sure that there are no holes or runs. Carry an extra pair in case you need to change them.
- Shoes should be in good repair and well polished. Avoid casual shoes, such as running shoes or sandals, and shoes with very high heels.

Conduct

- Arrive in the lobby 5 to 10 minutes before the interview.
- Do not bring anyone with you. If someone has driven you to the place, ask the person to wait outside.
- Do not carry your cellphone in your hand. Place it in your purse, pocket, or on a holster. Make sure it is shut off for the interview.
- Do not chew gum, smoke, or eat as you wait for the interviewer. Ensure that your clothing does not smell of tobacco.
- Do not ask to use the phone, talk on a cellphone, or text-message anyone while waiting.
- Do not talk with the receptionist unless that person starts the conversation.
- If you feel nervous, take deep breaths to calm yourself.

Interview Tips

Being adequately prepared should help you feel relaxed during the interview. If you feel calm, you are more able to focus on details that may help you get the job. Some of these are discussed below.

- ***Use a firm handshake.*** When you meet the interviewer, shake hands and smile. Use a firm handshake. A limp, clammy handshake makes a poor impression. Make sure your hands are dry. If your palms are perspiring, wipe them on a tissue as you wait in the lobby.

- ***Do not use the interviewer's first name.*** The exception is if you are asked by the interviewer to do so. However, do address the interviewer by name.
- ***Project a confident image.*** Whether sitting or standing, practise good posture, breathe deeply to relax, and avoid nervous habits such as picking at your fingernails or fiddling with your hair. Be aware of gestures and body language that might be perceived negatively, such as crossed arms. Look the interviewer in the eye, and keep your hands folded in your lap.
- ***Make appropriate eye contact when speaking*** (see Chapter 5).
- ***Listen carefully.*** If you listen carefully, you should be able to answer questions concisely and directly. Do not be afraid to ask the interviewer to repeat a question.
- ***Take your time.*** Some people talk quickly when they are nervous. Slow down, take a deep breath, and think about the question before you answer. An answer given too quickly may sound rehearsed.
- ***Answer questions honestly.*** You must be honest in your answers. If you do not understand a question or are unsure of an answer, say so. Do not try to hide aspects of your past that you think may disqualify you from the job. Instead, explain how you have learned from past mistakes. For example, if you were fired from your last position, explain the reason and give examples of how you have corrected the behaviour.
- ***Speak positively about your previous job.*** Do not demean, ridicule, appear upset with, or speak critically about your previous employer, regardless of the circumstances, as doing so may suggest a negative attitude or an aversion to authority.
- ***Use experiences to support opinions.*** When you are asked for your opinion, support your answer with examples from your experience. For instance, after saying, "I think it's important for support workers to know their scope of practice," describe a situation that illustrates this point. If you are inexperienced, use an example from your course of study.
- ***Ask the right questions.*** Most interviewers conclude by asking if you have any questions. The questions you prepared in advance may have been answered during the interview. Rather than trying to think up new questions, it is acceptable to say something like, "No, I don't have any questions. You have addressed all the questions that I had during our discussion." If you do have a question, make sure that it is appropriate. Do not ask questions about the salary, benefits, hours, and vacation times. It is suitable, though, to ask about these when you are offered the position.
- ***Concluding the interview.*** At the end of the interview, thank the interviewer for her time. Show confidence and enthusiasm by saying something like, "I am really interested in working for your facility, and I am sure I could be a productive member of your staff." Whatever you say, it is important to be genuine.

Follow-Up

Send a brief thank-you note after an interview. Write the note as soon as possible, no later than the day following the interview. The thank-you note will indicate that you are enthusiastic and courteous, and it might set you apart from other candidates.

The note can be handwritten or prepared on a computer. If you write the note by hand, use a plain white note card. Write at least one draft before you write the final copy. Ask someone else to read the note before you send it. Mail the note rather than sending it by email. This approach shows the employer you are prepared to make an effort.

Express your thanks for the interview and reinforce your interest in the position. Sign your name on the card (see **FIGURE 47–5** for a sample note).

THE EMPLOYMENT OFFER

You may be offered the position at the end of the interview or within a few days following the interview. Or you may wait weeks before hearing anything. Instead of sitting by the phone and waiting, continue to explore other opportunities. Even if you are not offered a job, the interview experience will have been worthwhile if you learn something from it. Review the interview process by asking yourself the questions in **BOX 47–4**.

October 03, 2016

Dear Ms. Frye,

Thank you for the interview on Wednesday morning. I appreciated the opportunity to meet you and to discuss your needs for the support worker position at Greenacres.

As I mentioned at the end of the interview, I am very interested in the position. I am sure that my recent experience in home care would enable me to make an immediate contribution to your care team.

Once again, thank you for your time and interest. I look forward to hearing from you.

All the best,

Sumi Ramarashan
(604) 432-7376

FIGURE 47–5 A sample thank-you note.

BOX 47–4 Learning From the Interview Experience

- Was I prepared enough? Did I practise my listening skills, relaxation techniques, and responses to potential questions?
- Did I arrive for the interview in plenty of time?
- Did I pay enough attention to my grooming, my clothing, and my conduct?
- Did I project a calm, professional, positive image?
- Did I present a portfolio that represented me in a professional manner?
- Did I listen attentively?
- Did I speak clearly and calmly?
- Did I answer all questions honestly?
- Did I use my experiences to support my opinions?
- Did I relate my skills and experience to the requirements of the job?
- Did I show enthusiasm for the job?
- Did I express interest in the job at the end of the interview?
- Did I send a thank-you note after the interview?

If you are not offered the job, contact the employer to find out why. Ask if you can talk to the person who interviewed you, either in person or on the phone. Most employers are willing to talk to people who are genuinely interested in improving their skills. Approach this conversation as a learning opportunity; do not sound angry, bitter, or accusatory.

Accepting an Offer

A conditional offer is often made in the form of a letter of hire, which your employer will show you at the end of the interview, during a subsequent meeting, or by mail. Signing the conditional offer (and emailing, faxing, or mailing it back) indicates that you have accepted the position. Before you accept an offer of employment, find out as much as you can about the terms of your employment. Find out if the offer is conditional and if the job begins with a trial period.

Terms of Employment

At the time of the job offer, make sure that you clarify your wages, your hours of work, requirements, and expectations. If, for example, a car is required for the position, find out the employer's policy on car mileage and repairs. Many employers publish procedure manuals that should address your questions.

If the job is a contract position, find out the length of the contract, the terms of the contract, and what is and is not included in the contract prior to accepting the offer.

If you are hired directly by a client or a client's family, you must specify the terms of your employment. The client may be required to contribute to Employment Insurance and Canada Pension Plan. The client may also be required to submit your taxes directly to the government. Before you accept employment directly with a client, read Revenue Canada's booklet *Employee or Self-Employed* (Catalogue Number RC4110), which is available online or at your local Canada Revenue Agency office.

Conditional Offer

In the health care field, an offer of employment is often conditional, meaning that you must meet certain conditions or requirements before you are hired. These conditions usually include a health report signed by your family physician that confirms that you are in good health and a police record check that shows that you do not have a criminal record. You are responsible for providing all required documents. Note that there may be a fee to obtain these documents. Some employers may also require that you have certain equipment necessary to perform the job. For example, in community settings, a cellphone may be essential.

Probation

Most employers hire new staff for a probationary (trial) period that lasts 3 to 6 months. During this time, both you and the employer can decide if you are the right fit for the job. Within this period, the employer can end your employment at any time or you can leave without the usual 2 weeks' notice, although giving notice will possibly get you a reference.

Benefits

Find out what you can about an employer's benefits package. Many employers have booklets that explain their benefit plan. Benefits do not usually begin until the end of the probationary period. If you work part-time, you may not be eligible for benefits. Be especially careful to find out about benefits if you are working directly for a client in the client's home.

How to Refuse or Leave a Job Without Leaving a Negative Impression

Occasionally, you might decide that you cannot work at an agency or facility (or you decide to leave the agency or facility). Quitting a job is a difficult thing to do, as it is important that the employer has a good impression of you. Many employers spend a lot of time and effort, both of which cost money, to train their employees and are understandably not happy when they leave, especially after a short period. Remember, you might want to return to that employer in the future! Ask to meet with your supervisor in person, and show up for this meeting dressed professionally. Remember, this meeting is the *last* chance you have to make a good impression!

It is important to give an employer adequate notice when you intend to leave. Two weeks' notice is considered to be the minimal amount of notice to give; most employers would prefer more time than that, if at all possible. Employers are more likely to provide a good reference when sufficient notice is given and the employee continues to be reliable through the duration of employment.

Refusing a job or leaving a job because you are going back to school, have been hired at another agency on a full-time basis (assuming your current position is part-time), are moving to another city, or are pregnant and have decided not to work for some time is easy to convey to an employer. It is important—whatever the reason—that you be honest, tactful, and pleasant to the employer.

If, however, you are leaving because you do not like the atmosphere of the workplace or you are unhappy with the agency or facility in any way, you need to be able to state your feelings tactfully as well! Prepare what you are going to say ahead of time. If necessary, write down your thoughts on small index cards so that you can refer to them. Always begin by stating what you *liked* about the workplace. Be as fair as possible, remembering that you wanted to work there once!

When stating what you do not like about the agency or facility, be as specific as possible. Instead of stating, "Well, I don't like the staff," you can be more specific (and therefore more helpful) if you can say, "I do not agree with the afternoon staff who put residents in bed by 6:30 p.m. I think the residents should have a say as to when they are put in bed, and their families should be involved in the decision process." Remember, you must always be honest. Do not lie or exaggerate a story to win favour with the supervisor!

Your statements inform the supervisor of the issues that exist in the agency or facility. If you are a valued employee, the supervisor might ask if you would reconsider your decision to leave. This is a choice only you can make. Regardless of whether your decision is to stay or leave, you should always be professional and pleasant when conveying it.

CHAPTER REVIEW

KEY POINTS

- Finding a job takes discipline, focus, and hard work. However, it can be done when you have good preparation and a sound plan.
- Resumé writing begins with (1) collecting necessary supplies and equipment and (2) identifying and setting your priorities and goals.
- In creating your resumé, you should ask yourself the following: (1) Is the information relevant? (2) Have I been completely honest? (3) Have I expressed myself clearly? (4) Is my resumé consistent? (5) Have I accounted for all of my time? (6) Is my resumé correct?
- The resumé should be accompanied by a letter of application (cover letter).
- In an interview, you need to (1) convey your qualities, skills, and experience in a positive manner and (2) make a good impression.
- Follow up an interview with a brief thank-you note.
- Learn from any and all interviews. If you are not being offered positions, you need to honestly ask yourself why.

CRITICAL THINKING IN PRACTICE

You are newly graduated and have been applying for various support worker jobs. A potential employer called you for an interview and then asked you to supply the names and contact information of three references. You forgot to inform one of your references that you used her name as a reference contact. The agency called her and, during the conversation, she informed the agency that you did not seek permission to use her name as a reference. As a result, you did not get this job. Is that fair to you? Is it important to ask your references each time you apply for a job? Why or why not?

REVIEW QUESTIONS

Answers to these questions are at the bottom of page 1097.

Circle T if the answer is true, and circle F if the answer is false.

1. **T F** It is best to prepare your resumé before you begin your job search.
2. **T F** A resumé is revised for each position applied for.
3. **T F** Every resumé should include an objective and a career profile.
4. **T F** A chronological resumé is best for those with a steady work history in their chosen field.
5. **T F** A functional resumé should not include employment history.
6. **T F** Resumés should make extensive use of graphics.
7. **T F** It is best to ask your references what they plan to say about you.
8. **T F** A letter of application should summarize the information from your resumé.
9. **T F** A solicited letter of application inquires about potential job openings.
10. **T F** A letter of application should list duties held in previous positions.
11. **T F** Most employers overlook small mistakes on letters, resumés, and applications.
12. **T F** It is acceptable to wear jeans to an interview as long as they are clean.
13. **T F** It is unacceptable to bring a friend to an interview, even if that person stays in the lobby.
14. **T F** The ability to listen is one of the most important skills for an interview.
15. **T F** It is a good idea to bring a prepared list of questions to an interview.

16. **T F** It is usually not necessary to practise answering questions before an interview.
17. **T F** Assume you can address the interviewer by that person's first name.
18. **T F** It is best not to ask about salary, benefits, and holidays during an interview.
19. **T F** Never admit in an interview that you have been fired from a previous position.
20. **T F** If an offer is conditional, it is usually firm.

Answers: 1.T, 2.T, 3.F, 4.T, 5.F, 6.F, 7.T, 8.F, 9.F, 10.F, 11.F, 12.F, 13.T, 14.T, 15.T, 16.F, 17.F, 18.T, 19.F, 20.F

Chapter opener image: garagestock/Shutterstock.com

Appendix

Support Workers From Across Canada

Province or Territory	Job Title(s)
British Columbia	Health Care Assistant
Alberta	Health Care Aide
Saskatchewan	Continuing Care Assistant
Manitoba	Health Care Aide
Ontario	Personal Support Worker Developmental Service Worker
Quebec	Home Health Aide Home Support Worker
New Brunswick	Personal Support Worker
Nova Scotia	Continuing Care Assistant
Prince Edward Island	Resident Care Worker
Newfoundland & Labrador	Home Support Worker/Personal Care Attendant
Yukon	Health Care Assistant
Northwest Territories	Personal Support Worker
Nunavut	Home Support Worker Community Support Worker

Glossary

abbreviation A shortened form of a word or phrase. *p. 196*

abduction Movement of a body part away from the midline of the body. *p. 539*

abrasion A partial-thickness wound caused by the scraping away or rubbing of skin. *p. 463*

absorption The process by which substances pass through the intestinal wall into the blood. *p. 570*

abuse Physical or mental harm caused by someone in a position of trust. *p. 253*

accessibility A principle of the *Canada Health Act* that states that people must have reasonable access to insured health care services. *p. 24*

accountability The willingness to accept responsibility and to explain one's actions, inactions or omissions, intentions, and decisions. *p. 91*

acquired brain injury (ABI) Damage to brain tissue caused by disease, medical condition, accident, or violence. Also known as **traumatic brain injury**. *p. 776*

acquired immune deficiency syndrome (AIDS) Immune system disease caused by human immunodeficiency virus (HIV). *p. 880*

act A specific law that has passed through the required legislative steps. *p. 131*

active immunity Natural acquisition of an illness, resulting in the body developing the antibodies to protect a person from getting it again. *p. 300*

active listening A nonjudgemental communication technique that focuses not only on understanding the content of what is being said but also on the underlying emotions and feelings conveyed by the sender. Active listeners concentrate fully on what is being said and pay attention to the client's nonverbal cues. *p. 71*

activities of daily living (ADLs) Self-care activities people perform daily to remain independent and to function in society. *p. 4*

acute care Health care that is provided for a relatively short time (usually days to weeks) and is intended to diagnose and treat an immediate health issue. *p. 35*

acute illness An illness or disability that appears suddenly and lasts for a short period, usually less than 3 months. *p. 35*

acute pain Sudden pain due to injury, disease, trauma, or surgery; it generally lasts less than 6 months. *p. 178*

acute stress A type of stress that is short in duration. *p. 101*

adduction Movement of a body part toward the midline of the body. *p. 539*

administrator The person appointed by the provincial courts to administer the estate of a client who has died without leaving a will. *p. 140*

admission Official entry of a client into a hospital or other health care facility. *p. 1036*

adolescence Ages approximately 12 to 18—the time between puberty and adulthood; a time of rapid growth and physical, sexual, psychological, and social maturity. *p. 312*

adult day centre See **community day program**. *p. 40*

adult day program See **community day program**. *p. 40*

advance care directive See **advance directive**. *p. 138*

advance directive A legal document in which a person states wishes about future health care, treatment, and personal care. Also known as an **advance care directive** or a **living will**. *p. 138*

adverse effect A dangerous or unwanted side effect of a medication. *p. 995*

advocate To speak or act on behalf of another person or group of people. *p. 3*

affect A person's feelings, emotions, and moods and the way the person demonstrates them. *p. 781*

afternoon care Routine care that occurs between lunch and the evening meal in a facility. *p. 613*

ageism Feelings of impatience, intolerance or prejudice based on negative attitudes and stereotypes toward a person or group of people because of their age. *p. 151*

age-related macular degeneration (AMD; ARMD) The breakdown (degeneration) of the macula (the light-sensitive part of the retina). AMD is a disease associated with aging that gradually destroys sharp, central vision. *p. 919*

allergy A sensitivity to a substance that causes the body to react with signs or symptoms. *p. 578*

alopecia Hair loss. *p. 651*

alternating pressure mattress A special type of mattress that has alternating areas of pressure of air, gel, or water baffles to reduce the risk for pressure sores. *p. 750*

alternative remedies Herbal or other "natural" products that do not require a physician's prescription. *p. 991*

Alzheimer's disease and related dementias (ADRD) A progressive, degenerative disease that gradually destroys nerve cells (neurons) in most areas of the brain and causes thinking and memory to become seriously impaired; the most common form of dementia. *p. 810*

ambulation The act of walking. *p. 545*

AM care Routine care given in a facility before lunch. AM care sometimes occurs before breakfast. Also known as **early morning care** and **morning care**. *p. 613*

amenorrhea Absence of at least three consecutive menstrual periods as normally expected to occur. *p. 788*

amputation The removal of all or part of an extremity. *p. 854*

amyotrophic lateral sclerosis (ALS) A degenerative disease characterized by loss of the motor neurons, with progressive weakness and atrophy of the muscles of the hands, forearms, and legs, spreading to involve most of the body and face. Also known as **Lou Gehrig's disease**. *p. 862*

anaesthesia The loss of feeling or sensation, produced by a medication that blocks pain impulses to the brain. *p. 1049*

anaphylaxis A severe allergic reaction that occurs rapidly and causes a life-threatening response involving the whole body. *p. 996*

anatomical position The body standing erect, with the feet shoulder-width apart, face forward, arms at the sides, and palms of the hands facing forward. *p. 273*

aneurysm A localized dilation of the wall of an artery or heart chamber. *p. 860*

angina pectoris Chest (*pectoris*) pain (*angina*) caused by ischemia, a lack of blood supply to the heart muscle, which is usually caused by an obstruction or spasm of the coronary arteries because of **coronary artery disease.** *p. 864*

anterior Located at or toward the front of the body or body part. Also called **ventral**. *p. 195*

anti-embolic stockings Close-fitting, circular, knitted, elastic stocking that are designed to prevent swelling in lower extremities or blood clots by increasing venous return to the heart. They are also called *compression stockings*, or *thromboembolic devices (TED)*. *p. 680*

antigen A substance, usually a protein, that the body recognizes as foreign and that can evoke an immune response. *p. 995*

anxiety A vague, uneasy feeling, often including a sense of impending danger or harm. *p. 104*

anxiety disorders A group of mental health disorders whose main symptom is **anxiety**, with fears and worries so disproportionate to the situation as to affect normal functioning. *p. 783*

apathy An absence of emotional feeling, which appears as indifference. *p. 807*

aphasia Partial or complete loss (*a*) of speech and language skills (*phasia*) caused by brain injury. *p. 903*

apnea The lack or absence (*a*) of breathing (*pnea*). *p. 932*

apraxia Impairment of the skilled motor system, resulting in the loss of being able to perform learned, purposeful movements, including activities of daily living (bathing, brushing teeth, and so on). *p. 809*

apraxia of speech Inability (*a*) to correctly move (*praxia*) the muscles used to speak. Apraxia is usually caused by a brain injury. *p. 904*

aquathermia pad A waterproof plastic or rubber pad that can be applied to areas of muscle sprain, edema, or mild inflammation in the place of a heating pad or cold pack. *p. 1022*

arrhythmia Abnormal (*a*) heart rhythm (*rhythmia*). *p. 867*

arterial ulcer An open wound on the lower legs and feet caused by poor arterial blood flow. *p. 475*

arteries Blood vessels that carry blood away from the heart. *p. 289*

arteriole The smallest branch of an artery. *p. 289*

arthritis Joint (*arthr*) inflammation (*itis*). *p. 855*

arthroplasty Surgical replacement (*plasty*) of a joint (*arthro*). *p. 855*

asepsis The practice of reducing or eliminating potential pathogens (bacteria, viruses, fungi, and parasites). There are two levels of asepsis: (1) **medical asepsis** and (2) **surgical asepsis**. *p. 432*

aspiration Inhalation of fluid or an object into the lungs. *p. 588*

assault Intentionally attempting to or threatening to touch a person's body without consent, causing the person to fear bodily harm. *p. 142*

assertiveness A style of communication in which thoughts and feelings are expressed positively and directly without offending others. *p. 79*

assessment The evaluation of information collected about the client through observation, reflection, and communication; a step in the care-planning process. *p. 202*

assigning Appointing someone to take on the responsibility to complete a task while providing client care or support. *p. 92*

assimilate Adopt the traditions of the larger society. *p. 150*

assisted-living facility A residential facility where residents live in their own apartments and are provided support services (also called **supportive housing facility**). A **retirement home** is one type of assisted-living facility. *p. 36*

asthma A respiratory disorder characterized by recurring episodes of paroxysmal dyspnea (intermittent spasms of shortness of breath); wheezing on expiration, inspiration, or both, caused by constriction (narrowing) of bronchi; coughing; and thick bronchial secretions of mucous. *p. 867*

athlete's foot A highly contagious fungal skin infection that causes the affected foot to peel, burn, itch, and turn red. *p. 848*

atrophy A decrease in size or wasting away of tissue. *p. 376*

attention-deficit/hyperactivity disorder (ADHD) A disorder that causes inappropriate levels of inattention as well as hyperactive and impulsive behaviour. *p. 896*

attitude A person's beliefs, values, or opinions toward engaging in healthy behaviours. *p. 53*

authority The legal right to do something. *p. 92*

autism spectrum disorder (ASD) A neuro-developmental disorder that impairs a person's ability to communicate and interact with others. It can include restricted repetitive behaviours, interests, and activities. *p. 897*

autonomy Having the freedom and choice to make decisions that affect one's life. Also known as **self-determination**. *p. 123*

bacteria Single-celled microbes that naturally occur on living, dead, or inanimate objects. *p. 423*

ball-and-socket joints Joints that allow movement in all directions. They are made up of the rounded end of one bone and the hollow end of another bone. The rounded end of one fits into the hollow end of the other. *p. 279*

base of support The area on which an object rests. *p. 494*

battery The touching of a person's body without the person's consent. *p. 142*

bed rails The metal or plastic sides of a hospital bed that are used to prevent a client from falling out of bed. *p. 397*

bedsore See **pressure ulcer**. *p. 465*

belief Conviction that something is true. *p. 118*

beneficence Doing or promoting good. *p. 123*

benefits Types of assistance that are provided through available insurance premiums. An example of a benefit is a dental procedure without any additional cost to the consumer. *p. 27*

benign Noncancerous. *p. 876*

benign prostatic hypertrophy (BPH) An enlarged prostate gland. *p. 873*

bias A point of view that prevents a person from being impartial. *p. 150*

biofilm A thin film that sticks to the teeth; it contains saliva, microbes, and other substances. *p. 613*

biohazardous waste Items that may be harmful to others because they are contaminated with blood, body fluids, secretions, or excretions; *bio* means life and *hazardous* means dangerous or harmful. *p. 453*

bipolar and related disorders A group of related brain disorders that cause unusual shifts in a person's mood, energy, and ability to function. *p. 779*

blanket warmers Warming cabinets designed to heat bed linens. *p. 1014*

blended family A couple with two or more children, one or more of whom is the natural child of both members of the couple and one or more of whom is the stepchild of one member of the couple. *p. 154*

blister pack A transparent moulded piece of plastic with multiple compartments, sealed to a sheet of cardboard with a foil backing, used to package individual-dose medications. Also known as a *bubble pack*. *p. 986*

blood pressure The amount of force exerted by the blood against the walls of an artery. *p. 250*

body alignment The way in which body parts (head, trunk, arms, and legs) are positioned in relation to one another, whether lying, sitting, or standing. Also known as **posture**. *p. 493*

body language An important part of nonverbal communication that can reveal a person's physical, mental, or emotional state through powerful messages such as gestures, postures, and facial expressions. *p. 72*

body mechanics The movement of the body. Proper body mechanics ensure the body moves in an efficient and careful way. *p. 493*

body temperature The amount of heat in the body; a balance between the amount of heat produced and the amount lost by the body. *p. 230*

boil See **furuncle**. *p. 848*

bony prominence An area on the body where the underlying bone seems to "stick out." *p. 465*

brace An apparatus worn to support or align weak body parts or to prevent or correct problems with the musculo-skeletal system; also called an **orthotic**. *p. 553*

Braden Scale A scale used to predict the likelihood of a client developing a pressure ulcer. *p. 467*

bradycardia A slow (*brady*) heart rate (*cardia*); a rate less than 60 beats per minute. *p. 237*

bradypnea Slow (*brady*) breathing (*pnea*); respirations are fewer than 12 per minute. *p. 932*

Braille A writing system for people who are visually impaired that uses raised dots for each letter of the alphabet. *p. 922*

bruise See **contusion**. *p. 463*

burnout A state of physical, emotional, and mental exhaustion that results in feelings of discouragement, negativity, and powerlessness. *p. 101*

Caesarean section A surgical incision into the abdominal and uterine walls; the baby is delivered through the incision. *p. 324*

call bell A safety device for clients in facilities that enables them to notify staff that they need assistance. *p. 407*

calorie A unit of measure of the energy produced as the body burns food. *p. 571*

Canada Health Act (1984) Federal legislation that clarifies the types of health care services that are insured; it outlines five principles (**comprehensiveness**, **universality**, **portability**, **accessibility**, and **public administration**) that must be met by provinces and territories to qualify for federal health funding. *p. 22*

Canadian Charter of Rights and Freedoms Part of the Canadian Constitution that lists the basic rights and freedoms to which all Canadians are entitled. *p. 130*

cancer A group of diseases characterized by out-of-control cell division and growth, which can occur in many body systems. *p. 876*

cannula A type of plastic tubing threaded over a needle; once in place in the vein, the needle is withdrawn, leaving the cannula in place. Also called a **catheter**. *p. 604*

capillaries The smallest form of blood vessels and the site of nutrient, gas, and waste exchange between cells and the bloodstream. *p. 289*

care conference See **family conference**. *p. 90*

care plan A document that details the care and services the client must receive. *p. 204*

care-planning process The method used by nurses and case managers to plan the client's care with the health care team. Also known as the **nursing process**. *p. 202*

caring Concern for clients' and their families' dignity, independence, preferences, privacy, and safety at all times. True *caring* requires honesty, sensitivity, comforting, discretion, and respect while showing this concern. *p. 16*

carriers Persons who are able to transfer a pathogen to others without getting an active infection themselves. *p. 427*

cartilage Connective tissue that cushions the joint so that bone ends do not rub together. *p. 279*

case manager A manager who assesses, monitors, and evaluates the needs of a client in a community care setting and also coordinates the services of the team. Also known as **team leader**. *p. 91*

cataract Clouding of the eye's lens. *p. 921*

catheter See **cannula**. *p. 604*

catheterization The process of inserting a catheter. *p. 702*

celiac disease Negative physical reaction to a gluten protein found in wheat or related grains such as barley, rye, and sometimes oats. *p. 585*

cell The basic functional unit of body structure and function. *p. 273*

centre of gravity The point in the body in which weight is evenly distributed or balanced on either side. *p. 493*

cerebral palsy (CP) A disorder affecting muscle control (*palsy*) caused by an injury or abnormality in the motor region of the brain (*cerebral*). *p. 892*

cerumen Ear wax. *p. 914*

cervical mucus A viscous discharge secreted by the glands in the cervix. *p. 323*

chart A legal document that details a client's condition or illness and responses to care. Also called a **record**. *p. 210*

charting See **documentation**. *p. 215*

chemical digestion The chemical breakdown of food into small nutrient parts that the body can absorb and utilize. *p. 294*

chemical restraints Medication that is ordered by a doctor and given to a client to control unsafe, undesirable, or bizarre behaviour or movement. *p. 396*

chest tube A hollow plastic tube surgically inserted into the chest cavity, which allows for the removal of trapped air (*pneumothorax*) and the drainage of blood or fluid (*hemothorax* or *pleural effusion*). *p. 956*

Cheyne–Stokes Respirations that gradually increase in rate and depth and then become shallow and slow; breathing may stop (*apnea*) for 10 to 20 seconds. *p. 932*

child abuse Mistreatment or neglect of a child by a parent, guardian, or caregiver. *p. 259*

child neglect Failure by a child's parents or other caregivers to meet the child's basic needs for emotional, psychological, and physical development. *p. 260*

cholecystitis Inflammation of the gallbladder. *p. 870*

chronic illness See **persistent illness**. *p. 35*

chronic obstructive pulmonary disease (COPD) A persistent lung disorder that obstructs (blocks) the airways; refers to chronic bronchitis and emphysema. *p. 868*

chronic pain See **persistent pain**. *p. 178*

chronic stress Ongoing stress that can lead to burnout. *p. 101*

chronic wound A wound that does not heal easily. *p. 463*

chronological resumé A resumé that highlights employment history, starting with the most current employment and working in reverse chronological order (backward) through earlier jobs. *p. 1078*

circulatory ulcer An open wound on the lower legs and feet caused by decreased blood flow through arteries or veins. Also known as **vascular ulcer**. *p. 473*

circumcision The surgical removal of foreskin from the penis. *p. 340*

cirrhosis Persistent liver disease characterized by normal liver cells being replaced by scar tissue. *p. 870*

civil laws Laws that deal with relationships between people. *p. 140*

clean-contaminated wound A wound occurring from the surgical portal of entry into the urinary, reproductive, or digestive system. *p. 460*

clean technique See **medical asepsis**. *p. 432*

clean wound A wound that is not infected; microbes have not entered the wound. *p. 463*

client A general term for any person receiving care or support services in a community setting: hospital patients, facility residents, and clients in the community. *p. 9*

clinical depression See **major depressive disorder**. *p. 781*

closed questions Questions that are structured so that the response can be restricted to one word such as *yes* or *no* or to a few words. *p. 74*

closed wound A wound in which tissues are injured but skin is not broken. *p. 463*

Clostridium difficile (C. difficile) A bacterium that causes diarrhea and colitis. It is the most common cause of infectious diarrhea in hospitalized people in the industrialized world and one of the most common infections in hospitals and long-term care facilities. *p. 425*

cognitive disability See **intellectual disability**. *p. 889*

cognitive function Brain function involving the memory, thinking, reasoning, understanding, judgement, and behaviour functions of the brain. *p. 805*

cognitive health Well-being in the intellectual dimension, achieved through an active, creative mind. *p. 51*

cognitive impairment The loss of the ability to remember, think, reason, understand, or live independently. *p. 805*

cold pack A commercial or homemade cold application; may be moist or dry. *p. 1026*

colitis Inflammation of the colon. *p. 870*

colonize To establish a habitat; for example, bacteria grow on or in specific regions of the body and survive as part of that person's **normal flora**. *p. 425*

colostomy An artificial opening (*stomy*) between the colon (*colo*) and the abdominal wall. *p. 739*

combining vowel A vowel added between two roots or between a root and a suffix to make pronunciation easier. *p. 193*

communicable disease A disease caused by microbes (disease-causing organisms) that spreads easily. Also known as **contagious disease**. *p. 426*

communicable phase The period when a person is infectious and can spread pathogens to others. *p. 427*

community-based services Health care and support services provided in a community setting, not in a facility setting. *p. 36*

community-based settings Places within the community that provide health care and support services. *p. 36*

community day program A daytime community-based program for people with physical or mental health issues or older adults who need assistance. Also known as **adult day program** or **adult day centre**. *p. 40*

compassion Awareness of the misfortune and suffering of another person and the desire to take action to reduce or eliminate the problem. *p. 165*

compassionate care Care that demonstrates concern for the dignity, independence, preferences, privacy, and safety (DIPPS) of clients and their families at all times. Also known as *person-centred care*. *p. 16*

competence The ability to do a job well. *p. 165*

complex continuing care Comprehensive inpatient care provided to people who are recovering from surgery, injury, an acute illness, or an exacerbation of a disease process. Also known as **sub-acute care**, *convalescent care*, or *transitional care*. *p. 35*

comprehensiveness A principle of the *Canada Health Act* that states that all necessary health services, including hospitalization and access to physicians and surgical dentists, must be insured. *p. 24*

compress A soft pad that is moistened and applied over a body area. *p. 1017*

compression bandage A bandage designed to provide pressure to a particular area. Also known as a *tensor bandage*. *p. 1026*

compulsion The uncontrollable urge to perform an act. *p. 786*

condom catheter A sheath that slides over the penis; tubing connects the catheter and drainage bag. *p. 713*

conduct Personal behaviour. *p. 119*

conduct disorder A disorder that causes the person to repeatedly violate the personal or property rights of others and the basic expectations of society. *p. 794*

condyloid joint A joint formed when the oval articular surface of one bone fits into the oval depression of the second articulating bone, such as at the wrist and the knuckles at the base of the fingers. *p. 280*

confidentiality Respecting, guarding, and using discretion in regard to personal and private information about another person. *p. 14*

conflict A clash between opposing interests and ideas. *p. 103*

confusion See **disorientation**. *p. 805*

congenital Present at birth. *p. 330*

congestive heart failure (CHF) An abnormal condition that occurs when the heart cannot pump blood normally. Blood backs up and causes an abnormal amount (congestion) of fluid in the tissues. Also known as *heart failure*. *p. 866*

conjunctivitis An inflammation of the clear membrane that covers the white part of the eye and lines the inner surface of the eyelids. The nonmedical term is **pink eye**. *p. 362*

consent Agreement or approval—for example, to medical treatment, health care, or personal care services. *p. 137*

constipation A condition in which bowel movements are less frequent than usual; the stool is hard, dry, and difficult to pass. *p. 733*

constrict To squeeze or make narrow. *p. 1026*

contagious disease See **communicable disease**. *p. 426*

contaminated wound A wound with a high risk for infection; microbes have entered the wound. *p. 463*

contamination The process of being exposed to microorganisms, including pathogens. *p. 435*

contracture The lack of joint mobility caused by abnormal shortening of a muscle. *p. 535*

controlled acts Tasks that must be performed only by those authorized to perform them. Controlled acts are considered to be harmful if performed by unqualified individuals. *p. 92*

contusion A closed wound caused by a blow to the body. Also known as a **bruise**. *p. 463*

coronary artery disease (CAD) A condition of impaired cardiac pumping due to narrowed or blocked arteries. *p. 683*

cover letter See **letter of application**. *p. 1083*

cradle cap (seborrheic dermatitis) A skin condition in which yellowish, scaly, or crusty patches, made up largely of oil and dead skin cells, appear on the scalp. *p. 328*

crime A violation of criminal law. *p. 140*

criminal laws Laws concerned with offences against the public and against society in general. *p. 140*

critical thinking The ability to think clearly and logically, using reflection and reason, based on knowledge obtained from experience, observation, or education. *p. 11*

Crohn's disease A persistent, inflammatory bowel disease of unknown origin, usually affecting the ileum, the colon, or another part of the gastrointestinal (GI) tract. *p. 870*

cross-contamination The spread of pathogens from one source to another. *p. 582*

cueing Providing of prompts in order to assist a client to complete a task. This prompting can be in the form of hand gestures, facial expressions, or verbal phrases. *p. 818*

cultural competence The ability to interact effectively with people from different cultures or socioeconomic backgrounds. *p. 153*

cultural conflict Negative feelings and conduct that can result when people from one culture try to impose their own set of values and behaviours on people from another culture. *p. 152*

culture The characteristics of a group of people, including the language, values, beliefs, customs, habits, ways of life, rules for behaviour, music, and traditions. *p. 149*

curriculum vitae (CV) A résumé that is lengthened to include a description of achievements, such as teaching experience, research, awards, publications, and degrees. *p. 1077*

cyanosis An abnormal condition, evidenced by bluish colour in the skin, lips, mucous membranes, and nail beds caused by a lack of oxygenated blood in the visible tissues. *p. 933*

cyst An abnormal, closed sac, which may contain air, fluids, or semi-solid material. *p. 848*

cystitis A bladder infection. *p. 872*

daily value (DV) How a serving fits into the daily diet of an adult; expressed as a percentage based on recommended daily intake. *p. 579*

dandruff Excessive amount of dry, white flakes that appear on the scalp, in the hair, or on the shoulders. *p. 652*

deconditioning The loss of muscle size, strength, and function (*muscle atrophy*) that results from immobility and inactivity. *p. 534*

decubitus ulcer See **pressure ulcer**. *p. 465*

deep Away from the surface or further into the body. *p. 273*

defamation The injuring of the name and reputation of a person by making false statements to a third person. *p. 143*

defecation The process of excreting feces from the rectum through the anus; bowel movement. *p. 731*

defence mechanisms A subconscious practice intended to either delay—or avoid altogether—uncomfortable feelings such as anxiety, guilt, stress, or embarrassment. These practices include **denial**, **displacement**, **fantasizing**, **projection**, **rationalization**, **regression**, **repression**, **suppression**, **passive-aggressiveness**, and **submissiveness**. *p. 78*

dehiscence The separation of wound layers along a surgical suture line. *p. 476*

dehydration The excessive loss of water from body tissues. *p. 593*

delegation A process by which a nurse authorizes another health care provider to perform certain tasks, including controlled acts. *p. 92*

delirium A state of temporary mental disorientation that can occur suddenly. *p. 806*

delusion A fixed, false belief that is not based on reality. *p. 778*

dementia A general term that describes the progressive loss of brain functions, which include cognitive and social functions. It is not a single disease but a group of illnesses that involve memory, behaviour, learning, and communication. Dementia is categorized as being either a mild or major **neuro-cognitive disorder**, depending on its symptoms. *p. 808*

denial An unwillingness to accept the truth or a certain reality. *p. 78*

dependence The state of relying on others for support; being unable to manage without help. *p. 166*

depressive disorders A group of disorders in which the client has sad, empty, or irritable moods accompanied by physical and thought changes that are severe enough to affect the client's ability to function. *p. 781*

dermatitis Inflammation of the skin caused by direct contact with an irritating or allergy-causing substance. *p. 845*

determinants of health The most important factors—such as lifestyle, environment, human biology, and health services—that determine health status in an individual or a community. *p. 54*

detoxification A process of allowing an abused substance to exit the body naturally or of removing the substance from the body medically; the person being detoxified may go into **drug withdrawal**. *p. 796*

development The maturation toward adulthood; usually characterized by physical changes and increased ability and functionality. *p. 305*

developmental disability A permanent disability that a person is born with or that begins before 18 years of age. *p. 887*

developmental task An activity that must be mastered during a stage of development. *p. 305*

diabetes A metabolic disorder characterized by hyperglycemia (high blood sugar levels) and resulting from low levels of insulin or a resistance to insulin's effect at a cellular level. *p. 894*

diabetic retinopathy A disorder (*pathy*) caused by diabetes, in which the blood vessels in the retina are damaged. *p. 920*

***Diagnostic and Statistical Manual of Mental Disorders*, fifth edition (*DSM-5*)** A manual published by the American Psychiatric Association that is used throughout North America to classify mental health disorders. *p. 772*

diarrhea The frequent passage of liquid stools. *p. 734*

diastole The period of heart muscle relaxation. *p. 241*

diastolic pressure The pressure in the arteries when the heart is at rest. *p. 241*

digestion The process of physically and chemically breaking down food into nutrients that can be absorbed for use by the cells. *p. 292*

dignity The state of feeling worthy, valued, and respected. *p. 16*

dilate To expand or open wider. *p. 1016*

dimensions of health All aspects of a person's health: physical, emotional, social, spiritual, cognitive. Holistic health considers all of these aspects. *p. 49*

diplegia Loss of ability to move (*plegia*) corresponding parts on both (*di*) sides of the body; both arms or both legs are affected. *p. 893*

DIPPS An acronym for the five principles of compassionate care (also known as *person-centred care*): *dignity*, *independence, preferences*, *privacy*, and *safety*. *p. 16*

dirty wound See **infected wound**. *p. 463*

disability The loss of physical or mental function. *p. 56*

discharge Official departure of a client from a hospital or other health care facility. *p. 1038*

discretion The use of responsible judgement to avoid causing distress or embarrassment to a person. *p. 14*

discrimination The unfair treatment of people on the basis of such aspects as their physical characteristics, health history, or group membership. *p. 60*

disease prevention Strategies that prevent the occurrence of disease or injury. *p. 28*

disinfection The process of destroying pathogens. *p. 441*

disorientation Mental confusion, or an impaired ability to recall people, time, or places as a result of (or any combination of) physiological changes to the brain, disease process, or substance-induced factors. Also known as **confusion**. *p. 805*

displacement A transfer of feelings (usually of anger) onto another person or item instead of onto the person who is the source of the anger. *p. 78*

disruptive, impulse-control, and conduct disorder Disorders in which the client displays difficult, disruptive, aggressive, or antisocial behaviours. *p. 793*

distal The part farthest from the centre or from the point of attachment. *p. 195*

distilled water Sterile and pure water that has been boiled and allowed to cool and condense. *p. 943*

distribution The path the drug takes from the bloodstream to the body tissues of the intended site of action. *p. 987*

diversity The state of different individuals and cultures coexisting. *p. 148*

diverticulosis The condition (*osis*) of having small pouches in the colon that bulge outward (*diverticulum*). *p. 871*

documentation Record of the care you have given the client and the observations you have made during care. Also called **charting**. *p. 215*

dorsal See **posterior**. *p. 196*

dorsiflexion Bending the toes and foot up at the ankle. *p. 539*

dosette Container that stores medications in separate compartments arranged by day or hour. Also known as *pillbox*. *p. 986*

Down syndrome (DS) A congenital disorder caused by an extra chromosome; DS results in varying degrees of intellectual disability. *p. 892*

droplet A drop of liquid. *p. 431*

drug antagonism An unusually weak drug effect that occurs when two or more drugs are taken at the same time. *p. 987*

drug interaction The combined action that a medication and another substance (such as another drug, alcohol, or food) has on the body. *p. 987*

drug synergism An unusually strong drug effect that occurs when taking two or more drugs at the same time. *p. 987*

drug tolerance The state at which the body gets accustomed to a substance, causing the individual to need larger and larger amounts of it to experience the same effect. *p. 795*

drug withdrawal A physical reaction that occurs when a person abusing a substance stops taking it. *p. 795*

dysarthria Difficulty (*dys*) speaking clearly (*arthria*), caused by weakness or paralysis in the muscles used for speech. *p. 904*

dysphagia Difficulty (*dys*) swallowing (*phagia*). *p. 377*

dyspnea Difficult, laboured, or painful breathing. *p. 377*

dysrhythmia An irregular rhythm of the pulse; beats may be unevenly spaced or skipped. *p. 237*

dysuria Painful or difficult (*dys*) urination (*uria*). *p. 692*

ear infection See **otitis media**. *p. 364*

early morning care See **AM care**. *p. 613*

eczema A persistent inflammatory condition of the skin that can include recurring skin rashes. *p. 845*

edema Swelling in tissues caused by an accumulation of fluid. *p. 473*

elective surgery Surgery that is scheduled but non-urgent. *p. 1043*

electronic communication The transfer of information through electronic media. *p. 69*

electronic privacy A person's right not to have his image, words, or character description or comments about his reputation made public by electronic means. *p. 136*

embolus An air bubble, blood clot (**thrombus**), or fat clot that travels through the vascular system until it lodges in a distant vessel. *p. 1051*

emergency surgery Surgery that must be done immediately to save a client's life or prevent permanent disability. *p. 1043*

emotional abuse Words or actions that cause mental harm, especially on a person's self-esteem. Also known as **psychological abuse**. *p. 254*

emotional health Well-being in the emotional dimension, achieved when people feel good about themselves. *p. 50*

emotional illness See **mental health disorder**. *p. 770*

emotional neglect Failure to meet a person's need to feel loved, wanted, safe, and worthy. *p. 260*

emotional pressure The feeling of being pushed beyond one's limits or abilities. *p. 102*

empathetic listening A nonjudgemental technique that requires the listener to be attentive to the sender's feelings. *p. 74*

empathy The ability to recognize, perceive, and have an understanding of another person's emotions by seeing things from his or her viewpoint. *p. 3*

end-of-life care See **palliative care**. *p. 35*

endospore The protective shell that surrounds dormant bacteria and viruses, which protects them from external harm. *p. 423*

enema The introduction of fluid into the rectum and lower colon. *p. 736*

engorged breasts Breasts that are overfilled with milk, which makes them swollen, hard, and painful. *p. 324*

enteral nutrition The giving of nutrients by way of the intestine (*enteral*). *p. 600*

environmental health According to the WHO, "all the physical, chemical, and biological factors external to a person and all the related factors impacting behaviours." *p. 55*

environmental restraints Barriers, furniture, or devices that prevent a client from having free movement. *p. 396*

epilepsy A group of neurological disorders characterized by recurrent episodes of convulsive seizures, sensory disturbances, abnormal behaviour, loss of consciousness, or some or all of the above. *p. 857*

episiotomy An incision made in the perineum to increase the size of the vaginal opening for the delivery of the baby. *p. 323*

equitable Fair, reasonable, and just. *p. 55*

estate trustee The person chosen by the now-deceased person to deal with his or her possessions, as stated in the will. Also known as **guardian of property** or **executor, executrix**. *p. 139*

ethical dilemma An apparent conflict between opposing moral choices; choosing one would result in going against another moral choice. *p. 121*

ethics The rules of conduct that guide us when deciding what is right and what is wrong, and what is good and what is bad. *p. 118*

ethnic identity The ethnic background a person feels a part of, based usually on similar language and customs. *p. 149*

ethnicity The sharing of a common history, language, geography, national origin, religion, or identity. *p. 149*

ethnocentrism The belief that one's own culture or ethnic group is better or more important than others'. *p. 149*

euphoria An exaggerated or abnormal expression of physical or emotional well-being that is not based on reality or truth. *p. 807*

eupnea Normal breathing. *p. 931*

eustachian tube The tiny drainage pipe in the middle ear. *p. 364*

eustress A type of stressor that is healthy and gives one a feeling of fulfillment or other positive feelings. *p. 101*

evaluation Assessing and measuring; a step in the care-planning process. *p. 205*

evening care See **HS care**. *p. 613*

evisceration Separation of the wound accompanied by protrusion of abdominal organs. *p. 476*

excretion Exiting from the body, especially through the stool, urine, lungs, or skin. *p. 987*

executor, executrix See **estate trustee**. *p. 140*

expressive aphasia Difficulty speaking or writing. *p. 903*

expressive–receptive aphasia Difficulty speaking and understanding language. Also known as **global aphasia**. *p. 904*

extension Straightening of a body part. *p. 539*

external rotation Turning of the joint outward. *p. 539*

face mask A mask used to deliver oxygen that covers the client's nose and mouth. *p. 941*

facility-based settings Workplaces that provide clients with accommodations, health care, and support services. *p. 37*

failure to thrive A term to describe infants, babies, or children who are below the norms for body weight, growth, or cognitive development. *p. 260*

false imprisonment Unlawful restraint or restrictions of a person's freedom of movement. *p. 142*

family A biological, legal, or social network of people who provide support for one another. *p. 168*

family conference A meeting attended by the health care team and family members to discuss the client's care. Also called **care conference**. *p. 90*

fan-fold To fold a sheet back and forth, in a form that resembles a fan. *p. 499*

fantasizing Daydreaming as an escape instead of dealing with reality. *p. 79*

febrile respiratory illness (FRI) A term used to describe a wide range of respiratory infections, such as colds, influenza, influenza-like illness (ILI), and pneumonia, spread through droplets. *p. 431*

fecal impaction The prolonged retention and accumulation of feces in the rectum. *p. 734*

fecal incontinence The inability to control the passage of feces and gas through the anus. Also known as *anal incontinence*. *p. 735*

feces The semi-solid mass of waste products in the colon. *p. 731*

feeding and eating disorders Altered body image perceptions that lead to disturbances in eating behaviours and an abnormal concern with body weight and shape. *p. 787*

fetal alcohol spectrum disorders (FASD) A group of physical and mental abnormalities that occur in children as a result of alcohol consumption by the mother during pregnancy. *p. 895*

fibromyalgia A condition associated with aching, stiffness, and fatigue in muscles, ligaments, and tendons. *p. 857*

financial abuse The misuse of a person's money or property. *p. 254*

fitted sheet A sheet (usually with elastic edges) tailored to fit a particular size of mattress. *p. 758*

flatulence The excessive formation of gas in the stomach and intestines. *p. 735*

flatus Gas or air from the stomach or intestines passed through the anus. *p. 735*

flexion Bending of a body part. *p. 539*

flowmeter A device that regulates the flow of oxygen to the nasal cannula or face mask. *p. 940*

flow rate The volume of a substance, such as oxygen or fluids, administered over a prescribed period. *p. 942*

focusing Limiting the conversation to a certain topic. *p. 76*

Foley catheter See **in-dwelling catheter**. *p. 702*

fomite Any nonliving object that is capable of carrying infectious organisms and that may serve as a mode of transmission. *p. 430*

foodborne illness An illness transmitted by contaminated food products. *p. 582*

footdrop The foot falls down at the ankle (permanent **plantar flexion**). *p. 536*

Fowler's position A semi-sitting to upright sitting position in bed. *p. 510*

fracture A broken bone. *p. 850*

fracture pan A small, thin, rimmed bedpan that is about 1 cm deep at one end. Also called a **slipper pan**. *p. 691*

fragile X syndrome The most common form of inherited developmental disorder. *p. 890*

friction Resistance that skin encounters when it rubs against another surface such as clothing, bedding, or another fold of skin. *p. 463*

frostbite A medical condition in which skin and other tissues are damaged by extreme cold. *p. 1026*

full-thickness wound A wound in which the dermis, epidermis, and subcutaneous tissue are penetrated; muscle and bone may be involved. *p. 463*

functional incontinence Urinary incontinence caused by physical conditions or environmental barriers that prevent the client from reaching the toilet in time. *p. 700*

functional resumé A resumé that highlights skills or functions and briefly lists positions held. *p. 1080*

fungi Microbes that live only on organic matter such as plants and animals. *p. 423*

furuncle A skin disorder caused by the infection of a hair follicle. Also called a **boil**. *p. 848*

gangrene A condition in which tissue dies and then decays. *p. 473*

gastroenteritis More commonly known as "stomach flu," this illness causes vomiting and diarrhea and can lead to dehydration, particularly in very young children and frail older adults. *p. 364*

gastro-esophageal reflux disease (GERD) A disorder of the digestive system that causes heartburn. *p. 869*

gastro-jejunostomy tube A combination device that includes access to both the stomach and the jejunum (the middle part of the small intestine). It is also known as a *GJ-tube*. *p. 600*

gastrostomy tube A tube inserted through an opening (*stomy*) into the stomach (*gastro*). It is also known as a *G-tube*. *p. 600*

gavage Tube feeding. *p. 600*

gel pack A commercially produced hot-and-cold pack designed to keep its temperature over a period. *p. 1022*

gender The roles, personality traits, attitudes, behaviours, values, and relative power and influence assigned to the sexes by society. *p. 56*

general anaesthesia Unconsciousness and the loss of feeling or sensation produced by a medication. *p. 1049*

generic name of a drug The name given to a drug approved by Health Canada. It is also known as the "official name" of a drug. *p. 992*

genetic endowment The genetic makeup that predisposes an individual to adopt certain behaviours that affect health status. *p. 56*

Gentle Persuasive Approaches (GPA) A program designed to train direct care providers in techniques to handle and reduce difficult responsive behaviours (e.g., grabbing, biting, and hitting) that are associated with dementias such as Alzheimer's disease to prepare the care providers for vulnerable care situations and for avoiding potential workplace injury. *p. 829*

geriatrics The branch of medicine that provides care for older adults. *p. 369*

gerontology The study of the aging process. *p. 369*

glaucoma An eye disease that causes pressure within the eye and vision loss. *p. 921*

gliding joint A joint formed by the interaction of the flat surfaces of the articulating bones, allowing for limited but complex gliding movements, such as in the wrist, ankle joints, and the vertebral column. *p. 280*

global aphasia See **expressive–receptive aphasia**. *p. 904*

glucosuria Glucose, a type of sugar (*glucos*) in the urine (*uria*). *p. 720*

gluten A protein that has come from wheat or related grains, such as barley, oats, rye, triticale, Kamut, or spelt. *p. 585*

gout A disease caused by the accumulation of uric acid in the cartilage of a joint, especially in the tendons. Also called *metabolic arthritis*. *p. 857*

grief The process of moving from deep sorrow caused by loss toward healing and recovery. *p. 1061*

grief counselling A support for people coping with the difficulties associated with the loss of a loved one. *p. 1061*

group home A residential facility in which a small number of people with physical or mental disabilities live together and are provided with supervision, care, and support services. *p. 39*

growth Increase in physical size and weight that occurs in a slow and steady manner. *p. 305*

guardian of property See **estate trustee**. *p. 139*

hallucination Seeing, smelling, hearing, tasting, or feeling something that is not real. *p. 778*

hand hygiene The process of cleaning hands. *p. 435*

handwashing The process of removing soil, dead skin cells, and excess microbes from the hands, using soap, friction, and running water. It is one form of **hand hygiene**. *p. 435*

harassment Troubling, tormenting, offending, or worrying a person through one's behaviour or comments. *p. 143*

hazardous material Any substance that presents a physical hazard or a health hazard in the workplace. *p. 411*

health A state of well-being in all dimensions of one's life. *p. 49*

health care–associated infection (HAI) An infection acquired while a person is a patient, client, or resident in a health care facility or while receiving care from a health care provider. This term has replaced the term **nosocomial infection**. *p. 427*

health care ethics The philosophical study of what is morally right and wrong when providing health care services. *p. 121*

health promotion A strategy for improving the population's health by providing the necessary information and tools for individuals, groups, and communities to make informed decisions that promote health and wellness. *p. 28*

heart attack See **myocardial infarction**. *p. 865*

hematoma The collection of blood under skin and tissues. *p. 476*

hematuria Blood (*hemat*) in the urine (*uria*). *p. 692*

hemiplegia Paralysis (*plegia*) of one side (*hemi*) of the body; the arm and leg, body organs, vision, the tongue, and the swallowing mechanisms on the affected side can all be compromised. *p. 859*

hemoglobin The substance in red blood cells that carries oxygen and gives blood its colour. *p. 287*

hemoptysis Bloody (*hemo*) sputum (*ptysis*, meaning "to spit"). *p. 931*

hemorrhage The excessive loss of blood within a short period. *p. 476*

hemorrhoids Swollen veins in the anal canal. *p. 734*

hepatitis Inflammation (*itis*) of the liver (*hepat*) that may be caused by bacterial or viral infection, parasitic infestation, alcohol, drugs, toxins, or transfusion of incompatible (not matching) blood type. *p. 870*

high Fowler's position A semi-sitting position in bed; the head of the bed is elevated 45 to 90 degrees. *p. 510*

hinge joints Joints that allow movement in one direction around a single axis (e.g., elbow joint). *p. 279*

hirsutism Excessive and increased hair growth. *p. 652*

hives See **urticaria**. *p. 845*

hoarding Collecting things and putting them away in a guarded manner. *p. 833*

holism A concept that considers the whole person; the whole person has physical, social, emotional, cognitive, and spiritual dimensions. *p. 49*

holistic health A state of well-being in all dimensions of one's life. *p. 49*

home care Health care and support services provided to people in their places of residence. *p. 28*

home management The cleaning and organizing of a home. *p. 962*

homeostasis A steady state or stable internal environment maintained when all of the organ systems in the human body work together. *p. 275*

homophobia Negative attitudes toward or intolerance of homosexuality or people who are identified or perceived as being lesbian, gay, bisexual, transgender, or questioning their sexuality (**LGBTQ**). *p. 152*

hormone A chemical substance produced by the cells of specialized glands and secreted into the bloodstream. *p. 298*

hospice A type of palliative care that provides home, residential, or inpatient care to a client who has a terminal diagnosis and is no longer seeking life-prolonging care. *p. 36*

hospital A facility for clients with acute illnesses or injuries who require admission and care on a relatively short-term basis, often not even overnight. *p. 37*

HS care Routine care given in a facility at bedtime (*HS* stands for "hour of sleep"). Also known as **evening care** or **PM care**. *p. 613*

humidified oxygen Oxygen that contains water vapour. *p. 943*

Huntington's disease An inherited neurological disorder that causes uncontrolled movements, emotional disturbances, and cognitive losses. *p. 861*

hyperextension Excessive straightening of a body part. *p. 539*

hypertension Persistent blood pressure measurements above the normal systolic (140 mm Hg) or diastolic (90 mm Hg) pressures. *p. 242*

hyperthyroidism A condition caused by an overactive thyroid gland. *p. 876*

hyperventilation Respirations that are more rapid (*hyper*) and deeper than normal. *p. 932*

hypotension A condition in which the systolic blood pressure is below 90 mm Hg and the diastolic pressure is below 60 mm Hg. *p. 242*

hypothyroidism A condition caused by an underactive thyroid gland. *p. 876*

hypoventilation Respirations that are slow (*hypo*), shallow, and sometimes irregular. *p. 932*

hypoxia A deficiency (*hypo*) of oxygen in the cells (*oxia*). *p. 932*

ileal conduit An artificial bladder made out of a section of the ileum. *p. 724*

ileostomy An artificial opening (*stomy*) between the ileum (small intestine; *ileo*) and the abdominal wall. *p. 740*

illness The loss of physical or mental health. *p. 56*

immobility An excessive lack of exercise and activity, which can cause serious health complications, affecting every system in the body. *p. 535*

immoral Conflicting with traditionally held moral principles; often regarded as indecent or deviant (not normal). *p. 118*

immunity Protection against a disease or condition. *p. 300*

impetigo A contagious skin disorder caused by bacteria. *p. 848*

implementation Carrying out or performing; a step in the care-planning process. *p. 205*

incident report A report submitted whenever an accident, error, or unexpected problem arises in the workplace. Also known as an **occurrence report**. *p. 411*

incision An open wound with clean, straight edges; usually intentionally created with a sharp instrument. *p. 463*

incontinence pad A pad placed in the centre of the bed on top of the bottom sheet to protect the bedsheets from body fluids. Also called an *absorbent pad* or *soaker pad*. *p. 755*

incubation period The time between exposure to a pathogenic organism and the appearance of signs and symptoms. *p. 427*

independence The state of not relying on others for control or authority. *p. 166*

in-dwelling catheter A tube (plastic, latex, or other material) that is inserted into the bladder through the urinary meatus and urethra. A balloon within the catheter that is inflated after insertion prevents the catheter from slipping out of the bladder. Also known as a **Foley** or **retention catheter**. *p. 702*

infancy The first year of life, during which the body undergoes rapid physical, psychological, and social growth and development. *p. 305*

infected wound A wound containing a large amount of bacteria and showing signs of infection. Also known as a **dirty wound**. *p. 463*

infection A disease state resulting from the invasion and growth of pathogens in the body. *p. 426*

infection control Policies and procedures to prevent the spread of infection within health care settings. *p. 422*

inferior Situated below another structure or toward the lower part of the body. *p. 273*

infiltration Intravenous fluids' entering surrounding tissues. *p. 606*

influenza ("the flu") A highly contagious infection of the respiratory tract by the causative (disease-causing) virus in airborne droplets. Symptoms include sore throat, cough, fever, muscular pains, and weakness. *p. 429*

informed consent Consent obtained under the legal condition whereby a person is first given complete, accurate, and relevant information so as to fully understand the action or procedure and its potential implications. *p. 137*

ingestion The process of taking food and fluids into the body. *p. 570*

ingrown hair A hair that curls into the side wall of the hair follicle or into the skin surface, which causes the skin to become inflamed. Also known as **razor bumps**. *p. 661*

ingrown nails Toenails that grow inward at the side of the nail bed. *p. 664*

inpatient A client who is assigned a bed and is admitted to stay in a facility overnight or longer. *p. 41*

insomnia A persistent condition in which the person cannot go to sleep or stay asleep throughout the night. *p. 185*

instrumental activities of daily living (IADLs) The complex skills needed to successfully live independently. *p. 4*

intake The amount of fluids taken in by the body. *p. 593*

intellectual disability Impaired ability to learn. Also known as **cognitive disability**. *p. 889*

intentional wound A wound created for treatment. *p. 463*

interdependence The state of relying on one another. *p. 166*

interdisciplinary team A team of health care providers from a variety of backgrounds and specialties who work together to meet the client's needs. Also known as a(n) *intradisciplinary team*, *interprofessional team*, *interprofessional health care team*, or *multidisciplinary team*. *p. 90*

internal rotation Turning of the joint inward. *p. 539*

interpersonal communication The exchange of information between two people, usually face to face. *p. 68*

intervention An action or measure taken by the health care team to help the client meet a goal in the care plan. *p. 204*

intravenous (IV) therapy Fluids given through a needle or catheter inserted into a vein; also referred to as *IV*, *IV therapy*, and *IV infusion*. *p. 604*

intubation The process of inserting an artificial airway. *p. 949*

invasion of privacy Violation of a person's right not to have his or her name, photograph, private affairs, health information, or any personal information made public without consent. *p. 142*

irritable bowel syndrome (IBS) A disorder of the bowel characterized by abdominal pain and changes in bowel habits. *p. 870*

isolation precautions Guidelines for preventing the spread of pathogens; include **Standard Practices** and **Transmission-Based Practices**. *p. 442*

jaundice A yellowing of the skin and the white part (sclera) of the eyes. *p. 331*

jejunostomy tube A tube inserted into the intestines through an opening (*stomy*) into the middle part of the small intestine (*jejunum*). It is also known as a *J-tube*. *p. 601*

justice Fair and equal treatment. *p. 123*

ketones A by-product of fatty acid metabolism. *p. 721*

Kussmaul respiration Deep, rapid respiration characteristic of diabetic acidosis or other conditions causing acidosis. *p. 932*

laceration An open wound with torn tissue and jagged edges. *p. 463*

lactation The process of producing and secreting milk from the breast. *p. 324*

laryngeal mirror An instrument used to examine the mouth, teeth, and throat. *p. 1039*

late adulthood Begins approximately at the age of 65 years. This stage is characterized by adjusting to decreased physical strength and loss of health, retirement, and reduced income; coping with the death of a partner; developing new friends and relationships; and preparing for one's own death. *p. 316*

late childhood Ages 9 to 12 years; characterized by becoming independent of adults; developing and keeping friendships with peers; understanding the physical, psychological, and social roles of one's identified gender; developing moral and ethical behaviour; developing greater muscular strength, coordination, and balance; and learning how to study. *p. 311*

lateral The farthest away from the midline of the body. *p. 195*

lateral position A side-lying position that uses pillows to support the back and separate the lower legs. *p. 511*

laundry care symbols Symbols on garment tags that indicate how to launder or care for specific garments. *p. 974*

legislation A body of laws that govern the behaviour of a country's residents. *p. 130*

letter of application A letter that is included with a resumé that summarizes the job applied for and reasons for applying for it; it can be solicited or unsolicited. Also called a **cover letter**. *p. 1083*

leukocytes White blood cells that are part of the blood; the cells are part of the immune system that fight infection. *p. 323*

LGBTQ An abbreviation that stands for the group of people who identify themselves as lesbian, gay, bisexual, transgender, or questioning their sexuality. *p. 152*

liable Legally responsible. *p. 140*

libel The making of false written statements that hurt the reputation of another person. *p. 143*

lice Small, insectlike parasites that live on the human body, most commonly on skin, hair, and the genital area. *p. 652*

licensed practical nurse (LPN) A health care provider licensed and regulated by the province or territory to carry out nursing techniques and provide client care. Known as a **registered practical nurse (RPN)** in Ontario. *p. 13*

lift Device used to move—or the action of moving—a client from one place to another, without the client's weight-bearing or assistance. *p. 524*

line of gravity An imaginary vertical line that extends from the centre of gravity to the base of support. *p. 493*

lithotomy position A back-lying position in which the hips are brought down to the edge of the examination table, the knees are flexed, the hips are externally rotated, and the feet are supported in stirrups. *p. 1040*

living will A document that lets the reader know one's preferences about care intended to sustain life. *p. 138*

local anaesthesia The loss of sensation in a small area, produced by a medication injected at the specific site or by a topical application. *p. 1049*

lochia Postpartum vaginal discharge that begins as a bloody discharge and then changes in colour and decreases in amount after 4 to 6 weeks. *p. 322*

log-rolling Turning the person as a unit, in alignment, with one motion. *p. 498*

long-term care Medical, nursing, and support services provided over the course of months or years to people who cannot care for themselves. Also known as *chronic care* or *continuing care*. In some provinces, this is also known as **complex continuing care**. *p. 35*

long-term care facility A facility that provides accommodations, 24-hour nursing care, and support services to people who cannot care for themselves at home but who do not need hospital care. Also known as *chronic care facility* or *continuing care facility*. In some provinces, it is called a *complex care facility* or *nursing home*. *p. 37*

Lou Gehrig's disease See **amyotrophic lateral sclerosis**. *p. 862*

low Fowler's position A semi-sitting position in bed; the head of the bed is elevated 15 to 30 degrees. *p. 510*

lunge (or stride) stance A position whereby you place one foot in front of the other foot, keeping both feet about a shoulder-width apart. *p. 494*

major depressive disorder A state of mind in which a person has severe feelings of worthlessness, self-blame, sadness, disappointment, and emptiness that last for weeks and interfere with the person's ability to perform activities of daily living; also known as **clinical depression**, although this term is not used anymore by physicians. *p. 781*

malignant Describes any condition in the body that, if untreated, may be a threat to health (e.g., malignant hypertension). Specifically, it describes a tumour that invades and destroys other cells or tissues. Also known as *cancerous*. *p. 876*

manual lift Physically picking up a client who cannot weight-bear, without the assistance of a mechanical lift. *p. 524*

marginalize The act of excluding people who are not part of the majority culture. *p. 56*

marginalized Prevented from having any power or control over one's life or health care because of language, life circumstances, or role in society, resulting in being shunned from mainstream society. *p. 257*

mastication The first step of digestion in which food is bitten, chewed, crushed, and ground by the teeth and muscles of the jaw. *p. 293*

mastitis An infection (*itis*) of the breast (*mast*). *p. 325*

mechanical digestion Physically breaking down large food particles into smaller pieces. *p. 293*

mechanical lift A device that can elevate and move the person while in a special body sling. *p. 515*

mechanical ventilation The use of a **ventilator** to move air into and out of the lungs. *p. 954*

medial The closest to the midline of the body. *p. 195*

medical asepsis Practices that reduce the number of pathogens and prevent their spread. Also known as **clean** technique. *p. 432*

medical diagnosis The identification of a disease or condition by a physician. *p. 203*

medicare Canada's national health care insurance system, which publicly funds the whole cost of medically necessary health services for permanent residents. *p. 21*

medication A drug or other substance used to prevent or treat disease or illness. *p. 987*

melena Dark, tarry stools containing decomposing blood. *p. 744*

menarche The time when menstruation first begins. *p. 312*

Ménière's disease An inner ear disorder that can affect both hearing and balance. *p. 914*

menopause The time when menstruation stops. *p. 315*

menstruation The process in which the lining of the uterus breaks up and is discharged from the body through the vagina. *p. 298*

mental disorder See **mental health disorder**. *p. 770*

mental health A state of mind in which a person copes with and adjusts to the stressors of everyday living in socially acceptable ways. *p. 770*

mental health care services Services provided to individuals and families confronting mental illness or disorders. Also known as **psychiatric care services**. *p. 36*

mental health disorder A disturbance in a person's ability to cope with or adjust to stress, affecting the person's thinking, mood, or behaviours and impairing functioning; also known as **mental illness**, **mental disorder**, **emotional illness**, or **psychiatric disorder**. *p. 770*

mental illness See **mental health disorder**. *p. 770*

mentor A person who shares her expertise and knowledge to create a safe, encouraging learning environment for the learner. *p. 88*

metabolism The chemical processes carried out by the cells of the body that create and use energy and produce cellular waste products as a result. *p. 987*

metabolization Chemical reactions that take place to convert a drug from smaller molecules into waste products before it can exit the body. *p. 299*

metastasis The spread of cancer to other parts of the body. *p. 876*

metered dose inhaler (MDI) A pressurized canister of medication that releases a single dose of medication as a mist. *p. 989*

methicillin-resistant *Staphylococcus aureus* (MRSA) A type of multidrug-resistant organism that is resistant to the antibiotic methicillin. *p. 425*

microbe See **microorganism**. *p. 422*

microorganism A form of life (*organism*) that is so small (*micro*) it can be seen only with a microscope. Also known as a **microbe**. *p. 422*

micturition See **urination**. *p. 690*

middle adulthood Ages approximately 40 to 65 years. This stage is characterized by seeing children growing up and moving away from home, adjusting to physical changes, developing leisure activities, and relating to aging parents. *p. 315*

middle childhood Ages 6 to 8 years; characterized by developing the social and physical skills needed for playing games; learning to get along with peers; learning behaviours and attitudes normative to one's gender; learning basic reading, writing, and arithmetic skills; developing a conscience and morals; and developing a good feeling and attitude about oneself. *p. 310*

midline An imaginary line that divides the body into right and left sides. *p. 273*

mildew The black discoloration caused by mould. *p. 972*

mobility The ability to move around. *p. 384*

morals The fundamental principles of behaviour each person believes to be *right or wrong for him- or herself* without concern for legalities or customs. *p. 118*

morning care See **AM care**. *p. 613*

mould A microscopic fungal parasite. *p. 972*

multidrug-resistant organism (MRO) A strain of bacteria that is very difficult to treat with common antibiotics. *p. 424*

multiple sclerosis (MS) A persistent, slowly progressive disease, in which the body's immune system attacks the protective myelin sheaths that surround the nerve cells of the brain and spinal cord (a process called *demyelination*), resulting in damaged areas that are unable to transmit nerve impulses. *p. 861*

muscle atrophy A decrease in size or a wasting away of muscle. *p. 535*

myocardial infarction (MI) Death (*infarction*) of heart tissue (*myocardium*) caused by lack of oxygen to the heart. Also known as **heart attack**. *p. 865*

nasal cannula A flexible tube inserted into the nares of the nose to deliver oxygen. *p. 940*

nasal speculum An instrument used to examine the inside of the nose. *p. 1039*

nasogastric (NG) tube A tube inserted through the nose (*naso*) into the stomach (*gastro*). It is also known as an *NG-tube*. *p. 600*

nasointestinal tube A tube inserted through the nose (*naso*) into the small intestine (intestinal). *p. 600*

necrotic tissue Localized tissue death as a result of disease or injury. *p. 482*

need (basic human) Something necessary or desirable for maintaining life and psychosocial well-being. *p. 174*

negative reinforcement Encouraging a behaviour by penalizing the person when that behaviour is not demonstrated. *p. 363*

neglect The state of being uncared for physically, emotionally, or psychologically. *p. 254*

negligence Failure to act in a careful or competent manner, resulting in harm to a person or damage to property. *p. 140*

neuro-cognitive disorder A significant decline in attention, functioning, learning, memory, language, deliberate motor movement, and social functioning. *p. 808*

newborn A baby, up to 28 days after birth; also called a *neonate*. *p. 305*

nocturia The need to urinate (*uria*) during the night (*noct*). *p. 185*

no-lift policy Agency regulations that prohibit workers from manually lifting clients and instruct them to use a mechanical lifting device instead. *p. 494*

nonmaleficence The ethical principle of doing no harm. *p. 124*

nonpathogen A microbe that does not usually cause infection or disease and is not harmful to humans. *p. 423*

nonspecific immunity The body's reaction to anything it does not recognize as a normal body substance. *p. 300*

nonverbal communication Messages sent without words. *p. 71*

normal flora The microorganisms (primarily bacteria and yeast) that are usually found on the surface of skin and mucous membranes and in the gastrointestinal tract. *p. 423*

nosocomial infection See **health care–associated infection (HAI)**. *p. 427*

nuclear family A family consisting of a father, a mother, and children. *p. 154*

nursing diagnosis A statement describing a health problem that is treated by nursing measures. *p. 203*

nursing process See **care-planning process**. *p. 202*

nutrients Substances that are ingested, digested, absorbed, and used by the body. *p. 571*

nutrition Processes involved in the ingestion, digestion, absorption, and use of foods and fluids by the body. *p. 570*

oath of confidentiality A pledge that promises that the signer will respect and guard personal and private information about a client, family, or agency. *p. 136*

obesity Excess fat accumulation that puts a person's health at risk. *p. 352*

objective data See **signs**. *p. 207*

observation The active process of using the senses to obtain information about the client's current condition. *p. 203*

obsession A persistent thought or desire. *p. 786*

obsessive–compulsive and related disorders Mental health disorders characterized by recurrent obsessions and compulsions that interfere with a person's daily life and relationships. *p. 786*

occurrence report See **incident report**. *p. 411*

OH&S (occupational health and safety) legislation Federal and provincial laws designed to protect employees from injuries and accidents in the workplace; these laws outline the rights and responsibilities of employers, supervisors, and workers. *p. 410*

oliguria Scant amount (*olig*) of urine (*uria*)—usually less than 500 mL in 24 hours. *p. 692*

open-ended questions Questions that invite a person to share thoughts, feelings, or ideas. *p. 75*

open wound A wound in which skin or the mucous membrane is broken. *p. 463*

ophthalmoscope A lighted instrument used to examine the internal structures of the eye. *p. 1039*

optimal health State of achievable maximum well-being in each of the five dimensions: physical, emotional, social, cognitive, and spiritual. *p. 52*

oral hygiene Measures performed to keep the mouth and teeth clean; mouth care. *p. 613*

organism Any single-celled or multicellular living thing. *p. 422*

organs Structures made of different tissues that are arranged to perform a specialized function. *p. 275*

organ systems Organs that work together to perform special functions. *p. 275*

orthopnea Shortness of breath (*dyspnea*) when lying in a flat or supine position; ability to breathe comfortably (*pnea*) only when sitting or standing (*ortho*). *p. 929*

orthopneic position Sitting up (*ortho*) and leaning over a table to breathe. *p. 933*

orthostatic hypotension A drop in (*hypo*) blood pressure when the client stands up (*ortho* and *static*). Also known as **postural** hypotension. *p. 536*

orthotic See **brace**. *p. 553*

osteoarthritis (OA) A type of arthritis that causes the cartilage that occupies the joints of the body to wear away, causing pain in and disfigurement to the joints. *p. 855*

osteomyelitis Inflammation or infection of the bone. *p. 852*

osteoporosis A bone disorder (*osteo*) in which the bone becomes porous and brittle (*poros*). *p. 855*

ostomy A surgically created opening that is used to drain wastes or to feed the client. *p. 600*

otitis media Infection (*itis*) of the middle (*media*) ear (*ot*), caused by either a virus or bacteria. Also known as **ear** infection. *p. 364*

otosclerosis A condition (*osis*) in which hardening (*sclero*) of the ossicles in the middle ear (*oto*) occurs, interfering with transmission of sound. *p. 914*

otoscope A lighted instrument used to examine the external ear and the eardrum (tympanic membrane). *p. 1039*

outpatient A client who does not stay overnight in a facility. *p. 41*

output The amount of fluids lost by the body. *p. 593*

overflow incontinence The leaking of urine when the bladder is too full. *p. 700*

over-the-counter (OTC) medication A medication that can be bought without a physician's prescription. *p. 990*

oxygen-conserving devices Devices that help reduce oxygen wastage. *p. 939*

palliative care Services for clients (and their families) living with or dying from a progressive, life-threatening illness. Also known as **end-of-life care**. *p. 35*

pandemic An epidemic that spreads quickly over a large region or even worldwide. *p. 429*

panic An intense and sudden feeling of fear, anxiety, terror, or dread for no obvious reason. *p. 783*

paralysis Complete or partial loss of ability to move a limb or muscle group. *p. 862*

paranoia Extreme suspicion about a person or a situation. *p. 778*

paraphrasing Restating someone's message in one's own words. *p. 74*

paraplegia Paralysis (*plegia*) from the waist down. *p. 862*

parasites Organisms that derive nourishment and protection from other living organisms, known as *hosts*. *p. 423*

Parkinson's disease Neurological disorder in which the cells in certain parts of the brain are gradually destroyed; causes tremors, muscle stiffness, slow movement, and poor balance. *p. 860*

partial-thickness wound A wound in which the dermis and epidermis of the skin are broken. *p. 463*

passive-aggressiveness The practice of expressing negative emotions, resentment, or anger toward others through passive, indirect ways (such as through procrastination or manipulation) instead of by verbalizing feelings in an assertive manner. *p. 79*

passive immunity A short-lived immunity passed from mother to fetus through the placenta and from the mother to the baby through breast milk. *p. 300*

pathogen A microbe that can cause harm, such as an infection or a disease. *p. 423*

patient A person receiving care in a hospital setting. Also known as a *client*. *p. 9*

pediculosis Infestation with **lice**. *p. 652*

pediculosis capitis Infestation of the scalp (*capitis*) with lice. *p. 652*

pediculosis corporis Infestation of the body (*corporis*) with lice. *p. 652*

pediculosis pubis Infestation of the pubic (*pubis*) hair with lice. *p. 652*

pelvic tilt A standing position whereby the pelvis is tilted by tightening the stomach muscles and flattening out the small of the back. *p. 494*

penetrating wound An open wound in which skin and underlying tissues are pierced. *p. 463*

percussion hammer An instrument used to tap body parts to test reflexes. Also known as a **reflex hammer**. *p. 1039*

percutaneous endoscopic gastrostomy (PEG) tube A tube inserted into the stomach (*gastro*) through a puncture wound (*stomy*) made through (*per*) the skin (*cutaneous*); a lighted instrument (*scope*) allows the physician to see inside the body cavity or organ (*endo*). *p. 601*

perineal care (pericare) Cleansing of the genital and anal areas. *p. 642*

peripheral Away from the centre of the body. *p. 273*

peristalsis The smooth muscle contraction that involuntarily pushes food forward in the digestive tract in one direction in a wavelike motion. *p. 293*

peri-wash A type of gentle soap for skin. It is used primarily as a cleanser and deodorizer of the perineal area soiled by urine and feces. *p. 480*

persistent illness An ongoing illness or disability, slow or gradual in onset, that may or may not grow worse over time. Also known as a **chronic illness**. *p. 35*

persistent pain Pain that lasts longer than 6 months; it may be constant or occur off and on. Also known as **chronic pain**. *p. 178*

personal empowerment Understanding and accepting that you can make your own healthy lifestyle choices, free from the influences of others. *p. 54*

personality disorders A group of disorders involving rigid and socially unacceptable behaviours. *p. 796*

personal protective equipment (PPE) Special clothing and equipment that act as a barrier between microbes and a person's hands, eyes, nose, mouth, and clothes; includes gloves, gowns, masks, and eye protection. *p. 441*

personal space The area immediately around one's body. *p. 156*

phantom limb pain Pain felt in a body part that is no longer there. *p. 179*

phlebitis An inflammation of a vein. *p. 867*

physical abuse The deliberate application of force to any part of another person's body, which may result in a nonaccidental injury and sometimes death. *p. 259*

physical health Well-being in the physical dimension, achieved when the body is strong, fit, and free from disease. *p. 49*

physical neglect Failure to adequately meet a dependant's need for food, clothing, shelter, cleanliness, medical care, and protection from harm. *p. 260*

physical restraints Garments or devices used to restrict movement of the whole body or parts of the body. *p. 396*

picture-frame dressing A type of dressing in which tape is applied to all four edges to reduce the likelihood of the dressing wrinkling or falling off. *p. 484*

pink eye See **conjunctivitis**. *p. 362*

pitting edema A type of edema that is evident by an impression left in the skin upon compressing the fingers into the swollen tissues and then removing the fingers. *p. 473*

pivot joints Joints that allow turning from side to side. *p. 280*

planning Establishing priorities and goals and developing measures or actions to help the client meet the goals; a step in the care-planning process. *p. 203*

plantar flexion The foot (*plantar*) is bent (*flexion*) with the toes pointed away from the leg. *p. 539*

PM care See **HS care**. *p. 613*

pneumonia Infection of the lung tissue. *p. 867*

podiatrist A physician who specializes in the evaluation and treatment of diseases of the foot. *p. 665*

pollutant A harmful chemical or substance in air or water. *p. 931*

polypharmacy The use of more medications by a client than is medically required. *p. 990*

polyuria The production of abnormally large amounts (*poly*) of urine (*uria*). *p. 692*

portability A principle of the *Canada Health Act* that states that residents continue to be entitled to coverage from their home province even when they live in a different province or territory or outside the country. *p. 24*

portfolio A binder containing the applicant's certificates, letters of recommendation, awards, proof of volunteering, or other pertinent information. *p. 1082*

positive reinforcement Encouraging a behaviour by rewarding the desired behaviour after it is demonstrated. *p. 363*

posterior The back surface of the body—often used to indicate the position of one structure to another. Also called **dorsal**. *p. 196*

postmortem care Care of the body after *(post)* death *(mortem)*. *p. 1070*

postoperative After surgery. *p. 1049*

postpartum After (*post*) childbirth (*partum*). *p. 322*

postpartum blues Feelings of sadness or mild depression in the mother during the first 2 weeks after childbirth; *baby blues*. *p. 325*

postpartum depression Major depression in the mother at any point during the first year after childbirth. *p. 326*

postpartum psychosis The most severe form of postpartum depression; the mother may experience delusions, hallucinations, and suicidal thoughts. *p. 326*

postural hypotension See **orthostatic hypotension**. *p. 536*

posture See **body alignment**. *p. 493*

power of attorney See **substitute decision maker for health care**. *p. 138*

prefix A word element placed at the beginning of a word to change the meaning of the word. *p. 191*

prejudice An attitude that forms an opinion about a person based on his or her membership in a group. *p. 150*

preoperative Before surgery. *p. 1045*

presbycusis The gradual hearing (*cusis*) loss associated with aging (*presby*). *p. 914*

presbyopia The gradual inability to focus (*opia*) on close objects; a condition associated with aging (*presby*). *p. 921*

preschool Ages 3 to 5 years; characterized by gaining an increasing ability to communicate and understand others, becoming able to perform self-care activities, learning the differences between the genders, learning to distinguish right from wrong, learning to play with others, and developing family relationships. *p. 308*

prescription (Rx) medication A medication that is prescribed by a physician and dispensed by a pharmacist. *p. 991*

pressure points Bony prominences that bear the weight of the body in certain positions and may lead to **pressure ulcers**. *p. 465*

pressure sore See **pressure ulcer**. *p. 465*

pressure ulcer Any injury caused by unrelieved pressure. Also known as **decubitus ulcer**, **bedsore**, or **pressure sore**. *p. 465*

primary caregiver A person—usually a family member or close friend—who assumes the responsibilities of caring for a dependent person, usually in the person's home. *p. 168*

primary care nurse A primary care nurse is responsible for the ongoing management of the health of a client. Duties include liaising with other health care team members, the client, and her or his family. *p. 13*

primary dementia Dementia that does not result from any other disease. *p. 810*

primary health care delivery The first point of contact people have with the health care system. It could be through a doctor, a nurse, or another health care provider or perhaps through phone- or computer-based services. *p. 25*

primary prevention strategies Strategies that are aimed at preventing a disease or illness by reducing its risk factors. *p. 56*

professional boundaries Appropriate limitations on behaviour, meant to protect the vulnerable client from the caregiver who has access to private knowledge about him or her. *p. 163*

professionalism An approach to work that demonstrates respect for others, commitment, competence, and appropriate behaviour. *p. 14*

prognosis The expected course of recovery, which may range from full recovery to death, based on the usual outcome of the illness. *p. 57*

projection Blaming someone else for one's own behaviour. *p. 79*

pronation Turning downward. *p. 539*

prone position A front-lying position on the abdomen, with the head turned to one side. *p. 512*

prostheses (singular, *prosthesis*) Artificial replacements for missing body parts. *p. 561*

proximal Nearest to the trunk of the body or the point of origin. *p. 196*

proxy See **substitute decision maker for health care**. *p. 138*

pseudo-dementia False (*pseudo*) dementia. Pseudo-dementia occurs when severe depression causes cognitive changes that mimic dementia. *p. 814*

psoriasis A persistent skin disorder that affects the skin and joints. It commonly causes red scaly patches to appear on the skin. *p. 848*

psychiatric care services See **mental health care services**. *p. 36*

psychiatric disorder See **mental health disorder**. *p. 770*

psychological abuse See **emotional abuse**. *p. 254*

psychosis A mental state in which a person's perception of reality is impaired. *p. 778*

psychosocial health Well-being in the social, emotional, intellectual, and spiritual dimensions of one's life. *p. 173*

psychotherapy A form of therapy in which a client explores thoughts, feelings, and behaviours with help and guidance from a mental health specialist. *p. 774*

puberty The period when the reproductive organs begin to function and secondary sex characteristics appear. *p. 312*

public administration A principle of the *Canada Health Act* that states that provincial health insurance must be administered by a public authority on a nonprofit basis. *p. 24*

pulse The beat of the heart felt at an artery as a wave of blood passes through the artery. *p. 236*

pulse oximeter A device that measures both a client's pulse rate and the oxygen level in the blood. *p. 239*

pulse rate The number of heartbeats or pulses felt in 1 minute. *p. 236*

puncture wound An open wound made by a sharp object; entry into skin and underlying tissues may be intentional or unintentional. *p. 463*

purulent drainage Thick drainage from a wound or body orifice, which may have a foul odour; purulent drainage is yellow, green, or brown and may indicate an infection. *p. 478*

pyelonephritis Inflammation of the kidney and renal pelvis because of bacterial infection. *p. 872*

quadriplegia Paralysis (*plegia*) of all four (*quad*) limbs and the trunk; paralysis from the neck down. *p. 862*

racism Feelings of superiority over, and intolerance or prejudice toward, a person or group of people who may have different physical appearances or cultural practices. *p. 149*

radiating pain Pain that is felt not just at the site of tissue damage but extends to nearby areas. *p. 178*

range of motion (ROM) Moving a joint to the extent possible without causing pain. *p. 538*

rationalization Justifying a behaviour or action by explaining it as being less harmful or hurtful than it really is. *p. 79*

razor bumps See **ingrown hair**. *p. 661*

reactive depression A term that some health care providers use to describe normal reactions, such as feelings of loss and sadness in response to what a person has just experienced. *p. 781*

receptive aphasia Difficulty understanding language. *p. 903*

record See **chart**. *p. 210*

reference A person who can speak to a potential employer about the applicant's skills, abilities, and personal qualities. *p. 1083*

referred pain Pain that is felt in a part of the body separate from the source of the pain. *p. 178*

reflective practice review A review and self-evaluation of care provided with the goal of identifying ways to improve clinical performance and caregiving. *p. 11*

reflex An involuntary movement in response to a stimulus. *p. 306*

reflex hammer See **percussion hammer**. *p. 1039*

reflex incontinence The loss of urine at predictable intervals. *p. 700*

regional anaesthesia The loss of sensation or feeling in a large area of the body, produced by the injection of a medication. *p. 1049*

registered nurse (RN) A health care provider who is licensed and regulated by the province or territory to maintain overall responsibility for the planning and provision of client care. *p. 11*

registered practical nurse (RPN) See **licensed practical nurse**. *p. 13*

registered psychiatric nurse (RPN) A nurse who is educated and registered in his or her own province to provide care specifically to individuals whose primary needs relate to mental, emotional, and developmental health. *p. 13*

regression A return to an earlier developmental stage as a way to escape from stress. *p. 79*

regulations Detailed rules that implement the requirements of a legislative act. *p. 131*

regurgitation The backward flow of food from the stomach into the mouth. *p. 603*

rehabilitation The process of restoring a person to the highest possible level of functioning through the use of therapy, exercise, or other methods. *p. 10*

rehabilitation services Methods, therapies, and educational programs used to restore or improve the client's independence and functional abilities. *p. 35*

relationship The connection between two or more people, shaped by the roles, feelings, and interactions of those involved. *p. 163*

remission A period when the signs and symptoms of a disease lessen or disappear. *p. 779*

renal calculi Kidney (*renal*) stones (*calculi*). *p. 872*

repression The involuntary action of blocking painful memories from the conscious mind. *p. 79*

reservoir The environment in which microbes live and grow; host. *p. 423*

resident A person living in a **residential facility** (often called a *long-term care facility*). *p. 9*

residential facility A facility that provides living accommodations and services; includes assisted-living facilities, long-term care facilities, group homes, and retirement residences. *p. 9*

respect Acceptance and regard for another person. *p. 165*

respiration The act of breathing air into (inhalation) and out of (exhalation) the lungs. *p. 240*

respiratory arrest Stoppage of breathing. *p. 930*

respiratory depression Slow, weak respirations at a rate of fewer than 12 per minute; respirations are not deep enough to bring enough air into the lungs. *p. 930*

respite care Temporary care of a person who requires a high level of support, care, and supervision; respite care gives caregivers a break from their duties. *p. 35*

restorative care Care that is aimed at re-establishing a client's sense of independence to its greatest potential. *p. 35*

restraint Any device, garment, barrier, furniture, or medication that limits or restricts freedom of movement or access to one's own body. *p. 388*

resumé A concise one- to two-page summary of experience, education, work-related skills, and personal qualities. *p. 1077*

retention catheter See **in-dwelling catheter**. *p. 702*

retinal detachment The separation of the retina from its supporting tissue. *p. 920*

retirement home A facility in which older adults who are independently mobile can live independently but receive hospitality services such as meals and housekeeping services (also known as an **assisted-living facility** or **supportive housing facility**). *p. 36*

Reye's syndrome A rare but potentially fatal disease causing inflammation of the brain, which can occur during the recovery stage of flu or chicken pox. It has been seen in children who take Aspirin. *p. 358*

RICE An acronym for "**R**est, **I**ce, **C**ompression, and **E**levate" as a method of treating recent injuries. *p. 1026*

right Something to which a person is justly entitled. *p. 130*

rigor mortis The stiffness or rigidity *(rigor)* of skeletal muscles that occurs after death *(mortis)*. *p. 1071*

root A word element containing the basic meaning of the word. *p. 193*

rotation Turning of the joint. *p. 539*

route How a medication enters and is absorbed by the body. *p. 987*

Routine Practices See **Standard Practices**. *p. 444*

saddle joint Joints that allow for a wide range of motion between two articulating saddle-shaped bones, such as at the base of the thumb. *p. 280*

same-sex family A family in which both adults who live together in a loving, intimate relationship are of the same gender. *p. 154*

sanguineous drainage Bloody drainage. *p. 478*

scabies A highly contagious skin infection caused by a mite. *p. 845*

schizophrenia spectrum disorders An extremely complex group of mental health disorders characterized by delusions, hallucinations, disturbances in thinking, and withdrawal from social activity. *p. 778*

scleroderma A progressive autoimmune disease that involves the hardening (*sclero*) of the skin (*derma*) and connective tissue throughout the body. *p. 849*

scope of practice The legal limits and extent of a health care worker's role. Scope of practice in a health care field varies from province to province and employer to employer. *p. 11*

seborrheic keratosis A noncancerous skin growth that is common in older adults. *p. 849*

secondary dementia Dementia that occurs as a result of a physical disease, ingestion of damaging substances, or injury. *p. 810*

secondary health care delivery An intermediate level of health care that includes diagnosis and treatment. It is performed in a hospital that has specialized equipment and laboratory facilities. *p. 25*

seizure Brief disturbance in the brain's normal electrical function; affects awareness, movement, and sensation. *p. 894*

self-actualization Realizing one's full potential. *p. 176*

self-awareness Understanding of one's own feelings, moods, attitudes, preferences, biases, qualities, and limitations. *p. 166*

self-determination See **autonomy**. *p. 123*

self-esteem Thinking well of oneself and being well thought of by others. *p. 167*

semi-Fowler's position A semi-sitting position in bed; the head of the bed is elevated 30 to 45 degrees. *p. 510*

serosanguineous drainage Thin, watery drainage that is blood-tinged (*sanguineous*). *p. 478*

serous drainage Drainage that is a clear and watery fluid. *p. 478*

sexism Feelings of intolerance or prejudice toward a person or group of people because of their gender. *p. 152*

sexual abuse Any nonconsensual sexual act (including touching) that results from a threat, coercion, or force. *p. 254*

sexual harassment Any conduct, comment, gesture, threat, or suggestion that is sexual in nature; a form of **sexual** abuse. *p. 254*

sexually transmitted infections (STIs) Diseases that are spread through sexual contact. *p. 881*

sharps Equipment or items that may pierce the skin; include needles, razor blades, and broken glass. *p. 446*

shearing Tearing of skin tissue caused when the skin sticks to a surface (usually the bed or chair) and deeper tissues move downward, exerting pressure on the skin. *p. 464*

shingles A viral infection causing a painful rash of raised blisters, which can appear anywhere on the body, usually on one side. It is caused by the same virus that causes chicken pox. *p. 845*

shock The condition that results when there is not enough blood supply to organs and tissues. *p. 476*

side effect A response to a medication that occurs in addition to the intended or main response. *p. 995*

signs Information about a client's health gained through observation and the use of other senses. Also known as *objective data*. *p. 207*

Sims' position A left-side-lying position; the right leg is sharply flexed so that it is not on the left leg, and the left arm is positioned along the client's back. *p. 512*

single-parent families Families in which the adult head of the household does not have a partner who shares the home. *p. 154*

sitz bath A shallow plastic bathtub, filled with warm water, designed to keep the buttocks and hips immersed while the person is in the sitting position. *p. 1020*

skin tear A break or rip in skin; the epidermis separates from the underlying tissue. *p. 463*

slander The making of false verbal statements that hurt the reputation of a person. *p. 143*

sleep–wake disorders Conditions in which repetitive disturbed sleep patterns lead to distress and impairment in that person's daytime functioning. *p. 790*

slider Item (including *slider sheet*, *slider board*, and *slider sheet system*) made of low-friction material with handles and used to move clients. *p. 498*

sliding pad See **turning pad**. *p. 497*

slipper pan See **fracture pan**. *p. 691*

SOB Acronym for "short of breath." *p. 929*

SOBOE Acronym for "short of breath on exertion." *p. 929*

social health Well-being in the social dimension, achieved when people have stable and satisfying relationships. *p. 50*

social media Websites and applications through which users create virtual communities or networks to share information, ideas, personal messages, and other content. *p. 69*

social reintegration See **social support**. *p. 4*

social support Equipping a person with the skills and knowledge necessary to successfully live independently outside an institution. Also known as **social reintegration**. *p. 4*

social support system An informal group of people who help each other or others outside the group. *p. 50*

solicited letter of application A letter of application that responds to an advertised position. *p. 1083*

spastic Uncontrolled contractions of skeletal muscle and smooth muscle. *p. 893*

specific immunity The ability of an organism to resist or overcome an infection or illness against a *certain* disease or infection caused by a pathogen or antigenic substance. *p. 300*

sphygmomanometer The instrument used to measure blood pressure. *p. 243*

spina bifida A congenital disorder caused by improper closing of the spine before birth. *p. 894*

spiritual health Well-being in the spiritual dimension achieved through the belief in a purpose greater than the self. *p. 51*

SpO_2 Peripheral capillary oxygen saturation; the reading given by a pulse oximeter for the percentage of oxygen-saturated hemoglobin that is dissolved in the blood. *p. 239*

spousal abuse Abuse of a partner by a partner in an intimate relationship such as a marriage or common-law relationship. *p. 256*

sputum Mucus from the respiratory system that is expectorated (expelled) through the mouth. *p. 946*

Standard Practices Guidelines to prevent the spread of infection from blood, body fluids, secretions, excretions, non-intact skin, and mucous membranes. Also known as **Routine Practices** or **Standard Precautions**. *p. 444*

Standard Precautions See **Standard Practices**. *p. 444*

stasis ulcer See **venous ulcer**. *p. 473*

stereotype An overly simple or exaggerated view of a group of people. *p. 151*

sterile Free of all microbes, both pathogens and nonpathogens, as well as their spores. *p. 435*

sterile field A work area free of all microbes, both pathogens and nonpathogens. *p. 455*

sterile technique See **surgical asepsis**. *p. 435*

sterilization The process of destroying *all* microbes. *p. 435*

Steri-Strip A proprietary type of adhesive bandage; thin strips are applied across a skin tear to bring the skin edges together and hold them together while the wound heals. *p. 464*

stethoscope An instrument used to listen to the sounds produced by the heart, lungs, and other body organs. *p. 244*

stigma Social disgrace associated with a particular circumstance, quality, or person that causes one to feel shame or embarrassment—for example, "the stigma of being fired from a job." *p. 60*

stoma A surgically created opening from a portion of the body cavity to the outside environment. *p. 724*

stool Excreted feces. *p. 731*

straight catheter A catheter that is inserted to drain the bladder and is then removed. *p. 702*

strep throat A throat that is infected with **streptococci**. *p. 362*

streptococci (singular, *streptococcus*) A type of bacteria that cause **strep throat** and other medical issues. *p. 364*

stress The emotional, behavioural, or physical response to an event or situation. *p. 101*

stress incontinence The leaking of urine during exercise and certain movements. *p. 700*

stressor An event or situation that causes stress. *p. 101*

stroke Sudden loss of brain function because of the disruption of blood supply to the brain. Also known as *cerebral vascular accident (CVA)*. *p. 515*

subacute care See **complex continuing care**. *p. 35*

subjective data See **symptoms**. *p. 207*

submissiveness A show of obedience, meekness, and compliance in the face of conflict or a difference of opinion, instead of assertiveness. *p. 79*

substance-related and addictive disorder The deliberate misuse of and inability to stop the abuse of prescription medications, illegal drugs, alcohol, or other substances. *p. 795*

substitute decision maker for health care A person authorized to make health care decisions on behalf of a living person who is unable to do so. Also called **power of attorney** for health care or **proxy** depending on the province. *p. 138*

substitute decision maker for property The person who would represent an incapable person's interests regarding his or her belongings. *p. 139*

suctioning The process of withdrawing or sucking up fluid (secretions). *p. 952*

sudden infant death syndrome (SIDS) The sudden, unexplained death of an apparently healthy infant under 1 year of age. *p. 329*

suffix A word element placed at the end of a root to change the meaning of the word. *p. 194*

suffocation A lack of oxygen that causes breathing to stop. *p. 402*

suicidal behaviour disorder A disorder whose main trait is recurrent thoughts about or a preoccupation with ending one's own life. *p. 791*

sundowning A condition in which the signs, symptoms, and behaviours of dementia increase at bedtime or during hours of darkness. *p. 830*

superficial Near the surface of the body. *p. 273*

superior Situated above another structure or toward the upper part of the body. *p. 273*

supervising Being responsible for monitoring and overseeing the activities of others on the health care team. *p. 91*

supination Turning upward. *p. 539*

supine position A back-lying position; the legs are together. Also called *dorsal recumbent position* or *horizontal position*. *p. 511*

supportive housing facility See **assisted-living facility**. *p. 36*

support worker A health care worker who provides services to people, both in facilities and in the community, who need help with their daily activities. *p. 3*

suppository A cone-shaped, solid medication that is inserted into a body opening. *p. 736*

suppression A conscious refusal to acknowledge a painful or upsetting situation. *p. 79*

suprapubic catheter A catheter that is surgically inserted into the bladder through the abdomen. *p. 702*

surgical asepsis Practices that keep equipment and supplies free of *all* microbes. Also known as **sterile technique**. *p. 435*

sympathy Feeling compassion for or understanding the difficulties of another person. *p. 165*

symptoms Information reported by a client that cannot be directly observed by others. Also known as **subjective** data. *p. 207*

syncope A brief loss of consciousness; fainting. *p. 536*

systole The period of heart muscle contraction. *p. 241*

systolic pressure The amount of force required to pump blood out of the heart and into the arterial circulation. *p. 241*

tachycardia A rapid (*tachy*) heart rate (*cardia*); a rate over 100 beats per minute in an adult. *p. 237*

tachypnea Rapid (*tachy*) breathing (*pnea*); respirations are 24 or more per minute. *p. 932*

tartar Hardened biofilm on teeth. *p. 613*

task A function, procedure, or activity that a support worker assists with or performs for the client. *p. 92*

team leader See **case manager**. *p. 91*

Telehealth Medical telephone call centres through which nurses give advice to callers about health concerns. *p. 25*

tertiary health care delivery The specialized, highly technical level of health care that takes place in large research and teaching hospitals. *p. 25*

therapeutic effect Causing a desired, positive effect in the body. *p. 995*

thrombus A blood clot that forms in a blood vessel, which has the potential to become an **embolus**. *p. 1050*

thrush A common yeast infection that resembles cottage cheese or milk curds and is found on the sides and roof of the baby's mouth and sometimes the tongue. *p. 330*

tinnitus Ringing in the ear. *p. 914*

tissue A group of similar cells with a common function. *p. 274*

toddlerhood Ages 1 to 3 years; characterized by tolerating separation from the primary caregiver, gaining control of bowel and bladder functions, using words to communicate, and starting to assert independence. *p. 307*

tonic–clonic seizure A seizure involving convulsions. *p. 894*

tort A wrongful act committed by an individual against another person or the person's property. *p. 140*

toxic shock syndrome (TSS) A rare, often life-threatening, illness that develops suddenly after an infection. *p. 323*

tracheostomy A surgically created opening (*ostomy*) through the neck into the trachea (*tracheo*). *p. 950*

trade name of a drug The name given to a drug by the manufacturer. Also known as the *proprietary name*. *p. 992*

transfer To move a person from one place to another, using the client's assistance with partial to full weight-bearing. *p. 514*

transfer belt A strong strap that is secured around the client's waist or hips to help and support the client to stand, sit, and walk. It is removed after the activity is completed. *p. 516*

transfer board A smooth board placed between two surfaces (e.g., a chair and a wheelchair) that allows the client to slide over more easily. *p. 518*

transfer of function A process by which a nurse authorizes another health care provider to perform certain tasks. *p. 92*

transgender A person's gender identity differing from that person's physical sex characteristics. *p. 152*

transient ischemic attack (TIA) A temporary interruption of blood flow to the brain. *p. 858*

Transmission-Based Practices Guidelines to contain pathogens within a certain area, usually the client's room. *p. 445*

trauma An accident or violent act that injures skin, mucous membranes, bones, or internal organs (*physical trauma*) or causes an emotionally painful, distressful, or shocking result (*emotional trauma*), which often leads to lasting mental and physical effects (*psychological trauma*). *p. 462*

traumatic brain injury See **acquired brain injury (ABI)**. *p. 776*

tuberculosis (TB) A persistent bacterial infection generally transmitted by the inhalation or ingestion of infected droplets and usually affecting the lungs, although infection of multiple organ systems occurs. *p. 432*

tumour A new growth of abnormal cells that could be **malignant** or **benign**. *p. 876*

tuning fork An instrument used to test hearing. *p. 1039*

turning pad A small pad or folded sheet placed on top of the bottom sheet and extending from the client's head to above the knees. Also known as a **sliding pad**, *turning sheet*, *transfer sheet*, or *lift pad*. A turning pad is sometimes (inaccurately) referred to as a *drawsheet*. *p. 497*

umbilical cord The structure that carries blood, oxygen, and nutrients from the mother to the fetus. *p. 339*

unethical Not morally correct. *p. 118*

unintentional wound A wound resulting from trauma. *p. 463*

universality A principle of the *Canada Health Act* that states that all residents are entitled to the same basic level of health care services across the country. *p. 24*

unregulated care providers (UCPs) A broad term applied to staff members who assist nurses and other health care providers in giving care. *p. 11*

unsolicited letter of application A letter of application that inquires about potential openings. *p. 1083*

upper respiratory infections (URIs) The medical term for colds and other viral illnesses that affect the throat, nose, and sinuses. *p. 363*

ureterostomy An artificial opening (*stomy*) between the ureter (*uretero*) and the abdomen. *p. 724*

urge incontinence The loss of urine in response to a sudden, urgent need to void. *p. 700*

urgent surgery Surgery that must be done soon to prevent further damage, disability, or disease. *p. 1043*

urinary frequency The need to urinate at frequent intervals. *p. 692*

urinary incontinence The inability to control the passage of urine from the bladder; the loss of bladder control. *p. 692*

urinary tract infection (UTI) An infection in the urinary system. *p. 871*

urinary urgency The need to void immediately. *p. 692*

urination The process of emptying urine from the bladder. Also known as **micturition** or **voiding**. *p. 690*

urticaria A common skin condition characterized by raised, usually itchy **wheals**. It is commonly caused by an allergic reaction to food, food additives, or drugs. Also known as **hives**. *p. 845*

vaccine A suspension containing a live (attenuated) or killed bacterium or virus that is administered for the purpose of inducing active immunity to a specific infectious disease. Vaccines are available in either oral or injectable suspensions. *p. 423*

vaginal speculum An instrument used to open the vagina so that it and the cervix can be examined. *p. 1039*

validate To acknowledge, recognize, or confirm the client's feelings. *p. 105*

validation therapy A type of therapy for people with dementia that focuses on empathy and advocates accepting the affected person's perception of reality. *p. 828*

values What an individual considers to be worthwhile or desirable qualities in a person. *p. 118*

vancomycin-resistant *Enterococcus* (VRE) A type of multidrug-resistant organism made up of bacterium. *p. 425*

vascular ulcer See **circulatory ulcer**. *p. 473*

vector An organism that spreads infection by transmitting pathogens from one host to another but is not the cause of the infection. *p. 430*

veins Blood vessels that carry blood back to the heart. *p. 289*

venous ulcer Open wounds on the lower legs and feet caused by poor blood return through the veins. Also known as **stasis ulcer**. *p. 473*

ventilator A machine used to provide airflow into and out of the lungs. *p. 954*

ventral See **anterior**. *p. 195*

venules The smallest form of veins. The venules drain blood from the capillaries and come together to form the veins. *p. 289*

verbal communication Messages sent through the spoken word. *p. 70*

verbal report A spoken account of care provided and observations made. *p. 209*

vertigo Dizziness. *p. 914*

viruses Infectious particles that are much smaller than bacteria and infect living cells to grow and multiply. *p. 423*

vital signs Temperature, pulse, respirations, and blood pressure (and SpO_2 if possible). *p. 225*

voiding See **urination**. *p. 690*

waterless, alcohol-based hand rubs Hand hygiene products that are rubbed into the hands and then allowed to dry completely, thereby killing most microbes on the skin's surface in seconds. Also called *waterless antiseptic handwash*. *p. 436*

weight-bear To shift body weight onto feet while attempting to stand. *p. 514*

wellness The achievement of the best health possible in all dimensions of one's life. *p. 52*

Wernicke–Korsakoff syndrome A brain disorder that is caused by lack of thiamine (vitamin B_1); affects the nervous system, including the brain; and is usually associated with heavy alcohol consumption over a long period. *p. 813*

wheal A circular, red, spongy lesion that evolves (develops) and changes over minutes to hours. It is usually surrounded by an area of redness called a *flare*. *p. 845*

wheat bag (or beanbag) A type of heating bag that provides dry heat and is heated in a microwave. *p. 1018*

will A legal document stating a person's wishes concerning the distribution or disposal of his or her property. *p. 139*

word element A part of a word. *p. 191*

workplace bullying Acts or verbal comments that could mentally "hurt" or isolate a person in the workplace. *p. 267*

workplace etiquette Professional, ethical, friendly, and respectful behaviour toward all staff and co-workers at all times. *p. 70*

Workplace Hazardous Materials Information System (WHMIS) A national system that provides safety information about hazardous materials; includes labelling, material safety data sheets (MSDSs), and employee education. *p. 411*

workplace violence Any physical assault or threatening behaviour that occurs in a work setting that is directed toward clients, members of the health care team, or both. *p. 413*

wound A break in the skin or mucous membrane. *p. 462*

young adulthood Ages approximately 18 to 40 years; characterized by choosing an education and an occupation, selecting and learning to live with a partner, becoming a parent and raising children, and developing a satisfactory sex life. *p. 314*

References

CHAPTER 1

1. The Association of Canadian Community Colleges and the Canadian Association of Continuing Care Educators. (2012). *Canadian educational standards for personal care providers.* Retieved from <https://www.collegesinstitutes.ca/wp-content/uploads/2014/05/Reference-Guide_Canadian-Educational-Standards-for-Personal-Care-Providers_ACCC.pdf>.
2. Kernisan, L., & Spencer Scott, P. (2014). *Activities of daily living: What are ADLs and IADLs?* Retrieved from <http://www.caring.com/articles/activities-of-daily-living-what-are-adls-and-iadls>.

CHAPTER 2

1. Payne, E. (2014). Could new approach to seniors save Canada's health-care system? Top doctor says yes. *Ottawa Citizen,* Retrieved from <http://ottawacitizen.com/news/national/could-new-approach-to-seniors-save-canadas-health-care-system-top-doctor-says-yes> November 18.
2. National Collaborating Centre for Aboriginal Health. (2011). *Access to health services as a social determinant of First Nations, Inuit, and Métis health.* Retrieved from <http://www.nccah-ccnsa.ca/docs/fact%20sheets/social%20determinates/Access%20to%20Health%20Services_Eng%202010.pdf>.
3. Health Canada. (2012). *First Nations health status report—Alberta region 2010–2011.* Retrieved from <http://publications.gc.ca/collections/collection_2012/sc-hc/H26-4-2011-eng.pdf>.
4. Health Canada. (2012). *Canada's health care system.* Retrieved from <http://www.hc-sc.gc.ca/hcs-sss/pubs/system-regime/2011-hcs-sss/index-eng.php#a5>.
5. Health Canada. (2008). Funded health programs and services. *First Nations & Inuit health.* Retrieved from <http://www.hc-sc.gc.ca/fniah-spnia/finance/agree-accord/prog/index-eng.php>.
6. Torrey, T. (2016). *Levels of medical care: Primary, secondary, tertiary and quaternary care.* Retrieved from <http://patients.about.com/od/moreprovidersbeyonddocs/a/Stages-Of-Care-Primary-Secondary-Tertiary-And-Quaternary-Care.htm>.
7. Canadian Centre for Occupational Health and Safety. (2012). *Aging workers.* Retrieved from <https://www.ccohs.ca/oshanswers/psychosocial/aging_workers.html>.
8. CBC News. (2013). *Officials seek solutions to chronic hospital bed shortage.* Retrieved from <http://www.cbc.ca/news/canada/thunder-bay/officials-seek-solutions-to-chronic-hospital-bed-shortage-1.1359672>.
9. Health Canada. (2015). *First Nations and Inuit health: Contribution agreements.* Retrieved from <http://www.hc-sc.gc.ca/fniah-spnia/finance/agree-accord/index-eng.php>.
10. Potter, P., Perry, A., Stockert, P., et al. (2014). *Canadian fundamentals of nursing* (5th ed.). Toronto, ON: Elsevier Canada.

CHAPTER 3

1. B.C. Seniors Living Association. (n.d.). *Frequently asked questions.* Retrieved from <http://www.bcsla.ca/about/faq/>.
2. Lilly, M. B. (2008). Medical versus social workplaces: Constructing and compensating the personal support worker across health care settings in Ontario, Canada. *Gender, Place & Culture, 15*(3), 285–299.

CHAPTER 4

1. World Health Organization. (1994). *Global strategy on occupational health for all: The way to health at work.* Retrieved from <http://www.who.int/occupational_health/publications/globstrategy/en/index2.html>.
2. Centre for Addiction and Mental Health. (2007). *Low-risk drinking guidelines.* Retrieved from <http://www.camh.ca/en/hospital/health_information/a_z_mental_health_and_addiction_information/alcohol/Pages/low_risk_drinking_guidelines.aspx>.
3. Nuu-chah-nulth Tribal Council. (2007). *Nuu-chah-nulth nursing program.* Retrieved from <http://www.nuuchahnulth.org/tribal-council/nursing.html>.
4. Lalonde, M. (1974). *Toward a healthy future: Second report on the health of Canadians.* Ottawa: Government of Canada. Retrieved from <http://publications.gc.ca/collections/Collection/H39-468-1999E.pdf>.
5. Public Health Agency of Canada. (2004). *What determines health?* Retrieved from <http://www.phac-aspc.gc.ca/ph-sp/determinants/index-eng.php#key_determinants>.
6. World Health Organization. (2016). Environmental health. *Health topics.* Retrieved from <http://www.who.int/topics/environmental_health/en/>.
7. Health Canada. (2009). *Environmental and workplace health.* Retrieved from <http://www.hc-sc.gc.ca/ewh-semt/index-eng.php>.
8. World Health Organization. (2015). *The right to health* [Fact sheet no. 323]. Retrieved from <http://www.who.int/mediacentre/factsheets/fs323/en/>.

CHAPTER 5

1. Bauerlein, M. (2009). Why Gen-Y Johnny can't read nonverbal cues. *Wall Street Journal.* Retrieved from <http://online.wsj.com/articles/SB10001424052970203863204574348493483201758>.
2. Tardanico, S. (2012). Is social media sabotaging real communication? *Forbes.* Retrieved from <http://www.forbes.com/sites/susantardanico/2012/04/30/is-social-media-sabotaging-real-communication/>.
3. *Mosby's dictionary of medicine, nursing and health professions* (9th ed., p. 495). (2013). St. Louis, MO: Elsevier, Mosby.
4. Hosley, J., & Molle, E. (2006). *A practical guide to therapeutic communication for health professionals* (pp. 117–119). St. Louis, MO: Elsevier, Mosby.

CHAPTER 6

1. *Regulated Health Professions Act*, S.O. 1991, c. 18. Retrieved from <http://www.ontario.ca/laws/statute/91r18>.
2. College of Nurses of Ontario. (2013). *Working with unregulated care providers.* Retrieved from <http://www.cno.org/Global/docs/prac/41014_workingucp.pdf>.
3. College of Nurses of Ontario standards representative, personal communication, October 27, 2014.

CHAPTER 7

1. Health Canada. (2013). *Activity plan #3 (adults): Setting SMART goals.* Retrieved from http://www.hc-sc.gc.ca/fn-an/food-guide-aliment/educ-comm/toolkit-trousse/plan-3b-eng.php.

CHAPTER 8

1. ALS Society of Canada. (2011). *Home page.* Retrieved from <http://www.als.ca/en>.

CHAPTER 9

1. Province of British Columbia. (2004). *Community care and assisted living update, order in Council No. 476/04.* Retrieved January 25, 2008, from <http://www.health.gov.bc.ca/ccf/ccal/ccalaupda.html>.
2. *Long-Term Care Homes Act* (1994, c. 26, s. 3(1)). Retrieved from <https://www.ontario.ca/laws/statute/07l08>.
3. Canadian Mental Health Association. (2016). *Informed consent to treatment.* Retrieved from <http://www.cmha.ca/public_policy/informed-consent-to-treatment/>.
4. *Canadian Elder Law.* (n.d.). Retrieved from <http://www.canadianelderlaw.ca/Power%20of%20Attorney.htm>.

5. Government of Canada. (2015). *Access to information and privacy*. Retrieved from <http://www.tbs-sct.gc.ca/atip-aiprp/index-eng.asp>.
6. *Canadian Centre for Occupational Health and Safety*. (2016). *OH&S legislation in Canada: Basic responsibilities*. Retrieved from <http://www.ccohs.ca/oshanswers/legisl/responsi.html>.
7. Government of Canada. (2007). *Workers' rights in Canada*. Retrieved from <http://www.servicecanada.gc.ca/eng/about/publication/workers_rights.shtml>.

CHAPTER 10

1. Canadian Museum of Immigration at Pier 21. (2016). *Canadian Multiculturalism Act, 1988*. Retrieved from <http://www.pier21.ca/research/immigration-history/canadian-multiculturalism-act-1988>.
2. Taylor, C., Peter, T., McMinn, T. L., et al. (2011). *Every class in every school: The first national climate survey on homophobia, biphobia, and transphobia in Canadian schools. Final Report*. Toronto, ON: Eagle Canada Human Rights Trust.
3. Kim (personal communication), September 22, 2015.
4. Sorrentino, S. (1998). *Mosby's textbook for nursing assistants* (5th ed., p. 102). St. Louis, MO: Mosby.
5. Davidhizar, R. E., & Giger, J. N. (1998). *Canadian transcultural nursing: Assessment and intervention* (p. 115). St. Louis, MO: Mosby.
6. Davidhizar, R. E., & Giger, J. N. (1998). *Canadian transcultural nursing: Assessment and intervention* (p. 29). St. Louis, MO: Mosby.
7. Sorrentino, S. (1998). *Mosby's textbook for nursing assistants* (5th ed., p. 98). St. Louis, MO: Mosby.
8. Potter, P. A., Perry, A., Ross-Kerr, J. C., et al. (2001). *Canadian fundamentals of nursing* (p. 119). Toronto, ON: Harcourt Canada.
9. Davidhizar, R. E., & Giger, J. N. (1998). *Canadian transcultural nursing: Assessment and intervention* (p. 51). St. Louis, MO: Mosby.
10. Davidhizar, R. E., & Giger, J. N. (1998). *Canadian transcultural nursing: Assessment and intervention* (p. 31). St. Louis, MO: Mosby.
11. Davidhizar, R. E., & Giger, J. N. (1998). *Canadian transcultural nursing: Assessment and intervention* (p. 30). St. Louis, MO: Mosby.
12. Davidhizar, R. E., & Giger, J. N. (1998). *Canadian transcultural nursing: Assessment and intervention* (p. 28). St. Louis, MO: Mosby.

CHAPTER 11

1. College and Association of Registered Nurses of Alberta. (2011). *Professional boundaries for registered nurses: Guidelines for the nurse–client relationship*. Retrieved from <http://www.nurses.ab.ca/content/dam/carna/pdfs/DocumentList/Guidelines/RN_ProfessionalBoundaries_May2011.pdf>.

CHAPTER 12

1. Broadmead Care Society. (2012). *Dementia care program*. Retrieved from <http://www.broadmeadcare.com/lodge-broadmead/dementia-care-program>.

CHAPTER 14

1. Potter, P. A., Perry, A. G., Ross-Kerr, J. C., et al. (2010). *Canadian fundamentals of nursing* (Revised 4th ed., p. 170). Toronto, ON: Elsevier Canada.

CHAPTER 16

1. Wathen, C. N., & MacMillan, H. L. (2003). Prevention of violence against women: Recommendation statement from the Canadian task force on preventive health care. *Journal de l'association médicale canadienne, 169*(6), 582–584.
2. Public Health Agency of Canada. (2016, May). *The health and social impacts of family violence*. Retrieved from <http://www.phac-aspc.gc.ca/sfv-avf/info/fv-social-impact-eng.php>.
3. Canadian Children's Rights Council. (n.d.). *Child abuse and neglect—Canada statistics*. Retrieved from <http://www.canadiancrc.com/Child_Abuse/Child_Abuse.aspx>.
4. Government of Canada, Department of Justice. (2015). *Risk factors for children in situations of family violence in the context of separation and divorce*. Retrieved from <http://www.justice.gc.ca/eng/rp-pr/cj-jp/fv-vf/rfcsfv-freevf/p4.html>.

5. Abusewatch.net. (2010). *Factors that contribute to child abuse and neglect.* Retrieved from <http://abusewatch.net/res_factors.php>.
6. Hockenbury, M., Wilson, D., Winkelstein, M., et al. (2011). *Wong's nursing care of infants and children* (9th ed.). St. Louis, MO: Mosby.
7. MacDonald, P. L., Hornick, J. P., Robertson, G. B., et al. (1991). *Elder abuse and neglect in Canada* (p. 29). Toronto, ON: Butterworths.
8. Public Health Agency of Canada. (2009). *Abuse of older adults: Department of Justice Canada overview paper.* Retrieved from <http://publications.gc.ca/collections/collection_2009/justice/J2-354-2009E.pdf>.
9. Canadian Centre for Occupational Health and Safety. (2014). *Bullying in the workplace.* Retrieved from <http://www.ccohs.ca/oshanswers/psychosocial/bullying.html>.
10. Canadian Nurses Association and Canadian Federation of Nurses Unions. (n.d.). *Joint position statement: Workplace violence and bullying.* Retrieved from <http://cna-aiic.ca/~/media/cna/page-content/pdf-en/Workplace-Violence-and-Bullying_joint-position-statement.pdf>.

CHAPTER 17

1. Cardoso, S. H. (2001). *Communication between nerve cells.* Retrieved from <http://www.cerebromente.org.br/n12/fundamentos/neurotransmissores/neurotransmitters2.htm>.

CHAPTER 19

1. Healthwise. (2015). *Mastitis while breast-feeding.* Retrieved from <https://myhealth.alberta.ca/health/Pages/conditions.aspx?hwid=hw98039>.
2. La Leche League Canada. (n.d.). *Do I have to stop breastfeeding if I have mastitis?* Retrieved from <http://www.lllc.ca/category/faq-categories/common-concerns-and-challenges/breast-pain>.
3. Health Canada. (2000). *Family-centred maternity and newborn care: National guidelines* (p. 6.19). Ottawa, ON: Minister of Public Works and Government Services.
4. Sword, W., Busser, D., Gannon, R., et al. (2007). *Care of women following referral for probable postpartum depression. Strategies in Women's Health Care.* Symposium of the 18th International Nursing Research Congress Focusing on Evidence-Based Practice.
5. Health Canada. (2000). *Family-centred maternity and newborn care: National guidelines* (p. 6.21). Ottawa, ON: Minister of Public Works and Government Services.
6. Health Canada. (2007). *Routine practices and additional precautions for preventing the transmission of infection in health care. Canadian communicable disease report.* Toronto, ON: Author.
7. MyHealth.Alberta.ca. (2015). *Umbilical cord care.* Retrieved from <https://myhealth.alberta.ca/health/pages/conditions.aspx?hwId=tp22060spec>.
8. MyHealth.Alberta.ca. (2015). *Circumcision: What to expect after surgery.* Retrieved from <https://myhealth.alberta.ca/health/pages/conditions.aspx?hwid=hw142449&#hw142484>.

CHAPTER 20

1. Eat Right Ontario. (2016). *Helping you support healthy eating for your kids at home and at school.* Retrieved from <http://www.eatrightontario.ca/en/Articles/School-Health/Articles/Helping-you-support-healthy-eating-for-your-kids-a.aspx#.VxJqHU0UXcs>.
2. Pless, B., & Millar, W. (2000). *Unintentional injuries in childhood: Results from Canadian health surveys.* Ottawa: Minister of Public Works and Government Services. Retrieved from <http://publications.gc.ca/pub?id=9.647646&sl=0>.
3. Statistics Canada. (2015). *Leading causes of death of children and youth, by age group, 2006 to 2008.* Retrieved from <http://www.statcan.gc.ca/pub/11-402-x/2012000/chap/c-e/tbl/tbl05-eng.htm>.
4. National Institute of Child Health and Human Development. (2003). Retrieved from <http://www.cnn.com/HEALTH/9905/03/infant.deaths/>; Fire Prevention Canada. (n.d.). *Burns: The need for caution.* Retrieved from <http://www.fiprecan.ca/burns-the-need-for-caution/>.
5. Health Canada. (2006). *Reye's syndrome.* Retrieved from <http://hc-sc.gc.ca/hl-vs/iyh-vsv/diseases-maladies/reye-eng.php>.
6. Health Canada. (2006). *Reye's syndrome.* Retrieved from <http://www.hc-sc.gc.ca/hl-vs/iyh-vsv/diseases-maladies/reye-eng.php>.

7. Baby Centre. (2011). *When is your child too sick for daycare?* Retrieved from <http://www.babycenter.ca/baby/health/whentoosicknursery/>; MediResource. (n.d.). *Strep throat.* Retrieved from <http://bodyandhealth.canada.com/channel_condition_info_details.asp?disease_id=121&channel_id=1020&relation_id=70907>.
8. Ontario Ministry of Health and Long-Term Care. (2015). *Immunizations: Measles, mumps and rubella (MMR) vaccine.* Retrieved from <http://www.health.gov.on.ca/en/public/publications/immune/mmr.aspx>.
9. Born, K., Yiu, V., & Sullivan, T. (2014). *Provinces divided over mandatory vaccination for school children.* Retrieved from "Health Debate" <http://healthydebate.ca/2014/05/topic/health-promotion-disease-prevention/mandatory-school-entry-vaccinations>.

CHAPTER 21

1. Government of Canada. (2013). *Addressing the challenges and opportunities of ageing in Canada.* Retrieved from <http://www.esdc.gc.ca/eng/seniors/reports/aging.shtml>.
2. Service Canada. (2015). *Old age security—Overview.* Retrieved from <http://www.servicecanada.gc.ca/eng/services/pensions/oas/pension/index.shtml>.
3. Harvard Health. (2014). *Depression in older adults and the elderly.* Retrieved from <http://www.helpguide.org/articles/depression/depression-in-older-adults-and-the-elderly.htm>.
4. Canadian Psychological Association. (2014). *"Psychology works" fact sheet: Depression among seniors.* Retrieved from <http://www.cpa.ca/docs/File/Publications/FactSheets/PsychologyWorksFactSheet_DepressionAmongSeniors.pdf>.

CHAPTER 22

1. Public Health Agency of Canada. (2014). *Seniors' falls in Canada: Second report.* Retrieved from <http://www.phac-aspc.gc.ca/seniors-aines/publications/public/injury-blessure/seniors_falls-chutes_aines/assets/pdf/seniors_falls-chutes_aines-eng.pdf>.
2. Health Canada. (2015). *Workplace Hazardous Materials Information System (WHMIS).* Retrieved from <http://www.hc-sc.gc.ca/ewh-semt/occup-travail/whmis-simdut/index-eng.php>.

CHAPTER 23

1. Public Health Ontario. (2014). *Best practices for hand hygiene in all healthcare settings* (4th edition). Retrieved from <http://www.publichealthontario.ca/en/eRepository/2010-12%20BP%20Hand%20Hygiene.pdf>.
2. Public Health Agency of Canada. (2014). *Cyclospora spp: Pathogen safety data sheet.* Retrieved from <http://www.phac-aspc.gc.ca/lab-bio/res/psds-ftss/cyclospora-eng.php>.
3. Public Health Agency of Canada. (2012). *Frequently asked questions: Pandemic influenza preparedness.* Retrieved from <http://www.phac-aspc.gc.ca/influenza/pp-faq-eng.php>.
4. Public Health Agency of Canada. (2015). *Flu (influenza).* Retrieved from <http://healthycanadians.gc.ca/diseases-conditions-maladies-affections/disease-maladie/flu-grippe/index-eng.php>.
5. Alberta Health. (2016). *Influenza is the flu.* Retrieved from <http://www.health.alberta.ca/health-info/influenza.html>.
6. Alberta Health Services. (2013). *Surgical aseptic technique and sterile field: Guidelines for asepsis for invasive surgical procedures conducted in community-based settings.* Retrieved from <http://www.albertahealthservices.ca/assets/wf/eph/wf-eh-surgical-aseptic-technique-sterile-field.pdf>.
7. Public Health Ontario: Provincial Infectious Diseases Advisory Committee. (2014). *Best practices for hand hygiene in all health care settings* (4th ed.). Retrieved from <http://www.publichealthontario.ca/en/eRepository/2010-12%20BP%20Hand%20Hygiene.pdf>.

CHAPTER 25

1. HME Mobility and Accessibility. (n.d.). *Sit to stand lifts.* Retrieved from <http://www.hmebc.com/product-category/sit-to-stand-lifts/>.

CHAPTER 26

1. Disability Credit Canada. (n.d.). *Obesity and osteoarthritis: The cruellest of combinations.* Retrieved from <http://disabilitycreditcanada

.com/obesity-and-osteoarthritis-the-cruellest-of-combinations/>.

2. MediResources Inc. (n.d.). *Osteoarthritis*. Retrieved from <http://bodyandhealth.canada.com/channel_condition_info_details.asp?disease_id=97&channel_id=2053&relation_id=108101>.

CHAPTER 28

1. Health Canada. *Eating well with Canada's food guide*. Retrieved from <http://www.hc-sc.gc.ca/fn-an/food-guide-aliment/-index-eng.php>.
2. Health Canada. (2010). *Eating well with Canada's food guide—First Nations, Inuit and Métis*. Retrieved from <http://www.hc-sc.gc.ca/fn-an/food-guide-aliment/fnim-pnim/index-eng.php>.
3. Health Canada. (2012). *Caffeine in food*. Retrieved from <http://hc-sc.gc.ca/fn-an/securit/addit/caf/food-caf-aliments-eng.php>.
4. Nordqvist, C. (2016). *Celiac disease: Symptoms, Causes, Treatments*. Retrieved from <http://www.medicalnewstoday.com/articles/38085.php>.
5. Alberta Health Services. (2015). *Preparing thick fluids: A training program for supportive living sites*. Retrieved from <http://www.albertahealthservices.ca/assets/info/nutrition/if-nfs-notes-pages-preparing-thick-fluids-a-training-program-for-supportive-living-sites.pdf>.

CHAPTER 31

1. Dellinger, M. M. (2007). *Caring for your African American or biracial child's hair*. Retrieved from <http://adoption.about.com/od/africanamericanhaircare/ss/blackhaircare_2.htm>.
2. The Muslim Girl. (n.d.). *Hair care tips for hijabis*. Retrieved from <http://themuslimgirl.com/hair-care-tips-for-hijabis/>.
3. Shavers.co.uk. (2015). *Keep your shaver in tip top condition*. Retrieved from <http://www.shavers.co.uk/shavermaintenance.php>.
4. Look Good, Feel Better. (n.d.). *New hair looks: Wig care*. Retrieved from <http://www.lookgood-feelbetter.org/women/hair_help/wig_care.htm>.

CHAPTER 34

1. Government of Ontario. (2011). *Public safety message from the chief coroner for Ontario*. Retrieved from <http://news.ontario.ca/mcscs/en/2011/02/public-safety-message-from-the-chief-coroner-for-ontario.html>.

CHAPTER 35

1. Canadian Mental Health Association. (2015). *Fast facts about mental illness*. Retrieved from <http://www.cmha.ca/media/fast-facts-about-mental-illness/>.
2. Health Canada. (2004). *Telemental health in Canada*. Retrieved from <http://publications.gc.ca/collections/Collection/H21-236-2004E.pdf>.
3. Mental Health Commission of Canada. (2013, November 18). *Opening minds: Interim report*. Retrieved from <http://www.mentalhealthcommission.ca/English/system/files/private/document/opening_minds_interim_report.pdf>.
4. Health Canada. (2002). *A report on mental illnesses in Canada*. Ottawa: Author.
5. North Simcoe Muskoka Acquired Brain Injury Collective. (n.d.). *Facts*. Retrieved from <http://www.abicollaborative.ca/facts.html>.
6. Niagara College Canada. (n.d.). *Disabilities and you—Mild acquired brain injury*. Retrieved from <http://www.niagaracollege.ca/cswd/abi_ovr.htm>.
7. Campbell, J. (2008). *Family life and brain injury*. Retrieved from <http://www.braininjurylondon.on.ca/index.php/News/2008-05-25>.
8. HubPages. (2013). *Self management skills in people with acquired brain injury (ABI)*. Retrieved from <http://hubpages.com/hub/Self-Management-Skills-in-Acquired-Brain-Injury>.
9. American Psychiatric Association. (2013). *Diagnostic and statistical manual of mental disorders*, 5th ed. (DSM-5) American Psychiatric Association: Arlington.
10. Schizophrenia Society of Canada. (n.d.). *Learn more about schizophrenia*. Retrieved from <http://www.schizophrenia.ca/learn_more_about_schizophrenia.php>.
11. Canadian Mental Health Association. (n.d.). *Post-traumatic stress disorder (PTSD)*. Retrieved from <https://www.cmha.ca/mental_health/post-traumatic-stress-disorder/>.

12. Kelty Mental Health Resource Centre. (n.d.). *Post-traumatic stress disorder (PTSD).* Retrieved from <http://keltymentalhealth.ca/mental-health/disorders/post-traumatic-stress-disorder#view-tabs-1>.
13. Smith, M., & Segal, J. (2016). *Anorexia nervosa: Signs, symptoms, causes, and treatments.* Help-Guide.org. Retrieved from <http://www.helpguide.org/articles/eating-disorders/anorexia-nervosa.htm>.
14. Ellis, C. R. (2016). *Pica: Practice essentials.* Medscape. Retrieved from <http://emedicine.medscape.com/article/914765-overview>.
15. Health Canada. (2002). *A report on mental illnesses in Canada* (p. 90). Health Canada Editorial Board Mental Illnesses in Canada. Retrieved from <http://www.phac-aspc.gc.ca/publicat/miic-mmac/index-eng.php>.
16. Heisel & Links. (2005). *Risk factors for suicide among older adults.* Cited from Canadian Coalition for Seniors Mental Health (2006). *National Guidelines for seniors' mental health: The assessment of suicide risk and prevention of suicide. Late Life Suicide prevention Toolkit.* <http://www.ccsmh.ca/en/projects/suicide.cfm>.
17. Canadian Medical Association. (2013). *Suicide rate among Canadian seniors on the rise.* Retrieved from <http://healthcaretransformation.ca/suicide-rate-among-canadian-seniors-on-the-rise/>.
18. Canadian Coalition for Seniors' Mental Health. (2006). *National guidelines for seniors' mental health: The assessment of suicide risk and prevention of suicide.* Retrieved from <http://canadiangeriatrics.ca/students/assets/File/NatlGuideline_Suicide(1).pdf>.
19. Young. (n.d.). *The shack.* Retrieved from <https://www.goodreads.com/quotes/110129-forgiveness-is-not-about-forgetting-it-is-about-letting-go>.
20. Centre for Addiction and Mental Health. (2011). *Canada's low-risk alcohol drinking guidelines.* Retrieved from <http://www.camh.net/About_Addiction_Mental_Health/Drug_and_Addiction_Information/low_risk_drinking_guidelines.html>.
21. Canadian Centre on Substance Abuse. (2015). *Collaborating for addiction and mental health care: Best advice.* Retrieved from <http://ccsa.ca/Resource%20Library/CCSA-Collaboration-Addiction-Mental-Health-Best-Advice-Report-2015-en.pdf>.

CHAPTER 36

1. Siberski, J. (2013). Dementia and DSM-5: Changes, cost, and confusion. *For the Record, 25*(1), 22. Retrieved from <http://www.fortherecordmag.com/archives/011413p22.shtml>.
2. Alzheimer's Association. (2014). *2014 Alzheimer's disease facts and figures.* Retrieved from <http://www.alz.org/downloads/facts_figures_2014.pdf>.
3. Alzheimer Society of Canada. (2015). *Alzheimer disease.* Retrieved from <http://www.alzheimer.ca/en/About-dementia/Alzheimer-s-disease>.
4. Diamond, J. (personal communication), Scientific Director, Alzheimer Society of Canada, Thursday, April 14, 2011.
5. Alzheimer Society of Canada. (2015). *Warning signs.* Retrieved from <http://www.alzheimer.ca/en/About-dementia/Alzheimer-s-disease/10-warning-signs> © September 2016. Alzheimer Society of Canada. All rights reserved. <www.alzheimer.ca>.
6. Alzheimer Society of Canada. (2016). *Vascular dementia.* Retrieved from <http://www.alzheimer.ca/en/About-dementia/Dementias/Vascular-Dementia>.
7. Alzheimer Society of Canada. (2015). *Frontotemporal dementia (FTD, Pick's disease).* Retrieved from <http://www.alzheimer.ca/en/About-dementia/Dementias/Frontotemporal-Dementia-and-Pick-s-disease>.
8. Alzheimer Society, Hastings–Prince Edward. (2014). *Mixed dementia.* Retrieved from <http://www.alzheimer.ca/en/bhq/About-dementia/Dementias/Mixed-dementia>.
9. Alzheimer Society of Canada. (2015). *Creutzfeldt–Jakob disease.* Retrieved from <http://www.alzheimer.ca/en/About-dementia/Dementias/Creutzfeld-Jakob-Disease>.
10. Alzheimer Society of Canada. (2015). *Wernicke–Korsakoff syndrome.* Retrieved from <http://www.alzheimer.ca/~/media/Files/national/Other-dementias/rarer_dementias_wernicke_korsakoff_e.pdf>.

11. Xiong, G. L., & Kenedi, C. A. (2016). *Wernicke–Korsakoff Syndrome.* Retrieved from <http://emedicine.medscape.com/article/288379--treatment>.
12. Alzheimer's Association. (2015). *Depression and Alzheimer's disease.* Retrieved from <https://www.alz.org/care/alzheimers-dementia-depression.asp>.
13. Alzheimer Society of Canada. (2016). *Stages of Alzheimer's disease.* Retrieved from <http://www.alzheimer.ca/en/About-dementia/Alzheimer-s-disease/Stages-of-Alzheimer-s-disease#end-of-life>.
14. Medina, L. (2013). *What happens if you absorb too much caffeine?* Livestrong. Retrieved from <http://www.livestrong.com/article/403231-the-side-effects-of-drinking-too-much-caffeine/>.
15. Fight Alzheimer's Save Australia. (n.d.). *Therapies and communication approaches.* Retrieved from <https://fightdementia.org.au/support-and-services/i-care-for-someone-with-dementia/therapies-and-communication-approaches>.
16. Mary-Lou van der Horst. (2011, April). *GPA—Gentle persuasive approaches in dementia care.* Abstract for Canadian Association of Continuing Care Educators National Conference, Vancouver, B.C., 2014.

CHAPTER 37

1. Canadian Skin Cancer Foundation. (2012). *About skin cancer.* Retrieved from <http://www.canadianskincancerfoundation.com/about-skin-cancer.html>.
2. Canadian Dermatological Association. (n.d.). *Malignant melanoma.* Retrieved from <http://www.dermatology.ca/skin-hair-nails/skin/skin-cancer/malignant-melanoma/>.
3. Buckley, R. (2016). *General principles of fracture care treatment & managment.* Retrieved from <http://emedicine.medscape.com/article/1270717-treatment>.
4. The Arthritis Society. (2015). *Arthritis in Canada: Facts and figures.* Retrieved from <https://arthritis.ca/getmedia/43e83e3e-1a54-4fda-81d5-042ffaf9983f/Arthritis-Facts-Figures-EN.pdf>.
5. Canadian Centre for Occupational Health and Safety. (2010). *Osteoarthritis.* Retrieved from <http://www.ccohs.ca/oshanswers/diseases/osteoart.html>.
6. Arthritis Society. (n.d.). *Rheumatoid arthritis.* Retrieved from <http://www.arthritis.ca/types%20of%20arthritis/ra/default.asp?s=1>.
7. Multiple Sclerosis Society of Canada. (n.d.). *About MS.* Retrieved from <https://mssociety.ca/about-ms>.
8. ALS Society of Canada. (n.d.). *The ALS Society of Canada.* Retrieved from <http://www.als.ca>.
9. Public Health Agency of Canada. (2015). *Cardiovascular disease.* Retrieved from <http://www.phac-aspc.gc.ca/cd-mc/cvd-mcv/index-eng.php>.
10. Heart and Stroke Foundation. (2016). Retrieved from <http://www.heartandstroke.com/site/c.ikIQLcMWJtE/b.3483991/k.34A8/Statistics.htm>.
11. Canadian Women's Health Network. (2014). *Short of breath: For Canadian women, COPD deaths surpass those from breast cancer.* Retrieved from <http://www.cwhn.ca/en/networkmagazine/shortofbreath?page=show>.
12. Healthwise, Incorporated. (2014). *Prostate enlargement/BPH health center.* WebMD. Retrieved from <http://www.webmd.com/men/prostate-enlargement-bph/benign-prostatic-hyperplasia-bph-topic-overview>.
13. Canadian Diabetes Association. (2016). *Are you at risk?* Retrieved from <https://www.diabetes.ca/about-diabetes/risk-factors/are-you-at-risk>.
14. Statistics Canada. (2015). *Leading causes of death, by sex: (Both sexes).* Retrieved from <http://www.statcan.gc.ca/tables-tableaux/sum-som/l01/cst01/hlth36a-eng.htm>.
15. Canadian Breast Cancer Foundation. (n.d.). *Breast cancer in Canada, 2015.* Retrieved from <http://www.cbcf.org/central/AboutBreastCancerMain/FactsStats/Pages/Breast-Cancer-Canada.aspx>.
16. Canadian Cancer Society. (2016). *Prostate cancer.* Retrieved from <https://www.cancer.ca/en/cancer-information/cancer-type/prostate/statistics/?region=on>.
17. Canadian Cancer Society. (2016). *What is childhood leukemia?* Retrieved from <https://www.cancer.ca/en/cancer-information/cancer-type/

leukemia-childhood/childhood-leukemia/?region=on>.

CHAPTER 38

1. Health Canada. (2002). *Congenital anomalies in Canada: A perinatal health report* (p. 2). Ottawa: Health Canada.
2. MentalHelp.net. (2016). *Introduction to attention-deficit hyperactivity disorder (ADHD)*. Retrieved from <https://www.mentalhelp.net/articles/introduction-to-attention-deficit-hyperactivity-disorder-adhd/>.
3. American Psychiatric Association. (2013). *Diagnostic and statistical manual of mental disorders* (5th ed., p. 99). Arlington, VA: Author.
4. Canadian Mental Health Association, British Columbia division. (2014). *Attention-deficit/hyperactivity disorder in children and youth.* Retrieved from <http://www.cmha.bc.ca/get-informed/mental-health-information/child-adhd>.
5. EatRight Ontario. (2016). *What you need to know about preservatives.* Retrieved from <http://www.eatrightontario.ca/en/Articles/Food-technology/Biotechnology/Novel-foods/What-you-need-to-know-about-preservatives.aspx>.
6. Geneva Centre for Autism. (n.d.). *Home page.* Retrieved from <http://www.autism.net>.
7. Canadian Press. (2013, July 11). *Autism gender bias clue found. CBC News.* Retrieved from <http://www.cbc.ca/news/health/autism-gender-bias-clue-found-1.1185572>.

CHAPTER 39

1. Joanette, Y., Lafond, D., & Lecours, A. R. (1993). *The client with aphasia. Living with aphasia: Psychosocial issues* (pp. 19–36). San Diego, CA: Singular Publishing Group.

CHAPTER 40

1. Telethon Speech & Hearing. (2011). *Causes, types and treatments of hearing loss/otitis media.* Retrieved from <http://www.doyouhear.org.au/causes-signs-symptoms/causes-types-and-treatment-of-hearing-loss-otitis-media>.
2. Starkey Hearing Technologies. (2015). *Hearing aid use & care.* Retrieved from <http://www.starkeycanada.ca/hearing-aid-use-and-care>.
3. CNIB. (2003). *Eye Connect: AMD.* Retrieved from <http://www.cnib.ca/amd/edu/amd_info.htm>.
4. Doctors of Optometry Canada. (n.d.). Retrieved from <http://doctorsofoptometry.ca/retinal-detachment/>.
5. Canadian Opthalmological Society. (n.d.). *Which lenses are right for you?* Retrieved from <http://www.cos-sco.ca/vision-health-information/conditions-disorders-treatments/cataract/which-lenses-are-right-for-you/>.

CHAPTER 42

1. Government of Canada. (2015). *Reduce humidity, moisture and mould.* Retrieved from <http://www.hc-sc.gc.ca/ewh-semt/air/in/poll/mould-moisissure/rid-debarrasser-eng.php>.
2. Innovation, Science and Economic Development's Office of Consumer Affairs. (n.d.). *Guide to apparel and textile care symbols.* Retrieved from <https://www.ic.gc.ca/eic/site/oca-bc.nsf/eng/ca02009.html>.

CHAPTER 46

1. Canadian Mental Health Association. (2015). *Grieving.* Retrieved from <https://www.cmha.ca/mental-health/your-mental-health/grief/Grieving>.
2. Reprinted from WHO Definition of Palliative Care, World Health Organization, <http://www.who.int/cancer/palliative/definition/en/>, Copyright 2015.

CHAPTER 47

1. Western Information and Privacy Officer. (2007). *Best practices: Electronic posting of student personal information.* Retrieved from <http://www.uwo.ca/tsc/resources/pdf/BestPracticesPersonalInformation.pdf>.

Index

Page numbers followed by *b*, *t*, and *f* indicate boxes, tables, and figures, respectively.

Procedures